Surgery Review Illustrated

NOTICE

Medicine is an ever-changing science. As new research and clinical experience broaden our knowledge, changes in treatment and drug therapy are required. The authors and the publisher of this work have checked with sources believed to be reliable in their efforts to provide information that is complete and generally in accord with the standards accepted at the time of publication. However, in view of the possibility of human error or changes in medical sciences, neither the authors nor the publisher nor any other party who has been involved in the preparation or publication of this work warrants that the information contained herein is in every respect accurate or complete, and they disclaim all responsibility for any errors or omissions or for the results obtained from use of the information contained in this work. Readers are encouraged to confirm the information contained herein with other sources. For example and in particular, readers are advised to check the product information sheet included in the package of each drug they plan to administer to be certain that the information contained in this work is accurate and that changes have not been made in the recommended dose or in the contraindications for administration. This recommendation is of particular importance in connection with new or infrequently used drugs.

Surgery Review Illustrated

Second Edition

Lisa M. McElroy, MD, MS

Resident Physician
Medical College of Wisconsin and Affiliated Hospitals
Milwaukee, Wisconsin

Travis P. Webb, MD, MHPE

Professor
Department of Surgery
Associate Dean for Curriculum
Vice Chair Trauma and Critical Care Surgery
Medical College of Wisconsin and Affiliated Hospitals
Milwaukee, Wisconsin

McGraw Hill Education

New York   Chicago   San Francisco   Athens   London   Madrid   Mexico City
Milan   New Delhi   Singapore   Sydney   Toronto

Surgery Review Illustrated, Second Edition

1 2 3 4 5 6 7 8 9   DSS   21 20 19 18 17 16

ISBN 978-0-07-1663298
MHID 0-07-166329-0

This book was set in Minion Pro by Cenveo® Publisher Services.
The editors were Brian Belval and Regina Y. Brown.
The production supervisor was Richard Ruzycka.
Project management was provided by Raghavi Khullar, Cenveo Publisher Services.
The cover designer was Dreamit, Inc.
RR Donnelley Shenzhen was printer and binder.

This book is printed on acid-free paper.

Names: McElroy, Lisa (Lisa M.), author. | Webb, Travis (Travis P.), author. |
    Tevar, Amit D. Surgery review illustrated. Preceded by (work):
Title: Surgery review illustrated / Lisa McElroy, Travis Webb.
Description: Second edition. | New York : McGraw-Hill Education, [2016] |
    Preceded by Surgery review illustrated / Amit D. Tevar, Rafael E. Azuaje,
    Larry T. Micon. c2005. | Includes bibliographical references and index.
Identifiers: LCCN 2016012502| ISBN 9780071663298 (paperback : alk. paper) |
    ISBN 0071663290 (paperback : alk. paper)
Subjects: | MESH: General Surgery | Surgical Procedures, Operative |
    Examination Questions
Classification: LCC RD37 | NLM WO 18.2 | DDC 617.0076—dc23 LC record
    available at http://lccn.loc.gov/2016012502

CONTENTS

CONTRIBUTORS

Isaac Josh Abecassis, MD
Resident Physician
Department of Neurological Surgery
University of Washington
Seattle, Washington

Zachary A. Abecassis, BS
Northwestern University
Feinberg School of Medicine
Chicago, Illinois

Elliot A. Asare, MD, MS
Resident Physician
Department of Surgery
Medical College of Wisconsin and Affiliated Hospitals
Milwaukee, Wisconsin

Leah Backhus MD, MPH
Associate Professor
Division of Cardiothoracic Surgery
Department of Surgery Division of Cardiothoracic Surgery
Department of Surgery of Cardiothoracic Surgery Stanford University
Palo Alto, California

Jonnae Y. Barry, MD
Resident Physician
Department of Otolaryngology
University of Arizona
Tucson, Arizona

Ronald Bays, MD
Assistant Clinical Professor
Division of Vascular Surgery
Department of Surgery
Central Michigan University
Mt. Pleasant, Michigan

Nicholas M. Bernthal
Assistant Professor and Attending Surgeon
Chief Division of Musculoskeletal Oncology
Department of Orthopaedic Surgery
David Geffen School of Medicine at UCLA
Los Angeles, California

David C. Borgstrom, MD, FACS
Associate Professor and Chief
Division of General Surgery
West Virginia University
Morgantown, West Virginia

Alexandra R. Brown, BS
Research Coordinator
Center for Healthcare Studies
Institute for Public Health and Medicine
Feinberg School of Medicine
Northwestern University
Chicago, Illinois

Aaron Carr, MD
Associate Professor
Division of Gastrointestinal Surgery Department of Surgery
University of California, Davis
Sacramento, California

Azzie A. Carr MD
Assistant Professor of Surgery
Division of Surgical Oncology
Medical College of Wisconsin
9200 W. Wisconsin Ave.
Milwaukee, Wisconsin

Alexander Chiu, MD
Professor and Chair
Department of Otolaryngology
University of Arizona
Tucson, Arizona

Kelly M. Collins, MD
Staff Surgeon
Transplant Institute
Henry Ford Health System
Detroit, Michigan

Waldo Concepcion, MD
Professor and Director
Pediatric Kidney Transplantation
Department of Surgery
Stanford University
Stanford, Arizona

Catherine M. Cosentino, MD
Pediatric Surgeon
Arizona Pediatric Surgery & Urology, Ltd.
Assistant Clinical Professor
Department of Surgery
Banner Health
University of Arizona College of Medicine
Tucson, Arizona

Elizabeth M. Coviello, DO
Resident Obstetrician/Gynecologist
Medstar Washington Hospital Center
Medstar Georgetown University Hospital
Washington, District of Columbia

Eleanor Curtis, MD
Resident Physician
Department of General Surgery
University of California, Davis and Travis Air Force Base
Sacramento, California

Neha Datta, MD
Resident Physician
Department of Surgery
University of California at Los Angeles
Los Angeles, California

Carley M. Davis, MD
Associate Professor
Department of Urology
Medical College of Wisconsin and Affiliated Hospitals
Milwaukee, Wisconsin

Tanya D. Davis, MD, Fellow
Division of Pediatric Urology Fellow
Children's National Health System
Washington, DC

Sepan Desai, MD
Assistant Professor
Division of Vascular Surgery
Department of Surgery
Southern Illinois University
Carbondale, Illinois

Peter B. Dorschner, BS
Medical Student Northwestern University
Feinberg School of Medicine
Chicago, Illinois

Anahita Dua, MD
Resident Physician
Department of Surgery
Medical College of Wisconsin and Affiliated Hospitals
Milwaukee, Wisconsin

J. Christopher Eagon, MD
Associate Professor
Department of Surgery
Washington University School of Medicine
Barnes-Jewish Hospital
St. Louis, Missouri

Audrey B. Erman, MD
Assistant Professor
Department of Otolaryngology
University of Arizona
Tucson, Arizona

Erynne A. Faucett, MD
Resident Physician
Department of Otolaryngology
University of Arizona
Tucson, Arizona

Andrew Feider, MD
Assistant Professor
Department of Anesthesiology Northwestern University
Feinberg School of Medicine
Chicago, Illinois

Cecily Anne Clark Ganheart, MD
Maternal Fetal Medicine Fellow
Department of Obstetrics and Gynecology
Medstar Washington Hospital Center
Medstar Georgetown University Hospital
Washington, Washington

David Greenhalgh, MD
Chief of Burns at Shriners Hospitals for Children
    Northern California
Professor of Surgery
University of California, Davis
Sacramento, California

Rachel A. Greenup, MD
Assistant Professor
Division of Surgical Oncology
Department of Surgery
Duke University Medical Center
Durham, North Carolina

O. Joe Hines, MD
Professor and Chief
Department of Surgery
David Geffen School of Medicine
University of California
Los Angeles, California

Andrew W. Hoel, MD
Assistant Professor
Division of Vascular Surgery
Department of Surgery
Northwestern University
Feinberg School of Medicine
Chicago, Illinois

Kristen A. Klement, MD
Craniofacial Fellow
Department of Plastic and Reconstructive Surgery
Medical College of Wisconsin and Affiliated Hospitals
Milwaukee, Wisconsin

Kathryn L. Jackson
Biostatistician
Institute for Public Health and Medicine, Feinberg School
    of Medicine
Northwestern University
Chicago, Illinois

Fabian M. Johnston, MD, MS
Assistant Professor of Surgery
Division of Surgical Oncology
Department of Surgery
Medical College of Wisconsin and Affiliated Hospitals
Milwaukee, Wisconsin

Stephen J. Kaplan, MD, MPH
Resident Physician
Department of Surgery
Virginia Mason Medical Center
Seattle, Washington

Ryan Kim, MD
Vascular Surgery Fellow
Division of Vascular and Endovascular Surgery
University of Missouri—Columbia
Columbia, Missouri

Karri Kluesner, MD
Resident Physician
Department of Plastic and Reconstructive Surgery
Medical College of Wisconsin and Affiliated Hospitals
Milwaukee, Wisconsin

Gregory Larrieux, MD
Resident Physician
Medical College of Wisconsin and Affiliated Hospitals
Milwaukee, Wisconsin

Amy Lee, MD
Assistant Professor
Department of Neurological Surgery
University of Washington
Seattle, Washington

Amy Lightner Hill, MD
Resident Physician
Department of Surgery
University of California
Los Angeles, California

Gina Lockwood, MD
Pediatric Urology Fellow
Connecticut Children's Medical Center/University of
    Connecticut
Hartford, Connecticut

John Logiudice, MD
Assistant Professor
Department of Plastic and Reconstructive Surgery
Medical College of Wisconsin and Affiliated Hospitals
Milwaukee, Wisconsin

Jorge Marcet, MD
Professor of Surgery
Division of Colon & Rectal Surgery
Department of Surgery
University of South Florida
Tampa General Hospital
Tampa, Florida

Lisa M. McElroy, MD, MS
Resident Physician
Department of Surgery
Medical College of Wisconsin and Affiliated Hospitals
Milwaukee, Wisconsin

Maria Michailidou, MD
Resident Physician
Department of Surgery
University of Arizona
Tucson, Arizona

John T. Miura, MD
Resident Physician
Department of Surgery
Medical College of Wisconsin and Affiliated Hospitals
Milwaukee, Wisconsin

Ravi Moonka, MD
Associate Professor
Department of Surgery, Virginia Mason Medical Center
Seattle, Washington

Lilah F. Morris, MD
Endocrine Surgeon
Northwest Medical Center
Tucson, Arizona

Rachel Morris, MD
Resident Physician
Department of Surgery
Medical College of Wisconsin and Affiliated Hospitals
Milwaukee, Wisconsin

Diana I. Ortiz, MD
Endocrine Surgery Fellow
Division of Surgical Oncology
Department of Surgery
Medical College of Wisconsin and Affiliated Hospitals
Milwaukee, Wisconsin

Lara Oyetunji, MD
Resident Physician
Department of Surgery
University of Washington
Seattle, Washington

Sherif Richman, MD
David Geffen School of Medicine
University of California at Los Angeles
Los Angeles, California

Margaret Riesenberg-Karges, MD
Resident Physician
Department of Surgery
Bassett Medical Center
Cooperstown, New York

Kathleen Romanowski, MD
Critical Care Fellow
Division of Critical Care
Department of Surgery
University of California, Davis
Sacramento, California

Jessica Rose, DO
Resident Physician
Institute for Reconstructive Surgery
Houston Methodist
Houston, Texas

Rachel Russo, MD
Resident Physician
Department of General Surgery
University of California, Davis
Sacramento, California

Carlos A. San Mateo, MD
Assistant Professor of Surgery
Division of Colon & Rectal Surgery
Department of Surgery
University of Miami Miller School of Medicine
Miami, Florida

Kathryn A. Schmidt, BS
Medical student
The Commonwealth Medical College
Scranton, Pennsylvania

Steven J. Schwulst, MD
Assistant Professor
Division of Trauma and Critical Care
Department of Surgery
Northwestern University
Feinberg School of Medicine
Chicago, Illinois

Michael B. Shapiro, MD
Professor and Chief
Division of Trauma and Critical Care
Department of Surgery
Northwestern University
Feinberg School of Medicine
Chicago, Illinois

Alexandra I. Stavrakis, MD
Resident Physician
Department of Orthopedic Surgery
University of California
Los Angeles, California

Mamta Swaroop, MD
Assistant (or Associate) Professor
Division of Trauma and Critical Care
Department of Surgery
Northwestern University
Feinberg School of Medicine
Chicago, Illinois

Thomas Wade, MD
Minimally Invasive Surgery Fellow
Department of Surgery, Washington University
School of Medicine
Barnes-Jewish Hospital
St. Louis, Missouri

Michael W. Wandling, MD, MS
Resident Physician
Department of Surgery
Northwestern University
Feinberg School of Medicine
Chicago, Illinois

Tracy S. Wang, MD, MPH
Associate Professor
Division of Surgical Oncology
Department of Surgery
Medical College of Wisconsin and Affiliated Hospitals
Milwaukee, Wisconsin

James Warneke, MD
Associate Professor
Department of General Surgery
University of Arizona
Tucson, Arizona

Travis Webb, MD
Professor
Department of Surgery
Associate Dean for Curriculum
Vice Chair Trauma and Critical Care Surgery
Medical College of Wisconsin and Affiliated Hospitals
Milwaukee, Wisconsin

Jason R. Wellen, MD, MBA
Assistant Professor of Surgery
Department of General Surgery
Washington University School of Medicine
St. Louis, Missouri

Campbell Williams, MD
Fellow
Department of Anesthesiology
Northwestern University
Feinberg School of Medicine
Chicago, Illinois

Kimberly C. Zamor, MD, MS
Resident Physician
Department of General Surgery
Boston University
Boston, Massachusetts

ACKNOWLEDGMENTS

The Authors and Publisher would like to thank the following individuals for their review of the page proofs:

Fadwa Ali, MD
Nicholas Berger, MD
Charles Fehring, MD
Rachel Landisch, MD
William Ragalie, MD

PREFACE

The practice of general surgery requires a broad base of knowledge and skills that is not static or based solely on what is taught in medical school, residency, or fellowship. Surgeons must adapt and learn new information as well as have foundational knowledge reinforced regularly in order to be able to practice at the highest level of performance. This text was developed to assist the surgical resident, fellow, and practicing physician in learning new concepts, as well as to reinforce previously learned material in a manner that will promote retention and continued expertise.

During medical school and residency, surgeons-in-training often use many textbooks and electronic media to achieve a strong foundational knowledge of topics in general surgery. However, when preparing for certification examinations, other manners of studying are also beneficial. The practice of answering board-style questions improves skills in answering questions as well as forces the learner to confront their own knowledge gaps. The comprehensive nature of this text makes it an excellent resource for surgeons taking the American Board of Surgery written and oral exams or the recertification examination.

The first edition of this book successfully provided an all-inclusive source for review of the broad expanse of general surgery. The question and answer format with brief referenced explanations proved popular with surgeons looking for a single resource to study for certification examinations. This second edition builds on the success of the previous edition. We have designed and extensively edited the text to cover the breadth of topics that are potentially tested on the licensure examinations and sought authors for each chapter who have expertise and academic interest in the topics. The information emphasizes the clinical science, but also contains basic science, including physiology, anatomy, and pathology.

We were impressed with the caliber of work each author contributed to this second edition. It should be emphasized that this review is not a replacement for the study of fundamental general surgery textbooks and journals in building a fund of knowledge. Instead, we present this text as a valuable resource for senior surgical residents and young surgeons preparing for their licensure examinations as well as for the seasoned practitioner wishing to periodically review the field of general surgery.

CHAPTER 1

CELL PHYSIOLOGY AND STRUCTURE

LISA M. MCELROY AND TRAVIS P. WEBB

1. What is the function of the various phospholipids that compose the lipid bilayer of cell membranes?
   (A) Separate the intracellular space from the extracellular space
   (B) Serve as substrates for the formation of signal transduction molecules
   (C) Serve as signals to induce the phagocytosis of apoptotic cells
   (D) Serve as a boundary between aqueous and nonaqueous components
   (E) All of the above

2. Which of the following plasma membrane molecules are exclusively located on the extracellular side of the lipid bilayer?
   (A) Glycolipids
   (B) Integral proteins
   (C) Peripheral proteins
   (D) Prenylated membrane proteins
   (E) A, B, and C

3. Which of these is *not* a function that is carried out by an integral membrane protein in a plasma membrane?
   (A) Receptor for growth factors
   (B) Pump for K^+
   (C) Channel for macromolecules
   (D) Structural protein
   (E) Determinant of membrane fluidity

4. Which of the following statements about osmolarity, electrochemical gradient, and membrane transport is *incorrect*?
   (A) Large intracellular macromolecules such as proteins do not make direct or indirect contributions to osmolarity.
   (B) The Donnan equilibrium states that nondiffusible and diffusible substances are distributed about the membrane so that the products of their concentrations are equal and ionic charges are balanced on both sides.
   (C) Treating a human cell with ouabain would cause the cell to swell and burst.
   (D) Ionophores can cause collapse of the electrochemical gradient in cells and can ultimately result in cell death.
   (E) Multidrug resistance (MDR) proteins can pump hydrophobic drugs out of the cell and are responsible for the resistance of cancer cells to certain chemotherapeutics.

5. Cystic fibrosis (CF) is an autosomal recessive disorder in which three nucleotides are deleted, resulting in the absence of a key amino acid in the CFTR chloride channel. Which of the following amino acids is deleted?
   (A) Phenylalanine
   (B) Glutamine
   (C) Lysine
   (D) Valine
   (E) Alanine

6. Which of the following are the calcium-dependent proteins responsible for intercellular adhesion and the segment of the junctional complex in which they are located?
   (A) Calcineurin at the zonula adherens
   (B) Calmodulin at the macula adherens
   (C) ZO-1 at the zonula occludens
   (D) Desmosomes at the macula adherens
   (E) Cadherins at the zonula adherens

7. Which of the following are classified as apical cytoskeletal specializations?
   (A) Cilia composed of microvilli
   (B) Stereocilia composed of actin microfilaments
   (C) Microvilli composed of actin microtubules
   (D) Microvilli composed of microfilament
   (E) All of the above

8. Which of the following is *not* a molecular motor protein?
   (A) Myosin
   (B) Kinesin
   (C) Dynein
   (D) Actin
   (E) Dynamin

9. Which of the following statements about receptors is true?
   (A) Ion channel–linked receptors activate the opening of an ion channel with the binding of ligand, which is the method of signaling used by most neurotransmitters.
   (B) G protein–linked receptors activate heterotrimeric GTPases in response to ligand-binding, such as in the action of neuropeptide Y.
   (C) Enzyme-linked receptors include receptor tyrosine kinases (RTKs) and receptor serine/threonine kinases, which are the receptors used by endothelial growth factor (EGF) and transforming growth factor-β (TGF-β).
   (D) Steroid hormone receptors are usually found in the cytosol, and the functions of vitamins A and D are dependent on this class of receptors.
   (E) All of the above

10. Which of the following motifs is important in steroid receptor structure?
    (A) Transmembrane domain
    (B) Zinc finger
    (C) Catalytic domain
    (D) Multiple C-terminal tyrosine residues
    (E) SH_2 domain

11. A eukaryotic cell is lysed and fractionated into plasma membrane, cytosolic, and nuclear fractions. Which of the following hormones would most likely be found in the nuclear fraction of the cell?
    (A) Human chorionic gonadotrophin
    (B) Glucagon
    (C) Aldosterone
    (D) Gastrin
    (E) Histamine

12. Which of the following statements about organelle function is *incorrect*?
    (A) The rough endoplasmic reticulum (rER) is the site of protein synthesis and the cotranslational modification of proteins.
    (B) The smooth endoplasmic reticulum (sER) is the site of phospholipid synthesis, steroid hormone synthesis, drug detoxification, and calcium store release.
    (C) The Golgi complex is the site of vesicular packaging of proteins, membrane component recycling, and posttranslational modification of proteins.
    (D) The mitochondrion functions in acetyl-CoA production, tricarboxylic acid (TCA) cycle, oxidative phosphorylation, and fatty acid oxidation.
    (E) The lysosome contains amino acid oxidase, urate oxidase, catalase, and other oxidative enzymes relating to the production and degradation of hydrogen peroxide and oxidation of fatty acids.

13. Which one of the following lysosomal storage diseases is X-linked recessive in inheritance?
    (A) Fabry disease
    (B) Krabbe disease
    (C) Gaucher disease
    (D) Niemann-Pick disease
    (E) Tay-Sachs disease

14. Cellular proteins processed mainly in the Golgi apparatus include all of the following *except*
    (A) Lysosomal enzymes
    (B) Peroxisomal enzymes
    (C) Membrane receptors
    (D) Secreted proteins
    (E) All of the above

15. Which of these cell types might be expected to have an extensive sER?
    (A) Adrenal zona glomerulosa cell
    (B) Adrenal chromaffin cell
    (C) Pancreatic acinar cell
    (D) Keratinocyte
    (E) Hepatic Küpffer cell

16. DNA fluorescent *in situ* hybridization of a cell isolated from human tissue displays an extremely long series of short tandem repeats (TTAGGG) at the end of the chromosomes. What type of cell would this most likely be?
    (A) Neuron
    (B) Kidney cell
    (C) Lymphocyte
    (D) Spermatozoa
    (E) Hepatocyte

17. Which of the following is *not* a mechanism of DNA mismatch repair or DNA excision repair?
    (A) When DNA is damaged by ultraviolet (UV) light, DNA mismatch repair proteins recognize and remove the altered nucleotides, followed by repair of the sequence with DNA polymerase and ligase.
    (B) Errors made by the DNA polymerase, which are missed by its proofreading exonuclease, are corrected by DNA mismatch repair proteins that recognize and degrade the mismatched base pair on the newly synthesized strand.
    (C) A single damaged purine base can be excised via nicks produced by AP endonuclease and a phosphodiesterase for removal of the damaged base, followed by repair with DNA polymerase and ligase.
    (D) When cytosines are spontaneously deaminated into uracils, they are recognized by uracil-DNA glycosidase; then repair proceeds with AP endonuclease, a phosphodiesterase, DNA polymerase, and DNA ligase.
    (E) Pyrimidine dimers are repaired by uvrABC enzymes, which excise a 12-residue sequence around the dimer, followed by repair with DNA polymerase and ligase.

18. Which is the shortest phase of the normal cell cycle?
    (A) G_1 phase
    (B) S phase
    (C) G_2 phase
    (D) M phase
    (E) All of the above are approximately equal in length.

19. Which of the following are *not* either proto-oncogene or oncogene products?
    (A) Vhl and Apc
    (B) Ras and Sis
    (C) Erb and Neu
    (D) Myc and Abl
    (E) Jun and Fos

20. A biopsy was performed on an aggressive tumor, and assays of various protein levels and enzyme activities were performed on the tumor cells. Which of the following proteins would likely *not* show either increased expression or activity?
    (A) Telomerase
    (B) Fas receptor
    (C) Myc
    (D) Ras
    (E) Bcl-2

21. Which protein is *not* involved in the stimulation and/or prolongation of the apoptosis pathway?
    (A) Cytochrome *c*
    (B) Bcl-X_L
    (C) Apaf-1
    (D) Bad
    (E) Bax

22. Which of these is *not* a function of heat shock proteins (HSPs)?
    (A) Aiding protein folding in intracellular compartments
    (B) Preventing protein aggregation
    (C) Facilitating the translocation of proteins across membranes
    (D) Facilitating the degradation of unstable proteins
    (E) Increasing the rate of protein synthesis

23. Which of the following statements about cellular metabolic pathways is *not* true?
    (A) Glycogenolysis in liver and muscle is responsible for supplying glucose to tissues in the first 8 h after a meal.
    (B) Gluconeogenesis in the liver supplies glucose from amino acid and fatty acid substrates 8–30 h after a meal.
    (C) Defects in protein metabolism can be due to organ dysfunction or inherited enzyme deficiencies.
    (D) Glucokinase is found throughout the body, whereas hexokinase is a high-capacity enzyme found only in the liver.
    (E) Even if the urine ketone test is negative, there can be a significant level of ketogenesis occurring in the liver.

24. Which glycogen storage disease (GSD) is a process that primarily affects glycogen storage in the muscles?
    (A) Type I GSD (Von Gierke disease)
    (B) Type II GSD (Pompe disease)
    (C) Type III GSD (Cori disease)
    (D) Type IV GSD (Andersen disease)
    (E) Type V GSD (McArdle disease)

25. Which of the following reactions is unique to gluconeogenesis in the liver and is *not* a directly reversed step of glycolysis?
    (A) Conversion of pyruvate to oxaloacetate by pyruvate carboxylase
    (B) Conversion of oxaloacetate to phosphoenolpyruvate (PEP) by PEP-carboxykinase (PEPCK)
    (C) Conversion of fructose-1,6-bisphosphate (F-1,6-BP) to fructose-6-phosphate (F6P) by fructose-1,6-bisphosphatase (F-1,6-BPase)
    (D) Conversion of glucose-6-phosphate to glucose by glucose-6-phosphatase
    (E) All of the above

26. Which intermediate is common to both cholesterol synthesis and ketogenesis?
    (A) Acetoacetate
    (B) B-hydroxybutyrate
    (C) B-hydroxy-β-methylglutaryl-CoA (HMG-CoA)
    (D) Mevalonate
    (E) None of the above

27. Which of the following statements about the urea cycle is *not* true?
    (A) The urea cycle is the main pathway responsible for the excretion of nitrogenous wastes derived from protein metabolism.
    (B) The nitrogens in urea are directly derived from ammonia, alanine, and glutamate via reactions of the urea cycle.
    (C) Urea cycle reactions occur in both the mitochondria and cytosol of hepatocytes.
    (D) The urea cycle uses ATP as energy in the formation of urea and is also known as the Krebs-Henseleit cycle or the Krebs ornithine cycle.
    (E) The fumarate byproduct of the urea cycle is converted into energy by the TCA cycle.

28. Which of the following statements is *not* true?
    (A) Selectins are Ca^{2+}-dependent cell–cell adhesion molecules in the bloodstream that mediate transient binding.
    (B) The extracellular matrix is made up primarily of GAGs and fibrous proteins.
    (C) Mutations in the fibrillin component of elastic fibers are responsible for Marfan syndrome.
    (D) TIMPs are proteases that break down the extracellular matrix for cell migration.
    (E) Serine protease MMPs are extracellular inhibitors protolytic enzymes

29. Which of the following statements about integrins is *not* true?
    (A) Integrins are structural proteins that function to anchor cells to the extracellular matrix and do not play a major role in signal transduction.
    (B) Integrins are the major receptors for binding extracellular matrix proteins such as collagens, laminins, and fibronectins, and they are dependent on extracellular divalent cations such as Ca^{2+} or Mg^{2+} for binding.
    (C) Integrins exist as transmembrane heterodimers with α and β subunits that are noncovalently associated.
    (D) Integrins serve as transmembrane linkers between the extracellular matrix and actin cytoskeleton but cannot directly activate cell shape changes.
    (E) All of the above are true.

30. Which of the following correctly describes a complement activation pathway?
    (A) The alternate pathway is activated by IgG or IgM bound to the surface of a microbe and involves the sequential activation of C1, C2, and C4.
    (B) The classic pathway involves the spontaneous activation of C3 by factors B and D.
    (C) Cleavage of C3 independently is the common point of the early cascade.
    (D) The lectin pathway cannot activate complement components
    (E) The final common pathway is the assembly of late complement components to form a membrane attack complex (MAC).

31. What is the role of the TLR pathway?
    (A) The TLR pathway mediates the inflammatory response to pathogenic substances such as LPS by activating the transcription of proinflammatory genes.
    (B) The TLR pathway is responsible for deactivating phagocytic cells after they have engulfed target pathogens.
    (C) The TLR pathway activates apoptosis in virus-infected cells as part of the innate and adaptive immune responses.
    (D) The TLR pathway is involved in signal transduction for activating inflammatory genes in response to hypoxia-inducible factors.
    (E) None of the above are correct.

32. Which of the following statements is *incorrect*?
    (A) There are two major isoforms of the cyclooxygenase (COX) enzyme, with COX-1 being constitutively expressed and COX-2 being inducible in inflammation.
    (B) Steroids block the arachidonic acid (AA) pathway at the level of PLA2.
    (C) Eicosapentaenoic acid (EPA) and aspirin inhibit the AA pathway in the same manner.
    (D) EPA is considered to be anti-inflammatory in its actions, while AA generally produces proinflammatory effects.
    (E) When EPA and AA are used as substrates for COX through the AA pathway, they result in different sets of prostanoid products.

33. Which of the following are considered proangiogenic factors?
    (A) Vascular endothelial growth factor (VEGF) and angiopoietin-1 (Ang1)
    (B) VEGF and angiopoietin-2 (Ang2)
    (C) Ang1 and Ang2
    (D) VEGF and angiostatin
    (E) All are proangiogenic factors

ANSWERS AND EXPLANATIONS

1. **(E)** Although phospholipids are commonly thought of only as the structural components of the cell membrane, they serve many signaling functions as well.

    The formation of the phospholipid bilayer plasma membrane results in the separation of the intracellular space from the extracellular space and controls the permeability of the cell to ions and molecules. The inclusion of cholesterol and glycolipids in the phospholipid bilayer additionally enhances the barrier properties and modifies the fluidity of the membrane. Thus, one of the main functions of phospholipids is to provide a fluid barrier between the cytosol and the extracellular environment.

    However, many phospholipids in the plasma membrane also serve as substrates for cell signaling, primarily in the conversion of extracellular signals to intracellular signals. Phosphatidylinositol 3′-kinase (PI3K) is a lipid kinase that phosphorylates inositol phospholipids, derivatives of phosphotidylinositol, to transmit intracellular signals in response to growth factors and cytokines. Phospholipases are another example of enzymes in the plasma membrane that are activated in response to a variety of extracellular ligands. Phospholipase A cleaves arachidonic acid (AA) or its relatives from the 2-position on membrane phospholipids to result in the eventual formation of inflammatory leukotrienes and prostaglandins. Phospholipase C cleaves an inositol phospholipid (i.e., PIP_2) on the cytosolic side of the plasma membrane to form two fragments 1,2-diacylglycerol (DAG) and IP_3. DAG remains in the membrane to activate protein kinase C (PKC), and cytosolic IP_3 stimulates the release of Ca^{2+} from the endoplasmic reticulum (ER). PKC remains bound to the cytosolic side of the plasma membrane where there is a concentration of negatively charged phosphatidylserines, which are necessary for its activity. PKC and cytosolic Ca^{2+} are involved in many signaling functions of the cell.

    The asymmetrical distribution of the charged phosphatidylserine molecules are also used to distinguish cells that have undergone apoptosis. Phosphatidylserines are normally maintained on the cytosolic side of the plasma membrane in living cells. The altered activities of phospholipid translocators in apoptotic cells results in the translocation of phosphotidylserines to the outer face of the cell membrane. The exposed phosphotidylserines serve as signals to induce the phagocytosis of apoptotic cells by macrophages.

BIBLIOGRAPHY

Alberts B, Johnson A, Lewis K, et al. Membrane structure. In: Alberts B, Johnson A, Lewis K, et al., eds. *Molecular Biology of the Cell.* 4th ed. New York, NY: Garland Science; 2002:583–592.

Aoki J, Nagai Y, Hosono H, et al. Structure and function of phosphatidylserine-specific phospholipase A1. *Biochim Biophys Acta* 2002;1582:26–32.

Mark Reeves. Cell biology. In: O'Leary JP, ed. *The Physiologic Basis of Surgery.* 4th ed. Baltimore, MD: Lippincott Williams & Wilkins; 2008:1–43.

2. **(E)** Glycosylated proteins are located exclusively on the extracellular side of the cell membrane, whereas membrane proteins are located only on the cytosolic or intracellular side. Lipid-linked proteins are synthesized first as proteins on free cytosolic ribosomes and are directed to the intracellular side of the plasma membrane by the attachment of the lipid group. Sugar residues are added to proteins or lipids in the lumen of the endoplasmic reticulum (ER) or Golgi apparatus, which are topologically analogous to the exterior of the cell. Vesicles that carry proteins or lipids from the ER or Golgi to the plasma membrane fuse with the lipid bilayer in a manner that results in the lumen of the vesicle becoming the extracellular face of the cell membrane. The sugar residues on glycolipids are important for modulating interactions with each other in lipid rafts and in altering the electrical effects in the membrane transport of ions.

    Most transmembrane proteins are actually glycoproteins; the glycosylation of these proteins is a post-transcriptional modification that adds an essential structural component for their various functions. Both glycolipids and glycoproteins are also important in cell–cell adhesion, as they bind to membrane-bound lectin or selectin molecules especially in the rolling interaction of neutrophils with the endothelium. Glycosylphosphatidylinositol (GPI) anchors are added to designated proteins in the ER, which are then associated with the extracellular side of the plasma membrane by a covalent linkage to PI. GPI-anchored proteins are important in immune function, and mutations in the GPI anchor are associated with immune dysfunctions such as paroxysmal nocturnal hemoglobinuria (PNH). PNH is the result of an acquired mutation in the phosphatidylinositol glycan A (*PIGA*) gene that is necessary for the synthesis of the GPI anchor. Since GPI-anchored proteins are necessary for the inactivation of complement, the mutation renders affected red blood cells (RBCs), granulocytes, and platelets hypersensitive to lysis by complement. Therefore, the significance of glycolipids, glycoproteins, and GPI-anchored proteins being located exclusively on the extracellular face of the cell membrane is a result of the topographic location of the glycosylation process and is related to their function.

    Peripheral proteins regulate receptor-mediated endocytosis. They are loosely bound to the cell membrane, most commonly the inner surface. Integral proteins are incorporated within the lipid bilayer via covalent bonds.

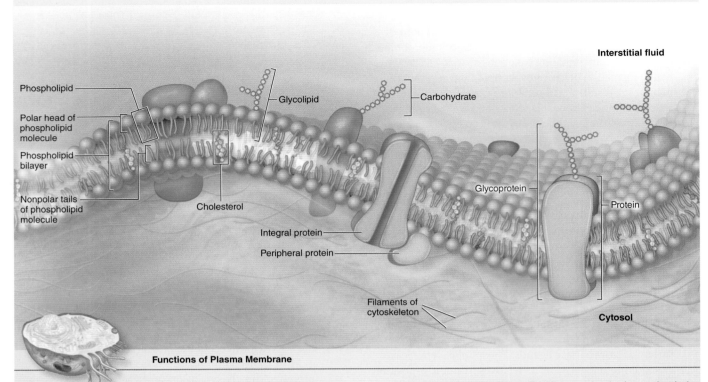

Functions of Plasma Membrane

1. **Physical barrier:** Establishes a flexible boundary, protects cellular contents, and supports cell structure. Phospholipid bilayer separates substances inside and outside the cell
2. **Selective permeability:** Regulates entry and exit of ions, nutrients, and waste molecules through the membrane
3. **Electrochemical gradients:** Establishes and maintains an electrical charge difference across the plasma membrane
4. **Communication:** Contains receptors that recognize and respond to molecular signals

FIGURE 1-1. The phospholipid bilayer and associated membrane proteins. From Mescher AL, ed. *Junqueira's Basic Histology.* 13th ed. New York, NY: McGraw-Hill; 2013: Chapter 2, Fig. 2-3.

BIBLIOGRAPHY

Alberts B, Johnson A, Lewis K, et al. Membrane structure. In: Alberts B, Johnson A, Lewis K, et al., eds. *Molecular Biology of the Cell.* 4th ed. New York, NY: Garland Science; 2002:592–589.
Mescher AL. The cytoplasm. In: Mescher AL (ed.), *Junqueira's Basic Histology.* 13th ed. New York, NY: McGraw-Hill; 2013: Chapter 2.

3. **(E)** Plasma membrane fluidity is determined by several factors: temperature, lipid composition involving phospholipid chain lengths, fatty acid chain saturation, and cholesterol content; it is not a function of integral proteins. Integral proteins are structures firmly embedded in the cell membrane via covalent bonds and are difficult to dissociate without the use of detergents. Transmembrane proteins are subtypes of integral proteins that physically span the entire lipid bilayer and often serve as receptor proteins to transduce outside-in or inside-out signaling pathways. Ion channels, transport proteins, and many receptors are integral proteins. In contrast to integral proteins, peripheral proteins are weakly associated with the membrane by covalent bonds or adaptor proteins and can be removed by altering the pH. Peripheral proteins can be found on either the intracellular or extracellular side of the cell membrane; hormone receptors are usually peripheral proteins.

Integral proteins have three general categories of function: (1) receptors, (2) channels or pumps, and (3) structural proteins. Receptor proteins can be subdivided by their methods of signal transduction into those linked to ion channels (i.e., neurotransmitter-gated, mechanical-gated, voltage-gated ion channels), G proteins (i.e., heterotrimeric GTP-binding proteins), or enzymes (i.e., tyrosine kinases, serine-threonine kinases). Integral proteins are also involved as receptors in immune function and in receptor-mediated endocytosis. Passive ion channels or active transport pumps are often integral proteins themselves. An example of structural function is the involvement of integral proteins with polysaccharide attachments in forming the glycocalyx layer on cell surfaces, which is involved in cell protection and lectin-mediated cell–cell adhesion.

BIBLIOGRAPHY

Gallagher PG. The red blood cell membrane and its disorders: Hereditary spherocytosis, elliptocytosis, and related diseases. In: Prchal JT, Kaushansky K, Lichtman MA, et al. (eds.), *Williams Hematology*, 8th ed. New York, NY: McGraw-Hill; 2010:Chapter 45.

Murray RK, Granner DK. Membranes: Structure & function. In: Bender DA, Botham KM, Weil PA, et al. (eds.), *Harper's Illustrated Biochemistry*, 29th ed. New York: McGraw-Hill; 2011:Chapter 40.

4. **(A)** Intracellular macromolecules contribute little to osmolarity directly because of their relatively low numbers and large sizes, but their indirect contribution is significant. The charges on intracellular macromolecules attract many small counterions, which then contribute to osmolarity and the Donnan effect. The tenets of the Donnan equilibrium are that nondiffusible and diffusible substances are distributed on the two sides of the membrane so that the products of their concentrations are equal and ionic charges are balanced on both sides. However, only the distribution of diffusible ions creates a potential difference across the membrane. The Donnan effect results in a higher concentration of diffusible ions intracellularly, and the membrane potential is maintained by the Na^+-K^+ ATPase pump. Treating human cells with ouabain or digitalis glycosides inhibits the Na^+-K^+ ATPase pump. At the cellular level, the prolonged inhibition of the pump results in the accumulation of intracellular Na^+, which causes the cell to swell and burst.

Polar or charged molecules have difficulty traversing cell membranes and must be transported by carrier or channel proteins. Channel proteins and some carrier proteins allow passive transport or facilitated transport down an electrochemical gradient. Some carrier proteins act in active transport to pump molecules against the electrochemical gradient. Ionophores are hydrophobic molecules released by microorganisms to form carriers or channels in host cell membranes to cause the rapid flow of ions down the electrochemical gradient. For example, gramicidin A is an antibiotic produced by certain bacteria that functions as a channel-forming ionophore to collapse the H^+, Na^+, and K^+ gradients of other bacteria sensitive to its effects. FCCP is a mobile carrier ionophore that dissipates the H^+ gradient across the mitochondrial inner membrane. Valinomycin dissipates K^+ gradients, and A23187 or ionomycin causes a massive influx of Ca^{2+} and can activate the apoptotic signaling pathway.

The automated blood counts (ABC) transporter superfamily consists of membrane channel proteins with two adenosine triphosphate (ATP)-binding cassettes or domains. The cystic fibrosis transmembrane conductance regulator (CFTR) is a member of the ABC transporter superfamily, whose members are also known as traffic ATPases. The binding of ATP to the domains leads to conformational changes that help transport molecules across the membrane, and ATP hydrolysis leads to dissociation of the domains to repeat the cycle. MDR proteins are ABC transporters that pump hydrophobic drugs out of the cytosol. MDR proteins are overexpressed in certain human cancer cells, making the cells resistant to many chemotherapeutic agents. An ABC transporter is also involved in many cases of *Plasmodium falciparum* infections, which are resistant to conventional malaria drugs such as chloroquine.

BIBLIOGRAPHY

Barrett KE, Barman SM, Boitano S, Brooks HL. Overview of cellular physiology in medical physiology. In: Barrett KE, Barman SM, Boitano S, Brooks HL (eds.), *Ganong's Review of Medical Physiology*. 24th ed. New York, NY: McGraw-Hill; 2012:Chapter 2.

Kipp H, Arias IM. Trafficking of canalicular ABC transporters in hepatocytes. *Annu Rev Physiol* 2002;64:595–608.

5. **(A)** The CF gene is 230 kb in length and codes for 1480 amino acids, yet a single phenylalanine deletion is usually the cause of dysfunction in the CFTR chloride channel. CFTR is an ATP-dependent transport protein that includes two membrane-spanning domains, two nucleotide-binding domains that interact with ATP, and one regulatory domain with several phosphorylation sites. This channel is located on the luminal plasma membrane of epithelial cells in many different tissues. In the regulation of Cl^- transport, CFTR is normally closed and only opens when it is phosphorylated by protein kinase A. There have been about 400 different mutations found in the CFTR gene since 1989; however, about 70% of individuals who have CF are linked to the deletion of three nucleotides encoding phenylalanine 508. The mutant CFTR is not glycosylated or transported to the cell surface, and the mutant CFTR eventually becomes degraded within the ER.

CF afflicts 1 in 2000 live births, making it the most common fatal inherited disease of whites. The disease affects exocrine glands in multiple organs, but its most devastating effects occur in the respiratory system. The thick, chloride-deficient mucus clogs airways and produces chronic infections. CFTR dysfunction also results in malabsorption and infertility. The lungs, pancreas, and bile ducts in CF demonstrate dysfunction in secreting Cl^-, resulting in a hyperviscous secretion product. In contrast, sweat glands are unable to reabsorb Cl^- properly before final secretion. The resulting increase in sweat NaCl content allows for diagnosis using the sweat chloride test with "a" Cl^- concentration above 50 mEq/L (children) or 60 mEq/L (adults) being positive.

BIBLIOGRAPHY

Boucher RC. Cystic fibrosis. In: Longo DL, Fauci AS (eds.), *Harrison's Principles of Internal Medicine*, 18th ed. New York, NY: McGraw-Hill; 2012:2147–2150.

6. **(E)** Cadherins are calcium-binding integral membrane glycoproteins crucial for cell–cell adhesion and are located at the zonula adherens. The cadherin family is divided into two major types: the classic cadherins associated with catenins intracellularly and the nonclassic cadherins unassociated with catenins. Classic cadherins are anchored to the actin cytoskeleton of the cell by intracellular intermediates called catenins. The major classic cadherins include E-cadherins (aka uvomorulin) on epithelial cells, N-cadherins on neural cells, VE-cadherins on vascular endothelial cells, and P-cadherins on several cell types. Cadherins undergo *cis*-dimerization with other cadherins on the same plasma membrane to form strand dimers and undergo calcium-dependent *trans*-dimerization with cadherins on adjacent plasma membranes to form adhesion dimers.

   The junctional complex consists of three major regions: zonula occludens, zonula adherens, and macula adherens. The zonula occludens is also called the tight junction because it is highly resistant to the passage of molecules and is composed of occludins, ZO-1, ZO-2, and claudins. The zonula adherens or belt desmosome is primarily composed of cadherins and, along with the zonula occludens, is highly tissue specific. The macula adherens is composed of desmosome proteins forming spot desmosomes and are distinct from the gap junctions, which are composed of connexons functioning in cell–cell communication. They are also distinct from hemidesmosomes, which anchor the cell to the basal lamina or basement membrane.

   ZO-1 and desmosomes are not calcium dependent, and neither calcineurin nor calmodulin is directly involved in cell–cell adhesion. Calcineurin is a calmodulin-binding protein found in the mammalian brain, which acts as a phosphatase in the regulation of calcium channels. Calmodulin is an intracellular protein that binds calcium and regulates various cell signaling functions, including phospholipase A_2 (PLA_2), actin cytoskeleton formation, various kinases, and adenylate and guanylate cyclases.

BIBLIOGRAPHY

Tan MCB, Goedegebuure PS, Eberlien TJ. Tumor biology and tumor markers. In: Townsend CM (ed.), *Sabiston: The Biological Basis of Modern Surgical Practice*, 18th ed. St. Louis, MO: Elsevier/Saunders; 2008:737–766.

7. **(E)** The cytoskeleton is a structural framework of three major components: actin, microtubules, and intermediate filaments, each of which is a protein polymer of repeating subunits held by noncovalent bonds.

   Epithelial cells can have apical cytoskeletal specializations such as cilia, stereocilia, or microvilli. Cilia are microtubule structures that function in motility using dynein ATPase to provide energy and are composed of the axoneme (i.e., a microtubule core of nine doublets circumferentially and two singlets centrally) attached at its base to a basal body (i.e., nine triplet microtubules circumferentially and none centrally). Cilia beat in waves to transport external materials in tissues such as the respiratory epithelium and oviducts.

   Stereocilia are long, irregular microvilli composed of actin microfilaments, functioning in signal transduction in hair cells of the inner ear or absorptive function in epididymal cells. Microvilli are composed of actin microfilaments anchored to the terminal web (i.e., apical actin network that connects to the zonula adherens) and greatly increase the surface area of cells important for absorption. Microvilli form the brush border of renal proximal tubular cells and the striated border of intestinal epithelial cells. In the intestinal epithelium, the microvilli are also coated with a glycocalyx layer that aids in carbohydrate digestion and physical protection.

BIBLIOGRAPHY

Reeves M. Cell biology. In: O'Leary JP (ed.), *The Physiologic Basis of Surgery*, 4th ed. Baltimore, MD: Lippincott Williams & Wilkins; 2008:1–43.

8. **(D)** Actin is a cytoskeletal filament and not a molecular motor protein; the rest are motor proteins. Molecular motor proteins are defined as proteins that bind to polarized cytoskeletal filaments (e.g., microtubules or actin) and use energy from ATP hydrolysis to move along the filament to generate unidirectional molecular level movements such as those involved in muscle contraction, the transport of intracellular cargo, cell division, and ciliary motion. Most motor proteins are associated with cytoskeletal filaments via a motor head domain, which binds and hydrolyzes ATP to undergo cycles of "walking" movements. For example, the myosin contraction cycle begins with the myosin head bound tightly to an actin filament in a *rigor* configuration (named for *rigor mortis*). The binding of an ATP molecule to the myosin head results in a conformational change that releases myosin from the actin filament. The hydrolysis of ATP occurs with an additional conformational change that cocks the myosin head to displace the head about 5 nm farther toward the plus end of the actin filament.

The force-generating power stroke is created by the weak binding of the myosin head to the new site on the actin filament associated with the release of inorganic phosphate from ATP hydrolysis and then the strong binding of the myosin head to actin associated with the release of ADP. The motor head domain resumes its prior conformation rebound at a portion of the cytoskeletal filament a few nanometers away to repeat the cycle. Other motor proteins such as kinesin and dynein undergo similar walking cycles coupling nucleotide hydrolysis with conformational changes, using two motor head domains that dimerize before alternately binding and unbinding cytoskeletal filaments.

Myosin was the first motor protein identified and was determined to be the skeletal muscle protein responsible for contraction. Myosin was later discovered to be present in nonmuscle cells and was found to function in different types of cell contraction in nonmuscle cells as well as in cytokinesis or cell division. This type of myosin consists of two heavy chains, each consisting of an N-terminal motor head domain and elongated C-terminal coiled-coil α-helical domain for dimerization; each heavy chain is associated with two different forms of light chains at its motor head region. This dimeric form of myosin was later renamed myosin II after the discovery of a monomeric form of myosin named myosin I in protozoa. Several additional monomeric and dimeric forms of myosin were later discovered and named myosin III through XVIII in order of discovery. There are about 40 myosin genes in humans with several structural classes being represented. Myosin is a conventional motor protein, using ATP hydrolysis to walk toward the plus ends of actin filaments; myosin VI is the only exception in that it moves toward the minus end.

Kinesin is a microtubule motor protein that belongs to the kinesin superfamily of kinesin-related proteins (KRPs). Kinesin contains an N-terminal motor domain, responsible for ATP-dependent transport toward the plus end of the microtubule, and a C-terminal coiled-coil domain responsible for dimerization and binding to cargo. The dimerization of kinesin allows the connection of two N-terminal "feet" that alternately bind and unbind to "walk" along the microtubule in an anterograde fashion.

The dyneins belong to a separate family of microtubule motors that mediate transport in the retrograde direction, toward the minus end of the microtubule. The *cytoplasmic dyneins* form homodimers with two motor domain heads and are responsible for vesicle trafficking and localization of the Golgi within the cell. The *axonemal dyneins* form heterodimers and heterotrimers responsible for the fast sliding movement of microtubules in the beating of cilia and flagella (see Fig. 1-2).

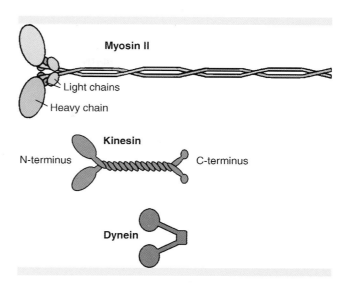

FIGURE 1-2. The structures of myosin, kinesin, and dynein.

BIBLIOGRAPHY

Reeves M. Cell biology. In: O'Leary JP (ed.), *The Physiologic Basis of Surgery*, 4th ed. Baltimore, MD: Lippincott Williams & Wilkins; 2008:1–43.

9. **(E)** Signaling molecules bind to specific receptors to activate signal transduction pathways inside target cells, which are then modified and terminated by complex feedback and regulatory mechanisms. The signal can also be terminated by ligand degradation, inactivation, or reuptake. Signal transduction is achieved by five general types of ligand-binding receptors: (1) ion channel–linked receptors, (2) G protein–linked receptors, (3) enzyme-linked receptors, (4) intracellular steroid hormone receptors, and (5) intracellular receptor guanylate cyclases. Signaling can also be accomplished without ligands in certain cases through direct voltage-gated or mechanical-gated ion channels.

Ion channel–linked receptors are multisubunit, single-pass transmembrane proteins that function by opening selective ion channels in response to ligand binding and include most of the major neurotransmitter receptors (NTRs). These include both excitatory NTRs (i.e., glutamate receptor, nicotinic acetylcholine receptor [nAChR], and serotonin receptor) and inhibitory NTRs (i.e., $GABA_A$ receptor and glycine receptor). As an example, the nAChR contains two ACh binding sites and is composed of five subunits that form an ion channel permeable to many cations (e.g., Na^+, K^+, Ca^{2+}). On binding of two ACh molecules, nAChR undergoes a conformational change to open the channel gate, primarily allowing the rapid influx of Na^+ ions to depolarize the postsynaptic membrane. At the neuromuscular junction, nAChR transmits the signal to contract from nerve cells to muscle cells. The glutamate NMDA receptor also forms an ion channel permeable to cations, but the NMDA receptor is blocked at resting membrane potential by extracellular Mg^{2+} ions. Both voltage-dependent membrane depolarization and glutamate binding are necessary to remove the Mg^{2+} plug and to open the channel gate, allowing the influx of Ca^{2+} ions important in long-term potentiation in the hippocampus. $GABA_A$ receptors are permeable to Cl^- ions, resulting in membrane hyperpolarization, and act as the major inhibitory NTR in the brain. Glycine receptors are also permeable to Cl^- ions and serve as the major inhibitory NTR in the spinal cord.

G protein–linked receptors (GPCRs) traverse the cell membrane seven times and are linked to heterotrimeric GTP-binding proteins with α-, β-, and γ-subunits. There are several known G proteins, which include G_s, G_i, G_o, G_q, and $G_{12/13}$. Ligand-binding results in dissociation of heterotrimeric G protein subunits and activation of downstream signaling, usually through the adenylate cyclase (AC) or PLC pathway. On binding of ligand, the associated G protein exchanges its GDP for GTP to become activated and is inactivated when its GTPase activity hydrolyzes the bound GTP to GDP. Activation of G_s protein results in the dissociation of the $α_s$-subunit, which stimulates AC and increases cAMP levels. Cholera toxin ADP-ribosylates the $α_s$-subunit to block its GTPase activity and overactivates AC activity to cause high cAMP levels and oversecretion in intestinal epithelium. In contrast, activation of G_i protein results in the dissociation of the $α_i$-subunit, which inhibits AC and decreases cAMP levels. Pertussis toxin ADP-ribosylates the $α_i$-subunit to block its dissociation from the other subunits and prevents AC inhibition to cause high cAMP levels and oversecretion in respiratory epithelium. Activation of G_q protein results in stimulation of PLC, which cleaves PIP_2 into DAG and IP_3 to activate PKC and elevation of cytosolic Ca^{2+}. Multiple G protein subtypes can be activated by a single GPCR, causing the activation of multiple signal transduction pathways. A number of ligands activate GPCRs including the adrenergic receptors, dopamine receptors, $GABA_B$ receptor, PAR-1 thrombin receptor, purinergic receptors (e.g., A-type adenosine receptor, P-type ATP receptor), glucagon receptor, neuropeptide receptors (e.g., NPY, VIP, opiate, bradykinin, ADH, oxytocin), and pituitary hormone receptors (e.g., TSH, ACTH, LH).

Enzyme-linked receptors have extracellular domains that bind ligand and intracellular domains that serve as enzymes to activate intracellular signaling. Enzyme-linked receptors are subdivided into RTKs (e.g., insulin receptor and various growth factor receptors), tyrosine kinase–associated receptors (e.g., GH receptor, prolactin receptor, and many cytokine receptors), receptor

serine-threonine kinases (e.g., TGF-β), receptor tyrosine phosphatases (e.g., CD45), and receptor guanylate cyclases (e.g., ANP receptor). RTKs oligomerize and autophosphorylate each other in response to binding oligomerized ligands. The phosphotyrosine residues interact with SH_2 domain-containing proteins, which activate son-of-sevenless (Sos) proteins, then Ras proteins, then Raf protein kinases, and finally the mitogen-activated protein kinase (MAPK) pathway to phosphorylate gene regulatory proteins (GRPs) in the nucleus. RTKs also activate the PLC-γ and PI3K pathways. Tyrosine kinase–associated receptors can phosphorylate other intracellular proteins such as Src to transduce its signal. Receptor serine-threonine kinases transmit their intracellular signal through the Smad pathway. Receptor tyrosine phosphatases dephosphorylate tyrosine residues in certain intracellular proteins to regulate their activities. Activation of receptor guanylate cyclases results in increased cGMP levels and activation of protein kinase G (PKG) to phosphorylate serine and threonine residues on certain intracellular proteins.

Intracellular steroid hormone receptors are distinctive in that their hydrophobic ligands can pass through the cell membrane to bind receptors in the cytosol and to induce nuclear translocation, activating the transcription of specific genes. Steroid hormone receptors are themselves GRPs that contain zinc finger motifs as their DNA-binding domains, which are composed of four cysteine residues bound to a zinc atom. Inactive steroid hormone receptors are complexed to the heat shock proteins Hsp90 and Hsp56 in the cytosol, which are released on binding of ligand to expose the DNA-binding region. The ligand–receptor complex translocates to the nucleus to activate the transcription of specific genes within 30 min, termed the primary response. The products of the primary response can then activate the transcription of other genes, termed the secondary response. Ligands for steroid hormone receptors include glucocorticoids, estrogen, progesterone, thyroid hormone, retinoic acid (vitamin A_1), and vitamin D_3.

Special intracellular receptor guanylate cyclases (aka soluble guanylyl cyclase [Sgc]) bind the unique gaseous ligand nitric oxide (NO) to activate cGMP production, PKG activation, and the phosphorylation of serine or threonine on intracellular proteins to activate signaling. NO is formed from arginine precursors by nitric oxide synthases (i.e., iNOS, eNOS, nNOS) with the half-life of NO being approximately 5 s. The gaseous nature of NO and its brief half-life mean that it only acts in a local fashion and is primarily regulated at the level of NOS activity. NO is an important neurotransmitter in the central and peripheral nervous systems, participates in the immune function of leukocytes, and causes blood vessel dilatation by smooth muscle relaxation. Many cardiovascular drugs for reducing blood pressure depend on the NO-cGMP pathway, including nitroglycerin and nitroprusside. Although originally studied as a drug for hypertension, sildenafil exploits the downstream portions of the NO-cGMP pathway in achieving penile erection by inhibiting PDE_5 (which normally breaks down cGMP in the corpus cavernosum) (see Fig. 1-3).

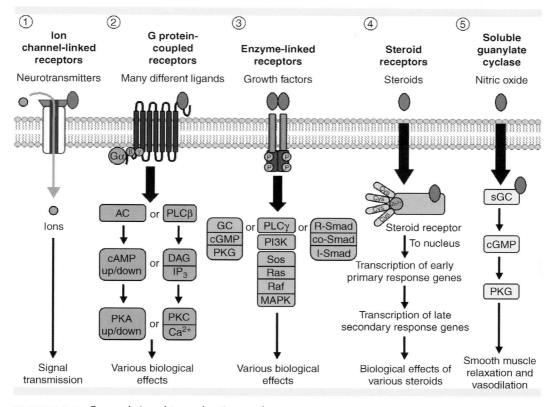

FIGURE 1-3. General signal transduction pathways.

BIBLIOGRAPHY

Ko TC, Evers BM. Molecular and cell biology. In: Townsend CM (ed.), *Sabiston: The Biological Basis of Modern Surgical Practice*, 18th ed. St. Louis, MO: Elsevier/Saunders; 2008:26–43.

10. **(B)** Steroid receptors exist as proteins floating freely in the cytosol, which translocate into the nucleus on binding of their substrate. Zinc finger motif is the specialized domain that steroid receptors use to recognize and bind DNA. These domains are known as Cys_2/Cys_2 fingers and have a primary amino acid sequence of $Cys-X_2-Cys-X_{13}-Cys-X_2-Cys$, in which X can be any amino acid. In the final folded structure of a single zinc finger, the four Cys residues form a tetrahedral structure with a Zn^{2+} atom in the middle. The intervening amino acids loop out to form an α-helix or beta-sheet, with one side of the helix making contact in the major groove of a DNA molecule conferring binding. A single steroid receptor molecule also has a second zinc finger that aids in dimerization with another receptor molecule when both have bound ligands. Since steroid molecules are hydrophobic and are able to freely pass through the phospholipid cell membrane, steroid receptors have no need for a transmembrane domain. Further, steroid receptors do not undergo signal transduction cascades as do membrane-bound receptors, eliminating the need for catalytic domains. Multiple C-terminal tyrosine residues are descriptive of membrane-bound RTKs, which use their catalytic domains to perform autophosphorylation on binding of oligomerized ligands. SH_2 domains are specialized regions of approximately 100 amino acids located on various intracellular proteins that bind to phosphorylated tyrosine residues on RTKs for signal transduction. Protein kinases (e.g., c-Src), adaptor molecules (e.g., Grb2), and regulatory subunits (e.g., p85 of PI3K) are examples of intracellular proteins with SH_2 domains.

Many hormones act on a cell by binding plasma membrane receptors, which in turn activate intracellular second messengers. Other hormones, such as the steroid hormones (i.e., testosterone, estrogen, aldosterone), thyroid hormones, vitamin D, and the retinoids are able to permeate the cell membrane and bind soluble receptors located in the cytosol or nucleus. Intracellular hormone receptors change their DNA-binding activity when they bind hormones. The binding of one of these hormones to its receptor causes dissociation of the receptor from a regulatory protein called Hsp90. This opens a DNA-binding domain on the receptor, and the receptor becomes a tissue factor. When this occurs, the hormone–receptor complex localizes to the nucleus and binds to response elements on certain genes that can lead to both activation and repression of specific genes involved in that cell's response to the hormone. Most of these receptors bind DNA as either homodimers or heterodimers.

11. **(C)** Human chorionic gonadotrophin, glucagon, gastrin, and histamine all act via plasma membrane receptors and would not be significantly present in the nuclear fraction of cell lysates. Steroid hormones generally have a two-phase effect on the target cell, which can vary between cell types and the specific hormone and receptor. The first response involves the increase in transcription of early-phase genes, which can then go on to activate the transcription of other proteins in a delayed fashion. In general, steroid hormones have a slower response than membrane receptors, sometimes taking 30 min to hours to exert their effects. Steroid hormones also have a much longer half-life in the body than water-soluble hormones, especially in the case of thyroid hormone. It has also been postulated that the metabolic enzymes involved in the production of these hormones in the body are able to communicate with the receptors to closely regulate the amounts of these hormones in the body.

BIBLIOGRAPHY

Paulsen DF. The plasma membrane & cytoplasm. In: Paulsen DF (ed.), *Histology & Cell Biology: Examination & Board Review*, 5th ed. New York, NY: McGraw-Hill; 2010:Chapter 2.

Reeves M. Cell biology. In: O'Leary JP (ed.), *The Physiologic Basis of Surgery*, 4th ed. Baltimore, MD: Lippincott Williams & Wilkins; 2008:1–43.

12. **(E)** Lysosomes are membranous organelles that contain acid hydrolases or lysosomal enzymes that include proteases, nucleases, lipases, and galactosidases that function at an acidic pH to degrade old intracellular organelles or phagocytosed substances (see Fig. 1-4). Organelles have a relatively rapid rate of turnover (e.g., liver mitochondria have a lifetime of 10 days) and are broken down in a process called autophagy. Old or damaged organelles are enveloped by an additional membrane to create an autophagosome, which fuses with a lysosome for degradation (see Fig. 1-5). For phagocytosed or endocytosed substances, these are taken up into early endosomes where some of the materials are recycled

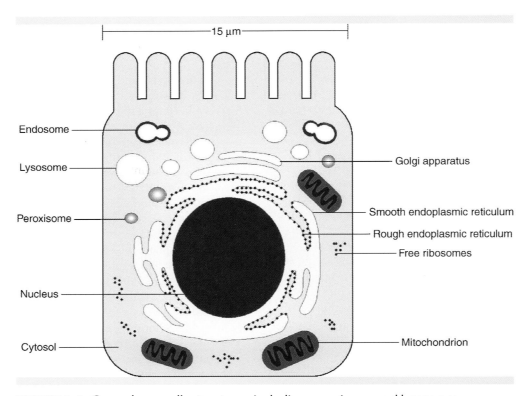

FIGURE 1-4. General organelle structures, including peroxisome and lysosomes.

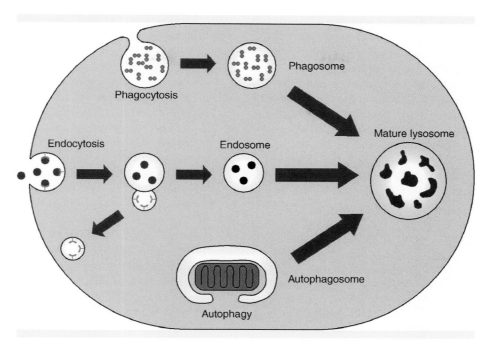

FIGURE 1-5. Lysosome formation.

back to the plasma membrane and others continue as late endosomes. Golgi hydrolase vesicles containing inactive lysosomal enzymes fuse with late endosomes to form mature lysosomes. There are numerous lysosomal storage diseases (e.g., Hunter, Hurler, Sanfilippo A, Tay-Sachs, Gaucher, Niemann-Pick, Pompe, I-cell, and Krabbe disease), each associated with mutations of different lysosomal enzymes and abnormal accumulation of undigested materials.

Peroxisomes are unique organelles in that they are surrounding only by a single membrane and contain amino acid hydrolase, hydroxyacid oxidase, urate oxidase, and catalase for the production and breakdown of hydrogen peroxide. The oxidative reactions performed by peroxisomes are important for the breakdown of toxic substances and fatty acid molecules. Peroxisomes are also essential for the production of certain phospholipid classes in myelin; therefore, many peroxisomal disorders result in neurologic disease. Peroxisomal dysfunction is the etiology of Zellweger syndrome (aka cerebrohepatorenal syndrome), which is an autosomal recessive neonatal syndrome characterized by incomplete myelinization of nervous tissue and muscular hypotonia, hepatomegaly, and small glomerular cysts of the kidney resulting in death shortly after birth. Adrenoleukodystrophy (ALD) is an X-linked recessive disorder involving the absence or dysfunction of peroxisomal enzymes essential for fatty acid β-oxidation. ALD results in the myelin degeneration in the nervous system and abnormal intracellular accumulation of lipids, manifesting

in progressive dementia, spastic paralysis, and adrenal insufficiency in children.

BIBLIOGRAPHY

Barrett KE, Barman SM, Boitano S, Brooks HL. Overview of cellular physiology in medical physiology. In: Barrett KE, Barman SM, Boitano S, Brooks HL (eds.), *Ganong's Review of Medical Physiology*, 24th ed. New York, NY: McGraw-Hill; 2012:Chapter 2.

Reeves M. Cell biology. In: O'Leary JP (ed.), *The Physiologic Basis of Surgery*, 4th ed. Baltimore, MD: Lippincott Williams & Wilkins; 2008:1–43.

13. **(A)** Lysosomal storage diseases are the result of a deficiency in one of many lysosomal enzymes and can be subdivided into nine forms of sphingolipidoses, five mucopolysaccharidoses (MPSs), and I-cell disease. It is also possible to include Pompe disease (type II glycogen storage disease) as a lysosomal disorder.

Lysosomal storage diseases should be considered in the differential diagnosis of patients with neurologic, renal, or muscular degeneration and/or unexplained hepatomegaly, splenomegaly. Of the nine forms of sphingolipidoses, the six major forms are Fabry, Krabbe, Gaucher, Tay-Sachs, Niemann-Pick, and metachromatic leukodystrophy. All are autosomal recessive in inheritance except for Fabry disease, which is X-linked recessive. Fabry disease occurs in 3 of 100,000 births, occurs due to a deficiency in α-galactosidase A, and causes an accumulation of ceramide trihexoside. Fabry is characterized by renal and cardiac failure, cerebrovascular complications, severe pain in the lower extremities, and angiokeratomas.

Krabbe is also known as globoid leukodystrophy, results in the deficiency of galactosylceramide β-galactosidase with galactocerebroside (aka galactosylceramide) accumulation in the brain, and leads to neurologic problems with early death. Gaucher disease is the most common sphingolipidosis occurring in 166 of 100,000 births, is caused by the deficiency of β-glucocerebrosidase, and results in the accumulation of glucocerebroside in the brain and reticuloendothelial system (RES). Enlarged Gaucher's cells with a characteristic "crinkled tissue paper" appearance is pathognomonic, and the most common type I form does not affect lifespans. To give a relative idea of the frequency of occurrence, Down syndrome has a prevalence of 125 in 100,000 births.

The next most common sphingolipidosis is Tay-Sachs, which occurs in 33 of 100,000 births. Tay-Sachs occurs because of a deficiency in hexosaminidase A, causes an accumulation of GM_2 ganglioside with death occurring before age 3, is associated with cherry-red spots on the maculae, and is especially prevalent in Ashkenazi Jews. Niemann-Pick disease is due to a deficiency in sphingomyelinase with accumulation of sphingomyelin in the RES, resulting in death before age 3. Cherry-red spots can also occur in Niemann-Pick although less frequently than in Tay-Sachs, which are because of lipid infiltration leading to the visualization of the red vascular choroids surrounded by white retinal edema. Metachromatic leukodystrophy is the deficiency of arylsulfatase A with accumulation of sulfatide in the brain, peripheral nerves, liver, and kidneys, resulting in spasticity and death before puberty. The minor sphingolipidoses include GM_1 gangliosidosis (resembling Tay-Sachs), Sandhoff disease (resembling a rapid form of Tay-Sachs), and Farber disease (a fatal accumulation of ceramide in joints and subcutaneous tissues).

BIBLIOGRAPHY

Grabowski GA, Hopkin RJ. Lysosomal storage diseases. In: *Harrison's Principles of Internal Medicine*. New York, NY: McGraw-Hill; 2012:3191–3197.

14. **(B)**

15. **(A) Explanations for 14 and 15.**

The Golgi works in conjunction with the ER for the production and processing of many proteins. The ER is a multifunctional contiguous intracellular membrane structure that encompasses many vital roles of the cell. The luminal compartment of the ER is a distinct cellular compartment that houses specific proteins and often a different chemo-osmotic milieu. One fluid membrane bilayer makes up at least three specific domains in the cell: the rER, the sER, and the outer nuclear envelope. Each domain has unique characteristics that are mainly determined by the proteins contained in each domain. During mitosis, these domains are lost and both daughter cells receive an equal portion of the ER. During interphase, the ER again subspecializes into its three domains as proteins become compartmentalized.

The rER has a granular appearance on electron micrographs because of the many ribosomes that are attached to the external portion of the membrane. These ribosomes contain a messenger RNA that is being actively transcribed into specific types of proteins found throughout the cell. Proteins translated in the rER include all transmembrane proteins, secreted proteins, and lysosomal enzymes; however, peroxisomal enzymes are imported from the cytosol directly into peroxisomes and are not synthesized in the rER. Only proteins translated in the rER can be shuttled to the Golgi for processing. Proteins to be translated in the rER contain a signal-recognition sequence of amino acids that is recognized during translation on a free ribosome by a protein called signal-recognition peptide (SRP). SRP halts cytosolic translation and brings the ribosome–mRNA complex to the rER, where there is a receptor for the SRP. The ribosome binds to a protein translocator pore on the external leaflet of the rER membrane, and translation is allowed to continue as the protein is fed through the pore into the ER lumen.

As proteins are fed into the ER, hydrophobic amino acid regions of the protein may remain embedded in the ER membrane. These will become membrane proteins and may localize to either the external plasma membrane or an intracellular organelle. Proteins that do not contain these membrane-spanning sequences will simply enter the ER lumen. Some proteins that contain multiple transmembrane sequences include ion channels and G protein–coupled receptors. Lipid vesicles, containing proteins from the rER, are shuttled to the *cis*-Golgi network, where they enter the Golgi apparatus. The Golgi modifies proteins it receives from the rER through addition and removal of sugar groups as well as phosphorylation and sulfation. The amino acid code of the protein will dictate its specific Golgi modifications. For example, lysosomal hydrolases are given an M6P group, which serves as a ligand for a Golgi receptor for M6P. This receptor binds these enzymes and carries them to lysosomes, where they are activated. In I-cell disease. This phosphorylation of mannose in the Golgi is defective, and these hydrolase enzymes cannot localize to lysosomes, so the lysosomal enzymes are mistakenly secreted by the cell.

Regions of a cell's ER that lack ribosomes and have a less coarse appearance on electron microscopy are called sER. The sER is not a major organelle in most cells but is pronounced in other types of cells that carry out specific processes. Some of these processes include steroid hormone synthesis (in adrenal cortex cells and Leydig cells of the testes), detoxification (in hepatocytes), and calcium sequestration (in muscle). The sER (called sarcoplasmic reticulum in muscle cells) contains integral membrane proteins called sER Ca^{2+}-ATPase pumps that shuttle Ca^{2+} ions into the ER lumen from the cytosol. Thus, the sER also serves as a Ca^{2+} storage compartment that can be released during certain signaling cascades.

BIBLIOGRAPHY

Reeves M. Cell biology. In: O'Leary JP (ed.), *The Physiologic Basis of Surgery*, 4th ed. Baltimore, MD: Lippincott Williams & Wilkins; 2008:1–43.

Steer ML. Exocrine pancreas. In: Townsend CM (ed.), *Sabiston: The Biological Basis of Modern Surgical Practice*, 18th ed. St. Louis, MO: Elsevier/Saunders; 2008:1589–1623.

16. **(D)** The series of short tandem repeats at the end of the chromosomes described is a telomere sequence. Telomeres are repeating DNA sequences (TTAGGG in humans) that are bound by specialized protein complexes, which confer stability and provide a protective role to the ends of chromosomes. Without these sequences, human chromosomes undergo progressive degradation of their ends because of the nature of DNA replication. Protection is also provided from nuclease attack, end-to-end joining of the chromosomes, and recombination. Eventually because of chromosomal instability, the replicative potential of these cells becomes limited, and the cells undergo apoptosis or enter a state of cellular senescence in which cells are neither dividing nor dying.

Telomerase is a ribonucleoprotein enzyme that functions in elongating telomere sequences at the ends of chromosomes through DNA reverse transcriptase activity. Telomerase expression is absent in most normal somatic cells but is present in germ cells and most cancers. Telomerase activity is high in germ cells such as a spermatozoa that are consistently being renewed and nearly absent in somatic cells. High telomerase activity results in long TTAGGG repeats on the chromosome ends of spermatozoa and allows indefinite replication without chromosome shortening. Low telomerase activity in somatic cells is believed to contribute to the aging process as the chromosomes progressively shorten with each round of replication. High telomerase expression and activity are also associated with cancer cells as they are able to replicate continuously at abnormally high frequencies. It is believed that inhibiting telomerase in cancer cells could be a prospective form of antineoplastic therapy.

BIBLIOGRAPHY

Ko TC, Evers BM. Molecular and cell biology. In: Townsend CM (ed.), *Sabiston: The Biological Basis of Modern Surgical Practice*, 18th ed. St. Louis, MO: Elsevier/Saunders; 2008:26–43.

17. **(A)** There are two major points at which DNA errors are repaired using two different repair processes: (1) DNA mismatch repair and (2) DNA excision repair. The DNA mismatch repair process corrects errors in DNA sequences that are produced during the replication process, whereas DNA excision repair is used to correct errors because of direct DNA damage. Therefore, in DNA damage induced by UV light, the DNA excision repair proteins are activated rather than the DNA mismatch repair proteins.

In DNA mismatch repair, DNA replication errors that occur during the action of DNA polymerase are initially corrected by the 3′-to-5′ proofreading exonucleolytic domain of the polymerase as it synthesizes new strands in the 5′-to-3′ direction. However, some mistakes escape this initial proofreading mechanism and are corrected by strand-directed DNA mismatch repair. New strands are initially marked with nicks that allow DNA mismatch repair proteins to recognize and correct any remaining errors. DNA mismatch repair proteins recognize and bind a mismatched base pair before activating degradation of the newly synthesized strand from the nearest nick back to the mismatch, and then the removed sequence is repolymerized.

Hereditary nonpolyposis colorectal cancer (HNPCC) is due to one inherited defective copy of any of four DNA mismatch repair genes (i.e., *hMSH2*, *hMLH1*, *hPMS1*, and *hPMS2*). Mutations can be detected by "microsatellite instability," which is the term for widespread alterations in the thousands of dinucleotide repeat sequences normally present in the human genome. Although one normal copy of mismatch repair genes can provide sufficient repair activity, the normal copy is susceptible to inactivating somatic mutations. Defects in mismatch repair result in a 1000-fold increase of the frequency of replication errors, which results in increased risk of colon cancer (especially cecum and proximal colon) even without extensive polyp formation.

The DNA excision repair process is used to correct DNA damage, which can be because of induced or spontaneous mutations unrelated to replication. DNA excision repair involves excision of the damaged sequence, synthesis of the proper sequence, and ligation. There are two major DNA excision repair pathways: base excision repair (BER) and nucleotide excision repair (NER). BER involves the removal of a single base and filling of the resulting nucleotide gap, whereas NER involves the removal of large portion of the nucleotide sequence followed by repair. The most common forms of DNA damage that occur are depurination of a single base, deamination of cytosine to uracil, or pyrimidine dimerization. Depurination involves the breaking of the *N*-glycosyl bond between the purine base and the deoxyribose sugar phosphate. The damaged purine is repaired by the BER pathway with excision by the AP endonuclease and a phosphodiesterase; DNA polymerase and ligase then restore the correct sequence. Deamination of cytosine occurs spontaneously about 100 times per day, and the conversion of C-G to U-A pairs would occur at replication in the absence of repair. Uracil-DNA glycosidase recognizes and removes the abnormal uracil in the DNA sequence, followed by repair through the BER pathway with AP endonuclease and a phosphodiesterase excising the remaining deoxyribose sugar phosphate. DNA polymerase and ligase restore the original sequence. Pyrimidine dimerization is caused by UV radiation, causing covalent linkage of neighboring pyrimidine bases, especially thymines. The uvrABC enzyme excises a 12-residue sequence that includes the pyrimidine dimer before DNA polymerase and ligase restore the correct sequence.

Genetic defects in DNA excision repair enzymes result in severe disorders that include xeroderma pigmentosum (XP), ataxia-telangiectasia (AT), Fanconi anemia, and Bloom syndrome. All are autosomal recessive in inheritance and result in high susceptibilities to cancers. XP results in UV radiation hypersensitivity with skin lesions, severe neurologic abnormalities, and high risk of skin malignancies causing early death. AT causes hypersensitivity to ionizing radiation with neurologic abnormalities, cerebellar ataxia, oculocutaneous telangiectasias, immunodeficiency, and susceptibility to lymphoid malignancies. Fanconi anemia is characterized by hypersensitivity to DNA cross-linking agents with pancytopenia, bone marrow hypoplasia, and congenital anomalies. Bloom syndrome causes hypersensitivity to many DNA-damaging agents and manifests in telangiectasia, immunodeficiency, growth retardation, and cancer predisposition.

BIBLIOGRAPHY

Kipps TJ. Composition and biochemistry of lymphocytes and plasma cells. In: Prchal JT, Kaushansky K, Lichtman MA, et al. (eds.), *Williams Hematology*, 8th ed. New York, NY: McGraw-Hill; 2010:Chapter 75.

Marti TM, Kunz C, Fleck O. DNA mismatch repair and mutation avoidance pathways. *J Cell Physiol* 2002;191:28–41.

Mescher AL. The nucleus. In: Mescher AL (ed.), *Junqueira's Basic Histology*, 13th ed. New York, NY: McGraw-Hill; 2013:Chapter 3.

Reeves M. Cell biology. In: O'Leary JP (ed.), *The Physiologic Basis of Surgery*, 4th ed. Baltimore, MD: Lippincott Williams & Wilkins; 2008:1–43.

18. **(D)** The cell cycle is subdivided into interphase and mitosis (M phase). Interphase consists of the G_0, G_1, and G_2 (gap) phases and the S phase between the G_1 and G_2 phases. The G_0 phase is a resting phase in which the cell cycle is suspended; many mature adult cells are in this phase, and this phase can last indefinitely. Organelle, RNA, and protein synthesis occurs during the G_1 phase (lasting for 5/16th of the cell cycle length) to prepare for cell division. This is followed by the G_1 checkpoint, at which progression of the cell cycle is regulated by cyclin-dependent kinase 2 (Cdk2). Cdk2-cyclin D and Cdk2-cyclin E are produced during G_1 to mediate the transition to the S phase. DNA replication occurs during the S phase (lasting for 7/16th of the cell cycle length) and doubles the number of chromosomes in the parent cell preparing the cell for division; centrosomes of the MTOC and histones also duplicate. ATP synthesis and Cdk1 production occur during the G_2 phase (lasting for 3/16th of the cell cycle length). Cdk1-cyclin A and Cdk1-cyclin B regulate the G_2 to M phase transition at the G_2 checkpoint.

The M phase is the shortest phase (lasting 1/16th of the cell cycle length) and is subdivided into prophase, metaphase, anaphase, and telophase. The MTOC consists of a centrosome complex that splits and moves to opposite poles of the cell during prophase. The mitotic spindle forms a network of microtubules between the centrosomes and connects to kinetochores on the centromeres of chromosome pairs. Chromosomes align at the central metaphase plate during metaphase, and the kinetochores separate to allow the split chromosome pairs to move to opposite poles during anaphase. The chromosomes decondense into chromatin as the nuclear envelopes and nucleoli reform at each pole during telophase. Cytokinesis occurs to divide the cytoplasmic contents at the cleavage furrow by the action of the contractile ring, composed of actin and myosin.

The M phase is very rapid in normal cells, and few cells can be caught in mitosis at any specific time point; however, cancer cells with altered cell cycles show increased frequency of mitosis and can often be seen in the M phase. Tumor suppressors such as p53 can arrest the cell cycle at the G_1 or G_2 checkpoints in cells with DNA damage by modulation of Cdk and cyclin production. The cells are suspended at the G_1 phase by p53 until DNA excision repair pathways can fix the damage. Apoptotic signaling can be activated in cells with irreparable DNA or organelle damage to prevent the uncontrolled proliferation of mutated or dysfunctional cells (see Figs. 1-6 and 1-7).

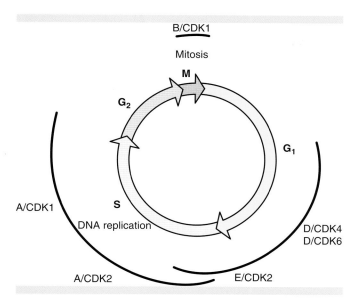

FIGURE 1-6. The cell cycle and its controls. From Feng X, Lin X. Molecular and genomic surgery. In: Brunicardi FC, Andersen DK, Billiar TR, et al. (eds.), *Schwartz's Principles of Surgery,* 9th ed. New York, NY: McGraw-Hill; 2010:Chapter 15, Fig. 15-7.

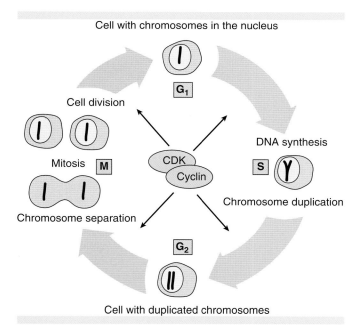

FIGURE 1-7. The cell cycle with chromosomes in the middle.

BIBLIOGRAPHY

Feng X, Lin X. Molecular and genomic surgery. In: Brunicardi FC, Andersen DK, Billiar TR, et al. (eds.), *Schwartz's Principles of Surgery,* 9th ed. New York, NY: McGraw-Hill; 2010:Chapter 15.

Ko TC, Evers BM. Molecular and cell biology. In: Townsend CM (ed.), *Sabiston: The Biological Basis of Modern Surgical Practice,* 18th ed. St. Louis, MO: Elsevier/Saunders; 2008:26–43.

19. **(A)** Proto-oncogenes encode proteins that normally stimulate the cell cycle, and tumor suppressor genes encode proteins that suppress the cell cycle. Oncogenes are mutated proto-oncogenes that are transcribed into oncoproteins, which alter the normal cell cycle, often causing cancer. Proto-oncogenes (e.g., c-*ras*) can become tumorigenic in four major ways: insertional mutagenesis by promoter or enhancer insertion, point mutation, chromosomal translocation, or gene amplification. By convention, proto-oncogenes and oncogenes are designated by three-letter abbreviations in italics with a prefix denoting its cellular or viral origin (e.g., c-*ras* and v-*ras*); the name of the protein product is not italicized and the first letter is capitalized (e.g., Ras). Tumor suppressor genes (e.g., *p53*, *Rb*, *BRCA-1*, *VHL*, *APC*, *DCC*, *NF-1*, *WT-1*) do not follow the same convention except that the gene is italicized and the protein is not, and their mutations result in a variety of familial cancer syndromes.

   Oncogenes encode four different types of signaling products to accelerate the cell cycle: (1) growth factor mimics, (2) mutant growth factor receptors, (3) altered signal transducers, and (4) altered nuclear TFs. For instance, the *sis* oncogene is a mutated form of PDGF that acts as a growth factor mimic to stimulate the formation of astrocytomas and osteosarcomas. The *erb* and *neu* oncogenes are mutated EGF receptors with increased activity compared to the wild-type, resulting in various cancers, especially breast cancer. At the intracellular signal transduction level, the *ras* oncogene encodes a p21 protein, which functions like a G protein except that the mutated form binds GTP irreversibly because of loss of GTPase activity, resulting in continuous stimulation of the cell cycle. The *abl* proto-oncogene, designated after a pediatrician named Abelson, also acts as an altered signal transducer when *abl* from chromosome 9 translocates to the major breakpoint cluster region *bcr* on chromosome 22. The t(9:22) translocation results in a fusion gene that encodes a constitutively active Bcr-Abl hybrid called *P210*, which is an abnormal intracellular tyrosine kinase found in chronic myelocytic leukemia (CML). Again at the signal transduction level, some forms of follicular lymphoma have a translocation of the immunoglobulin (Ig) heavy chain locus on chromosome 14 to the *bcl-2* locus on chromosome 18, resulting in increased expression of Bcl-2 and inhibition of apoptosis. At the TF level in the nucleus, the c-*myc* proto-oncogene encodes a helix-loop-helix TF, which can be mutated into an overactive form. The c-*myc* proto-oncogene on chromosome 8 can also be translocated to the Ig heavy chain locus on chromosome 14 in some forms of Burkitt lymphoma, resulting in Myc overexpression. Also at the transcriptional level, mutations of *jun* or *fos* proto-onco-genes can result in overactive leucine zipper TFs in their homodimeric forms or their heterodimeric form, the latter of which is also called activated protein-1.

Tumor suppressor genes usually encode GRPs or regulators of GRPs, which either inhibit the gene expression of products that stimulate the cell cycle or activate the expression of products that suppress the cell cycle. Therefore, tumor suppressors generally act at the transcriptional level. For instance, *p53* encodes a zinc finger GRP that increases the production of inhibitors of Cdk2-cyclin D and Cdk2-cyclin E, arresting cells with damaged DNA at the G_1 phase of the cell cycle. The *p53* gene is named for the molecular weight of its protein product and is mutated in the majority of known cancers. In retinoblastoma, the Rb protein product binds and inhibits a GRP, preventing the expression of certain gene products that stimulate the cell cycle. Rb is the prototype for the Knudson two-hit hypothesis, which states that two separate mutagenic events are necessary to induce alterations on both *rb* chromosomes. In familial forms of retino-blastoma, one defective *rb* chromosome is inherited and only one somatic mutation is needed. In sporadic cases of retinoblastoma, two somatic mutations are required to produce loss-of-function in both gene copies.

BIBLIOGRAPHY

Ko TC, Evers BM. Molecular and cell biology. In: Townsend CM (ed.), *Sabiston: The Biological Basis of Modern Surgical Practice*, 18th ed. St. Louis, MO: Elsevier/Saunders; 2008:26–43.

Stewart JH, Levine EA. Oncology. In: O'Leary JP (ed.), *The Physiologic Basis of Surgery*, 4th ed. Baltimore, MD: Lippincott Williams & Wilkins; 2008:188–217.

20. **(B)** All of the choices except for Fas receptor, which is involved in proapoptotic signaling, may have increased expression or activity in transformed cells. Telomerase activity allows for stabilization and prevention of degradation of chromosomal ends through continual cycles of replication of a cell, and high levels of telomerase expression have been shown in a wide variety of human tumors. The c-*myc* gene is termed an immediate-early gene encoding for a TF that can rapidly cause continual growth and replication of the cell on its overexpression. Such an example can be seen with Burkitt lymphoma, where a translocation between the Ig heavy chain locus on chromosome 14 and the c-*myc* gene on chromosome 8 leads to high levels of Myc protein expression. Ras, a monomeric G protein, commonly acts as an oncogene when point mutations occur which lower its GTPase activity. Thus, Ras being left in a constant "on" state leads to upregulation of signal transduction pathways causing increased expression of growth factors and tumor induction. Ras mutations can be seen in such cancers as

pancreatic adenocarcinoma and cholangiocarcinoma. The gene for *bcl-2* encodes an antiapoptotic factor, in which increased levels of Bcl-2 dimers in a cell favor cellular survival. B-cell lymphomas are examples of malignancies in which translocation of the *bcl-2* gene on chromosome 18 with the Ig heavy chain locus on chromosome 14 causes overexpression of the Bcl-2 protein, promoting cellular survival and growth of indolent tumors.

Apoptosis, also known as programmed cell death, is the regulated suicide of a cell in response to damage or stress in the absence of inflammation or involvement of neighboring cells. The function of apoptosis is to efficiently remove one's own cells that are unnecessary or may be a threat to overall health. The two main apoptotic pathways are the extrinsic pathway initiated by an extracellular ligand and the intrinsic pathway initiated by intracellular events. In both pathways, there are four main phases of apoptic progression: (1) the initial signal, (2) the control phase, (3) the execution phase, and (4) the removal of dead cell debris.

The initial signal can be triggered by various mechanisms such as decreased survival stimuli (e.g., decreased hormones, growth factors, or cytokines), receptor–ligand interactions (e.g., tumor necrosis factor receptor, Fas death receptor), or specific injurious agents (e.g., heat, radiation, or hypoxia). The control phase can involve the regulation of Fas receptor-Fas ligand signaling for targeted cell death by killer lymphocytes in the extrinsic pathway or can involve regulation of cytochrome *c* release by the Bcl-2 family in the intrinsic pathway.

The extrinsic pathway of apoptosis involves the production of Fas ligand by killer lymphocytes and the activation of Fas receptor. The activated Fas death receptor clusters and recruits adaptor proteins to activate procaspase-8 to initiate the caspase cascade and targeted cell death by cytotoxic T-lymphocytes. The intrinsic pathway of apoptosis involves the release of cytochrome *c* from mitochondria to bind to the adaptor protein Apaf-1, which activates procaspase-9 to trigger the caspase cascade and cell death.

21 **(B)**. In the intrinsic pathway, apoptotic signals increase the permeability of mitochondria by forming pores and stimulate the release of cytochrome *c* from the mitochondria. Especially at this step, the Bcl-2 family of intracellular proteins can promote or hinder the apoptotic process. Bcl-2 itself and Bcl-X_L are members of the Bcl-2 family that inhibit the apoptotic pathway partly by preventing the release of cytochrome *c*, while Bax and Bak are members that promote apoptosis by stimulating the release of cytochrome *c*. Bad is a member that also functions in promoting apoptosis by binding and inactivating inhibitory members of the Bcl-2 family.

The execution phase of apoptosis is regulated by caspases, which are involved in an amplifying intracellular proteolytic cascade to transmit the death signal throughout the cell. Caspases normally exist as inactive procaspases in the cytosol, which may be activated by adaptor proteins recruited by the initiating signal. The activation of a small number of initiator caspases leads to an amplifying cascade as each initiator caspase cleaves more procaspases, which in turn cleave other procaspases. Some activated caspases can eventually cleave downstream signaling proteins and are known as effector caspases. Members of the inhibitor of apoptosis (IAP) family can regulate the caspase cascade by binding to specific procaspases to prevent their activation and to caspases to inhibit their activity.

The final step in apoptosis is the removal of dead cellular debris by phagocytes. This process is fast and complete and does not leave any signs of inflammation (see Fig. 1-8).

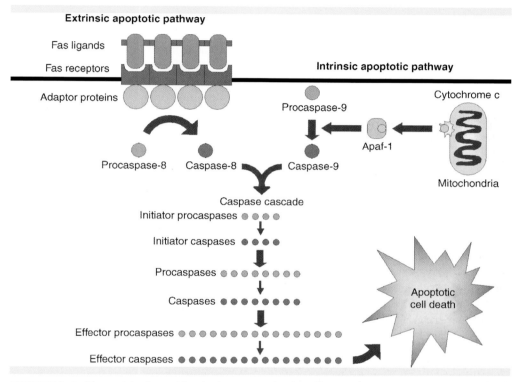

FIGURE 1-8. The extrinsic and intrinsic apoptotic signaling pathways.

BIBLIOGRAPHY

Brunicardi FC, Andersen DK, Billiar TR, et al. Oncology. In: Brunicardi FC, Andersen DK, Billiar TR, et al. (eds.), *Schwartz's Principles of Surgery*, 9th ed. New York, NY: McGraw-Hill; 2010:Chapter 10.

Jan BV, Lowry SF. Systemic response to injury and metabolic support. In: Brunicardi FC, Andersen DK, Billiar TR, et al. (eds.), *Schwartz's Principles of Surgery*, 9th ed. New York, NY: McGraw-Hill; 2010:Chapter 2.

Reeves M. Cell biology. In: O'Leary JP (ed.), *The Physiologic Basis of Surgery*, 4th ed. Baltimore, MD: Lippincott Williams & Wilkins; 2008:1–43.

22. **(E)** Heat shock proteins (HSPs) are a family of proteins involved in cellular protection during stress. HSPs, which tend to be activated by high temperatures or other stresses, are chaperone proteins that mainly function to aid the proper folding and unfolding of proteins inside the cell. HSP do not affect the rate of protein synthesis but aid proteins in reaching their complex conformations during and after synthesis. HSP are also involved in refolding proteins after they cross the membranes of certain organelles such as the ER or mitochondria. HSP perform other cytoprotective functions such as correcting misfolded proteins, preventing protein aggregation, facilitating the degradation of unstable proteins, and aiding the translocation of proteins across membranes. The protective nature of HSP is especially necessary in stressful situations such as recovery from light-induced damage to the retina and ischemia–reperfusion injury to various organs. HSP synthesis is increased dramatically in the liver after resuscitation involving cardiac shock.

Extracellular HSPs can interact with several receptors, but highly purified HSPs do not show any cytokine effects, suggesting HSP's role in antigen presentation and cross-presentation and in vitro cytokine functions may be attributable to molecules bound to or chaperoned by HSPs.

The HSP include the Hsp70 and chaperonin families. Both are significant contributors to protein folding during normal and adverse conditions. One of the important functions of the Hsp70 family in adverse conditions is thermotolerance. Organism's ability to become resistant to heat stress after a sublethal heat exposure. The cell can also develop tolerance for other stresses such as hypoxia, ischemia, acidosis, energy depletion, cytokines, and UV radiation. This heat tolerance will usually develop after a few hours and last approximately 3–5 days. Hsp70 chaperones promote the proper folding of proteins by blocking hydrophobic peptide segments around non-native polypeptides. In contrast, chaperonins enclose proteins within a central cavity to enhance efficient folding of certain proteins by shielding them from their local environments.

BIBLIOGRAPHY

Martindale RG, Zhou M. Nutrition and metabolism. In: O'Leary JP (ed.), *The Physiologic Basis of Surgery*, 4th ed. Baltimore, MD: Lippincott Williams & Wilkins; 2008:1–43.

Sauaia A, Moore FA, Moore EE. Multiple organ failure. In: Mattox KL, Moore EE, Feliciano DV (eds.), *Trauma*, 7th ed. New York, NY: McGraw-Hill; 2013:Chapter 61.

23. **(D)** Hexokinase is found in all cells and performs the first step of glycolysis by catalyzing the phosphorylation of glucose in position 6 by ATP. Glucokinase can also perform the first step of glycolysis but has a low affinity for glucose substrate and is predominantly found in the liver. Only hexokinase is inhibited by its glucose-6-phosphate product because the role of glucokinase is to provide a high-capacity system to rapidly breakdown glucose when excess exists.

Problems with cellular metabolic pathways such as glycolysis, glycogenolysis, gluconeogenesis, glycogen storage, protein metabolism, and fatty acid oxidation can be the result of organ dysfunction or rare inherited metabolic disorders. Defects in protein metabolism can specifically be the result of liver or kidney failure as well as inherited enzyme deficiencies such as phenylketonuria. When there are nutritional problems in specific pathways, the timing of the signs and symptoms may hint at the biochemical pathways affected. For instance, if a catabolic process such as glycolysis or β-oxidation were deficient, the patient would have neuromuscular symptoms unrelated to meals. If the defect was in glycogen storage, the patient could present with hepatomegaly and problems maintaining blood glucose levels for the first 8 h postprandial. Gluconeogenesis abnormalities result in a drop in blood glucose between 8 and 30 h postprandial.

Highly active tissues such as the brain, eyes, liver, muscles, RBCs, and kidneys need a continuous supply of glucose to survive. The brain, liver, and RBCs do not need insulin for glucose transport and utilization, whereas muscles and adipocytes have insulin-dependent glucose transporters inhibited by fasting. This serves to provide glucose to the most essential cells necessary for survival during periods of prolonged fasting. The breakdown of liver and muscle glycogen via glycogenolysis can supply the entire body for an average of 8 h (sometimes up to 18 h) without any carbohydrate intake. The Cori cycle cooperates with glycogenolysis as the glucose from glycogenolysis in the muscles is converted into lactate during muscular activity. The lactate is transported through the circulation to the liver, where it is converted into pyruvate and glycogen with the use of ATP. The pyruvate is converted into glucose to be transported back to the muscles through the circulation along with the glucose from glycogenolysis in the liver. After the glycogen stores are exhausted, the body relies on gluconeogenesis in the liver to provide glucose fuel from different substrates such as lactate, pyruvate, α-ketoacids, glycerol, and acetyl-CoA.

When gluconeogenesis occurs in the liver to provide glucose fuel for other organs, glycolysis is inhibited in the liver but not in other organs. Although a low level of gluconeogenesis can occur in the kidney and intestinal epithelia, the liver is the primary center for gluconeogenesis. Since the glycogen stores are exhausted, proteins and fats are primarily used as substrates to convert into glucose. One significant supply of pyruvate substrate for gluconeogenesis is the breakdown of branched chain amino acids (BCAAs) in muscles, which include leucine, isoleucine, and valine. Lactate, glutamine, and alanine can be transported to the liver from muscles to serve as substrates for gluconeogenesis. Glycerol and acetyl-CoA are derived from fatty acid breakdown to be converted into pyruvate for gluconeogenesis.

In extremely prolonged starvation, ketogenesis in the liver converts fatty acids and amino acids into acetoacetate. Acetoacetate is then reduced into β-hydroxybutyrate (β-HB) by the enzyme β-HB dehydrogenase, with the utilization of NADH. Some of the acetoacetate is spontaneously converted into acetone instead, which is responsible for the fruity breath odor in diabetic ketoacidosis (DKA). Ketone bodies can be used by the brain, heart muscle, and skeletal muscle in the absence of glucose or free fatty acids. The urine ketone test only detects acetoacetate and acetone in ketoacidosis, which can be misleading because the β-HB product is favored by high-redox states that produce an excess of NADH (see Figs. 1-9 and 1-10).

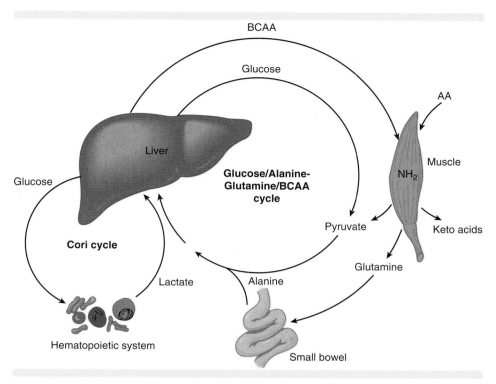

FIGURE 1-9. Preservation of metabolic intermediates during fasting. From Barbour JR, Barbour EF, Herrmann VM. Surgical metabolism & nutrition. In: Doherty GM (ed.), *Current Diagnosis & Treatment: Surgery,* 13th ed. New York, NY: McGraw-Hill; 2010:Chapter 10, Fig. 10-2.

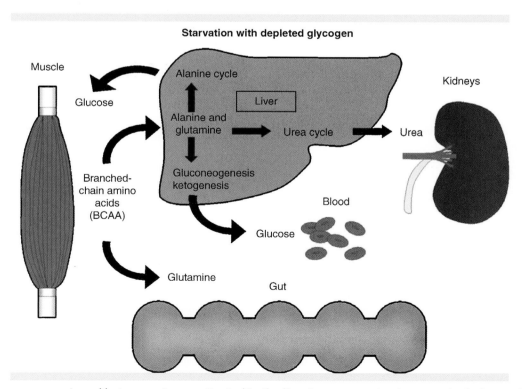

FIGURE 1-10. Gluconeogenesis and ketogenesis are activated in the liver in response to glycogen depletion and prolonged starvation.

BIBLIOGRAPHY

Barbour JR, Barbour EF, Herrmann VM. Surgical metabolism & nutrition. In: Doherty GM (ed.), *Current Diagnosis & Treatment: Surgery*, 13th ed. New York, NY: McGraw-Hill; 2010:Chapter 10.

van Solinge WW, van Wijk R. Disorders of red cells resulting from enzyme abnormalities. In: Prchal JT, Kaushansky K, Lichtman MA, et al. (eds.), *Williams Hematology*, 8th ed. New York, NY: McGraw-Hill; 2010:Chapter 46.

24. **(E)** Glycogen storage disease or glycogenosis is the result of defects in one or more enzymes involved in the synthesis or degradation of glycogen. Most often, the tissues that are affected by these abnormalities are the liver, heart, and muscle. The types of disorders are broken down into 12 subcategories based on the enzyme deficiency, but only types I through VIII will be briefly discussed.

Type I GSD (Von Gierke) is caused by a deficiency in the enzyme glucose-6-phosphatase. Glycogen accumulates in the liver and kidneys, enlarging these organs, and severe hypoglycemia with growth retardation is observed. No glucose can be released from the liver; instead, glucose-6-phosphate becomes a substrate for hepatic glycolysis and lactic acid production as occur in the muscles. This leads to the severe lactic acidemia often seen in these patients. Glycolysis and the pentose phosphate pathway (aka hexose monophosphate pathway) also increases phosphorylated intermediate compounds and inhibits the rephosphorylation of adenine nucleotides. This activates nucleic acid degradation into uric acid, causing hyperuricemia and gout. The hypoglycemia that results from this disorder stimulates epinephrine. This in turn activates lipoprotein lipase and free fatty acid movement to the liver for triglyceride synthesis; however, malonyl-CoA inhibits the fatty acids from entering the mitochondria and the β-oxidation of fatty acids to support the hypoglycemia does not occur.

Type II GSD (Pompe) is caused by a deficiency of α-1,4-glucosidase, which is usually found in lysosomes and can also be classified as a lysosomal enzyme disorder. Without this enzyme, there is a buildup of glycogen in almost all tissues, and the heart is especially affected, resulting in early death.

Type III GSD (Cori) is caused by a deficiency of the glycogen debranching enzyme, α-1,6-glucosidase. Only the outer branches of glycogen can be degraded by glycogen phosphorylase, resulting in the accumulation of glycogen with many short branches. Clinically, Cori disease can resemble Von Gierke but is usually less severe since gluconeogenesis is unaffected. The growth retardation is controllable with frequent ingestion of glucose sources to prevent hypoglycemia.

Type IV GSD (Andersen) is due to the deficiency of glucosyl α-4,6-transferase, resulting in the accumulation of glycogen with few long branches in the liver and spleen. Although infants may appear normal at birth, Andersen disease results in early death, usually before age two.

Type V GSD (McArdle) is caused by a deficiency in muscle glycogen phosphorylase, which is involved in removing 1,4-glucosyl groups to release glucose-1-phosphate. Although not lethal, the inability to breakdown muscle glycogen leads to painful cramps and myoglobinuria with strenuous exercise. Muscle enzymes such as creatine kinase and aldolase may also be elevated in these patients.

Type VI GSD (Hers) is because of the deficiency of liver glycogen phosphorylase, which is the rate-limiting enzyme of glycogenolysis, resulting in glycogen accumulation in hepatocytes and leukocytes. Type VII GSD is the deficiency of phosphofructokinase in muscle and blood cells, resulting in muscle cramps and myoglobinuria on extreme exertion; the clinical picture resembles the muscle specificity of McArdle disease. Type VIII GSD is the deficiency of phosphorylase kinase in the liver, which resembles Hers disease.

BIBLIOGRAPHY

Cross H. Appendix I. Biochemical basis of diseases. In: Janson LW, Tischler ME (eds.), *The Big Picture: Medical Biochemistry*. New York, NY: McGraw-Hill; 2012.

Kishnani PS, Chen Y. Glycogen storage diseases and other inherited disorders of carbohydrate metabolism. In: Longo DL, Fauci AS, Kasper DL, et al. (eds.), *Harrison's Principles of Internal Medicine*, 18th ed. New York, NY: McGraw-Hill; 2012:Chapter 362.

25. **(E)** For the most part, the gluconeogenesis pathway is just the reversal of glycolysis; however, there are three key steps in glycolysis that cannot be reversed and must be bypassed by four steps that are unique to gluconeogenesis. The first step that must be circumvented in gluconeogenesis is the irreversible conversion of phosphoenolpyruvate to pyruvate in glycolysis by the pyruvate kinase enzyme. To prevent both the forward glycolysis reaction and reverse gluconeogenesis reaction from occurring simultaneously in a futile cycle, liver pyruvate kinase is inactivated by protein kinase A–dependent phosphorylation during prolonged fasting. The lack of upstream F-1,6-BP reactant or the presence of excess ATP or alanine products also inhibits pyruvate kinase activity. Only the liver performs gluconeogenesis with the inhibition of glycolysis, and the other tissues such as the brain or RBCs continue glycolysis using the glucose supplied by the liver reactions.

The gluconeogenesis reaction at first step involves the carboxylation of pyruvate to form oxaloacetate or oxaloacetic acid (OAA) in liver mitochondria by pyruvate carboxylase with CO_2, biotin, Mg^{2+}, Mn^{2+}, and ATP. OAA is then reduced to malate because OAA is unable to cross the mitochondrial membrane to the cytosol. Once in the cytosol, malate is then converted back into OAA. OAA is then converted to PEP by PEPCK, using the energy of GTP hydrolysis. Pyruvate carboxylase is activated by the presence of acetyl-CoA from fatty acid breakdown, amino acid breakdown, or lactate metabolism.

The second step that must be bypassed in glycolysis is the irreversible rate-limiting reaction of phosphofructokinase-1 (PFK-1), which is activated by AMP or insulin-stimulated fructose-2,6-bisphosphate formation (by PFK-2) and inhibited by ATP or citrate. PFK-1 converts fructose-6-phosphate (F6P) into F-1,6-BP. The circumventing gluconeogenesis reaction at this step is performed by F-1,6-BPase in liver cytosol, which hydrolyzes F-1,6-BP into F6P. The third step that must be bypassed is the hexokinase reaction (glucokinase in liver) of glycolysis. To form free glucose molecules, glucose-6-phosphate is hydrolyzed by glucose-6-phosphatase in the liver cytosol (see Fig. 1-11).

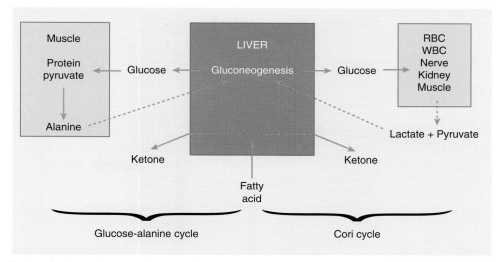

FIGURE 1-11. The Cori cycle. From Brunicardi FC, Andersen DK, Billiar TR, et al. (eds.), *Schwartz's Principles of Surgery,* 9th ed. New York, NY: McGraw-Hill; 2010:Chapter 2, Fig. 2-19.

BIBLIOGRAPHY

D'Angelica M, Fong Y. The liver. In: Townsend CM (ed.), *Sabiston: The Biological Basis of Modern Surgical Practice*, 18th ed. St. Louis, MO: Elsevier/Saunders; 2008:1463–1523.

Jan BV, Lowry SF. Systemic response to injury and metabolic support. In: Brunicardi FC, Andersen DK, Billiar TR, et al. (eds.), *Schwartz's Principles of Surgery*, 9th ed. New York, NY: McGraw-Hill; 2010:Chapter 2.

26. **(C)** Both cholesterol synthesis and ketogenesis occur in the liver mitochondria. Ketogenesis is the process by which the liver can take acetyl-CoA and produce ketone bodies for use by extrahepatic tissues such as brain, cardiac muscle, skeletal muscle, and renal cortex when glucose is unavailable. The compounds that are considered ketone bodies include acetoacetate, acetone, and β-hydroxybutyrate. The common steps of cholesterol synthesis and ketogenesis begin with the conversion of two acetyl-CoA molecules into one acetoacetyl-CoA molecule by the enzyme acetoacetyl-CoA thiolase. Acetoacetyl-CoA is converted by HMG-CoA synthase into HMG-CoA, which is the branching point where cholesterol synthesis and ketogenesis diverge. In cholesterol synthesis, the rate-limiting step is the conversion of HMG-CoA to mevalonate by HMG-CoA reductase, which is inhibited by statin drugs. In ketogenesis, HMG-CoA is cleaved into acetoacetate by HMG-CoA lyase. Some of the acetoacetate is reduced to β-hydroxybutyrate by the enzyme β-hydroxybutyrate dehydrogenase. This reaction is dependent on the NADH/NAD⁺ ratio. Some of the acetoacetate can also undergo spontaneous decarboxylation to acetone, but the amount of acetone produced is normally very small.

Under normal conditions, the body does not need significant ketogenesis; however, in times of severe starvation the amount of ketone body formation increases drastically. Carbohydrate depletion slows the entry of acetyl-CoA into the TCA cycle, and increased lipolysis and reduced systemic carbohydrate availability during starvation divert excess acetyl-CoA toward hepatic ketogenesis. A number of extrahepatic tissues, but not the liver itself, are capable of using ketones for fuel. Ketosis represents a state in which hepatic ketone production exceeds extrahepatic ketone utilization. This allows organs such as the heart and the skeletal muscles to conserve glucose to provide the central nervous system with enough fuel. As the process is prolonged, the higher levels of acetoacetate and β-hydroxybutyrate in the blood result in the additional utilization of ketone bodies by the brain. DKA is a condition marked by low insulin, excess glucagon, and excess ketone bodies. The overabundance of ketone bodies in this condition is the result of dysfunctional glucose transport in muscles and adipocytes, which are insulin dependent. The increased glucagon/insulin ratio additionally stimulates fatty acid oxidation and ketone body production. In normal starvation ketosis, insulin is present to antagonize the breakdown of fatty acids, but there is no mechanism in DKA to halt this process, leading to significant ketosis and dangerous acidosis (see Fig. 1-12).

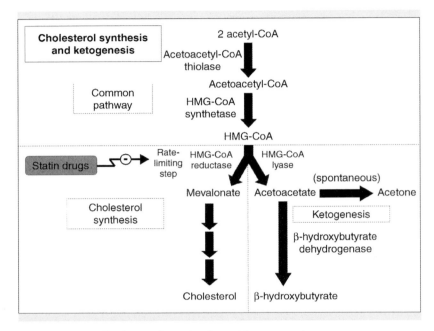

FIGURE 1-12. Cholesterol synthesis and ketogenesis.

BIBLIOGRAPHY

Jan BV, Lowry SF. Systemic response to injury and metabolic support. In: Brunicardi FC, Andersen DK, Billiar TR, et al. (eds.), *Schwartz's Principles of Surgery*, 9th ed. New York, NY: McGraw-Hill; 2010:Chapter 2.

27. **(B)** The urea cycle is a series of biochemical reactions performed by the liver to rid nitrogenous wastes from the body and accounts for about 90% of the nitrogen in urine. Urea is produced within the liver and is carried through the blood to the kidneys, where it is excreted. Dysfunction of the liver or kidneys can result in the accumulation of ammonia or urea and its metabolites, resulting in uremia and metabolic encephalopathy. The first nitrogen of urea is derived from ammonia, while the second nitrogen is from aspartate; both are products of protein metabolism. Transaminases or aminotransferases, glutamate dehydrogenase, and argininosuccinate synthetase are the enzymes responsible for supplying the nitrogen from ammonia and aspartate. Ammonia is the result of glutamate breakdown since most amino acids undergo transamination reactions linked with α-ketoglutarate. Aspartate is derived from oxaloacetate via a transamination reaction linked with glutamate.

The urea cycle begins with carbamoyl phosphate synthetase I using ATP and *N*-acetylglutamate to convert ammonia and CO_2 (or bicarbonate) to carbamoyl phosphate. This reaction occurs in the mitochondrial matrix of hepatocytes and is considered to be the rate-limiting step. Carbamoyl phosphate synthetase I in the mitochondria should not be confused with carbamoyl phosphate synthetase II in the cytosol, which is responsible for catalyzing the first step in pyrimidine synthesis. The second step of the urea cycle also occurs in the mitochondrial matrix and involves the combination of carbamoyl phosphate and ornithine into citrulline by ornithine transcarbamoylase. Citrulline is transported from the mitochondria to the cytosol (by the citrulline-ornithine exchange transporter) where it is combined with aspartate by the ATP-dependent argininosuccinate synthetase enzyme to form argininosuccinate. Argininosucci-nate is then broken down into fumarate and arginine by argininosuccinate lyase. Fumarate is recycled into energy by the TCA cycle (aka citric acid or Krebs cycle), whereas arginine is hydrolyzed into urea and ornithine. The urea molecule is excreted in the urine, and the

ornithine molecule is recycled to the urea cycle at the second step. Recycled ornithine is able to efficiently enter the mitochondrial matrix via the citrulline-ornithine exchange transporter, which also serves to transport citrulline out to the cytosol after the second step of the urea cycle (see Fig. 1-13).

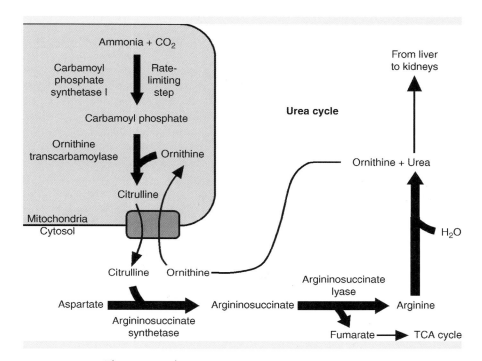

FIGURE 1-13. The urea cycle.

BIBLIOGRAPHY

D'Angelica M, Fong Y. The liver. In: Townsend CM (ed.), *Sabiston: The Biological Basis of Modern Surgical Practice*, 18th ed. St. Louis, MO: Elsevier/Saunders; 2008:1463–1523.

28. **(D)** Selectins or lectins are carbohydrate-binding pro-teins located on the surface of many different types of cells. There are at least three different types of lectins, which include E-selectin (on endothelial cells), L-selectin (on leukocytes), and P-selectin (on platelets and endo-thelial cells). Selectins are especially important in the binding of leukocytes to endothelial walls, which enables them to migrate from blood vessels into tissues. For instance, activated endothelial cells at sites of inflam-mation can express E-selectins for binding and slowing down leukocytes and platelets. Lymphocytes can express L-selectin to bind oligosaccharides on endothelial cells of lymphoid organs to result in the accumulation of lymphocytes. In the migration of white blood cells (WBCs) out of blood vessels, selectins and integrins act in sequence to modulate the weak rolling adhesion and firm binding adhesion, respectively. The Ig protein superfamily modulates Ca^{2+}-independent cell–cell adhe-sion, in contrast to cadherins, selectins, and integrins, which are dependent on Ca^{2+} or Mg^{2+}. There are several members of the Ig superfamily, which include the inter-cellular adhesion molecules (ICAMs) on endothelial cells and neural cell adhesion molecules (N-CAMs). ICAMs bind to integrins on WBCs for firm adhesion before migration, and N-CAMs bind cells together via homo-philic interactions.

The extracellular matrix is made up of two main classes of extracellular macromolecules: Glycosamino-glycans (GAGs) and fibrous proteins. GAGs are further subdivided into four main groups that include hyaluro-nan, heparan sulfate, keratan sulfate, and chondroitin or dermatan sulfate. GAGs are usually found covalently attached to core proteins in the form of proteoglycans, except hyaluronan. Fibrous proteins include collagen, elastin, fibronectin, and laminin. Collagen can be even further subdivided into at least 18 types with specific characteristics and tissue distributions. Collagen is the most important matrix protein for providing tensile strength and pliability to the extracellular matrix. Members of the fibroblast family of cells are mainly responsible for secreting matrix macromolecules, which are then assembled into an intricate network that interconnects cells within various tissues. The nature of the matrix molecules and the organization of the network determine the characteristics of the extracellular matrix in different tissues.

Elastin is the main component of elastic fibers and is similar to collagen except for the random coil structure and the lack of hydroxylysine or glycosylation. Elastic fibers are composed of elastin cores covered by microfibrils, which contain fibrillin. Mutations in the fibrillin gene are responsible for Marfan syndrome.

Fibronectin is a glycoprotein dimer that is a component of the extracellular matrix and is composed of domains or modules that occur commonly in many other ligands and receptors. For instance, the type III fibronectin repeat can bind integrins and is also found in many growth factor receptors. A crucial Arg-Gly-Asp (RGD) sequence is responsible for the binding properties of fibronectin, and snakes exploit this quality in their venom, which contains RGD sequence anticoagulants called disintegrins.

Extracellular proteolytic enzymes can degrade the extracellular matrix and can be divided into two general classes: matrix metalloproteases (MMPs) and serine proteases. MMPs exist in over 19 forms and depend on Ca^{2+} or Zn^{2+} for activity. MMPs and serine proteases work together to breakdown matrix proteins such as collagen, fibronectin, and laminin. Specific MMPs such as the collagenases are selective for certain matrix proteins. This allows the structure of the matrix to be retained while allowing cell migration through a cleared portion of the matrix. To localize the action of matrix proteases, many are secreted as inactive precursors, allowing their action to be confined to a local area and activated only when needed. Cell-surface receptors can also bind and localize protease to specific sites of action, and protease inhibitors such as tissue inhibitors of metalloproteases (TIMPs) and serine protease inhibitors (serpins) can also help limit the area of protease activation.

BIBLIOGRAPHY

Phelan HA, Eastman AL, Frota A, et al. Shock and hypoperfusion states. In: O'Leary JP (ed.), *The Physiologic Basis of Surgery*, 4th ed. Baltimore, MD: Lippincott Williams & Wilkins; 2008:87–111.

29. **(A)** Integrins are transmembrane heterodimers composed of noncovalently associated α- and β-subunits, dependent on divalent cations for binding ligands. They serve as the major receptors for extracellular matrix proteins and link the extracellular matrix to the actin cytoskeleton of cells without directly affecting cell shape changes. Integrins provide both structural and signaling functions through their extracellular ligand-binding and intracellular domains. The structural function of integrins is because of their transmembrane linking of extracellular matrix proteins and intracellular anchor proteins that are bound to the actin cytoskeleton at focal adhesions. However, the integrins also serve as signal transducers by activating outside-in and inside-out signaling. Integrins exist in large numbers on the cell surface and bind extracellular molecules with low affinity, activating intracellular signaling pathways that communicate to the cell the nature of the extracellular matrix to which the cell is bound, termed outside-in signaling. Integrins also must be activated by the cell before mediating adhesion, especially in platelets and leukocytes, termed inside-out signaling. Changes in integrin conformation can be promoted by signals coming from the cell, promoting stronger adhesion and binding.

Leukocyte adhesion deficiency is due to the absence of β_2-integrin subunits, resulting in the lack of LFA-1 (i.e., $\alpha_L \beta_2$ integrin), which mediates firm leukocyte binding to vessel walls and migration into the tissues. Patients with this deficiency suffer repeated bacterial infections and impaired healing. Glanzmann thrombasthenia is a bleeding disorder because of the deficiency of β_3 integrin, causing problems with platelet-fibrinogen. Typical features of leukocyte adhesion defects include recurrent serious infections, abscesses without pus formation, poor wound healing, and gingival or periodontal disease. The most severe phenotype manifests with infections in the neonatal period, including delayed separation of the umbilical cord with associated omphalitis. Laboratory evaluation often demonstrates a striking neutrophilia, and diagnosis of suspected cases is confirmed by flow cytometry analysis for CD18 (LAD I) or CD15s (LAD II). Treatment includes aggressive antibiotic therapy.

BIBLIOGRAPHY

Hauk PJ, Johnston RB Jr, Liu AH. Immunodeficiency. In: Hay WW Jr, Levin MJ, Deterding RR, et al. (eds.), *Current Diagnosis & Treatment: Pediatrics*, 21st ed. New York, NY: McGraw-Hill; 2012:Chapter 33.

30. **(C)** The complement system involves the interaction of serum proteins produced by the liver as a component of innate immunity. The complement system can assist the action of antibodies or contribute directly to pathogen elimination. The early complement components consist of C1, C2, and C4, with the cleavage of C3 complex being

the crucial and common point of the early cascade. The cascade of C3 activation through sequential proteolytic cleavage occurs through three different pathways: (1) the classic pathway, (2) the alternative pathway, and (3) the lectin pathway. The resulting fragments of complement such as C3a, C4a, and C5a act as chemoattractants that can recruit phagocytes to sites of infection or inflammation. The C3b component can bind covalently to pathogen surfaces and acts in opsonization to facilitate phagocytosis or to activate late complement activation.

The classic pathway is activated by IgG or IgM antibodies binding to microbe surfaces, resulting in the binding and cleavage of C1, C2, C4, and, eventually, C3. The alternative pathway involves the spontaneous activation of C3 with the assistance of complexes involving factors B and D. Human cells produce proteins that prevent this spontaneous reaction from proceeding on their surfaces, but pathogenic cells do not. Mannose binding lechtin (MBL) is also called mannose-binding protein (MBP) and recognizes carbohydrates such as mannose and N-acetylglucosamine on pathogen surfaces. MBL forms a complex with serine proteases called MBL-associated serine proteases (MASP) that proteolytically cleave C2, C4, and C3. Thus, MBL is able to activate the complement pathway through the MBL-MASP or lectin pathway independent of the classic and alternative pathways. The liver usually produces MBL, and MBL deficiency has been associated with many disease states.

The late complement components are activated by the cleavage of C5 by membrane-bound C3b. The fragment C5b remains on the cell surface and binds late complement components C6, C7, and C8 to form the C5678 complex. This complex can bind C9 to induce a conformational change in C9 to cause its insertion into the target cell membrane. The C9 molecule continues to bind other C9 molecules until a large transmembrane channel is formed, resulting in the lysis of the cell. The C5–C9 complex is also called the MAC. Deficiency in MAC results in increased susceptibility to bacterial infections, especially *Neisseria meningitidis*.

There are also several inhibitors and regulators of the complement pathways, including soluble control proteins (e.g., C1 inhibitor, factor H, factor I, C4b binding proteins, and protein S) and membrane regulatory proteins (e.g., CD55 or DAF, CD59, MCP). Deficiency in C1 inhibitor results in hereditary angioedema because of complement overactivation, and deficiency in GPI anchors for CD55 and CD59 results in paroxysmal nocturnal hemoglobinuria because of complement-mediated lysis of RBCs (see Fig. 1-14).

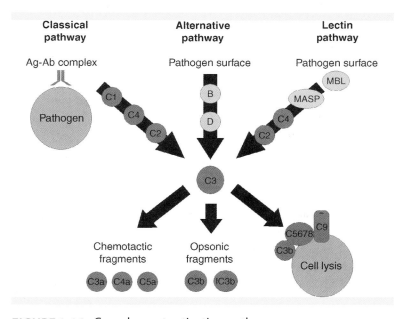

FIGURE 1-14. Complement activation pathways.

BIBLIOGRAPHY

Gupta S, Lawrence WT. Wound healing: Normal and abnormal mechanisms and closure techniques. In: O'Leary JP (ed.), *The Physiologic Basis of Surgery*, 4th ed. Baltimore, MD: Lippincott Williams & Wilkins; 2008:150–175.

31. (A) The TLR family of receptors activates host cell gene expression in response to pathogens. There are at least 10 TLRs, many of which play important roles in the innate immune system for the recognition of pathogenic particles such as LPS. Lipopolysaccharide (LPS) is bound by circulating LPS-binding protein (LBP), and the complex is recognized by CD14 on macrophage surfaces. The resulting complex can then stimulate TLR4 for the activation of nuclear factor–κB (NF-κB) through the adaptor proteins and signaling mediators of the MAPK pathway called MyD88, IRAK, TRAF6, and TAK1. NF-κB normally remains bound to inhibitory κB (IκB) until phosphorylated by IκB kinase (IKK), which is activated

by TAK1 in the TLR4 pathway. Phosphorylation of IκB induces its degradation and frees NF-κB. The activated NF-κB then translocates to the nucleus, as does the AP-1 TF (i.e., Jun and Fos heterodimer), which is activated in parallel to NF-κB by TAK1, and ERK/JNK. The final result is the activated transcription of genes involved in the inflammatory or immune response (see Fig. 1-15).

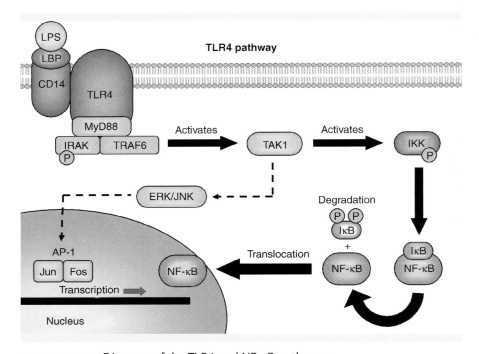

FIGURE 1-15. Diagram of the TLR4 and NF-κB pathways.

BIBLIOGRAPHY

Fry DE. Surgical infection. In: O'Leary JP (ed.), *The Physiologic Basis of Surgery*, 4th ed. Baltimore, MD: Lippincott Williams & Wilkins; 2008:218–257

32. **(C)** There are two major isoforms of the COX enzyme: COX-1 is constitutively and ubiquitously expressed in the human body, whereas the inducible COX-2 is upregulated by inflammatory stimuli. Corticosteroids and other steroidal anti-inflammatory agents block the arachidonate pathway at the level of PLA_2, aspirin irreversibly acetylates the COX enzyme, and other nonsteroidal anti-inflammatory drugs reversibly inhibit COX. While COX inhibitors and steroidal agents also block the formation of TXA_2, only EPA additionally produces PGI_3.

There are two essential fatty acids in the human diet, linoleic acid (C18:2; $\Delta^{9,12}$, ω-6 PUFA) and α-linolenic acid (C18:3; $\Delta^{9,12,15}$, ω-3 PUFA). In the human body, the

majority of linoleic acid is converted into AA, which is also known as eicosatetraenoic acid (C20:4; $\Delta^{5,8,11,14}$, ω-6 PUFA). Briefly, the fatty acid nomenclature indicates that AA contains 20 carbons and 4 double bonds at locations that are 5, 8, 11, and 14 bonds away from the carboxy end of the fatty acid, and the ω-6 designation signifies that the final double bond is 6 bonds away from the terminal ω-carbon. EPA (C20:5; $\Delta^{5,8,11,14,17}$, ω-3 PUFA) likewise contains 20 carbons but 5 double bonds with the fifth double bond located 17 bonds away from the carboxy end and 3 bonds away from the ω-carbon. In contrast to AA, EPA is not endogenously produced in humans; ω-3 or ω-6 PUFAs cannot be synthesized *de novo* and the two families cannot be interconverted in animals. Although phytoplankton and other relatively simple life forms have the ability to convert α-linolenic acid into EPA, human and most other animals lack the enzymes necessary to elongate and desaturate α-linolenic acid into the more biologically active longer chain species, EPA and docosahexaenoic acid. Marine animals derive their EPA from ingesting phytoplankton or other fish, while humans must ingest EPA in the form of fish oils (e.g., salmon, mackerel, cod liver oil, anchovy).

EPA acts at three levels of the arachidonate pathway: (1) membrane incorporation, (2) competitive inhibition of COX, and (3) conversion to a unique set of prostanoids. First, EPA competes with linoleic acid and AA to become incorporated into the 2-position of membrane phospholipids, from which they are liberated by PLA_2 to serve as a substrate for COX. Additionally, the administration of dietary fish oil led to the incorporation of EPA into the membranes of vascular endothelial cells in surgical patients. Second, EPA competes with AA for the membrane-bound COX enzymes but does not have the kinetic profile of a typical competitive inhibitor because of its slow release from the COX enzyme. The x-ray crystallographic structure of the interaction shows that EPA may bind within the COX active site and hairpin turn in a strained conformation because of the additional double bond (producing increased electron density and different structural *cis-trans* isomers), resulting in the slow release of EPA and the low observed rate of EPA oxygenation. Third, COX enzymes normally act to convert AA into prostaglandins of the 2-series, but COX converts EPA into prostaglandins of the 3-series. The 2-series prostaglandins include thromboxane A_2 (TXA_2), a potent vasoconstrictor and platelet agonist produced by platelet COX, and prostaglandin I_2 (PGI_2 or prostacyclin), an extremely potent vasodilator and platelet antagonist produced by endothelial COX. In contrast, many of the 3-series prostanoids (TXA_3, PGG_3, PGH_3) have no biological activity, with the exception of PGI_3, which is nearly as active as prostacyclin in its vasodilatory and platelet antagonistic activities. Thus, EPA products result in a shift of platelet function toward antiaggregation.

EPA has been shown to reduce the severity of tumors and other chronic inflammatory conditions. It is hypothesized that the effects of EPA on atherosclerosis, malignancies, and chronic inflammatory diseases may be linked. One argument links the three by pathogenic theory and postulates that the EPA's main effects are as an anti-inflammatory, antiproliferative agent.

BIBLIOGRAPHY

Alarcon LH, Fink MP. Mediators of the inflammatory response and metabolism. In Townsend CM (ed.), *Sabiston: The Biological Basis of Modern Surgical Practice*, 18th ed. St. Louis, MO: Elsevier/Saunders; 2008:44–68.

33. **(A)** VEGF was originally discovered in the 1980s as vascular permeability factor (VPF) and has dual effects of increasing blood vessel permeability and promoting angiogenesis. Ang1 was discovered in the mid-1990s as a proangiogenic factor that also decreases vascular permeability. Embryologic studies have shown that VEGF is necessary for vasculogenesis (i.e., the de novo formation of vessels) and the early morphogenic phase of angiogenesis (i.e., the formation of vessels from existing vessels). The blood vessels formed by VEGF compose a leaky, primitive vascular network of tubes without fine capillary branching. Ang1 acts on these primitive vessels to promote interactions between endothelial cells, pericytes, and smooth muscle cells, inducing extensive capillary branching and forming the tight vessels characteristic of normal mature vasculature. VEGF and Ang1 are both proangiogenic growth factors that act via tyrosine kinase receptors.

There are several isoforms and splice variants of VEGF that have been discovered since the original identification of VEGF-A_{165}. The isoforms VEGF-A through VEGF-D exist, and VEGF-A can be subdivided into five splice variants with different heparin-binding properties. The biological action of VEGF-A_{165} has already been described, much less is known about VEGF-B, and VEGF-C plus VEGF-D are known to be lymphangiogenic factors. References to VEGF in this discussion indicate the original VEGF-A. Most of the biological actions of VEGF are through the receptors VEGFR-1 and more importantly VEGFR-2. The neuropilin coreceptor can aid VEGF receptor binding, and VEGFR-3 is found on lymph vessels for the specific binding of VEGF-C and VEGF-D. VEGF gene transcription is upregulated by the activation of a gene regulatory protein called hypoxia-inducible factor 1 (HIF-1), which is activated by hypoxia in tissues.

Ang1 acts through the Tie-2 receptor (Tie-1 is an orphan receptor), which is endothelial cell specific. Ang1 remains constitutively bound to its receptor on mature vessels and is only displaced by Ang2, its natural antagonist, in areas of vessel damage and repair such as in wound healing, the female menstruation cycle, and in inflammation (including tumors). The displacement of Ang1 by Ang2 allows regression of the blood vessels to their leaky primitive state, which primes them for repair by VEGF and Ang1. Thus, VEGF has concerted action with the antiangiogenic factor, Ang2, in tumor angiogenesis. Ang2 is necessary to destabilize the normal host vasculature back to the primitive state, and VEGF is then immediately necessary to facilitate growth of the vessels toward the tumor. Ang1 can act on the blood vessels following VEGF, similar to their synergistic actions during embryologic angiogenesis. However, VEGF often acts alone during tumor angiogenesis, and tumor vessels tend to be more leaky than normal blood vessels. Without the immediate availability of VEGF, Ang2 alone causes the regression of vessels. So although the concerted action of

Ang2 and VEGF can be considered proangiogenic, Ang2 is really an antiangiogenic factor while VEGF is a pro-angiogenic factor. Ang1 and Ang2 do not show a similar synergistic relationship since they bind to the same receptor with comparable affinities and tend to directly antagonize each other.

Endostatin and angiostatin are endogenous antiangiogenic factors. Preclinical studies have shown that endostatin can cause the shrinkage of existing tumor vessels and inhibit tumor growth; however, angiogenic inhibitors such as angiostatin and endostatin can be activated by tumors to modulate angiogenesis both at the

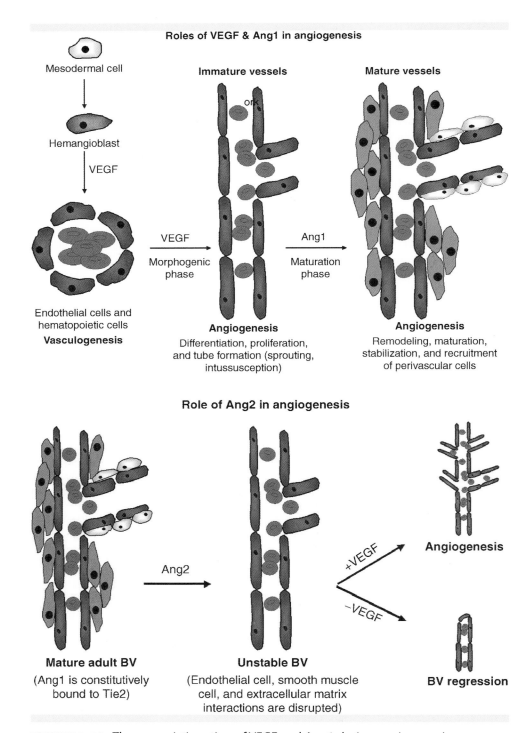

Roles of VEGF & Ang1 in angiogenesis

Mesodermal cell

Hemangioblast

VEGF

Endothelial cells and hematopoietic cells
Vasculogenesis

Immature vessels

VEGF
Morphogenic phase

Angiogenesis
Differentiation, proliferation, and tube formation (sprouting, intussusception)

Mature vessels

Ang1
Maturation phase

Angiogenesis
Remodeling, maturation, stabilization, and recruitment of perivascular cells

Role of Ang2 in angiogenesis

Mature adult BV
(Ang1 is constitutively bound to Tie2)

Ang2

Unstable BV
(Endothelial cell, smooth muscle cell, and extracellular matrix interactions are disrupted)

+VEGF

Angiogenesis

−VEGF

BV regression

FIGURE 1-16. The synergistic action of VEGF and Ang1 during angiogenesis.

primary site and at downstream sites of metastasis. This gave rise to the theory that removing the primary tumor could allow the enhanced growth of satellite lesions that were held in check by antiangiogenic factors secreted by the primary tumor. Therefore, instead of the theory that a tumor can only produce proangiogenic factors, the evolving idea is that a tumor can produce both antiangiogenic and proangiogenic factors to direct the flow of blood away from other tissues and toward itself. Besides directing the supply of nutrients, the guiding of blood vessel growth by tumor is also believed to be important in metastatic processes (see Fig. 1-16).

BIBLIOGRAPHY

Ethridge RT, Leong M, Philips LG. Wound healing. In: Townsend CM (ed.), *Sabiston: The Biological Basis of Modern Surgical Practice*, 18th ed. St. Louis, MO: Elsevier/Saunders; 2008:191–216

Brock CS, Lee SM. Anti-angiogenic strategies and vascular targeting in the treatment of lung cancer. *Eur Respir J* 2002;19:557–570.

Conti CJ. Vascular endothelial growth factor: regulation in the mouse skin carcinogenesis model and use in antiangiogenesis cancer therapy. *Oncologist* 2002;7(Suppl 3):4–11.

Ellis LM, Ahmad S, Fan F, et al. Angiopoietins and their role in colon cancer angiogenesis. *Oncology* 2002;16(Suppl 3):31–35.

Ferrara N. Role of vascular endothelial growth factor in physiologic and pathologic angiogenesis: therapeutic implications. *Semin Oncol* 2002;29(Suppl 16):10–14.

Folkman J. Role of angiogenesis in tumor growth and metastasis. *Semin Oncol* 2002;29(Suppl 16):15–18.

Guppy M. The hypoxic core: A possible answer to the cancer paradox. *Biochem Biophys Res Commun* 2002;299:676–680.

Jain RK. Tumor angiogenesis and accessibility: role of vascular endothelial growth factor. *Semin Oncol* 2002;29(Suppl 16):3–9.

Lie W, Reinmuth N, Stoeltzing O, et al. Antiangiogenic therapy targeting factors that enhance endothelial cell survival. *Semin Oncol* 2002;29(Suppl 11):96–103.

Qin LX, Tang ZY. The prognostic molecular markers in hepatocellular carcinoma. *World J Gastroenterol* 2002;8:385–392.

Ribatti D, Vacca A, Presta M. The discovery of angiogenic factors: a historical review. *Gen Pharmacol* 2000;35:227–231.

Thurston G. Complementary actions of VEGF and angiopoietin-1 on blood vessel growth and leakage. *J Anat* 2002;200:575–580.

CHAPTER 2

SURGICAL NUTRITION

LISA M. MCELROY AND TRAVIS P. WEBB

QUESTIONS

1. A 67-year-old woman is admitted to a general surgical floor with the diagnosis of a small bowel obstruction. Which of the following is the best initial nutritional assessment?
   (A) Serum transferrin
   (B) Serum prealbumin
   (C) Serum albumin
   (D) Serum glutamine
   (E) History and physical examination

2. A 34-year-old man is mechanically ventilated in the intensive care unit after a closed head injury. He is 5′11″ tall and weighs 176 lb. He has no burns, has not had surgery, and shows no signs of sepsis. Which of the following is his estimated caloric requirement per 24 h?
   (A) 1760 kcal
   (B) 1840 kcal
   (C) 2200 kcal
   (D) 2390 kcal
   (E) 2570 kcal

3. A 35-year-old trauma victim with malabsorption requires nutritional support. The patient's injuries include a stable nondisplaced fracture of the third thoracic vertebra, a closed head injury, multiple upper and lower extremity fractures, and bilateral pulmonary contusions requiring ventilatory support. Which of the following are the most appropriate site and type of venous access in this patient?
   (A) Bilateral antecubital fossa, 18-gauge peripheral intravenous catheters
   (B) Femoral vein, central venous catheter
   (C) Dorsum of one foot, 16-gauge peripheral intravenous catheter
   (D) Subclavian vein, central venous catheter
   (E) Unilateral antecubital fossa, 18-gauge peripheral intravenous catheter

4. Enteral nutrition is appropriate in which of the following conditions?
   (A) Major upper gastrointestinal bleed
   (B) Complete small bowel obstruction
   (C) Hemodynamic instability
   (D) Colonic fistula with 500 mL/day output
   (E) None of the above

5. A 45-year-old man has sustained a closed head injury and multiple rib fractures in a motor vehicle collision. The patient requires maximal ventilatory support because of bilateral pulmonary contusions and aspiration pneumonitis. His Glascow Coma Scale score is 5. Which of the following would be the most appropriate method of artificial nutrition?
   (A) Parenteral nutrition with a protein-sparing formula through a central venous catheter
   (B) Intragastric tube feeding
   (C) Parenteral nutrition through a peripheral venous catheter
   (D) Postpyloric tube feeding
   (E) Any of the above with appropriate calories

6. A 63-year-old man with end-stage renal disease requiring hemodialysis three times per week presents with bone pain and several pathologic fractures of the extremities. Which electrolyte abnormality is the most likely to be seen in this patient?
   (A) Hypokalemia
   (B) Hypernatremia
   (C) Hyperphosphatemia
   (D) Hypercalcemia
   (E) Hypochloremia

7. A 35-year-old male trauma patient is being considered for extubation after a 10-day course of ventilatory support following a motor vehicle crash in which he suffered a duodenal injury requiring an exploratory laparotomy. The patient has been receiving parenteral nutrition and currently has a tidal volume of 400 mL and a respiratory rate of 40 breaths/min. What changes in his supplemental nutrition may improve this patient's minute ventilation?
   (A) Adding long-acting insulin to the mixture
   (B) Increasing the proportion of glucose calories
   (C) Decreasing the total volume with a more concentrated solution
   (D) Increasing the proportion of fat calories
   (E) Adding fat-soluble vitamins A, D, E, and K

8. Which of the following would most accurately reflect the metabolic stress on a 45-year-old woman undergoing an elective open cholecystectomy?
   (A) Albumin of 3.6 g/dL
   (B) Weight loss of 400 g
   (C) Urine nitrogen loss of 8 g per day
   (D) Retinal-binding protein of 6 mg/dL
   (E) Urine nitrogen gain of 2g/day

9. A 28-year-old patient with a closed head injury requires ventilatory and nutritional support. The patient has no evidence of bowel obstruction, is receiving enteral feeds through a gastrostomy tube, and is found to have aspirated gastric contents. The patient has no immediate pulmonary compromise. Which of the following therapies is appropriate to treat this condition in the first 12 hours?
   (A) Corticosteroids
   (B) Oral and gastric suctioning
   (C) Empiric antibiotics
   (D) Gastric content culture
   (E) Endotracheal tube replacement

10. Which is the most commonly cultured hospital acquired organism in patients with aspiration pneumonia?
   (A) *Streptococcus pneumoniae*
   (B) *Staphylococcus aureus*
   (C) Anaerobic species
   (D) *Pseudomonas aeruginosa*
   (E) *Haemophilus influenzae*

11. What is the most appropriate single agent for empiric coverage of the above patient?
   (A) Metronidazole
   (B) Clindamycin
   (C) Piperacillin-tazobactam
   (D) Vancomycin
   (E) First-generation penicillin

12. Which of the following vitamins requires colonic bacteria for synthesis?
   (A) Vitamin A
   (B) Thiamine
   (C) Niacin
   (D) Vitamin D
   (E) Vitamin K

13. A 45-year-old man with alcoholic liver disease and short gut syndrome was previously on chronic parenteral nutrition. He has been switched to an elemental enteral diet for the past 6 months, which has been poorly tolerated. He has complained of generalized weakness for several months and now has erythematous, scaly and symmetrical lesions on his upper extremities, stomatitis, and glossitis. What is the most appropriate treatment for these symptoms?
   (A) Addition of fat-soluble vitamins A, D, E, and K
   (B) Thiamine replacement
   (C) Niacin replacement
   (D) Change to a lactose-free enteral feed
   (E) Addition of tincture of opium

14. Which of the following trace element deficiencies is associated with glucose intolerance and peripheral neuropathy?
   (A) Copper
   (B) Iron
   (C) Fluorine
   (D) Chromium
   (E) Selenium

15. Which of the following statements about vitamins is true?
   (A) Vitamins are essential and cannot be produced by the body.
   (B) Water soluble vitamin deficiency can result in anemia
   (C) Cholecalciferol is converted to calcitriol in the kidney and liver.
   (D) Fat-soluble vitamin deficiency can result in coagulopathy.
   (E) All of the above.

16. An adult man develops acute necrotizing pancreatitis after an endoscopic retrograde cholangiopancreaticogram. The patient requires ventilatory support and is in need of nutritional support. Which is the best route of providing nutrition?
   (A) Parenteral nutrition via peripheral access
   (B) Parenteral nutrition via central access
   (C) Enteral nutrition via jejunal feeding tube
   (D) Oral elemental supplementation
   (E) Enteral nutrition via gastric tube

17. A 35-year-old woman presents with a small bowel obstruction 9 months after a duodenal switch procedure. She has been unable to tolerate oral intake for 8 days. Parenteral nutrition is started and 48 h later she is noted to have paresthesias, ocular disturbances, and seizures. Which of the following is responsible for her neurologic changes?
    (A) Hyperkalemia
    (B) Hypophosphatemia
    (C) Vitamin B_1 deficiency
    (D) Hypokalemia
    (E) Hypomagnesemia

18. An 18-year-old man undergoes extensive small bowel resection after a gunshot wound to the abdomen. Despite his resultant short gut, his remaining colonic function allows him to subsist on an oral high-carbohydrate diet. What substrate is the preferred fuel for colonocytes?
    (A) Short-chain fatty acids (SCFAs)
    (B) Glutamate
    (C) Luminal oligopeptides
    (D) Ketones
    (E) Fructose

ANSWERS AND EXPLANATIONS

1. **(E)** The nutritional assessment of the surgical patient consists of a subjective (clinical) assessment combined with objective (biochemical) measures. The *history and physical examination* are the primary nutritional assessment tools. A thorough history should include recent weight loss, dietary intake, gastrointestinal symptoms, functional capacity, and symptoms focused on nutritional deficiency. Physical examination may reveal edema, poor wound healing, bruising, pale conjunctivae, or glossitis, among other signs.

   While many different *objective* measures of nutritional status have been shown to be accurate and reproducible in clinical studies, body mass index (BMI) and prealbumin concentration are the most commonly used. Their popularity lies in the fact that they are inexpensive, simple, and reasonably accurate.

   BMI is defined as weight (kg) divided by the square of height (m²). It is considered a more accurate indicator than ideal body weight (IBW) because it is less dependent on comparison to control populations. A BMI of less than 18.5 kg/m² is associated with increased morbidity in hospitalized patients.

   The serum albumin concentration correlates with global protein synthesis, degradation, and exchange between fluid compartments. However, albumin does not reflect acute changes in nutritional status because of its long half-life (18–21 days) and as a negative acute phase reactant it is decreased in acute inflammatory states, compared with prealbumin, which has a half-life of 48 hours. A serum albumin level of less than 3.5 g/dL

is associated with increased morbidity in hospitalized patients. A prealbumin of 5 to 10 mg/dL indicates moderate nutritional depletion.

Glutamine is an important nutrient for the maintenance of gut mucosa during stress; however, it has been proposed as an additive to feeding solutions, and not as a nutritional marker.

BIBLIOGRAPHY

Carney DE, Meguid MM. Current concepts in nutritional assessment. *Arch Surg* 2002;137:42–45.

Martindale RG, Zhou M. Nutrition and metabolism. In: O'Leary JP, ed. *The Physiologic Basis of Surgery*. 4th ed. Baltimore, MD: Lippincott Williams & Wilkins; 2008:112–149.

2. **(D)** Critically ill patients require accurate determination of nutritional needs to avoid the complications of both under- and overfeeding (Table 2-1).

   Nutritional needs are determined by measuring basal energy expenditure (BEE), and the most accurate method of quantifying BEE is by indirect calorimetry (IC). Unfortunately, IC is expensive, requires skilled personnel, and frequently overestimates BEE in stressed patients.

   A more common practice is the use of standardized equations to estimate BEE based on factors such as height, weight, age, and sex. Different equations have been developed for specific populations and clinical situations; in fact, over 200 have been published. The more notable of these include the Harris-Benedict, Frankenfeld, Swinamer, Penn State, and Ireton-Jones equations. The Harris-Benedict equation is the most frequently applied because of its ease of use and because of its good correlation with IC in diverse patient populations.

TABLE 2-1 Complications of Underfeeding and Overfeeding

Overfeeding	Underfeeding
Physiologic stress	Increased complications
Hyperosmolar state	Immune suppression
Hyperglycemia	Prolonged hospitalization
Hepatic dysfunction	Poor wound healing
Excessive cost	Nosocomial infection
Fluid overload	Respiratory compromise
Azotemia	Prolonged mechanical ventilation
Respiratory compromise	
Prolonged mechanical ventilation	

The Harris-Benedict equation provides an estimate of BEE as follows:
Men:

$$66.5 + [13.75 \times \text{weight (kg)}] + [5.0 \times \text{height (cm)}] - [6.78 \times \text{age (years)}]$$

Women:

$$655 + [9.56 \times \text{weight (kg)}] + [1.85 \times \text{height (cm)}] - [4.68 \times \text{age (years)}]$$

The calculated BEE is adjusted to simulate the patient's actual clinical state by multiplying by an estimated stress factor, which ranges from 1.25 to 1.75 depending on the clinical situation.

The calculation for our ventilated trauma patient is as follows:

$$\text{BEE} = 66.5 + [13.75 \times 80 \text{ kg}] + [5.0 \times 180 \text{ cm}] - [6.78 \times 34 \text{ years}] = 1836 \text{ kcal per day}$$

Multiplying by the stress factor of 1.3 for fracture/trauma, we obtain the answer of 2386 kcal per day.

BIBLIOGRAPHY

Cheng CH, Chen CH, Wong Y, Lee BJ, Kan MN, Huang YC. Measured versus estimated energy expenditure in mechanically ventilated critically ill patients. *Clin Nutr* 2002;21:165–172.

Jan BV, Lowry SF. Systemic response to injury and metabolic support. In: Brunicardi FC, Andersen DK, Billiar TR, et al., eds. *Schwartz's Principles of Surgery*. 9th ed. New York: McGraw-Hill; 2010:Chapter 2.

MacDonald A, Hildebrandt L. Comparison of formulaic equations to determine energy expenditure in the critically ill patient. *Nutrition* 2003;19:233–239.

Mahmoud N, Kulaylat MN, Dayton MT. Surgical complications. In: Townsend CM (ed.), *Sabiston: The Biological Basis of Modern Surgical Practice*, 18th ed. St. Louis, MO: Elsevier/Saunders; 2008:328–370.

3. **(D)** Parenteral nutrition requires central venous catheterization, which is performed using the Seldinger technique and a 15- to 17-cm polyurethane catheter with two or three lumens. All lines should be placed under maximal sterile precautions including hand wash, mask and cap, and sterile drapes, gowns, and gloves. Thorough insertion site cleansing should be undertaken as well, preferably with 2% chlorhexidine.

Site selection is important in minimizing the most commonly seen complications of central venous catheters (CVCs):

Infection. CVCs are estimated to account for more than 90% of all catheter-related bacteremias. Internal jugular or subclavian sites have had bacteremia rates of 1% to 5% and rates of significant colonization of the catheters (≥15 cfu on semiquantitative culture) ranging between 5% and 30%.

Patients with femoral vein catheters had a higher incidence of infectious complications (19.8% versus 4.5%; $p < 0.001$) and thrombotic complications (21.5% versus 1.9%; $p < 0.001$) compared with patients with subclavian catheters.

Venous thrombosis. Mechanical adverse events include arterial puncture, pneumothorax, hemothorax, mediastinal hematoma, malposition, and air embolism. The most common mechanical injuries include arterial puncture and minor bleeding. The complication of pneumothorax occurs in only 1.5% to 2.3% of subclavian CVC placements.

Risk factors for mechanical complications include increased time for insertion, nighttime placement, more than two needle passes for insertion, BMI greater than 30, and previous catheterization or surgery near the site of placement. Ultrasound guidance was not found to significantly decrease incidence of complications in subclavian vein catheterization.

Site selection for CVC placement is often based on the comfort level of the technician, rather than on the complication rates of the different sites. The Centers for Disease Control and Prevention recommends that, if not contraindicated, the subclavian vein should be used for the insertion of nontunneled CVCs in adult patients in an effort to minimize infection risk.

Several observational studies have found lower rates of infectious complications with subclavian catheters versus internal jugular catheters and a similar rate of mechanical complications. Ultrasonographic guidance of internal jugular vein catheterization has been associated with decreased rates of complications and increased rates of successful first insertion.

BIBLIOGRAPHY

Hind D, Calvert N, McWilliams R, et al. Ultrasonic locating devices for central venous cannulation: meta-analysis. *BMJ* 2003;327:361.

Leung J, Duffy M, Finckh A. Real-time ultrasonographically-guided internal jugular vein catheterization in the emergency department increases success rates and reduces complications: a randomized, prospective study. *Ann Emerg Med* 2006;48:540–547.

McConville JF, Kress JP. Intravascular devices. In: Hall JB, Schmidt GA, Wood LD (eds.), *Principles of Critical Care*, 3rd ed. New York: McGraw-Hill; 2005:Chapter 5.

Merrer J, Jonghe BD, Golliot F, et al. Complication of femoral and subclavian venous catheterization in critically ill patients. *JAMA* 2001;286:700–707.

4. **(D)** Patients who present with objective markers of malnutrition or will be unable to provide themselves with oral nutrition for 7 to 10 days benefit from supplemental nutrition. Enteral feeding has been found to have several key benefits over parenteral nutrition.

First, there are the decreased costs of providing long-term feeds via the enteral route. The solution itself is less expensive than parenteral nutrition solutions, daily electrolyte adjustments are not required, and administration costs are minimized.

Another benefit is the trophic effect of enteral feeds on small and large bowel mucosa. Parenteral nutrition can lead to intestinal mucosal atrophy and a resultant increase in bacterial translocation, which may contribute to the known increase in incidence of septic complications in parenterally fed patients.

Enteral nutrition also avoids the risks associated with intravenous access, including infection and vascular access complications.

Absolute contraindications to enteral nutrition are bowel obstruction, persistent intolerance (e.g., emesis, diarrhea), hemodynamic instability, major upper gastrointestinal bleed, and inability to safely access the gastrointestinal tract. The relative contraindications include high output intestinal fistula (>800 mL/day), acute inflammatory bowel disease, persistent ileus, and significant bowel-wall edema.

BIBLIOGRAPHY

MacFie J. Enteral versus parenteral nutrition. *Br J Surg* 2000;87:1121–1122.

Martindale RG, Zhou M. Nutrition and metabolism. In: O'Leary JP (ed.), *The Physiologic Basis of Surgery*, 4th ed. Baltimore, MD: Lippincott Williams & Wilkins; 2008:112–149.

Mendoza MC, Puyana JC. Nutritional support in the critically ill. In: Cameron JL (ed.), *Current Surgical Therapy*, 10th ed. Philadelphia, PA: Elsevier/Saunders; 2011:1284–1289.

5. **(D)** The enteral route should be used for nutritional supplementation whenever it is not contraindicated. The route of enteric feeds must be carefully chosen to provide adequate calories quickly while minimizing the risk for aspiration. Options include intragastric, postpyloric, gastrostomy, jejunostomy, and gastrojejunostomy tube feeding:

Nasogastric feeding is reserved for patients with intact mentation and protective laryngeal reflexes to minimize the risk of aspiration.

Small-bowel feeding via nasojejunal or nasoduodenal tubes have lower risks of aspiration pneumonia.

Percutaneous endoscopic gastrostomy (PEG) is indicated in patients with impaired swallowing or oropharyngeal or esophageal obstruction. In patients who cannot tolerate gastric feedings, PEG-jejunostomy and direct percutaneous endoscopic jejunostomy are feasible alternatives. Sugical gastrostomy or jejunostomy should be considered in patients undergoing complex abdominal or trauma surgery.

Generally accepted indications for postpyloric feedings include nasogastric tube output greater than 600 mL in 24 h, known history of aspiration, lack of adequate airway protection, severe pulmonary dysfunction, recent regurgitation, and inability to be maintained with the head of bed at 30°. If any of these contraindications exist, the patient should receive a postpyloric feeding tube, which can be placed under fluoroscopic guidance or using a bedside technique.

Early enteral nutrition is defined as being started within the first 48 h of intensive care unit admission. Benefits include decreased mortality and infection. Feedings should be started at a low volume and advanced to goal rate in the absence of signs of intolerance such as increased gastric residuals, osmotic diarrhea, and/or abdominal distention. Postpyloric feeds should be advanced in a manner similar to intragastric feeds, and patients should also be assessed for signs of feeding intolerance such as abdominal distention and/or diarrhea. Parenteral feeding is an option if the patient is unable to tolerate transpyloric catheter feeding.

Patients who will require enteral feeding for an extended period of time should be considered for gastrostomy tube placement. Those who cannot tolerate gastric feeding should be considered for gastrojejunal or jejunostomy tube placement.

BIBLIOGRAPHY

Jan BV, Lowry SF. Systemic response to injury and metabolic support. In: Brunicardi FC, Andersen DK, Billiar TR, et al. (eds.), *Schwartz's Principles of Surgery*, 9th ed. New York: McGraw-Hill; 2010:Chapter 2.

Mendoza MC, Puyana JC. Nutritional support in the critically ill. In: Cameron JL (ed.), *Current Surgical Therapy*, 10th ed. Philadelphia, PA: Elsevier/Saunders; 2011.

Niv E, Fireman Z, Vaisman N. Post-pyloric feeding. *World J Gastroenterol* 2009 Mar 21;15(11):1281–1288.

6. **(C)** The total body phosphate content of an average man is approximately 10 g/kg and 85% is found in the skeleton. The extracellular portion of total body phosphorus is less than 1% and 10% is protein bound with approximately 33% fixed to sodium, calcium, and magnesium. Daily intake of phosphate is 1000 to 1500 mg. The small bowel, primarily the jejunum, is responsible for absorption of 60% to 70% of phosphate intake. Fecal and urinary output is usually regulated to maintain a total body phosphate balance of zero.

Parathyroid hormone plays a key role in phosphate homeostasis in the renal failure patient. Hyperphosphatemia and the resultant decrease in the levels of ionized calcium act directly to increase the secretion of parathyroid hormone. Parathyroid hormone in turn stimulates osteoclast activity to promote bone resorption of calcium and phosphorus. In addition, there is greater metabolization of calcidiol to calcitriol, leading to improved small bowel absorption of calcium. Finally, parathyroid hormone acts directly on the renal tubules to increase calcium reabsorption and phosphate excretion, resulting in phosphaturia. The kidney is able to adequately maintain normal phosphate levels until the glomerular filtration rate is less than 25 mL/min.

Because excess phosphorus is effectively excreted, clinical cases of hyperphosphatemia are generally limited to patients with an acute phosphorus load, renal failure, and dysfunctional renal excretion of phosphorus.

Increased phosphorus load can be due to overdose of phosphorus or vitamin D, burns, fleet enemas, cell death (e.g., rhabdomyolysis, tumor lysis syndrome), or acidosis.

Decreased renal clearance of phosphorus leads to hypocalcemia due to binding of ionized calcium by phosphorus, and calcification of the soft tissues. Severe cases may result in acute renal failure and cardiac arrhythmias.

In patients with normal renal function, saline infusion and acetazolamide can induce natriuresis and increase renal clearance of phosphorus. In patients with abnormal renal function, or symptomatic hypocalcemia, dialysis is the most effective method of phosphorus removal.

Next in the treatment is the use of oral phosphate binding agents such as aluminum carbonate, calcium carbonate, and acetate. Aluminum salts remain the most effective phosphate binders, but there is still no satisfactory method to reliable reduce phosphate levels in the dialysis patient. The known increase in cardiovascular complications in those patients with chronically elevated phosphorus levels makes this an active avenue for continued research.

BIBLIOGRAPHY

Albaaj D, Hutchison A. Hyperphosphataemia in renal failure: causes, consequences and current management. *Drugs* 2003;63:577–596.

Blacher J, Guerin AP, Pannier B, et al. Arterial calcifications, arterial stiffness and cardiovascular risk in end-stage renal disease. *Hypertension* 2001;38:938–942.

Block GA, Port FK. Re-evaluation of risks associated with hyperphosphatemia and hyperparathyroidism in dialysis patients: recommendations for a change in management. *Am J Kidney Dis* 2000;35:1226–1237.

7. **(D)** A commonly used tool to determine substrate oxidation and utilization is the respiratory quotient. The respiratory quotient is determined by following formula:

$$\text{Respiratory quotient} = \frac{CO_2 \text{ produced}}{O_2 \text{ consumed}}$$

The respiratory quotient for protein oxidation is 0.85, fat oxidation is 0.7, glucose oxidation is 1.0, and lipogenesis is >1.0.

The patient represented above has a minute ventilation of 16 L/min, which is likely because of increased CO_2 production from the caloric distribution and quantity of the parenteral nutrition. The first hyperalimentation error is in providing too many nonprotein calories distributed as glucose. Glucose has a respiratory quotient of 1.0 versus fat's respiratory quotient of 0.7 and therefore causes greater production of CO_2. Compounding the problem, the excess nonprotein calories are converted into fat. The respiratory quotient of lipogenesis is greater than 1, contributing to elevated CO_2 and the compensatory increased minute ventilation.

The nutritional formula in this patient should be adjusted to provide fewer calories and a greater portion of those calories as lipid.

Clinicians should also perform a thorough evaluation for other potential nonmetabolic sources of failure to wean. An unfortunate complication of decreasing calories in a patient who may be undergoing continued metabolic stress from an evolving inflammatory process is inadvertent and unnecessary malnutrition.

BIBLIOGRAPHY

Martindale RG, Zhou M. Nutrition and metabolism. In: O'Leary JP (ed.), *The Physiologic Basis of Surgery*, 4th ed. Baltimore, MD: Lippincott Williams & Wilkins; 2008:112–149.

Moore FA, McQuiggan M. Nutritional support of the stressed intensive care unit patient. In: Hall JB, Freid EB (eds.), *Society of Critical Care Medicine and American College of Chest Physicians 4th Combined Critical Care Course*. New York, NY: SCCM/ACCP; 2002.

8. **(C)** Urine nitrogen balance is an excellent measure of metabolic stress. A negative nitrogen balance denotes that inadequate protein is being supplied to offset the nitrogen excreted as the breakdown product of protein metabolism. Nitrogen balance in the clinical setting is assessed by measuring 24-h urine urea output.

$$\text{Nitrogen balance} = \text{nitrogen (g)}_{\text{Intake}} - \text{nitrogen (g)}_{\text{Output}}$$

$$\text{Nitrogen balance} = \frac{\text{protein (g)}_{\text{Intake}}}{6.25 - \text{nitrogen (g)}_{\text{Output}}}$$

The goal of nutritional support should be to maintain neutral or positive nitrogen balance.

The measurement of serum albumin reflects long-term nutritional status (18 to 21 days) and therefore does not accurately measure the acute metabolic stress of surgery. Weight loss is also not an accurate measure of short-term stress; additionally, small fluctuations in body weight are readily attributable to changes in fluid status. While retinol binding protein (RBP) has been promoted as a measure of nutritional status, its ability to accurately reflect acute metabolic stress is limited by its variable response to other stimuli such as infection.

BIBLIOGRAPHY

Barbour JR, Barbour EF, Herrmann VM. Surgical metabolism & nutrition. In: Doherty GM (ed.), *Current Diagnosis & Treatment: Surgery*, 13th ed. New York: McGraw-Hill; 2010:Chapter 10.

Pingleton SK. Nutrition in chronic critical illness. *Clin Chest Med* 2001;22:149–163.

9. **(B)**

10. **(D)**

11. **(C)**

Explantations for questions 9–11

Aspiration is defined as the inhalation of either gastric or oropharyngeal contents into upper and lower airways. Aspiration may result in pneumonia or pneumonitis.

Aspiration pneumonitis, also known as Mendelson syndrome, is defined as acute lung injury after the inhalation of regurgitated gastric contents. This syndrome commonly occurs in patients who have a marked disturbance of consciousness such as that resulting from a drug overdose, seizures, a massive cerebrovascular accident, or the use of anesthesia. The risk of this adverse event is increased as the level of consciousness decreases, and the level of lung injury is proportional to the acidity of the gastric contents and the presence of particulate matter. Gastric acid prevents the growth of bacteria and therefore bacterial contamination in aspiration pneumonitis is less frequently a concern. The exception to this is when there is an elevation in the pH of gastric contents as occurs with proton pump inhibitors and H2 blockers and with increased colonization, which may be seen with small bowel obstruction.

The most appropriate initial treatment option for aspiration pneumonitis is immediate suctioning of the oropharynx to prevent further aspiration. Enteral feeds with a nasogastric tube or gastric tube should be held and the stomach aspirated. The use of empiric antibiotics in those who develop fever or leukocytosis in the first 24 h after an aspiration event is not necessary and likely leads to selection of more resistant organisms.

Antibiotic management is recommended for those who may have colonization of their gastric contents or for those who fail to improve after 48 h.

Aspiration pneumonia develops after the inhalation of colonized oropharyngeal material. Aspiration of colonized secretions from the oropharynx is the primary mechanism by which bacteria gain entrance to the lungs. The most common community acquired organisms are *Streptococcus pneumonia*, *Staphylococcus aureus*, *Haemophilus influenzae*, and *Enterobacter* species. Among hospitalized patients, *Pseudomonas aeruginosa* and other gram-negative species were the most common.

Prevention of aspiration in patients undergoing surgery is achieved by instituting measures that reduce gastric contents, minimize regurgitation, and protect the airway. For adults, a period of no oral intake, usually 6 hours after a night meal, 4 hours after clear liquids, and a longer period for diabetics, is necessary to reduce gastric contents before elective surgery.

A patient who sustains aspiration of gastric contents needs to be immediately placed on oxygen and have a chest radiograph to confirm the clinical suspicions. A diffuse interstitial pattern is usually seen bilaterally and is often described as bilateral, fluffy infiltrates. Antibiotic choices include third-generation cephalosporins, fluoroquinolones, and piperacillins. Both large trials showed there to be no patients who speciated to an anaerobic organism. It is not recommended to start an anaerobic antibiotic agent unless there is evidence of pulmonary abscess or periodontal disease. Commonly chosen single coverage antibiotics such as clindamycin and penicillin have inappropriate gram-negative coverage spectrums for hospitalized patients with aspiration pneumonia. Administration of antibiotics shortly after aspiration is controversial except in patients with bowel obstruction or other conditions associated with colonization of gastric contents. Administration of empirical antibiotics is also indicated in a patient with aspiration pneumonitis that does not resolve or improve within 48 h of aspiration. Corticosteroid administration does not provide any beneficial effects to patients with aspiration pneumonitis.

BIBLIOGRAPHY

Light BR. Pneumonia. In: Hall JB, Schmidt GA, Wood LD (eds.), *Principles of Critical Care,* 3rd ed. New York: McGraw-Hill; 2005.

Mahmoud N. Kulaylat MN, Dayton MT. Surgical complications. In: Townsend CM (ed.), *Sabiston: The Biological Basis of Modern Surgical Practice*, 18th ed. St. Louis, MO: Elsevier/Saunders; 2008:328–370.

Marik PE. Aspiration pneumonitis and aspiration pneumonia. *N Engl J Med* 2001;344:665–671.

12. **(E)** Vitamin A includes retinol, retinaldehyde, and retinoic acid, collectively termed retinoids. Vitamin A plays

a role in normal vision, growth, cell differentiation, iron utilization, and immunity.

Thiamine is referred to as vitamin B_1 because it was the first B vitamin to be identified. Thiamine plays a role in energy generation and peripheral nerve conduction.

Niacin is also known as vitamin B_3 and includes nicotinic acid, nicotinamide, and their biologically active derivatives. Nicotinic acid and nicotinamide serve as precursors of two coenzymes, nicotinamide adenine dinucleotide (NAD) and NAD phosphate (NADP), which are active in oxidation reduction reactions, DNA repair, and calcium mobilization.

Vitamin D plays a role in immune function, inflammation, cellular proliferation and differentiation, and calcium metabolism. The major source of vitamin D is synthesis in the skin, which is catabolized by UV-B exposure.

Vitamin K exists in two forms, K_1, which is obtained from vegetable and animal sources, and K_2, which is synthesized by bacterial flora and found in hepatic tissue. Broad-spectrum antibiotic treatment can precipitate vitamin K deficiency by depleting intestinal bacteria and inhibiting the metabolism of vitamin K.

Water-soluble vitamins include B_1, B_2, B_6, and B_{12}; vitamin C; niacin; folate; biotin; and pantothenic acid. These vitamins are obtained via diet and absorbed in the duodenum and proximal small bowel. Deficiency is relatively common, due to limited storage in the body. Vitamins A, D, E, and K are fat soluble and are absorbed in the proximal small bowel in association with bile salt micelles and fatty acids. After absorption, they are delivered to the tissues in chylomicrons and stored in the liver or subcutaneous tissue and skin.

BIBLIOGRAPHY

Russell RM, Suter PM. Vitamin and trace mineral deficiency and excess. In: Longo DL, Fauci AS, Kasper DL, et al. (eds.), *Harrison's Principles of Internal Medicine*, 18th ed. New York: McGraw-Hill; 2012:Chapter 74.

13. **(C)** This patient is suffering from niacin deficiency. Niacin (also known as nicotinic acid or vitamin B_3) is obtained from dietary sources and is primarily absorbed in the stomach and ileum. Animal protein breakdown remains the greatest source of natural dietary niacin (1.5% of tryptophan is converted into niacin). This conversion increases in deficiency states. Nicotinamide adenine dinucleotide (NAD^+) and nicotinamide adenine dinucleotide phosphate (NADPH) are both coenzymes that require niacin for production. These coenzymes are necessary for glycolysis, lipid synthesis, and oxidative phosphorylation. NAD is involved in the catabolism of carbohydrates, fats, proteins, and alcohol. NADP functions in anabolic reactions, for the synthesis of fatty acids and cholesterol. The reduced form NADP is converted to NADPH and is used

in reactions to detoxify reactive oxygen species and drugs. In addition, NAD is also involved in nonredox reactions such as cell signaling and DNA repair.

The U.S. Recommended Daily Allowance of niacin is 45 to 80 µg for men and 45 to 65 µg for women. During severe illness, niacin intake should be 200 mg per day.

The symptoms of niacin deficiency begin with nonspecific changes such as anorexia, weight loss, and weakness. Signs of later stages include the classic erythematous, scaly lesions of the extremities. Also commonly seen are stomatitis, glossitis, enteritis, and diarrhea. Malabsorption and diarrhea can facilitate greater niacin deficiency. Central nervous system symptoms include insomnia, amnesia, anxiety, depression, seizures, and psychosis. Peripheral paresthesias may also be noted.

The treatment of acute deficiency states is niacin replacement with doses of 100 mg per day. Symptoms completely and quickly resolve with correction of niacin stores.

BIBLIOGRAPHY

Tawa NE, Fischer JE. Metabolism in surgical patients. In: Townsend CM (ed.), *Sabiston: The Biological Basis of Modern Surgical Practice*, 18th ed. St. Louis, MO: Elsevier/Saunders; 2008.

Wan P, Moat S, Anstey A. Pellagra: a review with emphasis on photosensitivity. *Br J Dermatol* 2011;164:1188–1200. doi:10.1111/j.1365-2133.2010.10163.x. Epub 2011 May 5.

14. **(D)** Trace elements represent less than 0.1% of the average diet. Deficiencies are found mostly in malnourished patients and those receiving hyperalimentation without trace elements. Routine testing for trace element deficiency is not indicated. However, the clinician should be familiar with the function of each of the trace elements and the key signs of their deficiencies.

Zinc deficiencies develop in patients who have a persistently catabolic state or chronic or excessive diarrhea. From 3 to 6 mg of elemental zinc per day is required in patients with normal stool losses, and between 12 and 20 mg is required in patients with short-bowel syndrome or excessive diarrhea. Zinc deficiency has numerous manifestations, including alopecia, poor wound healing, immunosuppression, night blindness or photophobia, impaired taste or smell (anosmia), neuritis, and a variety of skin disorders (generalized eruptions, perioral pustular rash, darkening of the skin creases) and is similar to the syndrome of zinc deficiency seen in sheep (acrodermatitis enteropathica).

Selenium deficiency is a rare condition and may be associated with diffuse skeletal myopathy and cardiomyopathy (with abnormalities in basement and plasma membranes on muscle biopsy), loss of pigmentation, and erythrocyte macrocytosis.

Copper is a key component of intracellular and extracellular enzymes. Deficiency is seen in chronic parenteral nutrition patients without adequate replacement. Symptoms of deficiency are hypochromic microcytic anemia, pancytopenia, depigmentation, and osteopenia. The microcytic anemia may be mistaken for pyridoxine deficiency.

Chromium deficiency is almost always seen in patients on parenteral nutrition without appropriate replacement. The daily amount of chromium required in parenteral nutrition to avoid insufficient states is 15 to 20 μg per day. Chromium is necessary for adequate utilization of glucose, and deficiency is often manifested as a sudden diabetic state in which blood sugar is difficult to control, along with peripheral neuropathy and encephalopathy. To treat chromium deficiency, 150 mg of chromium per day is given for several days.

Calcium, iron, and other metals are absorbed in the duodenum. Consequently, duodenal bypass (as after a Billroth II gastrectomy) or resection (as after a Whipple procedure) often results in long-term deficiencies of these ions.

Classifications of iron deficiency include:

- Early (no anemia, serum Fe and ferritin decreased, transferrin increased),
- Intermediate (no anemia, transferrin saturation <15%, ferritin <12 μg/L),
- Late (hypochromic microcytic anemia).

The daily requirement for oral iron is 15 mg/day, but only 5% to 10% is absorbed, leaving the parenteral requirement at 1 to 2 mg/day. The ability to excrete parenteral iron is limited, and iron overload will develop in a significant number of patients given iron routinely.

Patients at increased risk of iron deficiency are premenopausal women (menstruation may increase Fe loss by an additional 1 mg/day), patients receiving more than 50% of their total caloric needs from TPN, patients with chronic gastrointestinal bleeding (e.g., Crohn disease in women), and patients maintained on hemodialysis (especially with concurrent erythropoietin therapy).

BIBLIOGRAPHY

Barbour JR, Barbour EF, Herrmann VM. Surgical metabolism & nutrition. In: Doherty GM (ed.), *Current Diagnosis & Treatment: Surgery*. 13th ed. New York: McGraw-Hill; 2010:Chapter 10.
Tawa NE, Fischer JE. Metabolism in surgical patients. In: Townsend CM (ed.), *Sabiston: The Biological Basis of Modern Surgical Practice*, 18th ed. St. Louis, MO: Elsevier/Saunders; 2008.

15. **(E)** Vitamins are essential elements of nutrition and cannot be synthesized by the body. The fat soluble vitamins are vitamins A, D, E, and K and are stored in body fat. Deficiencies in vitamin A (retinol) cause xerophthalmia and keratomalacia. Vitamin D (cholecalciferol) plays a key role in calcium absorption. It is converted to calcitrol in the kidney and liver; insufficient supply of vitamin D leads to rickets in children and osteomalacia in adults. Deficiency of vitamin E (α-tocopherol), an antioxidant, results in hemolytic anemia and neurologic changes. Vitamin K (naphthoquinone) plays a role in the function of certain coagulation factors (factors II, VII, IX, and X, protein C, and protein S).

The water-soluble vitamins include those in the B complex and vitamin C. Thiamine (vitamin B_1) deficiency leads to heart failure, beriberi, neuropathy, and fatigue. Riboflavin (vitamin B_2) is involved in oxidation-reduction reactions and glossitis and dermatitis are the most common features of its deficiency. Pyridoxal phosphate (vitamin B_6) deficiency leads to neuropathy, glossitis, and anemia. Dermatitis and alopecia are the features of biotin (vitamin B_7) deficiency. Folate (vitamin B_9) plays a role in DNA synthesis and its deficiencies are associated with megaloblastic anemia and glossitis. Cyanocobalamin (vitamin B_{12}) is involved in DNA synthesis and myelination and predictably megaloblastic anemia and neuropathy are the signs associated with its deficiency.

Vitamin C (ascorbic acid) hydroxylates proline in collagen synthesis. Scurvy is seen in those lacking artificial or organic supplies of vitamin C.

BIBLIOGRAPHY

Szeto WY, Buzby GP. Nutrition, digestion and absorption. In: Kreisel D, Krupnick AS, Kaiser LR (eds.), *The Surgical Review: An Integrated Basic and Clinical Science Study Guide*. Philadelphia, PA: Lippincott Williams & Wilkins; 2001:272–291.

16. **(C)** The controversy over the appropriate route for nutrition in the acute pancreatitis patient is still a topic of heated discussion. The physiologic insult resulting from acute and even chronic pancreatitis induces a state of stress metabolism. This is generally compounded with prehospitalization starvation because of poor oral intake secondary to gastroparesis, small bowel ileus, and/or nausea and vomiting. These factors all contribute to the importance of promptly starting and continuing nutritional support in these patients.

In the past, patients with episodes of acute pancreatitis requiring nutrition were given parenteral nutrition in order to avoid excess exocrine stimulation of the pancreas. The avoidance of enteral feeding has not been shown to improve patient outcomes, other than decreased pain. In addition, clinical studies have shown that jejunal feeds fail to result in pancreatic exocrine stimulation relative to feeds to more proximal segments of small bowel and the stomach.

In cases of severe acute pancreatitis, every attempt should be made to access the intestinal tract and enterally feed patients. Enteral feeding has been shown to enhance intestinal epithelial barrier function, reduce septic complications from severe acute pancreatitis, and, in some series, reduce mortality. Elemental enteral formulas have also been shown to decrease exocrine stimulation of the pancreas relative to intact protein formulas.

BIBLIOGRAPHY

Baron TH, Morgan DE. Acute necrotizing pancreatitis. *N Engl J Med* 1999;340:1412–1417.

Clancy TE, Ashley SW. Management of acute pancreatitis. In: Zinner MJ, Ashley SW (eds.), *Maingot's Abdominal Operations*, 12th ed. New York: McGraw-Hill; 2013.

Fink D, Alverdy JC. Exocrine pancreas. In: Townsend CM (ed.), *Sabiston: The Biological Basis of Modern Surgical Practice*, 18th ed. St. Louis, MO: Elsevier/Saunders; 2008:1589–1623.

17. **(B)** The patient is suffering from refeeding syndrome. This is a potentially morbid condition associated with electrolyte and fluid shifts that occur as a consequence of reintroduction of feeding after a period of starvation or fasting.

    Refeeding syndrome can be seen after the onset of parenteral or enteral feeding in any chronically malnourished patient, especially those in which there has been a greater than 15% weight loss over several months. Known risk factors include prisoners of war, prolonged fasting, weight loss in patients after obesity surgery, alcoholics, malnourished elderly, those undergoing chemotherapy, and patients with eating disorders.

    The physiology centers on the conversion of starvation lipid metabolism to refeeding carbohydrate metabolism. The insulin release causes intracellular uptake of glucose, phosphate, potassium, magnesium, water, and protein. Fluid balance abnormalities, vitamin B_1 deficiency, hypophosphatemia, hypomagnesemia, and hypokalemia are primary features.

    Changes in serum electrolytes affect the cell membrane potential, and impair function in nerve, cardiac, and skeletal muscle cells based on the type and severity of biochemical abnormality present. Subsequent symptoms range from nausea, vomiting, and lethargy to respiratory insufficiency, cardiac failure, hypotension, arrhythmias, delirium, coma, and death. The fluid disturbances center on dehydration and resultant prerenal azotemia. Compounding this problem is the glucose disturbance of hyperglycemia which can cause osmotic diuresis and hyperosmolar nonketotic coma.

Treatment of patients with electrolyte abnormalities secondary to refeeding syndrome should be prompt correction of deficiencies and frequent electrolyte monitoring. Patients that are at high risk for refeeding syndrome should have a gradual increase in feeds from 20 kcal/kg per day to goal over a period of 5 to 7 days, or until the patient is metabolically stable. All patients who are malnourished should have electrolytes corrected before starting feeding and should be monitored frequently after the start of either parenteral or enteral nutrition.

BIBLIOGRAPHY

Crook MA, Hally V, Panteli JV. The importance of the refeeding syndrome. *Nutrition* 2001;17:632–637.

Khan LU, Ahmed J, Khan S, MacFie J. Refeeding syndrome: a literature review. *Gastroenterology research and practice*, 2011.

Khan LU, Ahmed J, Macfie J. Refeeding syndrome: a literature review. *Gastroenterol Res Pract* 2011;2011. pii: 410971. doi: 10.1155/2011/410971. Epub 2010 Aug 25. PMID: 20886063; PMCID: PMC2945646

18. **(A)** Carbohydrates in the diet that reach the colon unabsorbed by the small bowel are fermented by anaerobic bacteria to form SCFAs. The most abundant SCFAs are butyrate, propionate, and acetate, with butyrate being the preferred substrate for the colonocyte. SCFAs are rapidly absorbed from the colonic lumen, and their oxidation inside the colonocyte is the major energy source of the colorectal epithelium.

    In patients with normal small bowel function, colonic SCFAs provide only 5% to 10% of daily calories; however, some studies have shown that the colon can be an energy salvage organ in patients with decreased small bowel function. In one study, preservation of half of colon length decreased parenteral energy requirements by half in patients with short gut syndrome.

    In addition to being an energy source, SCFAs have been proposed to be involved in various cell-signaling systems in the colonocyte. Impaired metabolism of SCFAs has been implicated in the pathogenesis of ulcerative colitis.

BIBLIOGRAPHY

Martindale RG, Zhou M. Nutrition and metabolism. In: O'Leary JP (ed.), *The Physiologic Basis of Surgery*, 4th ed. Baltimore, MD: Lippincott Williams & Wilkins; 2008:112–149.

Ohkusa T, Okayasu I, Ogihara T, et al. Induction of experimental ulcerative colitis by *Fusobacterium varium* isolated from colonic mucosa of patients with ulcerative colitis. *Gut* 2003;52:79–83.

CHAPTER 3

WOUND HEALING AND CARE

LISA M. MCELROY AND TRAVIS P. WEBB

1. Regarding Fig. 3-1, which of the following statements is correct?
   (A) Lymphocytes play a minor role during inflammation
   (B) Wound healing is complete by 6 months
   (C) Epithelialization occurs during maturation
   (D) Granulation tissue develops during proliferation
   (E) Myofibroblasts produce contracture of the wound during proliferation

2. A 39-year-old man underwent a ventral hernia repair with prosthetic mesh. The peak of collagen production in his wound will be achieved by day
   (A) 2
   (B) 7
   (C) 14
   (D) 21
   (E) 28

3. The maximum net collagen content for the patient in Question 2 will be achieved by day
   (A) 7
   (B) 14
   (C) 21
   (D) 42
   (E) 90

4. The greatest burst strength of a wound is achieved by
   (A) 1 week
   (B) 3 weeks
   (C) 6 weeks
   (D) 12 weeks
   (E) 6 months

5. The patient described in question 2 comes back for a 3-week follow-up visit. Figure 3-2 depicts the patient's wound after removal of the staples. Which of the following is the best option for the management of this patient's wound?
   (A) Primary closure of the skin with stitches
   (B) Mesh irrigation with antibiotic solution daily and closure of the wound by secondary intention
   (C) Wound debridement and placement of a new PTFE mesh
   (D) Removal of PTFE mesh and placement of polypropylene mesh
   (E) Removal of PTFE mesh and closure of the wound with Vicryl mesh

6. The same patient comes back to your office for a follow-up visit. His skin was left open after the second repair and he is placing wet-to-dry dressing changes with normal saline twice a day. It seems that the wound did not decrease in size since the last visit. An alternative to manage this patient's wound is to
   (A) Tell the patient that there is nothing else to do and continue to do dressing changes with normal saline twice a day
   (B) Increase the frequency of dressing changes to three times a day
   (C) Close the wound with stitches
   (D) Close the wound with staples
   (E) Place a vacuum-assisted device system (V.A.C.)

7. A 35-year-old woman underwent a ventral hernia repair around 6 months ago. She comes back complaining of a nodule at the incision site. The nodule is excised and microscopically revealed macrophages, collagen, and giant cells. In addition, a polarized refractile material is present in the nodule. What is the most likely diagnosis?
   (A) Normal wound healing
   (B) Abscess formation
   (C) Suture granuloma
   (D) Hypertrophic scar
   (E) Keloid

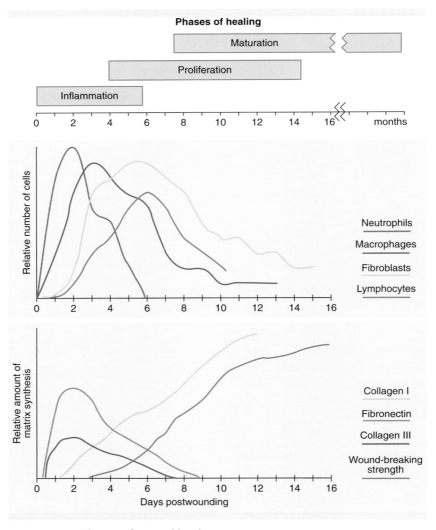

FIGURE 3-1. Phases of wound healing.

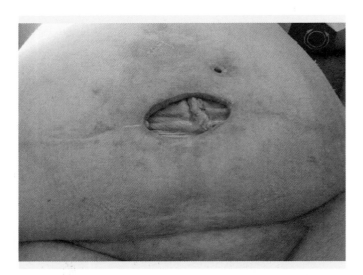

FIGURE 3-2. Abdominal wound with tissue defect.

8. A 60-year-old man underwent an elective, uncomplicated femoral hernia repair. Dense collagen deposition is most likely to be seen how long after the surgery?
   (A) 1 day
   (B) 2 days
   (C) 7 days
   (D) 14 days
   (E) 1 month

9. A 45-year-old man undergoes an exploratory laparotomy because of a perforated duodenal ulcer. Intraoperatively, 1.5 L of turbid fluid is found. After closing fascia the best management of his wound is
   (A) Closure of skin with staples
   (B) Interrupted skin closure
   (C) Closure of skin with Dermabond
   (D) Wound left open and local wound care
   (E) Subcuticular skin closure

10. A 5-year-old boy presents with a recurrent history of pyogenic infections. He has always had a normal white blood cell count. An analysis of the patient's neutrophils is performed and reveals a defect in neutrophil rolling. Which of the following is the most likely diagnosis?
    (A) Decreased neutrophil rolling, which is normal in children
    (B) Chronic granulomatous disease
    (C) Selectin deficiency
    (D) Integrin deficiency
    (E) Immunoglobulin deficiency

11. Patients with chronic granulomatous disease are more susceptible to infections. Which of the following is the mechanism responsible for their immunosuppression?
    (A) Defective lysosome release
    (B) Decreased synthesis of interleukin (IL)-1 and tumor necrosis factor-alpha (TNF-α)
    (C) Lack of opsonization
    (D) Lack of oxygen-dependent killing of bacteria by neutrophils
    (E) Deficiency of selectins

12. A 65-year-old man underwent a colectomy for colon cancer. Postoperatively, you find out he has been taking aspirin daily. Which one of the following features of the inflammatory response will be ablated in this patient?
    (A) Chemotaxis
    (B) Vasodilatation
    (C) Cytokine release
    (D) Collagen synthesis
    (E) Fibroblastic proliferation

13. A 45-year-old woman underwent a kidney transplant 6 months ago and has been taking cyclosporine and steroids. She developed cholelithiasis and requires a laparoscopic cholecystectomy. She wants to know if her chance to have a wound infection is increased. The best answer to her question is
    (A) No, steroids and cyclosporine do not increase the chance to have wound infection when used chronically
    (B) Yes, because of inhibition of collagen synthesis and fibroblast proliferation
    (C) Yes, because of persistent vasoconstriction and hypoxia
    (D) Yes, because of structural nuclear changes and decreased DNA synthesis
    (E) Yes, mainly because of cyclosporine, which blocks IL-2 and decreases migration of macrophages

14. You are concerned with adherence of the graft to the wound bed. Which of the following factors will down-regulate wound angiogenesis?

    (A) Lactate
    (B) Von Hippel–Lindau protein
    (C) Acidic pH
    (D) Fibroblast growth factor (FGF)-1
    (E) Prostaglandins

15. With regard to cytokines, which of the following statements is correct?
    (A) IL-1 is secreted mainly by lymphocytes and mediates inflammation.
    (B) IL-10 is involved in cell division and activation.
    (C) IL-8 is secreted by macrophages and promotes chemotaxis.
    (D) IL-2 is a major inhibitor of cell division.
    (E) Tumor necrosis factor is produced by T cells and is associated with a rise of immature neutrophils in the blood circulation.

16. Regarding growth factors, which one of the following statements is correct?
    (A) Epidermal growth factor (EGF) inhibits matrix metalloproteinases (MMPs).
    (B) Platelet-derived growth factor (PDGF) is a powerful chemoattractant and influence in the deposition of extracellular matrix.
    (C) FGF is secreted by lymphocytes and promotes angiogenesis.
    (D) Vascular endothelial growth factor (VEGF) promotes angiogenesis in healthy tissue only.
    (E) Transforming growth factor-beta (TGF-β) inhibits expression of PDGF in low doses.

17. What is the most common type of collagen in this wound (see Fig. 3-3)?
    (A) I
    (B) II
    (C) III
    (D) IV
    (E) V

18. In reference to Fig. 3-3, which one of the following statements is correct?
    (A) This tissue is rich in mature vessels.
    (B) Fibroblasts are scarce.
    (C) Excess granulation tissue will inhibit wound closure.
    (D) Reepithelialization occurs before granulation tissue formation.
    (E) After complete healing, the epithelialized skin will regain hair follicles.

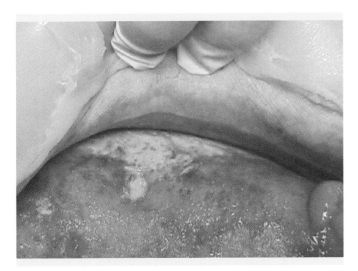

FIGURE 3-3. Healing wound with granulation tissue.

19. A 35-year-old woman with breast cancer underwent lumpectomy and radiation therapy. She had recurrence of the tumor and underwent a modified radical mastectomy. Regarding radiotherapy's effect on wound healing, all of the following statements are true, *except*:
    (A) It can cause fibroblast injury.
    (B) It decreases the amount of collagen deposition.
    (C) Effects are reversible after 1 year of last treatment.
    (D) Radiation therapy increases the risk of wound infection.
    (E) Wound healing is impaired because of vascular damage.

20. Regarding nitric oxide (NO), which one of the following statements is correct?
    (A) It has a long half-life.
    (B) Glutamine is a substrate for NO synthesis.
    (C) Inhibition of NO increases collagen deposition.
    (D) L-Arginine and NO can partially reverse the impaired healing of chronic diabetic ulcers.
    (E) NO increases cyclic adenosine monophosphate (cAMP).

21. A 32-year-old man comes back to your clinic for a 6-month follow-up after an appendectomy. He is an alcoholic, lives by himself, and states that since surgery he has eaten mostly fast food. On physical examination, his skin is dry with reddish spots. His appendectomy scar, which was healed 3 months after surgery, is dehisced. His gum is red, swollen, and shiny. Regarding this condition, which one of the following statements is correct?
    (A) Laboratory studies should be performed to confirm clinical diagnosis.
    (B) Leukopenia is associated in 30% of the cases.

(C) Abnormalities are not reversed by vitamin supplementation.
(D) Ingestion of dairy products can reverse this condition.
(E) Dehiscence of the wound was caused most likely by infection of the wound.

22. Which of the following patients is a suitable candidate to undergo hyperbaric oxygenation (HBO) therapy because of chronic nonhealing wound of the right thorax?
    (A) 56-year-old man with untreated pneumothorax
    (B) 35-year-old man receiving cisplatin for testicular carcinoma
    (C) 45-year-old female 35%-burn patient treated with sulfamylon
    (D) 55-year-old male alcoholic treated with disulfiram
    (E) 65-year-old woman status post chest radiation and heart transplant with wound dehiscence because of infection

23. Regarding Matrix Metalloproteinases (MMPs), which one of the following statements is correct?
    (A) MMPs are secreted in their active form.
    (B) MMPs are always present in chronic wounds.
    (C) Disruption of the basal the membrane is a critical determinant for collagenase activity.
    (D) Cytokines downregulate the activity of MMPs.
    (E) MMPs are stored intracellularly for long periods of time

24. Regarding the condition illustrated by Fig. 3-4, which of the following statements is correct?

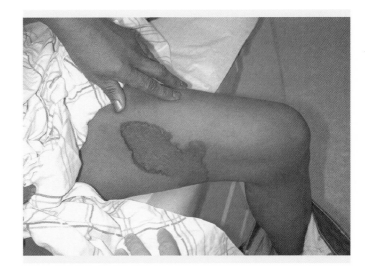

FIGURE 3-4. Hypertrophic scar.

(A) It is limited to the area of wound healing.
(B) It is preventable.

(C) It is most common on the lower extremities, lower back, and abdomen.

(D) Histologically, keloid scar and hypertrophic scar are not different.

(E) Collagen type I is the predominant type of collagen.

25. Regarding Fig. 3-5, which one of the following statements is *incorrect*?

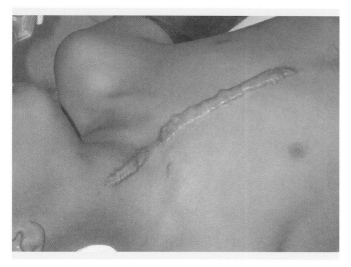

FIGURE 3-5. Sternal keloid.

(A) It is a preventable condition.

(B) Tension during closure is a contributory factor.

(C) Scar parallel to the underlying muscle may prevent this condition.

(D) Infection is a common cause for this condition.

(E) Fibroblasts have increased sensitivity to TGF-β1.

26. The differences between a keloid and a hypertrophic scar include all of the following *except*

(A) Presence of antinuclear antibodies against fibroblasts

(B) Levels of ATP

(C) Collagen bundles with a glazed appearance

(D) Scar limits

(E) The predominant collagen is type I

27. A 65-year-old white man sustained a severe burn to his right lower extremity during the Vietnam conflict. He is being seen in your clinic because of intermittent drainage from his chronic leg wound (see Fig. 3-6). The most appropriate management of this patient is

(A) Wet-to-dry dressing changes with normal saline and follow-up in 1 month.

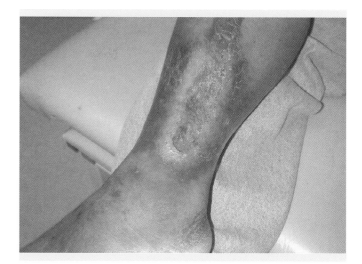

FIGURE 3-6. Nonhealing leg wound (Marjolin ulcer).

(B) Silvadene to the wound and follow-up in 1 month

(C) Radiograph of the lower extremity

(D) Biopsy of the wound

(E) Exploration of the wound

28. Which of the statements regarding fibroblasts is *incorrect*?

(A) This cell uses fibronectin as provisional stroma for ingrowth.

(B) Cell proliferation is non-cytokine dependent.

(C) Collagen synthesis by this cell starts around the third day postinjury.

(D) MMPs are secreted by this cell.

(E) Fibroblasts participate actively in wound contraction.

29. Regarding vitamins and wound healing, which one of the following statements is *correct*?

(A) Correction of vitamin C deficiency can be obtained with ingestion of 50 μg of ascorbic acid per day.

(B) Vitamin A potentiates the effects of steroids in wound healing.

(C) Zinc deficiency has no effect on bursting strength of the wound.

(D) Catabolic bioproducts of arginine can retard wound healing.

(E) Vitamin E has anti-inflammatory properties.

30. Regarding the inflammatory phase of wound healing, which one of the following statements is *correct*?
    (A) After initial injury, the first cells to arrive to the wound are neutrophils.
    (B) Immediate vasodilatation occurs in order to increase cellular inflow to the wound.
    (C) Neutrophils are essential for wound healing.
    (D) Lymphocytes play a major role in contaminated wounds.
    (E) IL-2 downregulates the initial inflammatory process.

31. At 8 days following a left hemicolectomy for adenocarcinoma, a 65-year-old man calls to report a sudden large amount of clear, salmon-colored fluid from his wound. His appetite and bowel function are normal, he reports well-controlled pain, and he denies fevers. His dressing from his hospital discharge is still in place. Which of the following is the most appropriate next step?
    (A) Ask him to take off his dressing and examine his wound.
    (B) Ask him to replace his saturated dressing with a dry one and call back in 2 days if the drainage continues.
    (C) Schedule him for a clinic visit the next morning.
    (D) Have him keep his routine, 10-day follow-up appointment.
    (E) Arrange to see him immediately in the emergency department or clinic.

32. Regarding biodegradation of suture material, which one of the following statements is *incorrect*?
    (A) Degradation of suture materials is mainly through hydrolysis.
    (B) Profile of strength loss always precedes the profile of mass or weight loss in sutures.
    (C) Variation of pH has little effect on suture biodegradation.
    (D) Gamma-irradiation accelerates loss of tensile strength of different sutures.
    (E) Because of the lack of hydrolyzable bonds, polyethylene and polypropylene are not subjected to hydrolytic degradation.

33. What is the predominant type of collagen in this wound (see Fig. 3-7)?
    (A) I
    (B) II
    (C) III
    (D) IV
    (E) V

34. What is most abundant type of collagen in the human body?
    (A) I
    (B) II
    (C) III

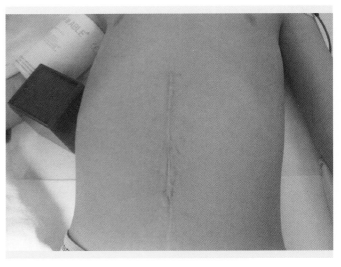

FIGURE 3-7. Healed abdominal wound.

    (D) IV
    (E) V

35. Regarding collagen, which one of the following statements is *correct*?
    (A) Collagen is a minor component of the extracellular matrix.
    (B) Collagen type III replaces collagen type I during maturation of the wound.
    (C) Deposition of collagen type I starts around the 14th day postinjury.
    (D) Hypoxia stimulates collagen production.
    (E) Exposure of fibrillar collagen to blood promotes aggregation and activation of platelets

36. Regarding collagen structure and synthesis, which one of the following statements is *correct*?
    (A) Collagen synthesis is inhibited by lactate.
    (B) Precursor forms are manufactured outside of the cell.
    (C) A-Ketoglutarate is a required cofactor for synthesis.
    (D) Fibroblasts actively secrete mature collagen molecules.
    (E) Prolyl hydroxylase is a byproduct of synthesis.

37. Regarding the process of apoptosis, which of the following statements is correct?
    (A) It is always a pathologic event.
    (B) Failure to exclude vital dye is observed.
    (C) There is an early disruption of membranes.
    (D) Ladder pattern of DNA fragments is observed.
    (E) Chromatin is loose and nucleolus is absent.

38. Which one of the following statements is *correct* about fibronectin?
    (A) Fibronectins are encoded by multiple genes.
    (B) Major functions are to mediate cellular adhesion and to promote cell migration.
    (C) Collagen usually serves as a template for fibronectin deposition.
    (D) Fibronectin matrix remains in the wound permanently.
    (E) Deposition of fibronectin inhibits chemotaxis.

39. Regarding proteoglycans, which one of the following statements is *correct*?
    (A) They contain a core glycosaminoglycan chain to which multiple proteins attach via hydrogen bonds.
    (B) They are located exclusively in the extracellular matrix.
    (C) Functions of these molecules include extracellular organization, promotion of growth factor receptor binding, and regulation of blood coagulation.
    (D) They inhibit fibril formation and wound healing.
    (E) Proteoglycan levels vary extensively during wound healing.

ANSWERS AND EXPLANATIONS

1. **(D)** Wound healing can be divided into three phases: inflammation, proliferation, and maturation. The inflammatory phase is characterized by hemostasis, inflammation and increased vascular permeability. Platelet aggregation and activation are stimulated by exposure to collagen and intravascular and extravascular proteins. Platelet adhesion to the endothelium is mediated through the interaction between high-affinity glycoprotein receptors and the integrin receptor glycoprotein IIb/IIIa. Platelet alpha granules contain histamine, serotonin, and other vasoactive amines that cause vasodilation and increased vascular permeability and cytokines including PDGF and TGF-α. Complement factors promote neutrophil chemotaxis and adhesion. Macrophages also play a key role during the inflammatory phase; cleaning debris, releasing cytokines, and promoting chemotaxis.

   A provisional extracellular matrix soon forms in the wound, composed primarily of fibrin and fibronectin, which form the scaffold for the migration of inflammatory, endothelia, and mesenchymal cells. By 48 h, the wound is completely epithelialized (and the surgical dressing can be safely removed). Cellular proliferation continues, as epidermis is reconstructed. The inflammatory phase resolves after 72 h, and macrophages begin to outnumber neutrophils.

   The appearance of fibroblasts marks the beginning of the proliferative phase, which predominate after 2 to 4 days. This phase is mediated by cytokines, including PDGF, epidermal growth factor, TGF-β, and insulin-like growth factor. Angiogenesis reconstructs damaged vasculature, stimulated by high lactate levels, acidic pH, and low oxygen tension mediated by FGF-1 and VEGF.

Collagen is produced by fibroblasts beginning 3 to 5 days after injury and gradually replaces fibrin in the wound. After 4 weeks, synthesis rates decline to match the rate of collagen degradation by collagenase. Granulation tissue formation is characteristic of the proliferative phase and serves as bridge for wound maturation, especially in open wounds. The migration and revascularization of endothelial cells are facilitated by the formation of a new extracellular matrix formation of new capillary vessels.

Wound contraction begins 4 to 5 days after injury, and maximal wound contraction continues for up to 15 days. Myofibroblasts are modified fibroblasts that interact with extracellular matrix, leading to wound contraction. It appears that wound contraction is more dependent on myofibroblasts than collagen synthesis.

Approximately 21 days after injury, maximal collagen content is reached and maturation begins. During the maturation phase (remodeling), fibroblasts and macrophages disappear and the wound collagen content stabilizes. Old collagen is broken and new collagen is synthesized in a denser, more organized fashion. The number of intermolecular cross-links between collagen molecules increased significantly. Slowly, as wound matures, collagen type III is replaced by collagen type I. By 6 weeks after injury, the wound has reached 80% to 90% of its eventual strength, and at approximately 6 months maximal strength is achieved, 80% to 90% of normal skin breaking strength.

BIBLIOGRAPHY

Ethridge RT, Leong M, Philips LG. Wound healing. In: Townsend CM, ed. *Sabiston: The Biological Basis of Modern Surgical Practice*. 18th ed. St. Louis, MO: Elsevier/Saunders; 2008:191–216.

Gupta S, Lawrence WT. Wound healing: normal and abnormal mechanisms and closure techniques. In: O'Leary JP (ed.), *The Physiologic Basis of Surgery*, 4th ed. Baltimore, MD: Lippincott Williams & Wilkins; 2008:150–175.

2. **(B)**

3. **(C)**

4. **(E)**

Explanations for questions 2 through 4

See Fig. 3-1.
Collagen secretion by fibroblasts begins 3 to 5 days after injury. Production of collagen increases rapidly, achieving its peak by 7 days and continuing at an accelerated rate for 2 to 4 weeks. After 4 weeks, the rate of collagen synthesis declines and a balance between the rates of collagen deposition–degradation will be achieved. The maximum net collagen deposition normally is achieved by 3 weeks.

Collagen synthesis involves the hydroxylation of lysine and proline moieties within the polypeptide chains. Hydroxylysine is required for covalent cross-link formation. This process requires oxygen, vitamin C, α-ketogluturate, and ferrous iron.

During scar remodeling, collagen deposition continues and MMPs degrade old collagen. The number of intramolecular and intermolecular cross-links between collagen fibers increases and wounds gradually increase their burst strength. After 3 weeks, wound burst/tensile strength is only 15%. After 6 weeks, the wound has reached 80% to 90% of its eventual strength, and at 6 months the wound is 80% to 90% of the strength of normal skin and its maximal strength.

BIBLIOGRAPHY

Gupta S, Lawrence WT. Wound healing: normal and abnormal mechanisms and closure techniques. In: O'Leary JP (ed.), *The Physiologic Basis of Surgery*, 4th ed. Baltimore, MD: Lippincott Williams & Wilkins; 2008:150–175.

5. **(E)** Many different techniques have been used to close abdominal wall defects. Primary repairs of ventral hernia have been associated with an incidence of recurrence of as high as 50%. Significantly better results have been achieved with mesh repairs with recurrence rates of around 6%. Although the use of mesh decreases the risk of recurrence, complications such as wound infection and intestinal fistula formation (see Fig. 3-8) occur more frequently when a foreign body material is used.

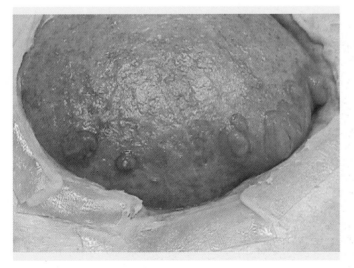

FIGURE 3-8. Open wound with multiple enterocutaneous fistuale.

Polyethylene terephthalate (Mersilene), polytetrafluoroethylene (PTFE), and polypropylene (Marlex, Prolene) are some of the commercially nonabsorbable materials available for hernia repair.

In case of wound infection, mesh exposure, or enteric fistula formation, the best alternative of treatment is removal of the foreign material and primary closure of the fascia when possible or placement of an absorbable mesh such as polyglactin 910 (see Table 3-1). The use of an absorbable mesh provides safe coverage of the abdominal contents, and decreases the incidence of abdominal compartment syndrome. Unlike permanent mesh, absorbable mesh does not chronically harbor infection, allowing local and systemic clearance of the infectious process. Unfortunately, the use of absorbable mesh will universally lead to ventral hernia recurrence, which will be cared for at a later date.

Table 3-1 Meshes Used in Incisional Hernia Repair

Proprietary Name	Composition
Prosthetic meshes	Parietex
Polyester/collagen film	Composix
Polypropylene/ePTFE	DualMesh, Dulex, MotifMESH
ePTFE	Prolene, Surgipro, ProLite
Polypropylene	Proceed
Polypropylene/polydioxanone	Sepramesh IP
Polypropylene/hyaluronate gel	C-Qur
Polypropylene/omega-3 fatty acid	TiMESH
Polypropylene/titanium	
Biologic meshes	Surgisis Gold
Porcine small intestine submucosa	AlloDerm
Human dermis	SurgiMend
Fetal bovine dermis	CollaMend
Porcine dermis	AlloMax
Human dermis	
Absorbable meshes	Gore Bio-A
Poly(glycolide:trimethylene carbonate)	Vicryl
Polyglactin	Dexon

ePTFE = expanded polytetrafluoroethylene.

BIBLIOGRAPHY

Scott DJ, Jones DB. Hernias and abdominal wall defects. In: Norton J, et al. (eds.), *Surgery, Basic Science and Clinical Evidence.* New York: Springer; 2001:814–817.

Seymour NE, Bell RL. Abdominal wall, omentum, mesentery, and retroperitoneum. In: Brunicardi FC, Andersen DK, Billiar TR, et al. (eds.), *Schwartz's Principles of Surgery*, 10th ed. New York: McGraw-Hill; 2015:Chapter 35.

6. **(E)** A novel approach to improve healing of open abdominal wounds is the application of negative pressure–assisted wound closure. Negative pressure therapy, such as the V.A.C. therapy system (see Fig. 3-9), consists of a computer-controlled therapy unit, a drainage canister, sterile plastic tubing, foam dressing, and clear adhesive. The foam dressing is placed into the wound. One end of the tube is connected to the foam, the other end to a canister that connects to the V.A.C. control unit. The wound area is sealed with the clear adhesive, similar to a large bandage (see Fig. 3-10). The V.A.C. system pulls infectious materials and other fluids from the wound through the tube and collects them inside the canister.

V.A.C. promotes healing by applying controlled negative pressure (vacuum) to the wound. It also helps to debride and to clean the contaminated wound bed. It does not replace sharp debridement of contaminated wounds and should not be used in wounds with necrotic or scar tissue.

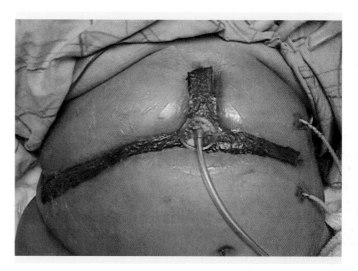

FIGURE 3-10. V.A.C. dressing place on an open wound.

Studies have demonstrated significant improvement in wound depth compared to traditional "wet-to-dry" dressings, as well as increase in capillary caliber and stimulated endothelial proliferation and angiogenesis.

The V.A.C system can be used in acute or subacute wounds, included in cases of dehiscence, flaps, and skin grafts. Chronic wounds (diabetic or pressure ulcers) and temporary abdominal wall closures are other applications.

BIBLIOGRAPHY

Ethridge RT, Leong M, Philips LG. Wound healing. In: Townsend CM (ed.), *Sabiston: The Biological Basis of Modern Surgical Practice*, 18th ed. St. Louis, MO: Elsevier/Saunders; 2008:191–216.

7. **(C)** Typically, giant cells are seen in the presence of foreign bodies. The polarizing refractile material, however, is diagnostic of a suture granuloma. No inflammatory infiltrate is seen, characteristic of abscess formation. Hypertrophic and keloid scars present normally with thickening of the scar and increased collagen deposition at the wound.

Suture granuloma is a well-recognized surgical complication that can mislead clinicians. Suture granulomas can be responsible for chronic open wounds or for persistent hematuria on kidney transplant recipients, or can be the cause of infection after a ventral hernia repair with mesh. Enterocutaneous fistula formation can also be attributed to suture granuloma.

Suture granulomas can lead to false-positive results when staging tumors with positron emission tomography (PET) scan because of the uptake by histiocytes of F2-fluoro-2-deoxy-D-glucose (FDG). The diagnosis of suture granuloma is clinical and the treatment consists of granuloma resection. Most of the symptoms associated

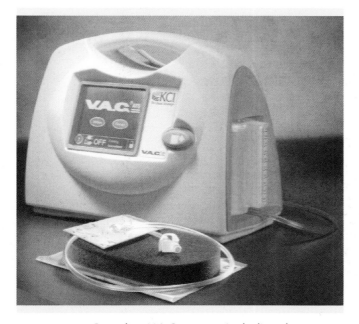

FIGURE 3-9. Complete V.A.C. system, including the computer-controlled unit, canister, plastic tubing, foam dressing, and clear tape dressing.

with suture granuloma will fade away after resection of the foreign body.

BIBLIOGRAPHY

Takahara K, Kakinoki H. Suture granuloma showing false-positive findings on FDG-PET. *Case Rep Urol* 2013;2013:472642.

8. **(E)** This patient underwent an elective procedure, with primary closure of the wound. After 1 month of the initial injury, dense collagen deposition can be seen.

On the first 24 h, an inflammatory infiltrate would be noticed. By 72 h, granulation tissue is seen followed by neovascularization. By the second to third week, collagen is prominent and inflammatory cells are seen but are scarce.

Intrinsic and extrinsic factors have a direct impact on how fast a wound will heal. Loss of tissue, bacteria contamination, and the presence of foreign body are all extrinsic factors that can limit the process of healing. Cardiovascular disease, renal failure, nutrition, and age are some of the intrinsic factors that can significantly retard wound healing.

Wound closure can be divided into three categories: primary, secondary, and tertiary. Primary or first-intention closures are wounds immediately sealed by suturing, stapling, skin grafting, or flap placement. Secondary closure involves no active sealing of the wound. The wound is left open because of gross contamination of the surgical field. Closure of the wound will be achieved by contraction and epithelialization. Wound closure by tertiary intention involves delayed closure of an infected wound after debridement, and local and systemic antibiotic treatment. It is also known as delayed primary closure.

BIBLIOGRAPHY

Gupta S, Lawrence WT. Wound healing: normal and abnormal mechanisms and closure techniques. In: O'Leary JP (ed.), *The Physiologic Basis of Surgery*, 4th ed. Baltimore, MD: Lippincott Williams & Wilkins; 2008:150–175.

9. **(D)** Secondary intention healing occurs because of the interaction of multiple forces. Wound contraction is the most important factor. Decreased edema, collagen synthesis, and deposition of granulation tissue are contributing factors. A wound left open will fill with granulation tissue and contraction will help to pull normal, healthy tissue to close the defect. Wounds are normally left open after gross contamination of the surgical field.

In 1964, the National Research Council (NRC) proposed the idea of using wound classification to predict risk for surgical site infection. Wounds were divided as

Table 3-2 Traditional Classification of Operative Wounds

Clean (class I)	Nontraumatic, uninfected wounds; no inflammation; primarily closed; no break in aseptic technique
Clean-contaminated (class II)	Alimentary, respiratory, or genitourinary tract entered under controlled conditions; no contamination; minor break in aseptic technique
Contaminated (class III)	Fresh traumatic wounds; gross spillage from gastrointestinal tract; acute, nonpurulent inflammation; major break in technique
Dirty-infected (class IV)	Traumatic wounds with retained devitalized tissue, foreign bodies or fecal contamination; perforated viscus; acute, purulent bacterial inflammation

being clean, clean-contaminated, contaminated, or dirty-infected (Table 3-2).

Wound infection rates for these four wound classes are 1.0% to 5.4% for clean, 2.1% to 9.5% for clean-contaminated, 6.4% to 13.2% for contaminated, and 3.1% to 12.8% for dirty-infected wounds.

BIBLIOGRAPHY

Napolitano LM. Surgical site infections. In: Cameron JL (ed.), *Current Surgical Therapy*, 10th ed. Philadelphia, PA: Elsevier/Saunders; 2011.

10. **(C)**

11. **(D)**

Explanations for questions 10 and 11

Chronic granulomatous diseases (CGDs) comprise a genetically heterogeneous group of diseases in which the reduced nicotinamide adenine dinucleotide phosphate–dependent oxide *enzyme* is deficient.

This defect impairs the intracellular killing of microorganisms, leading to defective neutrophil rolling, the first step for transmigration of neutrophils from the vasculature to the tissues. Rolling depends on the interaction between selectins and their sialylated ligand molecules. Selectins (CD11) mediate neutrophil binding, and beta$_2$-integrins (CD18) are required for further activation-induced firm sticking and emigration. CHD is characterized by reduced killing of ingested microbes because of a defective NADPH oxidase system. This system produces superoxide anions, essential for production of H_2O_2, OH, and HOCl.

Patients with CGD characteristically experience recurrent and often severe pyogenic infections, a granulomatous tissue response, and impaired phagocyte microbicidal activity because of the absence of respiratory burst oxidase activity. Patients usually present as children with multiple recurrent pyogenic infections and a normal white blood cell count and a normal differential. Clinically, patients develop recurrent infections such as pneumonia, lymphadenitis, hepatic abscess, and osteomyelitis. The most characteristic pathogens are *Staphylococcus aureus*, *Serratia marcescens*, *Pseudomonas cepacia*, and *Aspergillus* spp., although a wide variety of other catalase-positive bacteria and fungi may cause disease as well. The nitroblue tetrazolium reduction test is used to diagnose CGD. Normal neutrophils can reduce this compound, whereas neutrophils from affected patients do not, facilitating the diagnosis via a colorimetric test.

Occasionally, granulomas can lead to obstruction of the gastric antrum and genitourinary tracts and poor wound healing. Surgeons become involved when the patient develops infectious or obstructive complications.

Although initially described as an X-linked disorder, with men affected and mothers and sisters serving as heterozygous carriers, CGD can be transmitted with the inheritance pattern of either an autosomal or an X-linked disease, depending on the molecular defect.

The management of patients with CGD is based largely on the early recognition and aggressive treatment of infections. When CGD patients require surgery, a preoperative pulmonary function test should be considered because such patients are predisposed to obstructive and restrictive lung disease. Prophylactic use of antimicrobial agents is of well-established benefit in patients with CGD, and trimethoprim-sulfamethoxazole is generally preferred.

Wound complications, mainly infection, are common. Sutures should be removed as late as possible because the wounds heal slowly. Abscess drains should be left in place for a prolonged period until the infection is completely resolved.

BIBLIOGRAPHY

Barbul A, Efron DT. Wound healing. In: Brunicardi FC, Andersen DK, Billiar TR, et al. (eds.), *Schwartz's Principles of Surgery*. 9th ed. New York: McGraw-Hill; 2010:Chapter 9.
Kishiyama JL. Disorders of the immune system. In: McPhee SJ, Hammer GD (eds.), *Pathophysiology of Disease*. 6th ed. New York: McGraw-Hill; 2010:Chapter 3.

12. **(B)** Searching for a better anti-inflammatory medication for his father, Dr. Felix Hoffmann discovered acetylsalicylic acid (ASA) in 1897. ASA is hydrolyzed in the liver and excreted in the urine. As a result of the rapid hydrolysis, ASA levels are always low. The peak of salicylates level for uncoated ASA is 2 h. Prostaglandins are potent mediators of the inflammatory response. The first and committed step in the production of prostaglandins from arachidonic acid is the bis-oxygenation of arachidonate to prostaglandin, followed by reduction to PGH2. Both reactions are catalyzed by cyclooxygenase (COX), also known as PGH synthase. There are two isoforms of COX in animals: COX-1, which carries out normal, physiologic production of prostaglandins, and COX-2, which is induced by cytokines, mitogens, and endotoxins in inflammatory cells and is responsible for the production of prostaglandins in inflammation.

ASA is a nonselective inhibitor of COX that blocks the COX pathway of arachidonic acid metabolism, which results in decrease prostaglandin output. Prostaglandins promote vasodilatation at the inflammatory site. Cytokine release is partially ablated by the use of aspirin. Release of IL-1 and TNF-α will not be blocked. Collagen synthesis can start as early as 10 h of the initial injury. Collagen synthesis or fibroblast proliferation is not directly affected by the use of aspirin.

BIBLIOGRAPHY

Kumar V, Fausto N, Abbas AK. *Robbins and Cotran Pathologic Basis of Disease*, 8th ed. Philadelphia: Saunders/Elsevier; 2010.

13. **(B)** During the past two decades, the survival rate of solid organ recipients has improved dramatically. The major factor in improved clinical outcome is the decline in death secondary to infection. Currently, 1-year mortality caused by infection has decreased to less than 5% for renal transplant patients. Better immunosuppression and understanding by the clinician of drug pharmacodynamics and pharmacokinetics are responsible for decrease morbidity and mortality after solid organ transplantation.

Steroids reduce the inflammatory process blocking transcription of cytokine genes (especially IL-1) leading to nonspecific inhibition of T lymphocytes and macrophages. Steroids also reduce collagen synthesis and wound strength by inhibiting fibroblast migration. Topical steroids also inhibit wound healing. The effects of steroids used after the first 3 to 4 days postinjury are not as severe as when used immediately postinjury. Regardless of when administered, steroids inhibit epithelialization and contraction and increase rates of wound infection.

Cyclosporine is a calcineurin inhibitor and a common immunosuppressant used to prevent transplant rejection. Binding of the drug with its cytoplasmic receptor leads to calcineurin inhibition and impaired expression of several T-cell activation genes, suppressing T-cell activation.

Cyclosporine also inhibits lymphokine production and release of IL-2. Cyclosporine does not significantly affect hydroxyproline content and macrophage migration, although there is some evidence that cyclosporine impairs wound healing. Studies in rats have shown that activin-β expression and MMP activity by fibroblasts are reduced.

BIBLIOGRAPHY

Barbul A, Efron DT. Wound healing. In: Brunicardi FC, Andersen DK, Billiar TR, Dunn DL, et al. (eds.), *Schwartz's Principles of Surgery*, 9th ed. New York: McGraw-Hill; 2010:Chapter 9.

Humar A, Dunn DL. Transplantation. In: Brunicardi FC, Andersen DK, Billiar TR, Dunn DL, et al. (eds.), *Schwartz's Principles of Surgery*, 9th ed. New York: McGraw-Hill; 2010:Chapter 11.

14. **(B)** Angiogenesis is an important intermediate wound healing event. It occurs 2–4 days after the initial injury. It reconstructs the vasculature that was damaged locally. Small capillary sprouts initially develop on venules at the periphery of the devascularized area. Eventually these capillary sprouts will interconnect forming vascular loops.

Angiogenesis is stimulated directly by high lactate levels, acidic pH, decreased oxygen tension, cytokines (IL-1), and prostaglandins. Certain polypeptide growth factors are absolutely essential to angiogenesis, including basic fibroblast growth factor (bFGF) and vascular endothelial growth factor (VEGF).

Heparin appears to stimulate angiogenesis. Heparin also binds to angiogenic factors such as tumor angiogenesis factor, endothelial cell growth factor, retina- and eye-derived growth factor, and cartilage-derived growth factor. Also matrix components, such as fibronectin and hyalurinic acid can stimulate angiogenesis.

Hypoxia is an early stimulus for fibroblast and endothelial activation, and several growth factors, such as TGF-β1 and VEGF are induced by low oxygen tension.

The von Hippel-Lindau tumor suppressor protein competitively binds to the hypoxiainducible transcription factor 1 (HIF-1) complex in the presence of oxygen and down regulates VEGF transcription leading to inhibition of angiogenesis

BIBLIOGRAPHY

Falanga V, Iwamoto S. Mechanisms of wound repair, wound healing, and wound dressing. In: Goldsmith LA, et al., eds. *Fitzpatrick's Dermatology in General Medicine*. 8th ed. New York, NY: McGraw-Hill; 2012:Chapter 248.

15. **(C)** IL-8 is secreted by macrophages and is a potent chemotactic agent. IL-1 and TNF-α are cytokines that mediate the acute inflammatory phase. Their secretion by macrophages results in fever and rise of immature neutrophils in the blood circulation. IL-2 is responsible for cell division. It is produced by T cells and has as major targets T, B, and natural killer cells. IL-10 downregulates the immune response. It is produced by and immunomodulates T cells. (Table 3-3)

Table 3-3 Cytokine Sources and Effects

Cytokine	Source	Effect
IL-1	Macrophage	Inflammation
IL-2	Helper T	Cell division
IL-6	Helper T	Activation, differentiation
IL-8	Macrophage	Chemotaxis
IL-10	Helper T	Inhibit cellular immunity
TNF-α	Macrophage	Inflammation

BIBLIOGRAPHY

Christie JD, Lanken PN. Acute lung injury and the acute respiratory distress syndrome. In: Hall JB, Schmidt GA, Wood LD (eds.), *Principles of Critical Care*, 3rd ed. New York: McGraw-Hill; 2005:Chapter 38.

Phelan HA, Eastman AL, et al. Shock and hypoperfusion states. In: O'Leary JP (ed.), *The Physiologic Basis of Surgery*, 4th ed. Baltimore, MD: Lippincott Williams & Wilkins; 2008:87–111.

16. **(B)** Growth factors have effects on cell locomotion, contractility, and differentiation.

EGF is secreted by monocytes and macrophages and promotes reepithelialization and angiogenesis. EGF also promotes extracellular matrix turnover, stimulating collagenases.

Platelets, monocytes, macrophages, and endothelial cells secrete PDGF. PDGF is a powerful chemoattractant that promotes deposition of intracellular matrix.

Monocytes, macrophages, and endothelial cells produce FGF. FGF promotes reepithelialization and angiogenesis.

VEGF also promotes angiogenesis in cancer, chronic inflammatory states, and healing wounds.

TGF-β is secreted by platelets, endothelial cells, lymphocytes, and macrophages. In low concentrations, it induces the synthesis and secretion of PDGF and is thus indirectly mitogenic. In high concentrations, it is growth inhibitory, owing to its ability to inhibit the expression of PDGF receptors.

BIBLIOGRAPHY

Ethridge RT, Leong M, Phillips LG. Wound healing. In: Cameron JL (ed.), *Current Surgical Therapy*, 10th ed. Philadelphia: Elsevier/Saunders; 2011.

17. **(C)**

18. **(C)**

Explanations for questions 17 and 18

Granulation tissue is a red beefy tissue deposited by fibroblasts. The histologic features of granulation tissue are the formation of new small blood vessels (angiogenesis) and the proliferation of fibroblasts. These new vessels are leaky, allowing the passage of proteins and red cells into the extravascular space. Thus, new granulation tissue is often edematous. Type III collagen is the most common type of collagen present in granulation tissue.

An excessive amount of granulation tissue deposition is called exuberant granulation or proud flesh and inhibits wound healing.

Granulation tissue will allow reepithelialization of the skin. After complete scar maturation, hair follicles will not be regained.

BIBLIOGRAPHY

Adams CA Jr, Heffernan DS, Cioffi WG. Wounds, bites, and stings. In: Mattox KL, Moore EE, Feliciano DV (eds.), *Trauma*, 7th ed. New York: McGraw-Hill; 2013:Chapter 47.

Kulaylat MN, Dayton MT. Surgical complications. In: Cameron JL (ed.), *Current Surgical Therapy*, 10th ed. Philadelphia: Elsevier/Saunders; 2011.

19. **(C)** Patients undergoing radiation therapy may present a challenge to healing. The effects of radiation therapy are variable and depend on a number of factors, including dose, frequency, and location. Cells display differential sensitivity to radiation in various phases of the cell cycle. In general, cells are more sensitive in early S and in mitosis, while they are less sensitive in late S and G_2. Rapidly dividing cells are more susceptible to radiation.

Conversely, cells that do not divide rapidly, such as neurons or muscle cells, tend to be resistant to radiation.

Radiation damages the DNA of exposed cells. The radiation effects on DNA can be direct or indirect. The direct effect is particularly damaging to the DNA and often results in damage to both DNA strands. Far more often, the effects on DNA are indirect. The ionization cellular fluid by radiation produces hydroxyl radicals (OH•), peroxide (H_2O_2), hydrated electrons (e_{aq}), and oxygen radicals (O•). These radicals will react with DNA to disrupt the backbone of sugars or directly damage the pyrimidine and purine bases causing cell damage.

In previously irradiated tissue, decreased vascularity and increased fibrosis limit the access of inflammatory cells to the area. The resulting cytokine deficiency impairs cellular aspects of healing. Because of the diminished blood supply, irradiated tissue is predisposed to infection.

BIBLIOGRAPHY

Gupta S, Lawrence WT. Wound healing: normal and abnormal mechanisms and closure techniques. In: O'Leary JP (ed.), *The Physiologic Basis of Surgery*, 4th ed. Baltimore, MD: Lippincott Williams & Wilkins; 2008:150–175.

20. **(D)** NO is a short-lived free radical that is involved in many important biological functions. NO is formed from the terminal guanidino nitrogen atom of arginine. Macrophages are responsible for the presence of most of the NO in the inflammatory phase of wound healing. Fibroblasts, keratinocytes, and endothelial cells contribute to ongoing NO synthesis but to a lesser degree. Inhibition of NO decreases collagen deposition and breaks strength of the wounds. Studies have shown that when rats are fed an arginine-free diet, wound healing is impaired. Also animal model studies have shown that NO can partially reverse the impaired healing of diabetes.

NO activates soluble guanylate cyclase, which increases cellular cyclic guanosine monophosphate (cGMP) concentrations (see Fig. 3-11).

BIBLIOGRAPHY

Witte MB, Barbul A. Role of nitric oxide in wound repair. *Am J Surg* 2002;183:406–412.

21. **(B)** Scurvy is caused by the deficiency of vitamin C (ascorbic acid) intake. Ascorbic acid is present in vegetables and fruits and absent in dairy products, poultry, and eggs. In the United States, scurvy is seen primarily among the poor and elderly, in alcoholics who consume less than 10 mg/d of vitamin C, in individuals consuming macrobiotic diets, and in young

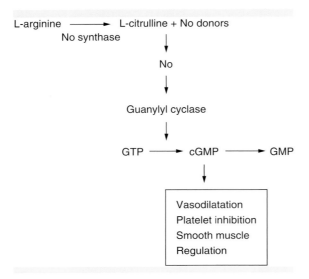

FIGURE 3-11. Schematic view of arginine and nitric oxide (NO) metabolism.

adults who eat severely unbalanced diets. In addition to generalized fatigue, symptoms of scurvy primarily reflect impaired formation of mature connective tissue and include bleeding into skin (petechiae, ecchymoses, perifollicular hemorrhages); inflamed and bleeding gums; and manifestations of bleeding into joints, the peritoneal cavity, the pericardium, and the adrenal glands. In children, vitamin C deficiency may cause impaired bone growth. Laboratory diagnosis of vitamin C deficiency is made on the basis of low plasma or leukocyte levels.

Diagnosis is primarily clinical. Mucocutaneous manifestations include change of skin color (pale), hyperkeratosis, reddish, bluish or black spots, gingival hypertrophy, and edema. Leukopenia is present in 30% of the patients. Treatment constitutes of initial replacement with 100 mg of vitamin C a day. Abnormalities are usually reversible, and complete recovery is achieved in most of the cases by 3 months.

Vitamin C is a required cofactor for collagen synthesis. Chronic nonhealing wounds, opening of well-healed wounds, and fascial dehiscence can be caused by deficiency of vitamin C.

BIBLIOGRAPHY

Russell RM, Suter PM. Vitamin and trace mineral deficiency and excess. In: Longo DL, Fauci AS, Kasper DL, et al. (eds.), *Harrison's Principles of Internal Medicine*, 18th ed. New York: McGraw-Hill; 2012:Chapter 74.

22. **(E)** HBO is a therapeutic modality that uses air or other gas mixtures at greater than atmospheric pressure for short intervals, over days or months, to treat various disease states. Gas gangrene, necrotizing fasciitis, osteomyelitis, decompression sickness, air or gas embolism, carbon monoxide and cyanide poisoning, radiation osteonecrosis, crush injury, selected nonhealing chronic wounds, and smoke inhalation are conditions shown to improve with HBO therapy.

Oxygen chambers are flooded with 100% oxygen with pressures varying from 3 to 6 ATA.

HBO effects are several, including

1. Decrease in the bubble size (governed by Boyle's law, which states that the volume of gas in an enclosed space is inversely proportional to the pressure exerted on it)

2. Increased leukocyte bactericidal and bacteriostatic function

3. Stimulation of fibroblast growth, which results in increased collagen formation and resultant neovascularization

4. Inhibition of neutrophil adherence to ischemic vessel walls

5. Reduction of postischemic vasoconstriction

6. Reduction of lipid peroxidation.

The most common adverse effects associated with HBO are barotrauma of the middle ear, cranial sinuses, teeth, or lungs.

Contraindications of HBO are patients receiving cisplatin, bleomycin, sulfamylon, or disulfiram and patients with untreated pneumothorax.

Other relative contraindications include pregnancy, known malignancy, emphysema, pneumonia, bronchitis, and hyperthermia.

BIBLIOGRAPHY

Clark JM, Thom SR. Oxygen under pressure. In: Brubakk AO, Neuman TS (eds.), *Bennett and Elliott's Physiology and Medicine of Diving*, 5th ed. London: Saunders; 2003:358–418.

Mulinde JM, Caplan ES. Hyperbaric oxygen. In: Mandell GL, Bennett JE, Dolin R (eds.), *Mandell: Principles and Practice of Infectious Diseases*, 5th ed. Philadelphia, PA: Churchill Livingstone; 2000:501–504.

23. **(C)** MMPs comprise a gene family of metal-dependent endopeptidases, including collagenases, gelatinases, stromelysins, matrilysin, and metalloelastase. These enzymes share important common properties. They are secreted as inactive zymogens, are rapidly secreted, and are not stored for long periods of time.

MMPs are upregulated by cytokines, especially TNF-α and IL-1, as well as growth factors, physical stresses, and drugs. They are downregulated by retinoic acid, gluco-corticoids, TGF-β, and specific and tissue-derived inhibitors (TIMPs).

MMPs play a key role in degradation of collagen but usually are not found in chronic wounds. The confinement of collagenase expression to the basal epidermal cells suggests that disruption of the basal membrane with subsequent exposure of keratinocytes is a critical determinant for epidermal collagenolytic activity.

BIBLIOGRAPHY

Mignatti P, Rifkin DB, Welgus HG, Parks WC. Proteinases and tissue remodeling. In: Clark RAF (ed.), *The Molecular and Cell Biology of Wound Repair*, 2nd ed. New York, NY: Plenum Press; 1996:427–461.

Reeves M. Cell biology. In: O'Leary JP (ed.), *The Physiologic Basis of Surgery*, 4th ed. Baltimore, MD: Lippincott Williams & Wilkins; 2008:1–43.

24. **(E)**

25. **(E)**

26. **(E)**

Explanations for questions 24 through 26

Hypertrophic scar (HTS) and keloids are both dermal fibrous lesions that develop at sites of prior dermal injury and wound repair. There are no known effective means of preventing keloid development. Keloid scars tend to occur above the clavicles, on the trunk, on the upper extremities, and on the face. They are often refractory to medical and surgical intervention.

HTSs usually develop within 4 weeks after trauma. The risk of HTSs increases if epithelialization takes longer than 21 days, independent of site, age, and race. Rarely elevated more than 4 mm above the skin level, HTSs remain within the boundaries of the wound. They usually occur across areas of tension and flexor surfaces, which tend to be at right angles to joints or skin creases. The lesions are initially erythematous and raised, and over time may evolve into pale, flatter scars.

A keloid scar extends beyond the limits of the original wound, different from hypertrophic scar that usually is contained within the limits of the original wound. Keloids are more likely familial than hypertrophic scars, and hypertrophic scars may subside in time, whereas this is rarely the case with keloids.

Histologically, Fibroblasts from keloid-prone patients have altered cytokine patterns and increased sensitivity

to transforming growth factor-β1 (TGF-β1). HTSs demonstrate increased epidermal thickness and an abundance of collagen and glycoprotein. Collagen bundles with a glazed appearance, presence of antinuclear antibodies against fibroblast, epithelial, and endothelial cells, and higher levels of adenosine triphosphate are found in keloid scar but not in HTS.

Collagen type I is the predominant type of collagen in both keloid scars and HTSs, different from a normal nonmature scar where the predominant type of collagen is type III.

BIBLIOGRAPHY

Barbul A, Efron DT. Wound healing. In: Brunicardi FC, Andersen DK, Billiar TR, et al. (eds.), *Schwartz's Principles of Surgery*, 9th ed. New York: McGraw-Hill; 2010:Chapter 9.

Ethridge RT, Leong M, Phillips LG. Wound healing. In: Cameron JL (ed.), *Current Surgical Therapy*, 10th ed. Philadelphia: Elsevier/Saunders; 2011.

Shaffer JJ, Taylor SC, Cook-Bolden F. Keloidal scars: a review with a critical look at therapeutic options. *J Am Acad Dermatol* 2002;46:563–597.

Vasconez HC, Habash A. Plastic and reconstructive surgery. In: Doherty GM, ed. *Current Diagnosis & Treatment: Surgery*, 13th ed. New York: McGraw-Hill; 2010:Chapter 41.

27. **(D)** Marjolin ulcers really reflect malignant degeneration arising within a preexisting cicatrix or scar. Squamous cell carcinoma is the most common cancer associated with Marjolin ulcer. Latency period for development of the cancer is variable ranging from 1 to 75 years.

Risk factors for Marjolin ulcer are burn scars, osteomyelitis tracts, pressure sores, hidradentitis, and other chronic wounds. The lesions are most commonly found in the lower extremity, especially the heel and plantar foot.

BIBLIOGRAPHY

Goodier CD, Hilarie H, Wise MW. Skin and subcutaneous tissue. In: O'Leary JP (ed.), *The Physiologic Basis of Surgery*, 4th ed. Baltimore, MD: Lippincott Williams & Wilkins; 2008:1–43.

Pekarek B, Buck S, Osher L. A comprehensive review on Marjolin's ulcers: diagnosis and treatment. *J Am Coll Cert Wound Specialists* 2011;3(3).

28. **(B)** Fibroblasts differentiate from resting mesenchymal cells in connective tissue and account for the delay between injury and the appearance of collagen in a healing wound (lag phase of wound healing). These cells are present by the third day postinjury in the wound and primarily function to synthesize collagen.

The migration and proliferation of fibroblasts are stimulated by chemotactic substances such as growth factors (PDGF, TGF-β), C5 fragments, thrombin, TNF-α, eicosanoids, elastin fragments, leukotriene B_4, and fragments of collagen and fibronectin. MMPs are secreted by fibroblasts and monocytes. These enzymes degrade elastin. Elastin turnover in nonwounded circumstances is extremely low, lasting the life of the individual.

Fibroblasts are also essential during wound contraction. When stimulated, they develop cytoplasmic actin-myosin contractile activity called myofibroblasts.

BIBLIOGRAPHY

Ethridge RT, Leong M, Philips LG. Wound healing. In: Townsend CM (ed.), *Sabiston: The Biological Basis of Modern Surgical Practice*, 18th ed. St. Louis, MO: Elsevier/Saunders; 2008:191–216.

29. **(E)** Vitamin C is essential for wound healing. Patients with ascorbic acid deficiency will require 100 mg orally daily for about 3 months to correct their deficiency.

Deficiency of vitamin A will impair monocyte activation, fibronectin deposition that further affects cellular adhesion, and impairment of the TGF-β receptors. Vitamin A contributes to lysosomal membrane destabilization and directly counteracts the effect of glucocorticoids. The recommended dietary allowance (RDA) of vitamin A is 900 retinol activity equivalents (RAE) for men and 700 RAE for women per day. This corresponds approximately to 3000 international units (IU) and 2300 IU, respectively. The Nutrition Advisory Group of the American Medical Association recommends 3300 IU of vitamin A for adult intravenous multivitamin formulations to prevent deficiency. Some investigators have recommended 25,000 to 50,000 IU per day orally and 10,000 IU intravenously for severely to moderately injured patients or for malnourished patients prior to and after elective surgery. The use of corticosteroids is associated with delayed wound healing and a higher risk of developing wound infection. Vitamin A supplementation antagonizes steroid-induced delays in wound healing. Studies with rabbits and rats have indicated that high doses of vitamin A reverse the anti-inflammatory effect of steroids and increase the tensile strength of the wound.

Zinc is an essential trace element required for protein synthesis and the function of several hundred zinc metalloenzymes and zinc finger proteins. Zinc is normally bound in the plasma; approximately 70% is bound loosely to albumin, 25% is more tightly bound to alpha$_2$-macroglobulin, and the remaining is bound to peptides and amino acids. The serum zinc concentration is the most frequently used method of assessing zinc status. Major food sources for zinc are proteins, such as red meat, and there is a direct correlation between dietary protein and dietary zinc intake. Patients with zinc deficiency will present with a wide variety of signs and symptoms, including diarrhea, impaired wound healing and impaired protein metabolism, hypogonadism, altered visual function, altered mental status, altered immune function, and impaired taste or anorexia. Zinc deficiency can be caused by chronic inflammatory states, poor zinc intake, poor absorption or increased excretion. Zinc deficiency can be associated with decreased wound burst strength.

Arginine may contribute to the wound healing process in multiple ways. When administered at pharmacologic levels it will cause secretion of anabolic hormones, insulin and growth hormone. Additionally, arginine present in the wound can be catabolized by immune cells to nitric oxide or ornithine. Nitric oxide is a powerful vasodilator, an autocrine stimulator of fibroblast-contractile and collagen-synthetic activities, and a mediator of macrophage-induced bacterial killing. Ornithine can be converted to proline and used for collagen synthesis, or converted to polyamines, which are important for cellular proliferation and differentiation.

Administration of arginine orally has been shown to enhance hydroxyproline deposition.

Vitamin E or tocopherol is an essential fat soluble vitamin. Vitamin E acts as an antioxidant in the human body and has become a popular nutrient in skin care products. It has anti-inflammatory properties, with a theoretical effect of inhibition of collagen deposition. Studies are still controversial regarding the true effect of tocopherol on wound healing.

BIBLIOGRAPHY

Ethridge RT, Leong M, Philips LG. Wound healing. In: Townsend CM (ed.), *Sabiston: The Biological Basis of Modern Surgical Practice*, 18th ed. St. Louis, MO: Elsevier/Saunders; 2008.

Scholl D, Langkamp-Henken B. Nutrient recommendations for wound healing. *J Intraven Nurs* 2001;24:124–132.

30. **(D)** After initial injury, vasoconstriction occurs followed by the entrapment of platelets. Platelets will degranulate, releasing several different substances, including homeostasis factors (i.e., von Willebrand factor, thrombospondin), growth factors (IGF-1, PDGF, TGF-β), proteases, and hydrolases that will cause protein and cell degradation. Vasodilatation occurs after homeostasis followed by inflow of neutrophils, monocytes, macrophages, and lymphocytes.

Although not essential for the wound-healing process, neutrophils scavenge necrotic tissue, foreign material, and bacteria.

Lymphocytes can play a major role in the resolution of the inflammatory process, especially in contaminated wounds. Lymphocytes produce interferon-λ, which decreases synthesis of prostaglandins and stimulates production of cytokines. T cells also stimulate IL-2 release, an upregulator of the immune system and inflammatory response, which directly stimulates monocytes to release free radicals against bacteria.

BIBLIOGRAPHY

Ethridge RT, Leong M, Philips LG. Wound healing. In: Townsend CM (ed.), *Sabiston: The Biological Basis of Modern Surgical Practice*, 18th ed. St. Louis, MO: Elsevier/Saunders; 2008:191–216.

31. **(E)** Dehiscence refers to the postoperative separation of the abdominal musculoaponeurotic layers of a wound. Risk factors include technical error in fascial closure, emergency surgery, intra-abdominal infection, advanced age, wound infection, hematoma/seroma, elevated intra-abdominal pressure, obesity, chronic corticosteroid use, previous wound dehiscence, malnutrition, radiation therapy and chemotherapy, and systemic disease (uremia, diabetes mellitus).

    Dehiscence occurs in 1% to 3% of patients, most commonly between postoperative days 7 and 10. Nearly one-fourth of patients present with sudden dramatic drainage of clear, salmon-colored fluid. Treatment is based on the size of the wound, size of the fascial defect or separation, and condition of the fascia. Short-term treatment may involve saline-moistened gauze and an abdominal binder, or placement of a negative pressure wound vacuum system. Evisceration warrants fluid resuscitation and operative exploration to rule out an infectious etiology. Successful fascial closure is achieved in 85% of patients.

BIBLIOGRAPHY

Kulaylat MN, Dayton MT. Surgical complications. In: Cameron JL (ed.), *Current Surgical Therapy*, 10th ed. Philadelphia, PA: Elsevier/Saunders; 2011.

32. **(C)** Degradation of suture materials is mainly through hydrolysis, although thermal, mechanical, ultraviolet radiation, and oxidation also can cause degradation of polymeric materials. Three important properties are used to describe biodegradation of suture materials: tensile strength, mass profile, and type of degradation products released into surrounding tissues. The profile of strength loss always occurs before the profile of mass or weight loss.

Variation of the pH has major impact on biodegradation of suture material. For example, in polyglactil 910 sutures (Vicryl), the curve of breaking strength has a convex shape with maximum retention strength at pH 7.0 and low retention strength at strong acidic or alkaline pH.

Gamma-irradiation causes loss of tensile strength of different sutures, with the amount of weaking proportional to the radiation dose.

Among nonabsorbable sutures, silk and cotton are the most susceptible to degradation. Because of the lack of hydrolysable bonds polyethylene and polypropylene are not subjected to hydrolytic degradation and retained their tensile strength *in vivo* for long periods of time.

BIBLIOGRAPHY

Gupta S, Lawrence WT. Wound healing: normal and abnormal mechanisms and closure techniques. In: O'Leary JP (ed.), *The Physiologic Basis of Surgery*, 4th ed. Baltimore, MD: Lippincott Williams & Wilkins; 2008:150–175.

33. **(A)**

34. **(A)**

35. **(E)**

36. **(C)**

Explanations for questions 33 through 36

Collagen is an essential component for wound healing and the main component of the extracellular matrix. Collagens are triple-helix structural proteins divided in XII subgroups or types. The most important types with their tissue distribution are shown below. Type I collagen is the most abundant form of collagen and accounts for a total of 90% of the total body collagen. It is present in all connective tissues, except cartilage and basal membranes. Collagen type III is initially deposited after an injury and will be replaced by collagen type I during maturation of the wound. Deposition of type I collagen starts by the seventh day postinjury. (Table 3-4)

During the inflammatory phase, the exposure of fibrillar collagen to blood promotes aggregation and activation of platelets.

During collagen synthesis (see Fig. 3-12), fibroblasts produce procollagen molecules (tropocollagen) within the cell, which are packed in the complex of Golgi and subsequently excreted. Once released to the extracellular space, cleavage of the nonhelical segments will occur. Prolyl hydroxylase is a rate-limiting enzyme for the synthesis of collagen and has as cofactors vitamin C, oxygen,

Table 3-4 Collagen Types

Type	Tissue Distribution
I	All connective tissues, except cartilage and basement membranes
II	Cartilage, vitreous humor, intervertebral disc
III	Skin, blood vessels, granulation tissue, internal organs
IV	Basement membranes

iron, and α-ketoglutarate. Lactate and hypoxia also indirectly stimulate prolyl hydroxylase synthesis.

BIBLIOGRAPHY

Barbul A, Efron DT. Wound healing. In: Brunicardi FC, Andersen DK, Billiar TR, Dunn DL, et al. (eds.), *Schwartz's Principles of Surgery*, 9th ed. New York: McGraw-Hill; 2010:Chapter 9.

37. **(D)** Death of a cell can be categorized in two groups: necrosis (incidental cell death) or apoptosis (programmed cell death).

Necrosis is characterized by loss of membrane function and abnormal permeability (observed by the cell's inability to exclude vital dye such as trypan blue). Disruption of organelles is seen early in the process. Most of the time, the effect of necrosis is seen in a large number of cells.

Apoptosis is precisely controlled, energy-dependent program of cell death. It is a physiologic event during which the cells shrink, condense, and fragment, forming membrane-bound apoptotic bodies for phagocytosis by neighboring cells and macrophages.

A key biochemical feature of apoptosis is internucleosomal cleavage of chromatin in a pattern indicative of endogenous endonuclease activation. This creates low-molecular-size fragments of DNA. A characteristic "ladder" pattern of DNA fragments is seen when DNA extracted from apoptotic cells is submitted to electrophoresis.

BIBLIOGRAPHY

Ko TC, Evers BM. Molecular and cell biology. In: Townsend CM (ed.), *Sabiston: The Biological Basis of Modern Surgical Practice*, 18th ed. St. Louis, MO: Elsevier/Saunders, 2008:191–216.

Reeves M. Cell biology. In: O'Leary JP (ed.), *The Physiologic Basis of Surgery*, 4th ed. Baltimore, MD: Lippincott Williams & Wilkins; 2008:1–43.

38. **(B)** Fibronectin is a cell adhesion protein found in blood and in matrices. Although encoded by a single gene, fibronectins exist in a number of different forms. Major functions include mediating cellular adhesion, promoting cell migration and chemotaxis, and regulating cell growth and gene expression.

Each fibronectin molecule consists of a series of structural and functional domains. Six or more peptides are present, and are capable of mediating cell adhesion. They are located in three general regions: the central cell-binding domain, the alternatively spliced IIICS region, and the heparin-binding domain.

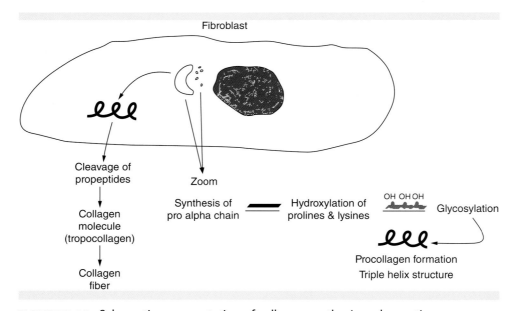

FIGURE 3-12. Schematic representation of collagen synthesis and excretion.

Fibronectin plays a major role in the capacity of cells to interact with fibrin, containing at least two fibrin-binding domains.

Fibronectin major fibrin-binding domain is homologous to the finger domain of TPA. Competition between TPA and fibronectin to bind on this homologous domain might be an important regulator of fibrinolysis.

Fibronectin is usually deposited before collagen, serving as matrix for further collagen deposition. Fibronectin matrix will be degraded by proteases as collagen is deposited and as the wound matures.

BIBLIOGRAPHY

Yamad KM, Clark RAF. Provisional matrix. In: Clark RA (ed.), *The Molecular and Cellular Biology of Wound Repair*, 2nd ed. New York, NY: Plenum Press; 1996:153–168.

39. **(C)** Proteoglycans are a heterogeneous group of protein–carbohydrate complexes containing at least one glycosaminoglycan chain covalently bound. Proteoglycans are named after the most prevalent glycosaminoglycan in the structure.

Proteoglycans are versatile molecules found in secretory granules, or as an intrinsic or extrinsic membrane protein, and in the extracellular matrix.

Many different functions are attributed to these molecules including blood coagulation regulators, promotion of extracellular organization, storage of growth factors, and promotion of growth factor receptor binding.

Chondroitin-4 sulfate occurs in high levels in granulation tissue, but it is not found in the mature scar. Levels of proteoglycans in general vary according to the degree of wound maturation.

BIBLIOGRAPHY

Gallo RL, Bernfield M. Proteoglycans and their role in wound repair. In: Clark RA (ed.), *The Molecular and Cellular Biology of Wound Repair*, 2nd ed. New York, NY: Plenum Press; 1996:475–488.

CHAPTER 4

HEMOSTASIS AND COAGULATION

LISA M. MCELROY AND TRAVIS P. WEBB

QUESTIONS

1. Which of the following is true regarding the intrinsic and extrinsic coagulation pathways?
   (A) In the classic model of coagulation, the extrinsic pathway initiates coagulation by interaction of circulating factors already within the blood.
   (B) In the classic model of coagulation, the intrinsic pathway initiates coagulation by interaction with subendothelial tissue factor.
   (C) Defects in the intrinsic pathway lead to elevations of the activated partial thromboplastin time (aPTT).
   (D) Defects in the intrinsic pathway lead to elevations of the prothrombin time (PT).
   (E) The intrinsic pathway requires the presence of factor VII and Ca^{2+}.

2. Which one of the following substances directly activates platelets during the process of clot formation?
   (A) Interleukin (IL) 3
   (B) IL-11
   (C) Epinephrine
   (D) Thrombopoietin
   (E) IL-6

3. Which of the following substances is primarily found in beta granules of platelets?
   (A) Platelet factor 4
   (B) Beta-thromboglobulin
   (C) Thrombospondin
   (D) Fibrinogen
   (E) Serotonin

4. In regard to coagulation *in vivo*, which of the following statements is true (see Fig. 4-1)?
   (A) Intrinsic pathway deficiencies are not associated with clinically significant bleeding.

   (B) Tissue factor (TF) is not a significant initiator of coagulation.
   (C) The intrinsic pathway is the initiator of events.
   (D) Tissue factor pathway inhibitor (TFPI) is present in large amounts.
   (E) Thrombin acts to activate further amounts of TF-VIIa, thus leading to a positive-feedback mechanism.

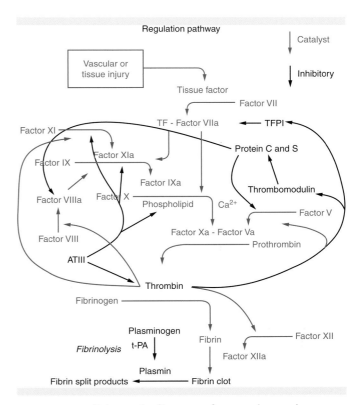

FIGURE 4-1. Schematic diagram of new enhanced coagulation scheme showing major role of tissue factor in activation of coagulation.

5. Which of the following statements is true regarding the physiology of the tissue factor pathway inhibitor TFPI?
   (A) Usually present in the plasma in small amounts.
   (B) Platelets carry the majority of the total TFPI in blood.
   (C) Heparin infusion *in vivo* decreases the circulating levels of TFPI.
   (D) Decreased levels can occasionally be seen in septicemia and disseminated intravascular coagulation (DIC).
   (E) Blocks the TF/VIIa/Va/Xa complex by binding to factor VIIa.

6. Which of the following statements concerning the regulation of the coagulation cascade (see Fig. 4-2) is true?

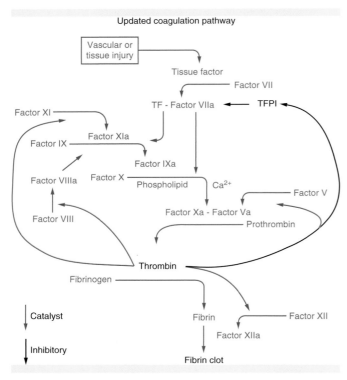

Updated coagulation pathway

FIGURE 4-2. Schematic representation of the physiologic cascade with regulation factors highlighted.

   (A) Antithrombin III (ATIII) activates factors IXa, Xa, and XIa.
   (B) Thrombomodulin changes the shape of thrombin and potentiates its ability to activate other proteins.
   (C) Proteins C and S are vitamin K-dependent factors responsible for inactivating factors Va and VIIIa.

   (D) Plasminogen acts to degrade the clot formation and prevent thrombosis.
   (E) Thrombin-activatable fibrinolysis inhibitor (TAFI) catalyzes the conversion of plasminogen to plasmin.

7. Low molecular weight heparin (LMWH) produces its primary effects because of its inhibition of which factor?
   (A) IIa
   (B) IXa
   (C) Xa
   (D) XIa
   (E) XIIa

8. von Willebrand's disease (vWD)
   (A) Is the second most common bleeding disorder after vitamin K deficiency.
   (B) Is caused by a quantitative or qualitative defect in a protein necessary for TF-VII interaction.
   (C) Inheritance of type I is autosomal recessive.
   (D) Results in an elevated PT.
   (E) Can be treated with cryoprecipitate.

9. All of the following drugs affect platelet function *except*
   (A) Nonsteroidal anti-inflammatory drugs (NSAIDs)
   (B) Warfarin
   (C) Nitroprusside
   (D) Furosemide
   (E) Abciximab

10. Which of the following statements regarding hemophilia is true?
    (A) Type A represents a deficiency in factor VIII and comprises 20% of all coagulation factor deficiencies.
    (B) Type B represents a deficiency in factor IX and is the second most common inherited coagulation disorder after vWD.
    (C) It is transmitted as an autosomal dominant disorder.
    (D) It results in an elevated PT.
    (E) Type A can be treated with DDAVP (desmopressin acetate) after mild trauma or before dental procedures.

11. A 21-year-old male presents with multiple gunshot wounds to both lower legs and right upper chest. He is taken emergently to the operating room, where his left lower leg is amputated below the knee and right middle and lower lobectomy is performed. Intraoperatively, he receives 12 units of packed red blood cells and postoperatively is sent to the intensive care unit and requires mechanical ventilation. Over the next several days, he develops acute respiratory distress syndrome, gram-negative pneumonia, and bacteremia.

He is started on appropriate antibiotics and maintained on mechanical ventilation and inotropic support. A week after admission, the patient develops a loss of palpable pulses distal to his popliteal artery on his right leg, although his dorsalis pedis can be located with Doppler. Labs reveal the patient to be in DIC.

Which of the following lab values is most sensitive for DIC?

(A) Slowly rising platelet count
(B) Selective deficiency of vitamin K factors
(C) Hypofibrinogenemia
(D) Prolonged bleeding time
(E) Presence of fibrin split products

12. Which of the following platelet function tests most resembles *in vivo* physiologic clotting?
(A) Aggregometry
(B) Flow cytometry
(C) Thromboelastography (TEG)
(D) Bleeding time
(E) All of the above

13. A 45-year-old female presents to the emergency department (ED) after a high-speed head-on collision with another vehicle. Primary survey reveals an intact airway with decreased breath sounds necessitating chest tube placement. Blood pressure is stable at 110/64 mm Hg. Secondary survey reveals abdominal tenderness. The computed tomographic (CT) scan is shown in Fig. 4-3.

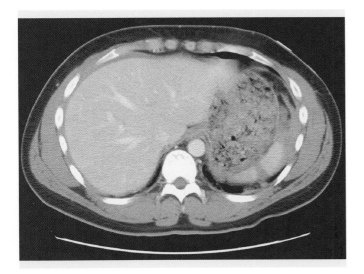

FIGURE 4-3. Abdomen CT with grade III splenic rupture.

Following admission to the ICU, the patient is noted to have continued draining of dark red blood from the chest tube at 100 mL/h. She becomes hemodynamically unstable and undergoes exploratory laparotomy and splenectomy; there is the appearance of generalized oozing within the peritoneal cavity. She is taken back to the ICU where she is warmed and resuscitated.

Over the next several days, she is noted to have continued oozing from her needlesticks with a slight decrease in hematocrit. Her chest tube output remains stable at approximately 50 mL/h and is still dark red in nature. She is taken back to the CT scanner, where fluid accumulation is noted around the liver and spleen bed.

If coagulation studies on this patient revealed a normal PT, fibrinogen, and platelet count and an elevated aPTT, all of the following statements are true *except*

(A) This could be caused by administration of heparin-containing substances and can be reversed with protamine.
(B) This could be caused by administration of LMWH that is being used for deep vein thrombosis (DVT) prophylaxis.
(C) If this picture is from heparin administration, then infusion of fresh frozen plasma (FFP) could enhance her anticoagulation.
(D) vWD can be associated with an elevation in the aPTT, leading to the possible use of DDAVP in this patient.
(E) Her prolonged bleeding could be caused by a factor deficiency.

14. Which of the following statements regarding factor V Leiden is true?
(A) The most common inheritable disorder of coagulation
(B) Associated with a defect in factor S activity
(C) Caused by a mutation in the gene for factor C
(D) Occurs in approximately 10% of people in the Western population
(E) Patients must be off anticoagulation for accurate diagnosis

15. A 68-year-old female presents to the ED with complaints of right-sided abdominal pain that began 12 h earlier. She has a history of polymyalgia rheumatica and takes prednisone daily.

   Physical examination revealed moderate right-sided tenderness without rebound tenderness. Mild hematuria is present on urinalysis, and mild elevated liver enzymes are noted. CT of the abdomen is shown in Fig. 4-4.

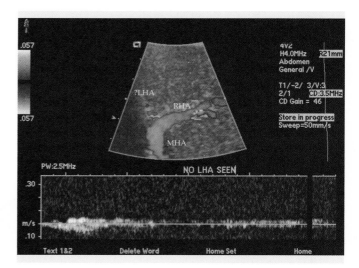

FIGURE 4-5. Hepatic ultrasound revealing flow through main hepatic artery into right hepatic artery without significantly measurable blood flow into left hepatic artery.

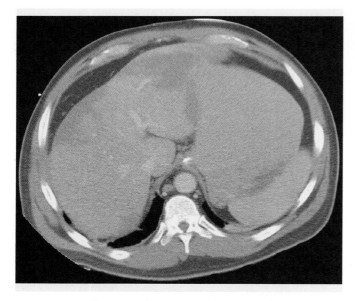

FIGURE 4-4. Computed tomographic image showing infarction of segments of the left lobe of the liver.

   This was followed by a hepatic ultrasound, shown above (see Fig. 4-5).

   Further workup revealed antibodies against phospholipid.

   Which of the following statements concerning the condition described above is true?
   (A) Patients must have detectable antibodies of immunoglobulin (Ig) E class against phospholipid membranes present in blood on several occasions to be classified as having antiphospholipid syndrome.
   (B) Anticardiolipin antibodies react with a β_2-glycoprotein I (β_2GI) protein found in plasma.
   (C) The Venereal Disease Research Laboratory (VDRL) test for syphilis is based on a non-complement-fixing antiphospholipid antibody.
   (D) Lupus anticoagulant antibodies can be ruled out by a single phospholipid-dependent coagulation assay.
   (E) Current protocols for detecting antiphospholipid antibodies use flow cytometric analyses.

16. Which of the following is true regarding elevated plasma levels of homocysteine?
   (A) Leads to an increase in coronary artery disease
   (B) Caused by a deficiency in B_6 intake
   (C) Is being treated with experimental drugs currently in clinical trials
   (D) Increases the risk of venous disease by a factor of 7
   (E) Is treated with folate supplementation in grains by the Food and Drug Administration (FDA)

17. Which of the following is true regarding the prothrombin G20210a substitution?
   (A) It is a common genetic mutation leading to hemophilia.
   (B) It is caused by a missense mutation.
   (C) It has a low relative risk of causing symptoms.
   (D) It leads to elevated levels of prothrombin.
   (E) It occurs in up to 4% of the population.

18. A 55-year-old previously healthy male is postoperative day 2 status post left hemicolectomy for Dukes B colon cancer. He is slow to regain mobility due to complaints of pain. All of the following are accepted treatment options for DVT prophylaxis *except*
   (A) Enoxoprin
   (B) Sequential compression devices (SCDs)
   (C) Elastic stockings (TED hose)
   (D) Clopidogrel
   (E) Warfarin

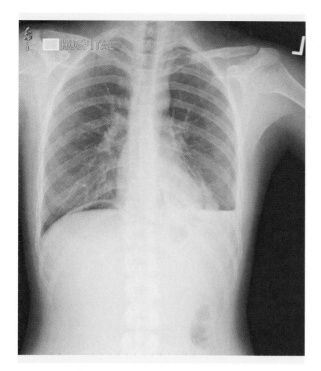

FIGURE 4-6. Chest x-ray (pneumoperitoneum).

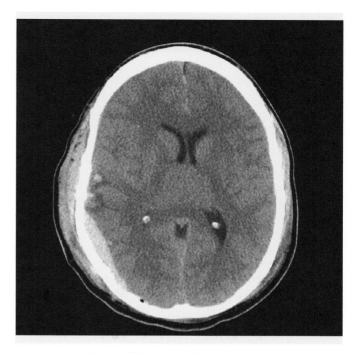

FIGURE 4-8. Head CT (subdural hematoma).

19. A 23-year-old female unrestrained driver was involved in a head-on collision with a pickup truck. She is confused (Glasgow Coma Scale [GCS] 8) and hypotensive on arrival to the ED. X-rays (see Figs. 4-6 through 4-9) are obtained.

She undergoes pelvic angiography with successful embolism for continued bleeding and external fixation of the femurs and pelvis. She is taken to the ICU intubated, sedated, and in critical condition. Forty-eight hours later, the patient's overall condition has not changed.

Which one of the following statements is true?
(A) The patient should be started on warfarin for DVT prophylaxis.
(B) Compression devices are contraindicated in this patient secondary to orthopedic fractures.
(C) Bedside inferior vena cava (IVC) filter placement requires fluoroscopic capability.
(D) Prophylactic IVC filter is not indicated.
(E) GCS score ≤ 9 is a known risk factor for developing venous thromboembolism.

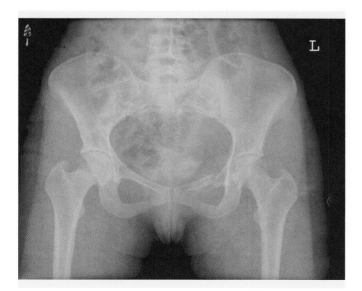

FIGURE 4-7. Pelvis x-ray.

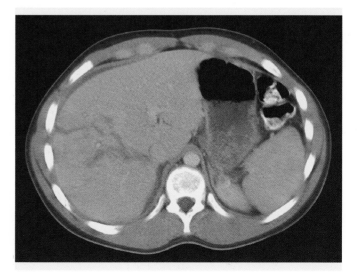

FIGURE 4-9. Abdominal CT (hepatic laceration).

20. If the patient in question 19 had been receiving therapeutic warfarin prior to her injury, her relative risk of mortality compared to a similarly injured person not on anticoagulation would be
    (A) 1
    (B) 1.5
    (C) 2
    (D) 3
    (E) 5

21. A 36-year-old male involved in a motor vehicle crash is admitted to the ICU for observation of a grade III liver laceration. He is transfused 2 units of packed RBCs because of a slow decline of hematocrit and blood pressure. He tolerates the first infusion without any difficulty; however, after 100 mL of the second infusion, the patient becomes profoundly hypotensive, develops chest pain, shortness of breath, and pain in his right arm. All of the following statements concerning this patient are correct *except*
    (A) This is a complement-derived destruction of RBCs.
    (B) It is often because of a clerical error.
    (C) It can lead to renal failure.
    (D) This would not happen if the blood was from an autologous source.
    (E) This presentation could have been delayed for days after the infusion.

22. Donated whole blood
    (A) Is routinely used in trauma situations.
    (B) Is more expensive for the hospital and the patient.
    (C) Is usually unavailable at most hospitals and blood banks.
    (D) Can be stored for 60 days in standard storage solutions.
    (E) Has a hematocrit > 80%.

23. Which of the following statements about blood processing and storage is *incorrect*?
    (A) Deglycerolized RBCs can be stored for up to 3 years.
    (B) Platelets are separated from the plasma component by centrifugation.
    (C) Plasma is stored at −18 to −30°C to preserve clotting factor function.
    (D) Packed RBCs contain essentially no platelets, and levels of factors V and VIII are stable.
    (E) Leukocyte concentrate can be obtained and used in patients who are profoundly granulocytopenic.

24. A patient receiving a standard unit of blood from a volunteer donor is at highest risk of contracting which virus?
    (A) Hepatitis A
    (B) Hepatitis B
    (C) Hepatitis C

    (D) Human immunodeficiency virus (HIV)
    (E) Parvovirus B19

25. Transfusion-related acute lung injury
    (A) Occurs in 1 in 1000 transfusions.
    (B) Can be caused by antibody formation to the blood donor cells.
    (C) Can be secondary to storage defects of the blood transfused.
    (D) Leads to death in greater than 35% of affected patients.
    (E) Usually manifests slowly and presents clinically several days after transfusion.

26. Regarding the transfusion of packed RBCs,
    (A) Transfusion is indicated if the hemoglobin is ≤ 7 g/dL.
    (B) Transfusion can be performed without involving the patient.
    (C) Transfusion should be two units at a time if indicated.
    (D) Transfusions can be used appropriately as a volume expander.
    (E) Transfusion should be based on clinical indications.

27. A 54-year-old patient is brought to the ED complaining of bleeding per rectum. The patient states she has lost approximately 25 lb in the last year and has had "sticky" bowel movements for months. Laboratory examination reveals hemoglobin of 6.5 g/dL after resuscitation. She is sent for colonoscopy, during which a large obstructing, fungating mass is noted in the sigmoid colon. She consents for the surgery but states that she is a Jehovah's Witness and will not accept any blood products.
    Which of the following statements is *correct*?
    (A) She is likely to refuse autologous blood as well.
    (B) She will refuse human albumin as a volume expander.
    (C) She should be cared for by someone who is sympathetic to her beliefs.
    (D) She will not accept immune globulin from animals.
    (E) She is at a high risk for complications without blood transfusion.

28. Acute normovolemic hemodilution
    (A) Is generally safe for elective cases in young healthy individuals.
    (B) Can be performed safely in patients with hematocrits ≤ 20%.
    (C) Decreases the risk of disease transmission.
    (D) Involves separating blood products prior to infusion.
    (E) Produces several physiologic changes, but the end result is less oxygen delivery to the tissues.

29. A 65-year-old man is seen in clinic for possible pancreaticoduodenectomy for pancreatic cancer. He is scheduled for surgery in 2 weeks. He asks you specifically about blood loss and that he wants to donate blood for himself. Which of the following statements concerning preoperative autologous blood transfusion is correct?
    (A) Preoperative blood transfusion is safe in patients with a hematocrit of 25%.
    (B) Blood can be donated up to 2 months prior to surgery.
    (C) Preoperative autologous blood transfusion prevents the risk of transfusion reactions.
    (D) Preoperative autologous blood transfusion is a cost-effective method to treat postoperative anemia.
    (E) Blood can be withdrawn as quickly as every 3–4 days.

30. A 45-year-old patient contracted hepatitis C from a blood transfusion in 1978. The patient underwent a successful liver transplantation, was given rabbit antithymocyte globulin on the day of surgery, and subsequently developed profound thrombocytopenia. Which of the following statements concerning platelet transfusion in this patient is *incorrect*?
    (A) If asymptomatic, a platelet count of $\leq 20,000/mm^3$ is an indication for transfusion.
    (B) Apheresis units have less human leukocyte antigen (HLA) to complicate this patient's immunosuppression.
    (C) Platelets are highly immunogenic.
    (D) Platelets should be withheld if the patient is symptomatic but hypothermic.
    (E) It is indicated for microvascular bleeding.

31. Red blood cell substitutes
    (A) Are currently approved by the FDA.
    (B) Are being produced by *Escherichia coli* through recombinant technology.
    (C) All showed decreased mortality in current trials.
    (D) Currently in use contain no human or bovine hemoglobin.
    (E) Include synthetic compounds based on polyethylene glycol.

32. Which of the following statements is correct regarding intraoperative and postoperative blood collection?
    (A) Cell-washing machines can process up to 10 units of blood per hour for infusion.
    (B) Cell-washing machines process blood intraoperatively and can be stored for up to 1 month.
    (C) Red cells obtained from cell-saver machines have longer half-life once infused than do allogenic cells.
    (D) Blood from devices such as chest tubes often contains high concentrations of hemoglobin (i.e., hematocrit).

(E) Blood from devices such as chest tubes and surgical drains can be reinfused without processing.

33. With regard to suture material, which one of the following statements is *incorrect*?
    (A) Suture material is categorized as absorbable versus nonabsorbable.
    (B) Steel produces the least amount of inflammation of all the suture material.
    (C) Steel suture materials are available in braided preparations.
    (D) Braided suture passes through tissue better than monofilament suture.
    (E) Surgical hemostasis begins with good surgical technique.

34. Which one of the following devices provides the least amount of adjacent tissue damage during normal usage?
    (A) Electrocautery on cutting mode
    (B) Electrocautery on coagulation mode
    (C) Harmonic scalpel
    (D) Argon beam coagulation
    (E) Nd-YAG laser

35. Fibrin preparations
    (A) Are commercially available in the United States by combining human thrombin and bovine cryoprecipitate.
    (B) As commercial sealants have been available in the United States for over 20 years.
    (C) Can be stabilized by the addition of aprotinin.
    (D) Are contraindicated in patients with vWD.
    (E) Require presence of thrombin from the patient for activation.

ANSWERS AND EXPLANATIONS

1. **(C)** Older textbooks divide the coagulation cascade into the intrinsic and extrinsic pathways. This traditional depiction is useful in interpreting coagulation test abnormalities, such as PT and aPTT. The intrinsic pathway can be activated without an extravascular source. The extrinsic pathway, in contrast, requires an extravascular component, such as tissue factor (TF), for activation. Both pathways are thought to be activated simultaneously to initiate and sustain clot formation (Fig. 4-10).

   Elevations in the aPTT arise from defects in the intrinsic pathway. This pathway begins with trauma to the blood vessel and exposure of blood to collagen in a damaged vascular wall, but as the name implies, it can also occur outside the vascular wall with most "wettable" surfaces, such as tables and glass. In response to these stimuli, factor XII (Hageman factor) is activated to form factor XIIa. Activated factor XII then activates factor XI to factor XIa. Activated factor XI converts factor IX to

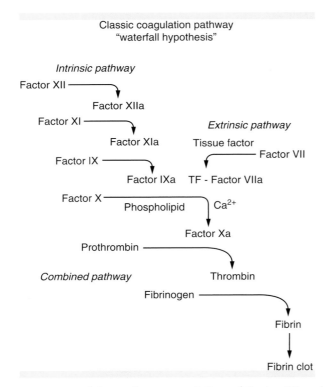

Classic coagulation pathway
"waterfall hypothesis"

Intrinsic pathway

Factor XII

Factor XIIa

Factor XI

Factor XIa

Extrinsic pathway

Factor IX

Tissue factor

Factor VII

Factor IXa   TF - Factor VIIa

Factor X

Phospholipid Ca^{2+}

Factor Xa

Prothrombin

Combined pathway

Thrombin

Fibrinogen

Fibrin

Fibrin clot

FIGURE 4-10. Schematic representation of the traditional coagulation scheme or "waterfall hypothesis."

factor IXa. Factor IXa then converts factor X to factor Xa. This activation of factor X is also greatly accelerated by factor VIIIa. Activated factor X converts the inactive molecule prothrombin to the active thrombin.

Elevations in the PT arise from defects in the extrinsic pathway. This pathway requires either a vascular wall to be penetrated or the presence of extravascular tissue. TF is found predominantly on most nonendothelial cells. Damage to vessel walls causes the plasma to be exposed to TF. TF combines with factor VII to form the TF-VIIa complex. TF-VIIa complex in the presence of Ca^{2+} and phospholipids can activate factor X to Xa, leading to thrombin formation.

Once thrombin has formed, it has numerous other jobs, including cleaving fibrinogen into the fibrin monomers. Fibrin monomers consist of fibrinopeptides A and B, which each undergo conformational changes to expose the active components and allow for polymerization. Polymerization of fibrin occurs by cross-linking the monomers forming a mesh-like substrate where the clot will form. In addition, thrombin is able, through a positive-feedback mechanism, to activate most of the components within the cascade, thereby leading to larger amounts of thrombin and fibrin.

BIBLIOGRAPHY

Choi K, Spence R, Shander A, et al. Hemostasis, thrombosis, anticoagulation, hematopoiesis and blood transfusion. In: O'Leary JP, Tabuenca A, Capote LR, eds. *The Physiologic Basis of Surgery.* Alphen aan den Rijn, the Netherlands: Wolters Kluwer Health; 2008:533–575.

Gonzalez EA, Jastrow KM, Holcomb JB, Kozar RA. Hemostasis, surgical bleeding, and transfusion. In: Brunicardi FC, Andersen DK, Billiar TR, Dunn DL, Hunter JG, Matthews JB, et al., eds. *Schwartz's Principles of Surgery.* 9th ed. New York, NY: McGraw-Hill; 2010: Chapter 4.

Wilmore D, Cheung L, Harken A, Holcroft J, Meakins J. Classic coagulation pathway "waterfall hypothesis." In: Soper N, ed. *ACS Surgery: Principles and Practice.* New York, NY: WebMD; 2002:77–90.

2. **(C)**

3. **(E)**

Explanations for questions 2 and 3

The primary role of platelets in the process of hemostasis is providing a phospholipid layer for which the coagulation activation sequences can progress. Platelets are found in the circulation as anucleate cellular particles with both alpha granules-which contain platelet factor 4, beta-thromboglobulin, thrombospondin, platelet-derived growth factor, fibrinogen, and von Willebrand's factor (vWF), and beta granules-which contain adenosine diphosphate (ADP), serotonin, and organelles. Their synthesis is primarily controlled by IL-3, IL-6, IL-11, and thrombopoietin. The cell surface contains several glycoprotein (GP) receptors responsible for hemostasis. GPIb interacts with vWF and causes adherence of the platelet to the injured vessel wall. GPIIb-IIIa serves as a receptor for fibrinogen and helps with platelet aggregation. After activation by substances such as adenosine triphosphate (ATP), ADP, epinephrine, thromboxane A_2, collagen, and thrombin, the platelets undergo shape changes, degranulate, and provide receptors for the coagulation factors.

Once released, the granules within platelets enhance the coagulation process. They act by further activating platelets, aiding with vasoconstriction, stimulating adherence of leukocytes, and providing microparticles essential in the formation of the platelet plug. Activated platelets also act as a surface by which the coagulation cascade can occur in the presence of Ca^{2+} and the phospholipid layer needed for factor activation.

As fibrin is formed, the platelets become intertwined within the cross-linking, helping to form the clot. Leukocytes are trapped as well, and they help initiate inflammatory responses necessary for wound healing. The final platelet plug is later replaced by endothelial cells and tissue repair occurs.

BIBLIOGRAPHY

Choi K, Spence R, Shander A, et al. Hemostasis, thrombosis, anti-coagulation, hematopoiesis and blood transfusion. In: O'Leary, JP, Tabuenca A, Capote LR, eds. *The Physiologic Basis of Surgery*. Alphen aan den Rijn, the Netherlands: Wolters Kluwer Health; 2008:533–575.

Owings J, Gosselin R. Bleeding and transfusion. In: Wilmore D, Cheung L, Harken A, Holcroft J, Meakins J, Soper N, eds. *ACS Surgery: Principles and Practice*. New York, NY: WebMD; 2002:77–90.

Rutherford E, Brecher M, Fakhry S, et al. Hematologic principles in surgery. In: Townsend C, Beauchamp RD, Evers BM, Mattox KL, eds. *Sabiston Textbook of Surgery: The Biological Basis of Modern Surgical Practice*. 18th ed. Philadelphia, PA: Elsevier Saunders; 2008:113–142.

4. **(A)** *In vitro*, two pathways exist by which coagulation could occur: the intrinsic pathway and the extrinsic pathway. The pathways converge to a final common pathway at factor X. The clinical relevance of the intrinsic pathway is not associated with clinically significant bleeding *in vivo*, although it does produce aberrations in tests of coagulation. TF is the important initiator of coagulation, and the extrinsic pathway requires exposure of tissue factor on the surface of the injured vessel wall to initiate the arm of the cascade beginning with factor VII. The TF-VIIa complex then proceeds similarly through the extrinsic pathway, leading to thrombin formation and eventually fibrin clot formation. Only limited amounts of thrombin are produced by this mechanism. Thrombin binds to and activates a protein called tissue factor pathway inhibitor that is present in small amounts usually, but more is released in the presence of heparin. This complex then inactivates the factor VII–TF complexes, thus inhibiting further synthesis of thrombin through this pathway, representing a negative-feedback system, thus controlling hemostasis.

The thrombin initially synthesized through the factor VII–TF complex pathway also has other functions that are procoagulant in nature. One of its main functions is to catalyze the activation of factors V, VIII, XI, and XIII; induce platelet aggregation; and induce expression of TF. In this manner, the intrinsic pathway is activated, leading to further clot production.

In summary, the extrinsic pathway is the initiator of events through the TF-VIIa complex. This in turn produces enough thrombin to activate the intrinsic pathway, leading to large amounts of clot-producing fibrin.

BIBLIOGRAPHY

Choi K, Spence R, Shander A, et al. Hemostasis, thrombosis, anti-coagulation, hematopoiesis and blood transfusion. In: O'Leary JP, Tabuenca A, Capote LR, eds. *The Physiologic Basis of Surgery*.

Alphen aan den Rijn, the Netherlands: Wolters Kluwer Health; 2008:533–575.

Owings J, Gosselin R. Bleeding and transfusion. In: Wilmore D, Cheung L, Harken A, Holcroft J, Meakins J, Soper N, eds. *ACS Surgery: Principles and Practice*. New York, NY: WebMD; 2002:77–90.

Rutherford E, Brecher M, Fakhry S, et al. Hematologic principles in surgery. In: Townsend C, Beauchamp RD, Evers BM, Mattox KL, eds. *Sabiston Textbook of Surgery: The Biological Basis of Modern Surgical Practice*. 18th ed. Philadelphia, PA: Elsevier Saunders; 2008:113–142.

5. **(A)** Tissue factor pathway inhibitor blocks the extrinsic TF-VIIa complex, eliminating this catalyst's production of factors Xa and IXa and blocking the production of thrombin. Most of the TFPI circulating in the plasma is bound to the lipoproteins, including low-density lipoprotein (LDL) and high-density lipoprotein (HDL). TFPI concentration in the plasma is quite low and is estimated at about 2 nM. Platelets carry only 10% of the total concentration of TFPI, and their release following stimulation is important in regulating the clot formation.

Experiments conducted with *in vivo* infusion of heparin show a two- to three-fold increase in the amount of circulating TFPI. This is not seen when heparin is infused *ex vivo*, leading to the hypothesis that a majority of TFPI is found in an extravascular source, likely the endothelium. This release after the infusion of heparin may augment the effects of heparin anticoagulation.

The infusion of TFPI has been studied as a possible treatment of sepsis-induced DIC. It is known that levels of TFPI do not rise in the face of DIC and sepsis, although the level of TF-VIIa complex is extremely elevated. This suggests that DIC in the face of sepsis is caused by an imbalance in the ratio of TFPI and TF-VIIa. Supraphysiologic doses of TFPI have been shown to stop DIC induced by TF in rabbits and decrease mortality in baboons.

BIBLIOGRAPHY

Choi K, Spence R, Shander A, et al. Hemostasis, thrombosis, anticoagulation, hematopoiesis and blood transfusion. In: O'Leary JP, Tabuenca A, Capote LR, eds. *The Physiologic Basis of Surgery*. Alphen aan den Rijn, the Netherlands: Wolters Kluwer Health; 2008:533–575.

Doshi SN, Marmur JD. Evolving role of tissue factor and its pathway inhibitor. *Crit Care Med* 2002;30(Suppl 5):S241–S250.

Gonzalez EA, Jastrow KM, Holcomb JB, Kozar RA. Hemostasis, surgical bleeding, and transfusion. In: Brunicardi FC, Andersen DK, Billiar TR, Dunn DL, Hunter JG, Matthews JB, et al., eds. *Schwartz's Principles of Surgery*. 9th ed. New York, NY: McGraw-Hill; 2010: Chapter 4.

6. **(C)** Regulation of the coagulation system is a complex process involving interactions of several proteins and

occurs simultaneously with the activation of the pro-coagulant and inhibitory factors mentioned previously. Just as thrombin is a major factor in formation of clot, it functions as the main downregulator.

Thrombomodulin is a membrane-bound molecule found on both normal and damaged endothelium. In the presence of thrombin, it binds to and changes the shape of thrombin. This conformational change causes the molecule to be a potent activator of proteins C and S, thus becoming a potent anticoagulant. This also keeps clot from forming on normal endothelium.

Proteins C and S are vitamin K-dependent molecules that, once activated by the thrombin-thrombomodulin complex, are potent inhibitors of factors VIIIa and Va, respectively. Formation of these two proteins highly regulates the formation of clots.

ATIII is a serine protease that requires no activation and is a slow inhibitor of thrombin and factors IXa, Xa, and XIa. Undamaged endothelium cells produce a membrane-bound receptor similar to the heparin molecule that will bind ATIII. This functions to reduce clot formation in the presence of normal endothelium.

Plasminogen is converted to plasmin through plasminogen activator (t-PA and u-PA) released from the endothelium. Once activated, plasmin is the primary fibrinolytic protein responsible for cleaving fibrin. Breakdown of fibrin prevents the obstruction of the blood flow within the vessel. Formation of plasmin is regulated by the protein called thrombin-activatable fibrinolysis inhibitor (TAFI). TAFI is activated by thrombin after it forms complexes with thrombomodulin, thus making the thrombomodulin-thrombin complex an inhibitor of fibrinolysis as well as a potent procoagulant.

BIBLIOGRAPHY

Owings J, Gosselin R. Bleeding and transfusion. In: Wilmore D, Cheung L, Harken A, Holcroft J, Meakins J, Soper N, eds. *ACS Surgery: Principles and Practice.* New York, NY: WebMD; 2002:77–90.

Rutherford E, Brecher M, Fakhry S, et al. Hematologic principles in surgery. In: Townsend C, Beauchamp RD, Evers BM, Mattox KL, eds. *Sabiston Textbook of Surgery: The Biological Basis of Modern Surgical Practice.* 18th ed. Philadelphia, PA: Elsevier Saunders; 2008:113–142.

7. **(C)** Both unfractionated heparin (UH) and LMWH exert direct effects by binding and catalyzing ATIII. This serine protease inhibitor forms a complex with heparin that is able to inhibit all of the procoagulation serine proteases listed but primarily thrombin and Xa. UH is approximately two to four times as big as LMWH. As the size of the molecule decreases, the complex is less able to inhibit factor IIa (thrombin) without losing its ability to inhibit factor Xa. LMWH-ATIII has complete ability to inhibit factor Xa but has lost its ability the inhibit IIa.

Laboratory monitoring of LMWH is largely unnecessary. LMWH has a much lower affinity for plasma proteins than does UH. This accounts for its 90% bioavailability after subcutaneous administration and less interpatient variability once dose is adjusted for weight. If monitoring is needed, then anti-Xa levels can be obtained. Peak response occurs 3–4 h after injection, and its plasma half-life is two to four times longer than UH.

Patients who require monitoring of LMWH include those with significant renal insufficiency or failure, pediatric patients, obese patients > 120 kg, and patients who are pregnant. Monitoring may be performed using anti-Xa activity assays. Side effects of LMWH are small and include a 1.3% change of developing thrombocytopenia, which is similar to UH. LMWH can also induce hemorrhage, which is most often seen as wound hematomas. It is not recommended to be used in patients with bacterial endocarditis, congenital or acquired bleeding disorders, active ulcerative and angiodysplastic gastrointestinal disease, or hemorrhagic stroke; shortly after brain, spinal, or ophthalmologic surgery; or in patients treated concomitantly with platelet inhibitors. There is a significant increase in risk of spinal and epidural hematoma after spinal/epidural anesthesia, which can lead to paralysis.

BIBLIOGRAPHY

Liem TK, Moneta GL. Venous and lymphatic disease. In: Brunicardi FC, Andersen DK, Billiar TR, Dunn DL, Hunter JG, Matthews JB, et al., eds. *Schwartz's Principles of Surgery.* 9th ed. New York, NY: McGraw-Hill; 2010: Chapter 24.

8. **(E)** vWD is the most common inherited bleeding disorder. It is an autosomal dominant disorder with a prevalence estimated at 1% of the population. vWF is found in specialized storage granules within endothelial cells and in alpha granules of platelets. Endothelial cells will secrete vWF, and their function is to assist in platelet aggregation as well as a carrier protein for factor VIII. Patients with vWD have low levels of factor VIII and present with symptoms of platelet dysfunction, such as mucosal bleeding, petechiae, epistaxis, and menorrhagia (see Table 4-1). vWD can also be acquired. Most acquired forms are seen in patients with lymphoproliferative disorders but can also be caused by drugs, malignancies, hypothyroidism, and autoimmune diseases. These patients produce antibodies directed at the vWF, leading to removal of the protein by the reticuloendothelial system.

The treatment of choice in patients with mild-to-moderate type 1, acquired vWD and some patients with type II is DDAVP. DDAVP is an analogue to vasopressin,

TABLE 4-1 Subtypes of von Willebrand's Disease

Type	Genetic	Phenotype
I	No abnormality in vWF but relative decrease in quantity and function. Autosomal dominant trait.	70–80% of cases. Mild excessive epistaxis, mucosal bleeding. Normal PT, mildly elevated aPTT.
II	Point mutations in the coding sequence of the vWF gene. Variable inheritance and penetration.	Subdivided in four types based on gene mutation and phenotype. Severity of bleeding is relative to type and location of mutation.
III	Complete absence of gene or catastrophic mutations lead to lack of formation of vWF. Autosomal recessive trait.	10% of cases. Present as severe bleeding. Normal PT, moderately elevated aPTT.
Platelet-type vWD	Mutation in platelet receptor for vWF.	Mild-to-moderate bleeding.

and it causes release of endogenous stores of vWF from the endothelial cells. Administration of DDAVP causes shortening in the bleeding time and normalization of factor VIII–vWF complex activities. DDAVP can only be used once every 48 h to allow re-formation of the used vWF and will have no effect in type III patients because they lack all forms of vWF.

Several other treatment options are available for patients who do not respond to DDAVP or have type III. Plasma-purified factor VIII concentrations usually have a sufficient quantity of vWF-VIII to be effective. Recombinant factor VIII does not contain any vWF and is ineffective. Cryoprecipitate also contains enough vWF to be effective. Several local preparations exist for ancillary treatment during dental procedures. These include aminocaproic acid elixir and tranexamic acid, which both can be administered as a mouthwash. These agents work by inhibiting fibrinolysis. Topical thrombin, Gelfoam®, and fibrin glue have also been used.

Major surgery can be performed in these patients if appropriate precautions are taken. In one review of over 64 major surgical cases performed on patients with vWD, no mortality was noted in these patients. These patients were treated with items listed for major bleeding, which occurred in only 6.7% of the population.

BIBLIOGRAPHY

Gonzalez EA, Jastrow KM, Holcomb JB, Kozar RA. Hemostasis, surgical bleeding, and transfusion. In: Brunicardi FC, Andersen DK, Billiar TR, Dunn DL, Hunter JG, Matthews JB, et al., eds. *Schwartz's Principles of Surgery*. 9th ed. New York, NY: McGraw-Hill; 2010: Chapter 4.

Owings J, Gosselin R. Bleeding and transfusion. In: Wilmore D, Cheung L, Harken A, Holcroft J, Meakins J, Soper N, eds. *ACS Surgery: Principles and Practice*. New York, NY: WebMD; 2002:77–90.

9. **(B)** Platelet disorders are generally broken up into quantitative defects (thrombocytopenia) or qualitative defects (thrombocytopathys). Inherited disorders include vWD and defects in the surface receptors GPIb and GPIIb-IIIa, thus preventing platelet aggregation. Acquired disorders are common occurrences and can usually be linked to food or drugs (see Tables 4-2 and 4-3).

TABLE 4-2 Common Inherited Diseases of Platelet Dysfunction

Disease	Characterization
von Willebrand's disease	Caused by a defect in vWF leading to decreased platelet aggregation.
Bernard-Soulier's syndrome	Glycoprotein IB is missing from the platelet membrane. Platelets are unable to bind to von Willebrand's factor.
Glanzmann's thrombasthenia	An abnormality of the glycoprotein IIb-IIIa complex on the cell membrane. Platelets do not bind fibrinogen properly and do not aggregate well.
Storage pool disorders	A deficiency or abnormality in the platelet granules or in their release mechanisms.
Gray platelet syndrome—alpha granules	
Delta storage pool deficiency—beta granules	

Thrombocytopenia is a quantitative defect of platelets defined when the count is less than 100,000/mm^3. Spontaneous bleeding may occur if platelet counts fall to less than 10,000/mm^3. Similar to vWD, this bleeding is manifested as mucosal bleeding, petechiae, gastrointestinal bleeding, and central nervous system (CNS) bleeding, which can

TABLE 4-3 Substances Known to Lead to Qualitative Defects in Platelet Functions

Fish oils	Aspirin	Antihistamines
Chocolate	Ibuprofen (NSAIDs)	Phenytoin
Red wine	Ticlopidine	Dipyridamole
Garlic	Penicillins	Ethanol
Herbs	Cephalosporins	Furosemide
Abciximab	Nitrofurantoin	Thiazide diuretics
Eptifibatide	Theophyllines	Halothane
Clopidogrel	Caffeine	Nitroprusside
Chemotherapy	Estrogen	Prostaglandins

sometimes be life threatening. Thrombocytopenia can also be seen in various autoimmune disorders, patients with acquired immunodeficiency syndrome (AIDS), and after massive volume resuscitation. The goal of treatment is replacement of the platelets with transfusion. One unit of platelets should raise the platelet count by 5000/mm³, with a goal of maintaining the count greater than 50,000/mm³. Treating the underlying cause of the thrombocytopenia, if known, will have greater benefit than transfusions. As more platelets are transfused, the patient is more likely to produce antibodies toward the platelets and decrease the half-life of the infusion.

A common cause of thrombocytopenia in the surgery patient is heparin-induced autoantibodies. These patients will generally present with a precipitous drop in the platelet count that returns to normal on discontinuation. Newer drugs derived from snake venom and leaches may be used in these patients if anticoagulation is necessary.

BIBLIOGRAPHY

Owings J, Gosselin R. Bleeding and transfusion. In: Wilmore D, Cheung L, Harken A, Holcroft J, Meakins J, Soper N, eds. *ACS Surgery: Principles and Practice*. New York, NY: WebMD; 2002:77–90.

Rutherford E, Brecher M, Fakhry S, et al. Hematologic principles in surgery. In: Townsend C, Beauchamp RD, Evers BM, Mattox KL, eds. *Sabiston Textbook of Surgery: The Biological Basis of Modern Surgical Practice*. 18th ed. Philadelphia, PA: Elsevier Saunders; 2008:113–142.

10. **(E)** The two most common genetically transmitted defects in the clotting factors are the absence of factor VIII (hemophilia type A) and factor IX (hemophilia type B). Both of these diseases are inherited as X-linked recessive disorders, with males almost exclusively affected. Hemophilias can have varying penetrance, with mild cases having 5% normal factor levels to a more severe form with levels less than 1%. In contrast to patients with platelet disorders, these patients will have spontaneous bleeding, deep bleeding, and hemarthroses.

Type A is the most common form and is seen in 70–80% of factor-deficient patients. These patients will have a prolonged aPTT with normal PT and bleeding times. DDAVP is effective for mild hemophilia A. As with vWD, administration of DDAVP will raise the levels of factor VIII. This is sometimes the only treatment needed for minor trauma or dental procedures. For more severe cases, the use of FFP, cryoprecipitate, or factor VIII concentrate is necessary. The use of FFP requires large volumes and is therefore a second-line treatment. Goal factor levels for minor surgery are usually 20–30% of normal, whereas 50–80% of normal levels are needed for major surgery. As with vWD, DDAVP is less effective if given repeatedly.

Type B or Christmas disease is the second most common clotting factor–deficient disorder and is seen is 15% of cases. Symptoms and laboratory findings with type B are identical to type A except for a decrease in factor IX levels. DDAVP will not be effective in this disorder. Standard treatment of type B bleeding is with prothrombin complex concentrate, which contains all of the vitamin K clotting factors, or factor IX concentrate, which is also available.

Defects in the production of other clotting factors have been noted and are generally secondary to point mutations and are extremely rare (<5%). Most cases, if diagnosed, can be treated effectively with FFP. Patients in hepatic failure will also have an acquired form with deficiencies in the vitamin K clotting factors. In contrast to hemophiliacs, they will have an elevated PT.

BIBLIOGRAPHY

Cogbill T. Abnormal operative and postoperative bleeding. In: Cameron J, ed. *Current Surgical Therapy*. 10th ed. Philadelphia, PA: Elsevier Saunders; 2011:1088–1091.

Owings J, Gosselin R. Bleeding and transfusion. In: Wilmore D, Cheung L, Harken A, Holcroft J, Meakins J, Soper N, eds. *ACS Surgery: Principles and Practice*. New York, NY: WebMD; 2002:77–90.

11. **(E)** DIC is characterized by widespread formation of thrombin with suppression of physiologic anticoagulant mechanisms and abnormal fibrinolysis. Several diseases are known to cause DIC (see Table 4-4). Tissue damage caused by burns releases TF, IL-1β, and TNF-α directly into the circulation and initiates the DIC pathway. Infection-related causes are generally thought to be caused by gram-negative bacteria, whereby lipopolysaccharide (LPS) and endotoxins from gram-positive

TABLE 4-4 Causes of Acute DIC

Sepsis and septic shock—generally an endotoxin- or exotoxin-related event

Obstetric accidents
   Amniotic fluid embolism—presence of mucus or meconium from the stressed fetus potentiates the thrombotic events
   Abruptio placentae—TF-like material is released from the placenta
   Retained fetus syndrome—necrotic fetal tissue activates the procoagulant system
   Abortion induced by hypertonic saline

Hematologic and oncologic diseases
   Solid tumors—activate procoagulant systems as they become necrotic
   Acute leukemias—caused by release of procoagulants from promyelocytes on administration of chemotherapy
   Intravascular hemolysis—release of ADP from red cells after transfusion reactions
   Myeloproliferative diseases—various anecdotal reports

Viremias (viral hepatitis, cytomegalovirus [CMV], and varicella)
Trauma
Thermal injury
Kasabach-Merritt's syndrome (giant cavernous hemangiomata)
Metabolic abnormalities—acidosis leads to sloughing of the endothelium with activation of coagulation

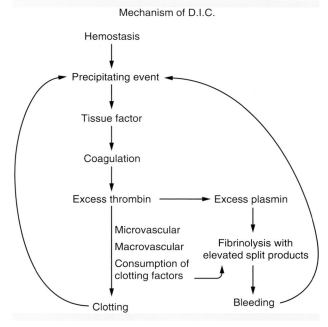

FIGURE 4-11. Mechanism of disseminated intravascular coagulation depicting activation of coagulation with excess thrombin formation. Thrombin leads to excess clotting in both micro- and macrovascular vessels, leading to end-organ damage and potentiating the effects of the cascade. Thrombin also leads to excess degradation of fibrin, leading to bleeding, hypotension, shock, and vascular permeability, resulting in worsening of the cascade.

BIBLIOGRAPHY

Cuff R. Coagulopathy in the critically ill patient. In: Cameron J, ed. *Current Surgical Therapy*. 10th ed. Philadelphia, PA: Elsevier Saunders; 2011:1169–1174.

Arruda VR, High KA. Coagulation Disorders. In: Kasper D, Fauci A, Hauser S, Longo D, Jameson J, Loscalzo J. eds. *Harrison's Principles of Internal Medicine*. 19th ed. New York, NY: McGraw-Hill; 2015.

organisms are known to activate the diffuse coagulation seen in DIC.

Thrombin induces the formation of tumor necrosis factor (TNF), IL-1, IL-6, endothelin, and selectin, inducing vascular permeability and end-organ damage. In addition to clot formation and subsequent unchecked fibrinolysis, thrombin leads to the activation of the complement cascade, which produces hypotension, shock, and further exacerbation of DIC (see Fig. 4-11).

Laboratory findings in DIC include the prolonged PT and/or aPTT, thrombocytopenia, schistocytes (fragmented red cells) in the blood smear, and elevated levels of fibrin split products. Of these, the most sensitive test for DIC is the presence of elevated levels of fibrin split products. The D-dimer test is more specific for detection of fibrin split products and indicates that the crosslinked fibrin has been digested by plasmin.

12. **(D)** Several commercially available tests are currently on the market for measurement of platelet function. The first and most often used test to measure platelet function is the peripheral platelet count. Modern equipment measures platelet counts through impedance measurements or through light-scattering properties, similar to a flow cytometer. These machines are generally easy to use and highly reproducible and require a small amount of whole blood in ethylene diaminetetraacetate (EDTA). They will often underestimate or overestimate the count in patients with certain diseases; smaller platelets are missed, or larger particles are counted separately. Newer protocols utilizing fluorochromes such as anti-CD61 with flow cytometry have led to more precise measurements of the platelet

count. The platelet count is a poor indicator of true platelet function. A patient may have a normal platelet count but a severe dysfunction of the platelets.

The most commonly used screening of *in vivo* physiologic clotting is assessment of the bleeding time. This is performed by making a standardized incision in the skin and accessing the length of time until clot formation. This test, although clinically useful, is highly operator dependent, poorly reproducible, and invasive and does not correlate with certain bleeding disorders. This test is being slowly replaced by better *in vitro* measurements that simulate *in vivo* bleeding.

The "gold standard" for platelet function is based on the aggregation properties of the platelets. This is formed by obtaining platelet-rich plasma after centrifugation. Platelets are then stimulated to aggregate, and as they adhere to one another, the properties of the light scattering are measured and recorded. Dysfunctional platelets cause the light scatter to change more slowly, and distinctive patterns will appear, leading to a diagnosis. Several commercially available products are available that use these properties for analyses.

Hemostasis is a combination of several different factors, including platelet function, interaction of clotting factors (both procoagulant and anticoagulant), and fibrin formation to effectively seal vessel injury and develop clots. The dynamics of these interactions are complex in nature, and faults in any step can lead to abnormal clot formation. Use of accurate bedside point-of-care tests, such as the thromboelastograph (TEG) and rotational thromboelastometry (ROTEM), avoids a number of the pitfalls associated with conventional laboratory-based hemostasis testing. Both systems mentioned measure the time to initial clot formation as well as fibrinogen and platelet function and fibrinolysis. The systems have been useful in management of patients undergoing liver transplantation and cardiac surgery and are increasingly used in trauma centers.

The TEG (Haemoscope Corporation, Niles, IL) system measures the clot's physical properties using a cylindrical cup that holds the blood as it oscillates through an angle of 4°45′ (see Fig. 4-12). Each rotation cycle lasts 10 s. The pin is suspended in the blood by a torsion wire and is monitored for motion. The torque of the rotating cup is transmitted to the immersed pin only after fibrin or fibrin-platelet bonding has linked the cup and pin together. The strength and rate of these fibrin or fibrin-platelet bonds affect the magnitude of the pin motion, such that strong clots move the pin directly in phase with cup motion. As the clot retracts, or lyses, these bonds are broken, and transfer of cup motion is diminished. A mechanical-electrical transducer converts the rotation of the pin into an electrical signal that can be monitored by a computer.

The resulting hemostasis profile (see Figs. 4-13 and 4-14) is a measure of the time it takes for the first fibrin

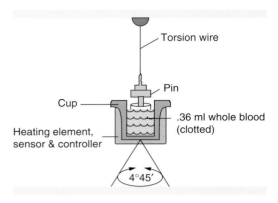

FIGURE 4-12. Cross-sectional view of the current TEG system (reproduced with permission, Haemoscope Corporation, Skokie, IL).

strand to be formed, the kinetics of clot formation, the strength of the clot (in either millimeters or in shear elasticity units of dyn/cm^2), and dissolution of clot. This profile is advantageous as it provides a numerical and graphic representation of coagulation and can differentiate between hyper- and hypocoagulable states. One of the disadvantages to the TEG is that it is not able to identify platelet dysfunction secondary to aspirin use as platelet adhesion is not tested with this system.

The TEG system has proved reliable in helping to diagnose patients with blunt trauma who are more likely to need a blood transfusion within the first 24 h. Approximately 85% of patients who have a hypocoagulable tracing will need blood products, compared to only 4% of patients who are hypercoagulable and almost no patients who have normal tracings. Although TEG has been used in research, it is underutilized by many clinicians in the clinical setting.

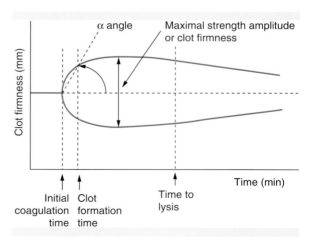

FIGURE 4-13. TEG system profile; R = reaction time; MA = maximum amplitude (reproduced with permission, Haemoscope Corporation, Skokie, IL).

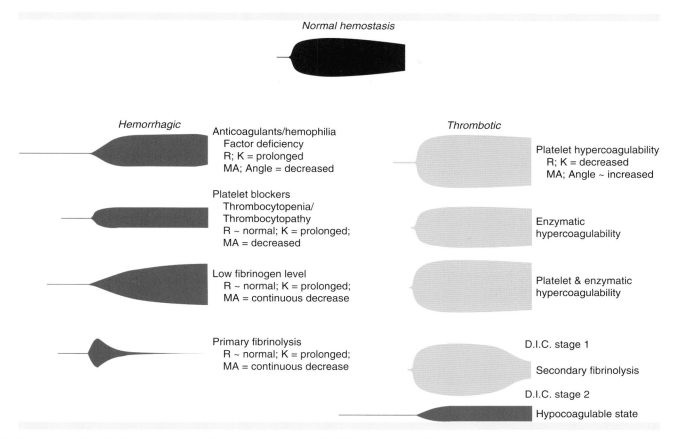

FIGURE 4-14. Qualitative interpretation of results from the TEG system. DIC = disseminated intravascular coagulation; R = reaction time; R + K = time to clot formation; MA (maximum amplitude) = millimeters of clot or strength of clot (reproduced with permission, Haemoscope Corporation, Skokie, IL).

BIBLIOGRAPHY

Streiff M, Haut E. Coagulopathy of trauma: pathogenesis, diagnosis and treatment. In: Cameron J, ed. *Current Surgical Therapy.* 10th ed. Philadelphia, PA: Elsevier Saunders; 2011:1014–1018.

13. **(B)** Patients who have continued bleeding after a surgical or traumatic procedure are usually evaluated with coagulation panels, which consist of PT (INR), aPTT, platelet counts, fibrinogen, and fibrin split product levels. Based on the results of these tests, a general hypothesis and treatment plan can be initiated.

An elevation of the aPTT without a concomitant rise in the PT is almost universally caused by administration of UH. Heparin half-life is approximately 1 h, and discontinuing heparin for 4–6 h will return levels to normal. LMWH does not elevate aPTT, and its activity can be tested with anti-Xa levels. Both UH and LMWH act by binding to ATIII and ultimately lowering thrombin levels. They can be reversed with the administration of protamine. Protamine is associated with anaphylactic reactions, hypotension, and pulmonary hypertension and should be used cautiously. FFP does not contain thrombin but does contain a sufficient amount of ATIII, which will likely potentate the effects of the heparin. vWD will commonly cause a slight elevation in the aPTT. This can be confirmed by performing platelet function analysis. Correction can be performed with DDAVP, cryoprecipitate, or purified (not recombinant) factor VIII.

The most common factor deficiencies are of IX and VIII. When factor levels fall below 40%, then the aPTT will start to be elevated. If mixing studies are performed, then the aPTT should normalize, revealing this to be a factor deficiency, not an inhibitor, causing the problem. Specific factor deficiency tests can be performed to determine which factor is missing, and appropriate therapy can be instituted. Hemophilia A and B are X-linked traits and are rare in females and would result in a passage of the allele through both X genes (see Table 4-5).

TABLE 4-5 Commercially Available Preparations for Treatment of Hemophilia and von Willebrand's Disease

Product Name	Origin
Alphanate, Monarc-M, Hermofil M, Humate, Koate-HP, Monoclate-P	Purified factor VIII from plasma; contains vWF for treatment of vWD
Recombinate, Kogenate, Bioclate, Helixate	Recombinant factor VIII; does not contain any vWF
Hyate:C	Porcine plasma
Autoplex T, Feiba VH Immuno, Mononine, AlphaNine-SD, Bebulin VH Immuno, Proplex T, Konyne 80, Profilnine SD	Purified factor IX from plasma
BeneFix	Recombinant factor IX
Novo Seven	Recombinant factors IX and VIII

BIBLIOGRAPHY

Cogbill T. Abnormal operative and postoperative bleeding. In: Cameron J, ed. *Current Surgical Therapy*. 10th ed. Philadelphia, PA: Elsevier Saunders; 2011:1088–1091.

14. **(A)** FVL was not recognized as an entity until 1994. It is caused by a single-point mutation in the gene for factor V production (FV:Q506 allele) and inherited as an autosomal dominant disorder with highly variable penetrance. Homozygous carriers are more affected than heterozygous individuals. FVL can be found in 4–6% of the general population and 10–33% of patients who develop venous thrombosis, with an overall prevalence in the Western population of about 5%. This incidence makes it the most common inherited disorder of coagulation. The carrier frequency in Hispanic, black, Asian, and native American populations is substantially less, but is existent.

    FVL mutation causes factor Va to be relatively resistant to inactivation by protein C (see Fig. 4-2). Activated protein C (APC) resistance ultimately leads to a hypercoagulable state, and individuals are prone to thrombosis. This is increased in individuals who are exposed to oral contraceptives, major surgery, or prolonged immobilization and relatively sedentary individuals.

    Clinically, FVL presents most commonly with DVT, although pulmonary embolism (PE) and superficial thrombophlebitis are common. Rarely does it present as arterial thromboses. Twenty percent of recurrent miscarriages in the second trimester are associated with FVL. It affects both sexes and all age groups equally.

Because of its high prevalence, it is often found in combination with other genetic defects, such as protein C, S, or ATIII deficiency or antiphospholipid syndrome. These individuals are at higher risk for thrombotic disease than with a single genetic defect.

FVL can be diagnosed with a simple mixing study to determine a patient's clotting time. The patient's blood, either anticoagulated or not, is mixed with plasma-deficient factor V to correct all other abnormalities. A standard aPTT is performed with the blood as well as with blood that has been supplemented with APC. A ratio of supplemented aPTT to unsupplemented aPTT is calculated. Patients with FVL will have a slower clotting time when APC is added compared to controls, leading to a ratio that is less than 2. Normal individuals will have a ratio greater than 2. This procedure is rapid, relatively cheap, and reproducible.

Treatment of patients with venous thrombosis secondary to FVL is with anticoagulation. Long-term preventive strategies have not been determined; however, most physicians will treat patients with recurrent DVTs with warfarin anticoagulation for life. Further studies are under way to determine the duration and type of anticoagulation needed.

BIBLIOGRAPHY

Middeldorp S, Meinardi JR, Koopman MM, et al. A prospective study of asymptomatic carriers of the factor V Leiden mutation to determine the incidence of venous thromboembolism. *Ann Intern Med* 2001;135(5):322–327.

Rutherford E, Brecher M, Fakhry S, et al. Hematologic principles in surgery. In: Townsend C, Beauchamp RD, Evers BM, Mattox KL, eds. *Sabiston Textbook of Surgery: The Biological Basis of Modern Surgical Practice*. 18th ed. Philadelphia, PA: Elsevier Saunders; 2008:113–142.

15. **(B)** The antiphospholipid syndrome is a collection of diseases resulting from antibodies against phospholipid membranes or associated binding cofactors in the blood. The syndrome was first noted in patients with syphilis who produce a complement-fixing antibody to mitochondrial phospholipids termed *cardiolipin*. This was later the basis for the VDRL test that is still used today.

    Several types of anticardiolipin antibodies have been discovered. These antibodies are primarily of the IgG or IgM types. Some react directly with cardiolipin, whereas others require the presence of the plasma phospholipid-binding protein β_2GI. This requirement for the presence of the binding protein is specific for patients with systemic lupus erythematosus but not with patients with syphilis. This has led to better tests to differentiate patients with syphilis from those with other noninfectious causes for anticardiolipin production.

Antiphospholipid antibodies are generally found among young healthy individuals, with a prevalence of 1–5%. Among patients with SLE, this can range as high as 12–30%. Affected patients are at a higher risk of venous thrombosis, myocardial infarction, strokes, miscarriages, thrombocytopenia, hemolytic anemia, livedo reticularis, and rarely arterial thrombosis. Renal involvement with hypertension is almost invariably present. Virtually any organ can be involved.

The diagnosis of antiphospholipid syndrome requires the presence of one clinical and one laboratory indicator.

Clinical manifestations required for diagnosis include one of the following:

- Documented episodes of arterial, venous, or small-vessel thrombosis in any tissue.
- One or more unexplained deaths of a morphologically normal fetus beyond the 10th week of gestation.
- One or more premature births of a normal neonate before the 34th week of gestation because of preeclampsia or eclampsia or severe placental insufficiency or three or more unexplained consecutive spontaneous abortions before the 10th week of gestation.

Laboratory diagnosis is based on enzyme-linked immunoassays that require β_2GI and IgM anticardiolipin antibodies. Several different tests and protocols exist; all must be negative to rule out the presence of disease.

Most individuals present with isolated thrombosis. Catastrophic antiphospholipid syndrome is a rare consequence of this disease, and patients will present with the acute and devastating syndrome of multiple thrombosis, usually leading to death. The kidney is the most common organ affected, followed by lungs, CNS, heart, and skin. Thromboses of small vessels tend to predominate, with a syndrome similar to DIC. The mortality rate is 50% and is secondary to multiple organ system failure. Treatment is aimed at removing the antibody with plasmapheresis and steroids as well as anticoagulation and fibrinolytic therapy.

Several studies have been performed looking at the prophylactic treatment of these patients. Aspirin has generally only been shown to help female patients with recurrent miscarriages. Anticoagulation with warfarin to an INR > 2.0 has been shown to reduce both venous and arterial thrombosis; however, discontinuation can lead to recurrent thrombosis and catastrophic antiphospholipid syndrome.

BIBLIOGRAPHY

Gonzalez EA, Jastrow KM, Holcomb JB, Kozar RA. Hemostasis, surgical bleeding, and transfusion. In: Brunicardi FC, Andersen DK, Billiar TR, Dunn DL, Hunter JG, Matthews JB, et al., eds. *Schwartz's Principles of Surgery.* 9th ed. New York, NY: McGraw-Hill; 2010: Chapter 4.

Levine JS, Branch DW, Rauch J. The antiphospholipid syndrome. *N Engl J Med* 2002;346(10):752–763.

Rand JH. Molecular pathogenesis of the antiphospholipid syndrome. *Circ Res* 2002;90(1):29–37.

16. **(A)** Homocysteine is a sulfur-containing amino acid that occurs in the body as a result of metabolism of methionine. These reactions are used in the body to methylate amino acids, for formation of adenosine and tetrahydrofolate, for conversion of thymidylate from uracil, and for conversion of glycine from serine. These reactions are summarized in Fig. 4-15. Any defect in these pathways can lead to an increase in homocysteine leading to homocystinuria or hyperhomocysteinemia.

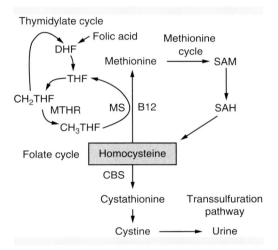

FIGURE 4-15. Methionine metabolism. DHR, dihydrofolate; CBS, cysthathionine beta-synthase; MS, methionine synthase; MTHR, methylenetetrahydrofolate reductase; SAH, S-adenosyl homocysteine; SAM, S-adenosyl methionine; THR, tetrahydrofolate.

Levels of homocysteine can be elevated for a variety of genetic and environmental factors. Enzyme deficiencies of cysthathionine beta-synthase (CBS), methylenetetrahydrofolate reductase (MTHR), and methionine synthase (MS), chronic renal failure, hypothyroidism, neoplasms, methotrexate, phenytoin, or theophylline are known to raise levels of homocysteine. Dietary or absorptional deficiencies of B_{12} can lead to elevation of homocysteine.

Mild hyperhomocysteinemia is often seen in patients with dietary, environmental, or heterozygote deficiency of MTHR or CBS. Unlike other prothrombotic diseases, there is strong evidence that links this disease with elevated risk of both arterial and venous thrombosis. There is a two- to four-fold increase in the risk of coronary artery disease (CAD) and DVTs. One meta-analysis showed that hyperhomocysteine was found in 21.7% of CAD, 26.6% of cerebrovascular accident (CVA), 32.8%

of peripheral vascular disease (PVD), and 13.8% of DVT patients.

Very high levels of homocysteine are found in patients devoid of either CBS or MTHR. These patients have a high level of arterial (usually CAD) and venous thrombosis as well as increased risks of skeletal and ocular problems as well as mental retardation/developmental delay. Prevalence in United States is not fully known but thought to be rare.

Mechanisms by which homocysteine causes thrombotic complications are not fully understood. One popular theory involves direct toxicity to the endothelium; however, homocysteine is known to potentiate the oxidation of LDL cholesterol, affect arachidonic acid metabolism, cause expression of thrombomodulin, activate factor V, and inhibit protein C.

Homocysteine levels are determined after fasting overnight. A postmethionine load test is often frequently performed. Homocysteine levels are determined 4–6 h after oral administration of 0.1 g/kg of methionine.

Treatment of homocysteine is accomplished by saturating the body of B_{12} and folate. This is designed to overcome the effects of mild enzyme deficiency and drive the pathway toward reducing homocysteine levels. No trials are currently under way looking at novel enzyme replacements or other drug replacement possibilities. Folate supplementation of grains by the FDA was done to lower levels of neural tube defects, and this supplementation level is too low to cause a significant decrease in homocysteine levels.

BIBLIOGRAPHY

Federman DG, Kirsner RS. An update on hypercoagulable disorders. *Arch Intern Med* 2001;161(8):1051–1056.
Seligsohn U, Lubetsky A. Hereditary thrombophilia. In: Prchal JT, Kaushansky K, Lichtman MA, Kipps TJ, Seligsohn U, eds. *Williams Hematology*. 8th ed. New York, NY: McGraw-Hill; 2010: Chapter 131.

17. **(D)** Prothrombin is a vitamin K-dependent protein that is the precursor to thrombin created during the coagulation cascade described previously. Prothrombin G20210a substitution, along with FVL, is one of the most common genetic disorders leading to thrombophilia. It is caused by replacement of G by A at nt 20210 in the 3′-untranslated region of the prothrombin gene, which augments translation and stability of prothrombin messenger ribonucleic acid (mRNA). This leads to decreased effectiveness of the prothrombinase complex to produce thrombin. As such, prothrombin levels are elevated. Heterozygous carriers were found to have approximately 30% higher levels than noncarriers. The change in ratio of

prothrombin to thrombin is thought to be the cause of this disease's thrombotic effects.

The prevalence of this mutation varies greatly among the world's population. It is almost entirely a disease of whites. The prevalence among healthy controls varies from 0.7 to 4.0%, whereas 4 to 8% of patients presenting with a first episode of thrombosis were found to have the mutation. This represents a relative risk of 2 to 7 compared with the general population.

BIBLIOGRAPHY

Federman DG, Kirsner RS. An update on hypercoagulable disorders. *Arch Intern Med* 2001;161(8):1051–1056.
Seligsohn U, Lubetsky A. Hereditary thrombophilia. In: Prchal JT, Kaushansky K, Lichtman MA, Kipps TJ, Seligsohn U, eds. *Williams Hematology*. 8th ed. New York, NY: McGraw-Hill; 2010: Chapter 131.

18. **(D)** General surgery patients can be classified into three groups based on their risk for DVT formation and on the risk factors listed in Table 4-6.

TABLE 4-6 Risk Factors for Developing DVT

History of DVT or PE	Prolonged immobility or paralysis	Cancer
Obesity (>20% IBW)	Varicose veins	Stroke or coma
Fractures of the pelvis, hip, or leg	Inflammatory bowel disease	Nephrotic syndrome
Hormone therapy	Hypercoagulable disorders	
IBW = ideal body weight; PE = pulmonary embolism.		

Prophylaxis of all patients includes early ambulation and the use of TED (antiembolism stockings) hose or SCDs from immediately before surgery until full ambulation is achieved. Moderate-risk patients can be treated with either subcutaneous heparin or LMWH, and the dose is adjusted depending on the risk factors. In both moderate- and high-risk patients, the addition of intravenous dextran can be considered. High-risk patients should be started on warfarin the day of or day after surgery, with dose adjusted to achieve an INR of 1.5–3 (see Table 4-7).

Major trauma patients are considered at high risk from thromboembolism. All patients should be started on a heparin-based regimen unless contraindicated.

TABLE 4-7 DVT Risk Stratification

Low risk—uncomplicated minor surgery (general anesthesia < 30 min) in patients < 40 years old with no clinical risk factors

Moderate risk
   Any surgery in patients 40–60 years old with no clinical risk factors
   Major surgery in patients < 40 years old with no additional risk factors
   Minor surgery in patients with risk factors

High risk
   Major surgery in patients > 60 years old with no additional risk factors
   Major surgery in patients 40–60 years old with additional risk factors
   Patients with myocardial infarction

Very high risk—Major surgery in patients > 40 years old with prior history of DVT, PE, cancer, or hypercoagulable state

SCDs or TED hose should be used until heparin is started. If a patient is at high risk for thromboembolism and has suboptimal prophylaxis, then an IVC filter should be considered.

Trials have been performed looking at the timing of starting LMWH. Most studies showed an inherent advantage of starting LMWH 2 h before operation. This has an added benefit of preventing DVTs during operation and in the immediate postoperative period. If bleeding is a concern, then the dose can be given up to 12 h prior to major operations.

Clopidogrel and other antiplatelet drugs have been shown to reduce DVT in the general surgery patients by as much as 37%; however, these studies appear misleading, and no consensus statement on the use of these drugs has been produced at this time.

BIBLIOGRAPHY

Freischlag J, Heller J. Venous disease. In: Townsend C, Beauchamp RD, Evers BM, Mattox KL, eds. *Sabiston Textbook of Surgery: The Biological Basis of Modern Surgical Practice.* 18th ed. Philadelphia, PA: Elsevier Saunders; 2008:2002–2019.

19. **(E)** Patients with multiple injuries are at a significant risk for venous thrombotic disease. Major risk factors for the development of venous thromboembolism include severe head injury (GCS ≤ 9), paralysis, major pelvic fracture, major lower extremity fracture, and repair of a major lower extremity vein. These factors are in addition to the preinjury risk factors listed in Table 4-6.

Patients who are considered high risk for thromboembolic complications should undergo prophylaxis with both SCDs and LMWH. Patients who are unable to undergo full prophylaxis should be considered for prophylactic IVC filter placement within 48 h of admission. Orthopedic fractures are not a contraindication for compression devices. Foot pumps can be used in this situation. Intracranial bleeding is a contraindication for both LMWH and warfarin use.

An IVC filter can be easily and safely placed in the ICU setting. Most filters are placed by experienced radiologists using fluoroscopy. IVC filters have also been deployed successfully with ultrasound guidance. The morbidity and mortality with vena caval filter insertion is extremely low. Several studies have examined both short-term and long-term complication rates of prophylactic IVC filter insertions. Complications include groin hematomas, arteriovenous (AV) fistulas, incomplete opening, and misplacement and occur in approximately 1.6–2% of patients. Long-term complications include caval penetration, 0–2%; migration, 1–5%; filter occlusion, 2–4%; and insertion site thrombosis, 2–6%. Prophylactic placement can offer up to a 98% protection rate from PE, which can be fatal. The safety and added benefit of prophylactic IVC filter placement should be considered in patients with major trauma who are unable to undergo full DVT prophylaxis.

BIBLIOGRAPHY

Freischlag J, Heller J. Venous disease. In: Townsend C, Beauchamp RD, Evers BM, Mattox KL, eds. *Sabiston Textbook of Surgery: The Biological Basis of Modern Surgical Practice.* 18th ed. Philadelphia, PA: Elsevier Saunders; 2008:2002–2019.

Henke P. Venous thromboembolism: diagnosis, prevention and treatment. In: Cameron J, ed. *Current Surgical Therapy.* 10th ed. Philadelphia, PA: Elsevier Saunders; 2011:867–873.

20. **(A)** Warfarin and its derivatives act by blocking the formation of the vitamin K–dependent clotting factors (II, VII, IX, and X and proteins C and S). The proteins lack the carboxyglutamic acid residue that is necessary to bind calcium. As such, the extrinsic pathway is primarily affected, with elevations seen in the PT and only slight elevations in the aPTT. Warfarin has a half-life of 40 h, and its effects can be reversed quickly with the use of FFP or slightly slower with vitamin K administration or by stopping the drug altogether.

Trauma in the face of anticoagulation with warfarin would intuitively seem to cause a greater tendency for bleeding, leading to increased mortality; however, several retrospective analyses have been done to see if preinjury warfarin use correlated with increased mortality. In two case-matched series, the use of warfarin did not have an adverse impact on mortality or length-of-stay outcomes in both head- and non–head-injured patients. It was noted that the warfarin-treated cohort without a head injury was less likely to be discharged home and needed skilled nursing or rehabilitation center assistance on discharge. This was not seen in the head-injured patients.

These studies, however, failed to compare mechanism of injury, which could show that patients on warfarin may have lower GCS scores, higher injury severity scores, and higher ASCOT (A Severity Characterization of Trauma) scores for the same type of mechanism.

BIBLIOGRAPHY

Kennedy DM, Cipolle MD, Pasquale MD, Wasser T. Impact of pre-injury warfarin use in elderly trauma patients. *J Trauma Injury Infect Crit Care* 2000;48(3):451–453.

Pieracci FM, Kashuk JL, Moore EE. Postinjury hemotherapy and hemostasis. In: Mattox KL, Moore EE, Feliciano DV, eds. *Trauma.* 7th ed. New York, NY: McGraw-Hill; 2013: Chapter 13.

Wojcik R, Cipolle MD, Seislove E, Wasser TE, Pasquale MD. Preinjury warfarin does not impact outcome in trauma patients. *J Trauma Injury Infect Crit Care* 2001;51(6):1147–1151; discussion: 1151–1142.

21. **(D)** Transfusion reactions can be categorized broadly into acute (<24 h) and delayed (>24 h) reactions. Hemolytic transfusion reactions occur secondary to the presence of antigens on the RBCs that are infused into a patient, who possesses or develops antibodies to the antigen. This activates a complement-mediated destruction of the RBCs, leading to cytokine release, hypotension, decreased renal blood flow, activation of the coagulation cascade, and ultimately DIC. Early signs and symptoms of a reaction are caused by the histamine release and present as pain and redness at the site of infusion, chest tightness, impending feeling of doom, and oozing from open skin sites. Laboratory evaluation includes urine analysis for hemoglobinuria, lactate dehydrogenase (LDH), haptoglobin, and indirect bilirubin. A direct Coombs test will be positive and is considered diagnostic.

Acute hemolytic reactions most often occur secondary to incompatibility with the major antigens A, B, O, and Rh. Clerical errors are the most common reason for mismatched blood transfusion. There are several steps along the way for errors to occur, from blood drawing and labeling specimens, laboratory processing, and matching of unit and patient prior to transfusions. Other minor antigens are also present on RBCs and can participate in reactions despite proper cross-matching and infusion of correctly assigned units.

When a reaction is suspected, the infusion should be stopped immediately and the unit returned to the blood bank along with a sample of the patient's blood for detection of major and minor antigens and to see if the correct unit of blood was infused. Treatment of the patient should begin immediately with infusion of antipyretics and histamine blockers. Supportive care should be given to the patient and signs and symptoms of DIC treated aggressively. Mainstays of treatment are fluid resuscitation to maintain renal blood flow and prevent renal tubular necrosis and diuresis following fluid resuscitation to maintain urine flow. Patients who develop DIC early are at greatest risk of mortality.

Delayed transfusion reactions occur 5 to 10 days after transfusion with symptoms of jaundice, fever, or precipitous fall in hematocrit. These nonhemolytic reactions are thought to be caused by recipient antibodies to infused donor plasma proteins One study also examined reactions given with autologous blood and noticed a reaction in 2.1% of all patients given autologous blood both in preoperative stored units and with blood salvaged during the operative procedure.

BIBLIOGRAPHY

Chen CL, Shapiro ML, Angood PB, Makary MA. Patient safety. In: Brunicardi FC, Andersen DK, Billiar TR, Dunn DL, Hunter JG, Matthews JB, et al., eds. *Schwartz's Principles of Surgery.* 9th ed. New York, NY: McGraw-Hill; 2010: Chapter 12.

Rutherford E, Brecher M, Fakhry S, et al. Hematologic principles in surgery. In: Townsend C, Beauchamp RD, Evers BM, Mattox KL, eds. *Sabiston Textbook of Surgery: The Biological Basis of Modern Surgical Practice.* 18th ed. Philadelphia, PA: Elsevier Saunders; 2008:113–142.

22. **(C)**

23. **(D)**

Explanations 22 and 23

Whole blood obtained from volunteers is rarely used in the United States, and many blood banks do not routinely store this product. Once a unit of whole blood is donated, it is quickly broken down into subcomponents for more efficient use of the blood and optimization of therapeutic potency. Whole blood can be stored in citrate phosphate dextrose adenine (CPDA) 1 or citrate phosphate dextrose (CPD), with a shelf life of approximately 35 days.

Packed RBCs are obtained by centrifugation of whole blood to separate the plasma and platelet components from the red cell mass. This process increases the hematocrit to approximately 80% and can be stored for 35 days in CPDA-1 or 42 days in AS-1 (Adsol) at 1–6°C. Solutions containing some combination of dextrose, adenine, sodium chloride, and either phosphate (AS-3) or mannitol (AS-1 and AS-5) extend the storage life of red cells, but longer storage decreases red cell viability. Packed RBCs contain essentially no platelets and levels of factors V and VIII are unstable.

The plasma component is then further centrifuged to pellet the platelets. It is then pooled with that of 6–10 other donors to provide one unit of pooled platelets. Alternatively, a single donor unit can be obtained by apheresis. This is especially useful for patients who have developed antibodies against specific platelet types and will help prevent immune destruction of donor cells. The plasma component is immediately frozen at –18 to –30°C to preserve clotting factor function (FFP). It can be thawed to 4°C to remove the cryoprecipitate component.

Each of these components can then be specialized to meet the needs of the patients. Leukocyte-reduced RBCs can be obtained to reduce the HLA components within the blood and reduce reactions and immunosuppression. Deglycerolized RBCs are available and can be stored frozen up to 3 years, allowing for stockpiling of rare blood units. Leukocyte concentrate can be obtained and used in patients with profound granulocytopenia; however, some blood banks and hospitals do not carry these special units secondary to cost and lack of support for their use (see Table 4-8).

BIBLIOGRAPHY

Chen CL, Shapiro ML, Angood PB, Makary MA. Patient safety. In: Brunicardi FC, Andersen DK, Billiar TR, Dunn DL, Hunter JG, Matthews JB, et al., eds. *Schwartz's Principles of Surgery*. 9th ed. New York, NY: McGraw-Hill; 2010: Chapter 12.

Rutherford E, Brecher M, Fakhry S, et al. Hematologic principles in surgery. In: Townsend C, Beauchamp RD, Evers BM, Mattox KL, eds. *Sabiston Textbook of Surgery: The Biological Basis of Modern Surgical Practice*. 18th ed. Philadelphia, PA: Elsevier Saunders; 2008:113–142.

24. **(E)** Transfusion of blood products is not without risk. Aside from transfusion reactions, blood products are potentially hazardous substances containing infectious agents. In the 1980s, one in ten patients transfused developed a hepatitis infection. Since learning of the risks of transferring diseases such as hepatitis and HIV in blood, blood banks began routinely screening donors and testing for viral components prior to infusion of the blood. This has led to a slow, steady decline in the risk of blood transfusion; however, some infected blood goes undetected, and the risk is still present.

Blood transfusion exposes the recipient to several immune products, which can lead to anywhere from graft-versus-host disease in an immunocompromised patient to increased immunosuppression in cancer patients, leading to recurrence of tumors and poorer prognosis. Gamma-irradiation and leukocyte depletion of blood products can decrease the risk of graft-versus-host disease.

BIBLIOGRAPHY

Chen CL, Shapiro ML, Angood PB, Makary MA. Patient safety. In: Brunicardi FC, Andersen DK, Billiar TR, Dunn DL, Hunter JG, Matthews JB, et al., eds. *Schwartz's Principles of Surgery*. 9th ed. New York, NY: McGraw-Hill; 2010: Chapter 12.

Goodnough LT, Brecher ME, Kanter ME, AuBuchon JP. Medical progress: transfusion medicine (first of two parts)—blood transfusion. *N Engl J Med* 1999;340(6):438–447.

Rutherford E, Brecher M, Fakhry S, et al. Hematologic principles in surgery. In: Townsend C, Beauchamp RD, Evers BM, Mattox KL, eds. *Sabiston Textbook of Surgery: The Biological Basis of Modern Surgical Practice*. 18th ed. Philadelphia, PA: Elsevier Saunders; 2008:113–142.

25. **(C)** Transfusion-related acute lung injury (TRALI) is caused by a number of factors, but usually occurs within 6 h of transfusion and clinically presents as noncardiac pulmonary edema. Patients develop mild dyspnea and pulmonary infiltrates secondary to leukoagglutination and pooling of granulocytes in the recipient's lungs. There are several mechanisms that exist to increase the permeability of the capillary membrane within the lung. One popular mechanism involves the infusion of antibody from the donor that attacks the patient's cells, primarily the neutrophils. Another leading theory involves the formation of lipid products on the donor cell membranes during storage. Patients are at greatest risk of developing acute lung injury in the setting of sepsis as neutrophils play an important role in the pathophysiology of this disease.

The incidence of acute lung injury is low, estimated as 1 in 5000 transfusions; however, some occurs subclinically or the patients die quickly and the disease is unrecognized. Despite this fact, almost 90% of patients recover.

BIBLIOGRAPHY

Luce JA. Anemia and blood transfusion. In: Hall JB, Schmidt GA, Wood LD, eds. *Principles of Critical Care*. 3rd ed. New York, NY: McGraw-Hill; 2005: Chapter 68.

TABLE 4-8 Summary of Available Blood Components

Whole blood	Platelets—single unit from whole blood
Packed RBCs	Platelets—apheresis unit
Leukocyte-reduced RBCs	Fresh frozen plasma
Deglycerolized RBCs	Solvent-/detergent-treated plasma
Leukocyte concentrate	Cryoprecipitate

26. **(E)**

27. **(C)**

Explanations 26 and 27

Blood utilization is an important aspect of surgical management. With the risks of transfusion reactions, disease transmission, and immunosuppression, it is imperative that blood is not infused without rational consideration of its need. Blood is primarily designed to deliver oxygen to the peripheral tissue from the lungs. Therefore, its transfusion should be aimed at raising the ability of the body to deliver oxygen to the peripheral tissue, not as a volume expander. The use of transfusion triggers based on hematocrit should be avoided. Instead, the patient should be evaluated for clinical symptoms of decreased oxygen concentration, such as tachycardia or increased cardiac output, hypoxia, or decreased venous saturation (VO_2) (see Table 4-9).

Hospital utilization reviews and indications for transfusion vary from hospital to hospital and from surgeon to surgeon. The science of blood transfusion and indications is not exact but is based on clinical knowledge and experience. Table 4-10 lists some suggested guidelines for red cell transfusion.

Several policies were set forth during a consensus conference on blood management and surgical practice guidelines in 1995 (see Table 4-11).

It is important to remember when dealing with patients who are Jehovah's Witnesses that their belief is based on their interpretation of the Bible regarding receipt of blood that is separated from the body, it is inherently evil and that they will be eternally doomed if they receive this blood. This includes all products that are derived from human or animal blood, including FFP, cryoprecipitate, and albumin. The clinician must ensure that the patient understands all of their options and is making decisions free of coercion to ensure the best outcomes.

Patients should be counseled on their increased risk of morbidity and mortality and their consent should contain this information as well; however, one must remember that courts have held physicians liable for transfusing these patients despite lifesaving attempts. If this is not agreeable to the surgeon, then the patient should be referred to another physician or center that is able to honor the patient's desire.

In the emergency situation, the physician is often faced with difficult decisions. If a patient has an advance directive, then this must be honored despite the patient's condition. If no advance directive is found, then lifesaving blood can be given; however, one must remember that the patient may not be happy with this after the fact. Most Jehovah's Witnesses would rather die with honor than lose their right for eternal life.

TABLE 4-9   Policies Set Forth by the Consensus Conference: Blood Management and Surgical Practice Guidelines on Surgical Red Blood Cell Transfusion Policies

Policy 1	Transfusion need should be assessed on a case-by-case basis.
Policy 2	Blood should be transfused one unit at a time, followed by an assessment of benefit and further need.
Policy 3	Exposure to allogeneic blood should be limited to appropriate need.
Policy 4	Perioperative blood loss should be prevented or controlled.
Policy 5	Autologous blood should be considered for use as an alternative to allogeneic transfusion.
Policy 6	Efforts should be made to maximize oxygen delivery in the surgical patient.
Policy 7	RBC mass should be increased or restored by means other than RBC transfusion.
Policy 8	The patient should be involved in the transfusion decision.
Policy 9	The reasons for and results of the transfusion decision should be documented contemporaneously in the patient's record.
Policy 10	Hospitals' transfusion policies and procedures should be developed as a cooperative effort that includes input from all those involved in the transfusion decision.
Policy 11	Transfusion practices, both individual and institutional, should be reassessed yearly or more often.

Source: Adapted with permission from Spence RK. Surgical red blood cell transfusion practice policies. *Am J Surg* 1995;170(6S):3S–12S. Copyright 1995, with permission from Excerpta Medica Inc.

TABLE 4-10 Suggested Transfusion Guidelines for Red Blood Cells

Hemoglobin ≤ 8 g/dL or acute blood loss in an otherwise-healthy patient with signs and symptoms of decreased oxygen delivery with two or more of the following:
Estimated or anticipated acute blood loss of ≥ 15% of total blood volume (750 mL in 70-kg male)
Diastolic blood pressure ≤ 60 mmHg
Systolic blood pressure drop ≥ 30 mmHg from baseline
Tachycardia (> 100 bpm)
Oliguria/anuria
Mental status changes
Hemoglobin ≤ 10 g/dL in patients with known increased risk of CAD or pulmonary insufficiency who have sustained or are expected to sustain significant blood loss
Symptomatic anemia with any of the following:
Tachycardia (> 100 bpm)
Mental status changes
Evidence of myocardial ischemia, including angina
Shortness of breath or dizziness with mild exertion
Orthostatic hypotension
Unfounded/questionable indications
To increase wound healing
To improve the patient's sense of well-being
7 ≤ hemoglobin ≤ 10 in otherwise-stable, asymptomatic patient
Mere availability of predonated autologous blood without medical indication

Source: Reprinted from Rutherford E, Brecher M, Fakhry S, et al. Hematologic principles in surgery. In: Townsend C, Beauchamp RD, Evers BM, Mattox KL, eds. *Sabiston Textbook of Surgery: The Biological Basis of Modern Surgical Practice.* 18th ed. Philadelphia, PA: Elsevier Saunders; 2008:113–142, with permission from Elsevier.

TABLE 4-11 Policies Set Forth by the Consensus Conference: Blood Management and Surgical Practice Guidelines on Surgical Management of Jehovah's Witnesses

Policy 1	Accept the limitation that allogeneic blood cannot be used.
Policy 2	Use alternatives to allogeneic blood whenever possible and appropriate.
Policy 3	Discuss consequences with the patient, including the potential for life-threatening hemorrhage and possible death if not transfused.
Policy 4	If unable or unwilling to treat a Jehovah's Witness patient, stabilize and transfer the patient to a sympathetic institution, such as a center for bloodless surgery.
Policy 5	Contact the local Jehovah's Witness liaison committee for information and help.
Policy 6	In an emergency or if a patient is unconscious, look for an advance directive.
Policy 7	Seek legal assistance when dealing with an unconscious or incompetent adult.

Source: Adapted with permission from Spence RK. Surgical red blood cell transfusion practice policies. Appendix 2. *Am J Surg* 1995;170(6S):14S–15S, with permission from Excerpta Medica Inc.

BIBLIOGRAPHY

Coimbra R, Doucet J, Bansal V. Principles of critical care. In: Mattox KL, Moore EE, Feliciano DV, eds. *Trauma*. 7th ed. New York, NY: McGraw-Hill; 2013: Chapter 55.

Cooper Z, Kelly E. Preoperative and postoperative management. In: Zinner MJ, Ashley SW, eds. *Maingot's Abdominal Operations*. 12th ed. New York, NY: McGraw-Hill; 2013: Chapter 2.

Rutherford E, Brecher M, Fakhry S, et al. Hematologic principles in surgery. In: Townsend C, Beauchamp RD, Evers BM, Mattox KL, eds. *Sabiston Textbook of Surgery: The Biological Basis of Modern Surgical Practice*. 18th ed. Philadelphia, PA: Elsevier Saunders; 2008:113–142.

28. **(A)** The act of ANH was proposed by Messemer in 1975. Briefly, it involves removal of the whole blood of a patient immediately before surgery and replacement of the blood volume with a colloid or crystalloid solution to maintain normovolemia. Performed after induction of anesthesia but before commencement of the operative procedure, ANH is tolerated well in most patient populations. The degree of hemodilution depends on the patient's medical status and type of operation performed. Hemodilution to a hematocrit level of 20% is generally safe without contraindications in patients less than 60 years of age. The operation is performed as usual, and the whole blood is reinfused with any massive blood loss after hemostasis is achieved. Contraindications include patients with coronary heart disease, severe aortic stenosis, left ventricular impairment, significant anemia, renal disease, severe hepatic disease, pulmonary emphysema, obstructive lung disease, severe hypertension, or clotting deficiencies.

Several physiologic conditions occur as a result of hemodilution. Mechanisms include a compensatory increase in cardiac output to maintain oxygen delivery, reduction in systemic vascular resistance, increased oxygen extraction, and shift of the oxygen dissociation curve to the right. These processes work together to maintain normal oxygen delivery even at profound (hematocrit < 20%) hemodilution.

Acute normovolemic hemodilution involves storing the whole blood in anticoagulated bags within the operating room. This reduces or nearly eliminates the worry concerning transfusion reactions; however, contamination of the blood can occur with poor aseptic techniques.

BIBLIOGRAPHY

Dorian RS. Anesthesia of the surgical patient. In: Brunicardi FC, Andersen DK, Billiar TR, Dunn DL, Hunter JG, Matthews JB, et al., eds. *Schwartz's Principles of Surgery*. 9th ed. New York, NY: McGraw-Hill; 2010: Chapter 47.

Rutherford E, Brecher M, Fakhry S, et al. Hematologic principles in surgery. In: Townsend C, Beauchamp RD, Evers BM, Mattox KL,

eds. *Sabiston Textbook of Surgery: The Biological Basis of Modern Surgical Practice*. 18th ed. Philadelphia, PA: Elsevier Saunders; 2008:113–142.

29. **(E)** With the knowledge of infectious disease transmission with transfusion, preoperative autologous blood transfusion has become more popular. Patients who are scheduled for elective operations for which the blood loss is expected to be greater than 1000 mL may be considered for autologous blood donation. Several states have made it mandatory that surgeons give patients the option of storing blood prior to surgery.

Before considering preoperative blood donations, patients should have good medical and nutritional status and a hematocrit ≥ 30% prior to undergoing phlebotomy. With monitoring, this procedure is safe even in patients with CAD. Predonation can occur up to 1 month prior to surgery, with blood withdrawn every 3–4 days. Iron supplementation and erythropoietin should be given to enhance erythropoiesis and prevent preoperative anemia.

Although the risk of disease transmission is diminished, this procedure does carry risks as several studies have shown that adverse events, including transfusion reactions, can occur after infusion of autologous blood. Surgeons should also be cautioned against transfusion of blood postoperatively just because the unit exists. Overtransfusion can lead to viscosity issues, pulmonary edema, ischemic events, clerical errors, and other medical problems.

Several controversies exist regarding the complete usefulness of preoperative blood donation. More blood is generally donated than used, making this procedure wasteful (discard rate of 20% to 73% of the units). Cost-effective models illustrate that the benefit-to-risk ratio of preoperative donation is low compared to volunteer donor units. Some studies have shown that preoperative autologous donation may appear to increase the risk of postoperative anemia, thus increasing the likelihood that transfusion will be necessary.

BIBLIOGRAPHY

Rutherford E, Brecher M, Fakhry S, et al. Hematologic principles in surgery. In: Townsend C, Beauchamp RD, Evers BM, Mattox KL, eds. *Sabiston Textbook of Surgery: The Biological Basis of Modern Surgical Practice*. 18th ed. Philadelphia, PA: Elsevier Saunders; 2008:113–142.

30. **(A)** The transfusion of platelets is indicated for patients who are at significant risk of bleeding from thrombocytopenia or platelet dysfunction. Older guidelines recommend transfusion of asymptomatic patients with counts ≤ 20,000/mm³; however, recent studies have determined this to be excessive, and patients can be watched if they

TABLE 4-12 Suggested Transfusion Guidelines for Platelets

Recent (within 24 h) platelet count ≤ 10,000/mm^3 (for prophylaxis)
Recent (within 24 h) platelet count ≤ 50,000/mm^3 with demonstrated microvascular bleeding ("oozing") or a planned surgical/invasive procedure
Demonstrated microvascular bleeding and a precipitous fall in platelet count
Patients in the operating room who have had complicated procedures or have required more than 10 U of blood and have microvascular bleeding; giving platelets assumes adequate surgical hemostasis has been achieved
Documented platelet dysfunction (e.g., prolonged bleeding time [>15 min], abnormal platelet function tests) with petechiae, purpura, microvascular bleeding (oozing), or surgical/invasive procedure

Unwarranted indications
    Empirical use with massive transfusion when patient is not having clinically evident microvascular bleeding (oozing)
    Prophylaxis in thrombotic thrombocytopenic purpura/hemolytic-uremic syndrome or idiopathic thrombocytopenic purpura
    Extrinsic platelet dysfunction (e.g., renal failure, vWD)

Source: Reprinted from Rutherford E, Brecher M, Fakhry S, et al. Hematologic principles in surgery. In: Townsend C, Beauchamp RD, Evers BM, Mattox KL, eds. *Sabiston Textbook of Surgery: The Biological Basis of Modern Surgical Practice.* 18th ed. Philadelphia, PA: Elsevier Saunders; 2008:113–142, with permission from Elsevier.

are asymptomatic. Suggested transfusion guidelines are summarized in Table 4-12.

Platelets are available in two types of preparations. Single-donor units are obtained from a single whole blood donation by one donor. Apheresis platelets are collected from single donors and contain a minimum of 3×10^{11} platelets in 250–300 mL plasma in the preparation. Although the unit is still immunogenic, the amount of HLA and the risk of disease transmission is less.

Pooled units come from separated whole blood from 6 to 10 different donors. These units are highly immunogenic and contain increased risk of disease transmission and antiplatelet antibody production. A six-pack of pooled or one apheresis unit of platelets should raise the patient's count by 30,000/mm^3.

BIBLIOGRAPHY

Rutherford E, Brecher M, Fakhry S, et al. Hematologic principles in surgery. In: Townsend C, Beauchamp RD, Evers BM, Mattox KL, eds. *Sabiston Textbook of Surgery: The Biological Basis of Modern Surgical Practice.* 18th ed. Philadelphia, PA: Elsevier Saunders; 2008:113–142.

31. **(A)** Within the last two decades, several pharmaceutical companies and academic departments have been extensively researching and developing alternatives to packed red cells. This has the potential of eliminating infectious risk, decreasing transfusion reactions, providing an unlimited supply of product, and possibly allowing Jehovah's Witnesses an alternative. Possible indications include trauma, hemorrhagic shock, perioperative blood losses, sepsis, stroke, myocardial infarction, cardiac arrest, and organ perfusion during transplantation, all aimed at increasing the oxygen carrying capacity currently available within the patient.

Products currently being tested generally fall into one of two categories: synthetic molecules, such as the porphyrins and the perfluorocarbon compounds, and molecules that incorporate hemoglobin in their structure, such as conjugated and polymerized stroma-free hemoglobin solutions. To be useful, these products must have the ability to carry as much oxygen as hemoglobin normally carries (1.34 mL of oxygen/g of hemoglobin), have a relatively good shelf life, have an acceptable half-life once infused, and have at least equal mortality compared to allogenic transfusions.

Hemoglobin-based oxygen carriers (HBOCs) are derived from human or bovine hemoglobin or through recombinant techniques. Red cells are lysed, and the hemoglobin is polymerized or pyridoxylated to decrease renal excretion. These solutions have the ability to carry oxygen and stay in the circulation for 4–5 days before clearance by the kidneys. Clinical trials are currently under way for several different preparations, which are being used principally in patients with acute trauma, cardiac surgery, or sepsis.

Perfluorocarbons can transport 40 to 50 mL of oxygen/100 mL of solution, greater than twice the amount of oxygen carried by saturated hemoglobin in an adult. However, human trials have showed limited success, largely due to differences in loading and unloading of oxygen, and the perfluorocarbons are not currently approved for use.

Numerous potential problems exist with red cell substitutes. Iron that is infused with these products enhances bacterial multiplication, leading to increased mortality in septic animal models. It is also taken up by macrophages, leading to an inflammatory response similar to allogeneic transfusions. These products increase nitric oxide metabolism, leading to vasoconstriction, increased pulmonary vascular resistance, oxidative damage, and platelet activation, and they interfere with standard photometric blood tests. A recent meta-analysis found increased rates of myocardial infarction and mortality with use of HBOCs. Other toxicities include renal and liver failure and stroke.

BIBLIOGRAPHY

McIntyre R, Moore F. Blood transfusion therapy. In: Cameron JL, ed. *Current Surgical Therapy*. 10th ed. Philadelphia, PA: Elsevier Saunders; 2010:1007–1013.

Natanson S, Kern SJ, Lurie P, et al. Cell-free hemoglobin-based blood substitutes and risk of myocardial infarction and death: a meta-analysis. *JAMA* 2008;299:2304–2312.

Rutherford E, Brecher M, Fakhry S, et al. Hematologic principles in surgery. In: Townsend C, Beauchamp RD, Evers BM, Mattox KL, eds. *Sabiston Textbook of Surgery: The Biological Basis of Modern Surgical Practice*. 18th ed. Philadelphia, PA: Elsevier Saunders; 2008:113–142.

32. **(A)** Intraoperative and postoperative recovery and reinfusion of patient's blood are two possible sources by which allogenic blood requirements can be diminished. Intraoperative blood recovery is performed by immediately adding heparin to the blood as it is recovered from the body. Pure erythrocytes are then washed, concentrated, and banked in saline free of heparin and returned to the bloodstream by infusion (cell-saver). Some devices have the ability to collect and process 10 units of blood per hour. Cells are not stored in appropriate media to allow for long-term storage and must be used within several hours of processing. Once infused, the red cells have a similar half-life to that of allogenic blood transfusions.

Cell washing does not sterilize the blood. Therefore, the cell-saver technique should not be used in the presence of bacterial contamination. Spreading of malignant cells is also considered a possibility and is generally contraindicated in the setting of cancer. Amniotic or ascitic fluid reintroduction can cause massive DIC and other unwarranted complications and should be avoided. Processed cells contain no plasma component and can precipitate dilutional coagulopathy.

Postoperative recovery of blood includes collections from such devices as chest tubes and surgical drains.

These collections are often diluted or hemolyzed and contain fragments of clots. Therefore, these collections must be used cautiously as the infusion of low-hematocrit fluid into the system may enhance the patient's blood deficit. Contraindications are similar to those for intraoperative cell-washing techniques.

BIBLIOGRAPHY

Goodnough LT, Brecher ME, Kanter ME, AuBuchon JP. Medical progress: transfusion medicine (second of two parts)—blood conservation. *N Engl J Med* 1999;340(7):525–533.

McIntyre R, Moore F. Blood transfusion therapy. In: Cameron JL, ed. *Current Surgical Therapy*. 10th ed. Philadelphia, PA: Elsevier Saunders; 2010:1007–1013.

Rutherford E, Brecher M, Fakhry S, et al. Hematologic principles in surgery. In: Townsend C, Beauchamp RD, Evers BM, Mattox KL, eds. *Sabiston Textbook of Surgery: The Biological Basis of Modern Surgical Practice*. 18th ed. Philadelphia, PA: Elsevier Saunders; 2008:113–142.

33. **(D)** The best method for preventing the need for blood transfusion is obviously good surgical technique and effective surgical hemostasis. Suture material should be chosen based on its properties and the result desired by the surgeon. Suture material is basically categorized as absorbable or nonabsorbable and whether it is monofilament or braided.

The choice of suture to use is based primarily on surgeon preference and by the properties of the suture compared to the task at hand. For short-term hemostasis and approximation of soft tissue, catgut, chromic, and polyglactic acid sutures work the best. They have the shortest tensile strength and are usually gone within 2–4 weeks. Monofilaments tend to slide better through tissue than does the braided; however, the knots will tend to unravel if not laid down correctly. Therefore, if tissue integrity is desired, then a monofilament is a better choice as it will not slice the tissue as it is passed.

All of the sutures listed in Table 4-13 have the ability to produce local and systemic irritation and inflammation. Suture made from animal products such as catgut and chromic tend to cause the highest rate of local irritation, whereas steel rarely causes any local or systemic reaction. Steel is also available in braided and single-strand preparations.

BIBLIOGRAPHY

Rutherford E, Brecher M, Fakhry S, et al. Hematologic principles in surgery. In: Townsend C, Beauchamp RD, Evers BM, Mattox KL, eds. *Sabiston Textbook of Surgery: The Biological Basis of Modern Surgical Practice*. 18th ed. Philadelphia, PA: Elsevier Saunders; 2008:113–142.

TABLE 4-13 Several Commercially Available Suture Products*

	Absorbable	Nonabsorbable
Braided	Polyglactic acid (Vicryl†) Polyglycolic acid (Dexon†)	Nylon (Surgilon†, Neurolon†) Polyester (Ti-Cron†, Ethibond†, Mersiline†) Silk Steel
Monofilament	Catgut Chromic Poliglecaprone 25 (Monocryl†) Polydioxanone (PDS II†) Gylocomer 631 (Biosyn†) Polyglyconate (Maxon†)	Nylon (Ethilon†) Polyester Polypropylene (Prolene†, SurgiPro†) Steel

*Products listed in the same categories do not necessarily have the same tensile properties.
†Brand names are copyright of Ethicon Inc. or United Surgical Steel and Davis and Geck Inc.

34. **(C)** Electrocautery is the method most used for obtaining hemostasis in the operative field. Standard operating room electrocautery can be used as either a bipolar or unipolar instrument. Bipolar settings do not require the patient to be "grounded," and electrons pass from one side of the instrument through the tissue and back through the other side, completing the circuit. Bipolar is used extensively in neurosurgical applications where passage of electrons through the brain tissue is not desired.

Unipolar settings require the patient to be grounded to the machine, and electrons are passed from the tip of the instrument through the adjacent tissue and diffuse through the patient to the grounding pad, completing the circuit. Typical machines can be set on "cutting," which provides a continuous current of electrons to desiccate the tissue but provides little hemostasis, or can be set to "coagulate," for which a sinusoidal pattern of electrons is passed to provide for dehydration and coagulation of vessels without cutting the tissue itself. Some machines allow for mixing or "blending" of these two modalities.

Ligasure (Valley Lab) is a brand of bipolar electrocautery that uses heat to denature proteins within the vessel wall, followed by a cool down under pressure, leading to vessel occlusion. It produces a thin-layer membrane that can easily be transected. Tests using this system showed that burst strengths are similar, if not superior, to clips and sutures.

An argon beam coagulator produces a high-flow stream of argon gas from the tip of the applicator. When placed in proximity to organ parenchyma, it spreads over the surface, blowing away debris and drying the field. Once activated, the argon transmits electricity from the top along the surface of the tissue, causing superficial coagulation of tissue to which the gas has spread. This is performed without excess heat or smoke.

Ultrasonic coagulation devices, such as the Harmonic Scalpel, use ultra-high frequency vibrations to provide cool cutting and coagulation of tissues with little damage to surrounding tissues. This device has found many uses in general surgery to include laparoscopic procedures and hemorrhoidectomy.

Also available are specialized devices that produce lasers, infrared photocoagulation, and radio-frequency ablation, which have their unique properties and uses.

BIBLIOGRAPHY

Neumayer L, Vargo D. Principles of preoperative and operative surgery. In: Townsend C, Beauchamp RD, Evers BM, Mattox KL, eds. *Sabiston Textbook of Surgery: The Biological Basis of Modern Surgical Practice.* 18th ed. Philadelphia, PA: Elsevier Saunders; 2008:251–279.

35. **(C)** Sealants derived from fibrin preparations have been used in Europe for over 20 years. Recently, the FDA approved for use in the United States one commercially available product (Tisseel VH; Baxter/Immuno AG, Vienna, Austria). Most fibrin preparations contain a combination of virally inactivated purified human fibrinogen and thrombin and can be applied in liquid or dried form to the area of injury. These two products are reconstituted in the operating room and are used within seconds to minutes of mixing together; they are applied as a thick liquid gel or aerosolized. Several products, including the US version, contain antifibrinolytic agents such as aprotinin or tranexamic acid (to increase clot stability) and factor XIII, which catalyzes cross-linking between fibrin molecules and cross-links several useful proteins. Addition of these two products to the stability of the sealant is still controversial.

Noncommercially available fibrin sealant is available and is often called "fibrin glue." It is made by mixing fibrinogen with thrombin, calcium chloride, and aprotinin to form a stable clot and applying this to the area of injury. This combination contains approximately 10% of the fibrin concentration of fibrin sealants and is not virally inactivated. Bovine thrombin has been known to cause antifactor V antibodies and severe hypotension on administration.

Fibrin sealants have many uses, including most applications where bleeding or seroma formation is an issue. Fibrin sealants have been used successfully in operative and reoperative cardiac surgery, carotid endarterectomy with polytetrafluorethylene patch angioplasty, circumcisions, bowel anastomosis, tooth extractions, orthopedic surgery, and dura mater closure after neurosurgical procedures to decrease cerebrospinal fluid leakage and to decrease seroma formation after soft tissue flap formation, as with mastectomies. The most useful application of fibrin sealants is in those patients with coagulopathies. Several studies have shown improved efficacy both inside and outside the operating room with patients with factor deficiencies.

BIBLIOGRAPHY

Carless PA, Anthony DM, Henry DA. Systematic review of the use of fibrin sealant to minimize perioperative allogeneic blood transfusion. *Br J Surg* 2002;89(6):695–703.

Fabian TC, Bee TK. Liver and biliary tract. In: Mattox KL, Moore EE, Feliciano DV, eds. *Trauma*. 7th ed. New York, NY: McGraw-Hill; 2013: Chapter 29.

CHAPTER 5

FLUIDS AND ELECTROLYTES

LISA M. MCELROY AND TRAVIS P. WEBB

QUESTIONS

1. A 70-year-old patient underwent transurethral resection of the prostrate. An irrigating solution (of 1.5% glycine) was used to distend the urethra and to obtain a clear surgical field. Postoperatively, he becomes agitated, begins to vomit, and develops muscle twitching, bradyarrythmias, hypertension, and respiratory failure. What is the most likely cause of his symptoms?
   (A) Hyperglycinemia
   (B) Urosepsis
   (C) Hyponatremia
   (D) Hypoxia
   (E) Hypertensive crisis

2. A 28-year-old male presents to the emergency room after falling while working in the yard. He complains of feeling weak and dizzy when he stands up. His supine blood pressure (BP) is 120/60 mmHg with a heart rate of 96 bpm. On standing, he has a BP of 85/30 mmHg and a heart rate of 120 bpm. He states he was fine earlier in the day and drank fluids to try to avoid dehydration. The rest of his examination is unremarkable except for a small laceration on his right elbow. X-rays did not reveal a fracture. His laboratory findings are as follows:

Na$^+$	137	WBC	8.4
K$^+$	5.0	Hgb	16.2
Cl$^-$	101	Hct	48
HCO$_3^-$	28	Plts	345
BUN	45	Urine Na$^+$	10
Cr	1.2	Urine Cr	120

Which of the following would *not* help assist in the diagnosis of volume depletion?
   (A) Urine creatinine
   (B) Serum urea nitrogen (BUN)/creatinine ratio
   (C) Urinary Na
   (D) Fractional excretion of Na
   (E) None of the above would aid in diagnosis

Questions 3 through 11 refer to the following scenario:
A 40-year-old woman with type 1 diabetes mellitus presents to the emergency room 3 days after developing a febrile illness with confusion, a systolic blood pressure of 90 mmHg, a regular heart rate of 120 bpm. Her examination reveals a purulent draining ulcer on the plantar surface of her right foot, and she is admitted to the surgery service. Her laboratory findings are as follows:

Na$^+$	120
K$^+$	7.5
Cl$^-$	86
HCO$_3^-$	10
BUN	40
Cr	1.3
Glucose	1000
Urine	ketones positive and 3+ proteinuria
ABG (arterial blood gas)	7.27/17/95

3. A bladder catheter is placed, and there is minimal urine output. What is the most appropriate intravenous fluid to administer at this time?
   (A) Ringer's lactate
   (B) 3% saline
   (C) 0.9% saline
   (D) 0.9% saline with 20 mEq/L of KCl
   (E) D$_5$W (5% dextrose in water) with three ampules of NaHCO$_3$

4. What is the initial acid-base disorder on the patient's arrival to the emergency room?
   (A) Metabolic acidosis
   (B) Respiratory acidosis
   (C) Metabolic acidosis and respiratory acidosis
   (D) Metabolic acidosis and respiratory alkalosis
   (E) Metabolic alkalosis and respiratory acidosis

5. What is the most likely cause of the hyponatremia?
   (A) Urinary salt wasting from diabetic kidney disease
   (B) Syndrome of inappropriate antidiuretic hormone (SIADH)
   (C) Hypovolemia
   (D) Hyperlipidemia
   (E) Dilutional

6. Which of the following would *least* likely explain the presence of hyperkalemia in this patient?
   (A) Decreased distal urinary flow
   (B) Metabolic acidosis
   (C) Insulin deficiency
   (D) Serum hyperosmolality
   (E) None of the above cause hyperkalemia

7. Which of the following does *not* lower serum K concentrations?
   (A) $CaCl_2$
   (B) Albuterol
   (C) Epinephrine
   (D) Insulin
   (E) Kayexalate

8. Which of the following is *least* effective in lowering the serum K concentration?
   (A) Albuterol
   (B) Hemodialysis
   (C) Bicarbonate
   (D) Insulin
   (E) Kayexalate

The patient from the preceding scenario receives 5 L of intravenous 0.9% saline and an insulin drip. Her vital signs stabilize, and her urine output increases to 50 mL/h. Her laboratory findings 4 h later are as follows:

Na^+	136
K^+	4.0
Cl^-	110
HCO_3^-	18
BUN	20
Cr	0.7
Glucose	300
PO_4^-	1.7
ABG	7.32/32/102

9. What is the patient's current acid-base disorder?
   (A) Metabolic acidosis with anion gap (AG)
   (B) Metabolic acidosis without AG
   (C) Metabolic acidosis with respiratory acidosis
   (D) Metabolic acidosis with respiratory alkalosis
   (E) Metabolic acidosis and alkalosis with respiratory alkalosis (triple disorder)

10. What is the most likely cause of the acid-base disorder?
    (A) Intravenous administration of sodium chloride solution
    (B) Loss of potential bicarbonate in the urine
    (C) Diabetic diarrhea
    (D) Low serum aldosterone levels associated with diabetic kidney disease
    (E) Renal tubular acidosis (RTA)

11. What is the most appropriate intravenous fluid to administer at this point?
    (A) 0.45% saline
    (B) D_5W 0.45% saline
    (C) D_5W 0.45% saline with 20 mEq KCl
    (D) D_5W 0.45% saline with 20 mM KPO_4
    (E) Ringer's lactate

12. Which of the following medications is mostly likely to cause hyponatremia?
    (A) Furosemide
    (B) Thiazide diuretic
    (C) Lithium
    (D) Demeclocyline
    (E) Lovastatin

13. Which of the following is *not* an action of angiotensin II?
    (A) Aldosterone secretion
    (B) Sodium absorption
    (C) Efferent arteriolar constriction
    (D) Arterial dilation
    (E) Nephrosclerosis in the kidney

14. All of the following symptoms are seen with hypermagnesemia *except*
    (A) Tachypnea
    (B) Depression of reflexes
    (C) Arrhythmias
    (D) Hypotension
    (E) Central nervous system depression

15. Which of the following is *not* a complication of hypophosphatemia?
    (A) Muscle weakness
    (B) Respiratory failure
    (C) Hemolysis
    (D) Seizures
    (E) Rhabdomyolysis

Questions 16 and 17 refer to the following scenario:
An 80-year-old man is admitted to the hospital from his nursing home for severe obtundation and possibly dehydration. He is diabetic and receiving tube feedings. The day before admission, he was found on the floor in his room, semicomatose. His urine volume was 1.5 L within the first 12 h. Some of his vitals and laboratory findings are as follows:

Blood pressure	128/60 mmHg
Na^+	170 mEq/L
Cl^-	130 mEq/L
Blood glucose	410 mg/dL
BUN	100 mg/dL
Creatinine	1.5 mg/dL
Serum osmolality	396 mOsm/L
Urine osmolality	408 mOsm/L

16. Which of the following statements is true?
    (A) He has simple central diabetes insipidus.
    (B) He has severe hyperchloremia and therefore resultant acidosis.
    (C) To be described as polyuric, he needs to make a minimum of 4.0 L per day of urine.
    (D) He has ongoing osmotic diuresis.
    (E) His well-preserved blood pressure shows that he is not severely volume depleted.

17. Given that he weighs 80 kg, his estimated water deficit is
    (A) 5 L
    (B) 10 L
    (C) 15 L
    (D) 18 L
    (E) Cannot be calculated

18. Which of the following reflects the composition of lactated Ringer's solution?
    (A) Na 140, K 3.5, Ca 3.0, Cl 110, lactate 25
    (B) Na 135, K 3.0, Ca 2.5, Cl 100, lactate 30
    (C) Na 130, K 3.0, Ca 3.0, Cl 100, lactate 30
    (D) Na 130, K 4, Ca 2.7, Cl 109, lactate 28
    (E) Na 140, K 4, Ca 2.5, Cl 110, lactate 25

19. Which of the following disorders is *not* associated with hypocalcemia?
    (A) Sarcoidosis
    (B) Vitamin D deficiency
    (C) Renal insufficiency
    (D) Hypoparathyroidism
    (E) Pancreatitis

20. A 50-year-old woman with chronic renal failure (baseline serum creatinine = 4.0) presents with diarrhea of 2 days duration. Her electrolyte panel reveals the following abnormalities:

Na^+	130 mEq/L
Cl^-	102 mEq/L
HCO_3^-	6 mEq/L
Arterial pH	7.18

What is her acid-base abnormality?
    (A) Severe high-AG metabolic acidosis
    (B) Mixed metabolic acidosis and respiratory alkalosis
    (C) Mixed high-AG metabolic acidosis and hyperchloremic metabolic acidosis
    (D) Severe hyperchloremic metabolic acidosis
    (E) Triple acid-base disorder

21. Which of the following hormones is produced by the kidney?
    (A) Calcitonin
    (B) Erythropoietin
    (C) 25-hydroxyvitamin D
    (D) Aldosterone
    (E) Antidiuretic hormone

22. A 44-year-old man is in the intensive care unit with sepsis from perforated diverticulitis. The patient has been treated for 1 week with aminoglycoside antibiotics and underwent an abdominal computed tomographic (CT) scan with contrast 2 days ago. The urine output has remained 50 mL/h, and a pulmonary wedge pressure by Swan-Ganz catheter is 18. The serum creatinine has increased from 1.0 to 1.8 mg/dL.

Which of the following has been shown to be effective in treating acute renal failure in such patients?
    (A) Low-dose dopamine
    (B) Atrial natriuretic peptide
    (C) Furosemide
    (D) *N*-acetyl-cysteine
    (E) None of the above

23. A 55-year-old male with benign prostatic hypertrophy is admitted to the urological service for acute renal failure. A Foley catheter is placed, and 2 L of urine are initially drained. He has no other medical history, and his baseline creatinine is 1. His initial laboratory findings are as follows:

Na$^+$	138
K$^+$	5.0
C Cl$^-$	118
HCO$_3^-$	24
BBUN	52
CCr	3.1

Which of the following abnormalities would *not* be expected to occur?
(A) Hyponatremia
(B) Hypernatremia
(C) Hyperkalemia
(D) Hypophosphatemia
(E) Hypomagnesemia

24. You are caring for a man with bladder cancer who has undergone cystectomy with urinary drainage via an ileal conduit. Which of the following is *not* a complication of urinary diversions?
(A) Metabolic acidosis
(B) Urolithiasis
(C) Cholelithiasis
(D) Hyperkalemia
(E) Adenocarcinoma

25. Hyperkalemia is associated with which of the following disorders?
(A) Type 1 distal RTA
(B) Type 2 proximal RTA
(C) Type 4 RTA
(D) Gitelman's syndrome
(E) Type 3 RTA

26. A 29-year-old male presents to your office after waking up the previous night with sudden right lower quadrant pain. He states that he vomited several times last night and has been unable to eat or drink. He feels weak and tired. He describes his pain as constant and nonradiating. He has no other past medical history. His vitals include a heart rate of 120 bpm, a BP of 94/56 mmHg, and a temperature of 100.7°F. Your physical examination is significant for guarding and a psoas sign. You suspect appendicitis and admit him to the hospital for an appendectomy. The patient's laboratory findings are the following:

Na$^+$	143	WBC	14.2
K$^+$	4	Hgb	15
Cl$^-$	101	Hct	46
HCO$_3^-$	23	Plts	250
BUN	38	Serum osmolarity	305
Cr	1.0	ABG	pH 7.47; PCO$_2$ 30; PO$_2$ 93
Ca^{2+}	9		
Alb	4		

What acid-base disorder does this patient have?
(A) Respiratory alkalosis
(B) Respiratory alkalosis and metabolic acidosis
(C) Respiratory alkalosis, metabolic acidosis, and metabolic alkalosis
(D) Respiratory acidosis and metabolic alkalosis
(E) Respiratory acidosis and metabolic alkalosis

27. A 65-year-old female is found to have an infrarenal abdominal aortic aneurysm by ultrasound during an evaluation for renal insufficiency. She is scheduled for a CT scan with intravenous contrast. Her only other medical condition is hypertension. Her creatinine clearance is 57 mL/min, with a creatinine of 1.2. She is taking the following medications:

- furosemide: 20 mg by mouth daily
- ramapril: 10 mg by mouth daily
- aspirin: 81 mg by mouth daily
- atrovastatin: 10 mg by mouth at bedtime

What recommendation will decrease the risk of contrast nephropathy?
(A) Hydration with normal saline 1 mL/kg/h for 12 h before and after CT
(B) Withdrawal of diuretic
(C) Acetylcysteine 600 mg by mouth twice daily for 2 days starting 1 day before the procedure
(D) Use of mannitol for forced diuresis
(E) None of the above are known to decrease contrast nephropathy

Questions 28 and 29 refer to the following scenario:
A 75-year-old man with diabetes and chronic obstructive pulmonary disease from tobacco use is in the surgical ICU with multiple injuries following a motor vehicle accident. He is mechanically ventilated and has developed multiple-organ dysfunction syndrome from sepsis. His laboratory findings are as follows:

Na^+	144
K^+	4.6
Cl^-	110
HCO_3^-	14
BUN	50
Cr	3.5
ABG	pH 7.00; PCO_2 60; PO_2 95

28. What is the patient's acid-base disorder?
    (A) AG metabolic acidosis
    (B) Non-AG metabolic acidosis
    (C) Respiratory acidosis
    (D) AG and non-AG metabolic acidosis
    (E) Metabolic acidosis and respiratory acidosis

29. Which of the following treatments will *not* worsen the patient's elevated PCO_2?
    (A) Bicarbonate
    (B) Citrate
    (C) Acetate
    (D) Lactate
    (E) *N*-tromethamine

30. Which ion channel does amiloride inhibit?
    (A) Sodium channel in the collecting tubule
    (B) Sodium-potassium-2 chloride channel in the thick ascending limb of the loop of Henle
    (C) Sodium-chloride channel in the distal convoluted tubule
    (D) Aquaporin 2 water channel in the collecting tubule
    (E) Potassium channels in the collecting tubule

31. Which of the following molecules does *not* aid in the secretion of acids by the kidney?
    (A) Ammonia
    (B) Urea
    (C) Phosphate
    (D) Sulfate
    (E) Ammonium

Questions 32 and 33 refer to the following scenario:
A 44-year-old man with a duodenal ulcer presents with intractable vomiting for 3 days. His laboratory findings are as follows:

Na^+	140 mEq/L	Urine pH	7.0
K^+	1.8 mEq/L	Urine Na^+	40 mEq/L
Cl^-	80 mEq/L	Urine K^+	80 mEq/L
HCO_3^-	44 mEq/L	Urine Cl^-	<10 mEq/L
Arterial pH	7.50		
Arterial PCO_2	52 mmHg		

32. What is the acid-base disorder, and what is the etiology of his hypokalemia?
    (A) Metabolic alkalosis with massive K^+ losses in his vomitus
    (B) Respiratory acidosis resulting from muscle fatigue
    (C) Metabolic alkalosis from vomiting and hypokalemia from renal K^+ losses
    (D) Hypokalemia as the result of intracellular shifts secondary to the alkalemia
    (E) Metabolic alkalosis and hypokalemia as the result of inadequate oral intake

33. Which of the following information regarding analysis of the urinary electrolytes is correct?
    (A) Euvolemia can be proven by his urine sodium concentration.
    (B) High urine pH would likely be related to a urinary infection.
    (C) If high urine pH is found, an error is most likely, and the test should be repeated.
    (D) Tubular dysfunction is responsible for potassium wasting in the presence of severe hypokalemia.
    (E) The urinary chloride concentration is a more reliable indicator of volume status than urinary sodium concentration.

34. A 69-year-old man is admitted for resection of squamous cell carcinoma of the lung. Laboratory values demonstrate a serum calcium level of 16. Which of the following will *not* lower the calcium level?
    (A) Gallium nitrate
    (B) Calcitonin
    (C) Furosemide
    (D) Hydrochlorothiazide
    (E) Bisphosphonates

35. Which of the following causes of acute renal failure is *not* associated with anuria (<50 mL per day urine output)?
    (A) Obstruction
    (B) Cortical necrosis
    (C) Aortic dissection
    (D) Glomerulonephritis
    (E) Contrast nephropathy

36. A 65-year-old woman is on postoperative day 7 following repair of an abdominal aortic aneurysm. Her hospital course has been complicated by intermittent episodes of hypotension necessitating fluid resuscitation and vasopressors. Because of persistent fevers, she is receiving cephalosporin and aminoglycoside antibiotics. She received intravenous radiocontrast on the day prior to surgery. She now has decreasing urine output associated with a rising serum creatinine level. On examination, BP is 130/68, pulse 110; heart and lung examination is normal; abdomen is mildly diffusely tender without rebound; bowel sounds are hypoactive; lower extremities have a nonraised, reddish rash with a reticular pattern. Laboratory findings are as follows:

BUN	60
Cr	4.5
WBC	15 (12% eosinophils)
ESR (erythrocyte sedimentation rate)	115
Bilirubin	0.8
LDH	150
AST/ALT (aspartate aminotransferase/alanine aminotransferase)	35/40
Amylase	900
Urinalysis (U/A)	10–20 RBC/HPF (red blood cells/high-power field)

What is the most likely cause of the acute renal failure?
(A) Contrast nephropathy
(B) Ischemic acute tubular necrosis (ATN)
(C) Aminoglycoside nephrotoxicity
(D) Allergic interstitial nephritis from cephalosporin
(E) Cholesterol emboli syndrome

37. All of the following segments of the nephron absorb magnesium *except*
(A) Proximal convoluted tubule
(B) Thin ascending segment of loop of Henle
(C) Thick ascending segment of loop of Henle
(D) Distal convoluted tubule
(E) None of the listed segments absorb magnesium

38. A 40-year-old man with end-stage renal disease is admitted to the hospital for elective creation of an arteriovenous (AV) fistula. His medications include calcium channel antagonists and angiotensin-converting enzyme (ACE) inhibitors for his high blood pressure, phosphate binders, a vitamin D analogue, and multivitamins. His serum calcium and phosphate levels are 11.4 and 5.8 mg/dL,

respectively. He complains of severe constipation since his surgery, and three doses of Fleet Phospho-Soda are administered in the course of the night. His morning laboratory data reveal hyperphosphatemia (18 mg/dL). What is the appropriate measure to take?
(A) Intravenous injection of 1,25-dihydroxy vitamin D_3 (Calcitriol)
(B) Intravenous infusion of alkali to facilitate intracellular shift of phosphate
(C) Obtain a nephrology consultation and have emergent dialysis started
(D) Follow serial phosphate levels closely; do not give any further enemas
(E) Normal saline bolus

39. During passage from the glomerular capillary to Bowman's space, what structure does the glomerular filtrate *not* pass through?
(A) Glomerular basement membrane
(B) Glomerular capillary fenestrated endothelium
(C) Bowman's visceral epithelial cells
(D) Vasa recta
(E) Renal podocytes

40. A 24-year-old male was admitted to the ICU after a motor vehicle crash 18 h ago. He was initially evaluated and found to have a compound fracture of the right femur, several fractured ribs, and multiple abrasions and was in a comatose state. A CT scan of his head was unremarkable at that time. His vital signs and fractures were stabilized, and he was placed on a ventilator. The nurse has noticed 4 L of urine output in the last hour. This is a change from the previous 12 h, when he had a total of 1 L of urine output. His intravenous fluid is 0.9% saline at 100 mL/h, and he is currently on no scheduled medications. His vitals include a BP of 135/82 mmHg, pulse of 90/min, temperature of 99.2°F, and respirations of 16. The following laboratory tests are ordered:

Admitting Labs		Current Labs			
Na$^+$	139	Na$^+$	150	Serum osmolarity	313
K$^+$	4	K$^+$	4.5	Urine osmolarity	50
Cl$^-$	105	Cl$^-$	110		
HCO$_3^-$	24	HCO$_3^-$	27		
BUN	12	BUN	30		
Cr	0.9	Cr	1.0		
Glu	98	Glu	110		

What is the most likely diagnosis?
- (A) Osmotic diuresis
- (B) Adrenal insufficiency
- (C) Central DI
- (D) Nephrogenic DI
- (E) Cerebral salt wasting

41. What segment of the nephron is responsible for the majority of sodium absorption?
    - (A) Proximal convoluted tubule
    - (B) Loop of Henle
    - (C) Distal convoluted tubule
    - (D) Collecting tubule
    - (E) Collecting duct

ANSWERS AND EXPLANATIONS

1. **(C)** Transurethral resection of the prostate (TURP) syndrome occurs from a combination of fluid overload, hyperosmolality, and hyponatremia following endoscopic surgical procedures. The syndrome has been reported in 1–2% of patients undergoing TURP and has a reported mortality rate of 0.2–0.8%.

   The syndrome is attributed to varying degrees of absorption of the irrigating fluid (300 mL to 4 L) via the exposed or open vascular bed of the prostate, resulting in electrolyte abnormalities based on the irrigation solution being used. The severity of the syndrome depends on the volume of solution absorbed as well as the nature of the irrigating solution. Early symptoms include parasthesia (prickling and burning sensation of the skin) of the face and neck, transient blindness, hypertension and chest pain, nausea, and vomiting, followed by signs of encephalopathy—confusion, apprehension, muscular twitching, and altered consciousness. Grand mal seizures, severe hypotension, bradyarrythmias, pulmonary edema, and cardiac arrest may supervene in the most severe cases.

   There is usually severe hyponatremia due to the inability to use physiologic saline during endoscopic procedures because of the interference of the ionic solution content with the electrocautery current. Therefore, the hyponatremia is dilutional and is seen in nearly all cases along with hyperglycemia. When glycine is used for irrigation, its metabolism results in hyperammonemia, which leads to more pronounced encephalopathy. Finally, hyperkalemia results from the transcellular fluid shifts and may contribute to the arrhythmias and hemodynamic instability in this syndrome.

BIBLIOGRAPHY

Hawary A, Mukhtar K, Sinclair A, Pearce I. Transurethral resection of the prostate syndrome: almost gone but not forgotten. *J Endourol* 2009;23(12):2013–2020.

2. **(A)** The serum chemistries and urine indices are a result of compensatory mechanisms to maintain volume status. The indices reflect relative handling of sodium, urea, and creatinine in a volume-depleted state. With volume depletion, there is an increase in the renin-angiotensin-aldosterone system (RAAS) and the sympathetic nervous system, leading to increased absorption of sodium along the nephron to increase volume status. The RAAS generates angiotensin II, which increases sodium absorption in the proximal tubule and promotes aldosterone secretion; aldosterone increases Na uptake in the collecting tubule. Sympathetic outflow to the kidney causes an increase in sodium absorption and renin release. Similarly, urea is absorbed along the nephron. Urea absorption is enhanced by volume depletion by a decreased glomerular filtration rate and antidiuretic hormone release. Renal handling of creatinine begins with filtration through the glomerulus, then excretion into the tubule along the nephron. There is some creatinine absorption, but this is minimal. The cumulative effects are a sodium-avid state with low urine sodium and increased sodium and urea uptake relative to creatinine. These are manifested in a fractional excretion of Na < 1%, low urine Na < 20, and BUN/Cr > 20 in patients with a volume-depleted state, all of which are present in this patient. Since renal creatinine handling is not significantly altered by volume depletion, it would not be helpful. It is important to note that other pathologic processes mimic these laboratory findings, requiring analysis of the entire patient and not just laboratory data to make a diagnosis.

BIBLIOGRAPHY

Phelan H, Eastman A, Frontan A, et al. Shock and hypoperfusion states. In: O'Leary JP, Tabuenca A, Capote LR, eds. *The Physiologic Basis of Surgery*. Alphen aan den Rijn, the Netherlands: Wolters Kluwer Health; 2008:87–111.

3. **(C)**

4. **(D)**

5. **(E)**

6. **(B)**

7. **(A)**

8. **(C)**

Explanation for questions 3–8

Diabetic ketoacidosis (DKA) is the life-threatening metabolic consequence of insulin deficiency and excess secretion of glucagon, catecholamines, glucocorticoids, and growth hormone. DKA is typically seen in patients with type 1 diabetes mellitus because of noncompliance with insulin therapy or acute illness or injury.

Symptoms include nausea, abdominal pain, excessive thirst, or fatigue. Clinical signs include Kussmaul breathing (rapid, deep respirations) and an acetone or fruity breath odor, hyperglycemia, AG metabolic acidosis, and ketosis.

The patient is volume depleted, as evidenced by the vital signs and lack of urine output. The volume depletion is a result of poor oral intake combined with polyuria induced by glycosuria. The urine produced during the osmotic diuresis of hyperglycemia is approximately half normal with respect to sodium content. Therefore, water deficits are in excess of sodium deficits. Although such patients are usually total body K^+ depleted, K^+ should not be administered until the establishment of good urinary flow. Lactated Ringer's solution contains K^+, as well as unnecessary alkali. Hypertonic saline is not indicated in the treatment of hyponatremia associated with DKA.

The low pH and low bicarbonate concentration indicate the patient has metabolic acidosis. The appropriate respiratory response should be a fall in the PCO_2 of 1.25 times the fall in bicarbonate, in this case 17.5. If the measured PCO_2 were 22.5, then the disorder would be pure metabolic acidosis with respiratory compensation. It would be incorrect to call it respiratory alkalosis because -osis implies a disorder rather than appropriate compensation. In this case, the PCO_2 of 17 is lower than mere compensation, so there is in fact a secondary disorder of respiratory alkalosis. In this patient, the metabolic acidosis is secondary to DKA, and the patient is also hyperventilating because of ketosis and Kaussmaul breathing.

Hyponatremia can develop in disorders associated with low, normal, or high serum osmolality. In severe hyperglycemia, the high serum osmolality draws water from the intracellular space into the serum and dilutes the serum sodium concentration. The serum sodium will fall approximately 2 mEq/L for every 100 mg/dL rise in serum glucose concentration. In this case, correction of hyperglycemia alone will correct the sodium concentration. SIADH is associated with hyponatremia and low serum osmolality. Hyperlipidemia at one time caused false hyponatremia (pseudohyponatremia) because of measuring technique. Newer assays for serum sodium measurements have alleviated this problem. Renal salt wasting is a rare disorder not associated with diabetic nephropathy.

Decreased distal urinary flow decreases renal excretion of potassium. Insulin deficiency allows potassium to leak out of cells. Serum hyperosmolality drags water out of cells along with intracellular potassium. The effect of metabolic acidosis on potassium shift is dependent on the type of acidosis. In mineral acidosis, such as infusion of HCl, chloride is restricted to the extracellular space, so that potassium must leave the cell as hydrogen ions enter to maintain electroneutrality. In organic acidosis, such as DKA or lactic acidosis, the anion accompanies hydrogen ion entering the cell so that potassium exchange is minimal. Although acidosis does contribute to the hyperkalemia, it is the least important of the choices.

$CaCl_2$ stabilizes cardiac membrane potential in the face of hyperkalemia and is the drug of first choice in treating hyperkalemia associated with changes on the electrocardiogram; however, it does not lower the potassium concentration. The other choices lower the potassium concentration either by shifting potassium into cells or by hastening its removal from the body.

Kayexalate and dialysis both lower potassium levels by removing it from the body. Insulin and inhaled albuterol are highly effective in temporarily lowering potassium concentrations by driving potassium into the intracellular compartment. As described, because of the minimal effect of organic acidosis on potassium concentrations, bicarbonate administration is the least-effective means.

BIBLIOGRAPHY

Adams C, Biffl W. Surgical critical care. In: Townsend C, Beauchamp RD, Evers BM, Mattox KL, eds. *Sabiston Textbook of Surgery: The Biological Basis of Modern Surgical Practice*. 18th ed. Philadelphia, PA: Elsevier Saunders; 2008:602–630.

Buse JB, Polonsky KS. Diabetic ketoacidosis, hyperglycemic hyperosmolar nonketotic coma, and hypoglycemia. In: Hall JB, Schmidt GA, Wood LD, eds. *Principles of Critical Care*. 3rd ed. New York, NY: McGraw-Hill; 2005:Chapter 78.

Weiner ID, Wingo CS. Hyperkalemia. In: DuBose TJ, Hamm L, eds. *Acid-Base and Electrolyte Disorders: A Companion to Brenner and Rector's The Kidney*. Philadelphia, PA: Saunders; 2002:406–407.

9. **(B)**

10. **(B)**

11. **(D)**

Explanation for questions 9–11

The pH and bicarbonate are both low, indicating metabolic acidosis. The anion gap (AG) is calculated to be 8, which is normal. The expected fall in PCO_2 is 1.25 × 6, or approximately 8. Because the PCO_2 has fallen appropriately to 32, this is a pure non-AG metabolic acidosis with respiratory compensation.

Although all of the listed conditions cause non-AG metabolic acidosis, it is the loss of potential bicarbonate in the urine in the form of ketones that is the most likely explanation. In DKA, the production of ketones leads to the generation of hydrogen ions and the consumption of bicarbonate. In the presence of insulin, metabolism of ketones results in the regeneration of bicarbonate. Any ketones lost in the urine during the polyuria associated with glycosuria are no longer available for regeneration of bicarbonate. Administration of insulin will correct the AG acidosis as the ketones present in the serum are converted to bicarbonate. The resulting non-AG acidosis represents the "bicarbonate" lost in the urine as ketones. The non-AG acidosis will correct over 3–4 days by generation of new bicarbonate by the kidneys.

Although the patient was initially hyperkalemic, it was the result of decreased distal urinary flow, hyperosmolality, and insulin deficiency. In fact, this patient is likely total body potassium depleted as the result of urinary losses of potassium incurred by the osmotic diuresis induced by the glycosuria. It was only masked by the aforementioned factors. Once good urinary flow is established and treatment with hydration and insulin is initiated, patients are at risk of developing severe hypokalemia. Therefore, potassium should be added to the intravenous fluids. Once the glucose falls to 300 mg/dL, glucose is required to avoid hypoglycemia. In addition, this patient's serum phosphorous is borderline low. Patients with DKA are typically phosphate depleted, which will be exacerbated by the infusion of insulin by driving phosphorous into cells. Therefore, to avoid the complications of hypophosphatemia, phosphate should also be provided.

BIBLIOGRAPHY

Adams C, Biffl W. Surgical critical care. In: Townsend C, Beauchamp RD, Evers BM, Mattox KL, eds. *Sabiston Textbook of Surgery: The Biological Basis of Modern Surgical Practice*. 18th ed. Philadelphia, PA: Elsevier Saunders; 2008:602–630.
Buse JB, Polonsky KS. Diabetic ketoacidosis, hyperglycemic hyperosmolar nonketotic coma, and hypoglycemia. In: Hall JB, Schmidt GA, Wood LD, eds. *Principles of Critical Care*. 3rd ed. New York, NY: McGraw-Hill; 2005:Chapter 78.

12. **(B)** Benzothiazides (thiazide diuretics) are a class of diuretics that inhibit the NaCl transport in the distal convoluted tubule (Fig. 5-1). Thiazide diuretics increase urine volume and the excretion of sodium, chloride, and potassium.

Proposed mechanisms for hyponatremia include (1) inhibition of dilution at the distal convoluted tubule,

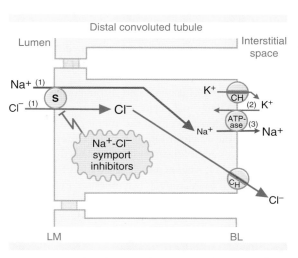

FIGURE 5-1. NaCl in the distal convoluted tubule (from Reilly RF, Jackson EK. Regulation of renal function and vascular volume. In: Knollmann BC, ed. *Goodman and Gilman's The Pharmacological Basis of Therapeutics*. 12th ed. New York, NY: McGraw-Hill; 2011:Chapter 25, Fig. 25-9.

leading to an increase in minimum urinary osmolarity; (2) a decrease in GFR, resulting in less tubular fluid (i.e., free water) reaching the collecting tubule to be excreted; (3) a volume-depleted state that increases ADH, causing free-water reabsorption; and (4) transcellular shifts of sodium to the intracellular space secondary to potassium losses. Other side effects of thiazide diuretics include hyperuricemia, decreased calcium excretion, enhanced magnesium loss, and hyperglycemia.

Loop diuretics (furosemide) have less frequently been documented to cause hyponatremia. Loop diuretics inhibit the Na-K-2CL transporter in the thick ascending limb in the loop of Henle, which is involved in both the diluting and concentrating system. Potassium, magnesium, and calcium excretion are increased in proportion to the increase in sodium excretion. Loop diuretics also act for short periods of time, limiting sodium loss. The most serious side effect is deafness, which may reflect electrolyte changes in the endolymph.

Lithium and demeclocycline are both known to cause DI, leading to hypernatremia. Hyponatremia is not a common side effect of lovastatin.

BIBLIOGRAPHY

Levy JH, Tanaka KA, Ramsay JG. Cardiac surgical pharmacology. In: Cohn LH, ed. *Cardiac Surgery in the Adult*. 4th ed. New York, NY: McGraw-Hill; 2012:Chapter 4.
Mevacor (Lovastatin). In: Sifton DW, ed. *Physicians Desk Reference*. 57th ed. Montvale, NJ: Thomson PDR; 2003:2036–2040.

Reilly RF, Jackson EK. Regulation of renal function and vascular volume. In: Knollmann BC, ed. *Goodman and Gilman's The Pharmacological Basis of Therapeutics.* 12th ed. New York, NY: McGraw-Hill; 2011:Chapter 25.

13. **(D)** Angiotensin II is generated through a cascade of enzymes. When renal perfusion pressures begin to fall, the juxtaglomerular cells of the afferent arterioles release renin into the systemic circulation. The presence of renin cleaves angiotensinogen (synthesized in the liver) to angiotensin I. Angiotensin I is cleaved further to obtain angiotensin II by ACE. ACE is synthesized in the lungs and released into the plasma. Angiotensin II binds to AT_1 receptors (see Chapter 38) in the zona glomerulosa that act via a G protein to activate phospholipase C. The resulting increase in protein kinase C fosters the conversion of cholesterol to pregnenolone (Fig. 5–2) and facilitates the action of aldosterone synthase, resulting in increased secretion of aldosterone.

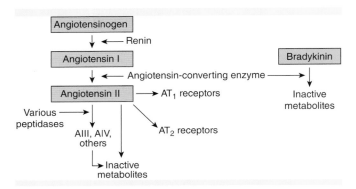

FIGURE 5-2. Renin angiotensin (from Barrett KE, Barman SM, Boitano S, Brooks HL, eds. *Ganong's Review of Medical Physiology.* 24th ed. New York, NY: McGraw-Hill; 2012: Chapter 38. Copyright © The McGraw-Hill Companies, Inc. All rights reserved).

The effects of angiotensin II are mediated mainly through its two receptors, AT_1 and AT_2. The effects of AT_1 and AT_2 are generally antagonistic. The AT_1 receptor is responsible for angiotensin II's effects on aldosterone secretion, arterial constriction, sodium reabsorption, glomerular efferent arteriolar constriction, nephrosclerosis in the kidney, and cardiac hypertrophy.

BIBLIOGRAPHY

Barrett KE, Barman SM, Boitano S, Brooks HL. The adrenal medulla and adrenal cortex. In: Barrett KE, Barman SM, Boitano S, Brooks HL, eds. *Ganong's Review of Medical Physiology.* 24th ed. New York, NY: McGraw-Hill; 2012:Chapter 20.

14. **(A)** Hypermagnesemia develops when magnesium intake exceeds excretion by the kidney. The most common cause of this is renal insufficiency, leading to decreased magnesium clearance. Magnesium-containing antacids and laxatives can produce toxic levels in patients with renal failure. Excess intake in conjunction with total parenteral nutrition, or rarely massive trauma, thermal injury, and severe acidosis, may be associated with symptomatic hypermagnesemia. Other situations in which hypermagnesemia has been documented are during its use as a tocolytic in obstetrics, use of antacids that contain magnesium, and excess absorption from the sigmoid colon when magnesium is used as a cathartic. Hypermagnesemia affects neurons, neuromuscular junctions, and muscles to produce its effect. Symptoms are related to the concentration of magnesium in the blood and range from hypotension to death. The initial signs and symptoms of hypermagnesemia are lethargy and weakness. Electrocardiographic changes resemble those in hyperkalemia (widened QRS complex, ST segment depression, and peaked T waves). When the serum level reaches 6 mEq/L, deep tendon reflexes are lost; with levels above 10 mEq/L, somnolence, coma, and death may ensue. The treatment of hypermagnesemia usually involves withholding magnesium intake and allowing for excretion to occur through the kidneys. In the presence of life-threatening symptoms, hypermagnesemia can be antagonized with calcium. If renal insufficiency is significant enough that magnesium excretion is hindered, then dialysis is the only option to decrease magnesium levels.

BIBLIOGRAPHY

Doherty GM. Fluid and electrolyte management. In: Doherty GM, ed. *Current Diagnosis and Treatment: Surgery.* 13th ed. New York, NY: McGraw-Hill; 2010:Chapter 9.

Shires GT III. Fluid and electrolyte management of the surgical patient. In: Brunicardi FC, Andersen DK, Billiar TR, Dunn DL, Hunter JG, Matthews JB, et al., eds. *Schwartz's Principles of Surgery.* 9th ed. New York, NY: McGraw-Hill; 2010:Chapter 3.

15. **(D)** Hypophosphatemia occurs secondary to a decrease in phosphorus intake, an intracellular shift of phosphorus, or an increase in phosphorus excretion.

Clinical manifestations of hypophosphatemia are related to adverse effects on the oxygen availability of tissue and to a decrease in high-energy phosphates and can be manifested as cardiac dysfunction or muscle weakness.

High-energy phosphate is needed by cells to provide adenosine triphosphate (ATP) for multiple functions. Lack of phosphate impairs muscle function and the ability of red cells to maintain cell membrane integrity.

Therefore, common complications of hypophosphatemia include muscle weakness with rhabdomyolysis and respiratory failure and hemolysis.

BIBLIOGRAPHY

Shires GT III. Fluid and electrolyte management of the surgical patient. In: Brunicardi FC, Andersen DK, Billiar TR, Dunn DL, Hunter JG, Matthews JB, et al., eds. *Schwartz's Principles of Surgery*. 9th ed. New York, NY: McGraw-Hill; 2010:Chapter 3.

16. **(D)** Hypernatremia (serum sodium > 145 mEq/L) reflects a water deficit relative to sodium levels. The source of water loss can be renal or extrarenal. Renal water loss occurs when the kidney is unable to concentrate urine due to either lack of antidiuretic hormone ADH or end-organ resistance to ADH, such as in diabetes insipidus.

    Early signs of hypernatremia include irritability, weakness, and lethargy that progresses to coma and death. If the patient is hypovolemic, circulating plasma volume should be corrected with isotonic fluids prior to correction of the free-water deficit to maintain perfusion. Diuretics may be administered to hypervolemic patients, as sodium excretion will be achieved along with the volume of free water lost. The equation for calculating free-water deficit is $0.6 \times$ weight (kg) $\times [([Na^+]/140) - 1]$.

    A urine output of 2.0 L per day can be described as polyuria. The urine osmolality of 408 mOsm/L is not consistent with simple central DI. There is an ongoing osmotic diuresis that is attributable to hyperglycemia, glycosuria, and azotemia. A measurement of his urine urea concentration should reveal a high level. He is not necessarily acidotic; rather, his high serum chloride is simply in keeping with the need for electrical neutrality, given a sodium of 170 mEq/L. He is likely to be severely volume depleted; this is camouflaged by a high serum osmolality, which helps to preserve intravascular fluid volume and therefore maintain a good blood pressure. This must be fully considered during treatment as too rapid a dilution of his serum back toward normal osmolality can cause a redistribution of body fluids that will result in severe hypovolemia and possibly even shock.

BIBLIOGRAPHY

Evans H, Maier R. Electrolyte disorders. In: *Current Surgical Therapy*. Morrison, L, Singer I. Hyperosmolal states. In: Narins RG, ed. *Maxwell and Kleeman's Clinical Disorders of Fluid and Electrolyte Metabolism*. 5th ed. New York, NY: McGraw-Hill; 1993:617–658.
Topf JM, Rankin S, Murray P. Electrolyte disorders in critical care. In: Hall JB, Schmidt GA, Wood LD, eds. *Principles of Critical Care*. 3rd ed. New York, NY: McGraw-Hill; 2005:Chapter 76.

17. **(B)** Water constitutes approximately 50 to 60% of total body weight. The relationship between total body weight and total body water (TBW) is primarily a reflection of body fat. Lean tissues such as muscle and solid organs have higher water content than fat and bone. In an average young adult male, 60% of total body weight is TBW, whereas in an average young adult female it is 50%.

    TBW is divided into three functional fluid compartments: plasma, extravascular interstitial fluid, and intracellular fluid (Fig. 5-3). The extracellular fluids (ECF), plasma, and interstitial fluid together comprise about one-third of the TBW and the intracellular compartment the remaining two-thirds.

% of Total body weight	Volume of TBW	Male (70 kg)	Female (60 kg)
Plasma 5%	Extracellular volume	14,000 mL	10,000 mL
Interstitial fluid 15%	Plasma	3500 mL	2500 mL
	Interstitial	10,500 mL	7500 mL
Intracellular volume 40%	Intracellular volume	28,000 mL	20,000 mL
		42,000 mL	30,000 mL

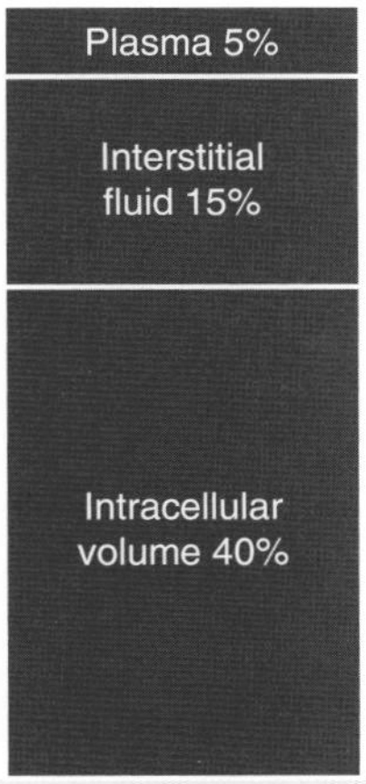

FIGURE 5-3. Functional body fluid components (from Shires GT III. Fluid and electrolyte management of the surgical patient. In: Brunicardi FC, Andersen DK, Billiar TR, Dunn DL, Hunter JG, Matthews JB, et al., eds. *Schwartz's Principles of Surgery*. 9th ed. New York, NY: McGraw-Hill; 2010:Chapter 3, Fig. 3-1. Copyright © The McGraw-Hill Companies, Inc. All rights reserved).

Given a weight of 80 kg, his TBW is approximately 60% of this (48 L). If we presume that this has a sodium concentration of 170 mEq/L, how much water will need to be added to dilute this to 140 mEq/L? If we assume that he has the same content of sodium, then the following equation should hold true: $170 \times 48 = 140 \times$ (new TBW).

Therefore, the new TBW $\times$ 170 = 48/140. The difference of new TBW and current TBW is the free-water deficit = $170 \times 48/140 - 48$ L ~ 10 L.

BIBLIOGRAPHY

Shires GT III. Fluid and electrolyte management of the surgical patient. In: Brunicardi FC, Andersen DK, Billiar TR, Dunn DL, Hunter JG, Matthews JB, et al., eds. *Schwartz's Principles of Surgery*. 9th ed. New York, NY: McGraw-Hill; 2010:Chapter 3.

18. **(D)** The compositions of common IV fluids are shown in Table 5-1.

BIBLIOGRAPHY

Fenves A, Rao A, Emmett M. Fluids and electrolytes. In: O'Leary JP, Tabuenca A, Capote LR, eds. *The Physiologic Basis of Surgery*. Alphen aan den Rijn, the Netherlands: Wolters Kluwer Health; 2008.

19. **(A)** Calcium homeostasis requires the kidney, the parathyroid gland, and vitamin D to maintain calcium levels. Failure of these mechanisms leads to hypocalcemia (Ca^{2+} < 8.4 mg/dL). Hypocalcemia occurs in hypoparathyroidism, hypomagnesemia, severe pancreatitis, chronic or acute renal failure, severe trauma, crush injuries, and necrotizing fasciitis; in critically ill patients with sepsis, burns, and acute renal failure; and in surgical patients after parathyroidectomy.

Renal insufficiency leads to hypocalcemia by the development of hyperphosphatemia, resistance to parathyroid hormone (PTH) by bone, and decreased synthesis of vitamin D. Hyperphosphatemia, a result of decreased GFR, is believed to cause hypocalcemia by the binding calcium and depositing it into tissues. PTH is secreted by the parathyroid gland when decreased ionized calcium is present. PTH is responsible for increased synthesis of 1,25-vitamin D, increased absorption of calcium and phosphate wasting by the kidney, and increased activity of osteoclasts in bones—all of which increase plasma calcium level. A deficiency in PTH by hypoparathyroidism or resistance of bone to PTH can lead to hypocalcemia. 1,25-Vitamin D, the most potent form of vitamin D, is a result of a series of enzymatic steps. The final step of synthesis occurs in the proximal tubules in the kidney. Vitamin D helps maintain calcium levels by increasing absorption of calcium from the gastrointestinal tract and augments the effects of PTH on bone. Hypocalcemia from pancreatitis has been ascribed to the action of pancreatic lipase on omental and retroperitoneal fat, with the release of fatty acids, which in turn bind calcium. Sarcoidosis, like other granulomatosis diseases, can produce excess quantities of vitamin D and can lead to a hypercalcemic state.

Clinical manifestations of acute hypocalcemia begin neuromuscular excitability (*tetany*). Tetany ranges from mild signs of perioral numbness and tingling, Trousseau sign (induction of carpopedal spasm with blood pressure cuff inflation), Chvostek sign (facial muscle spasm after

TABLE 5-1 Electrolyte Solutions for Parenteral Administration

Solution	Electrolyte Composition (mEq/L)						
	Na	**CL**	**K**	**HCO$_3^-$**	**Ca**	**Mg**	**mOsm**
Extracellular fluid	142	103	4	27	5	3	280–310
Lactated Ringer's	130	109	4	28	3		273
0.9% Sodium chloride	154	154					308
D$_5$ 0.45% Sodium chloride	77	77					407
D$_5$W							253
3% Sodium chloride	513	513					1026
D$_5$ = 5% dextrose; D$_5$W = 5% dextrose in water.							

stimulation of facial nerve), and muscle cramps to laryngeal spasm and seizures. Prolongation of the QT interval may progress to malignant arrhythmias such as torsades de pointes or heart block.

BIBLIOGRAPHY

Doherty GM. Fluid and electrolyte management. In: Doherty GM, ed. *Current Diagnosis and Treatment: Surgery.* 13th ed. New York, NY: McGraw-Hill; 2010:Chapter 9.
Evans H, Maier R. Electrolyte disorders. In: *Current Surgical Therapy.*

20. **(C)** This case illustrates how much information is obtainable from a close examination of serum electrolytes alone. The patient has an AG of 22 and therefore a high AG acidosis. Metabolic acidosis from increased acid production is associated with an AG exceeding 15 mEq/L. Conditions in which this occurs are renal failure, DKA, lactic acidosis, methanol ingestion, salicylate intoxication, and ethylene glycol ingestion. The lungs compensate by hyperventilation, which returns the hydrogen ion concentration toward normal by lowering the blood PCO_2. The increase in AG (from a normal of 10–12 mEq/L) is 10 mEq/L. If the acidosis were explained solely by the AG, then we should expect a diminution of bicarbonate of comparable degree, 8–12 mEq/L. The HCO_3 should be in the range of 14–18 mEq/L, and the patient's low HCO_3 suggests that there is a mixed acid-base disorder, with an additional abnormality that lowers the bicarbonate level from the expected 14–18 mEq/L to the actual 6 mEq/L. This may be a respiratory alkalosis or a hyperchloremic metabolic acidosis. The pH of 7.18 suggests the diagnosis of mixed AG metabolic acidosis and hyperchloremic metabolic acidosis. This is in concordance with the clinical history, with chronic renal failure as a cause of the high AG and diarrhea the cause of hyperchloremic acidosis.

BIBLIOGRAPHY

Doherty GM. Fluid and electrolyte management. In: Doherty GM, ed. *Current Diagnosis and Treatment: Surgery.* 13th ed. New York, NY: McGraw-Hill; 2010:Chapter 9.

21. **(B)** There are a variety of hormones synthesized in the kidney. Erythropoietin is made in the proximal cells of the kidney. It is deficient in patients with chronic kidney disease and leads to anemia. Fortunately, this hormone can be manufactured, and its administration is a major advance in the management of renal insufficiency. Other hormones that are produced in the kidney include 1,25-vitamin D, renin, and prostaglandins. Calcitonin is produced in the thyroid gland and regulates calcium

homeostasis. 25-Hydroxyvitamin D is synthesized from vitamin D_3 to 25-hydroxyvitamin D by 25-hydroxylase in the liver. Aldosterone is produced in the adrenal cortex and released in response to angiotensin II. The posterior pituitary is normally the site of synthesis of antidiuretic hormone, and it normally is released in volume depletion or hypertonic states.

BIBLIOGRAPHY

Lal G, Clark OH. Thyroid, parathyroid, and adrenal. In: Brunicardi FC, Andersen DK, Billiar TR, Dunn DL, Hunter JG, Matthews JB, et al., eds. *Schwartz's Principles of Surgery.* 9th ed. New York, NY: McGraw-Hill; 2010:Chapter 38.
Leavey SF, Weitzel WF. Endocrine abnormalities in chronic renal failure. *Endocrinol Metab Clin North Am* 2002;31(1):107–119.

22. **(E)** Low-dose dopamine, ANP, and furosemide are all effective in reversing acute renal failure in animal models. Clinical trials to determine the benefit of nutritional therapy with amino acids to improve renal failure show conflicting results. Although small trials and case series have also suggested benefits in clinical trials, large randomized controlled trials with these agents have shown none are effective in humans, and their use should be abandoned. Although studies suggest Mucomyst may decrease the risk of acute renal failure from administration of radiocontrast in high-risk patients when given as prophylaxis, there is no evidence it ameliorates established acute renal failure.

BIBLIOGRAPHY

Reddy B, Murray P. Acute renal failure. In: Hall JB, Schmidt GA, Wood LD, eds. *Principles of Critical Care.* 3rd ed. New York, NY: McGraw-Hill; 2005:Chapter 75.

23. **(C)** Relief from an obstructive nephropathy results in postobstructive diuresis. The increase in urine output is caused by an increase in volume status from obstruction, accumulation of solutes that generate an osmotic load (urea and the like), possible retained natriuretic compounds, and depressed salt and water reabsorption when urine flow is reestablished. Obstruction also impairs ion channels, which are responsible for the kidney's concentrating ability, sodium handling, and response to ADH, which all lead to further loss of free water and sodium. This unregulated relative loss of free water to sodium determines whether hyponatremia or hypernatremia develops. Tubular functions that are responsible for potassium, phosphorus, and magnesium balance are also affected and result in their respective loss.

BIBLIOGRAPHY

Curhan GC, McDougall WS, Zeidel ML. Urinary tract obstruction. In: Brenner BM, ed. *Brenner and Rector's The Kidney.* 6th ed. Philadelphia, PA: Saunders; 2000:1820–1844.

Seifter JL. Urinary tract obstruction. In: Longo DL, Fauci AS, Kasper DL, Hauser SL, Jameson JL, Loscalzo J, eds. *Harrison's Principles of Internal Medicine.* 18th ed. New York, NY: McGraw-Hill; 2012: Chapter 289.

24. **(D)** Metabolic acidosis with a normal AG results from exogenous administration of acid (HCl or NH_4^+), from loss of bicarbonate (e.g., diarrhea, fistulas, ureterosigmoidostomy), or from renal losses. Loss of bicarbonate is accompanied by a gain of chloride; thus, the AG remains unchanged. Reabsorption of urinary ammonium chloride by the intestinal segment causes a non-AG metabolic acidosis. Patients with urinary diversions have increased urinary calcium levels because metabolic acidosis causes dissolution of the skeleton. In addition, removal of the terminal ileum can lead to increased intestinal absorption of dietary oxalate. The resulting increased urinary calcium and oxalate levels can result in stone formation. With urinary diversions, there is an increased potential for the formation of gallstones, primarily related to ileal resection. Pigment stones are the predominant type. Ureterointestinal anastomoses such as ileal conduit, colon conduit, and the like are associated with a wide variety of cancers. The most commonly reported anastomosis associated with cancer is ureterosigmoidostomy. These cancers are usually diagnosed 10–20 years after surgery. Hypokalemia, rather than hyperkalemia, is typically seen with urinary diversions.

BIBLIOGRAPHY

Shires GT III. Fluid and electrolyte management of the surgical patient. In: Brunicardi FC, Andersen DK, Billiar TR, Dunn DL, Hunter JG, Matthews JB, et al., eds. *Schwartz's Principles of Surgery.* 9th ed. New York, NY: McGraw-Hill; 2010:Chapter 3.

25. **(C)** The clinical distinction between the different RTAs is based on the presence of hypokalemia or hyperkalemia, urinary pH, response to $NaHCO_3$, and serum aldosterone levels. Type 1 RTA is a disorder of the distal acidification process. It can be caused by a number of disorders, including hydrogen ATPase dysfunction, a sodium channel abnormality in the parietal cell, or back-diffusion of hydrogen. It usually manifests with hypokalemia, a urine pH > 5.5, and no change in fractional excretion of HCO_3 with $NaHCO_3$ loading. Proximal acidification defect presents with type 2 RTA. This disorder is usually seen with disturbances of other proximal tubular functions, such as phosphaturia and aminoaciduria. Proximal RTA presents with hypokalemia, urine pH

< 5, and an increase in fractional excretion of HCO_3 to $NaHCO_3$ load. Type 4 is usually a deficiency of aldosterone or resistance to its presence. Aldosterone promotes hydrogen ion and potassium secretion by enhancing sodium absorption and the hydrogen ATPase activity. Hyperkalemia, urine pH < 5, and a varying aldosterone level are the clinical features of type 4 RTA. Gitelman's syndrome presents with hypomagnesemia, hypokalemia, and metabolic alkalosis. It simulates activation of the thiazide-sensitive sodium chloride channel in the distal convoluted tubule.

BIBLIOGRAPHY

Barakat A, Rennert OM. Gitelman's syndrome (familial hypokalemia-hypomagnesemia). *J Nephrol* 2001;14:43–47.

Soriano R. Renal tubular acidosis: the clinical entity. *J Am Soc Nephrol* 2002;13(8):2160–2170.

26. **(C)** Examination of his ABG shows respiratory alkalosis. The pH is elevated with a decrease in PCO_2. In a respiratory alkalosis, a compensatory metabolic acidemia is generated by the kidney. Examination of this patient's electrolytes shows a normal HCO_3 as well as an elevated AG of 19, indicating metabolic acidosis. With an AG metabolic acidosis present, he must also have a metabolic alkalosis to have a normal HCO_3; thus, a triple disorder exists (respiratory alkalosis, metabolic acidosis, and metabolic alkalosis).

The etiology of this acid-base disorder can be understood from the patient's illness. Respiratory alkalosis occurs from an increase in respiratory drive with subsequent increase in minute ventilation and decreased PCO_2. The pain he is experiencing is most likely the cause of his respiratory alkalosis. Other reasons for respiratory alkalosis include anxiety, salicylate intoxication, central nervous system pathology, and primary pulmonary pathology. This patient also has an AG metabolic acidosis, caused by an acid after it disassociates leaving an unmeasured anion and a hydrogen ion that is buffered by HCO_3. The elevated AG is likely a combination of lactic acidosis (hypoperfusion and infection) and ketosis (starvation). To generate a metabolic alkalosis, hydrogen must be lost in excess of HCO_3 or HCO_3 must be added. In this case, the patient's vomiting has led to a loss of hydrogen and retention of bicarbonate, leading to metabolic alkalosis.

BIBLIOGRAPHY

DuBose TD. Acid-base disorders. In: Brenner BM, ed. *Brenner and Rector's The Kidney,* 6th ed. Philadelphia, PA: Saunders; 2000:925–997.

Kaufman D, Kitching AJ, Kellum JA. Acid-base balance. In: Hall JB, Schmidt GA, Wood LD, eds. *Principles of Critical Care*. 3rd ed. New York, NY: McGraw-Hill; 2005:Chapter 77.

27. **(A)** Contrast nephropathy is a multifactorial process. It is likely a combination of decreased blood flow resulting in ischemia to the medulla, the generation of reactive oxygen species leading to cellular injury, and atheroembolic phenomena. Contrast nephropathy usually manifests within 48 h. Hydration has been shown to decrease the risk of contrast nephropathy by increasing blood flow and possibly limiting the time that the tubular epithelium is exposed to contrast. In a recent study, normal saline has been shown to be superior to half-normal saline in diminishing the risk. Furthermore, intravenous hydration is superior to oral liquid intake. Acetylcysteine is a free radical scavenger that has been used to minimize the risks of contrast nephropathy. In a recent study, when acetylcysteine was added to hydration versus hydration alone, there was a relative risk of 10% of developing contrast nephropathy. The use of diuretics and mannitol to minimize the risk of contrast nephropathy has been unsuccessful and may actually heighten the risk. Withholding furosemide and avoiding the use of mannitol are recommended.

BIBLIOGRAPHY

Mintz E, Gruberg L. Radiocontrast-induced nephropathy and percutaneous coronary intervention: a review of preventive measures. *Expert Opin Pharmacother* 2003;4(5):639–652.

Mueller C, Buerkle G, Buettner HJ, et al. Prevention on contrast media-associated nephropathy: randomized comparison of 2 hydration regimens in 1620 patients undergoing coronary angioplasty. *Arch Intern Med* 2002;162(3):329–336.

Tepel M, van der Giet M, Schwarzfeld C, Laufer U, Liermann D, Zidek W. Prevention of radiographic-contrast-agent-induced reductions in renal function by acetylcysteine. *N Engl J Med* 2000;343:180–184.

Trivedi HS, Moore H, Nasr S, Aggarwal K, Agrawal A, Goel P, et al. A randomized prospective trial to assess the role of saline hydration on the development of contrast nephrotoxicity. *Nephron Clin Pract* 2003;93:C29–C34.

28. **(E)**

29. **(E)**

Explanation for questions 28 and 29

The pH and bicarbonate are low, so the patient has a metabolic acidosis. The AG is elevated. An appropriate respiratory response to the metabolic acidosis would be hyperventilation, resulting in a low PCO_2. Because this patient's PCO_2 is high, there is also a respiratory acidosis.

For bicarbonate to buffer a proton, water and CO_2 are produced and the lungs must exhale CO_2. Likewise, the by-product of converting citrate, lactate, or acetate into bicarbonate is CO_2. Retained CO_2 in a patient with COPD or fixed ventilation will accumulate CO_2, and the acidosis will worsen. N-tromethane on the other hand, is both a CO_2 and proton pump. It corrects both metabolic acidosis and respiratory acidosis. Its side effects include hypoventilation, hyperkalemia, hyperglycemia, and vascular necrosis.

BIBLIOGRAPHY

Kaufman D, Kitching AJ, Kellum JA. Acid-base balance. In: Hall JB, Schmidt GA, Wood LD, eds. *Principles of Critical Care*. 3rd ed. New York, NY: McGraw-Hill; 2005:Chapter 77.

30. **(A)** Amiloride inhibits the sodium channel located on the tubular epithelial surface of the collecting tubule. It is involved in volume balance, potassium, and acid excretion. The channel allows sodium to move intracellularly from the tubule. This absorption produces a negative transcellular electrical gradient that aids in potassium and hydrogen ion secretion. An activating mutation of this sodium channel causes Liddle's syndrome. Liddle's syndrome is manifested by hypertension, hypokalemia, metabolic alkalosis, and suppression of the RAAS. The disease is autosomal dominant, and patients often require renal transplantation. The manifestations of this syndrome can be treated with amiloride by blocking sodium absorption. The sodium-potassium-2 chloride channel and sodium chloride channel are inhibited by furosemide and thiazide diuretics, respectively. Aquaporins are water channels that are located throughout the course of the nephron. Aquaporin 2 is one of these channels located in the collecting tubule. Under the influence of ADH binding to its V_2 receptor, the channel is translocated from intracellular vesicles to the epithelial membrane, increasing water absorption. Inhibitors of V_2 receptor are under development and in clinical trials. They may become important for the treatment of hyponatremia.

BIBLIOGRAPHY

Elliott WJ, Kalahasti P, Lau SM, Nally JV, Gomez-Sanchez CE. Secondary hypertension. In: Lerma EV, Berns JS, Nissenson AR, eds. *Current Diagnosis and Treatment: Nephrology and Hypertension*. New York, NY: McGraw-Hill; 2009:Chapter 42.

Salant DJ, Gordon CE. Polycystic kidney disease and other inherited tubular disorders. In: Longo DL, Fauci AS, Kasper DL, Hauser SL, Jameson JL, Loscalzo J, eds. *Harrison's Principles of Internal Medicine*. 18th ed. New York, NY: McGraw-Hill; 2012: Chapter 284.

31. **(B)** The kidney excretes 50 mEq of hydrogen ions daily that are derived from metabolic processes. To meet the daily goal of acid secretion, titratable acids and ammonia are used because free hydrogen ion secretion is minimal. Phosphate and sulfate, derived from the metabolism of amino acids, are both titratable acids. Both molecules bind hydrogen that is secreted into the tubule and are excreted in the urine; however, they do not provide enough buffering capacity because of limited quantities. Ammonia provides a larger buffering capacity because it can be generated to meet demand. Ammonium is produced in the proximal tubules principally from the metabolism of glutamine (see Fig. 5-4 regarding renal ammonium formation). Ammonium enters the proximal tubule via a carrier transport protein; ammonia is then formed. Ammonia (NH_3) is freely permeable in cellular membranes because it carries no charge. Ammonia is trapped in the tubular lumen by the conversion to ammonium (NH_4^+) by combining ammonia with a secreted hydrogen ion, a process called "diffusion trapping." Through a mechanism of ammonia absorption, ammonium uptake, and recycling by the thick ascending limb, an increased concentration of ammonia is established in the medullary interstitium. In the inner medullar collecting tubule, ammonia is converted to ammonium as it diffuses from the high interstitium concentration into the tubule and trapped by the acidification process and finally excreted in the urine. Through this trapping mechanism and titrable acids, the kidney is able to excrete the acid load. Urea is not involved in acid secretion, but plays a significant role in water handling.

BIBLIOGRAPHY

Barrett KE, Barman SM, Boitano S, Brooks HL. Acidification of the urine and bicarbonate excretion. In: Barrett KE, Barman SM, Boitano S, Brooks HL, eds. *Ganong's Review of Medical Physiology*. 24th ed. New York, NY: McGraw-Hill; 2012:Chapter 39.

Unwin R, Shirley DG, Capasso G. Urinary acidification and distal renal tubular acidosis. *J Nephrol* 2002;15(S5):S140–S150.

32. **(C)** The patient has a metabolic alkalosis related to profuse and prolonged vomiting. The same abnormality occurs commonly in surgical practice as a result of prolonged nasogastric suction. Metabolic alkalosis results from the loss of acid (in this case via vomitus), volume depletion, and potassium depletion. For each proton that is secreted into the lumen of the stomach, a bicarbonate ion is added to the plasma. Normally, that proton passes on to the duodenum and reacts with a bicarbonate ion from pancreatic secretion. With vomiting or nasogastric suction, however, the proton is lost to the body. Thus, loss of gastric juice simultaneously results in a rise in serum bicarbonate concentration. The normal compensatory excretion of bicarbonate by the kidneys is compromised by their need to preserve volume by increasing tubular reabsorption of sodium and whatever anions are also filtered. There is a threshold of bicarbonate concentration above which the reabsorptive capacity of the proximal tubule is surpassed, at which time bicarbonate begins to "spill" into the urine. This spilled bicarbonate, which is only poorly reabsorbable in the distal nephron, "drags" out cations (principally, Na^+ and K^+) with it to maintain electrical neutrality. Gastric secretion has a potassium concentration comparable to plasma (4–5 mEq/L only). The potassium losses that result in this patient's profound hypokalemia occur at the kidney and are not the direct result of vomiting.

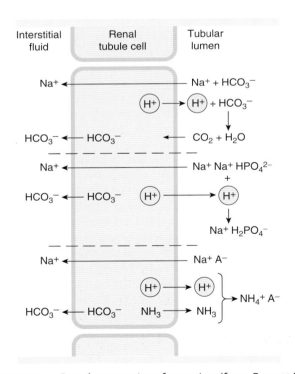

FIGURE 5-4. Renal ammonium formation (from Barrett KE, Barman SM, Boitano S, Brooks HL. Acidification of the urine and bicarbonate excretion. In: Barrett KE, Barman SM, Boitano S, Brooks HL, eds. *Ganong's Review of Medical Physiology*. 24th ed. New York, NY: McGraw-Hill; 2012:Chapter 39, Fig. 39-2. Copyright © The McGraw-Hill Companies, Inc. All rights reserved).

BIBLIOGRAPHY

Doherty GM. Fluid and electrolyte management. In: Doherty GM, ed. *Current Diagnosis and Treatment: Surgery*. 13th ed. New York, NY: McGraw-Hill; 2010:Chapter 9.

33. **(E)** When there is the excretion of an anion in urine (a poorly reabsorbable anion such as bicarbonate, ketoanions, some drugs), electrical neutrality dictates that the anion must be accompanied by cations (usually sodium and potassium). Thus, sodium excretion does not reflect volume status in this situation, and the urinary chloride more accurately reflects volume status. Conversely, when there is the excretion of a cation such as ammonium (in a state of metabolic acidosis), the ammonium ion will drag out with it anions such as chloride ions. The urinary chloride does not reflect volume status; rather, it is the urine sodium that is a more reliable indicator of volume status.

The patient's high urine pH suggests that there is ongoing bicarbonaturia and that the patient is not in a state of equilibrium as yet. An alternative explanation is if the patient has been receiving bicarbonate or some other base from an exogenous source. This patient admitted to having ingested large amounts of Tums to alleviate his vomiting prior to hospitalization.

BIBLIOGRAPHY

Doherty GM. Fluid and electrolyte management. In: Doherty GM, ed. *Current Diagnosis and Treatment: Surgery*. 13th ed. New York, NY: McGraw-Hill; 2010:Chapter 9.

34. **(D)** Inhibition of bone resorption can be achieved with gallium nitrate, calcitonin, and bisphosphonates. Bisphosphonates are highly effective in inhibiting osteoclast activity in the bones. Action of onset is delayed for 3–4 days, so a more immediate acting agent is usually administered. Calcitonin is also a potent inhibitor of osteoclast activity. Its effect on serum calcium levels occurs within hours of administration, so it is often combined with bisphosphonates. Its effect is transient. Tachyphylaxis develops in 2–3 days. Lasix increases the renal excretion of calcium. Hydrochlorothiazide, on the other hand, increases tubular reabsorption of calcium in the distal tubule and can cause hypercalcemia.

BIBLIOGRAPHY

Shires GT III. Fluid and electrolyte management of the surgical patient. In: Brunicardi FC, Andersen DK, Billiar TR, Dunn DL, Hunter JG, Matthews JB, et al., eds. *Schwartz's Principles of Surgery*. 9th ed. New York, NY: McGraw-Hill; 2010:Chapter 3.

35. **(E)**

36. **(E)**

Explanation for questions 35 and 36

Contrast nephropathy is defined as a rise in the serum creatinine within 48 h of contrast administration, so this is not the explanation. Ischemic ATN associated with her intermittent bouts of hypotension is a possibility, but it would not explain the peripheral eosinophilia, elevated amylase, or the lower extremity rash. Interstitial nephritis from the cephalosporin would cause renal failure, high eosinophil count, and a rash, but not the elevated amylase. All of the findings, however, are consistent with the diagnosis of cholesterol emboli syndrome. Often referred to as "pseudovasculitis," it develops days to weeks after an arterial vascular procedure. It causes renal failure, pancreatitis, intestinal ischemia, arthralgias, livedo reticularis, digital infarction, and cerebral infarction. Laboratory findings include high ESR and eosinophil counts and low complement levels. Therapy is supportive.

Contrast nephropathy is usually a nonoliguric form of acute renal failure. Oliguria does occur, but frank anuria would be rare. On the other hand, complete bilateral renal obstruction, acute cortical necrosis associated with septic abortions, aortic dissection occluding the renal arteries, and severe acute glomerulonephritis are all associated with anuria.

BIBLIOGRAPHY

Modi K, Rao V. Atheroembolic renal disease. *J Am Soc Nephrol* 2001; 12:1781–1787.
Singri N, Ahya S, Levin M. Acute renal failure. *JAMA* 2003;289: 747–751.

37. **(B)** Magnesium that is unbound to protein in plasma (~80%) is filtrated through the glomerulus. From there, it is absorbed at different parts of the nephron, each with its own mechanism. In the proximal convoluted tubule, magnesium uptake is by bulk transport along with sodium and water absorption. The thick ascending limb is the major segment for magnesium absorption. Magnesium moves through a paracellular pathway driven by a potential gradient. This gradient is established by the Na-K-2Cl channel, inward rectifying potassium channel (ROMK) and the chloride channel on the basolateral membrane. The gradient is established by the electrical neutral absorption of Na, K, and Cl by the Na-K-2Cl channel. Some of the absorbed potassium reenters the tubule through the ROMK channel, and chloride exits the cell into the basolateral space. The movement of potassium and chloride leads to a potential gradient that is positive in the lumen and negative in the basolateral space. Magnesium moves down this gradient to be

absorbed. The remaining magnesium is taken up in the distal convoluted tubule. The mechanism of absorption in the distal convoluted tubule is not fully understood but is connected to sodium and chloride absorption because it is inhibited by thiazide diuretics. The thin ascending segment on the loop of Henle is not significantly involved in magnesium absorption.

BIBLIOGRAPHY

Topf JM, Rankin S, Murray P. Electrolyte disorders in critical care. In: Hall JB, Schmidt GA, Wood LD, eds. *Principles of Critical Care.* 3rd ed. New York, NY: McGraw-Hill; 2005:Chapter 76.

38. **(C)** This case illustrates the danger of administration of Fleet Phospho-Soda enemas to patients with end-stage renal disease. There is significant absorption of phosphate in the colon. Colonic disease with inflammation and poor colonic motility can result in even greater potential to absorb phosphate administered by this route. Because patients with end-stage renal disease are unable to excrete such absorbed phosphate, there is the potential for severe and sometimes life-threatening hyperphosphatemia. Other possible sources of phosphate loads in these patients include poor dietary compliance with the phosphate-restricted diet, patients taking milk for the relief of dyspepsia, infants receiving cow's milk (which is richer in phosphate than human milk), blood transfusions, patients receiving vitamin D or its analogues, and tissue breakdown as in rhabdomyolysis or tumor lysis.

The most concerning consequences of severe hyperphosphatemia are the following:

1. Soft tissue (metastatic) calcifications, which can involve the skin, joints, blood vessels, heart, lungs, and kidneys.
2. Hypocalcemia/tetany resulting from the reciprocal relationship of serum phosphate and calcium, such that very high levels of phosphate are associated with low levels of calcium.

The most appropriate intervention is dialysis; whether intermittent or continuous depends on the severity of the hyperphosphatemia and if it is expected to resolve rapidly or would require prolonged treatment.

BIBLIOGRAPHY

Gennari FJ, ed. Diagnosis of acid-base disorders. In: *Medical Management of Kidney and Electrolyte Disorders.* New York, NY: Dekker; 2001:169–189.
Topf JM, Rankin S, Murray P. Electrolyte disorders in critical care. In: Hall JB, Schmidt GA, Wood LD, eds. *Principles of Critical Care.* 3rd ed. New York, NY: McGraw-Hill; 2005:Chapter 76.

39. **(D)** The structures that separate the glomerular capillary from Bowman's space are the glomerular capillary endothelium, basement membrane, and the Bowman's visceral epithelial cells, called podocytes. These structures limit not only the formed elements of blood but also loss of protein in the filtrate. Proteins are limited to the capillary space by their size and electrical charge. The generation of filtrate is governed by Starling's forces, as in other capillary beds. The vasa recta is formed from the glomerular efferent arteriole and plays an important role in salt and water balance.

BIBLIOGRAPHY

Pallone TL, Zhang Z, Rhinehart K. Physiology of the renal medullary microcirculation. *Am J Physiol Renal Physiol* 2003;284(2): F253–F266.
Tryggvason K, Wartiovaara J. Molecular basis of glomerular permselectivity. *Curr Opin Nephrol Hypertens* 2001;10(4):543–549.

40. **(C)** The laboratory data can be consistent with either central or nephrogenic DI, but in this male patient with a recent motor vehicle accident who is in a comatose state, central DI is the most likely diagnosis. Generally, to differentiate between central and nephrogenic DI, a water deprivation test is performed, where desmopressin is given. An increase in urine osmolarity and decrease in urine output signify central DI. Patients with a similar clinical picture have been described with pituitary stalk syndrome. The syndrome is usually seen in male patients in their 20s to 30s who are usually in a comatose state from motor vehicle accidents. The clinical picture has three phases. First, there is a phase of the cessation of AVP secretion that occurs acutely and may have an onset from 5 h to 6 days. There is the acute onset of polyuria and hypernatremia. Close monitoring of serum electrolytes is needed to promptly diagnose this complication. Spontaneous recovery is frequent. Delayed diagnosis, on the other hand, can result in hypernatremic brain injury, hypovolemia, shock, and ischemic brain injury. The second phase (antidiuretic) is the result of AVP release from injured axons. This may occur within 3–12 days after injury and can result in life-threatening hyponatremia, especially as the patient is receiving large volumes of hypotonic fluid at the time for the treatment of the hypernatremia of the first phase.

There are important differential diagnoses of the second phase to be considered; however, hyponatremia may be the result of the development of SIADH. Hyponatremia may also be the result of high AVP levels, resulting from volume depletion secondary to the previous polyuria or secondary to a cerebral salt-wasting syndrome. Cerebral salt wasting is manifested by hyponatremia, volume depletion, and intracranial pathology.

In the last two cases, water or fluid restriction would be inappropriate measures to take. These patients also may have abnormalities of other pituitary hormones, such as adrenocorticotropic hormone (ACTH), that lead to adrenal insufficiency, which can minimize the first phase of hypernatremia or worsen the hyponatremia of the second phase. The third phase is the final phase of complete recovery with return to normal posterior pituitary function or of partial recovery (partial central DI), or of no recovery (complete central DI). Spontaneous recovery is the more usual outcome. Osmotic diuresis from mannitol, glucose, and the like can lead to hypernatremia by loss of free water, but this patient's urine osmolarity does not support this diagnosis.

BIBLIOGRAPHY

Bichet DG. Nephrogenic and central DI. In Shrier RW, ed. *Diseases of the Kidney and Urinary Tract*. Baltimore, MD: Lippincott Williams & Wilkins; 2001:2549–2576.

Harrigan HR. Cerebral salt wasting syndrome. *Crit Care Clin* 2001;17(1):125–138.

Robinson AG, Verbalis JG. Posterior pituitary gland. In: Larsen PR, ed. *Williams Textbook of Endocrinology*. 10th ed. Philadelphia, PA: Saunders; 2003:281–329.

41. **(A)** All of the tubular segments listed contribute to sodium absorption. Sodium absorption is the primary mechanism of volume regulation because water absorption generally follows sodium absorption. It is the proximal convoluted tubule that does the majority of absorption, about 65–75% of sodium. In a decreasing order, the loop of Henle, distal convoluted tubule, and collecting tubule contribute to 25, 10, and 0–5% of sodium absorption, respectively.

BIBLIOGRAPHY

Andreoli TE. An overview of salt absorption by the nephron. *J Nephrol* 1999;12(S2):S3–S15.

CHAPTER 6

PREOPERATIVE EVALUATION

LISA M. MCELROY AND TRAVIS P. WEBB

QUESTIONS

1. What is the single most important test to perform to ascertain a patient's risk assessment and preparation prior to a surgical procedure?
   (A) History and physical exam
   (B) Serum electrolytes
   (C) Chest x-ray
   (D) Electrocardiogram
   (E) Stress test

2. Which of the following is a predictor of difficult intubation?
   (A) Prior neck injury with normal mobility
   (B) Interincisor distance >4 cm
   (C) Large underbite
   (D) Large thyromental distance
   (E) Inability to shift the lower incisors in front of the upper incisors

3. A 48-year-old Caucasian male with a history of hypertension, diabetes mellitus, and one block right lower extremity claudication presents for a preoperative evaluation. He smokes two packs of cigarettes per day. He works as a top executive in a major advertising firm. He has never had chest pain. Routine evaluation includes a resting ECG that reveals Q waves 0.04 s wide in V5 and V6 and one-half the height of the R waves. What should this be interpreted as?
   (A) Normal variation of a patient with hypertension
   (B) Coronary artery disease (CAD)
   (C) Normal variation of a patient with diabetes mellitus
   (D) Normal variation of a patient with Berger disease
   (E) No evidence of CAD because the patient has never had chest pain

4. Which of the following will immediately delay or cancel an elective surgical case if not obtained appropriately preoperatively?
   (A) Complete blood count (CBC)
   (B) Urinalysis
   (C) CXR
   (D) Informed consent
   (E) ECG

5. A 48-year-old Hispanic male with a history of gastroesophageal reflux disease refractory to medical management is advised to undergo an elective Nissen fundoplication. An extensive preoperative history and physical reveals no evidence of cardiac or pulmonary disease. What would be the most appropriate preoperative laboratory studies to obtain given the fact the patient has no significant past medical history?
   (A) CBC
   (B) CBC, ECG
   (C) CBC, ECG, blood glucose
   (D) CBC, ECG, CXR, basic metabolic panel, glucose
   (E) None

6. A 67-year-old Asian American male with a history of congestive heart failure, diabetes mellitus, hypertension, CAD, chronic renal insufficiency, and peripheral vascular disease presents for preoperative teaching prior to undergoing arteriovenous fistula creation. He has undergone all appropriate preoperative evaluation and testing. Of his current medications listed below, which should be stopped preoperatively?
   (A) Furosemide
   (B) Metformin
   (C) Atenolol
   (D) Aspirin
   (E) Digoxin

7. Which of the following preoperative conditions is *least likely* to be associated with significant extracellular fluid volume depletion in a surgical patient?
   (A) Enterocutaneous fistula
   (B) Small bowel obstruction
   (C) Peritonitis
   (D) Pancreatitis
   (E) Closed head injury

8. A 68-year-old African American female on dialysis presents 12 weeks after an episode of diverticulitis requiring percutaneous drainage of an abscess. An elective sigmoidectomy is now planned. If started now, which of the following medications would reduce her risk of perioperative myocardial infarction (MI)?
   (A) Metoprolol
   (B) Diltiazem
   (C) Hydrochlorothiazide
   (D) Lisinopril
   (E) Furosemide (Lasix)

9. Which of the following surgical procedures places a 55-year-old Caucasian male without history of chronic obstructive pulmonary disease (COPD) at highest risk for postoperative pulmonary complications?
   (A) Laparoscopic ventral hernia repair
   (B) Diaphragm repair after traumatic rupture 2 years ago
   (C) Total abdominal colectomy
   (D) Left radical nephrectomy
   (E) Coronary artery bypass graft

10. Which of the following does *not* help ameliorate cardiac stress perioperatively in high-risk patients?
   (A) Maintaining normal body temperature
   (B) Providing epidural anesthesia
   (C) Providing metoprolol perioperatively
   (D) Transfusing two units of packed red blood cells
   (E) Maintaining a perioperative heart rate of 50–60 bpm

11. Which of the following is true regarding preoperative renal risk assessment?
   (A) All patients should have preoperative blood urea nitrogen (BUN) and serum creatinine testing.
   (B) A reduced preoperative glomerular filtration rate does not increase the risk of postoperative renal dysfunction.
   (C) Body mass index (BMI) and serum creatinine are used to estimate creatinine clearance.
   (D) Dialysis patients should be routinely screened for anemia and nutritional status.
   (E) Proteinuria detected on urinalysis does not warrant further assessment.

12. When should parenteral antibiotics be given perioperatively?
   (A) The night before surgery
   (B) 6 h prior to surgery
   (C) 60 min prior to incision
   (D) At the time of incision
   (E) 60 min after incision

13. A 50-year-old woman with history of biliary colic and gallstones noted on ultrasound presents for elective laparoscopic cholecystectomy. What amount of operative time increases the risk of developing deep venous thrombosis?
   (A) 30 min
   (B) 60 min
   (C) 90 min
   (D) 120 min
   (E) 150 min

14. Coagulation studies would be indicated prior to which of the following operations?
   (A) Inguinal herniorrhaphy
   (B) Femoral-popliteal bypass graft
   (C) Right hemicolectomy
   (D) Total thyroidectomy
   (E) Laparoscopic appendectomy

15. A 64-year-old African American female with history of diabetes and left great toe amputation secondary to infection presents obtunded and febrile. On examination, the patient is noted to have an ulcer along the lateral aspect of her foot with cellulitis. No pus is expressible. Blood glucose is 843 mg/dL. Serum potassium is 4.0. Arterial blood gas (ABG) reveals pH of 7.28 and PCO_2 of 38 mmHg. White blood cell (WBC) is 15.4. Urine dip is positive for ketones and glucose. What is the next step in the management of this patient?
   (A) Surgical debridement in the operating room
   (B) Immediate amputation in the operating room
   (C) 1 L normal saline bolus
   (D) 1 L normal saline with 1 ampule of $NaHCO_3$
   (E) 10 units of regular insulin subcutaneously

16. A 40-year-old Caucasian female diagnosed with Crohn disease 3 weeks prior presents with 2 weeks of lower gastrointestinal bleeding for which she has required multiple blood transfusions. She has been treated with infliximab and high-dose steroids. She now experiences hypotension with continued bleeding and is taken urgently to the operating room, where she undergoes a total abdominal colectomy with ileostomy. Preoperatively, she only received antibiotics. Two hours after operation, the patient is persistently hypotensive in the 80/30s despite multiple boluses of 0.9% normal saline.

Her postoperative hematocrit is 30%. What is the best next step in this patient's management?
(A) Continue to give normal saline boluses
(B) Transfuse 2 units of packed red blood cells
(C) Start a dopamine drip at 5 µg/kg/min
(D) Give 100 mg IV of hydrocortisone
(E) Reexplore her immediately

17. Which of the following medications should be given first in the preoperative preparation of a patient with pheochromocytoma?
(A) Phenoxybenzamine
(B) Propranolol
(C) Nifedipine
(D) Lisinopril
(E) Hydrochlorothiazide

18. Which of the following is an independent risk factor for cardiovascular death after elective noncardiac and cardiovascular surgery?
(A) Renal insufficiency
(B) Hyperthyroidism
(C) Pheochromocytoma
(D) Adrenal insufficiency
(E) Hypertension

19. A 43-year-old Caucasian male with a history of Caroli disease and end-stage liver disease is to undergo an elective Nissen fundoplication. Which of the following would optimize the patient's liver function prior to the surgery?
(A) Hemodialysis
(B) Control of hypertension
(C) Right hepatic lobectomy
(D) Transjugular intrahepatic portal caval shunt (TIPS)
(E) None of the above

20. Which of the following is *not* a manifestation of thyroid storm?
(A) Fever
(B) Tachycardia
(C) Significantly elevated levels of T_4 and T_3 compared to hyperthyroidism
(D) Atrial fibrillation
(E) Seizures

21. Which of the following heart sounds noted during physical examination would require infective endocarditis prophylaxis prior to noncardiac surgery?
(A) Fixed splitting of S2
(B) Holosystolic murmur
(C) S3
(D) Loud A2
(E) A2 before P2 with increased splitting on inspiration

22. Which of the following is a contraindication to regional anesthesia?
(A) History of chronic headaches
(B) Previous surgical site infection
(C) Therapeutic anticoagulation
(D) Pulmonary hypertension
(E) Morbid obesity with obstructive sleep apnea

ANSWERS AND EXPLANATIONS

1. **(A)** A history and physical is diagnostic in 75–90% of patients. Diagnostically, the history is three times more productive than the physical examination and 11 times more effective than routine laboratory tests. Furthermore, "routine" preoperative testing is not cost-effective, may result in morbidity to the patient from further workup of false-positive results, and is less predictive of perioperative morbidity than the American Society of Anesthesiologists (ASA) status or American Heart Association (AHA)/American College of Cardiology (ACC) guidelines for surgical risk.

The preoperative medical history should include previous exposure to anesthesia, allergies including medication and foods, and family history of problems with anesthesia or surgical procedures. A detailed list of current medications should be fully explored for potential interactions, and patients should be counseled to continue medications up to the morning of surgery.

Review of systems with identification of comorbidities (history of myocardial infarction [MI], syncope, angina, anemia, orthostatic intolerance, pulmonary edema, valvular disease, hepatic and renal failure, diabetes) reveals areas for further testing. A baseline level of activity should be ascertained. Patients who are unable to achieve at least 4 METs (metabolic equivalents) of activity, which is defined as being able to climb two flights of stairs without stopping, or walking briskly for up to four city blocks, and those with BMI >35 are particularly prone to comorbidities that may seem unusual at an early age, including sleep apnea and ischemic heart disease.

The physical exam should be focused on the neurologic, cardiac, pulmonary, hepatobiliary, and renal systems.

BIBLIOGRAPHY

Dorian RS. Anesthesia of the surgical patient. In: Brunicardi FC, Andersen DK, Billiar TR, Dunn DL, Hunter JG, Matthews JB, Pollock RE eds. *Schwartz's Principles of Surgery* 9th ed. New York, NY: McGraw-Hill; 2010:Chapter 47.

Neumayer L, Vargo D. Principles of preoperative and operative surgery. In: *Sabiston Textbook of Surgery* 18th ed. Philadelphia, PA: Elsevier Saunders; 2008:251–279.

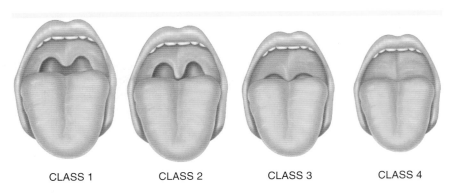

CLASS 1   CLASS 2   CLASS 3   CLASS 4

MALLAMPATI CLASSIFICATION
CLASS 1: Soft palate, fauces, uvula, pillars
CLASS 2: Soft palate, fauces, portion of uvula
CLASS 3: Soft palate, base of uvula
CLASS 4: Hard palate only

FIGURE 6-1. The Mallampati classification. From Dorian RS. Anesthesia of the surgical patient. In: Brunicardi FC, Andersen DK, Billiar TR, Dunn DL, Hunter JG, Matthews JB, Pollock RE eds. *Schwartz's Principles of Surgery* 9th ed. New York, NY: McGraw-Hill; 2010:Chapter 47, Fig. 47-2.

Shammash JB, Ghali WA. Preoperative assessment and perioperative management of the patient with nonischemic heart disease. *Med Clin North Am* 2003;87(1):137–152.

2. **(E)** An airway examination should be performed in all patients preoperatively so as to identify those patients in whom management of the airway and conventional endotracheal intubation may be difficult. The Mallampati classification is based on the amount of the posterior pharynx one can visualize with maximal mouth opening and tongue protrusion in the sitting position (see Fig. 6-1).

Predictors of difficult intubation include obesity, immobility of the neck, interincisor distance <4 cm in an adult, a large overbite, or the inability to shift the lower incisors in front of the upper incisors. The thyromental distance is the distance from the thyroid cartilage to the tip of the chin and should be >6.5 to 7 cm.

BIBLIOGRAPHY

Dorian RS. Anesthesia of the surgical patient. In: Brunicardi FC, Andersen DK, Billiar TR, Dunn DL, Hunter JG, Matthews JB, Pollock RE (eds.), *Schwartz's Principles of Surgery*, 9th ed. New York, NY: McGraw-Hill; 2010:Chapter 47.

3. **(B)** Preoperative cardiac evaluation should begin with a thorough history and physical exam. Risk factors for perioperative cardiac complications include diabetes mellitus, renal insufficiency, ischemic heart disease, congestive heart failure, and poor functional status. Noninvasive testing is recommended in any patient who reports a past medical history consistent with coronary artery disease or has three or more risk factors.

Patients with an abnormal resting ECG are three times more likely to have a fatal perioperative infarction. A Q wave of 0.04 s or wider and at least one-third the height of the R wave is evidence of a prior MI. Evidence of prior MI must be taken as evidence of CAD; however, a normal resting ECG does not rule out CAD. Further testing includes the following modalities.

Echocardiography (resting and stress) can estimate left ventricular ejection fraction (LVEF), which if reduced correlates with perioperative myocardial events. Also, wall motion abnormalities or thickening defines the presence of ischemia.

Radionuclide cardiac studies assess LVEF, which correlates with the incidence of perioperative infarction and severity of CAD. Myocardial perfusion imaging analyzes and distinguishes between areas of ischemia and scars from a previous infarction as well as between ischemic and nonischemic cardiomyopathy that has excellent correlation with risk of postoperative infarctions.

In patients with known or suspected CAD undergoing high-risk procedures, an ECG at baseline, immediately postoperatively, and on the first 2 days after surgery appears to be cost-effective. Postoperative markers should be reserved for the subset of patients with clinical, ECG, or hemodynamic evidence of cardiovascular dysfunction. Patients who sustain acute MIs in the perioperative period need to be followed closely secondary to increased risk of future cardiac events.

BIBLIOGRAPHY

Adams C, Biffle W, Cioffi W. Surgical critical care. In: *Sabiston Textbook of Surgery* 18th ed. Philadelphia, PA: Elsevier Saunders; 2008:602–630.

Cohn SL, Goldman L. Preoperative risk evaluation and perioperative management of patients with coronary artery disease. *Med Clin North Am* 2003;87(1):111–136.

Stonemetz J. Preoperative preparation of the surgical patient. In: Cameron JL, Cameron, AM (eds.), *Current Surgical Therapy*. Philadelphia, PA: Elsevier Saunders; 2010:1070–1073.

4. **(D)** Consent is permission, granted by the patient to the surgeon, to make a diagnostic or therapeutic intervention on the patient's behalf. For consent to be valid, it must be informed. The patient must be provided all relevant information. To be valid, it must also be voluntary, that is, as free from coercion as possible while recognizing that in extremis the patient's condition itself may be inherently coercive. The surgeon's ethical objective is to judiciously provide the patient sufficient information with which to decide what course to follow. This entails selectively presenting all information pertinent to the patient's condition regarding benefits, risks, and alternatives while avoiding overwhelming the patient with extraneous data. To walk the line between what is pertinent and what is extraneous requires prudent judgment.

Informed consent has become a baseline best-practice ethical standard in modern medical care. It is a necessary but insufficient condition for ethically sound patient care. More moral work remains to be done if the physician–patient relationship is to be more than a contractual arrangement for rendering services. The ultimate goal is to achieve the best outcome, not only in terms of adherence to ethical principles of practice but also in keeping with patients' moral values, with what matters most to patients in their relationships and their lives. Achieving this goal certainly entails the provision of information and the granting of consent, but this exchange must take place in the context of a conversation about how the proposed intervention will affect a particular patient's life.

Informed consent is ultimately the responsibility of the operating surgeon. It is not only a legal obligation, but grounded in the ethical principle of autonomy. It provides the patient a chance to ask questions, calm fears, and strengthen trust between the surgeon and the patient. Furthermore, well-informed patients require less analgesia in the postoperative period and experience less pain. Informed consent includes explaining the risks, benefits, alternatives, and outcomes of surgery. Include as many details as possible, and if possible, write them out. If the patient is not competent, then a surrogate must give informed consent in a nonemergent setting. In an emergent setting, institutions have several options for providing consent. A "three-doc consent"

is a popular version of this (in which three physicians agree that a procedure is needed in an emergent situation to prevent significant morbidity or mortality and indicate so in the chart). The patient's social support and rehabilitation needs should be assessed preoperatively. Home services or rehabilitation may be needed postoperatively. Inquiry regarding health care power of attorney and do-not-resuscitate (DNR) status should life-threatening complications arise should also be discussed.

BIBLIOGRAPHY

Baker RJ, Fischer JE. *Preparation of the Patient. Mastery of Surgery* 4th ed. New York, NY: Lippincott Williams & Wilkins; 2001:23–54.

Carson R. Ethics in surgery. In: *Sabiston Textbook of Surgery* 18th ed. Philadelphia, PA: Elsevier Saunders; 2008:21–25.

5. **(E)** A routine test is one that is obtained on an asymptomatic, apparently healthy patient in the absence of any specific clinical indication. In general, routine preoperative testing is not recommended; rather, specific testing should be considered for specific patients based on history and physical exam. The history and physical examination are the most reliable and cost-effective preoperative screening tools available. Laboratory examinations ordered in preoperative surgical patients should screen for asymptomatic disease that may affect the surgical result (e.g., unsuspected anemia or diabetes), diseases that may contraindicate elective surgery or require treatment before surgery (e.g., diabetes, heart failure), diagnose disorders that require surgery (e.g., hyperparathyroidism, pheochromocytoma), and evaluate the nature and extent of metabolic or septic complications. Healthy asymptomatic patients undergoing elective surgery do not require preoperative testing.

BIBLIOGRAPHY

Dunphy JE, Way LW. Approach to the surgical patient. In: Doherty GM (ed.), *Current Diagnosis & Treatment: Surgery*, 13th ed. New York, NY: McGraw-Hill; 2010:Chapter 1.

Fischer SP. Cost-effective preoperative evaluation and testing. *Chest* 1999;115(5):96S–100S.

King MS. Preoperative evaluation. *Am Fam Physician* 2000;62(2):387–396.

Smetana GW. The case against routine preoperative laboratory testing. *Med Clin North Am* 2003;87(1):7–40.

Smith R, Ng V, Twomey P, et al. Preoperative testing, planning, and risk stratification. In: *ACS Surgery: Principles & Practice*. Philadelphia, PA: Decker Publishing Inc.; 2013.

6. **(B)** Optimization of comorbid conditions such as CHF, diabetes, and HTN is essential. Most medications can be

safely continued through the perioperative period. Withdrawal of β-blockade is associated with unstable angina, tachyarrhythmias, MI, or sudden death. Digoxin should be continued with careful monitoring of levels and signs of toxicity (arrhythmias, nausea, vomiting, headache, dizziness, visual disturbance). Electrolytes and volume status should also be monitored as all classes of antihypertensives, and digoxin can cause disturbances in and be influenced themselves by these.

Oral hypoglycemic agents such as metformin and glyburide should be held for at least 8 hours preoperatively. Diuretics, such as furosemide and hydrochlorothiazide, and angiotensin converting enzyme (ACE) inhibitors/angiotensin receptor blockers, such as lisinopril and captopril, should be held the day of surgery unless prescribed for CHF, in which case patients should take their morning dose.

Monoamine oxidase inhibitors (MAOIs) such as isocarboxazid and phenelzine should be discontinued at least 2 weeks prior to elective surgery, because they may potentiate sympathomimetic amines leading to hypertensive crisis. MAOIs also prolong effects of central nervous system (CNS) depressants and can have severe interactions with narcotics (most notably meperidine) and tricyclic antidepressants.

Oral anticoagulants should be discontinued 5 to 7 days in advance of elective surgery and replaced with heparin if necessary. All herbal supplements should be stopped at least 24 hours prior to surgery.

β-Blockers, asthma medications, antireflux medications, and aspirin should be continued perioperatively. ACE/ARB inhibitors for hypertension should also be continued if hypertension is difficult to control without them.

Multiple factors may lead a surgical patient to experience extracellular fluid volume depletion: mechanical small bowel obstruction, fistula loss, vomiting, diarrhea, peritonitis, pancreatitis, and so on. Physical examination may reveal skin tenting, dry mucous membranes, tachycardia, oliguria, or postural hypotension. Operating on a patient prior to adequate volume resuscitation may lead to cardiovascular collapse.

Monitoring renal function via urine output measured through an indwelling bladder catheter is essential to assess adequate resuscitation. Normal hourly urine output is 0.5 mL/kg in an adult and greater than or equal to 1 mL/kg in children, depending on age (in patients not receiving diuretics or experiencing glycosuria). More invasive monitoring with central venous pressure (CVP) or pulmonary artery wedge pressure may be appropriate in select cases, although their role is controversial. Other guides that may assist in difficult resuscitations include arterial pH, lactate, and base deficit.

Rate of resuscitation is guided by the urgency of need for operation (replacement of deficits and ongoing losses may be necessary in the operating room). Resolution of clinical signs of volume deficit is the best indicator of response. Correction of electrolyte imbalances follows the same principles in emergent as in nonemergent situations. Maintenance fluid requirements can be estimated as 100 mL/kg/d for the first 10 kg, 50 mL/kg/d for the second 10 kg, and 10 mL/kg/d thereafter. If bolus is required, 1000 mL of Ringer's lactate may be given in less than an hour and safely repeated up to 3000–5000 mL with sodium replacement of 450–700 meq with careful urine output and CVP monitoring. Choosing the type of repletion solution depends on the source of existing abnormalities and ongoing losses.

BIBLIOGRAPHY

Backman SB, Bondy RM, Deschamps A, Moore A, Thomas Schricker T. Perioperative considerations for anesthesia. In: Souba WW (ed.), *ACS Surgery: Principles & Practice*, 6th ed. New York, NY: WebMD; 2008.

Stonemetz J. Preoperative preparation of the surgical patient. In: Cameron JL, Cameron, AM (eds.), *Current Surgical Therapy*. Philadelphia, PA: Elsevier Saunders; 2010:1070–1073.

7. **(E)** Preoperative fluid assessment is critical in a surgical patient. Often, the surgeon is required to make a rapid assessment of the patient's fluid and electrolyte imbalances and replete ongoing losses. Regardless of whether the patient is managed preoperatively in the trauma bay or the clinic setting, depleted intravascular volume is best established through a thorough history and physical examination.

BIBLIOGRAPHY

Baker RJ, Fischer JE. Preparation of the patient. In: *Mastery of Surgery* 4th ed. New York, NY: Lippincott Williams & Wilkins; 2001:23–54.

Sampliner JE. Postoperative care of the pancreatic surgical patient: the role of the intensivist. *Surg Clin North Am* 2001;81(3):637–645.

8. **(A)** Nearly 1 million patients each year experience a perioperative myocardial infarction. Major risk factors include diabetes and unstable angina (see Fig. 6-2). Women are underrepresented in the cohorts used to develop the ACC/AHA guidelines. Subsequent studies in gynecologic patients have shown that hypertension and previous MI are major predictors in women relative to men.

According to the ACC/AHA medium- to high-risk patients, perioperative risk for cardiovascular morbidity and mortality was decreased by 67% and 55%,

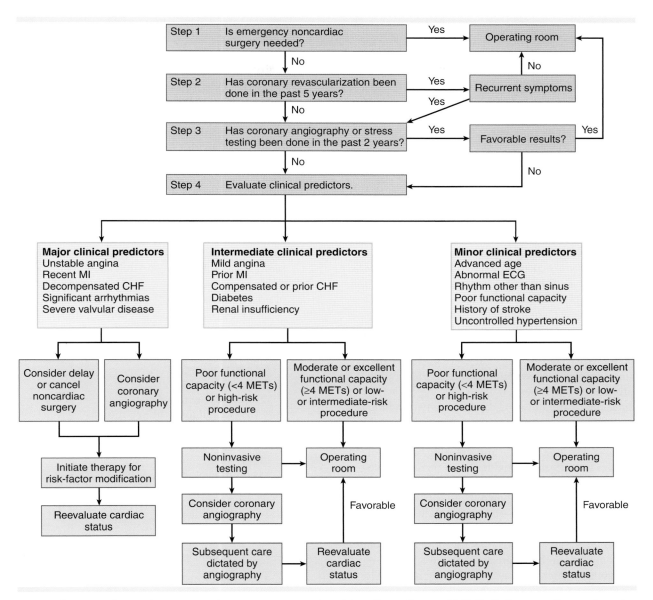

FIGURE 6-2. Preoperative and postoperative management algorithm. From Cooper Z, Kelly E. Preoperative and postoperative management. In: Zinner MJ, Ashley SW (eds.), *Maingot's Abdominal Operations*, 12th ed. New York, NY: McGraw-Hill; 2012:Chapter 2, Fig. 2-1.

respectively, for patients receiving β-blockers in the perioperative period versus those receiving placebo. The benefit was most noticeable in the 6 months after surgery, but event-free survival was significantly better in the group that received β-blockers up to 2 years after surgery.

The current AHA/ACC recommendations for medium- to high-risk patients are to start β-blocker therapy as early as possible preoperatively with a goal heart rate of 60 bpm.

BIBLIOGRAPHY

Cohn SL, Goldman L. Preoperative risk evaluation and perioperative management of patients with coronary artery disease. *Med Clin North Am* 2003;87(1):111–136.

Cooper Z, Kelly E. Preoperative and postoperative management. In: Zinner MJ, Ashley SW (eds.), *Maingot's Abdominal Operations* 12th ed. New York, NY: McGraw-Hill; 2012:Chapter 2.

Neumayer L, Vargo D. Principles of preoperative and operative surgery. In: *Sabiston Textbook of Surgery* 18th ed. Philadelphia, PA: Elsevier Saunders; 2008:251–279.

9. **(B)** As a rule, the closer the surgery is to the diaphragm, the higher the risk of pulmonary complications. Assessment of pulmonary function should be performed for all lung resection cases, for thoracic procedures requiring single-lung ventilation, and for major abdominal and thoracic cases in patients who are older than 60 years, have significant underlying medical disease, smoke, or have overt pulmonary symptomatology.

In patients who have a history of lung disease or those in whom a pulmonary resection is contemplated, preoperative assessment of pulmonary function is of great value secondary to increased risk of mortality from pulmonary complications postoperatively. Smoking, underlying chronic obstructive pulmonary disease (COPD), and poor exercise tolerance are the greatest risk factors for postoperative pulmonary complications. Physicians should ask about a history of smoking, decreased exercise capacity, dyspnea, and chronic cough. Examination should note pursed lip breathing, clubbing, and chest wall anatomy that could impair pulmonary function.

Arterial blood gas should be checked in high-risk patients. PaO_2 less than 60 mmHg correlates with pulmonary hypertension, and a $PaCO_2$ of greater than 45 mmHg is associated with increased perioperative morbidity.

Spirometry and diffusing capacity are two techniques used to evaluate preoperative pulmonary function. In general, patients with a preoperative forced expiratory volume in 1 second (FEV1) and diffusing capacity of the lungs for carbon monoxide (DLCO) greater than or equal to 80% predicted need no further pulmonary evaluation. Studies have shown that few postoperative pulmonary complications occurred in patients with an FEV1 greater than 2 L undergoing pneumonectomy, an FEV1 greater than 1.5 L for those undergoing lobectomy, and an FEV1 greater than 0.6 L for those undergoing segmentectomy. Additionally, a DLCO less than 60% predicted has been shown to increase mortality, whereas a DLCO greater than 60% but less than 80% has an increased risk of postoperative pulmonary complications.

Patients who do not meet initial preoperative requirements for lung resection should undergo predicted postoperative lung function testing. Although studies vary as to the exact values necessary for safe pulmonary resection, current recommendations are for exercise testing to be performed in patients with a postoperative FEV1 or DLCO less than 40%.

Cardiopulmonary exercise testing is useful in evaluating patients who are marginal candidates for pulmonary resection. Maximal oxygen consumption is a calculated value from this test that gives an indication of lung function. In general, patients with a preoperative maximal oxygen consumption of greater than 20 mL/kg/min

will tolerate lung resection without an increased risk of complications. Those with a value less than 10 mL/kg/min have been shown to be at a higher risk for postoperative complications and are deemed inoperable. Split-function studies along with a pulmonary perfusion scan can be used to evaluate patients with maximal oxygen consumption values between 10 and 20 mL/kg/min. This allows prediction of postoperative function with respect to the portion of the lung to be removed (i.e., the functional contribution of the portion of lung that is being resected).

Ideally, patients should quit smoking for 8 weeks prior to operation. This allows recovery of cilia, decreased secretions, and drop in blood carbon monoxide (CO) levels. Cessation for shorter periods may be associated with a hyperactive inflammatory response in the respiratory system. Patients who quit smoking more than 9 weeks prior to operation approach nonsmokers in terms of postoperative pulmonary complications.

Risk factors for pulmonary complications include the following:

- Upper abdominal and thoracic surgical procedure
- Emergency surgery
- Age > 50
- Decreased functional status
- > 10% weight loss within 6 months
- Chronic steroid use
- COPD
- FEV1 < 2 L
- Maximum voluntary ventilation <50% of predicted value
- Peak expiratory flow rate <100 L or 50% of predicted value
- PCO_2 > 45 mmHg
- PO_2 < 50 mmHg

BIBLIOGRAPHY

Beckles MA, Spiro SG, Colice GL, et al. The physiologic evaluation of patients with lung cancer being considered for resectional surgery. *Chest* 2003;123(1):105S–114S.

Neumayer L, Vargo D. Principles of preoperative and operative surgery. In: *Sabiston Textbook of Surgery* 18th ed. Philadelphia, PA: Elsevier Saunders; 2008:251–279.

Stephan F, Boucheseiche S, Hollande J, et al. Pulmonary complications following lung resection: a comprehensive analysis of incidence and possible risk factors. *Chest* 2000;118(5):1263–1270.

10. **(D)** Transfusion is not indicated unless a patient is anemic. It is possible to ameliorate cardiac stress perioperatively. Hypothermia causes an increase in catecholamine, cortisol, and stress hormone release. Keeping a patient

normothermic helps blunt this response. Epidural anesthesia blocks afferent nervous stimulation. This results in attenuation of sympathetic nervous system stimulation. Other maneuvers that ameliorate cardiac stress include control of heart rate and blood pressure with β-blockade.

BIBLIOGRAPHY

Grass JA. The role of epidural anesthesia and analgesia in postoperative outcome. *Anesthesiol Clin North Am* 2000;18(2):407–428.

Kehlet H, Wilmore DW. Multimodal strategies to improve surgical outcome. *Am J Surg* 2002;183(6):630–641.

Lee TW, Grocott HP, Schwinn D, et al. High spinal anesthesia for cardiac surgery: effects on beta-adrenergic receptor function, stress response, and hemodynamics. *Anesthesiology* 2003;98(2):499–510.

Smith R, Ng V, Twomey P, et al. Risk stratification, preoperative testing, and operative planning. In: Wilmore DW, Souba WW, Fink MP, et al. (eds.), *ACS Surgery: Principles & Practice.* New York, NY: WebMD; 2002.

11. **(D)** Although mild to moderate renal impairment is often asymptomatic, renal insufficiency is an independent risk factor for postoperative complications and requires careful adjustment of potential nephrotoxic agents. A detailed medical history may reveal symptoms indicative of renal impairment, such as fatigue, lower extremity swelling, and shortness of breath. Physical examination may reveal signs of fluid overload such as edema and pulmonary crackles.

Routine laboratory testing is not indicated in all patients. However, patients in whom there is a suspicion of renal impairment, or who are likely to be exposed to nephrotoxic agents or hypotension during the procedure, should undergo serum BUN and creatinine testing. Patients with a reduced glomerular filtration rate or a creatinine level greater than 2 mg/dL have an increased risk of postoperative renal dysfunction requiring dialysis compared with patients without renal disease. Creatinine clearance, determined from the patient's serum creatinine concentration, age, and weight, is a more accurate assessment of renal function than serum creatinine.

Urinalysis can also be used to test for asymptomatic renal disease, as well as urinary tract infections. Proteinuria is indicative of glomerular damage, and casts are associated with conditions such as acute interstitial nephritis, glomerulonephritis, and acute tubular necrosis. Urine sodium and creatinine, if included in the analysis of the urine, can be used to calculate the fractional excretion of sodium (FeNa) and aid the physician in distinguishing prerenal from postrenal causes of renal failure. Increased nitrites and white blood cells indicate an infection of the urinary tract. However, in the absence of clinical suspicion, a routine urinalysis is not cost-effective.

Patients with chronic renal dysfunction who require dialysis are at increased risk for postoperative mortality. All dialysis patients should undergo baseline laboratory testing to evaluate their degree of renal dysfunction and identify other risk factors such as anemia, ischemic heart disease, poor nutritional status, volume overload, and electrolyte abnormalities, the most common of which is hyperkalemia. Preoperative dialysis should be performed to optimize a patient's fluid and electrolyte levels, and early postoperative dialysis may also be required.

BIBLIOGRAPHY

Neumayer L, Vargo, D. Principles of preoperative and operative surgery. In: *Sabiston Textbook of Surgery* 18th ed. Philadelphia, PA: Elsevier Saunders; 2008:251–279.

Roy M, Zarebczan B, Weber S. Evaluation of surgical risk, including cardiac and pulmonary risk assessment. In: *ACS Surgery: Principles & Practice.* Philadelphia, PA: Decker Publishing Inc.; 2013.

12. **(C)** Antibiotic prophylaxis is the administration of an antimicrobial agent before initiation of surgery to reduce the number of microbes that enter the tissue. Prophylaxis is limited to the period before and during the procedure. In contrast, empiric therapy is the use of an antimicrobial agent when the risk of surgical infection is high due to either the disease process or the level of contamination. The first dose of antibiotics should be administered within 60 minutes prior to the surgical incision. For patients undergoing procedures that exceed the serum half-life of the antibiotic, repeat doses should be given. However, postoperative continuation has not been shown to provide any benefit.

The Surgical Care Improvement Project (SCIP) is a national effort toward improving the safety of surgical care through a reduction in postoperative complications. The guidelines developed as part of SCIP are monitored in every hospital. SCIP guideline 1 states that prophylactic antibiotics should be received within 1 hour before surgical incision, and guideline 3 indicates the discontinuation of prophylactic antibiotics within 24 hours after surgery completion (48 hours in cardiac patients).

BIBLIOGRAPHY

Beilman GJ, Dunn DL. Surgical infections. In: Brunicardi FC, Andersen DK, Billiar TR, Dunn DL, Hunter JG, Matthews JB, Pollock RE (eds.), *Schwartz's Principles of Surgery* 9th ed. New York, NY: McGraw-Hill; 2010:Chapter 6.

Neumayer L, Vargo D. Principles of preoperative and operative surgery. In: *Sabiston Textbook of Surgery* 18th ed. Philadelphia, PA: Elsevier Saunders; 2008:251–279.

13. **(A)** In general surgery populations, the incidence of pulmonary embolism (PE)/deep vein thrombosis (DVT) is 1.6% and 25%, respectively. The etiology of venous thromboembolism (VTE) is described by Virchow's triad: endothelial injury, stasis, and hypercoagulation. The highest incidence of venous thromboembolism occurs within 24 hours of operation. Most occur within 2 weeks of surgery. Pulmonary embolisms generally arise from lower extremity DVTs that have propagated from the calf into the popliteal vein (<20% of all DVTs). Two-thirds of deaths occur within 30 minutes of the embolic event.

Risk factors for the development of VTE may be acquired or inherited (see Table 6-1). Hereditary hypercoagulopathies occur in 1–20% of the population and increase the risk of VTE by 100–400%. There is also an increased risk of developing a DVT in any patient older than 40 undergoing general anesthesia for longer than 30 minutes.

The most commonly used measures of DVT prophylaxis in surgical patients are early ambulation, low-dose unfractionated heparin, low-molecular-weight heparin, sequential compression devices (SCDs), and elastic stockings. SCDs work through stimulation of endothelial cell fibrinolytic activity and should be placed prior to the start of an operation and continued until the patient begins ambulating. Heparin in its various forms binds antithrombin III and increases its activity 1000-fold.

BIBLIOGRAPHY

Henke P. Venous thromboembolism: diagnosis, prevention and treatment. In: Cameron JL, Cameron AM (eds.), *Current Surgical Therapy*. Philadelphia, PA: Elsevier Saunders; 2010:1070–1073.

Wakefield TW, Rectenwald JR, Messina LM. Veins & lymphatics. In: Doherty GM (ed.), *Current Diagnosis & Treatment: Surgery*, 13th ed. New York, NY: McGraw-Hill; 2010:Chapter 35.

14. **(B)** Surgeries that affect the coagulation system include peripheral vascular surgery, cardiopulmonary bypass procedures, and prostatectomy. Most other surgeries can safely rely on a careful history and physical examination to elucidate bleeding risks. History should include personal or family history of prior bleeding or thromboembolic events, hematologic, liver, or kidney diseases, and use of "blood thinners" (e.g., aspirin, warfarin, clopidogrel). A careful hematologic review of systems including hematuria, menorrhagia, gastrointestinal bleeds, easy bruising, epistaxis, and hemarthroses should uncover most occult hazards. Unusual dietary habits should be sought. Physical examination, especially of the skin and mucous membranes, should search for evidence of hematologic disorders or other organ system disorders that can lead to hemostasis problems. Petechiae, ecchymosis, venous stasis, lack of pulses, and stigmata of liver

TABLE 6-1 Risk Factors for Venous Thromboembolism

Acquired
Advanced age
Hospitalization/immobilization
Hormone replacement therapy and oral contraceptive use
Pregnancy and puerperium
Prior venous thromboembolism
Malignancy
Major surgery
Obesity
Nephrotic syndrome
Trauma or spinal cord injury
Long-haul travel (>6 hours)
Varicose veins
Antiphospholipid antibody syndrome
Myeloproliferative disease
Polycythemia
Inherited
Factor V Leiden
Prothrombin 20210A
Antithrombin deficiency
Protein C deficiency
Protein S deficiency
Factor XI elevation
Dysfibrinogenemia
Mixed Etiology
Homocysteinemia
Factor VII, VIII, IX, XI elevation
Hyperfibrinogenemia
Activated protein C resistance without factor V Leiden

(adenopathy, hepatosplenomegaly, jaundice, telangiectasias, gynecomastia) or renal disease provide clues. Patients with a normal bleeding history and physical examination who undergo low-risk procedures do not need preoperative coagulation screening.

Preoperative coagulation studies are indicated in patients with a history of abnormal bleeding, in patients who cannot provide a history, in high-risk procedures, or if the patient uses anticoagulants.

Further studies including prothrombin time (PT), activated partial thromboplastin time (aPTT), and platelet count may be clinically indicated in high-risk procedures, although these are often normal. At best, if the results are normal, they provide baseline values to monitor bleeding problems after cardiopulmonary bypass or anticoagulation. In a patient in whom there is high clinical suspicion of a hematologic abnormality, further tests are required prior to surgery, including fibrinogen and von Willebrand factor panel. The bleeding time does not correlate with surgical bleeding complications. Other studies that might be checked include thrombin time, platelet aggregation, α_2-antiplasmin, and factor XIII assays.

Prolonged PT results from a defect in the extrinsic pathway. This is usually caused by hepatic insufficiency, severe factor VII deficiency, or vitamin K deficiency (poor absorption, nutrition, cholestasis). Vitamin K deficiency may be corrected with a 10-mg injection if hepatic synthesis is intact.

Prolonged aPTT results from a defect in the intrinsic pathway. This is usually caused by deficiency of factor VIII (hemophilia A), IX (hemophilia B), XI, or XII; lupus anticoagulant; or von Willebrand disease. A 1:1 mixing of patient plasma and normal plasma is performed. If the PTT corrects, a factor deficiency is the likely culprit; if not, the presence of a factor inhibitor or lupus anticoagulant is more likely. Further specific factor assays are available to assess the deficiency.

Prolonged PT and PTT are seen with disseminated intravascular coagulation (DIC); deficiencies of factors II, V, or X; and coagulation factor inhibitor. Patients with DIC must have the etiology treated.

Presented below are several disorders with management options.

Von Willebrand disease is the most common inherited coagulation disorder with prevalence in the general population of 1%. von Willebrand factor is the serum carrier of factor VIII. It is produced by endothelial cells and megakaryocytes and stored intracellularly in Weibel-Palade bodies. It circulates as multimers and causes platelet adhesion to subendothelial collagen in regions of high shear and initiates platelet plug formation. von Willebrand disease occurs when von Willebrand factor is deficient or qualitatively abnormal. Type I is the most common, being autosomal dominant and characterized by decreased concentrations of qualitatively normal factor. Desmopressin (DDAVP) 0.3 µg/kg is recommended for diagnostic procedures and mucosal biopsies and causes an elaboration of factor VIII and von Willebrand factor from endothelial cells. About 48 hours must elapse for von Willebrand factor to reaccumulate. At this time, a second dose may be given with the same effect as the first. A factor VIII concentrate that contains a high concentration of high-molecular-weight von Willebrand factor is recommended for therapeutic procedures. Type II is caused by qualitative abnormality, and type III

(autosomal recessive), the most severe, is characterized by markedly reduced amounts of von Willebrand factor. Type II may be treated with cryoprecipitate. Types II and III both need the concentrate of factor VIII/von Willebrand factor noted above.

Hemophilias are classified according to factor levels: mild (6–30%), moderate (2–5%), and severe (1%). Patients with mild hemophilia A undergoing low-risk procedures may use DDAVP, which increases the release of von Willebrand factor and circulating levels of factor VIII, or recombinant factor VIII concentrates (with history of little exposure to blood products). Moderate or severe patients have a target of 100% factor VIII (plasma concentrates may be used) for the first 5–7 days postoperatively in major surgery and for 50% after postoperative day 1 in minor surgery. Hemophilia B patients may be treated with DDAVP or factor IX concentrates (contain small amounts of activated clotting factors) with the same guidelines as those with factor VIII deficiency. Antifibrinolytics should be avoided because of the increased risk of thrombosis. Hemophilia C patients (factor XI deficiency) can be corrected with fresh frozen plasma (FFP) or plasma-derived virally inactivated factor XI concentrate (potentially thrombogenic) to a target of less than 70%.

In patients with coagulation factor inhibitors, immunosuppression and repletion of the affected factors are required. Lupus anticoagulant relays an increased risk of thrombosis, not bleeding. Platelet count should be checked, and deep venous thrombosis prophylaxis initiated.

Thrombocytopenia is associated with pseudothrombocytopenia (platelet aggregation), splenic sequestration (normal total platelet mass without clinical bleeding), drugs, decreased production, and increased destruction. Treatment of patients with thrombotic thrombocytopenic purpura and hemolytic uremic syndrome (thrombocytopenia, microangiopathic hemolytic anemia, renal failure, and neurologic abnormalities) involves total plasma exchange with cryoprecipitate supernatant plasma in the replacement fluid. In idiopathic thrombocytopenia purpura, antiplatelet antibodies are treated with immunosuppression and occasionally splenectomy. A goal platelet count of 80,000–100,000 is sought preoperatively for this disorder. Cessation of any drugs that cause thrombocytopenia usually leads to the recovery of platelet counts. A platelet count of less than 20,000 is associated with spontaneous bleeding. The platelet count should be greater than 50,000 preoperatively and is an indication for transfusion. For a platelet count between 50,000 and 100,000, transfusion is indicated based on risk of bleeding. For a count greater than 100,000 or in disorders with increased platelet destruction, transfusion is rarely indicated.

Actively bleeding renal patients (platelet dysfunction) may be treated with correction of anemia, DDAVP (0.3 µg/kg IV or intranasally), cryoprecipitate, intravenous conjugated estrogens (0.6 mg/kg 4 or 5 days before surgery), or dialysis. Raising the hematocrit to 30% improves uremic bleeding. There is a decrease in aggregation and adhesiveness of platelets and in the levels of platelet factor II, with a resultant prolonged bleeding time. The nature of the lesion caused by renal insufficiency is unknown. Dialysis with heparin must be timed to have an appropriate coagulation profile prior to surgery.

BIBLIOGRAPHY

Cogbill T. Abnormal operative and postoperative bleeding. In: Cameron JL, Cameron AM (eds.), *Current Surgical Therapy*. Philadelphia, PA: Elsevier Saunders; 2010:1088–1091.

Joseph AJ, Cohn SL. Perioperative care of the patient with renal failure. *Med Clin North Am* 2003;87(1):193–210.

Neumayer L, Vargo D. Principles of preoperative and operative surgery. In: *Sabiston Textbook of Surgery* 18th ed. Philadelphia, PA: Elsevier Saunders; 2008:251–279.

O'Leary JP, Capote LR. *The Physiologic Basis of Surgery* 3rd ed. Philadelphia, PA: Lippincott Williams & Wilkins; 2002:536.

15. **(C)** Optimal control of diabetes is essential in preoperative patients who are at increased risk of developing infectious, metabolic, electrolyte, renal, and cardiac complications during and after surgery. The attendant immunosuppression seen in poorly controlled diabetics increases the risk for postoperative wound infections. Neutrophil phagocytosis and chemotaxis, as well as collagen synthesis, are adversely affected when the blood glucose levels are greater than 250 mg/dL. Wound infections, skin infections, pneumonia, and urinary tract infections (UTIs) account for two-thirds of all postoperative complications and 20% of all postoperative deaths in diabetics. Further, many surgical emergencies can give rise to diabetic emergencies such as diabetic ketoacidosis (DKA) or hyperglycemic hyperosmolar nonketotic coma (HHNC). The best method for tightly controlling diabetes mellitus during major surgery is with a continuous intravenous (IV) insulin and glucose infusion.

DKA arises from a combination of effects from insulin deficiency and increase in epinephrine, norepinephrine, cortisol, glucagons, and growth hormone with resultant insulin resistance. In addition, epinephrine causes a decrease in insulin secretion. The patient's metabolism is characterized by hyperglycemia, accelerated gluconeogenesis, reduced peripheral glucose utilization, catabolism of lean tissue and lipid stores, hyperosmolar, osmotic diuresis, volume depletion, paradoxical dilutional hyponatremia, acidemia, ketonemia, and inability to metabolize long-chain fatty acids via lipogenic pathways.

Precipitants giving rise to this state include infection, pregnancy, acute MI, trauma, acute psychiatric illness, major surgery, thyrotoxicosis, and pheochromocytoma. Signs and symptoms include dehydration, vomiting, tachypnea, severe abdominal pain, and obtundation. Blood glucose greater than 700 mg/dL, serum osmolarity greater than 340 mOsm/L, arterial pH less than 7.3 with PCO_2 ≤40 mmHg, ketonemia, and ketonuria are diagnostic of DKA.

The differential diagnoses are lactic acidosis, uremia, intoxication (including ethanol), sepsis, cerebrovascular accident, and intra-abdominal catastrophe.

Although HHNC and DKA may coexist, patients who have HHNC by definition do not have acidosis or ketonemia/ketonuria. They present obtunded, dehydrated, and azotemic with extremely elevated blood glucose levels. They can be as high as 1000 mg/dL. HHNC is instigated by many of the same culprits as DKA. Pancreatitis and certain medications (β-blockers, furosemide, parenteral nutrition, thiazides) are also implicated in HHNC. There is sufficient insulin present to suppress lipolysis, preventing ketosis. Therapy is similar to DKA. Resuscitation should be initiated immediately.

Treatment is manifold and includes aggressive fluid resuscitation (patients may have up to a 10-L deficit) with isotonic fluid. Five percent dextrose should be added when the blood glucose drops below 250 mg/dL to prevent hypoglycemia and cerebral edema. Potassium chloride should be added with the second liter or with the first if hypokalemic while acidemic on presentation. Bicarbonate is seldom required secondary to metabolism of ketones (acetoacetate and β-hydroxybutyrate); add 100 mEq of $NaHCO_3$ if pH <7.1, HCO_3 <10 mEq/dL, or to relieve Kussmaul respirations. Insulin therapy is as follows: 10–30 unit bolus; regular insulin drip at 5–10 units/h; discontinue drip when blood glucose ≤250 mg/dL; cover with subcutaneous regular insulin subsequently; address precipitating factor(s). In this case, the patient should be resuscitated prior to being taken to the operating room, if indicated.

BIBLIOGRAPHY

Adams C, Biffl W, Cioffl W. 2008. Surgical critical care. In: *Sabiston Textbook of Surgery* 18th ed. Philadelphia, PA: Elsevier Saunders; 2008:602–630.

Andreoli TE, Bennet JC, Carpenter CCJ, et al. *Cecil Essentials of Medicine* 4th ed. Philadelphia, PA: W.B. Saunders; 1997:533–545.

Scherpereel PA, Tavernier B. Perioperative care of diabetic patients. *Eur J Anaesthesiol* 2001;18:277–294.

Schiff RL, Welsh GA. Perioperative evaluation and management of the patient with endocrine dysfunction. *Med Clin North Am* 2003;87(1):175–192.

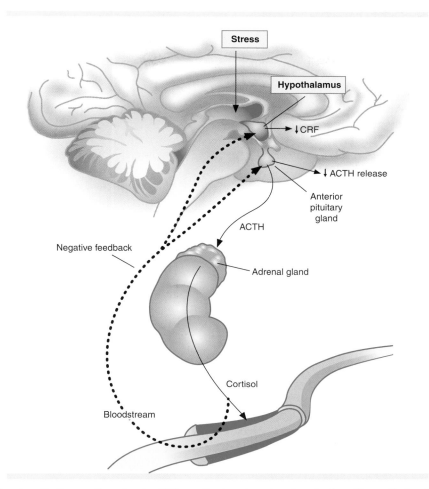

FIGURE 6-3. Hypothalamic-pituitary-adrenal axis. CRF, corticotropin-releasing factor. (From *Endocrine surgery* 4th edition fig. 6-4).

16. **(D)** The production of glucocorticoids by the adrenal cortex is regulated predominantly by adrenocorticotropic hormone (ACTH) secreted by the anterior pituitary under the influence of hypothalamic corticotropin-releasing hormone (CRH) (see Fig. 6-3).

   Patients with primary adrenal insufficiency (Addison disease) have defects in cortisol and aldosterone secretion. In secondary adrenal insufficiency (e.g., from previous steroid intake), aldosterone secretion is intact. Surgery is one of the most potent activators of the hypothalamic-pituitary-adrenal (HPA) axis, resulting in increased plasma ACTH and cortisol concentrations.

   The patient described is in addisonian crisis, a result of acute adrenal insufficiency, the consequences of which can be fatal if left untreated. Acute adrenal insufficiency may be caused by abrupt cessation of pharmacologic doses of chronic glucocorticoid therapy or surgical excision or destruction of the pituitary or adrenal gland.

   Symptoms of adrenal insufficiency are nonspecific, such as fatigue, weakness, anorexia, orthostasis, and abdominal pain. Clinical signs include hyponatremia,

hyperkalemia, acidosis, hypoglycemia or hyperglycemia, normocytic anemia, eosinophilia, and lymphocytosis.

   Diagnosis is made by administration of ACTH stimulation test (cosyntropin) with pre- and postcortisol levels. A baseline serum cortisol level greater than 19 mg/dL (525 nmol/L) rules out adrenal insufficiency, and a level less than 3 mg/dL (83 nmol/L) indicates its presence. Symptomatic patients below this level should be treated with steroids; however, this should not impede prompt therapy with hydrocortisone or equivalent (dexamethasone should not interfere with the stimulation test). Approximately 300 mg of hydrocortisone per day is required to treat a patient in crisis. In addition, repletion of volume and electrolytes is mandatory.

   Glucocorticoid prophylaxis should be administered preoperatively to patients currently on steroids or who received steroids within 6 months to 1 year of surgery. A stress dose of hydrocortisone (100 mg) may be given with induction of anesthesia. For minor surgical procedures, usual maintenance dose is continued postoperatively. For major surgical procedures, a stress dose (100 mg) is continued every 8 hours until stable or free of complications and then tapered to the usual maintenance dose.

Mineralocorticoid deficiency is rare and manifests with the above electrolyte imbalances. Glucocorticoid therapy typically exerts sufficient mineralocorticoid activity, but if the patient continues to be hypotensive, mineralocorticoid replacement may be indicated (deoxycorticosterone acetate or fluorohydrocortisone). Mineralocorticoid replacement does not need to be initiated until the dosage of hydrocortisone is less than 50 mg/d.

BIBLIOGRAPHY

Jabbour SA. Steroids and the surgical patient. *Med Clin North Am* 2001;85(5):1311–1317.

Kulaylat M, Dayton M. Surgical complications. In: *Sabiston Textbook of Surgery* 18th ed. Philadelphia, PA: Elsevier Saunders; 2008:328–370.

Marik PE, Zaloga GP. Adrenocortical insufficiency. In: Hall JB, Schmidt GA, Wood LD (eds.): *Principles of Critical Care*, 3rd ed. New York, NY: McGraw-Hill; 2005:Chapter 79.

Schiff RL, Welsh GA. Perioperative evaluation and management of the patient with endocrine dysfunction. *Med Clin North Am* 2003;87(1):175–192.

Stein S, Michelassi F. Crohn's disease of the small bowel-medical management. In: Cameron JL, Cameron AM (eds.), *Current Surgical Therapy*. Philadelphia, PA: Elsevier Saunders; 2010:97–100.

17. **(A)** Pheochromocytoma is a neuroendocrine tumor of the chromaffin cell that originates from the adrenal medulla and extra-adrenal paraganglia cells that most commonly produces hypertension and hypovolemia from release of catecholamines that can lead to a fatal hypertensive crisis or hypotension intraoperatively. When tumor veins are ligated during surgery, the sudden drop in circulating catecholamines can lead to vasodilatation. The catecholamine output of the contralateral adrenal may be suppressed from previous catecholamine excess. In the hypovolemic patient, this can lead to hypotension, shock, and death.

Pheochromocytoma has a varied presentation. Patients are volume-depleted. They also may complain of paroxysmal hypertension (up to 75% of patients) with or without headache, chest pain, abdominal pain, dyspnea, fever, seizures, end-organ damage in a pheochromocytoma crisis, insulin resistance, normal blood pressure, and persistent hypertension (50% of patients). Left ventricular hypertrophy, dysfunction, and cardiomyopathy may result.

Patients with pheochromocytoma are treated preoperatively for 2 to 4 weeks with α-blockade, such as phenoxybenzamine. The addition of β-blockade may prove necessary after institution of α-blockade, if hypertension is persistent or tachycardia ensues. Close intraoperative communication with anesthesiology colleagues cannot be overemphasized, with availability of sodium nitroprusside, phentolamine, and adrenergic agents following tumor removal to control blood pressure intraoperatively. The patient should be hospitalized for several days before the operation when postural hypotension is present, for observation and administration of intravenous fluid. Phenoxybenzamine's side effects include somnolence, orthostatic hypotension, stuffy nose, and an inability to ejaculate. Selective α₁-receptor blockers prazosin, doxazosin, or terazosin can be used if these are not tolerated. Metyrosine competitively inhibits tyrosine hydroxylase, the rate-limiting step in catecholamine biosynthesis, and may be added when other antihypertensive agents are not effective. Second-line agents include calcium channel blockers (calcium ion transport is essential for release of catecholamines from chromaffin cells) and angiotensin-converting enzyme inhibitors. β-Adrenergic blockade (propranolol, metoprolol, atenolol) should then be initiated if not contraindicated (asthma, CHF) to prevent the reflex tachycardia associated with nonselective α-receptor blockade, perioperative arrhythmias, and cardiac complications. β-Blockade should be begun several days after α-blockade and at least a few days prior to surgery, when adequate α-blockade is achieved or an unopposed α-effect of the catecholamine may occur, leading to block of β receptor–mediated vasodilatation in skeletal muscle with resultant vasoconstriction, hypertensive crisis, CHF, or pulmonary edema. Morphine and phenothiazines may precipitate hypertensive crisis and should be avoided preoperatively.

Anesthetic drugs that precipitate catecholamine secretion should be avoided (isoflurane, enflurane, nitroprusside, nitroglycerin, phentolamine). Cardiac arrhythmias are best managed with short-acting β-blockers (esmolol) or lidocaine perioperatively. Invasive monitoring is required, occasionally needing a Swan-Ganz catheter in patients with significant cardiac disease. Laparoscopic procedures are generally better tolerated.

Hypertension may persist for up to 2 weeks postoperatively. Urinary catecholamines should be checked to rule out residual disease. Twenty-five percent of patients have persistent hypertension from other etiologies. Hypoglycemia must be guarded against. If bilateral adrenalectomy is performed, steroid replacement will be required.

BIBLIOGRAPHY

Ellison T, Edil B. Laparoscopic adrenalectomy. In: Cameron JL, Cameron AM (eds.), *Current Surgical Therapy*. Philadelphia, PA: Elsevier Saunders; 2010:1274–1279.

Plouin PF, Duclos JM, Soppelsa F, et al. Factors associated with perioperative morbidity and mortality in patients with pheochromocytoma: analysis of 165 operations at a single center. *J Clin Endocrinol Metabol* 2001;86(4):1480–1486.

Prys-Roberts C. Phaeochromocytoma: recent progress in management. *Br J Anaesthesia* 2000;85(1):44–57.

Schiff RL, Welsh GA. Perioperative evaluation and management of the patient with endocrine dysfunction. *Med Clin North Am* 2003;87(1):175–192.

Townsend CM. The adrenal glands. In: *Sabiston Textbook of Surgery* 18th ed. Philadelphia, PA: Elsevier Saunders; 2008:997–1030.

18. **(A)** Renal insufficiency is an independent risk factor for cardiovascular death after elective general and cardiovascular surgery. One study found the following as predictive of perioperative MI: valvular disease, previous CHF, emergency surgery, general anesthesia, preoperative diagnosis of CAD, lower preoperative and postoperative hemoglobin concentrations, and increased intraoperative bleeding.

Preexisting renal insufficiency is a risk factor for the development of acute renal failure (ARF) postoperatively. ARF is broadly defined as a sudden deterioration of renal function resulting in retention of nitrogenous wastes including urea and creatinine. Other risk factors of postoperative ARF include cardiac dysfunction, sepsis, hypovolemia, cholestatic jaundice, advanced age (suspected without definitive data), trauma surgery, procedures on the heart, aorta, and peripheral arterial system, and hepatic transplantation.

Prerenal ARF results from diminished renal perfusion caused by volume depletion and/or hypotension. Intrinsic ARF patients have diminished baseline glomerular filtration rate (GFR) because of diabetes, hypertension, or vascular disease. Acute tubular necrosis is the most common mechanism of renal failure and occurs in the setting of critical surgical illness and multiple organ failure.

Postrenal ARF occurs as a result of of tubular obstruction (sulfonamide and acyclovir crystals or bladder dysfunction). Creatinine is a simple but rough estimation of GFR, which in turn is a rough estimate of renal function. Twenty percent of patients presenting with a creatinine between 1.5 and 3.0 mg/dL have coexisting cardiovascular disease. In a patient with previously unknown renal insufficiency, it must be worked up in conjunction with an internist or nephrologist before an elective operation.

Patients on dialysis should have their dialysis (within 24 hours of the procedure) and fluid management carefully managed by a multidisciplinary team consisting of the surgeon, nephrologist, anesthesiologist, cardiologist, endocrinologist, primary care physician, and nutritionist. During the postoperative period, dialysis patients undergo heparin-free dialysis for at least 24 hours. In patients with severe renal insufficiency (creatinine >3.0 mg/dL) not on dialysis, appropriate volume resuscitation should be guided by invasive monitoring, either by CVP or pulmonary wedge pressure. Uremic patients may have platelet dysfunction resulting in an increased bleeding tendency manifested by a prolonged bleeding time. An indwelling bladder catheter is required. Nephrotoxic agents or agents that impair renal blood flow autoregulation should be avoided. Examples of these agents include contrast dye, aminoglycosides, nonsteroidal anti-inflammatory drugs (NSAIDs), and angiotensin-converting enzyme inhibitors. Low-dose dopamine has been shown to increase urine flow rate in sick postoperative patients but confers no significant protection from renal dysfunction. It is suggested that the dose of low-molecular-weight heparins be decreased by 50% when the GFR is lower than 10 mL/min.

BIBLIOGRAPHY

Bellomo R, Chapman M, Finfer S, et al. Low-dose dopamine in patients with early renal dysfunction: a placebo-controlled randomized trial. Australian and New Zealand Intensive Care Society (ANZICS) Clinical Trials Group. *Lancet* 2000;36(9248):2139–2143.

Joseph AJ, Cohn SL. Perioperative care of the patient with renal failure. *Med Clin North Am* 2003;87(1):193–210.

Sprung J, Abdelmalak B, Gottlieb A, et al. Analysis of risk factors for myocardial infarction and cardiac mortality after major vascular surgery. *Anesthesiology* 2000;93(1):129–140.

Weldon BC, Monk TG. The patient at risk for acute renal failure. Recognition, prevention, and preoperative optimization. *Anesthesiol Clin North Am* 2000;18(4):705–717.

19. **(E)** Unlike renal or pulmonary insufficiency, there is no artificial means to support hepatic function. This patient population is prone to multiple complications including gastrointestinal hemorrhage, electrolyte abnormalities (hyponatremia), renal dysfunction (hepatorenal syndromes), and encephalopathy.

In a patient with suspected liver disease secondary to history and physical, the following liver function tests (LFTs) and synthetic function tests should be ordered: serum bilirubin, aspartate aminotransferase (AST or SGOT), alanine aminotransferase (ALT or SGPT), alkaline phosphatase, prothrombin time (PT), and serum albumin.

The Child-Pugh classification of cirrhosis indicates surgical risk, with even low scoring individuals having an increased complication risk. Patients treated medically with improvement of their Child's classification have proportionate improvement in survival (Child's C to Child's A or B).

	Bilirubin	Albumin	Nutrition	Encephalopathy	Ascites	Operative Mortality
A	<2	>3.5	Excellent	None	None	<5%
B	2–3	3.0–3.5	Good	Minimal	Easily controlled	<15%
C	>3	<3	Poor	Severe	Poorly controlled	≈33%

The Model for End-Stage Liver Disease (MELD) score is based on serum international normalized ratio (INR), bilirubin, and creatinine and has also been shown to predict morbidity in patients undergoing cholecystectomy, hepatectomy, and cardiac surgery. It has been recommended that patients with a MELD score greater than 15 not undergo elective surgery because the risk of a complication outweighs any surgical benefit. Mortality increases by approximately 1% for each MELD point up to 20 and by 2% for each point above 20. Although both scoring systems are in use, numerous studies have demonstrated the MELD score to be superior to the Child-Pugh score in predicting perioperative morbidity and mortality.

Further evaluation of sequelae of cirrhosis may be warranted including endoscopy, pulmonary function tests, CAD, CHF, and renal function.

BIBLIOGRAPHY

Geller DA, Tsung A. Liver. In: Brunicardi FC, Andersen DK, Billiar TR, Dunn DL, Hunter JG, Matthews JB, Pollock RE (eds.), *Schwartz's Principles of Surgery*, 9th ed. New York, NY: McGraw-Hill; 2010:Chapter 31.

Rikkers L. Surgical complications of cirrhosis and portal hypertension. In: Townsend CM (ed.), *Sabiston Textbook of Surgery*, 18th ed. Philadelphia, PA: Elsevier Saunders; 2008:1524–1546.

Roy M, Zarebczan B, Weber S. Evaluation of surgical risk, including cardiac and pulmonary risk assessment. In: *ACS Surgery: Principles & Practice*. Philadelphia, PA: Decker Publishing Inc.; 2013.

20. **(C)** Thyroid storm or thyrotoxicosis is a condition of hyperthyroidism accompanied by fever, central nervous system agitation or depression, and cardiovascular dysfunction that may be precipitated in patients who have underlying hyperthyroidism of any cause. The diagnosis is clinical, and therapy needs to be instituted prior to return of any lab values. Further, although thyroxine (T_4) and triiodothyronine (T_3) levels are elevated, they are not more so than in nontoxic hyperthyroidism. T_3 and T_4 exert direct inotropic and chronotropic effects on cardiac muscle with increased cardiac output that may limit cardiac reserves during surgery in the hyperthyroid patient. Atrial fibrillation is present in 10–20% of patients.

Treatment of thyroid storm involves four components:

1. Therapy to reduce the serum thyroid hormone levels
2. Therapy to reduce the action of the thyroid hormones on peripheral tissues
3. Therapy to prevent cardiovascular decompensation and to maintain normal homeostasis
4. Treatment of the precipitating event(s)

BIBLIOGRAPHY

Klein I, Ojamaa K. Mechanisms of disease: thyroid hormone and the cardiovascular system. *N Engl J Med* 2001;344(7):501–509.

McArthur JW, Rawson RW, Means JH, et al. Thyrotoxic crisis. *JAMA* 1947;132:868.

Schiff RL, Welsh GA. Perioperative evaluation and management of the patient with endocrine dysfunction. *Med Clin North Am* 2003;87(1):175–192.

Weiss RE, Refetoff S. Thyroid disease. In: Hall JB, Schmidt GA, Wood LD (eds.), *Principles of Critical Care*, 3rd ed. New York, NY: McGraw-Hill; 2005:Chapter 80.

21. **(B)** The cardiac sounds listed in the question are associated with atrial septal defect, mitral regurgitation or ventricular septal defect, left ventricular failure or volume overload (normal in children), systemic hypertension, and normal heart, respectively.

There is a significant prevalence of valvular heart disease among patients undergoing elective major noncardiac procedures. The American Heart Association has published guidelines for antibiotic prophylaxis for prevention of endocarditis, the need of which is dictated by both the cardiac abnormality and type of surgical procedure. There exist no published randomized trials demonstrating that prophylaxis lowers the risk of developing endocarditis. Nevertheless, the morbidity and mortality associated with infective endocarditis are used to justify prophylaxis for patients who have high- and intermediate-risk cardiac lesions and who are to undergo bacteremia-inducing procedures.

Knowledge of the pathogens associated with types of procedures is paramount in choosing the appropriate prophylaxis agent. The target for prophylaxis in procedures involving the oral cavity, respiratory tract, or esophagus is viridans streptococci. For genitourinary and gastrointestinal cases, there is a strong association with enterococcal endocarditis. Prophylaxis against *Staphylococcus aureus* is employed when incising and draining skin or soft tissue infections.

Procedures for which antibiotic prophylaxis is recommended include dental procedures that induce gingival or mucosal bleeding (especially extractions); tonsillectomy or adenoidectomy; gastrointestinal or respiratory mucosa; rigid bronchoscopy; esophageal varix sclerotherapy; esophageal dilatation; endoscopic retrograde cholangiography with biliary obstruction; gallbladder surgery; cystoscopy with urethral dilation; urethral catheterization if UTI present; urinary tract surgery, including prostate; and incision and drainage of infected tissue.

Procedures for which prophylaxis is recommended only if patients are at highest risk include flexible bronchoscopy, gastrointestinal endoscopy, and vaginal hysterectomy. Further, in the absence of infection, the following may need prophylaxis: urethral catheterization, dilatation and curettage, uncomplicated vaginal delivery, therapeutic abortion, insertion or removal of intrauterine devices, sterilization procedures, and laparoscopy.

The following procedures are not recommended for prophylaxis: dental procedures not likely to cause bleeding, shedding of primary teeth, tympanostomy tube insertion, endotracheal tube insertion, transesophageal echocardiography, cardiac catheterization, pacemaker implantation, incision or biopsy of scrubbed skin, Cesarean section, and circumcision.

Certain preexisting cardiac disorders are associated with relatively high risk of infective endocarditis, with the presence of prosthetic heart valves being the highest. Other disorders for which prophylaxis is recommended include patent ductus arteriosus, aortic regurgitation or stenosis, mitral regurgitation with or without stenosis, ventricular septal defect, coarctation of the aorta, postoperative intracardiac lesion with residual hemodynamic abnormality, or prosthetic device. Cardiac disorders with relatively high risk but not recommended for prophylaxis include previous infective endocarditis, cyanotic congenital heart disease, and surgically constructed systemic pulmonary shunts.

Intermediate-risk conditions include mitral valve prolapse with regurgitation (murmur) or thickened valve leaflets, mitral stenosis, tricuspid valve disease, pulmonary stenosis, asymmetrical septal hypertrophy, bicuspid aortic valve or calcific aortic sclerosis with minimal hemodynamic abnormality, degenerative valvular disease in elderly patients, and postoperative (<6 months) intracardiac lesion with minimal or no hemodynamic abnormality.

Cardiac disorders with very low or negligible risk for which prophylaxis is not recommended include mitral valve prolapse without regurgitation (murmur) or thickened valve leaflets, trivial valvular regurgitation on echocardiogram without structural abnormality, atrial septal defect (secundum), arteriosclerotic plaques, CAD, pacemaker or implanted defibrillators, postoperative (>6 months) intracardiac lesion with minimal or no hemodynamic abnormality, prior coronary bypass graft surgery, and prior Kawasaki disease or rheumatic fever without valvular dysfunction.

Penicillin-resistant flora may emerge among patients who are receiving continuous penicillin for prevention of rheumatic fever or repetitive doses for serial dental procedures. A regimen without penicillin is preferable in these patients. If prophylaxis is initiated several days before surgery, then organisms become resistant at the mucosal site.

BIBLIOGRAPHY

Braunwald E. *Heart Disease: A Textbook of Cardiovascular Medicine*, 6th ed. Philadelphia, PA: W.B. Saunders; 2001:1742–1745.
Shammash JB, Ghali WA. Preoperative assessment and perioperative management of the patient with nonischemic heart disease. *Med Clin North Am* 2003;87(1):137–152.

22. **(C)** Neuraxial (central) anesthesia involves the continuous or intermittent injection of anesthetic into the epidural or intrathecal space; the effect is sensory analgesia, motor blockade, and inhibition of sympathetic outflow. Peripheral nerve blockade results in inhibition of conduction in fibers of a single peripheral nerve or plexus (cervical, brachial, or lumbar) in the periphery. Intravenous regional anesthesia involves IV administration of a local anesthetic into a tourniquet-occluded extremity. In these settings, additional pain control may be achieved by administering local anesthetics into the wound cavity.

Contraindications to regional anesthesia include patient refusal or inability to cooperate during the procedure, elevated intracranial pressure, anticoagulation, vascular malformation or infection at the needle insertion site, severe hemodynamic instability, and sepsis. Preexisting neurologic disease is a relative contraindication. Procedures performed solely under infiltration may be associated with patient dissatisfaction caused by intraoperative anxiety and pain.

Although hemorrhagic complications can occur after any regional technique, bleeding associated with neuraxial blockade is the most serious of these because of the potentially devastating consequences. Spinal hematoma may occur as a result of vascular trauma from placement of a needle or catheter into the subarachnoid or epidural space or may occur spontaneously, even in the absence of antiplatelet or anticoagulant therapy. The reported incidence of spinal hematoma is estimated to be less than 1 in 150,000 for epidural anesthesia and 1 in 200,000 for spinal anesthesia. With such low incidences, it is difficult to determine whether any increased risk can be attributed to anticoagulation.

BIBLIOGRAPHY

Backman SB, Bondy RM, Deschamps A, et al. Perioperative considerations for anesthesia. In: Ashley SW, Klingensmith ME, Cance WG, et al. (eds.), *ACS Surgery: Principles & Practice*. Hamilton, Ontario: B.C. Decker; 2012.

CHAPTER 7

ANESTHESIA

CAMPBELL D. WILLIAMS AND ANDREW FEIDER

QUESTIONS

1. A 40-year-old male status post kidney transplant 2 years ago with history of diabetes mellitus and hypertension presents to an ambulatory surgery center for debridement of an atrioventricular (AV) fistula that was used in the past for dialysis. Despite tight glycemic control, the patient has diabetic retinopathy and neuropathy. His preoperative blood pressure is 172/95 mmHg. His renal function is normal, and he no longer requires hemodialysis. What is this patient's American Society of Anesthesiologists (ASA) physical status?
   (A) Class 1
   (B) Class 2
   (C) Class 2E
   (D) Class 3
   (E) Class 4

2. The patient in Question 1 is brought to the operating suite and preoxygenated. General anesthesia is induced with fentanyl, propofol, and rocuronium. The anesthesiologist makes an initial attempt at laryngoscopy but is unsuccessful. The patient is repositioned, and a different type of laryngoscope blade is used without success. The patient is unable to be mask ventilated. Oxygen saturation is 96%. What is the best approach at this juncture according to the emergency airway algorithm?
   (A) Attempt to reverse the rocuronium with neostigmine
   (B) Allow the patient to wake up
   (C) Attempt to ventilate through a laryngeal mask airway (LMA)
   (D) Perform a cricothyrotomy
   (E) Perform a retrograde intubation over a wire

3. Which of the following factors is *unique* to the pediatric airway?
   (A) Small occiput
   (B) Short, broad epiglottis
   (C) Narrowest part of the airway at the cricoid cartilage
   (D) Long trachea
   (E) Relatively small tongue

4. Which of the following is *true* concerning neonatal physiology in relation to adult physiology?
   (A) Larger functional residual capacity (FRC) increases oxygen reserve
   (B) Decreased respiratory rate
   (C) Larger tidal volume per kilogram than adults
   (D) Cardiac output is dependent on heart rate
   (E) Kidney function is normal by 2 months of age

5. A 74-year-old male is being evaluated 1 week prior to a scheduled carotid endarterectomy. His medical history includes three recent transient ischemic attacks, hypertension, and type 2 diabetes requiring insulin for control. He has a 50-pack-year history of tobacco use but has not smoked for 12 years. His home medications include lisinopril, metoprolol, and insulin. The patient swims 1500 yards three times per week and plays tennis two times per week. He denies shortness of breath, history of myocardial infarction (MI), chest pain, or congestive heart failure (CHF). A 12-lead electrocardiogram (ECG) performed 15 months ago by his primary care physician is included with his records and shows sinus rhythm, 71 bpm, no block, and no pathologic Q waves, but some nonspecific S-T changes in leads V1, V4, and V5. Which of the following cardiac tests or interventions should be performed prior to surgery?
   (A) Transthoracic echocardiogram
   (B) Treadmill stress testing
   (C) Dobutamine stress echo
   (D) Coronary angiography with subsequent intervention if stenotic lesions are detected
   (E) No further testing or intervention needed prior to surgery

6. Which of the following drugs is a depolarizing neuromuscular blocking agent?
   (A) Cisatracurium
   (B) Succinylcholine
   (C) Vecuronium
   (D) Rocuronium
   (E) Pancuronium

7. Which of the following is a potential effect of succinylcholine?
   (A) Hyperkalemia
   (B) Increased intraocular pressure
   (C) Malignant hyperthermia
   (D) Myalgias
   (E) All of the above

8. A 45-year-old male with end-stage renal disease (ESRD) on hemodialysis is scheduled for a pancreatoduodenectomy for pancreatic cancer. Preoperative potassium is 4.8 mEq/dL. He recently had surgery and was an easy intubation with a grade 1 view per the anesthesia record. What drug is most appropriate to maintain neuromuscular blockade during the procedure?
   (A) Rocuronium
   (B) Pancuronium
   (C) Cisatracurium
   (D) Vecuronium
   (E) Succinylcholine

9. If a trauma patient with a full stomach has a contraindication to succinylcholine and needs a rapid sequence intubation, what is the neuromuscular blocker of choice?
   (A) Rocuronium
   (B) Pancuronium
   (C) Cisatracurium
   (D) Atracurium
   (E) Mivacurium

10. During the fascial closure at the end of an exploratory laparotomy, a patient has one out of four twitches using the peripheral nerve stimulator to monitor the ulnar nerve. Approximately what degree of neuromuscular blockade remains?
    (A) 5%
    (B) 25%
    (C) 50%
    (D) 75%
    (E) 95%

11. A patient has undergone general anesthesia for an exploratory laparotomy. Rocuronium was used for muscle relaxation. At the end of the procedure, there is evidence of residual neuromuscular blockade with use of a nerve stimulator. What drug or combination of drugs should be used to reverse the neuromuscular blockade and limit side effects?
    (A) Edrophonium alone
    (B) Atropine/glycopyrrolate
    (C) Neostigmine/glycopyrrolate
    (D) Edrophonium/glycopyrrolate
    (E) Neostigmine alone

12. Which of the following best describes the mechanism of action of local anesthetics?
    (A) Binding of the cationic form of the local anesthetic molecule to extracellular calcium channels
    (B) Binding of the neutral (basic) form of the local anesthetic molecule to cytoplasmic sodium receptors
    (C) Binding of the cationic form of the local anesthetic molecule to transmembrane sodium receptors
    (D) Binding of the neutral (basic) form of the local anesthetic molecule to transmembrane potassium channels in the activated-open state
    (E) Binding of the local anesthetic molecule to acetylcholine receptors

13. Lipid solubility, protein binding, and pK_a of theoretical local anesthetic drugs are listed below. Which combination would create the most potent drug with the most rapid speed of onset and longest duration of action?
    (A) Lipid solubility: high; protein binding: high; pK_a: 7.8
    (B) Lipid solubility: high; protein binding: low; pK_a: 7.7
    (C) Lipid solubility: high; protein binding: high; pK_a: 8.9
    (D) Lipid solubility: low; protein binding: low; pK_a: 7.6
    (E) Lipid solubility: low; protein binding: high; pK_a: 8.5

14. An otherwise healthy, 80-kg 47-year-old male undergoes wide local excision of a suspected malignant melanoma along the right midaxillary line overlying the fifth rib. The incision is elliptically shaped, 10 cm long and 6 cm wide, and able to be closed primarily. Which of the following represents the best choice for local anesthetic infiltration to manage postoperative pain?
    (A) 30 mL of 2% lidocaine with 1:200,000 epinephrine
    (B) 40 mL of 1% lidocaine without epinephrine
    (C) 5 mL of 0.25% mepivacaine without epinephrine
    (D) 30 mL of 0.75% bupivacaine with 1:200,000 epinephrine
    (E) 20 mL of 0.5% bupivacaine with 1:200,000 epinephrine

15. A 56-year-old female with a long history of rheumatoid arthritis and hypertension is admitted through the emergency department with fever, malaise, and shortness of breath. She reports allergies to penicillin, sulfa drugs, and many cosmetics. Her vital signs are temperature (T) 102.3°F, heart rate (HR) 105 bpm, respiratory rate (RR) 29 breaths/min, and blood pressure (BP) 130/75 mmHg. Chest x-ray shows a left-sided pleural effusion. The decision is made to perform bedside thoracentesis with insertion of a chest tube. The patient complains of palpitations and increased malaise approximately 5 minutes after infiltration and intercostal block with a total of 5 mL of 1% lidocaine combined with 5 mL of 0.25% bupivacaine and 1:200,000 epinephrine. Repeat

measurement of vital signs shows HR 145 bpm and BP 175/110 mmHg. What is the most likely explanation of her symptoms?

(A) Allergic reaction to lidocaine
(B) Allergic reaction to bupivacaine
(C) Accidental intravascular injection resulting in cardiac toxicity from lidocaine
(D) Vascular absorption of the epinephrine
(E) Accidental intravascular injection resulting in cardiac toxicity from bupivacaine

Questions 16 and 17 refer to the following case scenario.

A 37-year-old white male with no medical history presents for left elbow surgery. A supraclavicular nerve block is performed using 40 mL of 0.5% bupivacaine with 1:200,000 epinephrine. The local anesthetic is injected in 5-mL doses with negative heme on aspiration between doses. During injection of the sixth injection, the patient complains of a metallic taste in his mouth and ringing in his ears. As the anesthesiologist is preparing to administer intravenous (IV) midazolam, the patient develops tonic-clonic seizures.

16. If the patient received an intravascular injection of high-dose bupivacaine, what is most likely to happen next?
(A) Systemic peripheral vasoconstriction
(B) Systemic peripheral vasodilation
(C) Cardiovascular collapse
(D) Disseminated intravascular coagulation
(E) Nothing; the central nervous system (CNS) excitation always spontaneously resolves

17. The patient now develops unstable ventricular tachycardia, and advanced cardiac life support (ACLS) is initiated. Besides supportive therapy, what drug is recommended to directly combat the etiology of this patient's condition?
(A) Epinephrine 1 mg bolus
(B) Diltiazem 20 mg bolus
(C) Lidocaine 2 mg/kg bolus
(D) Intralipid 20% 1.5 mL/kg bolus
(E) Propofol 3 mg/kg bolus

18. A 77-year-old male victim of abdominal penetrating trauma presents to the emergency room with a Glasgow coma scale (GCS) score of 13, HR 118 bpm, RR 26 breaths/min, and BP 73/30 mmHg. External bleeding is controlled, and the patient is resuscitated with 3 L normal saline and 2 units of packed red blood cells. On arrival to the operating room, his vital signs are now HR 105 bpm, RR 22 breaths/min, and BP 95/54 mmHg. Which of the following intravenous medications represents the best choice to induce general anesthesia and facilitate endotracheal intubation?

(A) Propofol 2 mg/kg with succinylcholine 1.5 mg/kg
(B) Propofol 4 mg/kg with succinylcholine 1.5 mg/kg
(C) Etomidate 0.2 mg/kg with succinylcholine 1.5 mg/kg
(D) Etomidate 2 mg/kg with succinylcholine 1.5 mg/kg
(E) Ketamine 0.2 mg/kg with succinylcholine 1.5 mg/kg

19. A 44-year-old man with a history of long-standing severe back pain following a car crash 20 years ago presents to the preoperative clinic. His current medication regimen includes a 100-µg/h fentanyl patch and one tablet of oxycodone 40 mg three times daily. Which of the following opiate side effects is the patient most likely to exhibit?
(A) Respiratory depression
(B) Constipation
(C) Mydriasis
(D) Nausea
(E) Sedation

20. A 38-year-old male presents with an open left femur fracture. There is no head or neck injury. The patient is able to relate that he has type 1 diabetes and chronic kidney disease. He denies previous operations, but states he had an uncle who died during a general anesthetic, and his younger brother spent 6 days in the intensive care unit following an elective knee arthroscopy. On further questioning, the patient states he believes he was told his brother had developed malignant hyperthermia during surgery. The decision is made to proceed to the OR but to perform a "trigger-free" anesthetic with continuous infusions of propofol and a narcotic. Select the narcotic from which complete recovery would be *most rapid* following a 5-hour continuous infusion.
(A) Morphine
(B) Fentanyl
(C) Sufentanil
(D) Remifentanil
(E) Meperidine

21. An anesthesiologist is ventilating a patient with 1.2% isoflurane and states that this equals one MAC of anesthesia. What is the definition of one MAC (minimum alveolar concentration) of a volatile anesthetic?
(A) The end-tidal anesthetic concentration that prevents movement in response to surgical stimulation in 50% of patients
(B) The end-tidal anesthetic concentration that prevents movement in response to surgical stimulation in 99% of patients
(C) The end-tidal anesthetic concentration at which 50% of patients are unresponsive to voice
(D) The end-tidal anesthetic concentration at which 99% of patients are unresponsive to voice
(E) The end-tidal anesthetic concentration at which all sympathetic reflexes are blunted

22. Which of the following is a physiologic effect of volatile anesthetics?
    (A) Increased tidal volume
    (B) Bronchoconstriction
    (C) Decreased respiratory rate
    (D) Bronchodilation
    (E) Increased sensitivity to the respiratory stimulant effects of carbon dioxide

23. Which of the following statements is true regarding anesthetic management of nonobstetric surgery during pregnancy?
    (A) Nonparticulate antacids such as sodium citrate for aspiration prophylaxis should be avoided.
    (B) High-dose nitrous oxide should be used for maintenance of anesthesia in all cases.
    (C) Nonemergent, necessary surgery should be performed during the second trimester.
    (D) Exposure to high FiO_2 should be minimized.
    (E) Patients should be placed in right uterine displacement position after 10 weeks' gestation.

24. Blood gas analysis of a patient with chronic obstructive pulmonary disease reveals pH 7.21, PCO_2 65, and PO_2 75 on room air. What is the primary acid-base disorder?
    (A) Metabolic acidosis
    (B) Metabolic alkalosis
    (C) Respiratory acidosis
    (D) Respiratory alkalosis
    (E) None of the above

25. A 63-year-old male with history of gastroesophageal reflux, asthma, and transient ischemic attack last year presents for right shoulder surgery. A left radial arterial line is placed for invasive blood pressure monitoring, and the appropriately sized blood pressure cuff on the left arm is set to cycle every 30 minutes. The patient is prepped and placed in a sitting position, and the surgery is started. The arterial line transducer is positioned at the level of the external auditory meatus, which is approximately 40 cm above the noninvasive cuff. One hour into the surgery, the mean arterial pressure (MAP) according to the noninvasive cuff is 80 mmHg. What should the MAP according to the arterial line read?
    (A) 50 mmHg
    (B) 65 mmHg
    (C) 80 mmHg
    (D) 95 mmHg
    (E) 110 mmHg

26. What is the most sensitive lead for detecting perioperative myocardial ischemia?
    (A) II
    (B) III
    (C) AVF

(D) V1
(E) V5

27. Which of the following is *true* regarding pulse oximetry?
    (A) Presence of carboxyhemoglobin can result in a falsely low or high pulse oximeter reading of around 85%.
    (B) Pulse oximetry uses a single wavelength of light to determine the hemoglobin oxygen saturation.
    (C) Presence of methemoglobin can result in a falsely low or high pulse oximeter reading around 85%.
    (D) Anemia with hemoglobin less than 6 g/dL will cause a decrease in pulse oximeter readings.
    (E) Pulse oximetry is a sensitive and accurate monitor of ventilation.

28. A 68-year-old male undergoes coronary artery bypass grafting. On postoperative day 3 in the intensive care unit (ICU), the following variables are noted by the use of a pulmonary artery catheter: cardiac index (CI) = 1.7 L/min/m², pulmonary capillary wedge pressure (PCWP) = 25 mmHg, SvO_2 = 50%, central venous pressure (CVP) = 10, systemic vascular resistance (SVR) 800 dynes · s · cm⁻⁵. Which of the following states best explains the above variables?
    (A) Hypovolemia
    (B) Hypervolemia
    (C) Left ventricular failure
    (D) Septic shock
    (E) Within normal limits

29. A 53-year-old woman receives a spinal anesthetic for a total knee replacement with 20 mg of 0.5% bupivacaine. Shortly afterward, she complains of tingling in her fingers and has 3/5 grip strength bilaterally. She is found to have numbness to pinprick at the C7 dermatome level bilaterally. Which of the following physiologic effects is most likely to occur?
    (A) Urinary incontinence
    (B) Dilated and relaxed small bowel
    (C) Decreased venous return
    (D) Tachycardia
    (E) Decreased inspiratory reserve volume

30. An 88-year-old man presents to the preoperative holding area for a right total hip arthroplasty. He has a complex medical history and has been an inpatient in the hospital for the past week. The surgery team would like the patient to receive spinal anesthesia. Under which of the following scenarios would performing a spinal anesthetic be safe according to the current American Society of Regional Anesthesia and Pain Medicine (ASRA) guidelines?
    (A) Last dose of clopidogrel 5 days ago
    (B) Last dose of therapeutic enoxaparin (Lovenox; 1 mg/kg) 13 hours ago

(C) Last dose of warfarin 6 days ago, current international normalized ratio (INR) 1.6

(D) Last dose of subcutaneous unfractionated heparin, 5000 mg 4 hours ago

(E) Last dose of ticlopidine 8 days ago

31. A 27-year-old woman had a vaginal delivery with epidural analgesia complicated by a dural puncture. On postoperative day 1, she complains of a severe frontal headache with tinnitus, photophobia, and nausea. The patient is unable to get out of bed and prefers to stay supine. She is afebrile. She also complains of localized lumbar back pain on palpation. Her neurologic exam is otherwise unremarkable. Treatment of this condition should include which of the following?

(A) Magnetic resonance imaging (MRI) of the spine

(B) Computed tomography (CT) scan of the spine

(C) Neurosurgery consult

(D) Epidural autologous blood patch

(E) Broad-spectrum antibiotics

32. Which of the following complications is most likely following massive transfusion of two blood volumes of packed red blood cells (pRBCs)?

(A) Hyperkalemia

(B) Hypokalemia

(C) Hypercalcemia

(D) Hyperthermia

(E) Right-shifted oxygen-hemoglobin dissociation curve

33. Which of the following statements regarding transfusion compatibility testing is true?

(A) Patients with A-negative blood will have anti-A antibodies in their plasma.

(B) Antibody screening is a check for anti-A and anti-B antibodies in donor serum.

(C) In previously transfused patients, nearly 15% have an irregular antibody other than anti-A or anti-B.

(D) Crossmatching of blood involves simulation of actual anticipated transfusion by mixing of recipient and donor blood.

(E) Transfusion with ABO-Rh–only compatible blood (i.e., typed only, not screened or crossmatched) results in a significant transfusion reaction about 10% of the time.

34. A 47-year-old female undergoing colonic resection requires intraoperative transfusion of packed red blood cells for unanticipated blood loss. Postoperatively, she has symptoms of fever, chills, chest pain, and nausea. Hemoglobinuria is later observed from the Foley catheter, and a hemolytic transfusion reaction is diagnosed. The transfusion is terminated, and blood and urine samples are sent to the laboratory. Which additional intervention is most appropriate in the immediate treatment of this type of transfusion reaction?

(A) Epinephrine

(B) Antihistamines

(C) Diuretics

(D) Hydrocortisone

(E) No treatment needed; reaction should resolve spontaneously

35. Which of the following statements regarding fluid management is *true*?

(A) Five percent dextrose is recommended for traumatic brain injury (TBI) patients.

(B) Lactated Ringer's (LR) solution is more acidic and contains more chloride than normal saline.

(C) Large doses of hydroxyethyl starch (>15 mL/kg) may cause a clinically significant coagulopathy.

(D) Colloids have been shown to be superior to crystalloids for intraoperative fluid resuscitation.

(E) A 100-kg patient with a 20% total body surface area burn should receive approximately 12 L of fluid over the first 24 hours according to the Parkland formula.

36. Which of the following statements regarding the laryngeal mask airway (LMA) is *true*?

(A) The patient must be kept breathing spontaneously.

(B) Muscle relaxant should be used routinely to facilitate placement.

(C) LMA placement secures the airway and prevents pulmonary aspiration.

(D) LMA placement is part of the ASA difficult airway algorithm in the case of cannot intubate, cannot ventilate.

(E) A laryngoscope is necessary for optimal LMA placement.

Questions 37 and 38 refer to the following scenario.

A 31-year-old female with a history of ulcerative colitis is admitted for exploratory laparotomy. Physical examination of the abdomen reveals right lower quadrant tenderness, high-pitched bowel sounds, and rebound tenderness. She has been actively vomiting at home.

37. The anesthesiologist decides to perform a rapid sequence induction (RSI) of anesthesia. Which of the following statements about an RSI is *true*?

(A) RSI involves mask ventilating the patient for only 30 seconds.

(B) RSI avoids the use of neuromuscular blocking agents.

(C) RSI can only be performed with succinylcholine.

(D) Use of cricoid pressure always prevents aspiration.

(E) RSI is recommended in patients with bowel obstructions or full stomachs.

38. During laryngoscopy, the anesthesiologist notes gastric contents in the oropharynx and trachea. A postoperative chest x-ray reveals diffuse bilateral infiltrates consistent with acute respiratory distress syndrome (ARDS). Which of the following statements regarding ARDS is *true*?
    (A) Diagnosis of ARDS requires a PaO_2/FiO_2 ratio of less than 100.
    (B) Positive end-expiratory pressure (PEEP) should be avoided because of risk of barotrauma.
    (C) Low tidal volumes (<6 mL/kg) have been shown to improve mortality.
    (D) Inhaled nitric oxide is contraindicated.
    (E) Plateau pressures should be maintained less than 40 cm H_2O.

39. A 38-year-old female with increased intracranial pressure is to undergo a craniotomy for tumor resection. Which of the following agents is most likely *contraindicated* for induction of general anesthesia?
    (A) Etomidate
    (B) Propofol
    (C) Fentanyl
    (D) Rocuronium
    (E) Ketamine

40. A 7-year-old male with no prior surgical history is induced for a procedure with propofol and succinylcholine and anesthesia is maintained with inhaled sevoflurane. Fifteen minutes into the procedure, he develops an acute elevation of end-tidal CO_2 and tachycardia, and his body temperature increases 3°C over the next 15 minutes. What therapy should be immediately administered to treat this disorder?
    (A) Dantrolene
    (B) Gastric lavage with cold saline
    (C) Calcium channel blockers
    (D) Mannitol
    (E) Rocuronium

41. A 25-year-old female presents to the preoperative clinic prior to a scheduled functional endoscopic sinus surgery. Given her history of severe motion sickness, she is concerned about postoperative nausea and vomiting (PONV) and asks how likely this is to occur after her upcoming surgery. In general, which of the following factors is *true* regarding a patient's risk of PONV?
    (A) Male gender increases the risk of PONV.
    (B) History of smoking decreases the risk of PONV.
    (C) Type of surgery has no effect on the incidence of PONV.
    (D) Younger age groups are at increased risk of PONV.
    (E) Type of intraoperative anesthesia has no effect on incidence of PONV.

ANSWERS AND EXPLANATIONS

1. **(D)** The American Society of Anesthesiologists (ASA) classification was developed in an effort to ensure that adequate comparisons between patient populations can be made between institutions for morbidity and mortality statistics. Notice the ASA classification is independent of the surgical procedure. Accordingly, it does not imply preoperative risk. Table 7-1 describes the different ASA classes.

   The patient in Question 1 is considered ASA class 3 because his diabetes is causing functional limitations (vision and nervous system), and his hypertension is not controlled.

TABLE 7-1 Summary of ASA Physical Classes

Class	Definition
1	Normal healthy patient
2	Patient with mild systemic disease (no functional limitations)
3	Patient with severe systemic disease (some functional limitations)
4	Patient with severe systemic disease that is a constant threat to life (functionality incapacitated)
5	Moribund patient who is not expected to survive without the operation
6	Brain-dead patient whose organs are being removed for donor purposes
E	If the procedure is an emergency, the physical status is followed by "E" (e.g., "2E")

BIBLIOGRAPHY

Butterworth JF IV, Mackey DC, Wasnick JD. Preoperative assessment, premedication, and perioperative documentation. In: Butterworth JF IV, Mackey DC, Wasnick JD (eds.), *Morgan & Mikhail's Clinical Anesthesiology*, 5th ed. New York, NY: McGraw-Hill; 2013:Chapter 18.

Butterworth JF IV, Mackey DC, Wasnick JD (eds.). *Morgan & Mikhail's Clinical Anesthesiology*, 5th ed. New York, NY: McGraw-Hill; 2013:297.

2. **(C)** The ASA established an algorithm in 1993 that describes a systematic approach to the patient with a difficult airway. A difficult airway is defined as the clinical situation in which a conventionally trained anesthesiologist experiences difficulty with face mask ventilation of the upper airway, difficulty with tracheal intubation, or both. The ASA difficult airway treatment plan algorithm is shown in see Fig. 7-1.

Difficult Airway Algorithm

1. Assess the likelihood and clinical impact of basic management problems.
   A. Difficult ventilation
   B. Difficult intubation
   C. Difficulty with patient cooperation or consent
   D. Difficult tracheostomy
2. Actively pursue opportunities to deliver supplemental oxygen throughout the process of difficult airway management.
3. Consider the relative merits and feasibility of basic management choices:

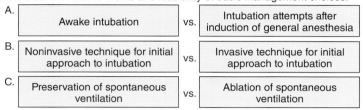

A. Awake intubation vs. Intubation attempts after induction of general anesthesia

B. Noninvasive technique for initial approach to intubation vs. Invasive technique for initial approach to intubation

C. Preservation of spontaneous ventilation vs. Ablation of spontaneous ventilation

4. Develop primary and alternative strategies.

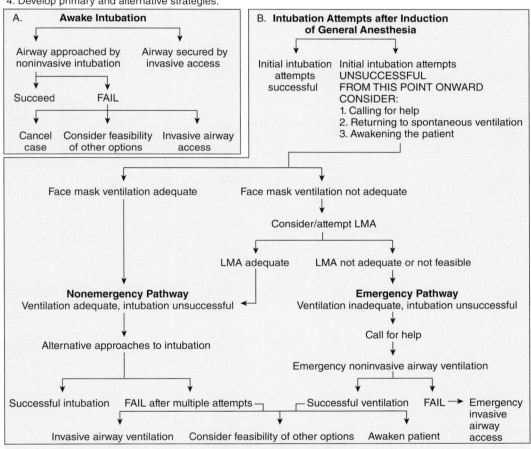

FIGURE 7-1. ASA difficult airway algorithm. From Butterworth JF IV, Mackey DC, Wasnick JD (eds.). *Morgan & Mikhail's Clinical Anesthesiology*, 5th ed. New York, NY: McGraw-Hill; 2013.

The case in the question is an unanticipated difficult airway after induction of general anesthesia, which is step 4, part B on the algorithm. The most important branch point of the algorithm is whether or not face mask ventilation is adequate. If mask ventilation is adequate, then a nonemergency pathway can be pursued.

If mask ventilation is *not* adequate, as in the case in question, then a supraglottic airway (SGA) such as an LMA should be placed. An observational study reports the LMA providing successful rescue ventilation in 94.1% of patients who cannot be mask ventilated or intubated. If ventilation with the SGA fails, then consider emergency invasive ventilation techniques such as percutaneous airway, jet ventilation, and retrograde intubation.

In the question stem, this patient was induced with rocuronium, which would make returning to spontaneous ventilation nearly impossible given the intermediate duration of action of rocuronium. Rocuronium is unable to be rapidly reversed with neostigmine immediately after giving an intubating dose. Cricothyrotomy and retrograde intubation may be potentially successful methods of securing this patient's airway, but LMA placement should be attempted first.

BIBLIOGRAPHY

Butterworth JF IV, Mackey DC, Wasnick JD. Airway Management. In: Butterworth JF IV, Mackey DC, Wasnick JD (eds.). *Morgan & Mikhail's Clinical Anesthesiology*, 5th ed. New York, NY: McGraw-Hill; 2013:Chapter 19.

Butterworth JF IV, Mackey DC, Wasnick JD (eds.). *Morgan & Mikhail's Clinical Anesthesiology*, 5th ed. New York, NY: McGraw-Hill; 2013:329.

3. **(C)** The pediatric airway differs from the adult airway in many aspects, requiring an understanding of these anatomical differences for proper mask ventilation and intubation.

Infants have a larger occiput, which puts the child's head in a naturally flexed position. The larynx is more cephalad and anterior in the neck (C3-C4) than in adults (C6). The epiglottis is omega-shaped and longer, which can make it harder to lift with a Macintosh laryngoscope blade. The vocal cords slant caudally at their insertion in the arytenoids. The narrowest part of the upper airway in children up to 5 years old is the cricoid cartilage. Thus, even if an endotracheal tube fits past the vocal cords, it may not be able to be advanced into the trachea. This is in contrast to adults, where the narrowest part of the airway is at the vocal cords. The trachea is also shorter, making placement of the endotracheal tube into the acute angle of the right mainstem bronchus easier to do. Infants have a relatively larger tongue volume in the mouth, creating less space for instrumentation. Because the trachea is relatively smaller, even small amounts of mucosal edema will have proportionately greater effect.

BIBLIOGRAPHY

Butterworth JF IV, Mackey DC, Wasnick JD (eds.). *Morgan & Mikhail's Clinical Anesthesiology*, 5th ed. New York, NY: McGraw-Hill; 2013:879.

Butterworth JF IV, Mackey DC, Wasnick JD. Pediatric anesthesia. In: Butterworth JF IV, Mackey DC, Wasnick JD (eds.). *Morgan & Mikhail's Clinical Anesthesiology*, 5th ed. New York, NY: McGraw-Hill; 2013:Chapter 42.

4. **(D)** The respiratory system of neonates is weaker and less efficient than that of adults. Respiratory rate is increased, although tidal volume and dead space per kilogram are nearly constant during development. The alveoli are not fully mature until approximately 8 years of age, which increases overall airway resistance. The immature alveoli also lead to reduced lung compliance. The ribcage is also more cartilaginous, making the chest wall more compliant. The compliant chest wall and less compliant lung tissue are more prone to collapse during inspiration. This leads to a decreased FRC and thus limited oxygen reserve, predisposing neonates to atelectasis and hypoxemia. This is exaggerated by their higher rate of oxygen consumption.

The neonatal heart undergoes significant changes over the first years of life. The volume of cellular mass in the neonatal heart dedicated to contractility is significantly less developed than in an adult heart. Because of this, the left ventricle is relatively noncompliant, making the cardiac stroke volume relatively fixed. Thus, cardiac output is entirely determined by heart rate. Basal heart rate is greater than in adults. The immature heart is more sensitive to depression by volatile anesthetics and to opioid-induced bradycardia. The sympathetic nervous system and baroreceptor reflexes are also not fully mature, causing neonates to not necessarily respond appropriately to hypovolemia or hypotension.

Other important physiologic changes to be aware of include an increased body surface area per kilogram, thin skin, and low fat content, which promotes greater heat loss to the environment. Hypothermia has been linked with cardiac irritability, decreased respiratory drive, elevated pulmonary vascular resistance, and an altered response to medications. Renal function does not approach normal value until 6 months of age and may be delayed until 2 years of age. The liver conjugates drugs and other molecules less readily early in life. Neonates also have reduced glycogen stores, which predisposes them to hypoglycemia. Percentage of total body water is also higher in neonates (80%).

BIBLIOGRAPHY

Butterworth JF IV, Mackey DC, Wasnick JD (eds.). *Morgan & Mikhail's Clinical Anesthesiology*, 5th ed. New York, NY: McGraw-Hill; 2013:878–881.

Butterworth JF IV, Mackey DC, Wasnick JD. Pediatric anesthesia. In: Butterworth JF IV, Mackey DC, Wasnick JD (eds.). *Morgan & Mikhail's Clinical Anesthesiology*, 5th ed. New York, NY: McGraw-Hill; 2013:Chapter 42.

5. **(E)** The American College of Cardiology (ACC) and American Heart Association (AHA) issued guidelines for perioperative cardiovascular examination for noncardiac

surgery in 1996 and updated them most recently in 2007. Recommendations are based largely on retrospective or observational data and knowledge of management of cardiovascular disorders in nonoperative settings. The guidelines provide a framework in which to consider cardiac risk in noncardiac surgery in a variety of situations using a stepwise approach. The overriding theme of the guidelines is that preoperative intervention is rarely indicated simply to lower the risk of surgery unless the intervention is indicated irrespective of the preoperative context. The goal of preoperative evaluation is not to give "cardiac clearance," but to identify the most appropriate treatment and testing strategies to optimize short- and long-term care of the patient.

Figure 7-2 shows the cardiac evaluation and care algorithm for noncardiac surgery based on active clinical conditions, known cardiovascular disease, or cardiac risk factors for patients 50 years of age or greater. In step 1, note that emergent surgery needs to proceed to the operating room (OR) irrespective of prior cardiac evaluation.

If the procedure is not an emergency, the first question is whether the patient has any active cardiac conditions. Active cardiac conditions include unstable coronary syndromes, decompensated heart failure, significant arrhythmias, and severe valvular disease. If present, the patient should be evaluated and treated per ACC/AHA guidelines. If no active conditions are present, then type of surgery should be considered. If the procedure is low risk, then the patient can proceed with surgery.

Noncardiac surgical procedures are stratified into three risk groups based on cardiac risk. High-risk surgeries with cardiac risk >5% include emergent major

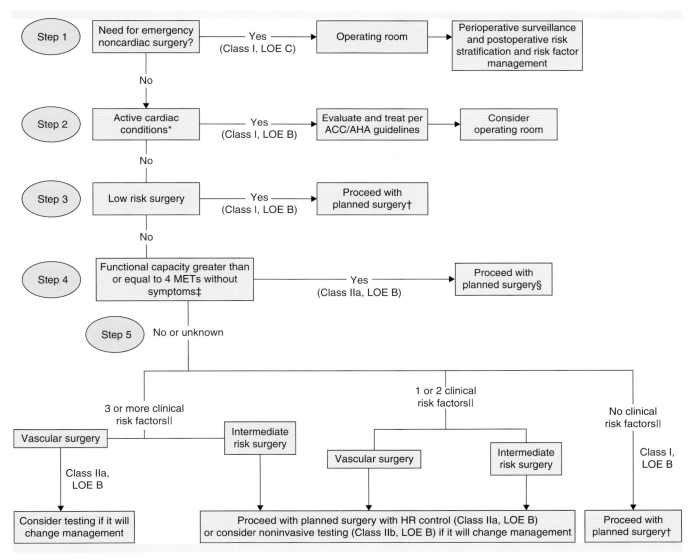

FIGURE 7-2. Cardiac evaluation and care algorithm for noncardiac surgery. LOE, level of evidence.

operations, aortic or other major vascular or peripheral vascular surgery, and long procedures with large blood loss or fluid shifts. Intermediate-risk surgeries with cardiac risk of 1–5% include procedures like carotid endarterectomy (CEA), head and neck, intrathoracic, intraperitoneal, prostate, and orthopedic surgeries. Low-risk procedures with cardiac risk <1% include procedures like endoscopic, superficial, cataract, or breast surgery.

If the procedure is intermediate or high risk, then the patient's functional capacity should be considered. If the patient's functional capacity is greater than 4 METs (e.g., light work around the house, climb a flight of stairs, walk a block on level ground at 4 mph), then he or she can proceed with surgery. If functional capacity is unknown or less than 4 METs, then clinical risk factors (ischemic heart disease, compensated heart failure, diabetes, renal insufficiency, and cerebrovascular disease) and type of surgery should be considered. If there are no risk factors, the patient can proceed with surgery. If one or more clinical risk factors are present, then testing should be considered based on the potential to change perioperative management.

In the question, the patient has two clinical risk factors (diabetes and cerebrovascular disease) and is going for an intermediate-risk surgery (CEA). He does not need emergency surgery, he has no active cardiac conditions, the procedure is not low risk, but his functional capacity is much greater than 4 METs, so he should be able to proceed with the CEA without further cardiac workup.

BIBLIOGRAPHY

Fleisher LA, Beckman JA, Brown KA, et al. ACC/AHA 2007 guidelines on perioperative cardiovascular evaluation and care for noncardiac surgery: a report of the American College of Cardiology/American Heart Association Task Force on Practice Guidelines (Writing Committee to Revise the 2002 Guidelines on Perioperative Cardiovascular Evaluation for Noncardiac Surgery). *Circulation* 116;2007:e418–e500.

6. **(B)** Neuromuscular blocking agents are divided into two classes: depolarizing and nondepolarizing. The only depolarizing drug used in clinical practice is succinylcholine. Nondepolarizing muscle relaxants (NDMRs) include atracurium, cisatracurium, vecuronium, rocuronium, and pancuronium. All of these drugs are quaternary ammonium compounds whose positively charged nitrogen imparts an affinity to nicotinic acetylcholine (Ach) receptors. Depolarizing muscle relaxants resemble Ach and readily bind to Ach receptors, generating a muscle action potential leading to end-plate depolarization. Therefore, succinylcholine binds to the nicotinic Ach receptor as an agonist and opens sodium

channels creating an action potential. Succinylcholine continues to bind to the receptor, making it unable to repolarize and generate another action potential. This is called a phase 1 block.

Nondepolarizing muscle relaxants function as competitive antagonists. These drugs bind Ach receptors and are incapable of inducing the conformational change necessary for sodium channel opening. They also prevent Ach from binding to the receptor, thus stopping development of an end-plate potential.

BIBLIOGRAPHY

Butterworth JF IV, Mackey DC, Wasnick JD (eds.). *Morgan & Mikhail's Clinical Anesthesiology*, 5th ed. New York, NY: McGraw-Hill; 2013:202–203.

Butterworth JF IV, Mackey DC, Wasnick JD. Neuromuscular blocking agents. In: Butterworth JF IV, Mackey DC, Wasnick JD (eds.). *Morgan & Mikhail's Clinical Anesthesiology*, 5th ed. New York, NY: McGraw-Hill; 2013:Chapter 11.

7. **(E)** Succinylcholine is a depolarizing neuromuscular blocking agent that acts at the postjunctional neuromuscular membrane to produce rapid skeletal muscle relaxation.

Succinylcholine stimulates all cholinergic autonomic receptors (nicotinic receptors on both parasympathetic and sympathetic ganglia). A prominent manifestation of the generalized autonomic stimulation is the development of cardiac dysrhythmias such as sinus bradycardia from stimulation of cardiac muscarinic receptors in the sinus node, junctional rhythms from relatively greater stimulation of the muscarinic receptors in the sinus node, and ventricular dysrhythmias likely secondary to a lowered threshold for catecholamine-induced dysrhythmias.

Succinylcholine administration causes an increase in plasma potassium level by about 0.5 mEq/dL in healthy patients. This is secondary to the depolarization of the muscle tissue. This increase may be exaggerated in patients with renal failure and patients who have proliferation of extrajunctional nicotinic receptors, which would include patients who have undergone denervation injury (i.e., patients with traumatic crush injury, unhealed third-degree burns, and upper motor neuron disease).

The incidence of myalgias after succinylcholine administration may be as high as 89%. It occurs most frequently following minor surgery in women and ambulatory patients. This may be secondary to muscle damage from unsynchronized contractions before the onset of paralysis.

Transient increased intraocular pressure after succinylcholine administration peaks at 2–4 minutes and subsides by 6 minutes. The mechanism is unknown. Despite this, it is safe for use for eye surgery unless the anterior chamber is open. Other potential side effects of succinylcholine include anaphylactic reaction and transient increases in intragastric pressure and intracranial pressure. It should also be noted that succinylcholine is one of the triggering agents for malignant hyperthermia and should be avoided in patients at risk for malignant hyperthermia.

BIBLIOGRAPHY

Miller RD. *Miller's Anesthesia*, 7th ed. Philadelphia, PA: Elsevier Churchill Livingstone; 2009:864–866.
Miller RD. Pharmacology of muscle relaxants and their antagonists. In: Miller RD (ed.), *Miller's Anesthesia*, 7th ed. Philadelphia, PA: Elsevier Churchill Livingstone; 2009:Chapter 29.

8. **(C)** The correct answer is cisatracurium, because it is primarily (77%) metabolized by Hoffman elimination in the blood, whereas renal clearance only makes up about 16% of elimination. In contrast, pancuronium is primarily (85%) eliminated by the kidney, and its active metabolite can accumulate in renal failure patients. Rocuronium is primarily (70%) eliminated by the liver with a somewhat significant concentration (10–25%) eliminated by the kidney. Vecuronium is eliminated by the kidney (40–50%) and the liver (50–60%). Succinylcholine, like mivacurium, is almost exclusively metabolized in the blood by butyrylcholinesterase, making it very short acting and inappropriate for maintenance of neuromuscular blockade for a procedure of this length.

BIBLIOGRAPHY

Miller RD. *Miller's Anesthesia*, 7th ed. Philadelphia, PA: Elsevier Churchill Livingstone; 2009:880.
Miller RD. Pharmacology of muscle relaxants and their antagonists. In: Miller RD (ed.), *Miller's Anesthesia*, 7th ed. Philadelphia, PA: Elsevier Churchill Livingstone; 2009:Chapter 29.

9. **(A)** If a patient has a contraindication to succinylcholine, such as history of malignant hyperthermia or a neuromuscular disease, then a nondepolarizing muscle relaxant (NDMR) should be used to facilitate intubation. If a rapid sequence intubation is desired, then time until maximum block is critical because the patient is an aspiration risk until the airway is secured with an endotracheal tube. Rocuronium is the most appropriate NDMR listed because it has a time to maximum block comparable to succinylcholine (approximately 0.9 minutes) when given at a dose of 1.2 mg/kg. Pancuronium, cisatracurium, atracurium, and mivacurium have a time to maximum block of at least 2.9, 1.9, 3.2, and 2.1 minutes, respectively.

BIBLIOGRAPHY

Miller RD. *Miller's Anesthesia*, 7th ed. Philadelphia, PA: Elsevier Churchill Livingstone; 2009:880.
Miller RD. Pharmacology of muscle relaxants and their antagonists. In: Miller RD (ed.), *Miller's Anesthesia*, 7th ed. Philadelphia, PA: Elsevier Churchill Livingstone; 2009:Chapter 29.

10. **(E)** Peripheral nerve stimulators are most commonly used by anesthesiologists to evaluate neuromuscular function after the use of neuromuscular blocking agents. Peripheral nerves such as the ulnar, medial, posterior tibial, common peroneal, and facial nerves are the most commonly monitored. Train of four (TOF) stimulation is frequently used. TOF involves four supramaximal stimuli given every 0.5 second (2 Hz). Each stimulus causes the muscle to contract, and the "fade" in the response provides basis for evaluation. The fade is often a subjective measure of the amplitude of the first response compared to the amplitude of the fourth response. If all four responses are the same, then the ratio is 1.0. During a nondepolarizing block, the ratio fades (decreases) and is inversely proportional to the degree of blockade.

    After an intubating dose of an NDMR, there are four phases of neuromuscular blockade that vary in length based on drug and dose. Intense neuromuscular blockade is the first phase, and there is no response to any pattern of nerve stimulation. Next is deep neuromuscular blockade characterized by no response to TOF, but presence of posttetanic twitches. Next is surgical blockade, which begins when the first response to TOF stimulation appears. The degree of neuromuscular blockade is 90–95% when only one twitch of four is detectable. One or two twitches in the TOF is usually sufficient relaxation for most surgical procedures. Four twitches present indicate about a 60–85% level of neuromuscular blockade. The final phase is recovery, which starts with return of the fourth twitch. This phase is highly variable, and a TOF ratio must exceed 0.8 or 0.9 to exclude residual muscle blockade.

BIBLIOGRAPHY

Miller RD. *Miller's Anesthesia*, 7th ed. Philadelphia, PA: Elsevier Churchill Livingstone; 2009:1525–1526.
Miller RD. Neuromuscular monitoring. In: Miller RD (ed.), *Miller's Anesthesia*, 7th ed. Philadelphia, PA: Elsevier Churchill Livingstone; 2009:Chapter 47.

11. **(C)** When neuromuscular blockade is no longer desired, such at the end of surgery, anticholinesterases can be given to antagonize nondepolarizing muscle relaxants (NDMRs). The anticholinesterase drugs clinically available are neostigmine, pyridostigmine, and edrophonium. They work by inhibiting acetylcholinesterase and thus increasing the concentration of Ach at the motor endplate, which can then compete with the residual NDMR for the Ach receptor.

Although edrophonium is more rapid acting, neostigmine is the anticholinesterase drug most commonly used in clinical practice because it is the most effective at antagonizing profound blockade of more than 90% twitch depression.

Because only the nicotinic effects of the anticholinesterases are desired, the muscarinic effects can be blocked by muscarinic antagonists such as atropine and glycopyrrolate. Edrophonium and atropine should be administered together because of their rapid onset times, while neostigmine and glycopyrrolate should be administered together because they are slower acting. Glycopyrrolate has the added advantage of being a quaternary amine, meaning it does not cross the blood-brain barrier like atropine and cause CNS changes.

BIBLIOGRAPHY

Miller RD. *Miller's Anesthesia*, 7th ed. Philadelphia, PA: Elsevier Churchill Livingstone; 2009:889–892.

Miller RD. Pharmacology of muscle relaxants and their antagonists. In: Miller RD (ed.), *Miller's Anesthesia*, 7th ed. Philadelphia, PA: Elsevier Churchill Livingstone; 2009:Chapter 29.

12. **(C)** Local anesthetics work by inhibiting voltage-gated sodium channels within the neuron, thus preventing activation and the sodium influx needed for membrane depolarization. The voltage-gated sodium channels are membrane-bound proteins composed of one large α subunit through which the sodium ions pass and one or two smaller β subunits. Local anesthetics bind to a specific region of the α subunit and inhibit the flow of sodium through the channel.

Local anesthetics exist in the tissue as two forms: neutral bases and charged cations. The ratio is determined by the pH of the tissue and the drug's pK_a. The neutral base form of the anesthetic most easily crosses the cell membrane while the sodium channel is open, but once intracellular, it is the cationic form of the molecule that binds to the closed conformation of the voltage-gated sodium channel. This binding stabilizes the channel and prevents return to the rested-closed state, which must be cycled through before the channel can again become activated-open (see Fig. 7-3).

BIBLIOGRAPHY

Butterworth JF IV, Mackey DC, Wasnick JD. Local anesthetics. In: Butterworth JF IV, Mackey DC, Wasnick JD (eds.). *Morgan & Mikhail's Clinical Anesthesiology*, 5th ed. New York, NY: McGraw-Hill; 2013:Chapter 16.

Butterworth JF IV, Mackey DC, Wasnick JD (eds.). *Morgan & Mikhail's Clinical Anesthesiology*, 5th ed. New York, NY: McGraw-Hill; 2013:263–266.

13. **(A)** Potency, duration of action, and onset of action are all important properties that differentiate local anesthetic drugs. Although many factors play a role in each of these properties, classically, potency has to do with lipid solubility (see Table 7-2). Compounds with a more hydrophobic (lipophilic) nature are more potent and produce longer lasting nerve blocks than more hydrophilic drugs. For example, bupivacaine is 8–10 times more

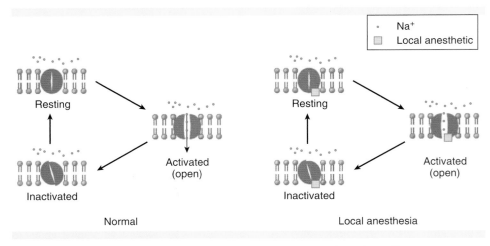

FIGURE 7-3. How local anesthetics bind to the voltage-gated sodium channels in the cell. From Butterworth JF IV, Mackey DC, Wasnick JD (eds.). *Morgan & Mikhail's Clinical Anesthesiology*, 5th ed. New York, NY: McGraw-Hill; 2013.

TABLE 7-2 Physiochemical Properties of Commonly Used Local Anesthetics

Local Anesthetic	Relative Lipid Solubility	pK_a	Protein Binding (%)
Bupivacaine	8	8.2	96
Etidocaine	16	8.1	94
Lidocaine	1	8.2	64
Mepivacaine	0.3	7.9	78
Ropivacaine	2.5	8.2	94
Chloroprocaine	2.3	9.1	NA
Cocaine	NA	8.7	91
Procaine	0.3	9.1	NA
Tetracaine	12	8.6	76

NA, not applicable.

lipid soluble than lidocaine, accounting for its increased potency.

Duration of action is determined by a complex combination of lipid solubility, potency, amount of drug, degree of vascularity of the tissue, and presence of vasoconstrictors to prevent vascular reuptake. Lipid solubility presumably plays a role because the drug diffuses more slowly away from a lipid-rich environment to the aqueous bloodstream. Lipid solubility of local anesthetics is correlated with plasma protein binding (local anesthetics primarily bind to α-1-acid glycoprotein and to a lesser extent albumin), which is commonly used as a marker for a local anesthetic's duration of action.

Onset of action is largely determined by the drug's pK_a, or the pH at which the fraction of ionized and nonionized drug is equal. Local anesthetics with a pK_a closer to physiologic pH have a greater fraction of nonionized base that more readily permeates the nerve cell membrane. A higher pK_a means more of the drug exists in the cationic form, and therefore, less nonionized base is available to cross the membrane resulting in a slower onset of action. However, one should note that despite having the highest pK_a, chloroprocaine has the fastest onset of action, perhaps secondary to the high concentration of drug delivered.

Therefore, a highly lipid-soluble drug with a high degree of protein binding and pK_a closest to physiologic pH will be the most potent with the most rapid onset and longest duration of action.

BIBLIOGRAPHY

Butterworth JF IV, Mackey DC, Wasnick JD. Local anesthetics. In: Butterworth JF IV, Mackey DC, Wasnick JD (eds.), *Morgan & Mikhail's Clinical Anesthesiology*, 5th ed. New York, NY: McGraw-Hill; 2013:Chapter 16.

Butterworth JF IV, Mackey DC, Wasnick JD (eds.). *Morgan & Mikhail's Clinical Anesthesiology*, 5th ed. New York, NY: McGraw-Hill; 2013:266–269.

Miller RD. Local anesthetics. In: Miller RD (ed.), *Miller's Anesthesia*, 7th ed. Philadelphia, PA: Elsevier Churchill Livingstone; 2009:Chapter 30.

Miller RD. *Miller's Anesthesia*, 7th ed. Philadelphia, PA: Elsevier Churchill Livingstone; 2009:913–916.

14. **(E)** All local anesthetics have a maximum recommended dose, which can be found in package inserts, drug indices, and databases (see Table 7-3). The purpose of these maximums is to limit or prevent systemic toxicity.

TABLE 7-3 Maximum Recommended Dosages of Local Anesthetics

Drug	Plain Solution			Epinephrine-Containing Solution	
	Concentration (%)	Max Dose (mg)	Duration (min)	Max Dose (mg)	Duration (min)
Short Duration					
Procaine	1-2	500	20-30	600	30-45
Chloroprocaine	1-2	800	15-30	1000	30
Moderate Duration					
Lidocaine	0.5-1	300	30-60	500	120
Mepivacaine	0.5-1	300	45-90	500	120
Prilocaine	0.5-1	350	30-90	550	120
Long Duration					
Bupivacaine	0.25-0.5	175	120-240	200	180-240
Ropivacaine	0.2-0.5	200	120-240	250	180-240

There are a number of factors that influence anesthetic activity in humans. The dose of local anesthetic can be increased by administering a larger volume or a higher concentration. Note that a higher volume of anesthetic solution likely influences spread of the medication (i.e., 20 mL of 1% lidocaine covers more area than 10 mL of 2% lidocaine). The addition of vasoconstrictors (usually epinephrine 5 µg/mL or 1:200,000) helps decrease the rate of vascular absorption, thus improving the depth and duration of anesthesia. There tends to be a greater increase in duration when epinephrine is added to short-acting agents like lidocaine compared to long-acting agents like bupivacaine. Care should be taken when attempting to combine local anesthetics because their toxicities are additive rather than independent.

In calculating the dose to be injected, one must consider both concentration and volume. For example, the maximum recommended dose of bupivacaine for infiltration in an adult is 175 mg. A 0.75% solution contains 7.5 mg/mL, whereas a 0.25% solution contains 2.5 mg/mL, so the maximum dose is reached with 70 mL of the latter but only 23.3 mL of the former. The most prudent method to decide what strength solution to use would be to consider what volume of solution will be needed to adequately infiltrate the entire area needing to be anesthetized, and then determine what strength solution will approach but not exceed the maximum dose in that volume. Note that the maximum dose of lidocaine for tumescent anesthesia is as high as 35–55 mg/kg and that levels do not peak until 8–12 hours after infusion.

For postoperative analgesia, bupivacaine is better than lidocaine and mepivacaine because of its long duration of action. A dose of 30 mL of 0.75% bupivacaine with 1:200,000 epinephrine exceeds the maximum recommended dose of bupivacaine.

BIBLIOGRAPHY

Miller RD. Local anesthetics. In: Miller RD (ed.), *Miller's Anesthesia*, 7th ed. Philadelphia, PA: Elsevier Churchill Livingstone; 2009:Chapter 30.

Miller RD. *Miller's Anesthesia*, 7th ed. Philadelphia, PA: Elsevier Churchill Livingstone; 2009:924–926.

15. **(D)** In the case described, the most likely explanation of both increased HR and blood pressure is the α-adrenergic effects of epinephrine, especially in the setting of an intercostal nerve block. Vascular absorption of drug varies greatly depending on the injection site. Blood concentration of anesthetic drug is highest after intercostal nerve blockade, followed in order of decreasing concentration by caudal, epidural, brachial plexus, lower extremity, and subcutaneous tissue infiltration.

Histamine-mediated anaphylaxis would result in tachycardia with hypotension from vasodilation. True allergic or anaphylactic reactions to local anesthetics are very rare. Although patients often experience a wide range of local and systemic symptoms, few of these reactions are confirmed allergic reactions. Aminoester drugs more commonly produce allergic-type reactions than aminoamide drugs. Some aminoester drugs are derivatives of para-aminobenzoic acid (PABA), which is a known allergen. Some aminoamides contain methylparaben as a preservative, which has a chemical structure similar to that of PABA. However, most aminoamides come in preservative-free solutions. In the rare patient with confirmed allergies to aminoamides and aminoesters, meperidine can be considered as an alternative for a spinal anesthetic.

Cardiac toxicity is unlikely to precede CNS symptoms and would not be expected to produce hypertension because toxicity results from cardiac depression. An intravascular injection of 50 µg epinephrine would result in immediate tachycardia and hypertension, not delayed.

BIBLIOGRAPHY

Miller RD. Local anesthetics. In: Miller RD (ed.), *Miller's Anesthesia*, 7th ed. Philadelphia, PA: Elsevier Churchill Livingstone; 2009:Chapter 30.

Miller RD. *Miller's Anesthesia*, 7th ed. Philadelphia, PA: Elsevier Churchill Livingstone; 2009:935.

16. **(C)** Local anesthetic systemic toxicity (LAST) primarily involves the CNS and the cardiovascular (CV) system. Generally the CNS is more susceptible than the CV system to the effects of local anesthetics, and CNS symptoms will arise at lower blood levels of local anesthetic than cardiovascular collapse. Note that negative aspiration for heme does not rule out intravascular injection.

CNS toxicity initially presents as lightheadedness and dizziness followed by visual and auditory disturbances such as difficulty focusing and tinnitus. This is followed by excitatory symptoms such as muscular twitching and tremors, and ultimately tonic-clonic seizures. In large enough doses, CNS excitation is followed by CNS depression. Respiratory and metabolic acidosis increase the risk for CNS toxicity from local anesthetics by increasing cerebral blood flow and decreasing intracellular pH, which facilitate conversion of drug to the cationic form, causing ion trapping.

Cardiovascular symptoms occur due to direct action by local anesthetics on both the heart and the peripheral blood vessels and indirect action through blockade of sympathetic and parasympathetic efferent activity.

Bupivacaine depresses the rapid phase of depolarization in Purkinje fibers and ventricular muscle to a greater extent than lidocaine. The rate of recovery is also slower with bupivacaine than lidocaine. High blood levels of local anesthetics prolong conduction time as indicated by prolonged PR interval and QRS duration. Very high levels depress spontaneous pacemaker activity causing sinus bradycardia and arrest. All local anesthetics exert dose-dependent negative inotropic action on cardiac muscle roughly proportional to their nerve blocking potency. Cocaine is the only local anesthetic shown to reliably produce vasoconstriction. Bupivacaine is the local anesthetic drug most likely to produce rapid and profound cardiovascular depression. The ratio of dosage required for cardiovascular collapse (CC) and the dosage required for CNS toxicity (CC/CNS ratio) is much lower for bupivacaine than for lidocaine.

BIBLIOGRAPHY

Miller RD. Local anesthetics. In: Miller RD (ed.), *Miller's Anesthesia*, 7th ed. Philadelphia, PA: Elsevier Churchill Livingstone; 2009:Chapter 30.

Miller RD. *Miller's Anesthesia*, 7th ed. Philadelphia, PA: Elsevier Churchill Livingstone; 2009:932–934.

17. **(D)** The treatment for LAST is different than for other cardiac arrest scenarios. According to the American Society of Regional Anesthesia and Pain Medicine, the initial focus is airway management, seizure suppression, and alerting the nearest cardiopulmonary bypass facility. Seizure suppression is preferably done with benzodiazepines and not propofol, especially in patients who have cardiovascular instability. Cardiac arrhythmias should be managed with ACLS. Vasopressin, calcium channel blockers, β-blockers, and additional local anesthetics should be avoided. There is no established role for antiarrhythmic drugs in the setting of LAST. Epinephrine should be given in reduced dosages of <1 μg/kg because even though standard, 1-mg ACLS dose epinephrine may restore circulation initially, it is highly arrhythmogenic, and animal studies have shown worse outcomes with this higher dosing.

The most important part of LAST treatment involves lipid emulsion therapy. Lipid emulsion therapy likely acts as a "lipid sink" that draws down the content of lipid-soluble local anesthetics from within the cardiac tissue. It should be given as an initial 1.5 mL/kg bolus followed by an infusion of 0.25 mL/kg/min. The bolus can be repeated once or twice for the unstable patient. The maximum dose is 10 mL/kg over the first 30 minutes. Failure to respond to lipid emulsion and vasopressor therapy should prompt initiation of cardiopulmonary bypass.

BIBLIOGRAPHY

Miller RD. Local anesthetics. In: Miller RD (ed.), *Miller's Anesthesia*, 7th ed. Philadelphia, PA: Elsevier Churchill Livingstone; 2009:Chapter 30.

Miller RD. *Miller's Anesthesia*, 7th ed. Philadelphia, PA: Elsevier Churchill Livingstone; 2009:933.

Neal JM, Bernards CM, Buterworth JF, et al. ASRA practice advisory on local anesthetic systemic toxicity. *Reg Anesth Pain Med* 2010;35:152–161.

18. **(C)** All of the intravenous anesthetics listed can be used to induce general anesthesia. However, etomidate and ketamine have the most favorable pharmacologic profile in this scenario.

Etomidate depresses the reticular activating system and mimics the inhibitory effects of GABA. Etomidate is a good drug for induction of anesthesia in this scenario because it is "cardiovascular stable" in the sense in that it does not greatly increase or decrease heart rate and blood pressure. The induction dose is 0.2–0.5 mg/kg IV. It is unique among the agents in producing dose-dependent adrenocortical suppression lasting 4–8 hours after induction. This suppression may be desirable or undesirable depending on the stress to which the patient is exposed in the perioperative period. There is a 30–60% incidence of myoclonus following etomidate induction.

Ketamine is an *N*-methyl-D-aspartate (NMDA) receptor antagonist with multiple effects throughout the CNS. It produces a "dissociative anesthesia" resembling a cataleptic state with unconsciousness, amnesia, and intense analgesia by "dissociating" the thalamus from the limbic system. It is one of the few IV anesthetic drugs that causes analgesia, amnesia, and unconsciousness. The induction dose is 1–2 mg/kg IV or 3–5 mg/kg intramuscularly (IM). The major advantage of ketamine in a trauma scenario is its effects on the cardiovascular system. A ketamine bolus causes increases in arterial blood pressure, heart rate, and cardiac output. These are indirect effects due to central stimulation of the sympathetic nervous system and inhibition of norepinephrine reuptake from nerve terminals. However, note that ketamine is also a direct myocardial depressant (generally overshadowed by sympathetic effects), probably from inhibition of calcium transients, which is unmasked by sympathetic blockade or exhaustion of catecholamine stores. Unique respiratory effects of ketamine include preservation of respiratory drive and potent bronchodilation. Ketamine may cause increased cerebral blood flow and intracranial pressure, so it should be used cautiously in patients with cranial space-occupying lesions. Also note that ketamine has an active metabolite, norketamine, which possess one-third to one-fifth the activity of ketamine, is renally excreted, and may contribute to prolonged effects following multiple doses or continuous infusion.

Propofol produces anesthesia by facilitating inhibitory neurotransmission mediated by γ-aminobutyric acid (GABA) receptor binding. An induction dose of propofol is 1–2.5 mg/kg. It causes a decrease in arterial blood pressure due to a drop in systemic vascular resistance (through inhibition of sympathetic vasoconstrictor activity), preload, and cardiac contractility. Large boluses of propofol markedly impair the normal arterial baroreflex response to hypotension. These changes are not ideal in the scenario with an acute trauma patient who is hypotensive and likely hypovolemic.

BIBLIOGRAPHY

Butterworth JF IV, Mackey DC, Wasnick JD. Intravenous anesthetics. In: Butterworth JF IV, Mackey DC, Wasnick JD (eds.), *Morgan & Mikhail's Clinical Anesthesiology*, 5th ed. New York, NY: McGraw-Hill; 2013:Chapter 9.

Butterworth JF IV, Mackey DC, Wasnick JD (eds.). *Morgan & Mikhail's Clinical Anesthesiology*, 5th ed. New York, NY: McGraw-Hill; 2013.

19. **(B)** Opioid side effects are numerous, which sometimes limits their use. All opioid agonists cause dose-dependent depression of ventilation, primarily through direct effects at brainstem respiratory centers; the apneic threshold rises, and the hypoxic drive decreases. They blunt the response to a carbon dioxide (CO_2) challenge, shifting the CO_2 response curve downward and to the right (i.e., at the same $PaCO_2$, alveolar ventilation will be less after a bolus of morphine than before). Nausea and vomiting can be caused by direct stimulation of dopamine receptors in the medullary chemoreceptor trigger zone in the floor of the fourth ventricle. Opioids can cause biliary smooth muscle spasm, decrease bowel peristalsis, and increase pyloric sphincter and bladder sphincter tone, explaining the side effects of biliary colic, constipation, delayed gastric emptying, and urinary retention. Tolerance develops to essentially all effects and side effects except constipation and miosis.

Opioids have few direct effects on the myocardial contractility when used alone. However, in clinical practice, combination of opioids with benzodiazepines or nitrous oxide may lower systemic blood pressure unlike when any of these drugs are used in isolation. Opioids themselves sometimes do cause a drop in arterial blood pressure as a result of vagus nerve–associated bradycardia (except meperidine, which causes tachycardia secondary to structural similarities to atropine), venodilation, and decreased sympathetic reflexes. Bolus doses of meperidine and morphine can cause enough histamine release to produce profound drops in SVR.

BIBLIOGRAPHY

Butterworth JF IV, Mackey DC, Wasnick JD. Analgesic agents. In: Butterworth JF IV, Mackey DC, Wasnick JD (eds.), *Morgan & Mikhail's Clinical Anesthesiology*, 5th ed. New York, NY: McGraw-Hill; 2013:Chapter 10.

Butterworth JF IV, Mackey DC, Wasnick JD (eds.). *Morgan & Mikhail's Clinical Anesthesiology*, 5th ed. New York, NY: McGraw-Hill; 2013:194–196.

20. **(D)** With the exception of remifentanil, opioids depend primarily on the liver for biotransformation and are then metabolized by the cytochrome P system, conjugated in the liver, or both. It should be noted that the end products of morphine and meperidine biotransformation are active and depend on renal elimination. The accumulation of morphine 6-glucuronide in patients with renal failure has been associated with prolonged narcosis and ventilator depression. The accumulation of normeperidine in patients with renal failure can produce seizures that are not reversed by naloxone.

Fentanyl, alfentanil, and sufentanil are very fast acting and have short duration because of high lipid solubility and redistribution. They have no active metabolites. However, as secondary tissue sites (fat, muscle) become saturated with repeat boluses or prolonged continuous infusion, return of drug from these sites to the plasma will keep plasma concentrations from falling rapidly after the drug is discontinued (see Fig. 7-4). In contrast, remifentanil contains an ester bond that is rapidly hydrolyzed by nonspecific plasma and tissue esterases. Consequently, termination of action of remifentanil remains constant and rapid regardless of length of infusion or the presence of hepatic or renal failure.

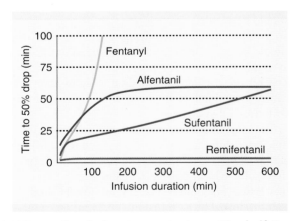

FIGURE 7-4. Graph showing context-sensitive half-times of various narcotics. From Butterworth JF IV, Mackey DC, Wasnick JD (eds.). *Morgan & Mikhail's Clinical Anesthesiology*, 5th ed. New York, NY: McGraw-Hill; 2013.

BIBLIOGRAPHY

Butterworth JF IV, Mackey DC, Wasnick JD. Analgesic agents. In: Butterworth JF IV, Mackey DC, Wasnick JD (eds.), *Morgan & Mikhail's Clinical Anesthesiology*, 5th ed. New York, NY: McGraw-Hill; 2013:Chapter 10.

Butterworth JF IV, Mackey DC, Wasnick JD (eds.). *Morgan & Mikhail's Clinical Anesthesiology*, 5th ed. New York, NY: McGraw-Hill; 2013:193–194.

21. **(A)** The standard measure of potency for inhaled anesthetics is the minimum alveolar concentration (MAC). MAC is defined as the end-tidal anesthetic concentration that prevents movement in response to surgical stimulation in 50% of patients. At 1.3 MAC, 95% of patients do not move in response to surgical stimulation. MAC values are additive (i.e., 0.5 MAC of nitrous oxide and 0.5 MAC of sevoflurane produce the same response to surgical stimulation as 1.0 MAC of isoflurane). MAC values are altered by physiologic and pharmacologic variables such as temperature, PaO_2, $PaCO_2$, blood pressure, electrolytes, pregnancy, and other drugs. It should be noted that there is a 6% decrease in MAC per decade of age.

BIBLIOGRAPHY

Butterworth JF IV, Mackey DC, Wasnick JD. Inhalation anesthetics. In: Butterworth JF IV, Mackey DC, Wasnick JD (eds.), *Morgan & Mikhail's Clinical Anesthesiology*, 5th ed. New York, NY: McGraw-Hill; 2013:Chapter 8.

Butterworth JF IV, Mackey DC, Wasnick JD (eds.). *Morgan & Mikhail's Clinical Anesthesiology*, 5th ed. New York, NY: McGraw-Hill; 2013:162–163.

22. **(D)** Commonly used inhaled anesthetics such as sevoflurane, desflurane, and isoflurane have very narrow margins of safety and require close monitoring of their physiologic effects. Concentrations that produce general anesthesia frequently cause significant CNS, cardiovascular, and respiratory depression.

Anesthetic doses of inhaled anesthetics lead to significant changes in respiration. Spontaneous breathing is typically rapid and shallow. This increased respiratory rate is unable to compensate for the decreased tidal volume, leading to reduced overall minute volume and elevated $PaCO_2$ levels. Also, the ventilatory responsiveness to carbon dioxide and arterial hypoxia is blunted. These depressant effects are typically treated by controlled ventilation during anesthesia. In addition, volatile anesthetics cause a decrease in airway resistance by relaxing bronchial smooth muscle. This bronchodilation may have a beneficial effect in patients with reactive airway disease. During induction, however, isoflurane and desflurane can irritate the airway. Both cause excessive secretions, coughing, and breath holding.

All volatile anesthetics depress the cardiovascular system. In general, blood pressure decreases as a result of a reduction in systemic vascular resistance and depressed myocardial contractility; however, the agents differ in the hemodynamic effects that lead to hypotension. Halothane decreases myocardial contractility and HR, whereas isoflurane, sevoflurane, and desflurane cause decreased blood pressure primarily through decreased systemic vascular resistance. In contrast, nitrous oxide produces little effect on systemic blood pressure.

CNS effects include increased cerebral blood flow and intracranial pressure. High concentrations >1.5 MAC may impair autoregulation of cerebral blood flow. One advantage is a decrease in cerebral metabolic oxygen requirements. Typically during neurosurgery cases, volatile anesthetics are titrated to 0.5 MAC to avoid undue increases in intracranial pressure.

BIBLIOGRAPHY

Butterworth JF IV, Mackey DC, Wasnick JD. Inhalation anesthetics. In: Butterworth JF IV, Mackey DC, Wasnick JD (eds.), *Morgan & Mikhail's Clinical Anesthesiology*, 5th ed. New York, NY: McGraw-Hill; 2013:Chapter 8.

Butterworth JF IV, Mackey DC, Wasnick JD (eds.). *Morgan & Mikhail's Clinical Anesthesiology*, 5th ed. New York, NY: McGraw-Hill; 2013:163–172.

23. **(C)** It is estimated that 2% of pregnant women undergo nonobstetric surgery in the United States annually. Aspiration prophylaxis should be administered to all pregnant patients beyond 14 weeks' gestation because physiologic changes at the lower esophageal sphincter enhance the risk of aspiration. A nonparticulate antacid such as sodium citrate should be administered immediately prior to induction of anesthesia to raise gastric pH. A histamine receptor antagonist like ranitidine and prokinetic agent like metoclopramide (Reglan) can be useful adjuncts as well but take up to an hour to take effect.

Nitrous oxide is a weak teratogen in rodents under certain conditions, even when normal homeostasis is maintained. The mechanism may be partially attributed to methionine synthetase inhibition. However, these studies were performed using high concentrations of nitrous oxide for prolonged periods of time, and no human studies have confirmed these effects. Whether nitrous oxide administration to humans during clinical anesthesia is teratogenic remains to be determined. Because there are a variety of other anesthetic agents available, nitrous oxide can generally be avoided.

The critical period of organogenesis occurs in the first 8 weeks of gestation. If at all possible, necessary surgery should be postponed until the second trimester to reduce the risk of teratogenic drugs. Elective surgery should be postponed until after delivery; however, if surgery is necessary, it is preferable to choose drugs with a long history of safety in pregnancy. These include thiopental, morphine, meperidine, muscle relaxants, local anesthetics, and volatile anesthetics. The use of nitrous oxide, as previously discussed, and benzodiazepines is controversial. Benzodiazepine use during the first trimester became controversial after an association was discovered between maternal diazepam ingestion and the incidence of infants with cleft palate. No evidence suggests that a single dose of benzodiazepine during the course of anesthesia is harmful to the fetus. Anesthetic management must take into account potential effects on the growing fetus as well as physiologic changes that occur during pregnancy.

Studies have suggested that isolated human placental vessels exposed to hyperoxia might cause uteroplacental vasoconstriction with potential impairment of fetal oxygen delivery. This fear has proven to be unfounded because studies in pregnant women have demonstrated better fetal oxygenation with increasing maternal PaO_2. Fetal PaO_2 never exceeds 60 mmHg, even when maternal PaO_2 increases to levels of 600 mmHg.

Left uterine displacement should be attained when the uterine size is equivalent to an 18- to 20-week gestation to avoid aortocaval compression. The right hip should be elevated 15 degrees off midline with a wedge of blankets or by tilting the bed.

BIBLIOGRAPHY

Chestnut D. Nonobstetric surgery during pregnancy. In: Chestnut D (ed.), *Obstetric Anesthesia: Principles and Practice*, 4th ed. St. Louis, MO: Mosby; 2009:Chapter 17.

Chestnut D. *Obstetric Anesthesia: Principles and Practice*, 4th ed. St. Louis, MO: Mosby; 2009:358–375.

24. **(C)** Measurement of arterial blood gas is used to assess ventilation, oxygenation, and acid-base status. Physiologic changes in H^+ are characterized by three phases including immediate chemical buffering, respiratory compensation, and a slower, but more effective, renal compensatory response. The major chemical buffering system in the blood is the bicarbonate/carbonic acid buffer.

The four primary acid-base disorders include respiratory acidosis, respiratory alkalosis, metabolic acidosis, and metabolic alkalosis. If the disorder primarily affects HCO_3^-, it is termed metabolic. If it primarily affects $PaCO_2$ (normal value 40 mmHg), it is termed respiratory. When one disorder occurs by itself, the acid-base disorder is termed simple. The presence of two or more primary processes indicates a mixed disorder.

In the case of a respiratory acid-base disorder, there is a primary increase or decrease in $PaCO_2$ leading to a decrease or increase in H^+ and a change in arterial pH. Respiratory acidosis, as represented by the blood gas in the question, is most likely secondary to hypoventilation because CO_2 production does not vary under most circumstances. Respiratory alkalosis is commonly secondary to central (e.g., pain, anxiety, infection) or peripheral (e.g., hypoxemia, severe anemia, pulmonary disease) stimulation and results in a decreased $PaCO_2$. Because the renal response to retain bicarbonate is relatively slow, the acute response to respiratory acid-base disorders is limited, and as a result, for approximately every 10-mmHg change in $PaCO_2$, the pH will change 0.08 units in the opposite direction. In this example, the pH change can be accounted for by the increase in $PaCO_2$.

The causes of metabolic disorders are more complex. A metabolic acidosis is defined as a primary decrease in HCO_3^- and is generally due to consumption of HCO_3^- by a strong acid, renal or gastrointestinal wasting of HCO_3^-, or rapid dilution of the extracellular fluid (ECF) compartment with a bicarbonate-free fluid. Most cases of metabolic alkalosis can be divided into those associated with NaCl deficiency and ECF depletion (chloride sensitive) and those with enhanced mineralocorticoid activity (chloride resistant). During metabolic disturbances, every 6-mEq change in HCO_3^- should change arterial pH by 0.1. If the change is greater or less than predicted, then a mixed disorder is likely present.

In evaluating oxygenation, the first thing to consider is whether hypoxemia is present. In most patients, hypoxemia exists if PaO_2 is less than 60 mmHg. This is the part on the oxyhemoglobin dissociation curve where the oxygen content of blood drops rapidly with small decreases in PaO_2. The patient in the question is not hypoxemic because PaO_2 is >60 mmHg on only room air.

BIBLIOGRAPHY

Butterworth JF IV, Mackey DC, Wasnick JD. Acid-base management. In: Butterworth JF IV, Mackey DC, Wasnick JD (eds.), *Morgan & Mikhail's Clinical Anesthesiology*, 5th ed. New York, NY: McGraw-Hill; 2013:Chapter 50.

Butterworth JF IV, Mackey DC, Wasnick JD (eds.). *Morgan & Mikhail's Clinical Anesthesiology*, 5th ed. New York, NY: McGraw-Hill; 2013:1141–1157.

25. **(A)** Blood pressure can be measured a variety of different ways, and understanding how these methods work is important to ensure these monitors are used properly.

Automated blood pressure monitors use oscillometry. Arterial pulsations create small oscillations in cuff pressure that are maximal at mean arterial pressure. A microprocessor uses algorithms to derive systolic and diastolic pressures. The sampling site can affect measurements, with greater systolic and diastolic differences the more distal the cuff is from the aorta. These differences are increased further by the use of vasodilating drugs such as nitroglycerin. Blood pressure measurements can also be altered by the presence of peripheral vascular disease. Care should be taken to avoid placing a blood pressure cuff on an extremity with any vascular abnormality, including dialysis access grafts.

Manual blood pressure readings are taken using Korotkoff sounds, which are the sounds of turbulent flow in an artery. The cuff is inflated to a pressure that collapses the underlying artery. Systolic pressure is noted at the appearance of sound after deflation of the cuff. Diastolic pressure is indicated by the muffling or disappearance of sound. Proper cuff size is assured with the cuff bladder extending at least halfway around a patient's arm. The width of the cuff should be 20–50% greater than the diameter of the extremity.

Arterial lines directly detect an arterial pressure wave that is transmitted through the tubing to a transducer. The transducer contains a diaphragm that is then distorted by the pressure wave and converted into an electrical signal. The transducer accuracy depends on correct zeroing procedure, which involves opening it to air and zeroing it at the desired level of measurement. During supine procedure, the transducer is typically zeroed at the midaxillary line. In a seated patient, the arterial pressure in the brain is significantly lower than the left ventricular pressure. Zeroing the transducer at the external auditory meatus approximates the arterial blood pressure at the circle of Willis.

The difference in blood pressure (mmHg) at two different sites is equal to the height of an interposed column of water (cmH$_2$O) multiplied by a conversion factor (1 cmH$_2$O = 0.74 mmHg). Thus, a 10-cm height difference between sampling sites results in an approximately 7.5-mmHg pressure differential, with the lower site having the greater pressure. Therefore, in the example, because the transducer is 40 cm *above* the noninvasive cuff, the arterial line should read a pressure of 30 mmHg *lower* (40 cm × 0.74 mmHg/cm). This puts the MAP at the circle of Willis around 50 mmHg, which is on the lower end of normal cerebral autoregulation.

BIBLIOGRAPHY

Butterworth JF IV, Mackey DC, Wasnick JD. Cardiovascular monitoring. In: Butterworth JF IV, Mackey DC, Wasnick JD (eds.), *Morgan & Mikhail's Clinical Anesthesiology*, 5th ed. New York, NY: McGraw-Hill; 2013:Chapter 5.
Butterworth JF IV, Mackey DC, Wasnick JD (eds.). *Morgan & Mikhail's Clinical Anesthesiology*, 5th ed. New York, NY: McGraw-Hill; 2013:87–91.

26. **(E)** All surgical patients undergo intraoperative monitoring of their ECG. The standard intraoperative ECG consists of five leads, consisting of the left arm, right arm, left limb, right limb, and V5 leads. This lead placement allows monitoring of any of the six limb leads (I, II, III, aVR, aVL, and aVF) and V5. The V5 lead can be moved to any of the precordial positions, especially V1 for special arrhythmia monitoring. Leads V3–V5 are preferred for ischemia monitoring.

During the perioperative period, ECG monitoring most commonly identifies stress-induced, ST-segment depression type ischemia. Because all 12 ECG leads are not being monitored perioperatively, selecting the most sensitive leads is very important. Studies have shown the single most sensitive lead for ischemia detection in high-risk patients undergoing noncardiac surgery is V5 (75%) followed by V4 (61%). Combining leads V4 and V5 is 90% sensitive, whereas the standard combination of II and V5 is 80% sensitive. If leads II, V4, and V5 could be monitored simultaneously, sensitivity would be increased to 98%. Lead II is routinely monitored because the axis of lead II parallels the atria, resulting in the greatest P-wave amplitude of any of the leads.

BIBLIOGRAPHY

Miller RD. Electrocardiography. In: Miller RD (ed.), *Miller's Anesthesia*, 7th ed. Philadelphia, PA: Elsevier Churchill Livingstone; 2009:Chapter 42.
Miller RD. *Miller's Anesthesia*, 7th ed. Philadelphia, PA: Elsevier Churchill Livingstone; 2009:1363–1364, 1378.

27. **(C)** An understanding of the technology behind pulse oximetry assures optimal care of patients. Pulse oximetry employs the Lambert-Beer law to noninvasively measure arterial blood oxygen saturation. This law states that oxygenated and deoxygenated hemoglobin absorb red and infrared light differently. A sensor containing light sources (two or three light-emitting diodes) and a light detector (a photodiode) are placed across any perfused tissue that can be transilluminated, such as a finger, toe, or earlobe.

The wavelengths used are in the red (660 nm) and infrared (940 nm) parts of the spectrum. Oxyhemoglobin absorbs more infrared light, whereas deoxyhemoglobin absorbs more red light. The difference in absorption during arterial pulsations is detected by the sensor, and resultant oxygen saturation is displayed. The ratio of absorptions is analyzed by a microprocessor to provide a SpO_2. A greater ratio of red/infrared absorption results in a lower SpO_2 value. Arterial pulsations are identified by plethysmography, which filters out light absorption from venous blood and other tissues.

The amplitude of the waveform produced can be used as a measure of tissue perfusion. Ear probes can detect changes in oxygen saturation sooner than finger probes by virtue of a shorter circulation time. Carboxyhemoglobin absorbs infrared light the same as oxyhemoglobin, leading to a falsely elevated reading. Methemoglobin absorbs the light of both red and infrared wavelengths equally, resulting in a 1:1 absorption ratio and corresponding SpO_2 reading of 85%. This reading is falsely low if the true saturation is greater than 85% or falsely high if the true saturation is lower than 85%. Carboxyhemoglobin and methemoglobin levels are best measured using co-oximetry. Anemia, even with a hemoglobin level as low as 2.3 g/dL, has little or no effect on SpO_2 values.

It is important to realize that pulse oximetry does not relay any information about a patient's ventilation status. Ventilation is monitored in the operating room using capnography, which gives an end-tidal CO_2 value. Capnographs rely on the absorption of infrared light by CO_2. There is a small gradient (2–5 mmHg) between $PaCO_2$ and $EtCO_2$, which reflects alveolar dead space.

BIBLIOGRAPHY

Butterworth JF IV, Mackey DC, Wasnick JD (eds.). *Morgan & Mikhail's Clinical Anesthesiology*, 5th ed. New York, NY: McGraw-Hill; 2013:124–125.

Butterworth JF IV, Mackey DC, Wasnick JD. Noncardiovascular monitoring. In: Butterworth JF IV, Mackey DC, Wasnick JD (eds.), *Morgan & Mikhail's Clinical Anesthesiology*, 5th ed. New York, NY: McGraw-Hill; 2013:Chapter 6.

Miller RD. *Miller's Anesthesia*, 7th ed. Philadelphia, PA: Elsevier Churchill Livingstone; 2009:1419–1429.

Miller RD. Respiratory monitoring. In: Miller RD (ed.), *Miller's Anesthesia*, 7th ed. Philadelphia, PA: Elsevier Churchill Livingstone; 2009:Chapter 44.

28. **(C)** The basic design of a pulmonary artery catheter consists of five lumens integrated into a 110-cm-long 7.5F catheter. The lumens consist of an air channel for inflation of the balloon, wiring for the thermistor probe for evaluation of cardiac output, a proximal port 30 cm from the tip (for infusions, CO injections, and central venous pressure [CVP] measurements), a ventricular port 20 cm from the tip for infusion of drugs, a distal port for aspiration, and a distal passage for mixed venous sampling and measurements of pulmonary artery pressure.

    Insertion is guided by a pressure waveform, as well as markings on the catheter. A central venous tracing

is seen at approximately 15 cm as the catheter enters the right atrium. An increase in the systolic pressure indicates passage of the catheter into the right ventricle. Entry into the pulmonary artery is signified by an increase in the diastolic pressure. A wedge pressure is identified by small-amplitude waves after minimal advancement into the pulmonary artery.

Hemodynamic variables derived from a pulmonary artery catheter include CVP, systemic vascular resistance (SVR), stroke volume (SV), cardiac output (CO), pulmonary artery pressure (PAP), and cardiac and ventricular indices. Pulmonary catheters allow more precise estimations of preload than central venous cannulation. The pulmonary capillary wedge pressure (PCWP) estimates left ventricular end-diastolic pressure (LVEDP). Estimations of LVEDP via PCWP may be inaccurate in the case of mitral valve disease or changes in left atrial or ventricular compliance. Cardiac output measurements are most commonly obtained by thermodilution technique, either through injection of a known volume and temperature of fluid into the proximal infusion port or by continuous measurement. The degree of temperature change is inversely proportional to cardiac output.

Certain conditions can be diagnosed with interpretation of the data collected from a pulmonary artery catheter. In the question stem, the patient has a normal CVP, suggesting euvolemia and adequate right heart function. The patient's low CI, elevated PCWP, low SVR, and low SvO_2 suggest left ventricular dysfunction and cardiogenic shock. Septic shock would likely present with an elevated CI, low SVR, and high SvO_2 secondary to shunting.

BIBLIOGRAPHY

Butterworth JF IV, Mackey DC, Wasnick JD. Cardiovascular monitoring. In: Butterworth JF IV, Mackey DC, Wasnick JD (eds.), *Morgan & Mikhail's Clinical Anesthesiology*, 5th ed. New York, NY: McGraw-Hill; 2013:Chapter 5.

Butterworth JF IV, Mackey DC, Wasnick JD (eds.). *Morgan & Mikhail's Clinical Anesthesiology*, 5th ed. New York, NY: McGraw-Hill; 2013:104–111.

29. **(C)** Spinal anesthesia is the placement of local anesthetic solution into the subarachnoid space. Direct injection of local anesthetic into cerebrospinal fluid (CSF) for spinal anesthesia allows a relatively small dose and volume of local anesthetic to achieve dense sensory and motor blockade. Many operations on the lower extremities, pelvis, and lower abdomen can be managed safely with spinal blocks alone, or they may be used simultaneously with general anesthesia for postoperative pain management. Adverse reactions do occur and range from

self-limited back pain to severe cardiovascular effects and even death.

Interruption of efferent autonomic transmission at the spinal nerve roots produces sympathetic blockade. Sympathetic preganglionic nerve fibers exit the spinal cord from T1–L2. Because the parasympathetic preganglionic fibers exit the spinal cord with cranial and sacral nerve roots, the physiologic responses of neuraxial blockade are from decreased sympathetic tone and/or unopposed parasympathetic tone.

Spinal anesthesia produces a consistent decrease in blood pressure and possible decrease in heart rate, with the degree depending on the extent of sympathectomy, because vasomotor tone is primarily determined by sympathetic fibers from T5–L1. Sympathectomy causes arterial and venous smooth muscle dilation, leading to pooling of blood in the viscera and lower extremities, causing a decreased circulating blood volume. The sympathetic cardiac accelerator fibers arise from T1–T4 and lead to bradycardia with a high spinal level. Unopposed vagal tone may explain the sudden cardiac arrest that sometimes is seen with spinal anesthesia. Therapy for spinal-induced hypotension includes fluids, head down position, and pharmacologic therapy with atropine, ephedrine, and other vasopressors as the situation dictates.

Alterations in pulmonary physiology are usually minimal because the diaphragm is innervated by the phrenic nerve, arising from C3–C5. Even with high thoracic levels, there is only a small decrease in vital capacity secondary to loss of the abdominal muscles' contribution to forced expiration.

Other effects of spinal anesthesia include vagal tone dominance in the gut causing a small, contracted gut with active peristalsis. There is little effect on renal function because renal blood flow is maintained through autoregulation. Both parasympathetic and sympathetic autonomic control of the bladder is lost, leading to urinary retention until the block wears off. Thus urinary catheter insertion is important in patients receiving spinal anesthesia. And finally, a T11 sympathectomy can block the adrenal response to surgical stress. This may be helpful by diminishing hyperglycemia, HTN, and catecholamine release.

BIBLIOGRAPHY

Butterworth JF IV, Mackey DC, Wasnick JD (eds.). *Morgan & Mikhail's Clinical Anesthesiology*, 5th ed. New York, NY: McGraw-Hill; 2013:945–947.

Butterworth JF IV, Mackey DC, Wasnick JD. Spinal, epidural, and caudal blocks. In: Butterworth JF IV, Mackey DC, Wasnick JD (eds.), *Morgan & Mikhail's Clinical Anesthesiology*, 5th ed. New York, NY: McGraw-Hill; 2013:Chapter 45.

30. **(D)** The actual incidence of neurologic dysfunction resulting from hemorrhagic complications associated with neuraxial blockade is unknown. The incidence cited in the literature is less than 1/150,000 with epidural anesthetics and less than 1/220,000 with spinal anesthetics. However, recent epidemiologic surveys suggest the frequency may be as high as 1/3000 in some populations. Because the incidence of spinal hematoma is so rare, a randomized controlled trial cannot be performed, so ASRA formed guidelines, most recently revised in 2010, regarding anticoagulation and neuraxial anesthesia from evidence-based reviews (Table 7-4).

TABLE 7-4 Guidelines for Performing Neuraxial Anesthesia (NA)

Drug	Time to Discontinue Prior to NA
Clopidogrel	7 d
Ticlopidine	10–14 d
Warfarin	INR <1.4
Unfractionated heparin	No contraindications for subcutaneous twice-a-day dose (but be aware of heparin-induced thrombocytopenia)
Low-molecular-weight heparin	12 h after prophylactic dose, 24 h after therapeutic dose
Aspirin	No contraindication

BIBLIOGRAPHY

Horlocker TT, Wedel DJ, Rowlingson JC, et al. Regional anesthesia in the patient receiving antithrombotic or thrombolytic therapy: American Society of Regional Anesthesia and Pain Medicine Evidence-Based Guidelines (Third Edition). *Reg Anesth Pain Med* 2010;35:64–101.

31. **(D)** The complications of neuraxial anesthesia range from bothersome to life threatening. Broadly, the complications can be classified into categories of adverse or exaggerated physiologic responses, complications related to needle/catheter placement, and drug toxicity. Adverse physiologic responses include urinary retention, high block, cardiac arrest, Horner syndrome, and anterior spinal artery syndrome. Complications related to instrumentation include backache, dural puncture, neural injury, spinal hematoma, catheter misplacement, arachnoiditis (inflammation of the arachnoid layer), and infection (meningitis or epidural abscess). Drug toxicity can lead to cauda equina syndrome, transient neurologic symptoms, and systemic local anesthetic toxicity.

The patient in the question has the signs and symptoms of a classic postdural puncture headache (PDPH). PDPH typically occurs hours to days after a dural puncture and is thought to result from a loss of CSF into the epidural space, leading to decreased hydrostatic pressure and traction on the meninges. Typically, PDPH is a bilateral, frontal, retro-orbital, or occipital headache that extends into the neck. It is commonly associated with photophobia and nausea. Occasionally cranial nerve palsies may be associated, usually with the abducens, oculomotor, or trochlear nerves. The hallmark is its association with body position. PDPH is aggravated by sitting or standing and relieved by lying supine.

PDPH can be treated conservatively with analgesics, caffeine, and hydration if the symptoms are not severe. For debilitating symptoms, an epidural blood patch can be effective. It involves injecting 15–20 mL of autologous blood into the epidural space at, or one level below, the level of dural puncture. It is believed to stop CSF leakage by either mass effect or coagulation. Approximately 90% of patients will respond to a single blood patch, and 90% of nonresponders will respond to a second blood patch.

When evaluating a patient for possible PDPH, it is important to rule out more catastrophic complications such as spinal or epidural hematoma, meningitis, arachnoiditis, and epidural abscess. Symptoms of spinal or epidural hematoma include sharp back and leg pain with motor weakness and/or sphincter dysfunction. When hematoma is suspected, immediate neuroimaging with MRI or CT and neurosurgery consultation are warranted. Meningitis may present with fever, headache, and neurologic symptoms, and an infectious workup should be pursued. Epidural abscesses often have a delayed presentation from 5 days to several weeks from neuraxial instrumentation. Localized back pain with radicular symptoms leading to motor and sensory deficits would be expected. Neuroimaging and surgery consult should also be immediately obtained.

The correct treatment for this patient's condition is an epidural autologous blood patch. All of her symptoms (tinnitus, photophobia, and positional frontal headache) can be explained by the history of dural puncture. The localized back pain without radicular symptoms can be explained by local needle trauma. She is otherwise neurologically intact and does not warrant any further imaging or surgery consultation.

BIBLIOGRAPHY

Butterworth JF IV, Mackey DC, Wasnick JD (eds.). *Morgan & Mikhail's Clinical Anesthesiology*, 5th ed. New York, NY: McGraw-Hill; 2013:960–972.
Butterworth JF IV, Mackey DC, Wasnick JD. Spinal, epidural, and caudal blocks. In: Butterworth JF IV, Mackey DC, Wasnick JD (eds.), *Morgan & Mikhail's Clinical Anesthesiology*, 5th ed. New York, NY: McGraw-Hill; 2013:Chapter 45.

32. **(A)** Massive transfusion is most often defined as the need to transfuse one to two times the patient's blood volume. The extracellular concentration of potassium in stored blood steadily increases with time as potassium moves out of RBCs. The potassium concentration may reach levels between 19 and 35 mEq/L in blood stored for 21 days. At rapid infusion rates up to 500–1000 mL/min, critical hyperkalemia leading to cardiac arrest can occur.

Citrate is added to pRBCs as a preservative to prevent clotting. Calcium binding by citrate can cause hypocalcemia and cardiac depression. However, this rarely occurs in clinical practice because patients with normal hepatic function are able to easily clear the citrate contained in 1 unit of pRBCs unless the transfusion rate exceeds 1 unit every 5 minutes.

Transfusion of 1 unit of pRBCs stored at 4°C will reduce the core temperature of a 70-kg patient by 0.25°C. Hypothermia should be minimized with use of fluid warmers.

Storage of pRBCs also leads to a progressive decrease in intracellular adenosine triphosphate (ATP) and 2,3-diphosphoglycerate (2,3-DPG), leading to a left-shifted oxygen-hemoglobin dissociation curve. Thus, transfusion of 2,3-DPG–depleted blood increases the patient's hemoglobin but results in less efficient oxygen delivery. 2,3-DPG levels return to normal over 12–24 hours.

Acidosis commonly occurs because the pH of blood stored for 21 days may be as low as 6.9 secondary to metabolism of glucose to lactate and the addition of the citrate phosphate dextrose preservative. Other concerns with massive transfusion include volume overload and dilutional coagulopathy. Coagulation studies and platelet counts should guide component transfusion with platelets, fresh frozen plasma, and cryoprecipitate.

BIBLIOGRAPHY

Butterworth JF IV, Mackey DC, Wasnick JD. Fluid management and blood component therapy. In: Butterworth JF IV, Mackey DC, Wasnick JD (eds.), *Morgan & Mikhail's Clinical Anesthesiology*, 5th ed. New York, NY: McGraw-Hill; 2013:Chapter 51.
Butterworth JF IV, Mackey DC, Wasnick JD (eds.). *Morgan & Mikhail's Clinical Anesthesiology*, 5th ed. New York, NY: McGraw-Hill; 2013:1175–1176.

33. **(D)** Type, screen, and crossmatch are compatibility tests used to detect harmful antigen-antibody interactions and prevent transfusion reactions. Determination of ABO-Rh types of both donor and recipient is the first and most

important step, because the most serious reactions are caused by accidental transfusion of ABO-incompatible blood. Anti-A and anti-B antibodies are formed when an individual lacks either or both of the A and B antigens. ABO typing is performed by testing RBCs for the A and B antigens and the serum for A and B antibodies. Thus, a patient with type A blood will make anti-B, and a patient with type B blood will make anti-A. Additional testing is performed for the Rh antigen because this is common and likely to produce immunization. After these tests, the patient is "typed."

The next step is the antibody screen. This is a test to determine the presence of abnormal red cell antibodies in recipient serum to clinically significant antigens. The antibody screen is carried out in three phases and is similar in time required to a crossmatch. The screen involves a trial transfusion between the recipient's serum and commercially supplied RBCs that are specifically selected to contain optimal numbers of RBC antigens or those antigens commonly implicated in hemolytic transfusion reactions. Examples of these antigens include D, C, E, c, e, Duffy, Kell, and Kidd. Now the patient is "screened." The type and screen is used most often when the patient is unlikely to require transfusion during the planned surgical procedure, but blood should be readily available.

The crossmatch is essentially a trial transfusion within a test tube where donor RBCs are mixed with recipient serum to detect a potential for serious transfusion reaction. There are three phases, including an immediate phase, an incubation phase, and an antiglobulin phase. In the first phase, conducted at room temperature, donor RBCs are mixed with the recipient's serum and examined for macroscopic agglutination. It tests for ABO incompatibilities and those caused by naturally occurring antibodies in the MN, P, and Lewis systems. In the second phase, the products of the first phase are incubated at 37°C in low ionic strength saline or albumin to enhance incomplete antibodies. This phase primarily detects antibodies in the Rh system. In the third and final phase, the indirect antiglobulin test, antiglobulin serum is used to detect antibodies that may be attached to donor RBCs. This phase detects antibodies in the blood Rh, Kell, Kidd, and Duffy blood group systems.

Routinely crossmatching blood for patients who have a low chance of getting transfused burdens the blood bank and makes the blood unavailable for use by others for 48–72 hours. The crossmatch-to-transfusion (C/T) ratio has been used to quantify this problem. It has been suggested that for surgical procedures in which the average number of units transfused per case is less than 0.5, determination of a type and screen should be adequate instead of a type and crossmatch. In previously transfused patients, only about 1 in 100 has an irregular antibody other than anti-A or anti-B. Of these irregular antibodies, some are only reactive at temperatures <30°C and therefore clinically insignificant. ABO-Rh typing alone results in a 99.8% chance of a compatible transfusion. The addition of an antibody screen increases safety to 99.94%, and a crossmatch increases this to 99.95%.

BIBLIOGRAPHY

Miller RD. *Miller's Anesthesia*, 7th ed. Philadelphia, PA: Elsevier Churchill Livingstone; 2009:1742–1744.
Miller RD. Transfusion therapy. In: Miller RD (ed.), *Miller's Anesthesia*, 7th ed. Philadelphia, PA: Elsevier Churchill Livingstone; 2009:Chapter 55.

34. **(C)** The patient in the question is clearly having a serious hemolytic transfusion reaction, and aggressive treatment is warranted. Transfusion reactions can be divided into allergic, hemolytic, and febrile. Most allergic reactions are mild and thought to be caused by the presence of foreign protein in the transfused blood. The most common symptoms are urticaria and itching. In severe cases, transfusion may need to be stopped. In most cases, however, patients can be treated symptomatically with diphenhydramine and the transfusion continued. Anaphylaxis most commonly occurs when immunoglobulin A (IgA)-deficient patients, who have formed anti-IgA, receive transfusion of IgA. These patients present with dyspnea, hypotension, laryngeal edema, chest pain, and shock. This can be prevented by transfusing IgA-deficient patients with "washed RBCs," a process that removes all traces of donor IgA.

Hemolytic transfusion reactions occur when incompatible blood is administered (often because of clerical errors) and is life threatening. Antibodies and complement in the recipient attack donor red blood cells, leading to hemolysis. The antibodies that commonly produce immediate hemolysis are anti-A, anti-B, Kell, Kidd, Lewis, and Duffy. Release of hemoglobin and cytokines leads to shock, disseminated intravascular coagulation (DIC), and acute renal failure. Many of the signs and symptoms of a hemolytic transfusion reaction may be masked by anesthesia. In an awake patient, signs include fever (most common), chills, chest/back pain, nausea, flushing, dyspnea, and headache; however, under general anesthesia, the only signs may be hemoglobinuria, bleeding diathesis, or hypotension. Unfortunately these are common in surgery, and the diagnosis is often not made until diffuse bleeding secondary to DIC or hemoglobinuria is noted later.

When a hemolytic transfusion reaction is suspected, the transfusion should be immediately discontinued, and blood and urine samples should be sent to the laboratory. The renal and coagulation systems are the primary therapy targets. High urine output (>75 mL/h) should be maintained with crystalloid solution and administration of furosemide or mannitol because renal failure is thought to occur from hemoglobin in the form of acid hematin precipitating in the distal tubules and causing mechanical blockage. Also, the use of sodium bicarbonate to alkalinize the urine has been suggested. DIC commonly occurs with hemolytic transfusion reactions, likely because RBC stroma is severed, releasing erythrocytin, which activates the intrinsic system of coagulation. This leads to consumption of platelets and factors I, II, V, and VII. Treat coagulopathy with appropriate products. Hypotension can be treated with fluids, vasopressors, and compatible blood if necessary.

Febrile reactions are more common and likely caused by pyrogenic cytokines and intracellular contents released by donor leukocytes. Patients often have fever only, but also may experience chills, myalgia, headache, nausea, or dyspnea. These reactions may be difficult to distinguish from a hemolytic reaction. There is no clear consensus on whether the transfusion should be terminated, but appropriate treatment consists of antipyretics and ruling out more serious reactions. These reactions can be prevented with the use of leukoreduced blood.

BIBLIOGRAPHY

Miller RD. *Miller's Anesthesia*, 7th ed. Philadelphia, PA: Elsevier Churchill Livingstone; 2009:1752–1755.
Miller RD. Transfusion therapy. In: Miller RD (ed.), *Miller's Anesthesia*, 7th ed. Philadelphia, PA: Elsevier Churchill Livingstone; 2009:Chapter 55.

35. **(C)** There are multiple different kinds of intravenous fluid (IVF) therapy with advantages and disadvantages to each different type. Knowing the composition of the different fluids is important and can help guide therapy. Five percent dextrose has an osmolarity of 252 mOsm/L, making it hypo-osmolar relative to plasma. This causes increased brain water and intracranial pressure (ICP), making it an undesirable choice for TBI patients. Hyperglycemia (>200 mg/dL) in TBI patients has also been proven to worsen morbidity and mortality.

Normal saline (NS) contains 154 mEq/L of both sodium and chloride and has a pH of 6.0. The low pH and high chloride content can contribute to non–anion gap, hyperchloremic metabolic acidosis when it is given in large quantities. Lactated Ringer's (LR) solution has a higher pH of 6.5 and is considered a balanced salt solution (130 mEq of Na^+/L). LR is more hypo-osmolar compared to NS (273 mOsm/L versus 308 mOsm/L) and contains less chloride (109 mEq/L). LR contains a buffer in the form of lactate, which is metabolized by the liver

into bicarbonate and can lead to a metabolic alkalosis. Also note that LR contains small amounts of potassium and calcium, which may limit its use in renal failure patients and when giving citrated blood products.

Hydroxyethyl starch (HES) is a synthetic colloid solution available as a 6% solution in 0.9% NaCl (Hespan). The pH is about 5.5, and the osmolarity is about 310 mOsm/L. HES solutions decrease levels of von Willebrand factor and associated factor VIII activity (acquired, type I von Willebrand–like syndrome), impair platelet function, and may induce platelet damage. The effects on coagulation are more significant in HES products with higher molar substitutions.

There has been an ongoing debate for decades on whether crystalloids or colloids are superior for perioperative volume replacement. Crystalloids are inexpensive and have few side effects. Colloids have better volume expanding properties and improve microcirculation. A review by the Cochrane Collaboration in critically ill patients showed that there is no evidence from randomized controlled trials that resuscitation with colloids reduces the risk of death, compared with crystalloid resuscitation, in patients with trauma or burns or after surgery.

Fluid management in an acutely burned patient focuses on restoration of plasma volume and a shift of the ECF volume into the burned but viable tissue. The Parkland formula prescribes fluids based on the percentage of body surface area burned (% BSA). The Parkland formula is mathematically expressed as: Fluid required in first 24 hours = 4 × body weight in kg × % BSA burned. Half of this amount should be given in the first 8 hours with the remaining amount given over the next 16 hours. Thus, a 100-kg patient with 20% BSA burned should receive 4 × 100 kg × 20% BSA = 8000 mL of fluid over the first 24 hours, with 4000 mL in the first 8 hours.

BIBLIOGRAPHY

Miller RD. Intravascular fluid and electrolyte physiology. In: Miller RD (ed.), *Miller's Anesthesia*, 7th ed. Philadelphia, PA: Elsevier Churchill Livingstone; 2009:Chapter 54.
Miller RD. *Miller's Anesthesia*, 7th ed. Philadelphia, PA: Elsevier Churchill Livingstone; 2009:1733–1734, 2798–2802.
Miller RD. Postoperative intravascular fluid therapy. In: Miller RD (ed.), *Miller's Anesthesia*, 7th ed. Philadelphia, PA: Elsevier Churchill Livingstone; 2009:Chapter 88.

36. **(D)** Periglottic devices, such as the laryngeal mask airway (LMA), are designed to form a seal in the pharynx between the respiratory and digestive tracts. They provide an intermediate between the face mask and tracheal tube in terms of anatomic position, invasiveness, and security. During routine use, the patient is anesthetized, often with propofol and sevoflurane, before the LMA is blindly inserted until

definite resistance is felt. Neuromuscular blocking agents are not required and are rarely used for placement. The cuff is then inflated, and gentle manual ventilation should result in lung expansion and bilateral breath sounds. Two tests that correlate with optimum position are the ability to generate an airway pressure of 20 cmH$_2$O and the ability to ventilate manually. An effective seal depends on the size and position of the LMA, inflation of the cuff, low airway resistance, and high pulmonary compliance.

The seal achieved by LMAs provides less protection against pulmonary aspiration than a properly inserted cuffed endotracheal tube. LMA malposition in which the upper end of the esophagus lies within the opening of the LMA (reported in up to a third or more of patients) increases the risk of pulmonary aspiration. Both positive-pressure and pressure support modes of ventilation can be used safely with an LMA in place, although higher pressures increase the risk for gastric insufflation and thus regurgitation.

The LMA is a key device at several places in the difficult airway algorithm (see Table 7-1). There are many reports of successful LMA rescue when tracheal intubation has failed, including the "cannot intubate, cannot ventilate" scenario. It should be noted that the LMA is not a secured airway, and there is still risk of airway obstruction or LMA malposition.

BIBLIOGRAPHY

Miller RD. Airway management in the adult. In: Miller RD (ed.), *Miller's Anesthesia*, 7th ed. Philadelphia, PA: Elsevier Churchill Livingstone; 2009:Chapter 50.

Miller RD. *Miller's Anesthesia*, 7th ed. Philadelphia, PA: Elsevier Churchill Livingstone; 2009:1581–1584.

37. **(E)** Induction of general anesthesia in patients with full stomachs or incompetent lower esophageal sphincters can result in aspiration of gastric contents. High-risk groups include obese patients, parturients, diabetics with gastroparesis, and patients with gastroesophageal reflux. Clinically significant aspiration can occur when pH is <2.5 or gastric volume is >25 mL. The goal of rapid sequence induction (RSI) is to limit the time in which the airway is unprotected after induction. During an RSI technique, mask ventilation is not performed because it can fill the stomach with air and increase the risk of aspiration even further. Therefore, proper preoxygenation is important because it allows most apneic patients to maintain oxygen saturation while waiting for neuromuscular blockade to occur. An RSI is performed by administering an intravenous anesthetic followed immediately by a neuromuscular blocker with a rapid onset, such as succinylcholine or high-dose (1.2 mg/kg) rocuronium. Cricoid pressure is generally held and direct laryngoscopy is performed when neuromuscular blockade is confirmed. Cricoid pressure theoretically occludes the esophageal lumen, preventing the passage of gastric contents into the pharynx. Cricoid pressure is contraindicated in actively vomiting patients (possibility of esophageal perforation), cervical spine fracture, and laryngeal fracture. Cricoid pressure is controversial because it can be ineffective, especially if not properly applied, and can cause the undesired effects of potentially increasing the risk of regurgitation and failed tracheal intubation.

The risk of an RSI is that intubation may not be successful and the ability to mask ventilate the patient is not established prior to giving muscle relaxant. Thus, a failed RSI can lead to a paralyzed patient who cannot be ventilated or intubated. If the patient is expected to have a difficult airway, then an awake technique that maintains airway reflexes and spontaneous ventilation or an RSI with surgical backup immediately available is advised.

BIBLIOGRAPHY

Flint PW, Haughey BH, Lund VJ, et al. *Cummings Otolaryngology Head and Neck Surgery*, 5th ed. Philadelphia, PA: Mosby; 2010:112–113.

Flint PW, Haughey BH, Lund VJ, et al. General considerations of anesthesia and management of the difficult airway. In: Flint PW, Haughey BH, Lund VJ, et al. (eds.), *Cummings Otolaryngology Head and Neck Surgery*, 5th ed. Philadelphia, PA: Mosby; 2010:Chapter 9.

38. **(C)** Acute respiratory distress syndrome (ARDS) is an inflammatory response of the lungs to both direct and indirect insults defined according to the following criteria: acute onset, presence of bilateral infiltrates on chest radiography, pulmonary artery wedge pressure <18 mmHg, and hypoxemia with a PaO$_2$/FiO$_2$ ratio <200. Patients meeting these criteria but with PaO$_2$/FiO$_2$ ratio <300 are diagnosed with acute lung injury (ALI). ARDS is characterized by abnormal mechanical properties of the lungs with hallmark features of reduced FRC and reduced static compliance of the respiratory system.

Large tidal volumes (TV) of 10–15 mL/kg were used in the past to normalize pH and PaCO$_2$. However, a large, multicenter, randomized controlled trial carried out by ARDSNet comparing TVs of 12 mL/kg to TVs of 6 mL/kg in ARDS patients had to be stopped early after accrual of 861 patients when an interim analysis revealed a 22% lower mortality rate in the low-TV group. These beneficial results occurred in all patient groups including septic and nonseptic patients. The lower TVs allow a lower static (plateau) airway pressure to be maintained (goal <30 cmH$_2$O) and may prevent barotrauma. This is the only intervention that has been unequivocally proven to reduce mortality in patients with ARDS.

Because ARDS is marked by high intrapulmonary shunt, hypoxemia is relatively unresponsive to oxygen therapy. Thus, positive end-expiratory pressure (PEEP) therapy is an important component in the treatment of ARDS. PEEP improves oxygenation by decreasing FRC and dead space ventilation and increasing lung compliance. Recent investigations testing the effects on mortality of "higher" PEEP titration have not shown any improvement in survival rate, although they have shown benefit in terms of ventilator-free days and need for nonconventional therapy. The optimal level of PEEP and best method to set PEEP have not been definitively established.

Inhaled nitric oxide (iNO) is a potential option for rescue therapy in patients with severe ARDS and refractory hypoxemia. iNO is a selective pulmonary vasodilator that might improve gas exchange and reduce pulmonary hypertension leading to better ventilation/perfusion matching.

BIBLIOGRAPHY

Barash PG. *Clinical Anesthesia*, 6th ed. Philadelphia, PA: Lippincott Williams & Wilkins; 2009:1458–1459.
Barash PG. Critical care medicine. In: Barash PG (ed.), *Clinical Anesthesia*, 6th ed. Philadelphia, PA: Lippincott Williams & Wilkins; 2009:Chapter 56.
de Durante G, del Turco M, Rustichini L, et al. ARDSNet lower tidal volume ventilatory strategy may generate intrinsic positive end-expiratory pressure in patients with acute respiratory distress syndrome. *Am J Respir Crit Care Med* 2002;165(9):1271–1274.

39. **(E)** The goal of anesthetic management for patients with increased intracranial pressure (ICP) is to minimize changes in cerebral blood flow (CBF) and thus minimize changes in ICP. Because the cranial vault is a rigid structure composed of brain (80%), blood (12%), and CSF (8%), any increase in one component must be offset by an equivalent decrease in another in order to prevent a rise in ICP. Factors that can alter CBF include mean arterial pressure, $PaCO_2$, temperature, and anesthetic drugs. The CBF remains relatively constant between mean arterial pressures of 60–160 mmHg because of autoregulation. This autoregulation may be impaired in the presence of a tumor or anesthetic agents. CBF is linearly related to $PaCO_2$ between tensions of 20 and 80 mmHg (i.e., as CO_2 increases, so does CBF and vice versa). CBF changes 5–7% per 1°C change in temperature. Hypothermia decreases both cerebral metabolic rate (CMR) and CBF, whereas hyperthermia has the reverse effect.

Etomidate decreases the CMR, CBF, and ICP. It decreases CMR in the cortex more than the brainstem. Etomidate also decreases production and increases absorption of CSF. Propofol also reduces CBF and CMR similar to etomidate, but the decreases in CBF may exceed the decrease in metabolic rate. Propofol is the most common induction agent for neuroanesthesia. Opioids such as fentanyl have minimal effects on CBF, CMR, and ICP unless $PaCO_2$ rises secondary to respiratory depression. Opioids are a useful adjunct for induction because they decrease the hemodynamic response to laryngoscopy. Neuromuscular blocking agents lack direct action on the brain. Succinylcholine can increase ICP, possibly as a result of cerebral activation, but the increase is minimal and clinically unimportant if an adequate dose of propofol is given. Nondepolarizing drugs such as rocuronium have minimal effect on the brain.

Ketamine is the only IV anesthetic that dilates cerebral vasculature and increases CBF (50–60%). Total CMR does not change because certain areas are activated while others are depressed. Ketamine may also impede absorption of CSF without affecting formation. Because other agents, such as propofol are readily available, ketamine is often avoided for neurosurgical procedures.

Volatile anesthetics such as sevoflurane produce dose-dependent decreases in CMR and increase CBF. Isoflurane decreases CMR the most, whereas halothane has the least effect. Sevoflurane produces the least cerebral vasodilation, whereas halothane has the greatest effect.

Other methods used to decrease intracranial pressure include changes in head position to facilitate venous drainage, hyperventilation, induced hypothermia, and surgical decompression or drainage of CSF. Other drugs used to decrease ICP include osmotic diuretics such as mannitol, loop diuretics, and corticosteroids.

BIBLIOGRAPHY

Butterworth JF IV, Mackey DC, Wasnick JD (eds.). *Morgan & Mikhail's Clinical Anesthesiology*, 5th ed. New York, NY: McGraw-Hill; 2013:580–586.
Butterworth JF IV, Mackey DC, Wasnick JD. Neurophysiology and anesthesia. In: Butterworth JF IV, Mackey DC, Wasnick JD (eds.), *Morgan & Mikhail's Clinical Anesthesiology*, 5th ed. New York, NY: McGraw-Hill; 2013:Chapter 26.

40. **(A)** Malignant hyperthermia (MH) is a rare (1:15,000 pediatric patients and 1:40,000 adult patients) and inherited disorder characterized by hypermetabolism of skeletal muscle. It is autosomal dominant with variable expression and is more common in males and the pediatric population. Susceptibility to MH is increased in central core disease and King-Denborough syndrome. The pathophysiology of MH is thought to involve the ryanodine receptor, which is an ion channel responsible for calcium release in the sarcoplasmic reticulum of skeletal muscle. The characteristic signs and symptoms commonly appear with exposure to inhaled volatile anesthetics and succinylcholine (called triggering agents).

Interestingly, prior uneventful anesthesia procedures are unreliable predictors of susceptibility to MH. Untreated, this disorder has an 80% mortality; however, the use of dantrolene has lowered this rate to below 10%.

Onset of clinical signs may immediately follow the introduction of a trigger, but also may be significantly delayed. The earliest signs of MH during anesthesia are muscle rigidity, tachycardia, and hypercarbia. Hyperthermia may be a late sign, but once it occurs, core temperature can rise up to 1°C every 5 minutes. Dark-colored urine reflects myoglobinemia and myoglobinuria. Laboratory testing typically reveals mixed metabolic and respiratory acidosis, hyperkalemia, and reduced mixed venous oxygen saturation. Acute kidney failure and DIC rapidly ensue if the patient survives the first few minutes.

Treatment of an MH episode is directed at terminating the episode and treating complications. The triggering agent should be immediately discontinued. The mainstay of therapy is dantrolene, which directly interferes with muscle contraction by binding the Ryr1 receptor and inhibiting calcium ion release from the sarcoplasmic reticulum. The dose is 2.5 mg/kg IV every 5 minutes until the episode is terminated. After initial control of symptoms, 1 mg/kg of dantrolene is given every 6 hours for 24–48 hours to prevent relapse.

While dantrolene is being administered, secondary therapy includes cooling measures such as cooling blankets and cold lavages. Hyperkalemia should be aggressively treated with insulin, calcium, and bicarbonate. Metabolic acidosis should be managed with sodium bicarbonate. Diuresis should be established with furosemide to prevent acute renal failure secondary to myoglobinuria. Note that dantrolene contains 3 g mannitol per 20-mg bottle. Calcium channel blockers should be avoided because they can cause hyperkalemia in patients receiving dantrolene. There is a 24-hour MH hotline that can be contacted at 1-800-MH-HYPER for assistance with treatment.

BIBLIOGRAPHY

Butterworth JF IV, Mackey DC, Wasnick JD (eds.). *Morgan & Mikhail's Clinical Anesthesiology*, 5th ed. New York, NY: McGraw-Hill; 2013:1185–1190.

Butterworth JF IV, Mackey DC, Wasnick JD. Thermoregulation, hypothermia, and malignant hyperthermia. In: Butterworth JF IV, Mackey DC, Wasnick JD (eds.), *Morgan & Mikhail's Clinical Anesthesiology*, 5th ed. New York, NY: McGraw-Hill; 2013: Chapter 52.

41. **(B)** Postoperative nausea and vomiting (PONV) occurs in 20–30% of patients and is a major contributor to delays in discharge and unanticipated admissions following outpatient surgery. Patients' "willingness to pay" out of pocket for effective antiemetic treatment of PONV, as measured by well-designed studies, is $56 in the United States.

Patient-related independent predictors for PONV include female gender (strongest individual predictor in adults), not smoking, history of PONV, motion sickness or migraines, and age (PONV decreases with age in adults). Anesthesia-related independent predictors include dose of intraoperative opioids, need for postoperative opioids, general anesthesia with volatile anesthetics, and long duration of anesthesia. Type of surgery is also important, but association needs to be distinguished from causality (e.g., long abdominal procedures have high incidence of PONV, but are also associated with long exposure to anesthesia, postoperative opioids, etc.). Procedures that tend to lead to a higher incidence of nausea include laparoscopy; ear, nose, and throat surgery; lithotripsy; breast surgery; ophthalmologic procedures; and any surgeries that lead to blood in the stomach or peritoneal irritation.

Because PONV is multifactorial, a patient's risk can be best estimated using several independent predictors simultaneously. A simplified risk score for adults exists that consists of four predictors and gives a score of 0 to 4 that predicts risk of PONV. The four predictors include female gender, nonsmoking status, history of PONV, and need for postoperative opioids. Each predictor that is present warrants 1 point. If none, one, two, three, or four of these risk factors are present, the incidence of PONV is predicted to be approximately 10%, 20%, 40%, 60%, and 80%, respectively.

In high-risk patients, many pharmacologic agents have been used preoperatively or intraoperatively to prevent PONV. Most of these act as antagonists of the major receptor types implicated in nausea and vomiting. These include dopamine, acetylcholine (muscarinic), histamine, and serotonin receptors. Dopamine antagonists such as promethazine are effective and are associated with sedation, which also can be helpful. Another dopamine antagonist, droperidol, has limited use because of significant side effects such as extrapyramidal symptoms, anxiety, and potential serious proarrhythmogenic effects (torsades de pointes). Serotonin antagonists such as ondansetron have been shown to be effective with minimal adverse effects. Anticholinergic medications include scopolamine or atropine. In addition, dexamethasone has been shown to decrease postoperative nausea and vomiting, especially in the pediatric population after tonsillectomy.

BIBLIOGRAPHY

Miller RD. *Miller's Anesthesia*, 7th ed. Philadelphia, PA: Elsevier Churchill Livingstone; 2009:2733–2743.

Miller RD. Postoperative nausea and vomiting. In: Miller RD (ed.), *Miller's Anesthesia*, 7th ed. Philadelphia, PA: Elsevier Churchill Livingstone; 2009:Chapter 86.

CHAPTER 8

TRAUMA

KIMBERLY C. ZAMOR AND ANDREW W. HOEL

1. A 33-year-old male is transported to your facility following a single stab wound to the anterior abdomen at the umbilicus. Initial vital signs are blood pressure 93/67 mmHg, heart rate 125 bpm, and respiratory rate 28 breaths/min. Intraoperatively, a large midline retroperitoneal hematoma is explored, and transection of the superior mesenteric artery (SMA) is identified posterior to the pancreas. Appropriate operative management of the mesenteric artery includes
   (A) Ligation only if proximal arterial injury
   (B) Ligation only if distal arterial injury
   (C) Proximal arterial ligation with bypass graft originating at the infrarenal aorta
   (D) End-to-end anastomosis with polytetrafluoroethylene (PTFE) graft
   (E) End-to-end anastomosis with saphenous vein graft

2. Following a motor vehicle crash, a 23-year-old trauma patient undergoes a contrast-enhanced computed tomography (CT) scan of the abdomen that reveals a large right perinephric hematoma with associated contrast extravasation, failure of the right kidney to uptake contrast, and a normal-appearing left kidney. The patient is hemodynamically normal and has no other intra-abdominal injuries. Appropriate management of the right kidney is
   (A) Admit for observation of residual renal function
   (B) Retroperitoneal exploration
   (C) Exploration through Gerota's fascia to exclude a parenchymal injury
   (D) Radiologic vascular stent placement
   (E) Nephrostomy tube and N-acetylcysteine

3. A 19-year-old male involved in a motor vehicle crash presents to the emergency department (ED) with hematuria. He is hemodynamically normal and undergoes a contrast-enhanced CT scan of the abdomen. He is found to have a grade V injury to the left kidney and a normal-appearing right kidney. Appropriate management of the injured kidney is
   (A) Nephrostomy tube placement
   (B) Renal artery bypass or graft
   (C) Observation with exploration for hemodynamic instability
   (D) Nephrectomy
   (E) Renal artery stent

4. A 20-year-old male presents to the ED with a stab wound to the right lower abdomen. On exploration, he has a 2-cm cecal laceration with gross contamination as well as a laceration to the right iliac vein. The best treatment option with regard to the iliac vein is
   (A) Primary repair
   (B) Ligation
   (C) Repair with PTFE
   (D) Extra-anatomic bypass graft
   (E) Repair with autogenous vein

5. Which of the following management options for suprarenal inferior vena cava injury is directly associated with renal failure?
   (A) Ligation
   (B) Lateral venorrhaphy
   (C) Spiral saphenous vein graft
   (D) Extra-anatomic bypass
   (E) Panel graft using saphenous vein

6. Following blunt abdominal trauma, mandatory exploration is indicated for a nonexpanding hematoma identified on CT scan in which of the following areas?
   (A) Right perinephric
   (B) Midline inframesocolic
   (C) Lateral pelvic
   (D) Retrohepatic
   (E) Left perinephric

7. Following a gunshot wound to the lower extremity, signs and symptoms that mandate exploration include which of the following?
   (A) History of significant hemorrhage at the scene, although no longer actively bleeding
   (B) Deficit in anatomically related nerve
   (C) Hypotension
   (D) Small, stable, nonpulsatile hematoma
   (E) Palpable thrill

8. The earliest symptoms of compartment syndrome are a result of tissue intolerance to hypoxia. Which of the following structures is the most sensitive to hypoxia?
   (A) Skin
   (B) Bone
   (C) Unmyelinated nerve
   (D) Myelinated nerve
   (E) Skeletal muscle

9. One day following fixation of a complex femur fracture sustained in a motor vehicle crash (MVC), a 24-year-old male complains of severe pain along the ipsilateral thigh. On examination, he is hemodynamically normal with a heart rate of 104 breaths/min, oxygen saturation of 94%, and blood pressure of 140/78 mmHg. He has no urinary catheter and no recorded urine output. Laboratory studies at that time include hemoglobin of 8.1 (down from 12.3 preoperatively) and potassium of 5.8 (up from 3.4 preoperatively). Which of the following would be included in the next steps in management?
   (A) Placement of a central venous catheter
   (B) Transfer to the intensive care unit
   (C) Obtain family history for bleeding disorders
   (D) Fasciotomy
   (E) Observation

10. Which of the following is *correct* regarding fasciotomy of the lower extremity for compartment syndrome?
   (A) A four-compartment fasciotomy cannot be performed using a single incision.
   (B) A four-compartment fasciotomy may be performed using anterolateral and posteromedial incisions.
   (C) Compartment syndrome involving the thigh may be treated by decompression of the quadriceps compartment or hamstring compartment.
   (D) The superficial branch of the tibial nerve is especially vulnerable when extending the fascial incision proximally in the superficial posterior compartment.
   (E) The most common cause of acute compartment syndrome in the lower extremity is thromboembolism.

11. Which of the following veins is most amenable to ligation?
   (A) Infrarenal vena cava
   (B) Suprarenal vena cava
   (C) Common femoral vein
   (D) Popliteal vein
   (E) Innominate vein

12. Which of the following statements is *true* regarding the incidence of contrast nephropathy (CN)?
   (A) The incidence in overall healthy patients is 5%.
   (B) The most important risk factor is dehydration.
   (C) In patients with a normal serum creatinine, contrast doses in excess of 200 mL of 300 mg/mL solution are considered a significant risk factor.
   (D) Mannitol has been shown to decrease the risk of CN.
   (E) The most important prophylactic maneuver is hydration.

13. Three months following a MVC in which she suffered a grade III liver laceration, a 34-year-old female presents with hematemesis. She has no history of peptic ulcer disease and denies nonsteroidal anti-inflammatory drug use. Following initial stabilization, the next most appropriate step would be
   (A) Upper endoscopy
   (B) Contrast-enhanced CT of the abdomen
   (C) Abdominal ultrasonography (US)
   (D) Admission for observation
   (E) Angiography

14. Which of the following vessel injuries can be safely ligated in an unstable trauma patient?
   (A) SMA
   (B) Internal iliac artery
   (C) Suprarenal inferior vena cava (IVC)
   (D) Infrarenal abdominal aorta
   (E) Simultaneous radial and ulnar arteries

15. The most appropriate management of an isolated radial artery injury with no clinical evidence of hand ischemia is
   (A) Primary repair
   (B) Ligation
   (C) Repair with vein graft
   (D) Repair with PTFE graft
   (E) Shunt

16. A 20-year-old male suffers a gunshot blast to the right neck. Initial workup reveals stable vital signs, an intact airway, and no active bleeding from the multiple small entrance sites visible along the right neck. As part of his workup, the arteriogram below is obtained (see Fig. 8-1).

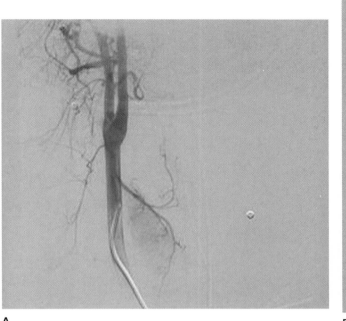
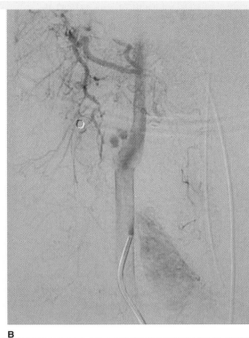

A   B

FIGURE 8-1. A and B Right carotid arteriogram.

This arteriogram demonstrates
(A) Normal arteriogram with no evidence of injury
(B) Right internal carotid artery–jugular vein fistula
(C) Right common carotid artery injury
(D) Right internal carotid artery injury
(E) Right external carotid artery injury

17. The patient described in Question 16 remains hemody-
namically normal and has a Glasgow Coma Scale score
of 15. The next step in the management of the patient is
(A) Median sternotomy and neck exploration
(B) Admission and observation alone
(C) Neck exploration
(D) Tracheobronchoscopy, esophagram, esophagoscopy,
and observation
(E) Admission and anticoagulation therapy

18. A left neck exploration is performed for a stab injury to
the neck in an otherwise healthy male. The left internal
jugular vein is found to be completely transected with
significant bleeding and hemodynamic instability. No
other vascular injury is identified. Appropriate management of the internal jugular vein is
(A) Primary repair
(B) Interposition saphenous vein graft
(C) Interposition with 6-mm PTFE
(D) Ligation of the left internal jugular vein
(E) External jugular vein transposition

19. A 33-year-old female was the unrestrained driver in a
high-speed motor vehicle crash. Emergency medical
services (EMS) reported significant steering wheel deformity. Primary and secondary surveys revealed a Glasgow
Coma Scale score of 15, heart rate of 79 bpm, respiratory
rate of 12 breaths/min, blood pressure of 134/76 mmHg,
a deformed left femur without open wound, and the
upright chest x-ray shown in Fig. 8-2.

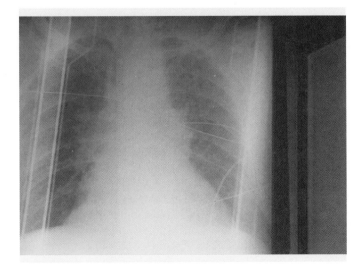

FIGURE 8-2. Chest x-ray.

The next step in management of this patient is
(A) X-ray of the left femur
(B) Admit and observe
(C) Cervical spine x-ray series
(D) Spiral CT scan of the chest
(E) Flat and upright abdominal x-ray

20. The patient described in Question 19 subsequently develops weakness in her right arm and hand. The following arteriogram was performed (see Fig. 8-3).

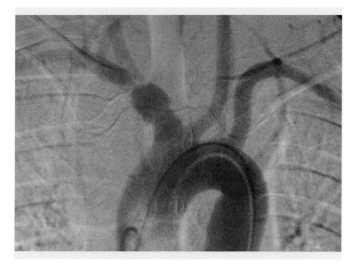

FIGURE 8-3. Aortic arch arteriogram.

This arteriogram demonstrates
(A) No injury
(B) Cardiac contusion
(C) Sternal fracture
(D) Aortic tear
(E) Innominate artery pseudoaneurysm

21. After arteriogram, the next step in the management of the patient described in Questions 19 and 20 is
(A) Anticoagulation with heparin and blood pressure control
(B) Repair of the injury via right anterolateral thoracotomy
(C) Repair of the injury via left anterolateral thoracotomy
(D) Repair of the injury via median sternotomy
(E) Admission and observation

22. A 62-year-old male is brought to the ED after being involved in a motor vehicle collision. Vital signs include Glasgow Coma Scale score of 15, heart rate of 78 bpm, respiration rate of 12 breaths/min, and blood pressure of 195/110 mmHg. Radiologic workup includes the arteriogram shown in Fig. 8-4.

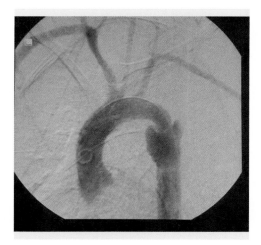

FIGURE 8-4. Aortic arch arteriogram.

This study demonstrates
(A) Ascending aortic injury
(B) Descending aortic injury
(C) Normal study; no injury demonstrated
(D) Subclavian artery injury
(E) Pericardial tamponade

23. After stabilization and full workup, the patient in Question 22 is found to have no other significant injuries. The next step in management of this patient is
(A) Admit and observe on cardiac monitor
(B) Operative repair of the aorta
(C) Endovascular repair of the subclavian artery
(D) Esophagogastroduodenoscopy (EGD) and bronchoscopy
(E) Emergency thoracotomy

24. A 22-year-old male presents to the ED after sustaining a stab wound to the left chest. The injury is 2 cm left of the sternum at the level of his nipple. Initial vital signs include a heart rate of 88 bpm, Glasgow Coma Scale score of 15, respiratory rate of 12 breaths/min, and blood pressure of 139/74 mmHg. Initial management of this patient should be
(A) Chest x-ray (CXR)
(B) Pericardiocentesis
(C) Left chest tube thoracostomy
(D) Esophagram
(E) Echocardiogram

25. An arteriogram is performed on the patient described in Question 24, and an injury to the proximal left subclavian artery is identified. The patient remains hemodynamically stable. The next step in the management of this patient is

(A) Admit and observe
(B) Subclavian repair through a median sternotomy
(C) Subclavian repair through a supraclavicular incision
(D) Subclavian repair through an anterolateral thoracotomy
(E) Exploratory laparotomy

26. A 19-year-old male presents to the ER following a self-inflicted gunshot wound to the left shoulder. His initial vital signs are heart rate of 100 bpm, respiratory rate of 12 breaths/min, blood pressure of 122/83 mmHg, and a Glasgow Coma Scale score of 15. Physical examination reveals absent pulses in the left brachial, radial, and ulnar arteries. Neurologic examination of the left hand and arm reveals no gross motor or sensory deficit. Following complete examination, an arteriogram is obtained (see Fig. 8-5).

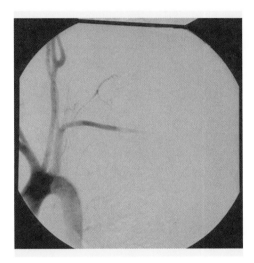

FIGURE 8-5. Arteriogram.

The arteriogram reveals an injury to the
(A) Left subclavian artery
(B) Left axillary artery
(C) Left brachial artery
(D) Left carotid artery
(E) Left internal mammary artery

27. Management of the vascular injury described in Question 26 includes
(A) Admit for observation and anticoagulation
(B) Repair the axillary artery with PTFE
(C) Repair the axillary artery with reversed saphenous vein graft
(D) Fracture stabilization with intramedullary (IM) rodding
(E) Permanent shunting of the vascular injury followed by fracture stabilization

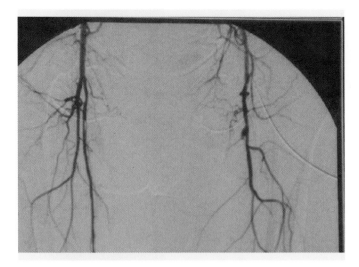

FIGURE 8-6. Arteriogram.

28. A 27-year-old male is transported to the ER following a gunshot wound to the left thigh. Physical examination reveals an entrance wound on the medial aspect of the left thigh and an exit wound on the lateral aspect of the left thigh. There is no pulse or Doppler signal in his left foot.

The patient's arteriogram is shown in Fig. 8-6 and reveals a
(A) Normal arteriogram
(B) Left common femoral artery injury
(C) Left profunda femoris artery injury
(D) Left superficial femoral artery injury
(E) Left external iliac artery injury

29. The next step in the management of the vascular injury presented in Question 28 is
(A) Admit and heparin anticoagulation
(B) Reversed saphenous vein interposition
(C) Endovascular stent placement
(D) Immediate above knee amputation
(E) Reversed saphenous vein bypass graft

30. A 37-year-old unrestrained driver is involved in an MVC where he is struck on the driver's side. The patient arrives at the ED hemodynamically normal but complaining of left-sided abdominal pain. An abdominal CT is performed. Based on the CT (see Fig. 8-7), what is the most appropriate management of this patient?
(A) Observe in the ED overnight and discharge to home in the morning if remains hemodynamically normal
(B) Observe in the intensive care unit with serial hematocrits and abdominal exams
(C) Perform angiography and embolization
(D) Perform exploratory laparotomy
(E) Discharge to home

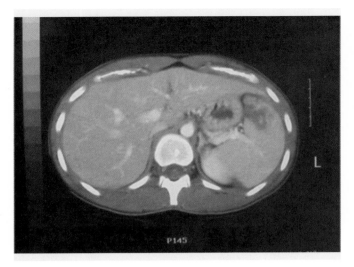

FIGURE 8-7. CT depicting grade III splenic laceration.

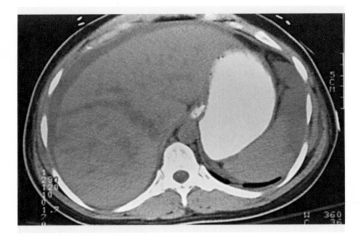

FIGURE 8-8. CT depicting liver laceration.

31. A patient is taken to the operating room after a failed attempt at nonoperative management for a splenic laceration. The surgeon enters the peritoneum, packs all four quadrants, and notes on initial survey that there is active bleeding from the left upper quadrant. What is the first step in mobilizing the spleen?
    (A) Divide the splenocolic ligament
    (B) Clamp and tie off the short gastric vessels
    (C) Mobilize the spleen and tail of the pancreas from lateral to medial
    (D) Divide the splenorenal and splenophrenic ligaments

32. A 26-year-old male presents with vague abdominal pain following a high-velocity MVC. Although hemodynamically normal during transport, his blood pressure on arrival to the ED is 65/30 mmHg and heart rate is 130 bpm. Focused assessment with sonography for trauma (FAST) examination is inconclusive. Diagnostic peritoneal lavage (DPL) is performed and is positive for >10 mL gross blood. The patient is taken to the operating room for immediate exploratory laparotomy. Upon entry into the peritoneum, massive hematoma is encountered in the right upper quadrant, and a liver injury is suspected. The patient's blood pressure remains 65/30 mmHg. What is the most appropriate next step?
    (A) Continue with abdominal exploration
    (B) Pringle maneuver
    (C) Direct suturing of any noticeable lacerations
    (D) Pack the abdomen and allow anesthesia to provide adequate resuscitation before further exploration
    (E) Pack the abdomen and return to the intensive care unit for resuscitation

33. A 48-year-old restrained male passenger involved in an MVC is brought to the ED. The patient is hemodynamically normal and complaining of vague abdominal pain. CT of the abdomen is performed (see Fig. 8-8). He is admitted for observation in the ICU. Approximately 24 hours after admission, the patient is complaining of increasing abdominal pain. The next morning, he is noted to be hypotensive and acidotic with peritoneal signs on examination. What is the most likely diagnosis?
    (A) Infected hepatic hematoma
    (B) Missed bowel injury
    (C) Liver hemorrhage
    (D) Pulmonary embolus
    (E) Hypoxia

34. A 41-year-old male who was shot in the abdomen multiple times undergoes an exploratory laparotomy with multiple bowel resections. Following surgery, he is taken to the ICU for further resuscitation. Which of the following signs is consistent with the development of an abdominal compartment syndrome?
    (A) Decreased central venous pressure
    (B) Decreased systemic vascular resistance
    (C) Increasing cardiac output
    (D) Decreasing PCO_2
    (E) Decreasing urine output

35. A 65-year-old male who was involved in an all-terrain vehicle (ATV) crash presents to the ED complaining of epigastric abdominal pain. Initial labs demonstrate an elevated amylase level. Abdominal CT demonstrates peripancreatic fluid without contrast extravasation. What is the most appropriate next step?
    (A) Observation and repeat amylase level
    (B) Exploratory laparotomy
    (C) Emergent endoscopic retrograde cholangiopancreatography

(D) Paracentesis to evaluate the intraperitoneal amylase level
(E) Magnetic resonance cholangiopancreatography

36. A 21-year-old male with a stab wound to the abdomen presents to the ED in stable condition. On local wound exploration, there is evidence of anterior fascia penetration and omental evisceration. The patient is taken to the operating room for an exploratory laparotomy. A complete transection of the ascending colon near the hepatic flexure with minimal contamination is identified. The most appropriate surgical management would be
(A) Ileostomy with Hartmann's pouch
(B) Colostomy with mucous fistula
(C) Debridement and ileocolostomy
(D) Debridement and primary anastomosis
(E) Right colectomy with primary anastomosis

37. A 36-year-old female is ejected during an MVC. She is found to have a pelvic fracture and hematuria. Cystogram is performed demonstrating the presence of an extraperitoneal bladder rupture. An indwelling bladder catheter is placed. After 14 days, a repeat cystogram identifies a persistent extraperitoneal leak. What is the most appropriate management?
(A) Remove the bladder catheter and observe the patient
(B) Continue the bladder catheter for 7–10 days longer and repeat cystogram
(C) Cystoscopy to evaluate the extent of the rupture
(D) Exploratory laparotomy and repair of extraperitoneal rupture

38. A 29-year-old male restrained passenger is brought to the ED in stable condition following an MVC. He is admitted for observation following an abdominal CT demonstrating a spleen laceration and a moderate amount of free fluid in the pelvis. Within 48 hours, the patient develops worsening abdominal pain and undergoes exploratory laparotomy. A small bowel perforation is identified (see Fig. 8-9). Which of the following statements regarding small bowel injuries is *correct*?
(A) They only occur when the bowel is crushed against the spine.
(B) They are frequently associated with Chance fractures.
(C) There has been a decreased incidence since the mandatory seat belt laws.
(D) Ninety percent of patients with blunt intestinal perforation have no other injuries.
(E) Laboratory studies and CT are used to localize the site of bowel injury.

39. An 18-year-old female unrestrained driver is involved in a head-on collision. Paramedics at the scene note

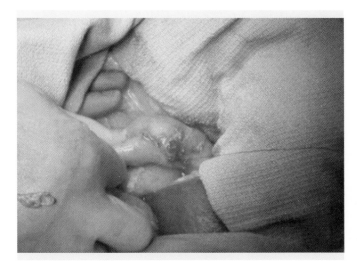

FIGURE 8-9. Small bowel perforation following motor vehicle crash.

extensive steering wheel and windshield damage. The patient is hemodynamically normal and complaining of head and abdominal pain. Head and abdominal CT are initially read as negative. After observation overnight, the patient is discharged to home. Approximately 72 hours later, the patient presents to the ED complaining of nausea and bilious emesis. Findings on repeat abdominal CT are shown in Fig. 8-10. What is the most appropriate management?
(A) Conservative management with nasogastric suction and total parenteral nutrition
(B) Esophagogastroduodenoscopy to evaluate severity of duodenal injury
(C) Exploratory laparotomy with evacuation of hematoma
(D) Angiography and embolization
(E) Percutaneous drainage by interventional radiology

40. A 16-year-old unrestrained driver is involved in a rollover head-on collision. Extensive damage to the vehicle and prolonged extrication time was noted. The patient was hemodynamically unstable upon extrication and was transported by air to a level I trauma center. While in transport, the patient became severely hypotensive and unresponsive, with impending respiratory distress. Which of the following is considered a life-threatening injury in this patient that warrants immediate intervention?
(A) Pneumothorax secondary to rib fractures
(B) Aortic intimal tear
(C) Diaphragm rupture
(D) Tension pneumothorax
(E) Myocardial contusion

(C) Underlying pulmonary contusion
(D) Pneumothorax
(E) Splinting from chest wall pain

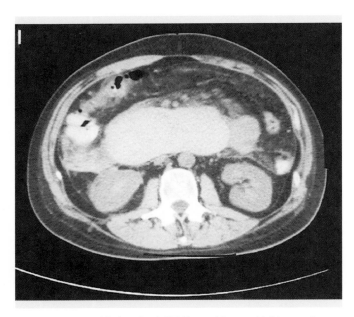

FIGURE 8-10. Abdominal CT. From Mattox K, Moore E, Feliciano D (eds.). *Trauma*, 7th ed. New York, NY: McGraw-Hill; 2012.

41. An unrestrained 23-year-old male drag racer involved in a high-speed motor vehicle crash presents to the ED with intense pain in the right chest. The primary survey demonstrates decreased breath sounds over the right hemithorax with noted paradoxical motion of the right chest wall during respiration (see Fig. 8-11). The major pathologic sequela of this injury is
(A) Disruption of ventilation because of paradoxical motion of the chest wall
(B) Bleeding from disruption of intercostal vessels

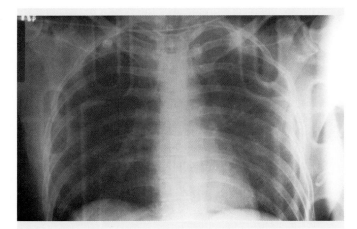

FIGURE 8-11. Chest x-ray. From Knoop KJ, Stack LB, Storrow AB, Thurman RJ. *The Atlas of Emergency Medicine*, 3rd ed. New York, NY: McGraw-Hill; 2009.

42. A 65-year-old male restrained driver involved in a high-speed MVC suffered a severe blow to the epigastrium and presents to the ED with abdominal pain out of proportion to the apparent injury. The patient is intubated, and a nasogastric tube is placed on arrival. The primary survey reveals decreased left-sided breath sounds. After assuring proper endotracheal tube placement, a chest tube is placed on the left side. Initial chest tube output is 50 mL of blood; then particulate matter is noted inside the chest tube. The usual mechanism of this injury is
(A) Laceration of the esophagus by a portion of a fractured rib
(B) Inappropriate nasogastric tube placement
(C) Sudden deceleration resulting in shear stress to the esophagus
(D) Compression of the esophagus against the vertebral column
(E) Forceful compression of the stomach

43. A restrained 52-year-old female presents to the ED following a high-speed MVC during which she suffered a side door impact. On arrival, primary survey reveals airway stridor and severe respiratory distress. A pneumothorax is suspected. Chest x-ray reveals massive pneumomediastinum. The patient is resuscitated and remains stable. Further evaluation of the chest radiograph reveals the right lung appearing to fall laterally and posteriorly away from the hilum. The next step in management should be
(A) Observation for 48 hours
(B) Tube thoracostomy
(C) Immediate bronchoscopy
(D) Exploratory thoracotomy
(E) Place patient on humidified air

44. A 35-year-old female involved in a restrained MVC presents to your ED. Initial chest radiograph is shown in Fig. 8-12.

The next step in management is
(A) CT scan of the abdomen
(B) Delayed thoracotomy
(C) Video-assisted thoracoscopy
(D) Barium swallow
(E) Nasogastric tube insertion

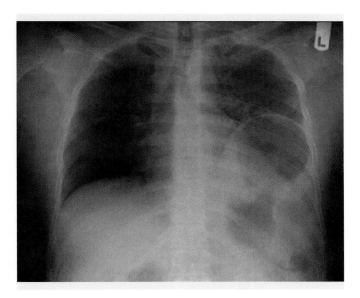

FIGURE 8-12. Chest x-ray.

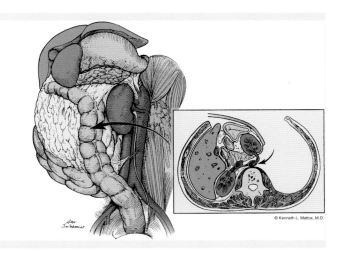

FIGURE 8-13. Mattox maneuver. From Skandalakis JE, Colborn GL, Weidman TA, et al. *Skandalakis' Surgical Anatomy*. New York, NY: McGraw-Hill; 2004.

ANSWERS AND EXPLANATIONS

1. **(C)** Operative management of the SMA is determined by the anatomic location of SMA injury, as described by Fullen et al (Table 8-1). The injury in the presented case is a Fullen zone I injury (posterior to the pancreas). Proper exposure and subsequent vascular control can be achieved by two methods, either by division of the pancreas or by medially rotating the left-sided abdominal viscera (Mattox maneuver; see Fig. 8-13). Repair should proceed with end-side anastomosis with saphenous vein graft or prosthetic graft, at the level of the infrarenal aorta. Such distal origin of the graft is preferred to avoid suture line in close proximity to pancreas or other upper abdominal injuries. Although the SMA has collateral blood supply, in the setting of trauma, there is often concomitant vasoconstriction that limits adequate collateral blood flow for bowel viability, and thus, ligation alone is not a plausible approach (choices A and B).

BIBLIOGRAPHY

Demetriades D, Inaba K. Vascular trauma: abdominal. In: Rutherford RB (ed.), *Vascular Surgery*, 7th ed. Philadelphia, PA: W.B. Saunders; 2010.

Dente CJ, Feliciano DV. Abdominal vascular injury. In: Mattox KL, Moore EE, Feliciano DV (eds.), *Trauma*, 7th ed. New York, NY: McGraw-Hill; 2012:Chapter 34.

2. **(B)** Hemorrhage or hematoma in the lateral perirenal region often represents renal artery, vein, or parenchymal injury. Exploration of the kidney should be avoided if the preoperative workup includes a normal

TABLE 8-1 Fullen Zones of Superior Mesenteric Artery (SMA) Injury

Fullen Zone	Description	Exposure	Treatment
I	Posterior to pancreas	Medial visceral rotation	Infrarenal bypass (saphenous vein or polytetrafluoroethylene [PTFE])
II	Between the pancreaticoduodenal artery and the middle colic artery branches	Transection of pancreas	Infrarenal bypass (saphenous vein or PTFE)
III	Distal to middle colic artery	-	Repair (may include microsurgery); if repair not possible, then colon resection
IV	Enteric branches	-	Repair (may include microsurgery); if repair not possible, then colon resection

intravenous pyelogram, renal arteriogram, or contrasted CT of the involved kidney. If the hematoma is not rapidly expanding and there is no free intraperitoneal bleeding, control of the renal artery may be obtained in the midline at the base of the mesocolon (see Fig. 8-14). On the right, this necessitates mobilization of the c-loop of the duodenum. If there is active bleeding from the renal parenchyma through a break in Gerota's fascia, the injury may be directly controlled through this laceration. In the setting of vascular injury, repair . . . options include lateral arteriorrhaphy or end-to-end anastomosis if possible. Interposition grafts using either vein or PTFE are

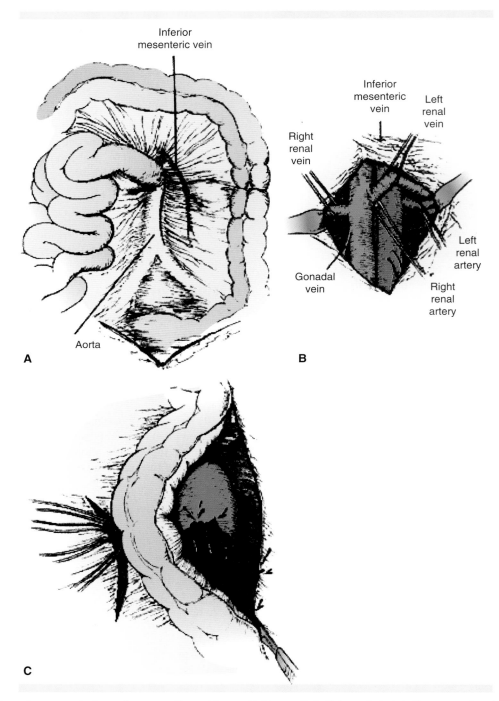

FIGURE 8-14. Vascular control of renal trauma. From Mattox K, Moore E, Feliciano D (eds.). *Trauma*, 7th ed. New York, NY: McGraw-Hill; 2012.

indicated only if there appears to be reasonable hope of renal salvage. In patients with significant renovascular injuries, multiple intra-abdominal injuries, or a long pre-operative ischemic period, nephrectomy is likely a more reasonable choice.

BIBLIOGRAPHY

Demetriades D, Inaba K. Vascular trauma: abdominal. In: Rutherford RB (ed.), *Vascular Surgery*, 7th ed. Philadelphia, PA: W.B. Saunders; 2010.

Dente CJ, Feliciano DV. Abdominal vascular injury. In: Mattox KL, Moore EE, Feliciano DV (eds.), *Trauma*, 7th ed. New York, NY: McGraw-Hill; 2012:Chapter 34.

Schuerer DJ, Brandes SB. Retroperitoneal injuries. In: Cameron JL, Cameron AM (eds.), *Current Surgical Therapy*, 10th ed. Philadelphia, PA: Elsevier Saunders; 2010:Chapter 204.

3. **(C)** Renal injuries account for 1–5% of all traumas. These are often challenging cases because nearly 90% of patients will have associated injuries. Of patients with grade IV or V renal injuries, nearly three-quarters will have associated abdominal injuries. Treatment options include observation, nephrectomy, primary vascular repair, and vascular repair using graft. Hematuria is a hallmark of renal injury, but it is not specific and does not predict injury severity. Only 50% patients with proximal renal vascular injury have hematuria. An important guiding principle when managing renal injury is to determine patient hemodynamic stability, mechanism of injury, ischemia time, and presence of a normal contralateral kidney. In this case, the patient was hemodynamically normal with grade V renovascular injury, and studies suggest that revascularization is a controversial approach and should be reserved for bilateral injury or solitary kidney. Typically attempts at vascular repair in grade V injuries are not warranted and, when attempted, are more likely to result in a poor outcome such as impaired renal function, renal failure, delayed nephrectomy, or new-onset hypertension. High-grade injuries (grades IV and V) should be reevaluated with contrast CT imaging every 3–5 days (Table 8-2).

BIBLIOGRAPHY

Dente CJ, Feliciano DV. Abdominal vascular injury. In: Mattox KL, Moore EE, Feliciano DV (eds.), *Trauma*, 7th ed. New York, NY: McGraw-Hill; 2012:Chapter 34.

Schuerer DJ, Brandes SB. Retroperitoneal injuries. In: Cameron JL, Cameron AM (eds.), *Current Surgical Therapy*, 10th ed. Philadelphia, PA: Elsevier Saunders; 2010:Chapter 204.

4. **(A)** Penetrating injuries that involve the iliac vessels commonly involve the overlying viscera. Cecum, ileum, sigmoid colon, ureters, bladder, and rectum are all at risk. Preferred exposure is via medial rotation of the cecum and ileum on the right and sigmoid colon on the left. Following proximal and distal control, repair of the common or external iliac artery is usually accomplished using 4.0–5.0 polypropylene. Resection with mobilization to allow end-to-end repair is possible for injuries less than 2 cm in length. Injuries to the iliac veins are approached in a similar fashion as arteries with proximal and distal control prior to exploration of the hematoma. Most injuries can be treated with primary repair via lateral venorrhaphy. If needed, the iliac vein may be ligated but has a risk of . . . venous thrombosis and chronic leg swelling. Because a large percentage will have associated gastrointestinal (GI) or genitourinary (GU) injuries, autogenous material should be used whenever possible, although prosthetic grafts have been tried with success in certain groups.

TABLE 8-2 Renal Injury Scale

Grade		Description
I	Contusion	Microscopic or gross hematuria; normal urologic studies
	Hematoma	Subcapsular, nonexpanding without parenchymal laceration
II	Hematoma	Nonexpanding perirenal hematoma confined to renal retroperitoneum
	Laceration	<1.0 cm parenchymal depth of renal cortex without urinary extravasation
III	Laceration	>1.0 cm parenchymal depth of renal cortex with collecting system rupture or urinary extravasation
IV	Laceration	Parenchymal laceration extending through renal cortex, medulla, and collecting system
	Vascular	Main renal artery/vein with contained hemorrhage
V	Laceration	Completely shattered kidney
	Vascular	Avulsion of renal hilum that devascularizes kidney

BIBLIOGRAPHY

Burlew CN, Moore EE. Trauma. In: Brunicardi F, Andersen DK, Billiar TR, et al (eds.), *Schwartz's Principles of Surgery*, 10th ed. New York, NY: McGraw-Hill; 2014.

Demetriades D, Inaba K. Vascular trauma: abdominal. In: Rutherford RB (ed.), *Vascular Surgery*, 7th ed. Philadelphia, PA: W.B. Saunders; 2010.

Dente CJ, Feliciano DV. Abdominal vascular injury. In: Mattox KL, Moore EE, Feliciano DV (eds.), *Trauma*, 7th ed. New York, NY: McGraw-Hill; 2012:Chapter 34.

5. **(A)** Overall, injuries to the IVC carry a mortality rate of greater than 50%, and this rate is even higher in the setting of suprarenal vena cava injuries. Exposure of the suprarenal vena cava can be achieved with a generous Kocher maneuver mobilizing the duodenum and ascending colon to the midline. Initial vascular control is accomplished with manual compression of the vena cava using sponge sticks, finger pressure, or balloon occlusion.

   Repair options are similar to those of the infrarenal vena cava, although ligation of the suprarenal vena cava is discouraged because of its high mortality rate and risk of renal failure.

   Options include lateral venorrhaphy as long as the diameter is not narrowed greater than 50%. Large defects are repaired with saphenous vein or panel grafts. Entire segment damage can be repaired with spiral vein grafts dependent on patient stability. Extra-anatomic bypass is generally not done in the acute setting because of associated injuries.

BIBLIOGRAPHY

Demetriades D, Inaba K. Vascular trauma: abdominal. In: Rutherford RB (ed.), *Vascular Surgery*, 7th ed. Philadelphia, PA: W.B. Saunders; 2010.

Dente CJ, Feliciano DV. Abdominal vascular injury. In: Mattox KL, Moore EE, Feliciano DV (eds.), *Trauma*, 7th ed. New York, NY: McGraw-Hill; 2012:Chapter 34.

6. **(B)** The retroperitoneal space is the area of the posterior abdominal wall that is located between the parietal peritoneum and the deep or internal surface of the transversalis fascia. The retroperitoneum is divided into three anatomic zones: zone 1: midline retroperitoneum, supramesocolic region, and inframesocolic region; zone 2: upper lateral retroperitoneum; and zone 3: pelvic retroperitoneum (see Fig. 8-15).

   A midline (supramesocolic or inframesocolic) hematoma (zone 1), regardless of whether it is a result of blunt or penetrating trauma, requires exploration to evaluate the significant vascular structures located in this area. Exposure is best accomplished using the Mattox

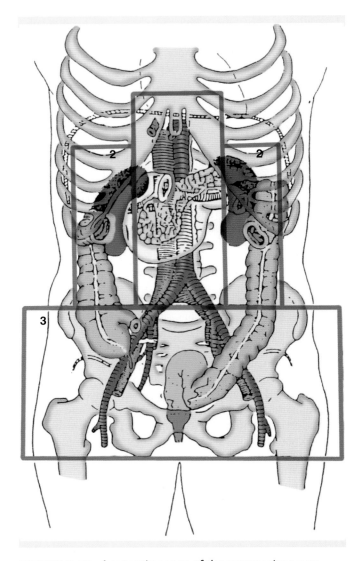

FIGURE 8-15. Anatomic zones of the retroperitoneum. From Skandalakis JE, Colborn GL, Weidman TA, et al. *Skandalakis' Surgical Anatomy*. New York, NY: McGraw-Hill; 2004.

maneuver, medially rotating the left-sided abdominal viscera including the left colon, spleen, tail of pancreas, and gastric fundus. (The kidney may sometimes be included in this mobilization.) The infrarenal aorta is exposed by lifting the transverse colon onto the lower chest and eviscerating the midgut to the right. Exposure of the inferior vena cava is done by combining a Kocher maneuver for duodenal mobilization with elevation of the right colon to the midline. Hematomas in the lateral retroperitoneum (zone 2) or perinephric region require exploration following penetrating injuries; however, in blunt trauma, a normal-appearing kidney on preoperative contrast-enhanced CT scan or a normal renal arteriogram does not mandate exploration because a significant vascular injury is unlikely. A lateral . . . pelvic area (zone 3) hematoma from penetrating trauma should be explored through a midline incision over the aortic bifurcation. In patients with blunt trauma, pelvic retroperitoneal hematoma found on CT or incidentally on celiotomy is not an indication for exploration unless it is rapidly expanding, ruptured, pulsatile, or associated with an injury to the iliac vessels, male urethra, or bladder. Hematoma or hemorrhage in the porta hepatis should be explored using a Pringle maneuver for vascular control with complete dissection of the porta structures. A hematoma in the retrohepatic retroperitoneum is not explored unless it is rapidly expanding or has ruptured with ongoing hemorrhage. A stable hematoma can be managed by perihepatic packing and damage control laparotomy techniques.

BIBLIOGRAPHY

Burlew CN, Moore EE. Trauma. In: Brunicardi F, Andersen DK, Billiar TR, et al (eds.), *Schwartz's Principles of Surgery*, 10th ed. New York, NY: McGraw-Hill; 2014.

Demetriades D, Inaba K. Vascular trauma: abdominal. In: Rutherford RB (ed.), *Vascular Surgery*, 7th ed. Philadelphia, PA: W.B. Saunders; 2010.

Dente CJ, Feliciano DV. Abdominal vascular injury. In: Mattox KL, Moore EE, Feliciano DV (eds.), *Trauma*, 7th ed. New York, NY: McGraw-Hill; 2012:Chapter 34.

Piper GL, Peitzman AB. Chapter 196. Blunt Abdominal Trauma. In: Cameron JL, Cameron AM. Current Surgical Therapy, 10th ed. Philadelphia, PA: Elsevier Saunders; 2010.

7. **(E)** Management of penetrating injuries with vascular trauma continues to be controversial with regard to mandatory exploration, workup, and observation with serial examination. The presence of "hard signs" in penetrating trauma mandate immediate exploration. However, the presence of "soft signs" requires further imaging and surveillance, but surgery is less frequent. Although the management protocol should be based on resources and experience specific to individual institutions, the consensus is that any "hard sign" is an indication for surgical exploration (Table 8-3).

BIBLIOGRAPHY

Burlew CN, Moore EE. Trauma. In: Brunicardi F, Andersen DK, Billiar TR, et al (eds.), *Schwartz's Principles of Surgery*, 10th ed. New York, NY: McGraw-Hill; 2014.

Patel KR, Rowe VL. Vascular trauma: extremity. In: Rutherford RB (ed.), *Vascular Surgery*, 7th ed. Philadelphia, PA: W.B. Saunders; 2010.

Sise MJ, Shackford SR. Peripheral vascular injury. In: Mattox KL, Moore EE, Feliciano DV (eds.), *Trauma*, 7th ed. New York, NY: McGraw-Hill; 2012:Chapter 41.

TABLE 8-3 Physical Signs of Vascular Injury

Hard signs of vascular injury
- Active pulsatile bleeding
- Distal pulse absent
- Observed expanding or pulsatile hematoma
- Palpable thrill
- Audible bruit
- Signs of ischemia (pallor, paresthesia, pain, paralysis, pulselessness, poikilothermia)

Soft signs of vascular injury
- History of moderate hemorrhage
- Injury in proximity to bony injury or penetrating wound
- Diminished pulse, compared to contralateral limb
- Peripheral nerve deficit

Stahel PF, Smith WR, Hak DJ. Lower extremity. In: Mattox KL, Moore EE, Feliciano DV (eds.), *Trauma*, 7th ed. New York, NY: McGraw-Hill; 2012:Chapter 40.

8. **(C)** The earliest symptoms of compartment syndrome are neurologic because unmyelinated type C sensory fibers are most sensitive to oxygen deprivation. These nerve fibers carry fine touch and mediate symptoms such as paresthesias. Tissue intolerance to hypoxia increases from unmyelinated to myelinated nerves, to skeletal muscle, to the most resistant, skin and bone.

Classically, pain is described as out of proportion to the clinical findings and worsens despite appropriate care of the injury (i.e., fracture stabilization). Important neurologic symptoms are of distal motor and sensory dysfunction, characteristically weakness and numbness in the distribution of the affected nerve(s). The peroneal nerve in the lower extremity is commonly affected, leading to weakness on dorsiflexion and numbness in the first dorsal web space. The median nerve of the upper extremity is most often affected with weakness in wrist extension and numbness in the first web space.

BIBLIOGRAPHY

Modrall JG. Compartment syndrome. In: Rutherford RB (ed.), *Vascular Surgery*, 7th ed. Philadelphia, PA: W.B. Saunders; 2010.

Thomas BJ, Fu FH, Muller B, et al. Orthopedic surgery. In: Brunicardi F, Andersen DK, Billiar TR, et al (eds.), *Schwartz's Principles of Surgery*, 10th ed. New York, NY: McGraw-Hill; 2014.

Vogel TR, Jurkovich GJ. In: Ashley SW, Cance WG, Chen H, et al. *Scientific American Surgery*. Ontario, Canada: Decker Intellectual Properties; 2007.

9. **(D)** The key to treatment of compartment syndrome is early recognition and treatment. This requires a high

index of suspicion whenever treating injuries historically at high risk for developing elevated compartment pressures. Classically, compartment syndrome in trauma is seen following major extremity trauma such as crush injury, closed fractures, or with reperfusion following acute arterial injuries with a prolonged ischemic time. Once suspected, compartment pressures should be measured using commercially available devices or simple insertion of an intravenous (IV) catheter into the compartment with pressure transduction using standard monitoring equipment. Pressures greater than 30–40 mmHg are generally indications that fasciotomy should be performed emergently. Immediate complications of compartment syndrome result from muscle necrosis and include hyperkalemia, renal failure because of myoglobinuria, infection, and possibly limb loss.

The patient in this case is demonstrating signs of early compartment syndrome and must be treated aggressively. Management should include measurement of compartment pressures, placement of a bladder catheter to allow frequent measurement of urine output, measurement of creatine kinase levels, and four-compartment fasciotomy in the event of true compartment syndrome. Rhabdomyolysis should be treated aggressively with fluid resuscitation using a crystalloid solution to maintain a urine output >100 mL/h. There is no indication to transfuse blood products in this patient based on the given information.

BIBLIOGRAPHY

Modrall JG. Compartment syndrome. In: Rutherford RB (ed.), *Vascular Surgery*, 7th ed. Philadelphia, PA: W.B. Saunders; 2010.
Sise MJ, Shackford SR. Peripheral vascular injury. In: Mattox KL, Moore EE, Feliciano DV (eds.), *Trauma*, 7th ed. New York, NY: McGraw-Hill; 2012:Chapter 41.
Srinivasan RC, Tolhurst S, Vanderhave KL. Orthopedic surgery. In: Doherty GM (ed.), *Current Diagnosis & Treatment: Surgery*, 13th ed. New York, NY: McGraw-Hill; 2010:Chapter 40.
Stahel PF, Smith WR, Hak DJ. Lower extremity. In: Mattox KL, Moore EE, Feliciano DV (eds.), *Trauma*, 7th ed. New York, NY: McGraw-Hill; 2012:Chapter 40.
Thomas BJ, Fu FH, Muller B, et al. Orthopedic surgery. In: Brunicardi F, Andersen DK, Billiar TR, et al (eds.), *Schwartz's Principles of Surgery*, 10th ed. New York, NY: McGraw-Hill; 2014.

10. **(B)** The most common cause of extremity acute compartment syndrome in trauma patients is the tibial fracture. The lower extremity has four compartments bound by muscle fascia. A complete fasciotomy of the calf requires decompression of the anterior, lateral, deep, and superficial compartments (see Fig. 8-16). To decompress the anterior and lateral compartments, a lateral incision between the tibial crest and fibula is made. A short transverse incision is then made through the leg fascia

allowing access to the lateral intramuscular membrane, which is then divided. The superficial branch of the peroneal nerve is especially vulnerable when opening the lateral compartment because the membrane is divided proximally as it lies posterior to this septum and must be avoided. The posterior compartments are exposed through a medial incision made 2 cm posterior to the posterior tibial crest. Care is taken to avoid the saphenous nerve and vein. A transverse incision through the enveloping fascia allows identification of the septum between the deep and superficial compartment for division. Alternatively, all four compartments may be released through a single lateral incision with or without a fibulectomy.

BIBLIOGRAPHY

Modrall JG. Compartment syndrome. In: Rutherford RB (ed.), *Vascular Surgery*, 7th ed. Philadelphia, PA: W.B. Saunders; 2010.
Owings JT, Kennedy JP, Blaisdell FW. Injuries to the extremities. In: Wilmore DW, American College of Surgeons (eds.), *ACS Surgery: Principles & Practice*. New York, NY: WedMD; 2002.
Thomas BJ, Fu FH, Muller B, et al. Orthopedic surgery. In: Brunicardi F, Andersen DK, Billiar TR, et al (eds.), *Schwartz's Principles of Surgery*, 10th ed. New York, NY: McGraw-Hill; 2014.

11. **(A)** The most commonly injured veins are the superficial femoral vein, popliteal vein, and common femoral vein. When these veins are injured, repair should be attempted via primary end-to-end anastomosis, lateral venorrhaphy, or interposition graft. Areas of questionable collateral flow, such as the innominate, common femoral, and popliteal veins and suprarenal vena cava, should always have repair attempted. Other venous injuries can be safely ligated should attempted repair be too dangerous because of the patient's associated injuries.

BIBLIOGRAPHY

Burlew CN, Moore EE. Trauma. In: Brunicardi F, Andersen DK, Billiar TR, et al (eds.), *Schwartz's Principles of Surgery*, 10th ed. New York, NY: McGraw-Hill; 2014.
Demetriades D, Inaba K. Vascular trauma: abdominal. In: Rutherford RB (ed.), Vascular Surgery, 7th ed. Philadelphia, PA: W.B. Saunders; 2010.
Sise MJ, Shackford SR. Peripheral vascular injury. In: Mattox KL, Moore EE, Feliciano DV (eds.), *Trauma*, 7th ed. New York, NY: McGraw-Hill; 2012:Chapter 41.

12. **(E)** Contrast nephropathy is the third most common cause of acute renal failure in hospitalized patients. The mechanism for the pathogenesis of contrast nephropathy is complex and is believed to be due to renal vasoconstriction and oxidant injury. The effect of contrast media on renal blood flow is biphasic. A very brief increase in

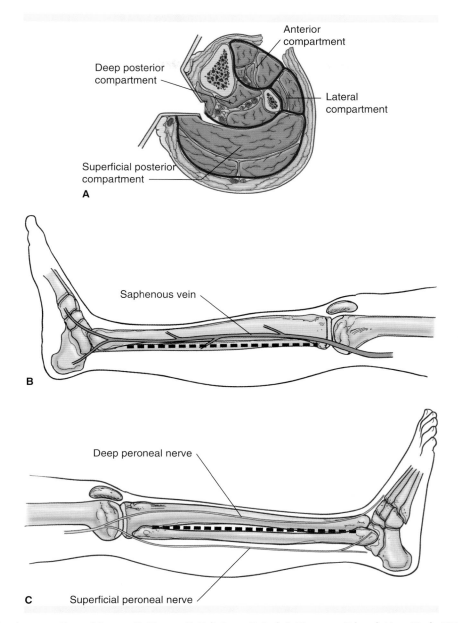

FIGURE 8-16. Calf fasciotomy. From Mattox K, Moore E, Feliciano D (eds.). *Trauma*, 7th ed. New York, NY: McGraw-Hill; 2012.

renal blood flow is followed by a sustained decrease in renal blood flow. This is unique to the kidney as contrast media induces vasodilatation in all other vascular beds. Contrast media exerts a low but significant chemical toxicity on several nephric enzyme systems, intracellular adenosine triphosphate, and isolated tubular cells.

Intravenous (IV) administration of contrast media represents a very low risk for contrast nephropathy in otherwise healthy patients (1%). Risk factors are advanced age, decreased baseline renal function, mode of administration (arterial worse than venous), diabetes, hypovolemia, use of nonsteroidal anti-inflammatory medications, type of contrast, and contrast dose. Adequate hydration is the most important preventive measure against contrast nephropathy. Studies have failed to show an effect with prophylactic treatment with mannitol or furosemide, whereas studies using *N*-acetylcysteine and sodium bicarbonate have shown conflicting results.

BIBLIOGRAPHY

13. **(E)** Biliary injury is common in both blunt and penetrating abdominal trauma. Eighty percent to 90% of blunt

liver injuries can be successfully managed nonoperatively in hemodynamically normal patients. However, higher grade injuries have increased failure rates. Complications of biliary injury include hemorrhage, hypoglycemia, coagulopathy, bile duct injury, peri- or intrahepatic abscesses, and hemobilia.

The popularity of observation for blunt liver trauma has led to a decrease in the incidence of hemobilia. Although not common and often difficult to recognize, it should be included in the differential in any patient with GI bleeding following a liver injury. Hemobilia usually presents as jaundice, right upper quadrant pain, and/or GI bleeding, although all three may not be present. Following blunt liver trauma, arteries, veins, and bile ducts are often injured without rupture of the liver capsule. Healing in this area is inhibited by bile stasis as well as tissue necrosis as a result of the injury. This can subsequently erode into hepatic blood vessels resulting in bleeding into the biliary tree. Evaluation of a patient suspected of having hemobilia depends on presentation as well as suspected etiology. Angiography is the definitive diagnostic study and identifies the vascular abnormality in over 90% of cases. Transarterial embolization is the treatment of choice for hemobilia. Studies have shown a success rate of 80–100% with a morbidity and mortality rate lower than that of surgery.

BIBLIOGRAPHY

Jaszczak N, Efron DT. Liver injury. In: Cameron JL, Cameron AM (eds.), *Current Surgical Therapy*, 10th ed. Philadelphia, PA: Elsevier Saunders; 2010:Chapter 199.

Wisner DH, Galante JM, Dolich MO, Hoyt DB. Abdominal trauma. In: Mulholland MW, Lillemoe KD, Doherty GM, et al (eds.), *Greenfield's Surgery: Scientific Principles & Practice*, 5th ed. Philadelphia, PA: Lippincott Williams & Wilkins; 2010.

14. **(B)** Major abdominal vascular injuries are most often due to penetrating trauma. Frequently these patients present in hypovolemic shock with multiple associated injuries. In theory, the proximal SMA could be ligated with bowel viability maintained through collateral circulation. In practice, however, the mortality rate from SMA injuries remains approximately 50%, most likely secondary to the profound hypovolemia these patients invariably suffer contributing to overall visceral ischemia as well as associated injuries. Injuries to the inferior mesenteric artery, on the other hand, can be safely ligated in the majority of patients without significant morbidity. The internal iliac artery may be safely ligated without significant sequelae. Ligation of the suprarenal vena cava is discouraged because of the associated high mortality rate and risk of renal failure. Without evidence of acute ischemia, either the radial or ulnar artery may be safely ligated, but not both simultaneously.

BIBLIOGRAPHY

Burlew CN, Moore EE. Trauma. In: Brunicardi F, Andersen DK, Billiar TR, et al (eds.), *Schwartz's Principles of Surgery*, 10th ed. New York, NY: McGraw-Hill; 2014.

Demetriades D, Inaba K. Vascular trauma: Abdominal. In: Rutherford RB (ed.), *Vascular Surgery*, 7th ed. Philadelphia, PA: W.B. Saunders; 2010.

Sise MJ, Shackford SR. Peripheral vascular injury. In: Mattox KL, Moore EE, Feliciano DV (eds.), *Trauma*, 7th ed. New York, NY: McGraw-Hill; 2012:Chapter 41.

Stahel PF, Smith WR, Hak DJ. Lower extremity. In: Mattox KL, Moore EE, Feliciano DV (eds.), *Trauma*, 7th ed. New York, NY: McGraw-Hill; 2012:Chapter 40.

15. **(B)** Laceration of the radial or ulnar artery is often clinically silent. Injuries to the ulnar artery are often accompanied by injuries to the ulnar nerve, which may be the only clinical finding. Isolated injury to the ulnar or radial artery may be safely ligated if there is a complete palmar arch and no history of prior radial or ulnar trauma/ligation. In the event of injury to both the ulnar and radial artery, the ulnar artery should be repaired because it is larger and the predominant artery to the hand. The radial artery is the smaller of the two arteries that supply the hand, and in the absence of obvious ischemia along its distribution, it may be ligated safely (see Fig. 8-17).

BIBLIOGRAPHY

Parnes N, Ben-Galim P, Netscher D. Upper extremity. In: Mattox KL, Moore EE, Feliciano DV (eds.), *Trauma*, 7th ed. New York, NY: McGraw-Hill; 2012:Chapter 39.

Patel KR, Rowe VL. Vascular trauma: extremity. In: Rutherford RB (ed.), *Vascular Surgery*, 7th ed. Philadelphia, PA: W.B. Saunders; 2010.

Sise MJ, Shackford SR. Peripheral vascular injury. In: Mattox KL, Moore EE, Feliciano DV (eds.), *Trauma*, 7th ed. New York, NY: McGraw-Hill; 2012:Chapter 41.

16. **(D)** Penetrating neck trauma is a potentially complex entity and demands a thorough understanding of anatomy and treatment algorithms in order to avoid missed injuries. Essential to this is recognition of the three arbitrary zones of the neck (see Fig. 8-18).

Zone I—From clavicle to cricoid cartilage and includes the great vessels, lungs, trachea, esophagus, thoracic duct, spinal cord, and nerve trunks.

Zone II—From cricoid cartilage to the angle of the mandible and includes the common carotid arteries and its branches, vertebral arteries, jugular veins, trachea, esophagus, spinal cord, and larynx.

Zone III—From angle of the mandible to the base of the skull and includes the pharynx, jugular veins, vertebral arteries, and distal internal carotid arteries.

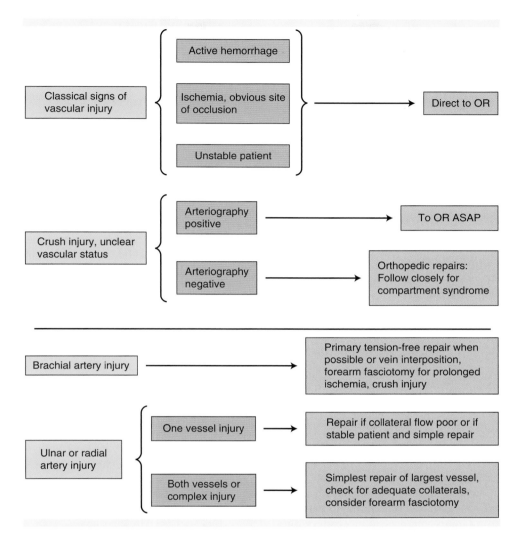

FIGURE 8-17. Upper extremity arterial injury management. OR, operating room. From Mattox K, Moore E, Feliciano D (eds.). *Trauma*, 7th ed. New York, NY: McGraw-Hill; 2012.

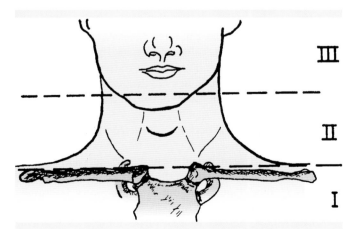

FIGURE 8-18. Zones of the neck. (Used with permission from Monson DO, Saletta JD, Freeark RJ. Carotid vertebral trauma. *J Trauma*. 1969;9:987.)

In the hemodynamically *unstable* patient, a neck exploration is mandatory regardless of the entrance site. In a hemodynamically normal patient, most authors agree that penetrating injuries to zone I or III should be evaluated by arteriography, tracheobronchoscopy, esophagram, and esophagoscopy. Currently, the management of zone II injuries is debated. Previously a mandatory neck exploration was recommended for all zone II injuries penetrating the platysma. This has been challenged, and many authors now recommend arteriogram, tracheobronchoscopy, esophagram, and esophagoscopy.

This patient has a "blush" around the right common carotid artery bifurcation with careful examination revealing a laceration to the right internal carotid artery.

BIBLIOGRAPHY

Arthurs ZM, Starnes BW. Vascular trauma: head and neck. In: Rutherford RB (ed.), *Vascular Surgery*, 7th ed. Philadelphia, PA: W.B. Saunders; 2010.

Feliciano DV, Vercruysse GA. Neck. In: Mattox KL, Moore EE, Feliciano DV (eds.), *Trauma*, 7th ed. New York, NY: McGraw-Hill; 2012:Chapter 22.

17. **(C)** For penetrating injuries to the carotid artery, level of consciousness is a key determinant of treatment decisions. This patient was described as hemodynamically normal with a normal level of consciousness. He should undergo right neck exploration and repair of the carotid artery injury. Because of the high incidence of associated injuries, tracheobronchoscopy and esophagoscopy should also be considered.

This injury is best approached through an anterior neck incision along the sternocleidomastoid muscle. Methods for arterial repair include primary repair, patch angioplasty, internal-to-external carotid artery transposition, and interposition grafting with saphenous vein or prosthetic conduit. Many authors advocate the use of shunts during the repair if the stump pressure is less than 60 mmHg or if there is minimal back bleeding. Unless there is an absolute contraindication (intracranial bleed, abdominal hemorrhage), systemic heparinization should be used.

Controversy exists regarding the appropriate management of similar patients with an associated neurologic defect. There are anecdotal reports of conversion of ischemic infarction to hemorrhagic infarction after revascularization. Carotid artery ligation is reserved for patients who sustain a carotid injury and present in a coma with no prograde flow in the internal carotid artery, uncontrollable hemorrhage, and when temporary shunt placement is technically not possible. In all other patients with neurologic deficit, the outcome is better if repair is performed.

The final population is patients with distal internal carotid artery (ICA) lesions. These are most often inaccessible and can be treated with ligation and anticoagulation, but this approach has a mortality rate of 45%.

BIBLIOGRAPHY

Arthurs ZM, Starnes BW. Vascular trauma: head and neck. In: Rutherford RB (ed.), *Vascular Surgery*, 7th ed. Philadelphia, PA: W.B. Saunders; 2010.

Feliciano DV, Vercruysse GA. Neck. In: Mattox KL, Moore EE, Feliciano DV (eds.), *Trauma*, 7th ed. New York, NY: McGraw-Hill; 2012:Chapter 22.

18. **(D)** The initial management of penetrating neck trauma is determined by hemodynamic stability. In the unstable patient, the diagnostic test of choice is immediate operative neck exploration. In the stable patient, many vascular injuries may be diagnosed with duplex ultrasound studies, arteriogram, or even complete physical examination.

The operative approach is via an oblique incision along the anterior border of the sternocleidomastoid muscle. Bleeding from the internal jugular vein may be easily controlled with digital pressure while control of the injured vessel is obtained. Lateral venorrhaphy may be performed for wall defects, but if the vein has been transected, primary repair will significantly compromise the lumen and ligation is the treatment of choice. In cases of bilateral internal jugular vein injury, attempts should be made for unilateral repair.

BIBLIOGRAPHY

Arthurs ZM, Starnes BW. Vascular trauma: head and neck. In: Rutherford RB (ed.), *Vascular Surgery*, 7th ed. Philadelphia, PA: W.B. Saunders; 2010.

Feliciano DV, Vercruysse GA. Neck. In: Mattox KL, Moore EE, Feliciano DV (eds.), *Trauma*, 7th ed. New York, NY: McGraw-Hill; 2012:Chapter 22.

19. **(D)** Mechanism of injury is a significant part of any trauma patient's history because it may suggest an increased risk for specific injuries. The history of a steering wheel deformity implies a significant deceleration force to the thoracic aorta and great vessels. This is further suggested by the supplied CXR, which demonstrates a widened mediastinum. The next step in evaluating this hemodynamically normal patient is spiral CT of the chest.

Blunt injury of the thoracic aorta and the intrathoracic great vessels is a complex and life-threatening entity. Shearing stress because of rapid deceleration leads to rupture of the aorta at sites of fixation. The most common site is the descending aorta at the level of the ligamentum arteriosum. Injuries of the great vessels occur, but they occur as a result of direct contact with the anterior chest wall.

There are clinical findings associated with traumatic rupture of the thoracic aorta and intrathoracic great vessel injury. These include flail chest, a fractured first or second rib, pulse deficits in the upper extremity, hoarseness or voice changes without laryngeal injury, fractured sternum, and history of high-speed deceleration. Any of these should increase your suspicion for a thoracic aortic disruption. Neurologic changes should initiate a search for intracranial injury, cervical carotid artery injury, and intrathoracic great vessel injury.

Radiographic findings associated with traumatic thoracic aortic tears include mediastinal widening (>8 cm on supine films), esophagus and tracheal deviation to the right, obliteration of the aortopulmonary window, apical cap, and obscuring of the aortic knob.

It should be noted that many authors argue the use of chest CT in this setting and would proceed directly to arteriogram. However, this remains controversial as more and more institutions are using chest CT as a screening tool with arteriogram reserved for patients with positive findings on CT. Benefits of performing a spiral CT of the chest include a negative predictive value of 99.9%.

BIBLIOGRAPHY

Brinkman WT, Bavaria JE. Vascular trauma: thoracic. In: Rutherford RB (ed.), *Vascular Surgery*, 7th ed. Philadelphia, PA: W.B. Saunders; 2010.

Mattox KL, Wall MJ Jr, Tsai P. Heart and thoracic vascular injuries. In: Mattox KL, Moore EE, Feliciano DV (eds.), *Trauma*, 7th ed. New York, NY: McGraw-Hill; 2012:Chapter 26.

20. **(E)** The diagnosis of thoracic aortic injury requires a high index of suspicion based on clinical findings and mechanisms of injury. Once suspected, the initial evaluation shifts from angiography to spiral CT as a screening tool. However, angiography remains the gold standard for diagnosis of aortic injury.

Aortic injuries are described using multiple classification systems, all based on anatomic features of the disruption. Involvement of the ascending aorta is the single most important anatomic determinant related to clinical behavior of the injury.

The presented angiogram demonstrates a normal aorta, left common carotid artery, and left subclavian artery. Close evaluation of the innominate artery reveals a pseudoaneurysm extending beyond the bifurcation into the common carotid and subclavian arteries.

This patient's CT scan was used as a screening test and revealed blood in the mediastinum but was not diagnostic. The patient's progressive neurologic changes are explained by the extension of the pseudoaneurysm along the subclavian artery and subsequent vascular compromise.

BIBLIOGRAPHY

Brinkman WT, Bavaria JE. Vascular trauma: thoracic. In: Rutherford RB (ed.), *Vascular Surgery*, 7th ed. Philadelphia, PA: W.B. Saunders; 2010.

Mattox KL, Wall MJ Jr, Tsai P. Heart and thoracic vascular injuries. In: Mattox KL, Moore EE, Feliciano DV (eds.), *Trauma*, 7th ed. New York, NY: McGraw-Hill; 2012:Chapter 26.

21. **(D)** With the diagnosis of an innominate pseudoaneurysm and neurologic changes, the patient requires appropriate preoperative evaluation for concomitant injuries and stabilization with aggressive blood pressure control, followed by surgical management of the pseudoaneurysm.

The approach to the innominate artery is via a median sternotomy. A partial occlusion clamp is then placed along the ascending aorta proximal to the pseudoaneurysm. A Dacron graft is then placed end-to-side on the ascending aorta. The median sternotomy can be extended to the right neck or the medial head of the clavicle can be resected for increased exposure of the distal pseudoaneurysm. At this point, the pseudoaneurysm can then be resected and the aortic stump oversewn.

In this case, a bifurcated graft was used for distal anastomosis to both the subclavian and common carotid arteries.

BIBLIOGRAPHY

Brinkman WT, Bavaria JE. Vascular trauma: thoracic. In: Rutherford RB (ed.), *Vascular Surgery*, 7th ed. Philadelphia, PA: W.B. Saunders; 2010.

Mattox KL, Wall MJ Jr, Tsai P. Heart and thoracic vascular injuries. In: Mattox KL, Moore EE, Feliciano DV (eds.), *Trauma*, 7th ed. New York, NY: McGraw-Hill; 2012:Chapter 26.

22. **(B)** CT scan of the chest revealed blood in the mediastinum and what appeared to be an injury at the aortic isthmus. Arteriogram confirms this diagnosis and demonstrates an aortic tear just opposite the ligamentum arteriosum.

Injuries to the aortic isthmus are the most common cause of death because of aortic injury secondary to blunt thoracic trauma. In comparison to the remainder of the aorta, the aortic isthmus is inherently weak and acts as a point of fixation, allowing for the transmission of deceleration forces onto the vessel wall. Those injuries that are contained within a mediastinal hematoma may survive to reach the hospital where they must be recognized early based on mechanism of injury.

After establishing the diagnosis of an aortic transection, the patient should be stabilized and concomitant injuries evaluated. One should closely monitor the cardiac rhythm, urine output, oxygen saturation, and blood pressure. Antihypertensives are often needed to maintain a systolic blood pressure less than 120 mmHg.

As in this case, based on CXR and mechanism of injury, a CT of the chest is often used as a screening tool; however, the arteriogram remains the gold standard for diagnosing aortic injuries (see Fig. 8-19).

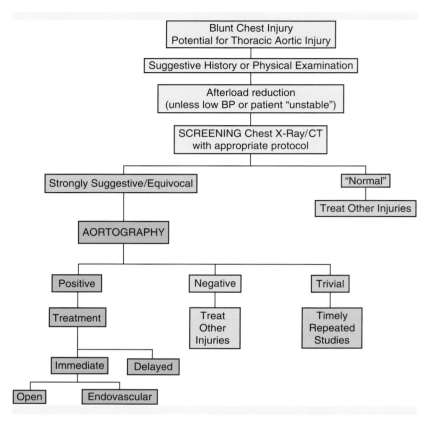

FIGURE 8-19. Approach to patient with suspected blunt aortic injury. BP, blood pressure; CT, computed tomography. From Mattox K, Moore E, Feliciano D (eds.). *Trauma*, 7th ed. New York, NY: McGraw-Hill; 2012.

BIBLIOGRAPHY

Brinkman WT, Bavaria JE. Vascular trauma: thoracic. In: Rutherford RB (ed.), *Vascular Surgery*, 7th ed. Philadelphia, PA: W.B. Saunders; 2010.

Mattox KL, Wall MJ Jr, Tsai P. Heart and thoracic vascular injuries. In: Mattox KL, Moore EE, Feliciano DV (eds.), *Trauma*, 7th ed. New York, NY: McGraw-Hill; 2012:Chapter 26.

Varghese TK. Chest trauma. In: Mulholland MW, Lillemoe KD, Doherty GM, et al (eds.), *Greenfield's Surgery: Scientific Principles & Practice*, 5th ed. Philadelphia, PA: Lippincott Williams & Wilkins; 2010.

23. **(B)** Although there are multiple approaches to the repair of an aortic isthmus injury, the primary concern is prevention of rupture prior to repair and then prevention of postoperative paraplegia secondary to spinal ischemia. Paraplegia develops with a rate of 2–20% in emergency situations.

The injured aorta is approached through a left posterolateral thoracotomy in the fourth intercostal space with the patient in a right decubitus position. From this approach, the aortic arch, left carotid, and left subclavian arteries can be controlled to allow repair of the injured segment. Only 20% of injuries can be repaired primarily, with the remainder requiring prosthetic graft placement via one of several methods.

The "clamp and sew" method is useful when the hematoma has ruptured and does not require bypass. Unfortunately the surgeon has less than 30 minutes of aortic cross-clamp time in which to complete the repair and return blood flow, because this method offers no spinal protection. If the injury extends to the arch and ascending aorta, this method is inadequate.

A second method uses cardiopulmonary bypass from the right atrium to the distal arterial bed. This allows repair of the aortic tear and any extension of the injury. It also provides cerebroperfusion through the intercostal arteries and protects the spinal cord from ischemia. In rare cases, it can be converted to total cardiopulmonary bypass with cardiac arrest if necessary. Unfortunately this requires full anticoagulation and is contraindicated in patients with associated injuries at high risk for bleeding.

Another method uses left heart bypass from the left atrium to the femoral artery. A centrifugal pump is used, which does not require an oxygenator or systemic anticoagulation. This method offers the spinal protection of cardiopulmonary bypass without the risks associated with anticoagulation.

The final method is the use of endovascular thoracic aortic stents, which has gained significant popularity in the past decade. The endovascular approach has been associated with decreased operative time, length of stay, morbidity, and mortality. More studies need to be performed to evaluate long-term outcomes, but the ability to dramatically decrease postoperative complications makes this approach promising.

BIBLIOGRAPHY

Brinkman WT, Bavaria JE. Vascular trauma: thoracic. In: Rutherford RB (ed.), *Vascular Surgery*, 7th ed. Philadelphia, PA: W.B. Saunders; 2010.

Mattox KL, Wall MJ Jr, Tsai P. Heart and thoracic vascular injuries. In: Mattox KL, Moore EE, Feliciano DV (eds.), *Trauma*, 7th ed. New York, NY: McGraw-Hill; 2012:Chapter 26.

24. **(A)** Many patients suffering penetrating trauma to the chest present initially as hemodynamically normal only to decompensate acutely. Such patients must be carefully evaluated with attention to subtle clinical findings that may be the only warning of impending instability. Standard advanced trauma life support protocols should be followed including evaluation for a patent airway and adequate respirations, as well as adequate vascular access with two large-bore peripheral IVs.

The location of the injury will determine structures at risk. Abdominal injuries must be considered because the diaphragm can elevate to the level of the nipples anteriorly and the tip of the scapula posteriorly. With an injury between the areas bordered by the nipples laterally, the heart, lungs, aorta, great vessels, trachea, thoracic duct, phrenic nerve, and esophagus are all at risk of injury.

A CXR is essential to assess for pneumothorax, hemothorax, widened mediastinum, and pneumoperitoneum.

Tube thoracostomy is often needed because of respiratory compromise secondary to pneumothorax and/or hemothorax. A chest tube also allows for quantification of the bleeding into the chest and the presence of large air leaks suggestive of injury to the bronchial tree.

Acute pericardial effusion of <30 mL may cause pericardial tamponade. Echocardiogram is often useful in detecting small amounts of pericardial hemorrhage prior to the development of tamponade. Signs often present with cardiac tamponade include jugular venous distention, muffled heart sounds, narrowed pulse pressure, and pulsus paradoxus. Pericardiocentesis is a useful maneuver that may buy the time needed until a surgical team is assembled. Repeated aspiration may be needed; however, this should never delay operative intervention.

Esophagram may be indicated based on the clinical symptoms such as dysphagia or location of the injury (i.e., penetrating zone I or midline neck). However, this is not done as part of the initial assessment.

BIBLIOGRAPHY

Brinkman WT, Bavaria JE. Vascular trauma: thoracic. In: Rutherford RB (ed.), *Vascular Surgery*, 7th ed. Philadelphia, PA: W.B. Saunders; 2010.

Mattox KL, Wall MJ Jr, Tsai P. Heart and thoracic vascular injuries. In: Mattox KL, Moore EE, Feliciano DV (eds.), *Trauma*, 7th ed. New York, NY: McGraw-Hill; 2012:Chapter 26.

Smith RS, Dort JM. Chest wall trauma, hemothorax and pneumothorax. In: Cameron JL, Cameron AM (eds.), *Current Surgical Therapy*, 10th ed. Philadelphia, PA: Elsevier Saunders; 2010:Chapter 195.

Varghese TK. Chest trauma. In: Mulholland MW, Lillemoe KD, Doherty GM, et al (eds.), *Greenfield's Surgery: Scientific Principles & Practice*, 5th ed. Philadelphia, PA: Lippincott Williams & Wilkins; 2010.

25. **(D)** Penetrating injuries to the great vessels are life-threatening emergencies. Although many will exsanguinate prior to arrival in the ED, others will present hemodynamically normal only to rapidly decompensate in the ED. Early diagnosis and prompt treatment are key to decreased morbidity and mortality.

Additional injuries contribute significantly to overall morbidity of great vessel injuries and should be assessed at the time of the initial operation through direct visualization, bronchoscopy, and/or esophagoscopy of the lungs, heart, diaphragm, thoracic duct, trachea, and esophagus.

The location of subclavian artery injury guides the operative incision required; thus when possible, preoperative imaging is important. Injuries to the subclavian artery can be approached though a median sternotomy, which will provide access to all of the great vessels with the exception of the proximal left subclavian artery. Injuries in the proximity of the proximal left subclavian artery are best approached through an anterolateral thoracotomy through the third or fourth interspace. If the vascular injury extends distally, a "trapdoor" incision (combining a limited sternotomy and a supraclavicular incision with resection of the medial clavicle) may be performed giving access to the distal left subclavian artery.

Once proximal and distal vascular control is obtained, small lacerations may be debrided and repaired primarily, whereas larger defects require saphenous vein or prosthetic material for graft. In patients who are hemodynamically unstable, the subclavian artery may be ligated, with low risk of upper extremity ischemia.

BIBLIOGRAPHY

Arthurs ZM, Starnes BW. Vascular trauma: head and neck. In: Rutherford RB (ed.), *Vascular Surgery*, 7th ed. Philadelphia, PA: W.B. Saunders; 2010.

Brinkman WT, Bavaria JE. Vascular trauma: thoracic. In: Rutherford RB (ed.), *Vascular Surgery*, 7th ed. Philadelphia, PA: W.B. Saunders; 2010.

Mattox KL, Wall MJ Jr, Tsai P. Heart and thoracic vascular injuries. In: Mattox KL, Moore EE, Feliciano DV (eds.), *Trauma*, 7th ed. New York, NY: McGraw-Hill; 2012:Chapter 26.

Mattox KL, Wall MJ Jr, Tsai P. Trauma thoracotomy: principles and techniques. In: Mattox KL, Moore EE, Feliciano DV (eds.), *Trauma*, 7th ed. New York, NY: McGraw-Hill; 2012:Chapter 24.

26. **(B)** The left subclavian artery originates at the aortic arch. The subclavian artery then becomes the axillary artery as it crosses the lateral border of the first rib. The axillary artery then becomes the brachial artery at the lateral border of the teres major muscle.

In the axilla, the pectoralis minor muscle crosses anterior to the axillary artery, dividing the vessel into three segments. The first segment of the axillary artery is medial to the pectoralis minor muscle and lateral to the clavicle. It gives off only the superior thoracic artery. The second segment lies beneath the pectoralis minor muscle and gives off the thoracoacromial and lateral thoracic arteries. The third segment of the axillary artery is lateral to the pectoralis minor muscle and gives rise to the subscapular and the anterior and posterior circumflex humeral arteries.

The vascular injury demonstrated on the arteriogram is to the axillary artery.

BIBLIOGRAPHY

Parnes N, Ben-Galim P, Netscher D. Upper extremity. In: Mattox KL, Moore EE, Feliciano DV (eds.), *Trauma*, 7th ed. New York, NY: McGraw-Hill; 2012:Chapter 39.

Patel KR, Rowe VL. Vascular trauma: extremity. In: Rutherford RB (ed.), *Vascular Surgery*, 7th ed. Philadelphia, PA: W.B. Saunders; 2010.

Sise MJ, Shackford SR. Peripheral vascular injury. In: Mattox KL, Moore EE, Feliciano DV (eds.), *Trauma*, 7th ed. New York, NY: McGraw-Hill; 2012:Chapter 41.

27. **(C)** In the presented patient, the arteriogram reveals an axillary artery injury. Proximal control is obtained through a transverse infraclavicular incision with extension into the anterior axilla for distal control. The pectoralis minor tendon may be divided for complete exposure of the middle section of the axillary artery (see Fig. 8-20). Once controlled both proximally and distally, the artery is then debrided at the injury site with primary repair if possible. For significant tissue loss or

destruction, a vein graft is ideal for axillary artery injury as opposed to prosthetic graft. Because of the risk of irreversible cellular damage, warm ischemia time should not exceed 6 hours. If extensive orthopedic manipulation at the site of the vascular injury is required, temporary vascular shunting may be used while the fracture is stabilized. Following fracture repair, the vascular repair may then be performed without the risk of disruption by subsequent bone manipulation. Lastly, the extremity is at risk for compartment syndrome, and fasciotomy should be considered at the time of the initial surgery based on the length of the ischemia time.

BIBLIOGRAPHY

Parnes N, Ben-Galim P, Netscher D. Upper extremity. In: Mattox KL, Moore EE, Feliciano DV (eds.), *Trauma*, 7th ed. New York, NY: McGraw-Hill; 2012:Chapter 39.

Patel KR, Rowe VL. Vascular trauma: extremity. In: Rutherford RB (ed.), *Vascular Surgery*, 7th ed. Philadelphia, PA: W.B. Saunders; 2010.

Sise MJ, Shackford SR. Peripheral vascular injury. In: Mattox KL, Moore EE, Feliciano DV (eds.), *Trauma*, 7th ed. New York, NY: McGraw-Hill; 2012:Chapter 41.

28. **(D)** The external iliac artery becomes the common femoral artery as it passes beneath the inguinal ligament. In the leg, the common femoral artery divides into the superficial femoral artery and the deep femoral (profunda femoris) arteries. The superficial femoral artery becomes the popliteal artery that then divides below the knee to form the posterior tibial, anterior tibial, and peroneal arteries. Significant collateral blood supply is found at the level of the knee through various geniculate branches from the profunda femoris, superficial femoral, and popliteal arteries. This collateral circulation may develop to supply the distal extremity in patients with chronic peripheral vascular disease but fails to provide sufficient blood flow in the acutely injured extremity.

The absence of contrast filling the superficial femoral artery in this arteriogram indicates an injury to the superficial femoral artery.

BIBLIOGRAPHY

Patel KR, Rowe VL. Compartment syndrome. In: Rutherford RB (ed.), *Vascular Surgery*, 7th ed. Philadelphia, PA: W.B. Saunders; 2010.

Sise MJ, Shackford SR. Peripheral vascular injury. In: Mattox KL, Moore EE, Feliciano DV (eds.), *Trauma*, 7th ed. New York, NY: McGraw-Hill; 2012:Chapter 41.

Stahel PF, Smith WR, Hak DJ. Lower extremity. In: Mattox KL, Moore EE, Feliciano DV (eds.), *Trauma*, 7th ed. New York, NY: McGraw-Hill; 2012:Chapter 40.

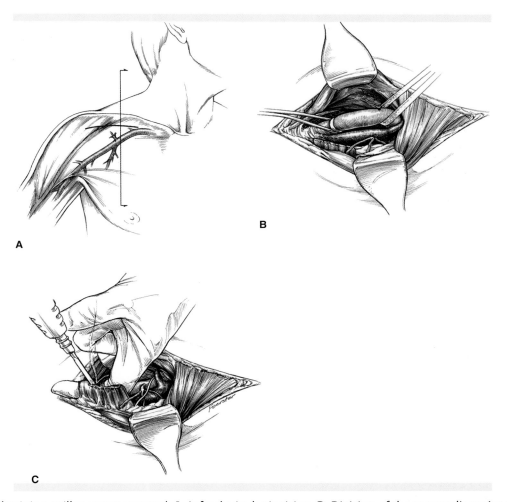

FIGURE 8-20. Obtaining axillary artery control. **A.** Infraclavicular incision. **B.** Division of the pectoralis major muscle. **C.** Axillary artery exposure and control. Reproduced with permission from Rutherford RB, ed. *Atlas of Vascular Surgery: Basic Techniques and Exposures.* Philadelphia: WB Saunders; 1993. © Elsevier.

29. **(B)** The initial approach to vascular injury is proximal control of the injured vessel to minimize blood loss. Proximal control of the lower extremity is best obtained in the inguinal region at the common femoral, profunda femoris, and superficial femoral arteries. Once isolated, the superficial femoral artery should be sharply debrided. Thrombectomy is then performed using a balloon-tipped catheter and heparin solution both proximally and distally. Primary anastomosis is often possible with minimal vessel destruction and with modest proximal and distal vessel immobilization. With significant tissue destruction, however, a reverse saphenous vein graft should be placed. Because of increased risk for concurrent deep venous injury in the setting of arterial injury, saphenous vein should be harvested from the contralateral extremity. Devitalized muscle and tissue are often present and should be debrided prior to closure of the wound. The extremity is at risk for compartment syndrome, and fasciotomy should be considered at the

time of the initial surgery based on the length of the ischemia time.

BIBLIOGRAPHY

Patel KR, Rowe VL. Compartment syndrome. In: Rutherford RB (ed.), *Vascular Surgery*, 7th ed. Philadelphia, PA: W.B. Saunders; 2010.
Sise MJ, Shackford SR. Peripheral vascular injury. In: Mattox KL, Moore EE, Feliciano DV (eds.), *Trauma*, 7th ed. New York, NY: McGraw-Hill; 2012:Chapter 41.
Stahel PF, Smith WR, Hak DJ. Lower extremity. In: Mattox KL, Moore EE, Feliciano DV (eds.), *Trauma*, 7th ed. New York, NY: McGraw-Hill; 2012:Chapter 40.

30. **(B)** Splenic injuries are extremely common in blunt abdominal trauma. The American Association for the Surgery of Trauma (AAST) developed a grading scale to describe these injuries (see Table 8-4 and Fig. 8-21).

Based on the AAST grading scale, Fig. 8-7 is a grade III splenic laceration. The decision for nonoperative

TABLE 8-4 American Association for the Surgery of Trauma Splenic Organ Injury Scale

Grade[a]		Injury Description
I	Hematoma	Subcapsular, <10% surface area
	Laceration	Capsular tear, <1 cm parenchymal depth
II	Hematoma	Subcapsular, 10–50% surface area, <5 cm in diameter
	Laceration	1–3 cm parenchymal depth that does not involve a trabecular vessel
III	Hematoma	Subcapsular, >50% surface area or expanding; ruptured subcapsular or parenchymal hematoma; intraparenchymal hematoma >5 cm or expanding
	Laceration	>3 cm parenchymal depth or involving trabecular vessels
IV	Laceration	Laceration involving segmental or hilar vessels producing major devascularization (>25% of spleen)
V	Laceration	Completely shattered spleen
	Vascular	Hilar vascular injury that devascularizes spleen

[a]Advance one grade for multiple injuries up to grade III.
From Mattox K, Moore E, Feliciano D (eds.). *Trauma*, 7th ed. New York, NY: McGraw-Hill; 2012.

management is based mainly on two factors: hemodynamic stability and abdominal examination. Hemodynamically unstable patients with blunt abdominal trauma will require further diagnostic interventions, diagnostic peritoneal lavage (DPL), focused abdominal sonography for trauma (FAST) examination, or less commonly, operative exploration.

The stable blunt abdominal trauma patient with suspected spleen injury should undergo abdominal CT with IV contrast, with careful attention also paid to the left kidney and distal pancreas (see Fig. 8-22). If there is evidence of active extravasation of contrast or "blush," ongoing bleeding is likely, and further evaluation with either angiography or repeat CT scanning is needed. If there is no sign of bleeding, observe the patient in the ICU (grade II or greater) with serial abdominal examinations and hematocrit. During this time, urine output should also be closely monitored, and vaccines to prevent streptococcal, meningococcal, and *Haemophilus* infections should be given in case of the need for urgent splenectomy. The majority of failures of nonoperative management will occur between 6 and 8 days.

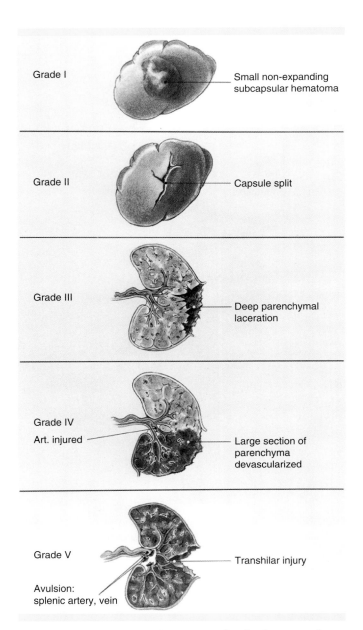

FIGURE 8-21. American Association for the Surgery of Trauma splenic injury grades. From Mattox K, Moore E, Feliciano D (eds.), *Trauma*, 7th ed. New York, NY: McGraw-Hill; 2012.

BIBLIOGRAPHY

Burlew CN, Moore EE. Trauma. In: Brunicardi F, Andersen DK, Billiar TR, et al (eds.), *Schwartz's Principles of Surgery*, 10th ed. New York, NY: McGraw-Hill; 2014.

Moore EE, Cogbill TH, Jurkovich GJ, et al. Organ injury scaling: spleen and liver (1994 Edition). *J Trauma* 1995;38:323.

Wisner DH. Injury to the spleen. In: Mattox KL, Moore EE, Feliciano DV (eds.), *Trauma*, 7th ed. New York, NY: McGraw-Hill; 2012:Chapter 30.

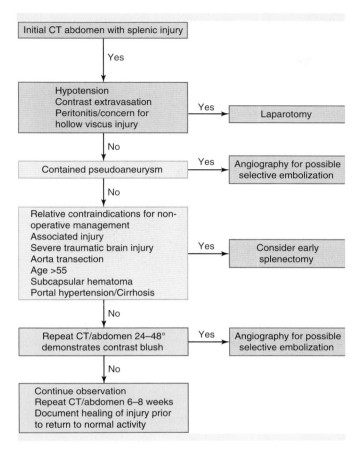

FIGURE 8-22. Treatment algorithm for splenic injury. CT, computed tomography. From Zinner MJ, Ashley SW. *Maingot's Abdominal Operations*, 12th ed. New York, NY: McGraw-Hill; 2013.

31. **(D)** The mobilization of the spleen is performed in a stepwise approach to avoid further injury and provide improved visualization of the left hemidiaphragm, left kidney, and posterior distal pancreas and spleen (see Fig. 8-23). The first step is to divide the splenorenal and splenophrenic ligaments initially by sharp dissection and continue with sharp and blunt dissection. Once these lateral attachments are divided, mobilizing the spleen and tail of the pancreas medially is the next step.

The two structures should be moved as a unit to avoid any injuries to either structure. The next step is to clamp and tie off the short gastric vessels. Avoid dividing these vessels with only scissors or Bovie electrocautery because of the risk of delayed bleeding. The last step is to divide the splenocolic ligament. If bleeding is encountered during removal of the spleen, digital compression is preferred. Mass clamping of the hilum should be reserved for instances of extreme hemorrhage because of the increased risk for damage of the tail of the pancreas during this maneuver.

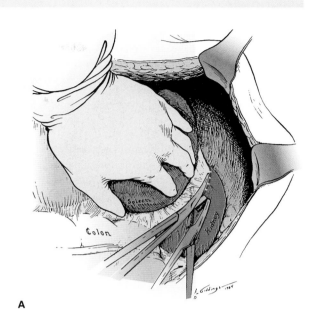

A

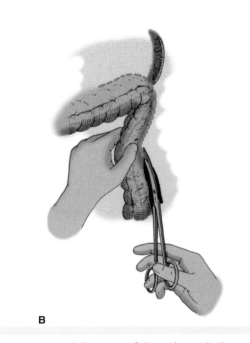

B

FIGURE 8-23. Mobilization of the spleen. **A.** From Mattox K, Moore E, Feliciano D (eds.). *Trauma*, 7th ed. New York, NY: McGraw-Hill; 2012. **B.** From Skandalakis JE, Colborn GL, Weidman TA, et al. *Skandalakis' Surgical Anatomy*. New York, NY: McGraw-Hill; 2004.

BIBLIOGRAPHY

Skandalakis JE, Colborn GL, Weidman TA, et al. Adrenal (suprarenal) glands. In: Skandalakis JE, Colburn GL, Weidman TA, et al. (eds.), *Skandalakis' Surgical Anatomy*. New York, NY: McGraw-Hill; 2004:Chapter 27.

Wisner DH. Injury to the spleen. In: Mattox KL, Moore EE, Feliciano DV (eds.), *Trauma*, 7th ed. New York, NY: McGraw-Hill; 2012:Chapter 30.

32. **(D)** Patients with hemodynamic instability and evidence of positive DPL require exploratory laparotomy. A positive DPL is described as aspiration of gross blood >10 mL or gastrointestinal (GI) contents, or lavage fluid with >100,000 red blood cells/μL (for blunt trauma), >500 white blood cells/μL, or Gram stain with bacteria present. DPL is warranted to rule out abdominal hemorrhage in hemodynamically abnormal patients without an identified source of blood loss.

The FAST examination has largely replaced DPL at major trauma centers to determine hemoperitoneum. Volumes of less than 250 mL are rarely visualized with FAST examinations, and the method cannot reliably determine the source of hemorrhage. Therefore, patients who are hemodynamically normal with a positive FAST exam should undergo CT scan.

Patients with suspected hepatic injury who undergo exploratory laparotomy may experience worsening hypotension upon entry into the peritoneum and evacuation of hemoperitoneum. Manual compression of the liver may be attempted to control hemorrhage by placing both hands over the anterior surface of the liver and applying pressure. Prior to exploration, the anesthesia team should be allowed to catch up with fluid loss and correct any coagulopathy. If there is an obvious source of major hemorrhage from the liver, the Pringle maneuver should be performed. The porta hepatis is clamped using either the finger or a non-crushing clamp. If significant bleeding persists, perihepatic packing should be considered. Less commonly, partial hepatectomy and veno-veno bypass are performed. If bleeding is controlled after the Pringle maneuver, direct suturing, as well as omental packing may be performed.

BIBLIOGRAPHY

Fabian TC, Bee TK. Liver and biliary tract. In: Mattox KL, Moore EE, Feliciano DV (eds.), *Trauma*, 7th ed. New York, NY: McGraw-Hill; 2012:Chapter 29.

33. **(B)** Liver injuries are graded similarly to splenic injuries (Table 8-5).

Nonoperative management of blunt hepatic injury is the standard of care in most trauma centers provided the patient remains hemodynamically normal. High-grade injury, large hemoperitoneum, and active extravasation

TABLE 8-5 American Association for the Surgery of Trauma Hepatic Organ Injury Scale

Grade[a]		Injury Description
I	Hematoma	Subcapsular, nonexpanding <10 cm surface area
	Laceration	Capsular tear, nonbleeding; ≤1 cm parenchymal depth
II	Hematoma	Subcapsular, nonexpanding, 10–50% surface area; intra-parenchymal nonexpanding ≤10 in diameter
	Laceration	Capsular tear, active bleeding; 1–3 cm parenchymal depth. <10 cm in length
III	Hematoma	Subcapsular, >50% surface area or expanding; ruptured sub-capsular hematoma with active bleeding; intraparenchymal hematoma >10 cm or expanding
	Laceration	>3 cm parenchymal depth
IV	Hematoma	Ruptured intraparenchymal hematoma with active bleeding
	Laceration	Parenchymal disruption involving 25–75% of hepatic lobe or 1–3 Couinaud segments within a single lobe
V	Laceration	Parenchymal disruption involving >75% of hepatic lobe or >3 Couinaud segments within a single lobe
	Vascular	Juxtahepatic venous injuries (i.e., retrohepatic vena cava/central major hepatic veins)
VI	Vascular	Hepatic avulsion

[a]Advance one grade for multiple injuries, up to grade III.
[b]International Classification of Diseases, 9th Revision.
[c]Abbreviated Injury Scale, 1990.
Adapted from Mattox K, Moore E, Feliciano D (eds.). *Trauma*, 7th ed. New York, NY: McGraw-Hill; 2012.

are not contraindications for nonoperative management; however, these factors increase the chances for failure during nonoperative management. The presence of fluid in the pelvis in the setting of solid organ injury requires observation. Significant transfusion requirements or hemodynamic instability should warrant operative exploration.

Peritonitis may indicate missed hollow viscus injury. Free fluid in the pelvis on CT scan may be a result of the

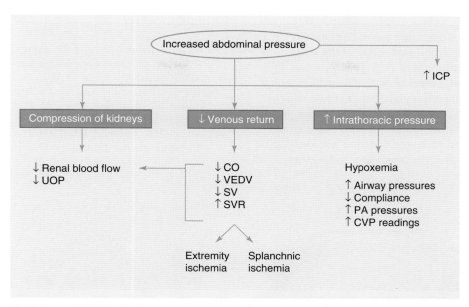

FIGURE 8-24. Pathophysiology of abdominal compartment syndrome. CO, carbon monoxide; CVP, central venous pressure; ICP, intracranial pressure; PA, pulmonary artery; SV, stroke volume; SVR, systemic vascular resistance; UOP, urine output; VEDV, ventricular end-diastolic volume. From Brunicardi F, Andersen DK, Billiar TR, et al. (eds.), *Schwartz's Principles of Surgery*, 10th ed. New York, NY: McGraw-Hill; 2014.

solid organ injury; however, a mesenteric or bowel injury may still exist. As a result, these injuries are occasionally missed. Other useful findings suggestive of small bowel injury on abdominal CT include pneumoperitoneum, focal bowel wall thickening, mesenteric hematoma, mesenteric fat streaking, or extravasation of oral or intravenous contrast. Surgeons should be suspicious of unexplained tachycardia, leukocytosis, hypotension, metabolic acidosis, and changes in the abdominal examination in patients managed nonoperatively for solid organ injuries.

BIBLIOGRAPHY

Moore EE, Cogbill TH, Jurkovich GJ, et al. Organ injury scaling: spleen and liver (1994 Edition). *J Trauma* 1995;38:323.

Fabian TC, Bee TK. Liver and biliary tract. In: Mattox KL, Moore EE, Feliciano DV (eds.), *Trauma*, 7th ed. New York, NY: McGraw-Hill; 2013:Chapter 29.

Fakhry SM, Watts DD, Luchette FA, EAST Multi-Institutional HVI Research Group. Current diagnostic approaches lack sensitivity in the diagnosis of perforated blunt small bowel injury: analysis from 275,557 trauma admissions from the EAST multi-institutional HVI trial. *J Trauma* 2003;54:295–306.

34. **(E)** Abdominal compartment syndrome (ACS) is the adverse clinical consequence of an acute increase in intra-abdominal pressure following trauma. The generally accepted parameters for defining this syndrome include an increase in intra-abdominal pressure above 20 cmH$_2$O, peak airway pressure of greater than 40 cmH$_2$O, oxygen saturation of less than 90% on 100% oxygen, and oxygen delivery index of less than 600 mL/m^2/min, as well as oliguria of less than 0.5 mL/kg/min (Fig. 8-24).

ACS is seen in a variety of clinical situations including abdominal trauma and severe sepsis and leads to decreased urine output, increased pulmonary inspiratory pressures, decreased cardiac preload, and increased cardiac afterload.

Leaving the fascia open prevents ACS in high-risk patients. These include patients with extensive intra-abdominal injuries, prolonged surgical intervention, and massive resuscitation efforts. Placing catheters into the bladder, stomach, or inferior vena cava allows indirect measurements of intra-abdominal pressures. Based on these measurements, recommendations regarding management have been proposed (Table 8-6).

TABLE 8-6 Grading of Abdominal Compartment Syndrome

Grade	Bladder Pressure (mmHg)	Recommendation
I	10–15	Maintain normovolemia
II	16–25	Hypervolemic resuscitation
III	26–35	Decompression
IV	>35	Decompression and reexploration

Treatment for ACS is decompressive laparotomy, either in the ICU or operating room. Once the abdomen is reopened and decompressed, many of the ventilation, cardiac, and renal findings of ACS quickly reverse. Further operative management of ACS may include several techniques. The simplest is placement of towel clips to close the skin along the midline incision, leaving the fascia open. Commonly, temporary silos and vacuum-assisted wound closure devices are used (see Fig. 8-25). Others include zippers, open packing, and meshes.

BIBLIOGRAPHY

Ali J. Torso trauma. In: Hall JB, Schmidt GA, Wood LH (eds.), *Principles of Critical Care*, 3rd ed. New York, NY: McGraw-Hill; 2005:Chapter 95.

Burlew CN, Moore EE. Trauma. In: Brunicardi F, Andersen DK, Billiar TR, et al (eds.), *Schwartz's Principles of Surgery*, 10th ed. New York, NY: McGraw-Hill; 2014.

Cheatham ML, Malbrain ML, Kirkpatrick A, et al. Results from the international conference of experts on intra-abdominal

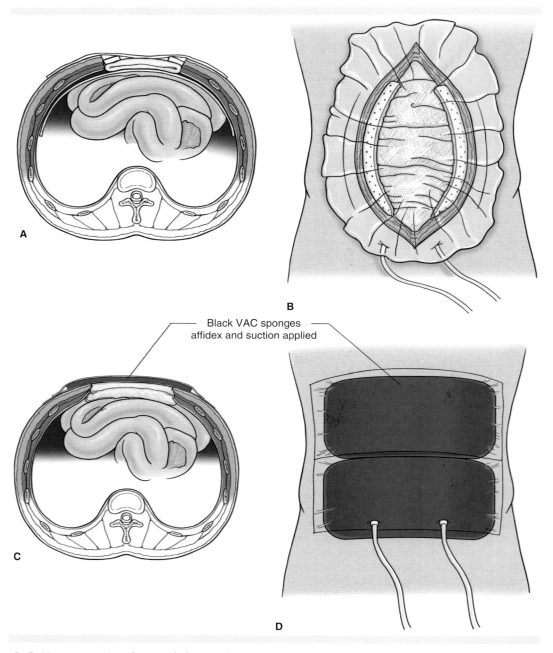

Black VAC sponges affidex and suction applied

FIGURE 8-25. A–D. Vacuum-assisted wound closure device. From Mattox K, Moore E, Feliciano D (eds.). *Trauma*, 7th ed. New York, NY: McGraw-Hill; 2012.

hypertension and abdominal compartment syndrome. II. Recommendations. *Intensive Care Med* 2007;33:951–962.

35. **(C)** Hyperamylasemia is not a reliable marker for pancreatic injury due to its poor sensitivity and specificity. However, in a patient with epigastric pain after blunt abdominal trauma, hyperamylasemia should prompt further investigation with abdominal CT. Abdominal CT findings suspicious for pancreatic injury include parenchymal fracture or hematoma, active hemorrhage from the gland or blood between the pancreas and splenic vein, and edema or hematoma of the parenchyma (see Fig. 8-26).

Diagnosis by CT remains difficult, with sensitivity for pancreatic ductal injury of approximately 50%. In hemodynamically stable patients with subtle CT findings and without clinical indications for laparotomy, MRCP and ERCP can be used to evaluate pancreatic duct injury. If a high suspicion of pancreatic injury remains, surgical exploration is warranted. Patients who are hemodynamically abnormal or have pancreatic injury diagnosed intraoperatively can undergo intraoperative pancreatography for ductal assessment.

BIBLIOGRAPHY

Biffl WL. Duodenum and pancreas. In: Mattox KL, Moore EE, Feliciano DV (eds.), *Trauma*, 7th ed. New York, NY: McGraw-Hill; 2013:Chapter 32.

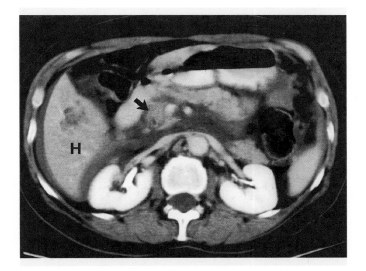

FIGURE 8-26. Computed tomography scan of pancreas, demonstrating subtle early signs of injury, including irregularity of the neck of the pancreas (*arrow*), peripancreatic fluid, and intrahepatic hematoma (H). Reproduced with permission from Smith DR, Stanley RJ, Rue LW III: Delayed diagnosis of pancreatic transection after blunt abdominal trauma. *J Trauma* 40:1009, 1996.

TABLE 8-7 American Association for the Surgery of Trauma Colon Injury Scale

Grade	Injury Description
I	(a) Contusion or hematoma without devascularization
	(b) Partial-thickness laceration
II	Laceration ≤50% of circumference
III	Laceration >50% of circumference
IV	Transection of the colon
V	Transection of the colon with segmental tissue loss

Reproduced with permission from Blumgart LH, ed. *Surgery of the Liver and Biliary Tract.* New York: Churchill Livingstone; 1988. © Elsevier.

Fisher M, Brasel, K. Evolving management of pancreatic injury. *Curr Opin Crit Care.* 2011;17:613–617.

36. **(D)** The colon is the second most common organ injured in victims of abdominal gunshot wounds and the most common organ injured in victims of posterior stab wounds. Diagnosis is frequently made via intraoperative assessment at the time of laparotomy; all paracolic hematomas should be explored in patients with penetrating trauma to the abdomen (Table 8-7). CT with IV contrast also has a 96% sensitivity, and findings include free gas, unexplained free peritoneal fluid, and thickened colonic wall.

Nondestructive injuries include those involving <50% of the bowel wall and without devascularization. Multiple prospective, randomized studies have demonstrated safe routine primary repair of all nondestructive colon injuries (Table 8-8). Destructive colon injuries include those with loss of more than 50% of the bowel wall circumference or with devascularization and that require a segmental colonic resection. In these settings, diversion is considered for patients with shock, significant associated injuries, peritonitis, or underlying disease. However, relative risk of abdominal septic complications is similar between both patient groups.

BIBLIOGRAPHY

Demetriades D, Inaba K. Colon and rectal trauma. In: Mattox KL, Moore EE, Feliciano DV (eds.), *Trauma*, 7th ed. New York, NY: McGraw-Hill; 2012:Chapter 33.

Demetriades D, Murray JA, Chan L, et al. Penetrating colon injuries requiring resection: diversion or primary anastomosis? An AAST prospective multicenter study. *J Trauma* 2001;50(5): 765–775.

TABLE 8-8 Primary Repair Versus Diversion: Prospective Randomized Studies With No Exclusion Criteria

| Study | Primary Repair | | Diversion | |
	No. of Patients	Abdominal Septic Complications	No. of Patients	Abdominal Complications
Chappuis et al.	28	4 (14.3%)	28	5 (17.9%)
Sasaki	43	1 (2.3%)	28	8 (28.6%)
Gonzalez	89	16 (18%)	87	18 (21%)
Total	160	21 (13.1%)	143	31 (21.7%)

Adapted from Mattox K, Moore E, Feliciano D (eds.). *Trauma*, 7th ed. New York, NY: McGraw-Hill; 2012.

Miller PR, Fabian TC, Croce MA, et al. Improving outcomes following penetrating colon wounds. *Ann Surg* 2002;235(6):775–781.

37. **(B)** Bladder rupture may result from sudden compression of the full bladder, shear forces, or a pelvic fracture and is generally accompanied by lower abdominal pain, an inability to void, and suprapubic or perineal ecchymoses. Over 80% of patients with blunt bladder ruptures have associated pelvic fractures, and over 95% of patients with bladder rupture have gross hematuria on presentation.

The diagnosis is made using stress cystography. The bladder is filled with 300–400 mL of contrast, and a plain abdominal radiograph or abdominal CT is taken. Underfilling the bladder may result in false-negative studies. The extravasation pattern determines whether the bladder rupture is intraperitoneal or extraperitoneal (see Fig. 8-27).

The standard treatment for extraperitoneal bladder ruptures is catheter drainage for 10–14 days followed by repeat cystogram. On repeat cystogram, over 85% of extraperitoneal ruptures will have resolved. If there is evidence of a persistent extraperitoneal bladder rupture, then continued catheter drainage for an additional 7–10 days is recommended followed by repeat cystogram. After additional drainage, persistent extraperitoneal ruptures are rare, and CT or cystoscopy is performed to evaluate for foreign bodies. With rare exception, intraperitoneal bladder perforations are uniformly repaired with operative management.

BIBLIOGRAPHY

Burlew CN, Moore EE. Trauma. In: Brunicardi F, Andersen DK, Billiar TR, et al (eds.), *Schwartz's Principles of Surgery*, 10th ed. New York, NY: McGraw-Hill; 2014.

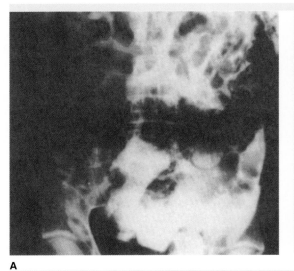
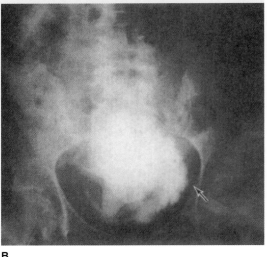

A   B

FIGURE 8-27. A. Intraperitoneal bladder rupture. Cystogram shows contrast surrounding loops of bowel. **B.** Extraperitoneal bladder rupture. Extravasation (at *arrow*) seen outside the bladder in the pelvis on cystogram. From McAninch J, Lue TF. *Smith and Tanagho's General Urology*, 18th ed. New York, NY: McGraw-Hill; 2012.

Coburn M. Genitourinary trauma. In: Mattox KL, Moore EE, Feliciano DV (eds.), *Trauma*, 7th ed. New York, NY: McGraw-Hill; 2013:Chapter 36.

38. **(B)** Small bowel injuries secondary to blunt abdominal trauma are increasing in incidence because of high-velocity motor vehicle crashes and mandatory seat belt laws.

The proposed mechanisms of injury include (1) crushing of bowel against spine, (2) tearing of bowel from mesentery by sudden deceleration, and (3) rupture of a closed loop of bowel under high intraluminal pressure.

A physical finding of ecchymoses along the anterior abdominal wall is referred to as the "seat belt sign" and may indicate underlying small bowel injuries. The "seat belt syndrome" refers to the complex of injuries including lumbar fractures, abdominal or chest wall ecchymoses, and small bowel injuries.

Isolated small bowel injury is found in up to 70% of patients who are ultimately found to have blunt small bowel injury.

BIBLIOGRAPHY

Diebel LN. Stomach and small bowel. In: Mattox KL, Moore EE, Feliciano DV (eds.), *Trauma*, 7th ed. New York, NY: McGraw-Hill; 2012:Chapter 31.
McNutt MK, Chinapuvvula NR, Beckmann NM, et al. (2015). Early surgical intervention for blunt bowel injury: the Bowel Injury Prediction Score (BIPS). *J Trauma Acute Care Surg* 2015;78(1):105–111.

39. **(A)** The CT image demonstrates a large duodenal hematoma without contrast extravasation. Approximately one-third of duodenal hematomas present with signs of obstruction 48 hours or more following blunt abdominal trauma (Table 8-9). This is likely caused by fluid shifts causing expansion of the hematoma. Radiographic findings include the presence of retroperitoneal hematoma on abdominal CT and narrowing of the duodenum on upper GI radiograph.

The management of duodenal hematomas is generally nonsurgical. Conservative management consisting of nasogastric suction, and total parenteral nutrition is recommended until the obstruction resolves. Serial upper GI studies should be performed at regular intervals of 5–7 days if obstruction is not resolving. If there is no resolution of symptoms by 2 weeks, surgical exploration with evacuation of hematoma may be appropriate to evaluate for pancreatic injury, duodenal perforation, or stricture. One study reviewing conservative management of duodenal hematomas reported an average hospitalization of 16 days (and 9 days of total parenteral nutrition) until resolution of symptoms.

TABLE 8-9 American Association for the Surgery of Trauma Duodenum Organ Injury Scale

Grade		Injury Description
I	Hematoma	Involving single portion of duodenum
	Laceration	Partial thickness, no perforation
II	Hematoma	Involving more than one portion
	Laceration	Disruption <50% of circumference
III	Laceration	Disruption 50–75% circumference of D2
		Disruption 50–100% circumference of D1, D3, D4
IV	Laceration	Disruption >75% circumference of D2
		Involving ampulla or distal common bile duct
V	Laceration	Massive disruption of duodenopancreatic complex
	Vascular	Devascularization of duodenum

From Mattox K, Moore E, Feliciano D (eds.). *Trauma*, 7th ed. New York, NY: McGraw-Hill; 2012.

BIBLIOGRAPHY

Bendinelli C, Yoshino O. Surgical treatment of duodenal trauma. In: *Trauma Surgery*. Milan, Italy: Springer; 2014:135–149.
Biffl WL. Duodenum and pancreas. In: Mattox KL, Moore EE, Feliciano DV (eds.), *Trauma*, 7th ed. New York, NY: McGraw-Hill; 2013:Chapter 32.

40. **(D)** Injuries that interfere with breathing should be detected during the primary survey—they include tension pneumothorax, flail chest, open pneumothorax, and massive hemothorax. Tension pneumothorax caused by either penetrating or blunt trauma develops when air continuously enters pleural space from the lung, bronchi, or trachea or through the chest wall and cannot escape and causes the lung to collapse. Eventually, intrapleural pressure increases and causes shifting of the mediastinum, which decreases venous return and results in decreased cardiac output.

Clinically, a sense of impending death, marked by respiratory distress, deviated trachea, distended neck

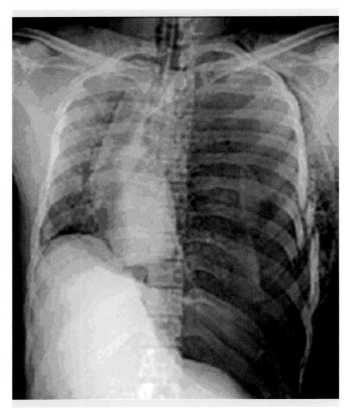

FIGURE 8-28. Chest x-ray demonstrating tension pneumothorax. From Sugarbaker D, Bueno R, Krasna M, Mentzer S. *Adult Chest Surgery*. New York, NY: McGraw-Hill; 2009.

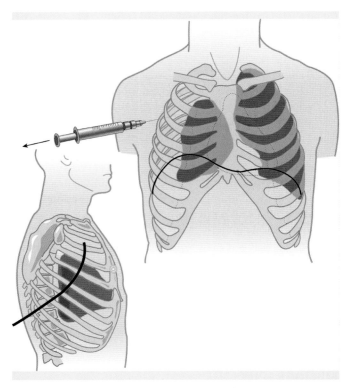

FIGURE 8-29. Needle decompression of tension pneumothorax. From Doherty GM (ed.). *Current Diagnosis & Treatment: Surgery*, 13th ed. New York, NY: McGraw-Hill; 2010.

veins, unilateral absence of breath sounds, cyanosis, and hypotension, may be seen. Diagnosis is generally clinical and not radiographic (see Fig. 8-28).

Treatment requires immediate decompression with a needle thoracentesis using a 14-gauge catheter over a needle inserted in the second intercostal space, midclavicular line. A rush of air escaping the catheter confirms diagnosis (see Fig. 8-29). This converts the tension component to a simple pneumothorax. Absence of rush of air suggests misdiagnosis or insertion of the needle into the wrong hemithorax.

If the diagnosis of tension pneumothorax still seems likely, the initial catheter is left in the chest, and the opposite hemithorax is punctured. When the needle thoracentesis confirms the presence of tension pneumothorax, tube thoracostomy should follow to provide immediate definitive treatment.

BIBLIOGRAPHY

Ali J. Torso trauma. In: Hall JB, Schmidt GA, Wood LH (eds.), *Principles of Critical Care*, 3rd ed. New York, NY: McGraw-Hill; 2005:Chapter 95.

Moore E, Feliciano D, Mattox K. *Trauma*, 5th ed. New York, NY: McGraw-Hill; 2004.

Salomone JP, Salomone JA III. Prehospital care. In: Mattox KL, Moore EE, Feliciano DV (eds.), *Trauma*, 7th ed. New York, NY: McGraw-Hill; 2012:Chapter 7.

Taylor JT, Smith MA. Benign pleural disorders. In: Yuh DD, Vricella LA, Yang SC, Doty JR (eds.), *Johns Hopkins Textbook of Cardiothoracic Surgery*, 2nd ed. New York, NY: McGraw-Hill; 2014.

41. **(C)** A flail chest occurs when three or more adjacent ribs are each fractured in two or more locations (see Fig. 8-30). This causes an unstable or floating segment of chest wall that moves paradoxically during respiration. A pneumothorax or hemothorax may be present. A more significant injury, however, is associated with pulmonary contusion leading to hemorrhage and edema of the injured lung. A chest wall injury of this magnitude is also associated with significant pain, and respiratory efficiency is reduced. In addition to increased work of breathing, flail chest is associated with pulmonary contusion, which results in decreased pulmonary compliance and increased shunt fraction.

Initial chest x-rays in patients with flail chest may be normal or show minimal pulmonary contusion, which progresses over the first 12 hours after injury. Treatment

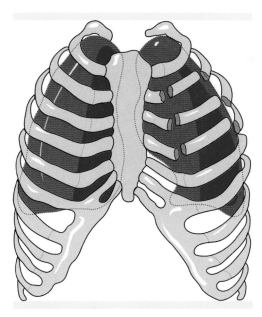

FIGURE 8-30. Flail chest. From Doherty GM (ed.). *Current Diagnosis & Treatment: Surgery*, 13th ed. New York, NY: McGraw-Hill; 2010.

is directed toward reversing hypoventilation caused by the pain and hypoxia caused by the associated pulmonary contusion. Careful monitoring of ventilation and oxygenation is required, and intubation and ventilatory support may be indicated in 20–40% of patients. Control of pain caused by multiple rib fractures by using regional anesthetic techniques such as intercostal nerve block, insertion of intrapleural catheter, or insertion of an epidural catheter is important to improve respiratory mechanics. A recent meta-analysis showed reduced ventilator and ICU days, as well as decreased mortality and need for tracheostomy, in patients with flail chest who underwent surgical fixation versus supportive ventilation and analgesia. However, most studies to date have been small retrospective analyses.

BIBLIOGRAPHY

Leinicke JA, Elmore L, Freeman BD, Colditz GA. Operative management of rib fractures in the setting of flail chest: a systematic review and meta-analysis. *Ann Surg* 2013;258:914–921.

Moore E, Feliciano D, Mattox K. *Trauma*, 5th ed. New York, NY: McGraw-Hill; 2004.

Slobogean GP, MacPherson CA, Sun T, Pelletier ME, Hameed SM. Surgical fixation vs nonoperative management of flail chest: a meta-analysis. *J Am Coll Surg* 2013;216:302–311.

42. **(E)** Blunt esophageal trauma is uncommon but may result from a direct blow to the organ, usually in the neck, or from increased intraluminal pressures against a closed glottis causing a bursting-type injury. Intrathoracic esophageal injuries tend to occur just proximal to the esophagogastric junction on the left side where the esophagus has less protection by the pleural lining and heart. This injury is thought to be a result of increased intra-abdominal pressure transmitted to the stomach. The resulting mediastinitis and immediate or delayed rupture into the pleural space may be lethal if unrecognized.

For blunt trauma, determining which victims need further study for esophageal injury is a vexing task. Esophageal injury should be considered for any patient who (1) has a left pneumothorax or hemothorax or pleural effusion without a rib fracture, (2) has received a severe blow to the lower sternum or epigastrium and is in pain or shock out of proportion to the apparent injury, or (3) has particulate matter in the chest tube after the blood begins to clear. Presence of a pneumomediastinum also suggests the diagnosis.

Treatment entails placement of a tube thoracostomy for drainage. If output is suggestive of gastric contents or an injury is otherwise clinically suspected, a contrast study or an upper GI endoscopy is indicated to evaluate for the esophageal injury (see Fig. 8-31).

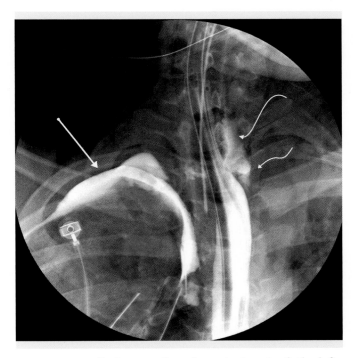

FIGURE 8-31. Barium swallow shows leak on both the left side of the cervical esophagus (*curved arrows*) and the right thoracic esophagus (*straight arrow*). From Mattox K, Moore E, Feliciano D (eds.). *Trauma*, 7th ed. New York, NY: McGraw-Hill; 2012.

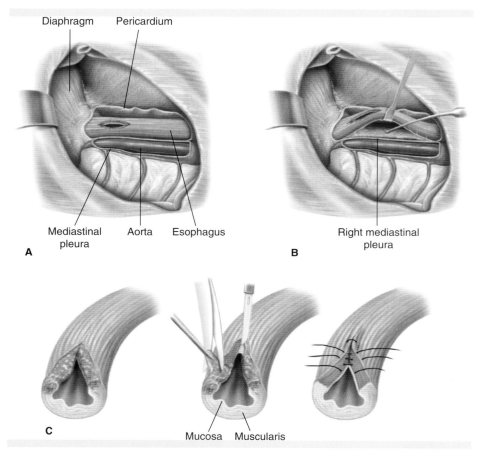

FIGURE 8-32. Repair of esophageal injury. Reproduced with permission from Maurice Hood R, ed. *Thoracic Surgery: Techniques in General Thoracic Surgery.* Philadelphia: WB Saunders Company; 1985.

Surgical repair entails local debridement, wide drainage, primary repair of the perforation, and buttressing with a pedicle flap for viable muscle (see Fig. 8-32).

BIBLIOGRAPHY

DuBose JA, O'Connor JV, Scalea TM. Lung, trachea, and esophagus. In: Mattox K, Moore E, Feliciano D (eds.). *Trauma*, 7th ed. New York, NY: McGraw-Hill; 2012:Chapter 25.

Paul S, Chang MY. Blunt and penetrating esophageal trauma. In: Sugarbaker DJ, Bueno R, Krasna MJ, Mentzer SJ, Zellos L (eds.), *Adult Chest Surgery.* New York, NY: McGraw-Hill; 2009: Chapter 41.

43. **(B)** Injury to the tracheobronchial tree is a rare but well-recognized complication of both penetrating and blunt chest trauma. Most victims die prior to emergency care from associated injuries to vital structures, hemorrhage, tension pneumothorax, or respiratory insufficiency from lack of adequate airway. The reported incidence of injury to the trachea or bronchus varies from 0.2 to 8%. Greater than 80% of tracheobronchial ruptures occur within 2.5 cm of the carina.

The presentation of thoracic tracheobronchial injury depends on whether the injury is confined to the mediastinum or communicates with the pleural space. Thoracic tracheobronchial injuries confined to the mediastinum usually present with massive pneumomediastinum. Injuries that do perforate into the pleural space usually create an ipsilateral pneumothorax. If the pneumothorax persists despite adequate placement of a chest tube and has a continuous air leak, it is suggestive of a tracheobronchial injury and bronchopleural fistula. A pathognomonic radiographic feature termed "fallen lung sign" includes the affected lung falling away from the hilum, laterally and posteriorly, in contrast to the usual pneumothorax, which collapses toward the hilum.

Evaluation of a patient with a tracheobronchial injury involves immediate tube thoracostomy. If persistent atelectasis, collapse, or massive air leak is noted, a bronchoscopy is the most reliable means of establishing the diagnosis and determining the site, nature, and extent of tracheobronchial disruption. Lesions selected for observation must involve less than one-third the circumference of the tracheobronchial tree

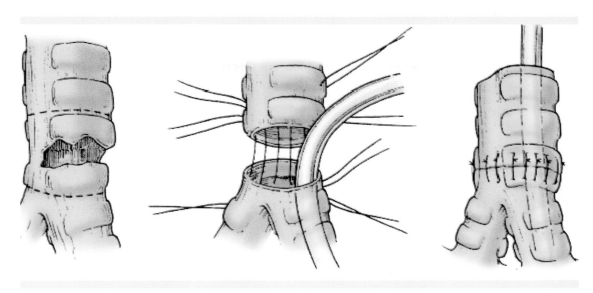

FIGURE 8-33. Repair of tracheal injury. From Yuh DD, Vricella LA, Yang SC, Doty JR (eds.). *Johns Hopkins Textbook of Cardiothoracic Surgery*, 2nd ed. New York, NY: McGraw-Hill; 2014.

with well-opposed edges and no tissue loss. Tube thoracostomy must fully expand the lung, and air leaks stop soon after insertion of the tube. There must be no associated injuries and no need for positive-pressure ventilation. Prophylactic antibiotics, humidified oxygen, voice rest, frequent suctioning, and close observation for sepsis and airway obstruction are required. If the aforementioned criteria are not met, operative repair is warranted. Optimal repair includes adequate debridement of devitalized tissue, including cartilage, and a tension-free primary end-to-end anastomosis of clean tracheal or bronchial ends with a buttressed vascularized pedicle (see Fig. 8-33).

BIBLIOGRAPHY

DuBose JA, O'Connor JV, Scalea TM. Lung, trachea, and esophagus. In: Mattox KL, Moore EE, Feliciano DV (eds.), *Trauma*, 7th ed. New York, NY: McGraw-Hill; 2013:Chapter 25.

Kaiser AC, O'Brian SM, Detterbeck FC. Blunt tracheobronchial injuries: treatment and outcomes. *Ann Thorac Surg* 2001;71(6):2059.

Koenig GJ Jr, Efron DT. Thoracic trauma. In: Yuh DD, Vricella LA, Yang SC, Doty JR (eds.), *Johns Hopkins Textbook of Cardiothoracic Surgery*, 2nd ed. New York, NY: McGraw-Hill; 2014.

44. **(E)** A traumatic diaphragmatic rupture typically results from the rapid increase in intra-abdominal pressure related to an episode of blunt trauma with subsequent rupture of the diaphragm. The diagnosis may be difficult in part because the force of injury is likely to result in multiple organ damage. A traumatic diaphragmatic rupture is more commonly diagnosed on the left side, and the stomach is the most common organ involved. Right diaphragmatic injuries are rarely diagnosed in the early postinjury period as the liver often prevents herniation of other abdominal organs into the chest.

The diagnosis of diaphragm rupture will often be missed initially because of misinterpretation of chest x-ray as showing an elevated diaphragm, acute gastric dilatation, a loculated pneumohemothorax, or subpulmonary hematoma. Often the chest radiograph will show opacification within the affected pleural cavity, air fluid levels, and mediastinal shift (see Fig. 8-34).

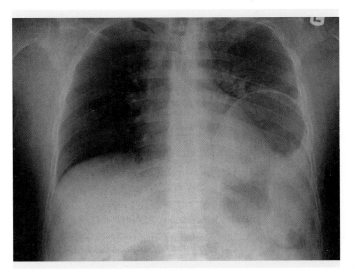

FIGURE 8-34. Chest x-ray showing diaphragmatic rupture. From Mattox K, Moore E, Feliciano D (eds.). *Trauma*, 7th ed. New York, NY: McGraw-Hill; 2012.

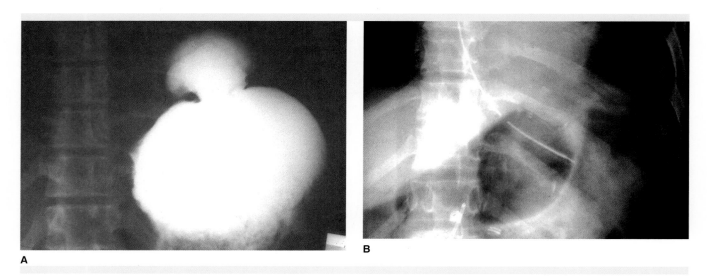

FIGURE 8-35. **A.** Diaphragmatic rupture on upper gastrointestinal imaging demonstrates a narrow area of barium entering the chest. **B.** Scout film shows compression of the gastric shadow. From Mattox K, Moore E, Feliciano D (eds.). *Trauma*, 7th ed. New York, NY: McGraw-Hill; 2012.

If a laceration of the left diaphragm is suspected, a nasogastric tube should be inserted. If the nasogastric tube appears in the thoracic cavity on the chest film, the need for contrast studies is eliminated and the patient should undergo immediate laparotomy. An upper GI contrast study should be performed if the diagnosis is not clear (see Fig. 8-35). Treatment for acute cases involves exploratory laparotomy for reduction of the herniated contents, inspection for other intra-abdominal injury, and diaphragm repair.

BIBLIOGRAPHY

Ali J. Torso trauma. In: Hall JB, Schmidt GA, Wood LH (eds.), *Principles of Critical Care*, 3rd ed. New York, NY: McGraw-Hill; 2005:Chapter 95.

Schuster KM, Davis KA. Diaphragm. In: Mattox KL, Moore EE, Feliciano DV (eds.), *Trauma*, 7th ed. New York, NY: McGraw-Hill; 2013:Chapter 28.

CHAPTER 9

BURNS

ELEANOR CURTIS, KATHLEEN ROMANOWSKI, RACHEL RUSSO, AND DAVID GREENHALGH

QUESTIONS

1. Which of the following cell types are found in the dermis?
   - (A) Fibroblasts
   - (B) Langerhans
   - (C) Keratinocytes
   - (D) Merkel cells
   - (E) Melanocytes

2. Platelet microthrombus formation and vascular constriction occur in which of the zones of burn injury?
   - (A) Zone of hyperemia
   - (B) Zone of stasis
   - (C) Zone of coagulation
   - (D) Zone of necrosis

3. Early increased microvascular permeability is caused by release of which mediator?
   - (A) Thromboxane A_2
   - (B) Histamine
   - (C) Catecholamines
   - (D) Oxygen free radicals
   - (E) Interleukin (IL)-6

4. An 11-month-old white female pulled a pot of hot grease off the stove and sustained burns to her chin, chest, and abdomen. On initial evaluation in the emergency room (ER), her wounds are noted to be dark red and dry in the central portion of the wound. This patient has most likely sustained a
   - (A) First-degree burn
   - (B) Superficial partial-thickness burn
   - (C) Fourth-degree burn
   - (D) Full-thickness burn

5. Burn edema is multifactorial, influenced by systemic and local cell mediators. Which of the following statements regarding burn edema is *true*?
   - (A) It is maximal after 48 hours.
   - (B) It decreases water and protein loss from the capillaries.
   - (C) It occurs in burned and unburned tissues.
   - (D) It is improved with excessive fluid resuscitation.

6. A 52-year-old man weighing 70 kg sustained a 65% total body surface area (TBSA) burn. What volume accurately represents his fluid requirements?
   - (A) 8000 mL in 24 h
   - (B) 18,200 mL in 16 h
   - (C) 12,800 mL in 24 h
   - (D) 9100 mL in 8 h

7. A 10-kg child with 0.5 m² TBSA pulled a pot of hot water off the stove and sustained a 30% TBSA burn. What volume best represents the child's calculated fluid requirements for the first 24 hours?
   - (A) 1200 mL in 24 h
   - (B) 2200 mL in 24 h
   - (C) 2000 mL in 24 h
   - (D) 1500 mL in 24 h

8. A 65-year-old chronic smoker presents with 2% TBSA facial burns after smoking on his porch while wearing oxygen by nasal cannula. His carboxyhemoglobin was 10% on admission. Which of the following is true?
   - (A) He most likely suffered a severe inhalation injury and should be intubated immediately.
   - (B) He has a moderate inhalation injury and should be placed on 100% nonrebreather until his carboxyhemoglobin normalizes.
   - (C) This is a normal carboxyhemoglobin level for a chronic smoker. He should continue nasal oxygen at his home dose and be monitored in the hospital until he can independently manage wound care.
   - (D) This carboxyhemoglobin is abnormally low for a smoker of his age and the number should be repeated.

9. A 4-year-old child was brought in with burns. Which of the following would make you suspect the child may have an inhalation injury?
   (A) A flash burn from a campfire with singed eyebrows and arm burns
   (B) Splash pattern burns on the nose, chin, and anterior chest from hot beverage spill
   (C) Cigarette burns on extremities
   (D) Structural fire in which the patient was found unconscious and rescued by emergency medical services (EMS)

10. What is the gold standard for diagnosing inhalation injury?
    (A) Chest x-ray
    (B) Computed tomography (CT) scan
    (C) Bronchoscopy
    (D) Burns to face

11. In a 45-year-old man with a 25% TBSA full-thickness burn to the trunk, arms, neck, and face, which of the following is an indication for escharotomy?
    (A) Circumferential burns of the forearm with interstitial tissue pressure of 35 mmHg
    (B) Mean airway pressures to 28 mmHg H$_2$O
    (C) Swelling of lips and tongue
    (D) Loss of radial pulse

12. Which of the following would make you suspect child abuse?
    (A) "V" shape scald burns extending from the chin to the umbilicus from pulling hot water off a stove
    (B) Flame burn to volar forearm from camp fire
    (C) Burn to chest and underarm from candle setting shirt on fire
    (D) Stocking distribution to lower legs and feet from bathing self

13. A 3-year-old child with a 40% TBSA burn to the trunk, arms, and scalp is brought to the operating room in preparation for a tangential excision of approximately 20% TBSA. Which of the following measures is most important in assuring a safe procedure?
    (A) Placement of a new subclavian vein catheter
    (B) Measurement of serum lactate level
    (C) Increasing ambient operating room temperature near or above 108°F
    (D) Transfusion of platelets and fresh frozen plasma in the preoperative period

14. A 30-year-old firefighter sustained 55% TBSA burns 6 days ago. Which of the following assessments demonstrates adequate nutritional support?
    (A) Low serum retinol-binding protein
    (B) Indirect calorimetry with a calculated respiratory quotient (RQ) of less than 0.8

    (C) Serum albumin of 2.5
    (D) Prealbumin of 20

15. Which of the following is *true* regarding burn hypermetabolism?
    (A) The patient's homeostatic thermostat remains unchanged.
    (B) There are decreased levels of circulating catecholamines.
    (C) Patients prefer to set the ambient room temperature to 65°F.
    (D) There is protein catabolism in skeletal muscles.

16. Enteral feeding is preferred to parenteral feeding in the burn patient for which of the following reasons?
    (A) Provision of carbohydrate calories
    (B) Avoidance of gastric ileus
    (C) Replacement of trace minerals
    (D) Reduced complications compared to total parenteral nutrition
    (E) Decreased risk of diarrhea

17. Deficiency of which of the following results in impaired collagen synthesis secondary to deficient hydroxylation of lysine and proline?
    (A) Selenium
    (B) Zinc
    (C) Ascorbic acid
    (D) Iron
    (E) Vitamin E

18. Anemia in the burn patient is frequently secondary to
    (A) Idiopathic reaction to silver sulfadiazine
    (B) Decreased circulating erythropoietin
    (C) Depletion of bone marrow progenitor cells
    (D) Increased erythrocyte fragility
    (E) Microthrombus formation

19. A 42-year-old man is intubated 1 week after a 53% TBSA burn with inhalation injury. The patient has had two operative excisions with grafting and currently has an increasing white blood cell (WBC) count to 20, temperature spikes to 103°F, oliguria, and hypotension. The most common source of sepsis in this patient is
    (A) Invasive burn wound infection
    (B) Urosepsis from indwelling catheters
    (C) Pneumonia
    (D) Central line–associated bloodstream infection

20. A decrease in cardiac output immediately following thermal injury is due in part to
    (A) Decreased systemic vascular resistance
    (B) Decreased venous return
    (C) Increased left ventricular distensibility
    (D) Norepinephrine release

21. Match the topical antimicrobial to its side effect.
    (A) Silver sulfadiazine (a) nephrotoxicity
    (B) Silver nitrate   (b) leukopenia
    (C) Mafenide   (c) metabolic acidosis
    (D) Bacitracin   (d) hyponatremia, hypochloremia

22. A 40-year-old electrical lineman is injured on an electric pole and is brought to the emergency department unconscious. He has an area on his left hand that is charred, evidence of thermal injury to the arm, and an exit wound on his right knee. Which of the following interventions is the first priority?
    (A) Escharotomy of the left arm
    (B) CT scan of the abdomen and pelvis
    (C) Endotracheal intubation
    (D) CT scan of the head and neck
    (E) Measurement of serum creatinine phosphokinase levels

23. A 24-year-old petroleum worker presents with a burn to his leg approximately 6% TBSA when hydrofluoric acid spilled onto his clothing. In addition to irrigation of the wound with saline, what therapy is indicated?
    (A) Irrigation with dilute sodium hydroxide (NaOH) solution
    (B) Application of dimethyl sulfoxide (DMSO) to the wound area
    (C) Topical application of calcium gluconate solution
    (D) Systemic infusion of magnesium sulfate

24. What initial treatment of frostbite has been shown to preserve limb function/viability?
    (A) Quickly reheating the limb to normal body temperatures
    (B) Intra-arterial tissue plasminogen activator (tPA)
    (C) Intravenous administration of warmed fluids
    (D) Heparin injection

25. The site of injury in toxic epidermal necrolysis syndrome (TENS) and Stevens-Johnson syndrome (SJS) is
    (A) The Nikolsky body
    (B) Superficial to basement membrane
    (C) The dermoepidermal junction
    (D) The endoplasmic reticulum

26. A critical factor in the "take" of a skin autograft is
    (A) Presence of elastin fibers in the graft
    (B) Diffusion of metabolites from wound bed to skin graft
    (C) The patient's intraoperative body temperature
    (D) Securing the graft with sutures or staples

27. Which of the following has a major risk of hypertrophic scar formation?
    (A) Third-degree burn grafted within a week
    (B) Partial-thickness burn that heals at 3 weeks
    (C) Split-thickness donor site that heals within 12 days
    (D) Partial-thickness wound that heals in 10 days

28. A 36-year-old man sustained a 20% TBSA hot water scald burn to his abdomen, genitalia, and right leg. One referral criterion that this patient meets for transfer to a burn center is
    (A) Burn of 20% TBSA or greater
    (B) Patient age
    (C) Scald burns
    (D) Patient sex

29. A 27-year-old lineman was on duty and came in contact with over 12,000 volts. He was found at the scene to be obtunded with obvious deformities in his hands. He was immediately intubated and then transported to the emergency department. What injury is commonly associated with this mechanism of burn?
    (A) Splenic laceration
    (B) Ruptured bowel
    (C) Cervical spine injury
    (D) Ruptured tympanic membrane

30. Which of the following public health interventions has caused the largest reduction in burn injuries?
    (A) Educating children on stop, drop, and roll
    (B) Recommending flame-resistant mattresses for children
    (C) Discussing burn prevention with mothers of infants prior to their children ambulating
    (D) Laws requiring smoke detectors in homes

31. What percentages best represent the TBSA burns of an adult patient with burns to bilateral lower extremities and groin and of an infant with a scald to the entire head?

Adult	Infant
(A) 37%	20%
(B) 49%	10%
(C) 49%	20%
(D) 37%	10%

32. An electrician exposed to 12,000 volts in a rural area is transferred to your facility 8 hours after initial injury. His urine is red-brown. How would you treat his condition?
    (A) Do escharotomies of all limbs
    (B) Increase fluids so that urine output is 100 mL/h
    (C) Start furosemide drip
    (D) Do nothing; the damage has already been done

33. A 19-year-old roofer presents with pain and tar on his legs after slipping on a roof. How would you best examine his wounds?
    (A) Carefully peel tar off wounds
    (B) Use water-based solvent to soften and cool tar to remove
    (C) Use petroleum dressings, changed every 2 hours, until the tar dissolves
    (D) Wait until the skin sloughs off; tar rarely causes deep burns

ANSWERS AND EXPLANATIONS

1. **(A)** The skin is the largest organ of the body and is composed of three distinct layers: the epidermis, the dermis, and the subcutaneous tissue. The epidermis is the most superficial layer and is composed of four separate layers: the basal layer, the stratum spinosum, the stratum granulosum, and the dead epidermis, the stratum corneum.

   The basal layer is the innermost layer and contains mitotically active keratinocytes. Melanocytes are found within the basal layer and provide ultraviolet radiation protection. In the stratum spinosum, the keratinocytes become more differentiated and are joined together by gap junctions that allow for cellular communication. The stratum granulosum is the most highly differentiated layer of the epidermis and is where most keratin production occurs. Most superficial is the stratum corneum, the outside nonliving layer, which is composed of keratin and provides the major barrier to the environment. Found scattered throughout the epidermis are Langerhans cells, which are important in antigen-processing cells, and Merkel cells, which serve as touch receptors.

   The epidermis and dermis are separated by the basement membrane zone. Anchoring fibrils connect these two layers. The dermis consists of a superficial thin layer called the papillary dermis and a deep, dense layer called the reticular dermis. The primary cell of the dermis is the fibroblast that produces the collagen, elastic fibers, and ground substance that compose the bulk of the dermis. Inflammatory cells migrate through the ground substance beneath the dermis, a large plexus of arterioles and venules called the subdermal plexus. This plexus further branches into superficial smaller vessels called the papillary plexus. The skin appendages, sebaceous glands, sweat glands, and hair follicles all lie within the dermis.

   The subcutaneous layer lies beneath the dermis. This layer contains fat cells that serve as an insulating layer for the body and supports blood vessels and nerves that travel into the dermis (see Fig. 9-1).

BIBLIOGRAPHY

Lewis G, Heimbach D, Gibran N. Evaluation of the burn wound: management decisions. In: Herndon D (ed.), *Total Burn Care*, 4th ed. London, United Kingdom: W.B. Saunders; 2012:125–135.

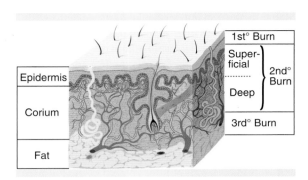

FIGURE 9-1. Layers of the skin. From Demling RH. Burns and other injuries. In: Doherty GM (ed.), *Current Diagnosis & Treatment: Surgery*, 13th ed. New York, NY: McGraw-Hill; 2010:Chapter 14.

Watson K. Structure of the skin. In: Hall J, Hall B (eds.), *Sauer's Manual of Skin Diseases*, 10th ed. Philadelphia, PA: Lippincott Williams & Wilkins; 2010:1–8.

2. **(B)** In 1953, Jackson published "The Diagnosis of the Depth of Burning" in the *British Journal of Surgery*. In this paper, Jackson describes three distinct zones of burn injury, the zones of coagulation, stasis, and hyperemia.

   The zone of coagulation is the area that is in direct contact with the offending agent. In this zone, cellular proteins have denatured and coagulated, cellular necrosis has occurred, and eschar is formed. This tissue has been irreparably damaged extending in both horizontal and vertical dimension. This can happen with 1 second of exposure at 69°C or after an hour at 45°C.

   The zone of stasis lies lateral and deep to the zone of coagulation. In this zone, the cells are injured and dermal capillary stasis occurs. There is a mix of viable and nonviable cells, with capillary vasoconstriction and ischemia. The damage in this region may progress to necrosis or may reverse and allow cellular recovery.

   The outermost zone is the zone of hyperemia. In this zone, cellular injury is minimal, in part because of its distance from the offending agent. Vasodilation occurs in this region because of the inflammatory process. All cells in this region will recover unless infection, further dehydration, or edema occurs (see Fig. 9-2).

BIBLIOGRAPHY

Jackson D. The diagnosis of the depth of burning. *Br J Surg* 1953;40:588–589.

Lewis G, Heimbach D, Gibran N. Evaluation of the burn wound: management decisions. In: Herndon D (ed.), *Total Burn Care*, 4th ed. London: W.B. Saunders; 2012:125–135.

3. **(B)** Histamine is released by mast cells in the thermally injured skin immediately following injury. Histamine causes

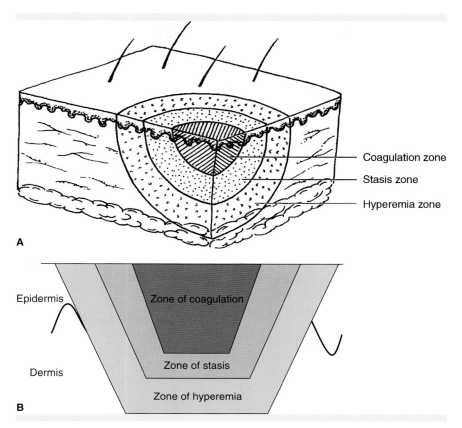

FIGURE 9-2. Zones of burn injury. From Lee J, Herndon D. Burns and radiation. In: Mattox K, Moore E, Feliciano D (eds.), *Trauma*, 7th ed. New York, NY: McGraw-Hill; 2012:Chapter 48.

transient formation of large endothelial gaps as a result of contraction of venular endothelial cells. These actions are only temporary but contribute to wound edema.

Thromboxane A$_2$ is produced locally by platelets. It is a potent vasoconstrictor that can increase edema formation at the site of burn but also plays an important role in the zone of stasis where it can convert a partial-thickness wound to a deeper full-thickness wound with increased ischemia.

Catecholamines are released in massive amounts after burn injury. They constrict arterioles, which can counteract wound edema and can partially inhibit histamine- and bradykinin-induced capillary permeability. Catecholamines can also have deleterious effects on the zone of stasis with increased ischemia.

Activated neutrophils release oxygen radicals after inflammation or reperfusion of ischemic tissue. This can take hours to days and does not play a role in early edema. These radicals can cause oxidation of lipids and proteins, causing proteolysis and creating higher vascular permeability, which contributes to bacterial dissemination. Some clinical trials have suggested a benefit of treatment with antioxidants (vitamin C and E). The use

of very-high-dose vitamin C decreased the fluid requirements of some patients in select trials.

IL-6 is the most consistently elevated cytokine after a burn; however, its function still remains unclear.

BIBLIOGRAPHY

Kramer G. Pathophysiology of burn shock and burn edema. In: Herndon D (ed.), *Total Burn Care*, 4th ed. London, United Kingdom: W.B. Saunders; 2012:103–114.

Murphy E, Sherwood E, Toliver-Kinsky. The immunological response and strategies for intervention. In: Herndon D (ed.), *Total Burn Care*, 4th ed. London, United Kingdom: W.B. Saunders; 2012:265–276.

4. **(D)** Burn wounds are now categorized as superficial or deep. The superficial burn consists of first-degree and superficial partial-thickness (superficial second-degree) burns. A first-degree burn is usually red-pink in appearance. The epidermis has been damaged and may exfoliate in approximately 7 days but has healed underneath by the time of slough. An example of a first-degree burn is a mild sunburn.

A partial-thickness burn implies that damage has occurred to the dermis. These burns can be further subdivided into superficial or deep partial-thickness burns. The superficial partial-thickness burn extends into the papillary dermis. It is characterized by blister formation, and on removal of the blister, the wound is noted to be pink and moist. The burn wound is extremely painful and will blanch easily when compressed. The hair follicles are intact. In a favorable environment, these wounds will heal within a 2- to 3-week period. The injured area is reepithelialized by the epithelial cells lining the dermal appendages: hair follicles and sebaceous glands.

Deep burns consist of deep partial-thickness burns and third-degree burns. These extend into the reticular dermis and below. These burns can be mottled and will likely form an eschar. Eschar is the product of coagulated proteins from the injured skin. The capillary refill of these wounds is slow, and the hair follicles are usually not intact. These wounds may heal in greater than 3 weeks and will most likely produce an unfavorable scar if treated nonsurgically.

Full-thickness or third-degree burn injuries involve the entire thickness of skin. No dermal appendages are viable for reepithelialization. These wounds contain necrotic tissue, and the eschar is usually dry and white or charred in appearance. These wounds may even be dark red in appearance as a result of intravascular coagulation, but they do not blanch with pressure and are generally insensate.

Fourth-degree burns consist of structures burned beneath skin such as muscle, bone, or tendon.

The dermis of small children is proportionally thinner than that of adults and does not reach adult thickness until approximately age 5. The elderly, on the other hand, undergo dermal atrophy starting after age 50. It is therefore more likely that a scald burn will be deeper in the very young and elderly and require surgical treatment, usually excision and skin grafting (see Figs. 9-3 and 9-4).

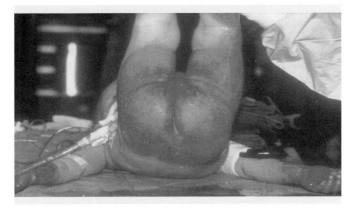

FIGURE 9-3. Scald injury in a young child.

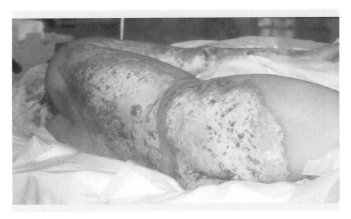

FIGURE 9-4. Scald injury in an elderly adult.

BIBLIOGRAPHY

Lewis GM, Heimbach DM, Gibran N. Evaluation of the burn wound: management decisions. In: Herndon D (ed.), *Total Burn Care*, 4th ed. London, United Kingdom: W.B. Saunders; 2012:125–130
Milner S, Asuku M. Burn wound management. In: Cameron J, Cameron A (eds.), *Current Surgical Therapy*, 11th ed. Philadelphia, PA: Saunders; 2014:1128–1131.

5. **(C)** The pathophysiology of burn edema is multifactorial. The primary cause is the disruption of capillary membranes and the leakage of intravascular fluid into the extravascular space. This leakage occurs in both the burned and unburned tissues. The edema formation is biphasic in nature with an early rapid and late gradual phase. Maximal edema occurs by approximately 12 hours in small burns and up to 24 hours in larger burns.

In the early phase, burn edema is seen only in the burn wound; this edema extends into surrounding tissue with time. The microvascular changes that occur with burn edema, apart from an increase in the separation of capillary intercellular junctions, include changes in the capillary and interstitial pressures. The interstitial hydrostatic pressure increases, drawing fluid from the intravascular space into the interstitium by generating oncotic pressure. In addition, through leaking capillaries, protein-rich plasma enters the interstitium. The plasma colloid osmotic pressure is decreased and the interstitial colloid osmotic pressure is increased, which further stimulates edema formation. Capillary pressure in the burned tissues significantly increases initially and slowly decreases over the next several hours.

BIBLIOGRAPHY

Kramer G. Pathophysiology of burn shock and burn edema. In: Herndon D (ed.), *Total Burn Care*, 4th ed. London, United Kingdom: W.B. Saunders; 2012:103–114.

Warden G. Fluid resuscitation and early management. In: Herndon D (ed.), *Total Burn Care*, 4th ed. London, United Kingdom: W.B. Saunders; 2012:115–124.

6. **(D)** The goal of fluid resuscitation of the burn victim is to preserve systemic tissue perfusion often in the setting of burn shock—a mix of hypovolemic and cellular shock. This goal is made difficult because of the "capillary leak" that occurs in the burned and unburned tissues. It is also known that plasma and blood volumes are decreased and extracellular fluid volume is increased, leading to substantial hemodynamic shifts and oliguria. Peripheral vascular resistance is increased. Cardiac output, although initially decreased, over the ensuing 18–24 hours, returns to or exceeds normal limits. Demling has experimentally shown that 8 hours after burn, the plasma protein content can be maintained. In other words, the "leak" will start to resolve.

There are numerous resuscitation formulas that have been described. The goal of each of these formulas is tissue perfusion. This perfusion can be verified by an adequate urine output of 0.5 mL/kg/h, reversal of acidosis, adequate mentation, and adequate filling pressures in adults. These resuscitation formulas aim for adequate hydration with avoidance of over- or underresuscitation.

The widely accepted Parkland formula is a lactated Ringer's (LR) solution of 4 mL/kg/% TBSA burn given over 24 hours. One-half of the calculated volume is delivered in the first 8 hours following the burn, and the remainder is delivered over the ensuing 16 hours. LR solution is used because it is isotonic in nature and has a decreased chloride load that prevents hyperchloremic metabolic acidosis. Because colloid solutions are "leaked" from the capillaries, creating increased osmotic pressure in the interstitium, crystalloid solutions are best for massive resuscitation.

Hypertonic saline solutions have also been described for use in large burns (>40% TBSA) and pulmonary injury and converted to LR after 8 hours. Colloid resuscitation is another accepted form of resuscitation. The Brooke and Evans formulas use colloid for one-quarter to one-half of the resuscitation volume. Other institutions initiate colloid after 8–12 hours, once the "capillary leak" has begun to resolve. Formulas using albumin, plasmalyte, low-molecular-weight dextran, and fresh frozen plasma have all been described (see Fig. 9-5).

BIBLIOGRAPHY

Warden G. Fluid resuscitation and early management. In: Herndon D (ed.), *Total Burn Care*, 4th ed. London, United Kingdom: W.B. Saunders; 2012:115–124.

7. **(B)** The burned child is not the equivalent of the burned adult. Resuscitation of a child requires careful consideration to adequately meet the needs of end-organs. In 1986, Merrell and colleagues established that children need approximately 2 mL/kg/% TBSA more fluid resuscitation than adults with similar size burns. Merrell also noted that children require resuscitation for smaller body surface area burns than do adults.

Physiologically, children have a greater proportion of body surface area to weight than do adults. In addition, because of the larger surface area of their heads, the standard "Rule of Nines" chart does not accurately assess a child's burned surface area. Children have proportionately larger evaporative losses than adults because of their larger surface areas. For instance, a 20% TBSA burn in an adult will lead to an 1100-mL fluid loss (22% of blood volume loss), whereas the same TBSA in a 10-kg child will lead to a 475-mL loss, or 59% of their circulating volume. Children less than 2 years of age have decreased glycogen stores and may, therefore, become hypoglycemic easily. The child's heart is also less compliant and may be more prone to volume overload. Careful consideration of these factors will mitigate over- and underresuscitation.

Several resuscitative formulas have been devised for the pediatric patient. The simplest formula uses the Parkland formula of 4 mL/kg/% TBSA burned and adds the child's normal maintenance fluid. Pediatric maintenance fluid rate is calculated based on weight: 4 mL/kg/h for the first 10 kg plus 2 mL/kg/h for the next 10 kg and 1 mL/kg/h for body mass over 20 kg. One-half of the total fluid volume indicated by the Parkland formula is infused over the first 8 hours, with the remainder infused over the ensuing 16 hours, in addition to an hourly maintenance fluid. The Parkland solution is LR, and the maintenance fluid may be LR or, in children under 2 years, LR in 5% dextrose (D5LR).

The Shriner's Hospital in Galveston, Texas, employs a formula based on the child's body surface area. This formula is 5000 mL/m^2 body surface area burned plus 2000 mL/body surface area over the first 24 hours. One-half of this solution is given over the first 8 hours, and the remainder is given over the ensuing 16 hours.

In children, resuscitation is titrated to maintain a urine output of 1–1.5 mL/kg/h. Acid-base balance, mentation, and vital signs are all monitored to aid in resuscitation.

BIBLIOGRAPHY

Lee J, Norbury W, Herndon D. Special considerations of age: the pediatric burn patient. In: Herndon D (ed.), *Total Burn Care*, 4th ed. London, United Kingdom: W.B. Saunders; 2012:405–414.

Merrell S, Saffle J, Sullivan J, et al. Fluid resuscitation in thermally injured children. *Am J Surg* 1986;152:664–669.

Warden G. Fluid resuscitation and early management. In: Herndon D (ed.), *Total Burn Care*, 4th ed. London, United Kingdom: W.B. Saunders; 2012:115–124.

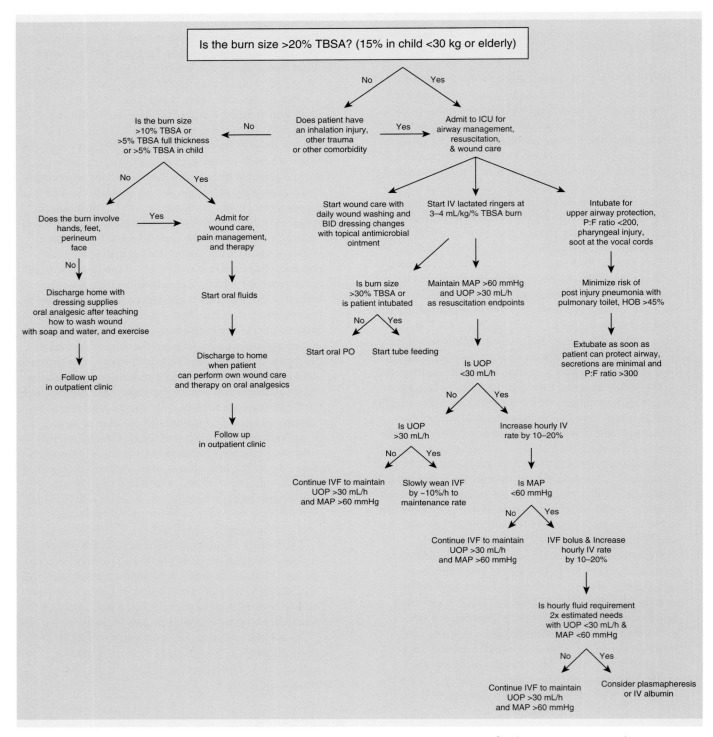

FIGURE 9-5. Burn algorithm. BID, twice a day; ICU, intensive care unit; IVF, intravenous fluid; MAP, mean arterial pressure; TBSA, total body surface area; UOP, urine output. From Brunicardi F. (ed.). *Schwartz's Principles of Surgery*, 9th ed. San Francisco, CA: McGraw-Hill Medical; 2010.

8. **(C)** Carbon monoxide (CO) is an odorless, colorless gas that is produced by incomplete combustion of many fuels. CO toxicity remains one of the most frequent causes of death after burn injury. The predominant effect of CO is its binding to hemoglobin to form carboxyhemoglobin (COHb). The affinity of CO for hemoglobin is 200 times higher than that of oxygen. The competitive binding of CO to hemoglobin reduces delivery of

oxygen to tissues, leading to severe hypoxia, especially of the most vulnerable organs such as brain and heart, where oxygen extraction is considerably higher than in most other organs. The oxygen–hemoglobin dissociation curve loses its sigmoid shape and is shifted to the left, thereby further impairing tissue oxygen availability.

If inhalation injury is suspected, arterial blood gas and COHb level should be obtained, and the patient should be placed on 100% oxygen. Signs of potential inhalation injury include facial burns, singed nasal vibrissae, carbonaceous sputum, abnormal mental status, respiratory distress, or COHb level above 10–15%. A normal COHb level for nonsmokers is less than 1.5%. Smokers can have COHb levels between 3–15%. The true COHb level should be estimated from the time the admission lab was drawn, calculating back to the time of the burn injury for a more accurate measure of the extent of inhalational injury. COHb levels greater than 10% may cause headaches and mild confusion. At levels of 30–40%, nausea and vomiting, altered mental status, and dizziness develop. At levels greater than 40%, cardiovascular and respiratory complications occur that can include tachycardia or arrhythmias, increased or decreased respirations, obtundation, and even death. A carboxyhemoglobin level greater than 60% has a greater than 50% chance of mortality. On 100% oxygen, the half-life of carboxyhemoglobin is 40 minutes. This short half-life may make it difficult to determine accurately the amount of carbon monoxide inhaled, since the 100% oxygen is routinely administered to patients as soon as they are extricated from the fire. The length of time that the patient has been treated with 100% oxygen must be considered when evaluating a patient's carboxyhemoglobin level.

BIBLIOGRAPHY

Light A, Grass C, Pursley D, Krause J. Carboxyhemoglobin levels in smokers vs. non-smokers in a smoking environment. *Respir Care* 2007;52(11):1576.

McCall JE, Cahill TJ. Respiratory care of the burn patient. *J Burn Care Rehabil* 2005;26:200–206.

Mlcak RP, Suman OE, Herndon DN. Respiratory management of inhalation injury. *Burns* 2007;33:2–13.

Woodson L, Talon M, Traber DL, Herndon DN. Diagnosis and treatment of inhalation injury. In: Herndon D (ed.), *Total Burn Care*, 4th ed. London, United Kingdom: W.B. Saunders; 2012:229–238.

9. **(D)** Inhalation injury is the leading cause of death in burn patients, with a reported mortality as high as 60%. History of being within a burning structure, loss of consciousness, or significant smoke inhalation should invoke suspicion. Physical findings of facial burns, singed nasal hairs, soot in the nose or mouth, oropharyngeal edema, hoarseness, stridor, or wheezing all should alert the clinician to the possibility of inhalation injury and prompt more thorough evaluation. Inhalation injury is generally separated into three components: carbon monoxide poisoning and injury above and injury below the glottis.

Prolonged exposure to smoke in an enclosed environment increases the risk for carbon monoxide poisoning and inhalational injury. Inspection of the oropharynx can reveal injuries above the glottis. The oropharynx can absorb a great amount of heat without permanent damage; however, edema develops rapidly and may cause temporary airway obstruction, especially in children. Even when initial evaluation demonstrates no edema, intubation may be prudent because resuscitation will result in significant tissue edema and possible upper airway obstruction. Facial and neck burns may also cause airway compromise. Patients with these injuries should be carefully considered for elective intubation if any signs of compromise become apparent.

Bronchoscopy is necessary to evaluate for injury below the glottis. Injuries below the glottis can be divided into thermal injury or injury as a result of the inhalation of the byproducts of combustion. Thermal injury occurs when superheated air is inhaled (i.e., steam burns). This is a rare occurrence because of the tremendous heat exchange of the upper airways. The byproducts of combustion cause a chemical pneumonitis and an acute hypersensitivity reaction: bronchorrhea and subsequent obstruction by mucus and atelectasis (see Figs. 9-6 and 9-7).

BIBLIOGRAPHY

Cancio LC. Airway management and smoke inhalation injury in the burn patient. *Clin Plast Surg* 2009;36(4):555–567.

Traber D, Herndon D, Enkhbaatar P, Maybauer M, Maybauer D. The pathophysiology of inhalation injury. In: Herndon D (ed.), *Total Burn Care*, 4th ed. London, United Kingdom: W.B. Saunders; 2012:219–229.

Woodson L, Talon M, Traber DL, Herndon D. Diagnosis and treatment of inhalation injury. In: Herndon D (ed.), *Total Burn Care*, 4th ed. London, United Kingdom: W.B. Saunders; 2012:229–238.

10. **(C)** Bronchoscopy is the current "gold standard" for the diagnosis of inhalation injury. This procedure allows for visualization of the upper airways and the tracheobronchial tree. Bronchoscopic findings often include erythema and/or edema of the airways, carbonaceous material, blistering, hemorrhage, and ulceration or necrosis of the mucosa; however, patients who are hypotensive or hypovolemic may not exhibit these findings initially until after resuscitation. Late bronchoscopy, 36–48 hours after injury, may show damage due to systemic inflammatory response rather than direct thermal injury.

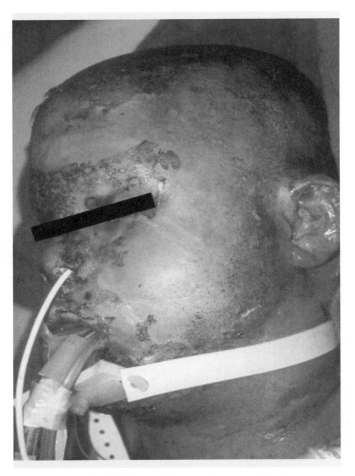

FIGURE 9-6. Scald injury with oropharyngeal edema.

Chest x-rays are not helpful in determining whether an inhalation injury has occurred. Most initial chest x-rays are normal in appearance, or if abnormal, this may be attributable to some other cause. CT scans are also inadequate.

Xenon-133 scanning has been used to aid in the diagnosis of smoke inhalation. This scan shows areas of the lungs that are ventilated. Areas in the lung with small airway obstruction will be revealed; however, this test is not specific for inhalation injury and must be used to complement other diagnostic tests. Inhalation injury remains a leading cause of morbidity and mortality in burn patients. High suspicion, accurate diagnosis, and prompt treatment of this injury are critical to early treatment (see Figs. 9-8 and 9-9).

BIBLIOGRAPHY

Endorf F, Gibran N. Burns. In: Brunicardi F (ed.), *Schwartz's Principles of Surgery*, 9th ed. San Francisco, CA: McGraw Hill Medical; 2010:197–208.

Greenhalgh DG, Saffle JR, Holmes JH, et al. American Burn Association consensus conference to define sepsis and infection in burns. *J Burn Care Res.* 2007;28:776–790.

Milner S, Asuku M. Burn wound management. In: Cameron J, Cameron A (eds.), *Current Surgical Therapy*, 11th ed. Philadelphia, PA: Saunders; 2014:1128–1131.

Traber D, Herndon D, Enkhbaatar P, Maybauer M, Maybauer D. The pathophysiology of inhalation injury. In: Herndon D (ed.), *Total Burn Care*, 4th ed. London, United Kingdom: W.B. Saunders; 2012:219–229.

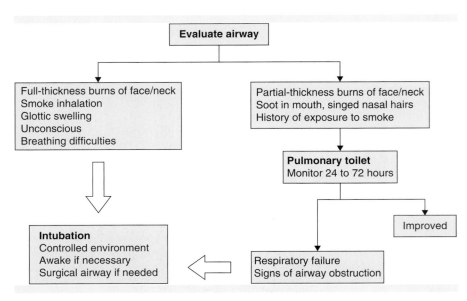

FIGURE 9-7. Airway management of the burned child.

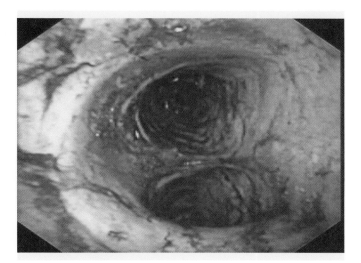

FIGURE 9-8. Airway inflammation from burn injury.

Woodson L, Talon M, Traber DL, Herndon D. Diagnosis and treatment of inhalation injury. In: Herndon D (ed.), *Total Burn Care*, 4th ed. London, United Kingdom: W.B. Saunders; 2012:229–238.

11. **(A)** Full-thickness circumferential or near-circumferential burns of the extremities may cause vascular compromise to the affected extremity. This occurs because the burned skin with the subsequent interstitial edema is relatively inelastic. As tissue edema increases, especially in the first 12–48 hours after burn, tissue pressures rise, which may lead to further ischemia of the underlying tissue. The clinical manifestations of compartment syndrome (i.e., pain, pallor, paresthesias, paralysis, and pulselessness) are not always easy to interpret in the burned extremity. Other methods must be used to determine whether a patient is at risk for tissue ischemia. Inability to palpate a pulse does not always imply a lack of perfusion in a burned extremity. Pulses may be hard to evaluate in older patients and patients with severe swelling, other anatomical differences, and eschar over the area. Evaluation of arterial flow by Doppler should be done in the event of an absent pulse. An escharotomy should be performed if arterial Doppler signal is absent.

The most reliable indicator of compartment syndrome is measurement of interstitial tissue pressure with a needle and fluid column or commercially available Stryker device. Pressures greater than 30 mmHg suggest tissue ischemia. An escharotomy should be performed if repeat pressures of 30 mmHg or greater are measured.

Escharotomies can be performed at either the bedside with sedation or in the operating room. The patient is placed in the anatomic position, and longitudinal incisions are made in the mid-lateral or mid-medial positions using either a knife or electrocautery. The incision is made through the inelastic burned skin, extending into the subcutaneous tissue. Particular care must be exercised at joints and near superficial nerves.

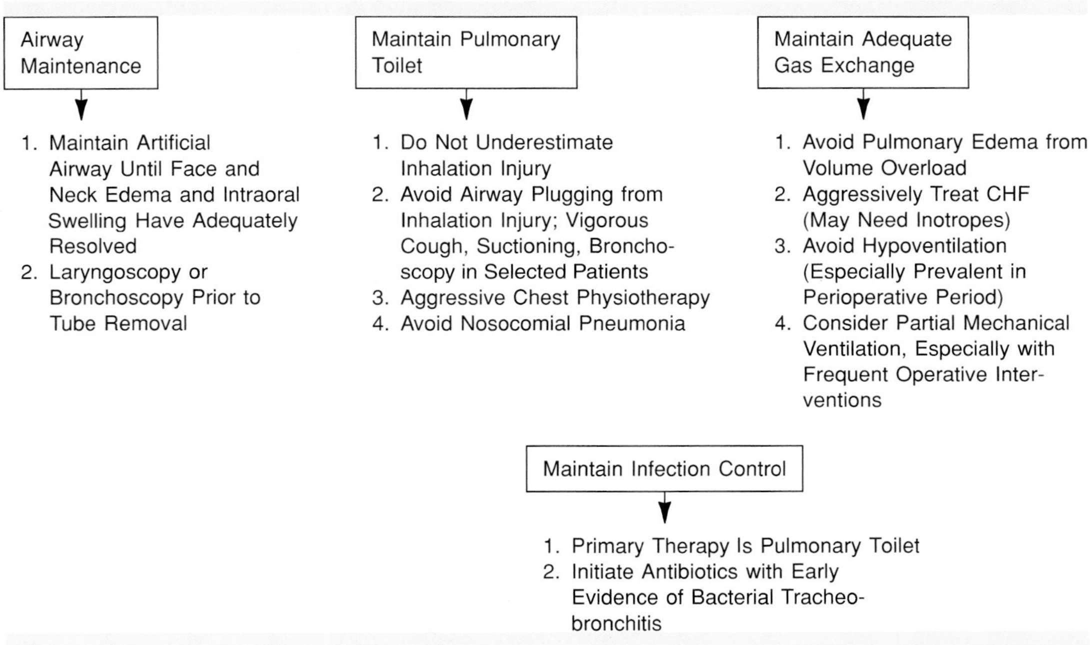

Airway Maintenance	Maintain Pulmonary Toilet	Maintain Adequate Gas Exchange
1. Maintain Artificial Airway Until Face and Neck Edema and Intraoral Swelling Have Adequately Resolved 2. Laryngoscopy or Bronchoscopy Prior to Tube Removal	1. Do Not Underestimate Inhalation Injury 2. Avoid Airway Plugging from Inhalation Injury; Vigorous Cough, Suctioning, Bronchoscopy in Selected Patients 3. Aggressive Chest Physiotherapy 4. Avoid Nosocomial Pneumonia	1. Avoid Pulmonary Edema from Volume Overload 2. Aggressively Treat CHF (May Need Inotropes) 3. Avoid Hypoventilation (Especially Prevalent in Perioperative Period) 4. Consider Partial Mechanical Ventilation, Especially with Frequent Operative Interventions

Maintain Infection Control

1. Primary Therapy Is Pulmonary Toilet
2. Initiate Antibiotics with Early Evidence of Bacterial Tracheobronchitis

FIGURE 9-9. Early treatment of pulmonary abnormalities in burn patients. CHF, congestive heart failure. From Hall JB, Schmidt GA, Wood LDH. *Principles of Care*, 3rd ed. New York, NY: McGraw-Hill; 2005.

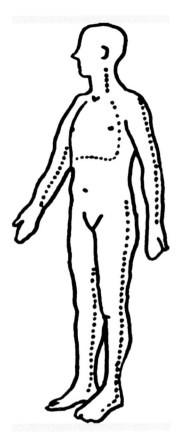

FIGURE 9-10. Sites of escharotomy.

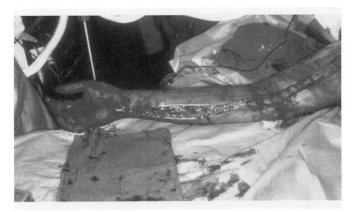

FIGURE 9-11. Upper extremity escharotomy.

Occasionally, trunk escharotomies need to be performed because of circumferential full-thickness trunk burns (see Fig. 9-10). These burns can interfere with chest excursion, increasing the mean airway pressure necessary to expand the chest, especially in young children, and cause difficulties with ventilation. Prophylactic escharotomies are performed in patients with circumferential or near-circumferential burned extremities and large body surface area burns. These patients will receive large volumes of fluid resuscitation with concomitant tissue edema formation (see Fig. 9-11).

BIBLIOGRAPHY

Endorf F, Gibran N. Burns. In: Brunicardi F (ed.), *Schwartz's Principles of Surgery*, 9th ed. San Francisco, CA: McGraw Hill Medical; 2010:197–208.

Milner S. Asuku M. Burn wound management. In: Cameron J, Cameron A (eds.), *Current Surgical Therapy*, 11th ed. Philadelphia, PA: Saunders; 2014:1128–1131.

Mlcak R, Buffalo M, Jimenez C. Pre-hospital management, transportation, and emergency care. In: Herndon D (ed.), *Total Burn Care*, 4th ed. London, United Kingdom: W.B. Saunders; 2012:93–102.

12. **(D)** Nonaccidental scalds can compose up to 2% of children admitted to burn centers. Inconsistent history and physical exam with burn should be a first indication. Circumferential extremity injuries and symmetrical burns to a child's buttocks and perineum are examples that should raise suspicion of abuse. Others that imply that the child may have an intentional burn include a scald in the absence of splash marks, symmetric bilateral burns in a glove or stocking pattern, uniformity of burn, and in a case involving submersion, joints or skinfolds may have sparing. Unintentional cigarette burns are usually superficial and ill defined. Intentionally inflicted cigarette burns are distinct and circular or oval with hyperpigmented edges. If abuse is expected, then looking for concurrent and previous injuries is required. This search should include a skeletal series looking for previous or current fractures. Child Protective Services in your state should be involved if abuse is suspected.

BIBLIOGRAPHY

Lewis GM, Heimbach DM, Gibran N. Evaluation of the burn wound: management decisions. In: Herndon D (ed.), *Total Burn Care*, 4th ed. London, United Kingdom: W.B. Saunders; 2012:125–130.

Ojo P, Palmer J, Garvey R, et al. Pattern of burns in child abuse. *Am Surg* 2007;73:253–255.

Tropez-Arceneaux L, Tropez-Sims S. Intentional burn injuries. In: Herndon D (ed.), *Total Burn Care*, 4th ed. London, United Kingdom: W.B. Saunders; 2012:689–697.

13. **(C)** Thermoregulation of the burn patient in the operating room is very difficult. Evaporative losses, blood losses, the infusion of cool solutions or blood products, and large exposed body surface areas will cause a rapid fall in the patient's body temperature. Every effort should be made to warm all solutions and warm the ambient room temperature. Cardiac dysfunction and coagulopathy can greatly complicate an already hazardous operation if the patient becomes hypothermic. Because of a child's large body surface area–to–volume ratio and somewhat immature homeostatic mechanisms, small children are particularly vulnerable to hypothermia. Operating rooms are heated up to 108°F.

Adequate intravenous access is essential for any burn procedure but more particularly for tangential excision and grafting because patients may lose from 25 to 250 mL of blood per body surface area excised and grafted. The smaller grafting procedures can be performed with only peripheral access; however, larger procedures require large-bore intravenous lines for rapid infusion of blood and fluids. Central lines and arterial catheters are helpful for patient monitoring. This patient would likely have central venous access and would not require a placement of a new subclavian line just for the procedure.

Debridement and grafting procedures for the burned patient may require a large volume of blood to be transfused. Platelets, packed red blood cells, and fresh frozen plasma may be necessary during the procedure depending on the patient's preoperative condition and the anticipated blood loss. Massive transfusions (>10 units of packed red cells) can cause coagulopathies due to the depletion of clotting factors and thrombocytopenia. Citrate, used as an anticoagulant in blood storage, binds with calcium to prevent activation of the coagulation cascade. This may result in a drop in ionized calcium, which in turn may result in cardiac abnormalities and hypotension. Serial monitoring of the patient's hemoglobin, chemistries, and coagulation profile is necessary.

BIBLIOGRAPHY

Lee J, Norbury W, Herndon D. Special considerations of age: the pediatric burn patient. In: Herndon D (ed.), *Total Burn Care*, 4th ed. London, United Kingdom: W.B. Saunders; 2012:405–414.

Lippman M, Myhre B. Hazards of massive transfusion. *J Am Assoc Nurse Anesth* 1975;43:269–277.

Woodson L, Sherwood E, Aarsland A, Talon M, Kinsky M, Morvant E. Anesthesia for burned patients. In: Herndon D (ed.), *Total Burn Care*, 4th ed. London, United Kingdom: W.B. Saunders; 2012:173–198.

14. **(D)** Accurate nutritional assessment of the burn patient is essential. The burn wound creates an acute stress state with marked catabolism and protein utilization. Inadequate nutritional support can lead to sepsis, immune dysfunction, and poor wound healing.

There are several methods available for nutritional monitoring. Indirect calorimetry is the best available means to measure energy expenditure. Indirect calorimetry measures whole-body oxygen consumption and carbon dioxide production while the patient is at rest. The produced values are entered into the Weir equation, and a resting energy expenditure (REE) is calculated. This value is then multiplied by a stress factor. A respiratory quotient (RQ) can be calculated using indirect calorimetry. An RQ less than 0.8 is consistent with fat and protein oxidation and, therefore, underfeeding. A value of 0.8–0.95 suggests an appropriate mix of fat, protein, and carbohydrate oxidation. An RQ of greater than 1.0 is suggestive of overfeeding and the need to decrease caloric consumption. However, indirect calorimetry is operator and equipment dependent; the values may be inaccurate because of mechanical dysfunction, operator error, or improper calibration.

Visceral proteins can be measured in the burned patient. Serum albumin, which has a half-life of 3 weeks, falls sharply after burn injury. Serum albumin levels can be falsely elevated by infusions of albumin and are not an accurate measure of nutritional status. Prealbumin has a short half-life of 2–3 days and is not affected by the infusion of albumin. Trends should be followed with a goal to achieve a normal prealbumin of 12 or greater. Prealbumin is not a perfectly accurate measurement of nutritional status, however, because large-volume resuscitation and frequent operative procedures can artificially lower these levels. Serum transferrin and retinol-binding protein are also markers of protein synthesis that are somewhat useful in trending nutritional status, but are relatively nonspecific.

BIBLIOGRAPHY

Gauglitz GG, Finnerty CC, Herndon DN, Williams FN, Jeschke MG. Modulation of the hypermetabolic response after burn injury. In: Herndon D (ed.), *Total Burn Care*, 4th ed. London, United Kingdom: W.B. Saunders; 2012:355–360.

Manelli J, Badett C, Botti G, Goldstein M, Bernini V, Bernard D. A reference standard for plasma proteins is required for nutritional assessment of adult burn patients. *Burns* 1998;24:337–345.

Saffle J, Graves C, Cochran A. Nutritional support of the burned patient. In: Herndon D (ed.), *Total Burn Care*, 4th ed. London, United Kingdom: W.B. Saunders; 2012:333–354.

Saffle J, Medina E, Raymond J, Westenskow D, Kravitz M, Warden G. Use of indirect calorimetry in the nutritional management of burned patients. *J Trauma* 1985;25:32–39.

15. **(D)** Postburn hypermetabolism is not completely understood. Burn patients often have an elevated core and skin temperature. The "resetting" of their homeostatic thermostat causes the patient's metabolic rate to increase. The burn patient with a large body surface area injury has enormous fluid losses from evaporation that require energy of 0.6 cal/mL of water. In patients with large TBSA burns, this can require greater than 2000 cal/d. Some causes of caloric expenditures from hypermetabolism can be mitigated through the use of dressings on burn wounds to prevent fluid loss, along with increasing the ambient temperature of patient rooms to prevent shivering.

Increased levels of circulating catecholamines, such as epinephrine, cortisol, and glucagon, result in alterations in the metabolism of carbohydrates, lipids, and proteins (see Fig. 9-12). Although carbohydrate metabolism is increased significantly, glucose intolerance is commonly seen in burned patients. This finding is likely because of increased circulating cortisol and glucagon. Serum insulin levels are increased in burn injury but not to the extent of gluconeogenesis. The endogenous carbohydrate stores are depleted so rapidly that amino acids are released from muscle tissue for gluconeogenesis. In addition to muscle protein catabolism, proteolysis has been documented.

Lipid metabolism is also affected by the burn injury. There is an increase in lipolysis, which results in elevated serum free fatty acids. Free fatty acids are precursors for cytokines such as prostaglandins and thromboxanes. These cytokines influence immunosuppression and inflammation.

Endotoxin and infection are further factors that contribute to burn hypermetabolism. The excision of necrotic tissue and the treatment of infection may decrease hypermetabolism by removing a source of bacteria and their toxins as well as decreasing release of catabolic enzymes from neutrophils in the burn wound. Coverage of the burn wound with allograft will improve the metabolic status of the patient, diminishing the hypermetabolic state. Attaining complete healing of the burn wound, however, whether by grafting or reepithelialization, dramatically reduces hypermetabolism and catabolism and allows for protein synthesis, although patients may remain relatively hypermetabolic for prolonged periods after healing.

Pharmacologic manipulations attempting to decrease the hypermetabolic and catabolic states have used β-blockade agents such as propranolol to lessen the effects of circulatory catecholamines on carbohydrate metabolism. Strict glucose control with insulin in diabetic patients may decrease protein catabolism and reduce rates of infection in intensive care unit patients. Anabolic steroids such as oxandrolone may hasten protein synthesis and mitigate, to some degree, the hypermetabolic state.

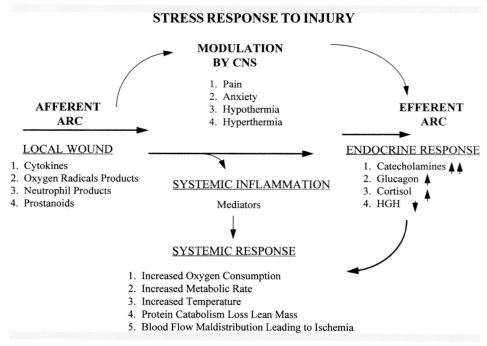

FIGURE 9-12. Stress response to injury. CNS, central nervous system; HGH, human growth hormone. From Hall JB, Schmidt GA, Wood LDH. *Principles of Care*, 3rd ed. New York, NY: McGraw-Hill; 2005.

BIBLIOGRAPHY

Baxter C. Metabolism and nutrition in burned patients. *Compr Ther* 1987;13:36–42.

Gauglitz GG, Finnerty CC, Herndon DN, Williams FN, Jeschke MG. Modulation of the hypermetabolic response after burn injury. In: Herndon D (ed.), *Total Burn Care*, 4th ed. London, United Kingdom: W.B. Saunders; 2012:355–360.

Mayes T. Enteral nutrition for the burned patient. *Nutr Clin Pract* 1997;12:S43–S45.

Saffle J. What's new in general surgery: burns and metabolism. *J Am Coll Surg* 2003;196:267–285.

Van den Berghe G, Wouters P, Weekers F, et al. Intensive insulin therapy in critically ill patients. *N Engl J Med* 2001;345:1359–1367.

Waymack J, Herndon D. Nutritional support of the burned patient. *World J Surg* 1992;16:80–86.

Yu Y, Tompkins R, Ryan C, Young V. The metabolic basis of the increase in energy expenditure in severely burned patients. *J Parenter Enteral Nutr* 1999;23:160–168.

16. **(D)** Patients with large body surface area burns and patients who cannot eat should have a feeding tube placed to aid in nutritional support. Enteral feeds should always be used over parenteral feeding because enteral feeds allow the gut mucosa to remain intact, which may decrease gut-related sepsis. Parenteral nutrition is associated with elevated serum insulin levels, hypernatremia, hyperosmolarity, and line-related complications. Parenteral nutrition has been noted to have an adverse effect on immune function with an increase in tumor necrosis factor (TNF) secretion. Therefore, if the gut can be used, enteral nutrition is the route of choice for burned patients. Enteral feeding should be initiated within 24 hours after the burn to decrease the incidence of gastric ileus; however, if gastric ileus does occur, placing the feeding tubes past the pylorus ensures that feeds are well tolerated and the risk of aspiration is decreased.

BIBLIOGRAPHY

Lee JO, Norbury WB, Herndon D. Special considerations of age: the pediatric burned patient. In: Herndon D (ed.), *Total Burn Care*, 4th ed. London, United Kingdom: W.B. Saunders; 2012:405–414.

Raff T, Hartman B, Germann G. Early intragastric feeding of seriously burned and long-term ventilated patients: a review of 55 patients. *Burns* 1997;23:19–25.

Saffle J, Graves C, Cochran A. Nutritional support of the burned patient. In: Herndon D (ed.), *Total Burn Care*, 4th ed. London, United Kingdom: W.B. Saunders; 2012:333–354.

17. **(C)** Burn injury may also cause alterations in several micronutrients needed to enhance wound healing and immunity. Some of the micronutrients that are regularly replaced are listed below:

- Vitamin A aids in wound healing and helps maintain epithelial integrity. Vitamin A functions as an antioxidant and has a positive effect on immune function.
- Vitamin C, or ascorbic acid, is an antioxidant and aids in the antibacterial function of the white blood cells (WBCs). Vitamin C is involved in the hydroxylation of proline and lysine, which is necessary for collagen synthesis. It is essential for wound healing and allows for tensile strength in wounds.
- Vitamin E serves as an antioxidant and aids in immune function. Vitamin E inhibits thromboxane and prostaglandin synthesis and stimulates fibroblasts.
- Zinc has an important role in wound healing. DNA and RNA replication, protein synthesis, and collagen formation are all influenced by zinc. Zinc is also important for immune function because it has a positive effect on lymphocyte function and cellular and humoral immunity.
- Selenium protects membrane lipids from free radical damage and is important in the function of lymphocytes.
- Iron is necessary for oxygen transport in the blood (hemoglobin) or muscles (myoglobin). Iron is a cofactor in many enzyme systems and is necessary for cell replication and DNA synthesis.

There are many other nutrients that are affected by a burn injury; however, these are the most commonly supplemented.

BIBLIOGRAPHY

Gamliel Z, DeBiasse M, Demling R. Essential micro minerals and their response to burn injury. *J Burn Care Rehabil* 1996;17:264–272.

Jeschke M, Finnerty CC. The hepatic response to a thermal injury. In: Herndon D (ed.), *Total Burn Care*, 4th ed. London, United Kingdom: W.B. Saunders; 2012:301–312.

Mancoll J, Phillips J. Delayed wound healing. In: Eriksson E (ed.), *Plastic Surgery Indications, Operations, and Outcomes*, vol. 1. St. Louis, MO: Mosby; 2000:65–78.

Saffle J, Graves C, Cochran A. Nutritional support of the burned patient. In: Herndon D (ed.), *Total Burn Care*, 4th ed. London, United Kingdom: W.B. Saunders; 2012:333–354.

18. **(D)** Burn injuries greater than 15% TBSA can have a profound effect on red blood cell (RBC) production and the coagulation cascade of the burn patient. These major burn patients develop anemia, which usually persists until their wounds are closed. There are various reasons for this loss. The burn patient can lose as much as 18% of his or her RBCs in the first 24 hours after a major burn injury. The RBC morphology changes, and the cell membrane can become fragile, making destruction easier. The patient undergoes frequent blood draws and multiple surgical excisions and grafting, which further contribute to anemia. The burn patient has a decrease

in the bone marrow production of RBCs. There is an increase in circulating erythropoietin in these patients, but the progenitor cells within the bone marrow do not respond appropriately. Therefore, RBC production is not increased to compensate for losses. Burn patients also have decreased serum iron levels and total iron binding capacity, which may further decrease erythropoiesis.

BIBLIOGRAPHY

Deitch E, Sittig K. A serial study of the erythropoietic response to thermal injury. *Ann Surg* 1993;217:293–299.

Lawrence C, Atac B. Hematologic changes in massive burn injury. *Crit Care Med* 1992;20:1284–1288.

Posluszny JA Jr, Gamelli R, Shankar R. Hematologic and hematopoietic response to burn injury. In: Herndon D (ed.), *Total Burn Care*, 4th ed. London, United Kingdom: W.B. Saunders; 2012:277–288.

19. **(C)** Infection is the leading cause of morbidity and mortality in burn patients. Awareness of the potential sources of infection in the burn patient leads to prompt treatment and prevention of complications. A partial list of possible infectious sources is listed.

- *Pneumonia.* Pneumonia is a common infectious complication in the burn patient. These infections usually start as infections of the tracheobronchial tree and spread to the distal lung periphery. Factors that increase the patient's susceptibility to pneumonia are aspiration, inhalation injury, burn size, and the presence of an endotracheal or nasal tracheal tube. Patients who have persistent fever without a known source should have a chest x-ray and sputum culture performed.
- *Wound infection.* The burn wound is a potential source of systemic infection until complete healing is accomplished. Frequent clinical inspection of the wound itself and correlation with the clinical picture and quantitative tissue biopsy of suspicious lesions are necessary to alert the clinician to deterioration. Early excision of the burn wound and grafting with allograft or autograft can avert invasive wound infection. All burns that have not yet been grafted or that have not healed primarily are heavily colonized with bacteria that reflect the ambient environment. More than 100,000 bacteria/g of burned tissue constitutes invasive infection. Burn wound sepsis must be treated with surgical excision, not simply antibiotics, and other causes of sepsis must be ruled out.
- *Urosepsis.* Urinary tract infections are common because of the necessity of indwelling urinary catheters to monitor systemic perfusion. Meticulous insertion and daily care of urinary catheters and removal as early as possible may decrease the incidence of urosepsis.

- *Central line–associated bloodstream infection.* Burn patients with significant body surface area involvement often require central venous access or arterial lines for monitoring. The venous catheters are frequent sources of infection because of their proximity to the burn wound and their "seeding" as a result of the necessity of frequent operative procedures such as burn wound debridements. These catheters should be meticulously placed and cared for and changed on a regular basis with the insertion site rotated routinely. Showers of bacteria from manipulation of these lines can cause rapid clinical deterioration and a picture of acute sepsis. Bacteremia can occur from any infected site including the wound. In patients with long hospitalizations or severe injury, endocarditis or valvulitis must be considered if a picture of recurrent bacteremia presents. Septic thrombophlebitis must also be considered, and present and past intravenous sites must be carefully examined for the presence of pus.
- *Sinusitis.* Sinusitis is a frequently overlooked cause of infection in the burn patient. Obstruction of the drainage of the paranasal sinuses because of long-term nasal intubation with tracheal or gastric tubes causes overgrowth of bacteria and invasive infection. Because the patient is sedated, clinical signs and symptoms may be difficult to elicit. Patients with sinusitis may have purulent nasal drainage, but the absence of this drainage does not preclude the infection. If suspected, x-rays or sinus CT scans are usually diagnostic. Surgical drainage may be necessary to obtain an accurate culture to guide antibiotic therapy. Removal of all nasal tubes, institution of appropriate antibiotics, and the use of nasal decongestants may be helpful.
- *Cholecystitis.* Cholecystitis, frequently acalculous, is a complication of critical illness, trauma, or major surgery. Fever, abdominal pain and tenderness, leukocytosis, and elevated liver function tests are seen; however, these signs and symptoms are relatively nonspecific, and because many patients are heavily sedated and difficult to examine, a high index of suspicion should lead to the liberal use of abdominal ultrasound. Distended or thickened gallbladder wall, the presence of "sludge" or stones themselves, and fluid around the gallbladder are all indicative of cholecystitis, which will usually require cholecystectomy to prevent necrosis, perforation, or other intra-abdominal catastrophe. Obviously, any other intra-abdominal event such as appendicitis or diverticulitis may occur in the burn patient, but these are considerably less frequent.
- Clostridium difficile *colitis.* Antibiotics alter the normal colonic flora and allow overgrowth of *C difficile* bacterium. The resulting diarrhea is profuse, watery, and foul smelling; diagnosis should be achieved by sending the stool for toxin polymerase chain reaction (PCR) or enzyme assays. Complications include

toxic megacolon and perforation. Although diarrhea is common in burn patients for many reasons, a high index of suspicion is necessary. Treatment includes specific antibiotic therapy usually with intravenous or oral metronidazole and oral or rectal vancomycin.

BIBLIOGRAPHY

Bullard Dunn KM, Rothenberger DA. Colon, rectum and anus. In: Brunicardi F (ed.), *Schwartz's Principles of Surgery*, 10th ed. New York, NY: McGraw-Hill; 2014:1175–1240.

Gallagher JJ, Branski LK, Williams-Bouyer N, Villarreal C, Herndon DN. Treatment of infection in burns. In: Herndon D (ed.), *Total Burn Care*, 4th ed. London, United Kingdom: W.B. Saunders; 2012:137–156.

Pham TH, Hunter JG. Gallbladder and extrahepatic biliary system. In: Brunicardi F (ed.), *Schwartz's Principles of Surgery*, 10th ed. New York, NY: McGraw-Hill; 2014:1309–1340.

Pruitt B, McManus A. Opportunistic infections in severely burned patients. *Am J Med* 1984;76:146–154.

20. **(B)** Thermal injury has the dramatic effect of decreasing the patient's cardiac output during the first 8–12 hours after burn, followed by a hyperdynamic state if therapy is adequate. The cause of the decrease in cardiac output is multifactorial including decreased venous return secondary to the capillary leak and fluid sequestration in the extracellular space, an increase in systemic vascular resistance, and decreased left ventricular distensibility as demonstrated on echocardiogram. This diastolic dysfunction decreases the amount of blood pumped out with each heartbeat. There is considerable evidence suggesting a systemic increase in cytokines, such as TNF-α and nuclear factor-κB, which serve as direct myocardial depressants that decrease contractility despite adequate intravascular volume replacement. A myocardial depressant factor has been described but not identified, although recent studies have shown that transient endotoxemia may play a role in myocardial dysfunction.

The systemic hormonal cascade triggered by trauma is dramatically present in any significant burn injury. Epinephrine is released immediately and gradually decreases. Norepinephrine peaks on day 2 and gradually decreases. Angiotensin II hormone is gradually elevated until it peaks on day 3. Vasopressin acts to increase vascular smooth muscle tone, increase systemic vascular resistance, and activate parasympathetic pathways of the heart. Vasopressin is immediately elevated and gradually diminishes over subsequent days. Atrial natriuretic peptide is initially decreased and begins to elevate by day 2. This cascade was reported to be associated with an increased stroke volume and cardiac output and a decreased systemic vascular resistance.

BIBLIOGRAPHY

Fagan SP, Bilodeau M, Goverman J. Burn intensive care. *Surg Clin North Am* 2014;94:765–779.

Muthu K, Shankar R, Gamelli R. Significance of the adrenal and sympathetic response to burn injury. In: Herndon D (ed.), *Total Burn Care*, 4th ed. London, United Kingdom: W.B. Saunders; 2012:289–300.

Saffle J. What's new in general surgery: burns and metabolism. *J Am Coll Surg* 2003;196:267–285.

21. **(A – b, B – d, C – c, D – a)** Topical antimicrobials have been used as the first-line burn wound treatment for many years (see Table 9-1).

TABLE 9-1 Commonly Used Topical Agents

	Bactericidal	Bacteriostatic	Pain	Gram Positive (g+)/Gram Negative (g–)	Eschar Penetration
SSD	+		–	g+/g–	Poor
Silver nitrate		+	–[a]	g+/g–	Poor
Sulfamylon		+	++	g+/g–	Excellent
Bacitracin		+	–	g+/g–	Poor
Bactroban (Mupirocin)	+		–	g+	Poor
Furacin	+		–	Some g+, mostly g–	Poor
Betadine	+		–	g+/g–	Poor

[a]If kept moist.
Adapted from: Heggars J, Hawkins H, Edgar P, Villareal C, Herndon D. Treatment of infection in burns. In: Herndon D (ed.), *Total Burn Care*, 2nd ed. London, United Kingdom: W.B. Saunders; 2002:109–119.

- Silver sulfadiazine (SSD) is a frequently used topical agent in burn care. SSD is a broad-spectrum bactericidal agent that has action against both gram-positive and gram-negative bacteria and, to some degree, yeast. SSD is relatively painless to apply but has poor eschar penetration. Side effects include transient leukopenia; argyria, which is a slate-gray or bluish discoloration of the skin or deeper tissues; interstitial nephritis; and rarely, methemoglobinemia.
- Silver nitrate solution (0.25–0.5%) is a bacteriostatic solution with both gram-positive and gram-negative spectrum. Silver nitrate has poor eschar penetration and is painless to apply. This solution leaches sodium and chloride from the wound and must be kept continuously wet to avoid precipitation in the wound and mechanical interference with wound healing by epithelialization. Side effects include hyponatremia, hypochloremia, argyria, and methemoglobinemia. Silver nitrate solution is extremely labor intensive to use because of the need for frequent reapplication and its characteristic staining of the bed linens, floors, and dressings a dark brown to black color.
- Mafenide acetate (Sulfamylon cream and 5% solution) is a broad-spectrum bacteriostatic topical antimicrobial with excellent eschar penetration. Sulfamylon is painful to apply, especially in the cream form, but is better tolerated by patients in solution or slurry. Side effects include being a potent cationic anhydrase inhibitor, especially when applied over a large surface area. This results in a hyperchloremic metabolic acidosis that may result in hyperventilation and respiratory alkalosis.
- Silver-impregnated dressings are applied topically to the burn wound. Body fluid and water activate the bacteriostatic silver ions. The dressings theoretically can be left in place up to 5–7 days, making nursing care simpler and decreasing pain for the patient. No significant toxicity has been reported with this product; however, with fewer dressing changes, festering infections could cause a delay in diagnosis.
- Bacitracin ointment is a broad-spectrum bacterial topical antimicrobial that is an adequate prophylactic agent but should not be used for controlling wound infections. Bacitracin is nontoxic to skin grafts and does not impede epithelialization of the wound as much as other topical antibacterial agents. Side effects include contact dermatitis that is very common with protracted use, nephrotoxicity, and ototoxicity when applied to large surface areas.
- Nitrofurantoin (Furacin) is a bactericidal topical ointment that is effective against gram-negative organisms and some gram-positive organisms. Side effects include possible severe contact dermatitis and nephrotoxicity.
- Povidone iodine (Betadine) is a broad-spectrum bactericidal and fungicidal topical antimicrobial that is not efficacious against *Pseudomonas*. Side effects include renal dysfunction, thyroid dysfunction (which is rare), and inactivation by the wound exudate.

BIBLIOGRAPHY

Barret J, Herndon D. Wound care. In: Barret J, Herndon D (eds.), *Color Atlas of Burn Care*. London, United Kingdom: W.B. Saunders; 2001:5.25–5.38.

Carroughers G. Burn wound assessment and topical treatment. *Burn Care and Therapy*. St. Louis, MO: Mosby; 1998:145–147.

Gallagher JJ, Branski LK, Williams-Bouyer N, Villarreal C, Herndon DN. Treatment of infection in burns. In: Herndon D (ed.), *Total Burn Care*, 4th ed. London, United Kingdom: W.B. Saunders; 2012:137–156.

Lewis GM, Heimbach DM, Gibran NS. Evaluation of the burn wound: management decisions. In: Herndon D (ed.), *Total Burn Care*, 4th ed. London, United Kingdom: W.B. Saunders; 2012:125–130.

Trofino R. Basics of burn care. *Nursing Care of the Burn-Injured Patient*. Philadelphia, PA: FA Davis; 1991:44–50.

22. **(C)** When evaluating a burn patient, there are four critical assessments: airway management, evaluation of other injuries, estimation of burn size, and diagnosis of carbon monoxide or cyanide poisoning. One should always start with the primary survey, taking into account the possibility of inhalational injury. The burn patient should be first and foremost considered a trauma patient, especially when details of the incident are uncertain. Intubation of the unconscious patient is immediately indicated.

Linemen with electrical burns may have sustained a fall or have been thrown away from a transformer with acceleration–deceleration injury. It is important to apply a cervical collar or use inline stabilization until spinal cord injury and head injury have been ruled out.

Cardiac arrhythmia, in particular ventricular fibrillation, is the most common cause of death at the scene and occurs soon after the burn injury. An electrocardiogram (ECG) should be obtained in the emergency department because myocardial injury can occur similar to myocardial contusion. Cardiac markers and serial ECGs should be obtained if myocardial injury is suspected.

The patient with an electrical injury is at significant risk of developing compartment syndrome. The damaged or necrotic muscle swells within the overlying fascia producing dangerously elevated tissue pressures. Serial measurements of compartment pressures are essential to avoid unnecessary muscle necrosis. If compartment syndrome is suspected, prompt fasciotomies should be performed. All four compartments in the lower leg and two in the forearm should be released. Release of the thigh and upper arm compartments may be necessary.

BIBLIOGRAPHY

Arnoldo BD, Hunt J, Sterling JP, Purdue G. Electrical injuries. In: Herndon D (ed.), *Total Burn Care*, 4th ed. London, United Kingdom: W.B. Saunders; 2012:433–440.

Hunt J, Mason A, Masterson T, Pruitt B. The pathophysiology of acute electrical injuries. *J Trauma* 1976;16:335–340.

McCauley R, Barret J. Electrical injuries. In: Achauer B (ed.), *Plastic Surgery Indications, Operations, and Outcomes*, vol. 1. St. Louis, MO: Mosby; 2000:375–385.

Nichter L, Bryant C, Kenney J, et al. Injuries because of commercial electrical current. *J Burn Care Rehabil* 1984;5:124–137.

23. **(C)** Although chemical burns make up a small percentage of the burns treated at a burn center, prompt initial treatment is important to prevent severe tissue damage. Chemical burns vary in severity depending on the type of offending agent and its manner of reactivity, the concentration or strength of the agent, the quantity of the agent in contact with the tissue, the duration of exposure, and the amount of tissue penetration of the agent.

Like thermal burns, chemical burns cause protein denaturation that results in protein coagulation. The great majority of chemicals involved in burns are either acids or alkalis, although solvents and hydrocarbons may also be occasionally involved. Acid chemicals cause a more "superficial" burn, resulting in a coagulation necrosis. Alkali substances produce a liquefaction necrosis and tend to penetrate deeper into the tissues.

The initial treatment of all chemical burns begins with protection of the rescuer by avoiding contact with the offending agent. The patient's clothing should be immediately removed and copious irrigation with water begun. The water should be made to drain or flow away from the patient, thereby diluting the concentration of the chemical and avoiding further injury by the dissolved chemical. Irrigation should continue for at least 30 minutes, and ocular injuries should likewise be irrigated. Neutralizing agents should not be used because of the exothermic reactions these agents can produce when they come in contact with the offending agent. Hydrofluoric acid is an agent used commonly in petroleum production and glass etching and requires therapy in addition to irrigation. In addition to the coagulative necrosis caused by the low pH, the fluoride ion, once in contact with the cells, combines with the positively charged ions of calcium and magnesium acting as a metabolic poison. Until the fluoride ion is completely neutralized by calcium or magnesium, the acid will continue to penetrate deeper into the tissues and cause further protein denaturation. Topical applications of calcium gluconate are necessary in addition to irrigation. These treatments are used four to six times per day until the patient has relief from the significant pain that is the cardinal symptom. Because of the attendant coagulation and necrosis, these wounds often require debridement and grafting as well.

Systemic toxicity may also occur with these chemical agents. Petroleum, formic acid, phenol, and nitrates cause systemic toxicity including pneumonitis, pulmonary edema, hemolysis, renal failure, and even death. Resuscitation and wound debridement of these patients are identical to a thermal burn. An accurate identification of the offending agent is important for tailoring the appropriate therapy (see Fig. 9-13).

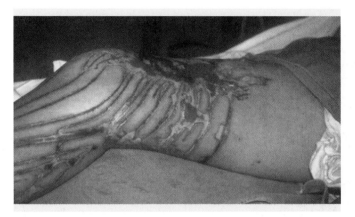

FIGURE 9-13. Lower extremity chemical burn.

BIBLIOGRAPHY

Elijah IE, Sanford AP, Lee JO. Chemical burns. In: Herndon D (ed.), *Total Burn Care*, 4th ed. London, United Kingdom: W.B. Saunders; 2012:455–460.

Leonard L, Scheulen J, Munster A. Chemical burns: effects of prompt first aid. *J Trauma* 1982;22:420–423.

Moran KD, O'Reilly T, Munster A. Chemical burns: a ten-year experience. *Am Surg* 1987;53:652–653.

Mozingo D, Smith A, McManus W, Pruitt B, Mason A. Chemical burns. *J Trauma* 1988;28:642–647.

24. **(A)** Frostbite injury is commonly seen in the northern states. Frostbite injury occurs because of a multitude of factors. There may be peripheral vasoconstriction and decreased blood flow to the extremities because of a drop in core body temperature and the homeostatic response of mandatory heat for the viscera at the expense of the extremities. Impaired patient recognition of impending injury is often because of alcohol, drugs, or psychological disorders. Other factors, such as homelessness, improper clothing, diabetes with neuropathy, and significant wind chill, may predispose a patient to frostbite. After prolonged or rapid exposure to cold depending on the temperature, rapid intracellular ice formation causes cell death. At more gradual cooling rates, osmotic shifts produce cellular dehydration and eventual cell death. Further tissue ischemia occurs because of vasoconstriction of the microcirculation. After this initial

vasoconstriction, the capillaries dilate for a short period of time, and microemboli are formed because of the damage to the endothelium. Tissue edema leads to further vascular resistance and progression to thrombosis, ischemia, and tissue necrosis suggestive of reperfusion injury.

The severity of frostbite cannot be assessed until rewarming of the affected part is complete. In most cases, there is initial insensitivity, followed by significant pain and hyperesthesia. First-degree frostbite demonstrates either erythema or pallor of the affected area but no blister formation. Second-degree frostbite involves some dermal injury and the formation of "white" blisters. Third-degree frostbite is a deeper injury that manifests with the formation of hemorrhagic blisters that evolve to eschar formation. Fourth-degree injury involves muscle or bone.

The treatment of frostbite injury begins with rapid rewarming of the affected part with warm water and environment (40–42°C). White blisters are debrided and treated with aloe vera, and hemorrhagic blisters are left intact. Extremities are elevated, and arteriography should be done. Tissue plasminogen activator should be used if arteriograms show impaired flow to the affected area. Thus far, this has been the only intervention to decrease the number of digits and limbs amputated and is currently undergoing standardization procedures.

Other adjuncts to rewarming have been investigated including hyperbaric oxygen, and intra-arterial vasodilators have been tested, although currently without any known benefit. Amputation of dry necrotic areas is generally performed after there is complete demarcation of the affected part (see Figs. 9-14 and 9-15).

BIBLIOGRAPHY

Bruen KJ, Ballard JR, Morris SE, Cochran A, Edelman LS, Saffle JR. Reduction of the incidence of amputation in frostbite injury with thrombolytic therapy. *Arch Surg* 2007;142:546–553.

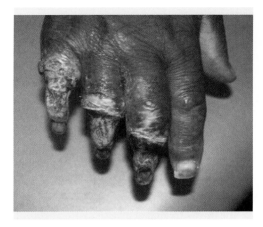

FIGURE 9-15. Frostbite of the hand.

Cochran A, Morris SE, Saffle JR. Cold-induced injury: frostbite. In: Herndon D (ed.), *Total Burn Care*, 4th ed. London, United Kingdom: W.B. Saunders; 2012:449–454.

Johnson AR, Jensen HL, Peltier G, DelaCruz E. Efficacy of intravenous tissue plasminogen activator in frostbite patients and presentation of a treatment protocol for frostbite patients. *Foot Ankle Spec* 2011;4:344–348.

Murphy J, Banwell P, Roberts A, McGrouther DA. Frostbite: pathogenesis and treatment. *J Trauma* 2000;48:171–178.

25. **(C)** Stevens-Johnson syndrome (SJS) (see Fig. 9-16) and toxic epidermal necrolysis syndrome (TENS) (see Fig. 9-17) are exfoliative skin disorders that are often treated in burn units. SJS generally involves an area of 10% TBSA or less. TENS affects an area of 30% or greater. The most common etiology is a rapid immune response to a foreign agent, most frequently a drug. Occasionally, SJS may be attributable to a viral or mycoplasmal infection. The most common causative agents are antibiotics or anticonvulsants.

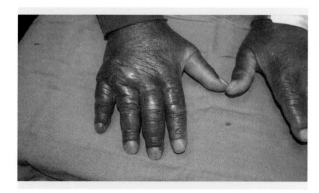

FIGURE 9-14. Frostbite of the hand.

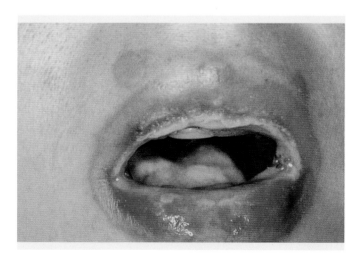

FIGURE 9-16. Stevens-Johnson syndrome.

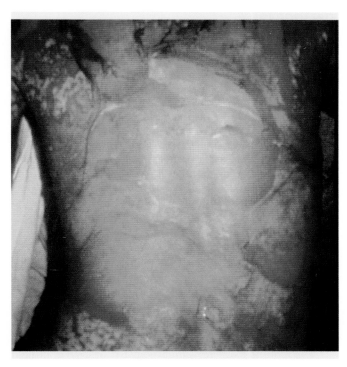

FIGURE 9-17. Toxic epidermal necrolysis.

These skin disorders are usually preceded by a prodromal phase, which includes fever and malaise. Skin tenderness and an erythematous rash follow this prodromal phase and are often suggestive of common viral infections with a viral exanthem. Next, however, large blisters develop in the erythematous area and epidermolysis follows. These blisters represent separation of the dermis and epidermis, and the definitive diagnosis of these syndromes is the positive Nikolsky sign, which manifests when light finger pressure causes the epidermis to desquamate in sheets. Mucosal involvement is common, especially in the oropharynx, anal, and ocular mucosa. Diagnosis is confirmed by skin biopsy, which reveals a dermoepidermal separation with areas of epidermal detachment. Epidermal necrosis is seen with TENS.

The treatment of SJS/TENS begins with the removal of the offending agent. The wounds in SJS/TENS are superficial and, if treated conservatively, will heal spontaneously. Topical antimicrobials may be used, but special care must be taken not to use agents that contain components of the initial causative agent (e.g., sulfa in any systemic, topical, or ophthalmic application). Intravenous fluids are administered to maintain adequate urine output and avoid renal failure. Nutritional support is initiated immediately to facilitate wound healing, particularly when oral mucosal damage has occurred. Corticosteroids, especially with large body surface area involvement, are contraindicated. Recently, studies have been published demonstrating some benefit to the administration of high-dose intravenous immunoglobulins with inhibition of skin slough and a survival rate of 88% at day 45. Further investigation of this treatment is ongoing.

Ocular involvement necessitates frequent ocular examinations by an ophthalmologist. Oral mucosal involvement may extend into the esophagus causing severe dysphagia. Gastrointestinal mucosal slough may occur with massive hemorrhage. Pulmonary tree sloughing may also occur with resultant airway obstruction. Sepsis is the most common cause of death in these patients, although acute respiratory failure is occasionally seen when pulmonary mucosal involvement occurs.

BIBLIOGRAPHY

Fagan S, Chai J, Spies M, et al. Exfoliative and necrotizing diseases of the skin. In: Herndon D (ed.), *Total Burn Care*, 4th ed. London, United Kingdom: W.B. Saunders; 2012:471–482.

Halebian P, Madden M, Finklestein J. Improved burn centre survival of patients with toxic epidermal necrolysis managed without corticosteroids. *Ann Surg* 1986;204:503–512.

Halebian P, Shires G. Burn unit treatment of acute, severe exfoliating disorders. *Ann Rev Med* 1989;40:137–147.

Prins C, Kerdel F, Padilla S, et al. Treatment of toxic epidermal necrolysis with high-dose intravenous immunoglobulins. *Arch Dermatol* 2003;139:26–32.

26. **(B)** A skin graft or skin autograft is the autologous transfer of dermis, epidermis, and component structures to another site on the organism after complete separation of the graft from its original site and blood supply. After transplantation occurs, the skin graft must adhere to the wound bed and become revascularized. This process is referred to as skin graft "take." There are three phases of skin graft take: plasmatic imbibition, inosculation, and revascularization.

Immediately after a skin graft is placed on a wound bed, a network of fibrin mesh is formed between the graft and the wound bed, allowing for graft adherence and setting the stage for the phase of graft nutrition that depends solely on diffusion. In the first 24 hours, the graft imbibes plasma like a sponge passively from bed to cells in the graft both by passive osmotic gradient and cell membrane transport. During this time, the graft becomes edematous and increases 40–50% in weight. This action, referred to as plasmatic imbibition, sustains the graft until revascularization occurs. The grafts are adherent but pale in appearance during this phase, which persists from 12–36 hours.

The next phase of graft take is inosculation. This term is used to describe the alignment or "kissing" of vessels from the wound bed with patent vessels remaining in the graft after harvest. There is controversy over whether the capillary buds project from the wound bed into the preexisting vessels or from new vessel formation by angiogenesis. This inosculation phase occurs from approximately 36–48 hours and gradually replaces the phase of plasmatic imbibition as the method of nutrition.

Revascularization continues after grafting for approximately 3–7 days. Initially, all of the vessels are unidirectional into the graft. Over time, these vessels differentiate into afferent and efferent vessels, and revascularization is complete. In this phase, the grafts appear pink and blanch with compression. Lymphatic flow is reestablished by postgraft day 5. Reinnervation of skin grafts depends on the graft thickness and the wound bed that the graft was placed on. The sensation to the graft is not normal; however, it does obtain some of the nervous characteristics of the adjacent skin and wound bed. The nerves grow into the skin graft from the wound base and periphery through the empty graft neurilemmal sheaths. Pain sensation returns first, followed by light touch and temperature. Reinnervation of the graft stops from 12–24 months. Split-thickness skin grafts have a faster rate of reinnervation, whereas full-thickness grafts have a more complete reinnervation.

Full-thickness skin grafts are grafts in which the full thickness of the skin, the epidermis, and the entire dermis are taken. The donor site must be closed primarily, by split-thickness skin grafting or by flap. Full-thickness skin grafts have a greater distance of diffusion in the phase of plasmatic imbibition and slower rate of revascularization. Full-thickness skin grafts are used for areas where graft contraction must be kept to a minimum, such as the face or hands, and are limited by the amount of donor skin available without compromising function at the donor site. Split-thickness skin grafts are used to cover large surfaces, may be reharvested multiple times, and can be meshed to cover larger surfaces (see Fig. 9-18).

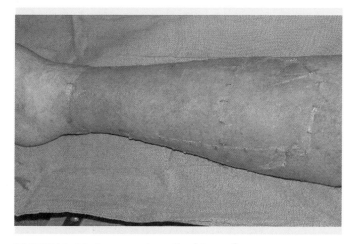

FIGURE 9-18. Lower extremity skin graft.

BIBLIOGRAPHY

Kelton P. Skin grafts. *Select Readings Plast Surg* 1995;8:2–18.
Ratner D. Skin grafting: from here to there. *Dermatol Clin.* 1998;16(1):75–90.
Scherer-Pietramaggiori SS, Pietramaggiori G, Orgill DP. Skin grafts. In: Neligan PC (ed.), *Plastic Surgery*, 3rd ed. Philadelphia, PA: W.B. Saunders; 2012:318–338.
Skouge J. Full thickness skin grafting. In: *Skin Grafting*. New York, NY: Churchill Livingstone; 1991:47–63.
Skouge J. Split thickness skin grafting. In: *Skin Grafting*. New York, NY: Churchill Livingstone; 1991:5–45.
Vasconez H. Skin grafts. In: Cohen M (ed.), *Mastery of Plastic and Reconstructive Surgery*, vol. 1. Boston, MA: Little, Brown & Company; 1994:45–55.

27. **(B)** Hypertrophic scar formation is common after burns when it takes more than 14 days for a burn to heal. Hypertrophic scars are often elevated, inelastic, erythematous, and pruritic. More commonly, they are associated with deeper burns, infection, or other causes of poor wound healing. Hypertrophic scars can also form contractures, leading to significant postburn morbidity and requiring scar revision by Z-plasty or even grafting if the burn encompasses a large area or inhibits movement. Hypertrophic scars do not extend beyond the borders of the original wound and are found often in Hispanics, Caucasians, and those of African descent. Keloids, which grow beyond the borders of the original wound, are more common in those with darkly pigmented skin and can occur in response to many wound types including punctures. Hypertrophic scars can enlarge for a period of months after the burn and then may regress to flat after a few years. Often, changes in pigmentation are permanent. Fibroblasts are responsible for creating the extracellular matrix, namely collagen, within a scar. Fibroblasts found within the deep dermis are most similar to those found in hypertrophic scars and create disorganized connective tissue with irregular collagen bundles. Current research is focused on these fibroblasts and cytokine actors and how they might be modified to create more normal scar tissue.

BIBLIOGRAPHY

Hawkins H, Finnerty C, Pathophysiology of the burn scar. In: Herndon D (ed.), *Total Burn Care*, 4th ed. London, United Kingdom: W.B. Saunders; 2012:507–516.
Kwan P, Desmouliere A, Tredget E. Molecular and cellular basis of hypertrophic scarring. In: Herndon D (ed.), *Total Burn Care*, 4th ed. London, United Kingdom: W.B. Saunders; 2012: 495–505.

28. **(A)** On arrival to the emergency department, the burn patient should have their airway, breathing, and

circulation assessed. The patient should be intubated if necessary, and supplemental oxygen of 100% FiO$_2$ should be provided. Complete exposure of the patient should be performed and secondary surveys undertaken to assess the extent of injury and rule out associated trauma. Evaluations of circumferential burns to the limbs or thorax should be completed to assess the need for escharotomy. Arterial blood gas, carboxyhemoglobin levels, a complete blood count, serum electrolytes, glucose, blood urea nitrogen (BUN), and creatinine laboratory evaluations should be obtained for major burn patients. Chest x-ray and any other radiologic examinations are to be performed as deemed necessary.

A complete history should be completed with details of the accident of particular importance. The patient should have intravenous access established and Ringer's lactate solution infused per Parkland formula. An indwelling urinary catheter should be placed, a tetanus immunization given, and gastric decompression with a nasogastric tube performed if necessary. The patient must be kept warm with warmed intravenous solutions and blankets. Transportation should be via ground or air depending on the stability of the patient and the travel distance.

There are established criteria for transferring patients to a burn center. These criteria include greater than 10% TBSA partial-thickness burns; full-thickness burns; burns involving specialty areas such as the face, perineum, genitalia, hands, feet, and joints; chemical and electrical burns; and patients with inhalation injury. Patients with preexisting medical conditions that would adversely affect patient management should be transferred. Any patient with associated trauma in whom the burn injury poses the greatest threat should also be transferred.

BIBLIOGRAPHY

American Burn Association. *Advanced Burn Life Support Providers Manual*. Chicago, IL: American Burn Association; 2011.

Bueno R, Demling R. Management of burns in the multiple trauma patient. *Adv Trauma* 1989:165–178.

Mlcak R, Buffalo M. Pre-hospital management, transportation, and emergency care. In: Herndon D (ed.), *Total Burn Care*, 4th ed. London, United Kingdom: W.B. Saunders; 2012:93–102.

Rosenkranz K, Sheridan R. Management of the burned trauma patient: balancing conflicting priorities. *Burns* 2002;28: 665–669.

29. **(C)** The burn patient should be first and foremost considered a trauma patient, especially when details of the incident are uncertain. One should always start with the primary survey, taking into account the possibility of inhalational injury. On secondary survey, the obvious hand deformities in this patient suggest a possible

contracture or posturing on the part of the patient. It is important to apply a cervical collar or use inline stabilization until spinal cord injury has been ruled out. Patients with electrical injuries can sustain such strong tetanic muscle contractions that compression fractures may occur. These patients may also fall from heights or be thrown and sustain further trauma. Extensive evaluation of these patients in the emergency department is imperative (see Fig. 9-19).

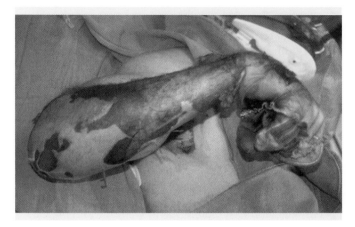

FIGURE 9-19. Upper extremity contracture.

BIBLIOGRAPHY

Endorf F, Gibran N. Burns. In: Brunicardi F (ed.), *Schwartz's Principles of Surgery*, 9th ed. San Francisco, CA: McGraw Hill Medical; 2010:197–208.

Mlcak R, Buffalo M, Jimenez C. Pre-hospital management, transportation, and emergency care. In: Herndon D (ed.), *Total Burn Care*, 4th ed. London, United Kingdom: W.B. Saunders; 2012:93–102.

30. **(D)** Many states have laws requiring residences to have working fire alarms. From the National Institute of Standards and Technology executive summary:

The home smoke alarm is credited as the greatest success story in fire safety in the last part of the 20th century. As inhalational injury remains the most common cause of fire-related death, the smoke alarm serves to alert occupants of a house fire and the presence of noxious smoke early enough to evacuate. The smoke alarm represents a highly effective fire safety technology that was rapidly adopted, now with nearly universal usage, in a remarkably short time. U. S. home usage of smoke alarms rose from less than 10% in 1975 to at least 95% in 2000, while the number of home fire deaths was cut nearly in half. Other highly effective fire safety technologies either affect a smaller share of the fire related deaths (e.g., child-resistant lighter, cigarette-resistant mattress or upholstered furniture) or have yet to see more than token usage (e.g., home fire sprinkler, reduced ignition-strength cigarette). A seminal component underpinning this success was the existence of a comprehensive, independent set of tests conducted in 1975-76 that clearly demonstrated the potential of smoke alarms to save lives. These were the so-called Indiana Dunes tests sponsored by The National Institute of Standards and Technology, NIST, (then the National Bureau of Standards) and conducted by Illinois Institute of Technology Research Institute and Underwriters Laboratories.

More recent tests with different types of alarms, including carbon monoxide detectors, were conducted in a similar manner to the Indiana Dunes tests. These continue to suggest that smoke alarms and other associated alarms have the potential to save lives.

BIBLIOGRAPHY

Hunt JL, Arnoldo BD, Purdue GF. Prevention of burn injuries. In: Herndon D (ed.), *Total Burn Care*, 4th ed. London, United Kingdom: W.B. Saunders; 2012:47–55.

US Fire Administration. Smoke Alarm Outreach Material. http://www.usfa.fema.gov/prevention/outreach/smoke_alarms.html. Updated September 26, 2014. Accessed September 28, 2014.

US Fire Administration. State-by-State Residential Smoke Alarm Requirements. FEMA, 2010. http://www.thewfsf.org/sap_usa_files/FEMA_StateSmokeAlarmRequirementsMay2010.pdf. Accessed November 9, 2015.

31. **(A)** The "Rule of 9s" is a way to estimate TBSA of a burn injury on an adult and can be modified to fit children. Only burns that are deeper than first-degree, partial- or full-thickness burns should be counted when assessing the percent burn in a patient. The 9's come from most areas of the body being divisible by 9 in the adult: the head is 9%, each arm is 9%, the legs are each 18%, and trunk anterior and posterior are each 18%. The neck accounts for the remaining 1%. The TBSA of children differs as they age, as seen in Fig. 9-20. The head, for example, can be up to 20% TBSA of an infant and less than 10% TBSA of an adult. This consideration is important when determining the management strategy and fluid requirements for a patient, because only burns involving greater than 20% TBSA are accounted for in the Parkland formula.

BIBLIOGRAPHY

Micak R, Buffalo M, Jimenez C. Pre-hospital management, transportation and emergency care. In: Herndon D (ed.), *Total Burn Care*, 4th ed. London, United Kingdom: W.B. Saunders; 2012: 93–102.

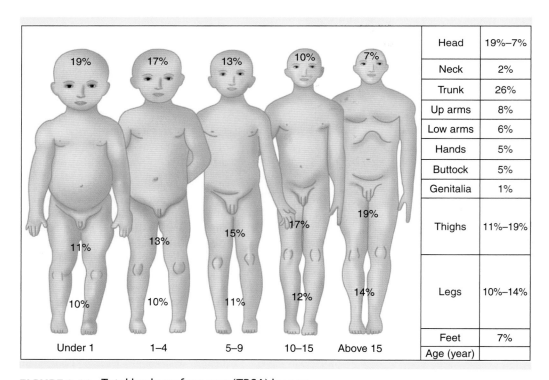

Head	19%–7%
Neck	2%
Trunk	26%
Up arms	8%
Low arms	6%
Hands	5%
Buttock	5%
Genitalia	1%
Thighs	11%–19%
Legs	10%–14%
Feet	7%
Age (year)	

FIGURE 9-20. Total body surface area (TBSA) by age.

32. **(B)** The pathophysiology of electrical burns is related to the resistance of the contact point, the amperage involved, the time of contact, and the type of current. Electricity is converted into heat within the body. Joule's law is described as

$$P(\text{power} = \text{heat}) = I^2(\text{amperage})R(\text{resistance})$$

The areas of greatest resistance are the skin and bone; however, once the electricity overcomes the resistance of the skin, the body acts as a volume conductor of heat. The tissue destruction is highest when the current enters an area with a small cross-sectional diameter and tends to be dissipated when a larger surface is crossed. Maximal tissue destruction occurs in the areas adjacent to the contact spots and is decreased as distance from these points increases. Often, the electrical burn patient will have normal-appearing skin with muscular tissue destruction beneath.

Acute muscle destruction, either from the immediate electrical burn or from the following compartment syndrome, causes a release of myoglobin from the damaged muscle cells. The myoglobin is then excreted in the urine, turning urine pink to muddy brown. These pigments can cause acute renal failure by obstructing the distal convoluted renal tubules. The patient's intravenous fluid should be increased to maintain an elevated urine output between 75 and 100 mL/h or 1–2 mL/kg/h until the myoglobin is cleared. The urine can be alkalinized to prevent precipitation of myoglobin in the renal tubules. Mannitol may be used for a rapid osmotic diuresis to allow the elevated urine output to continue. Although alkalinization and mannitol have not been supported by level I evidence, they are used in many burn centers across the United States.

BIBLIOGRAPHY

Arnoldo BD, Hunt JL, Sterline JP, Purdue GF. Electrical injuries. In: Herndon D (ed.), *Total Burn Care*, 4th ed. London, United Kingdom: W.B. Saunders; 2012:47–55.

Loiacono LA, Price LA. Electrical and lightning injury. In: Cameron J, Cameron A (eds.), *Current Surgical Therapy*, 11th ed. Philadelphia, PA: Saunders; 2014:1143–1152.

33. **(C)** Tar and asphalt create scald wounds. They are often heated to 400–500°F (>200°C) in the reservoir of the tar truck. The tar cools as it is spread over a roof or driveway; however, it can still cause deep burns because it remains in contact with the skin until removed. Removal of tar without causing further damage to the skin beneath can be challenging. No burn assessment can be made until the wound is clean. Removing the tar can be done using petroleum-based ointment, with or without vitamin E, under a dressing. The dressing should be changed every 2–4 hours until the tar has dissolved. Sprays exist that can help dissolve tar without further injury to the skin. Tar is not water soluble, so water-based solvents will not work.

BIBLIOGRAPHY

Lewis G. Heimbach D, Gibran N. Evaluation of the burn wound: management decisions. In: Herndon D (ed.), *Total Burn Care*, 4th ed. London, United Kingdom: W.B. Saunders; 2012: 125–135.

Ng K, Dalen D, Rhine D. Management of hot tar burn using vitamin E ointment containing petroleum and polyoxyethylene sorbitan. *Can J Emerg Med* 2013;15:307–310.

CHAPTER 10

INFLAMMATION AND SHOCK

ZACHARY ABECASSIS, PETER DORSCHNER, AND STEVEN SCHWULST

QUESTIONS

1. Cells of the monocyte-macrophage lineage recognize antigens by which of the following mechanisms?
   - (A) Lipid A
   - (B) Toll-like receptors (TLR)
   - (C) T-cell receptor
   - (D) Immunoglobulin G
   - (E) Interleukin (IL)-2

2. The cell type most characteristic of chronic inflammation is the
   - (A) Macrophage
   - (B) B cell
   - (C) Natural killer cell
   - (D) Neutrophil
   - (E) Eosinophil

3. The resolution of an acute inflammatory process is mediated by which of the following?
   - (A) Apoptosis
   - (B) Anti-inflammatory cytokines
   - (C) Angiogenesis
   - (D) Corticosteroids
   - (E) All of the above

4. In the alternative pathway of the complement cascade, the stimulus for the production of C3 convertase is provided by which of the following?
   - (A) Antibody-antigen complex
   - (B) Virus-infected cells
   - (C) Mannin-binding lectin
   - (D) IL-3

5. A 35-year-old man develops a fever of 38.9°C 24 hours after being involved in a motor vehicle crash in which he sustained multiple lower extremity fractures. This febrile response stems from which of the following mediators?
   - (A) IL-1
   - (B) IL-2
   - (C) Interferon (IFN)-α
   - (D) IL-10
   - (E) IL-4

6. Which molecule is a precursor of nitric oxide?
   - (A) Citrulline
   - (B) Arginine
   - (C) Tryptophan
   - (D) Alanine
   - (E) Leucine

7. The severity of hypovolemic shock has been found to correlate with
   - (A) Hematocrit
   - (B) Pulmonary capillary wedge pressure (PCWP)
   - (C) Lactic acid
   - (D) PaO_2
   - (E) White blood cell count

Questions 8 and 9

An 80-year-old male undergoes pancreatic debridement. On postoperative day 6, the patient begins a regular diet, and subsequently, the output from the drains also markedly increases. Two days later, the patient develops hypotension and tachycardia, accompanied by oliguria and confusion.

8. The first organ affected by the compensatory mechanisms of hypovolemic shock is the
   - (A) Heart
   - (B) Kidney
   - (C) Gastrointestinal tract
   - (D) Skin
   - (E) Spleen

9. The initial compensatory mechanism to hypovolemic shock is the release of
   (A) Aldosterone
   (B) Norepinephrine
   (C) Renin
   (D) Vasopressin
   (E) Angiotensinogen

10. A 22-year-old male presents to the emergency department after sustaining a gunshot wound to the right upper quadrant of his abdomen. On arrival, the patient is lethargic. His systolic blood pressure is 85 mmHg with a heart rate of 130 bpm. Fluid resuscitation is initiated. Which of the following is the most appropriate resuscitation fluid?
   (A) 0.9% sodium chloride
   (B) Albumin
   (C) Dextran
   (D) 5% dextrose in 0.45% sodium chloride
   (E) 3% sodium chloride

11. A 41-year-old woman presents to the emergency department after sustaining a gunshot wound to the abdomen, with injuries to the liver and large bowel. Despite successful resuscitation and operative intervention, the patient dies 2 weeks later of multisystem organ failure in the intensive care unit. Which organ most likely first experienced dysfunction?
   (A) Liver
   (B) Gastrointestinal tract
   (C) Lung
   (D) Kidney
   (E) Heart

12. A 23-year-old man presents to the emergency department after an altercation in which he sustained trauma to his head and neck. On arrival, the patient is found to have a systolic blood pressure of 65 mmHg with a heart rate of 50 bpm. His Glasgow Coma Scale score is 5. A head computed tomography (CT) reveals a large epidural hematoma, whereas a cervical spine CT demonstrates bilateral vertebral facet dislocations at the level of C4. What is the likely cause of his hypotension?
   (A) Head trauma
   (B) Hypovolemia
   (C) Massive vasodilatation
   (D) Alcohol intoxication
   (E) Blunt cardiac injury

13. The most common mechanism of spinal cord injury is
   (A) Distraction
   (B) Transection
   (C) Impact with persisting compression
   (D) Impact alone
   (E) Laceration

14. In which category of shock is the Trendelenburg position considered a viable treatment option?
   (A) Cardiogenic
   (B) Neurogenic
   (C) Hypovolemic
   (D) Septic
   (E) Cardiac compressive

15. A 74-year-old previously healthy woman is admitted to the hospital and undergoes an uneventful open appendectomy for a ruptured appendix. On postoperative day 1, the patient reports crushing substernal chest pain with radiation to the left arm. She appears pale, anxious, and diaphoretic. Her extremities are cold. Initial vital signs reveal a systolic blood pressure of 75 mmHg and a heart rate of 101 bpm. An electrocardiogram (ECG) is consistent with an acute anterior myocardial infarction. What factor predicts the development of cardiogenic shock in the setting of an acute myocardial infarction (MI)?
   (A) ST elevations on presenting ECG
   (B) Age less than 75 years old
   (C) Posterior infarction
   (D) Pulmonary rales on physical examination
   (E) Inferior infarction

16. The patient in Question 15 is transferred to the intensive care unit, and judicious fluid resuscitation and vasopressor support are initiated. A pulmonary artery catheter is placed to guide therapy. What readings are characteristic of cardiogenic shock?

	Cardiac Output	Systemic Vascular Resistance	PCWP	Central Venous Pressure
(A)	Low	High	High	Normal to high
(B)	Low	High	Low	Low
(C)	High	Low	Low	High
(D)	Low	High	Low	High
(E)	High	Low	Low	Low

17. A transthoracic echocardiogram is obtained and demonstrates new-onset mitral regurgitation. An angiogram is immediately performed, showing acute left main coronary artery occlusion. What is the next step in management?
   (A) Thrombolytic therapy
   (B) Emergent coronary artery bypass graft (CABG) with mitral valve repair
   (C) Emergent percutaneous coronary intervention (PCI) (angioplasty with stenting)

(D) Medical stabilization followed by delayed PCI

(E) Placement of an intra-aortic balloon pump (IABP)

18. A 69-year-old woman with a history of hypertension presents to the emergency department with complaints of sudden-onset crushing chest pain. On physical examination, she is ill-appearing, hypotensive, and tachycardic. An ECG reveals ST elevations in the V3 and V4 leads. What is a characteristic finding on echocardiogram in this condition?

(A) Tricuspid regurgitation

(B) Left ventricular hypokinesis

(C) Mitral regurgitation

(D) Left ventricular dilatation

(E) Aortic root dilatation

19. Which of the following are the typical measurements demonstrated by a Swan-Ganz catheter placed in the 69-year-old woman described in Question 18?

	Central Venous Pressure	PCWP	Cardiac Index
(A)	Normal	High	Low to normal
(B)	High	Low to normal	Low to normal
(C)	High	High	Low
(D)	Low	Low	High
(E)	Normal	Low	High

20. Which is true about an intra-aortic balloon pump?

(A) It increases perfusion at the expense of elevated oxygen consumption.

(B) It inflates during late diastole and deflates in late systole.

(C) It is complicated by vascular damage and bleeding in 5–20% of patients.

(D) It significantly improves mortality in early revascularization candidates.

(E) It is contraindicated for use in patients with mitral regurgitation.

21. Inflation of the intra-aortic balloon pump occurs at which point on an ECG?

(A) T wave

(B) P wave

(C) PR interval

(D) R wave

(E) QRS complex

22. A 30-year-old man is involved in an altercation in which he was stabbed in the left thoracoabdominal flank. Prior to his arrival at the emergency department by ambulance, the patient is hemodynamically normal without signs of respiratory compromise. On arrival to the trauma bay, the blood pressure is 82/45 mmHg and heart rate is 100 bpm. Fluid resuscitation is initiated with only transient increases in the blood pressure. On examination, breath sounds are equal bilaterally. No abdominal tenderness is elicited. A chest x-ray is unremarkable, and focused assessment with sonography for trauma (FAST) exam demonstrates cardiac tamponade. The patient develops pulseless electrical activity. What is the next step in management while in the emergency department?

(A) Continued intravenous hydration

(B) Emergency department thoracotomy

(C) Subxiphoid pericardial window

(D) Pericardiocentesis

(E) Placement of a pulmonary artery catheter

23. What readings would a pulmonary artery catheter have demonstrated in the patient described in Question 22 prior to the advent of the pulseless electrical activity?

(A) High cardiac output

(B) Equalization of the systolic pressures among the cardiac chambers

(C) Equalization of the diastolic pressures among the cardiac chambers

(D) High systemic vascular resistance

(E) High PCWP

24. A 65-year-old man presents to the emergency department in obvious respiratory distress following a seafood dinner. On arrival, the patient is intubated. His vital signs are significant for marked tachycardia and hypotension. Urticarial lesions are identified. What is the mediator of this condition?

(A) Immunoglobulin (Ig) A

(B) IgG

(C) IgE

(D) IgM

(E) IgD

25. The patient in Question 24 has been taking β-blocking medications for treatment of hypertension. Epinephrine was given at the standard dosage for treatment of anaphylaxis without any improvement in his condition. What agent should be used next for treatment of his current hypotension?

(A) Epinephrine in a higher dosage

(B) Glucagon

(C) Hydrocortisone

(D) Ranitidine

(E) Norepinephrine

26. An example of an anti-inflammatory cytokine is
    (A) IL-2
    (B) IFN-γ
    (C) Lymphotoxin-α (LT-α)
    (D) IL-4
    (E) Tumor necrosis factor-α (TNF-α)

27. Which of the following is a biological function of TNF-α in inflammation?
    (A) Initiation of the coagulation cascade
    (B) Increased insulin sensitivity
    (C) Inhibition of macrophage phagocytosis
    (D) Stimulation of muscle growth

28. Which of the following is true of tissue oxygenation in septic shock?
    (A) Oxygen delivery is elevated while oxygen extraction is decreased.
    (B) Oxygen delivery is reduced while oxygen extraction is increased.
    (C) Arterial-venous oxygen difference is increased.
    (D) Both oxygen delivery and extraction are increased.
    (E) Mixed venous oxygen is decreased.

29. Glucocorticoids influence the inflammatory response by which of the following?
    (A) Enhanced production of IkB
    (B) Increased neutrophil aggregation
    (C) Increased production of cyclooxygenase (COX)
    (D) Increased IL-2 levels
    (E) Enhancement of inducible nitric oxide synthase production

30. A 46-year-old woman develops septic shock following an open cholecystectomy for a gangrenous gallbladder. She remains intubated after surgery but exhibits persistent hypoxia with maximal ventilator support. The diagnosis of acute respiratory distress syndrome (ARDS) is suggested. This condition is defined by which of the following criteria?
    (A) $PaO_2/FiO_2 < 200$ and PCWP < 18 mmHg
    (B) $PaO_2/FiO_2 > 200$ and PCWP < 18 mmHg
    (C) $PaO_2/FiO_2 < 200$ and PCWP > 18 mmHg
    (D) $PaO_2/FiO_2 > 200$ and PCWP > 18 mmHg

31. Positive end-expiratory pressure (PEEP) is added to the ventilatory support of the patient in Question 30 with an improvement in her oxygenation. Which of the following describes the mechanism by which PEEP improves oxygenation?
    (A) Reduction in the rate of pulmonary edema formation
    (B) Improvement in the reabsorption of edema fluid
    (C) Inhibition of the opening of collapsed alveoli

    (D) Prevention of the collapse of alveoli
    (E) Enhancement of surfactant production

32. A 75-year-old man with a history of steroid-dependent chronic obstructive pulmonary disease undergoes a left hemicolectomy for treatment of cancer. The operation is complicated by an anastomotic dehiscence, requiring reexploration and the creation of a colostomy. Following surgery, the patient becomes febrile and exhibits a decline in his systolic blood pressure. The nitric oxide–induced vasodilatation exhibited by this patient is mediated by which intracellular messenger?
    (A) Cyclic adenosine monophosphate (cAMP)
    (B) Cyclic guanosine monophosphate (cGMP)
    (C) Inositol 1,4,5-trisphosphate (IP_3)
    (D) Diacylglycerol (DAG)
    (E) Inosine 5-monophosphate (IMP)

33. The effects of nitric oxide inhibition include
    (A) Pulmonary hypertension
    (B) Decreased neutrophil adhesion
    (C) Increased peroxynitrite production
    (D) More pronounced inhibition of mitochondrial respiration
    (E) Elevated cardiac output

34. A pulmonary artery catheter measures which of the following parameters directly?
    (A) Cardiac index
    (B) Systemic vascular resistance
    (C) Mixed venous oxygen saturation
    (D) Left ventricular end diastolic pressure
    (E) Pulmonary vascular resistance index

35. The variable directly measured by gastric tonometry is the
    (A) Gastric mucosal pH
    (B) Gastric mucosal PCO_2
    (C) Gastric mucosal PO_2
    (D) Gastric mucosal bicarbonate
    (E) Splanchnic hypoperfusion

ANSWERS AND EXPLANATIONS

1. **(B)** Phagocytic cells such as macrophages, monocytes, and neutrophils compose the innate immune system. Innate immunity represents a preexisting resistance to antigens, not requiring a prior exposure. This contrasts with acquired immunity, which depends on repeated contact with the antigen to augment the immune response. Although the innate immune system commences an inflammatory reaction, its interaction with the T and B cells of acquired immunity propagate and strengthen the response.

The specificity of the response to an antigen is mediated by the toll-like receptors (TLRs), a family of pattern recognition molecules. This family of transmembrane protein receptors, present on the surface of macrophages and monocytes, binds various antigenic products such as bacterial flagellin and DNA. Each of the 10 known TLRs detects a particular antigen; for example, TLR-3 and TLR-4 bind viral double-stranded DNA and lipopolysaccharide (LPS), respectively. Following the attachment of LPS to the LPS-binding protein, TLR-4, in conjunction with MD2 and the soluble protein CD14, activates a cascade of intracellular proteins, including the toll/IL-1 receptor–associated protein and the mitogen-activated protein (MAP) kinases, ultimately resulting in activation of nuclear factor-κB (NF-κB) (see Fig. 10-1). This transcription factor promotes the expression of numerous inflammatory mediators.

Lipid A is the toxic moiety of LPS, the characteristic outer membrane component of gram-negative bacteria. The T-cell receptor detects antigens in the context of antigen-presenting cells, phagocytic cells that expose antigenic components on their surface. Immunoglobulin G is generated by B cells in response to a specific antigen; this antibody may appear on the surface membrane of B cells or free within the blood. IL-2 is a cytokine product of the inflammatory process.

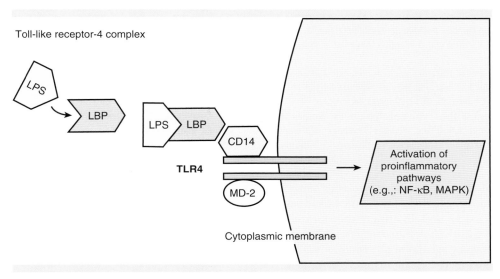

FIGURE 10-1. The toll-like receptor (TLR) binds lipopolysaccharide (LPS). LBP, lipopolysaccharide-binding protein. From Brunicardi FC, Andersen DK, Billiar TR, et al. (eds.), *Schwartz's Principles of Surgery*, 9th ed. New York, NY: McGraw-Hill Professional; 2009:Fig. 2-13.

BIBLIOGRAPHY

Beutler B, Poltorak A. Sepsis and evolution of the innate immune response. *Crit Care Med* 2001;29(7):S2–S6.

Henneke P, Golenbock DT. Innate immune recognition of lipopolysaccharide by endothelial cells. *Crit Care Med* 2002;30(5):S207–S213.

Jan BV, Lowry SF. Systemic response to injury and metabolic support. In: Brunicardi F, Andersen DK, Billiar TR, et al (eds.), *Schwartz's Principles of Surgery*, 9th ed. New York, NY: McGraw-Hill; 2010:Chapter 2.

Kumar V, Abbas AK, Fausto N, Aster JC, Perkins JA. Acute and chronic inflammation. In Kumar V, Abbas AK, Aster JC (eds.), *Robbins and Cotran Pathologic Basis of Disease, Professional Edition*, 8th ed. Maryland Heights, MO: W. B. Saunders; 2010:Chapter 2.

Levinson W. Cellular basis of the immune response. In: Levinson W (ed.), *Review of Medical Microbiology & Immunology*, 12th ed. New York, NY: McGraw-Hill; 2012:Chapter 58.

Zigarelli B, Sheehan M, Wong HR. Nuclear factor-κB as a therapeutic target in critical care medicine. *Crit Care Med* 2003;31(1):S105–S111.

2. **(A)** Chronic inflammation represents the persistence of an acute inflammatory process. It may occur in the setting of multiple episodes of acute inflammation at a single site or the incomplete eradication of an initial inflammatory focus. The predominant cell type involved in chronic inflammation is the macrophage, its activity promoted by tumor necrosis factor-α (TNF-α) and interferon-γ (INF-γ). Mediators released from activated macrophages affect fibroblast activity and vascular formation, resulting in scarring. The prototypical lesion resulting from these factors is the granuloma—a collection of inflammatory cells encased in a fibrotic shell. Granulomata are especially associated with intracellular

bacteria and inorganic pathogens, as with tuberculosis or berylliosis. These lesions confine bacteria to a single area, restrict bacterial reproduction, and limit nutrition and oxygen to the pathogens within.

Although lymphocytes also take part in the chronic inflammatory process, macrophages serve as the predominant cell type. Neutrophils act in acute inflammation. The natural killer cell destroys tumor cells as well as virus-infected cells. Eosinophils are involved in allergic reactions and helminthic parasite infections.

BIBLIOGRAPHY

Kumar V, Abbas AK, Fausto N, Aster JC, Perkins JA. Acute and chronic inflammation. In Kumar V, Abbas AK, Aster JC (eds.), *Robbins and Cotran Pathologic Basis of Disease, Professional Edition*, 8th ed. Maryland Heights, MO: W. B. Saunders; 2010:Chapter 2.

Levinson W. Cellular basis of the immune response. In: Levinson W (ed.), *Review of Medical Microbiology & Immunology*, 12th ed. New York, NY: McGraw-Hill; 2012:Chapter 58.

Winchester R. Principles of the immune response. In: Humes HD, DuPont HL, Gardner LB (eds.), *Kelley's Textbook of Internal Medicine*, 4th ed. Philadelphia, PA: Lippincott. Williams & Wilkins; 2000:14–21.

3. **(E)** A number of anti-inflammatory cytokines participate in the downregulation of the acute inflammatory process, including IL-4, IL-10, and transforming growth factor (TGF)-β. IL-4, in particular, initially acts as a pro-inflammatory agent, but ultimately counters production of the superoxide anion and IL-6. Programmed cell death, apoptosis, may also contribute to the resolution of inflammation. TNF-α has been shown to induce apoptosis by binding to its receptor, TNFR1, thus activating its death domain. Several other mediators demonstrate similar effects: the eicosanoids, IL-10, and the antioxidants. Attention has also focused on the hypothalamic-pituitary-adrenocortical axis, with the realization that glucocorticoids, as immunosuppressants, may moderate the inflammatory response. In studies, observations have been made of increases in adrenocorticotropic hormone (ACTH) and corticosterone in animals injected with IL-1, IL-6, and TNF-α. Finally, the mediators responsible for wound healing and angiogenesis, among them TGF-α and -β, endothelial cells, epidermal growth factor, and platelet-derived growth factor, are also subjects of study for their role in the downregulation of inflammation.

BIBLIOGRAPHY

Choi K, Spence RK, Shander A, Scott-Connor CEH. Hemostasis, thrombosis, anticoagulation, hematopoiesis, and blood transfusion. In: O'Leary JP (ed.), *The Physiologic Basis of Surgery*, 4th ed. Philadelphia, PA: Lippincott Williams & Wilkins; 2008:533–575.

Kumar V, Abbas AK, Fausto N, Aster JC, Perkins JA. Acute and chronic inflammation. In Kumar V, Abbas AK, Aster JC (eds.), *Robbins and Cotran Pathologic Basis of Disease, Professional Edition*, 8th ed. Maryland Heights, MO: W. B. Saunders; 2010:Chapter 2.

Levinson W. Cellular basis of the immune response. In: Levinson W (ed.), *Review of Medical Microbiology & Immunology*, 12th ed. New York, NY: McGraw-Hill; 2012:Chapter 58.

4. **(B)** There are three pathways by which complement is activated: the classical, alternative, and mannan-binding lectin pathways (see Fig. 10-2). The classical pathway is initiated by antibody-antigen complexes, whereas the alternative pathway begins in the absence of antibody with virus-infected cells, parasites, or LPS. The mannan-binding lectin pathway commences in the presence of lectin, a protein that binds to mannan, a carbohydrate found on certain microorganisms. Despite their disparate beginnings, the three pathways converge with C_3, which is cleaved into C_{3a} and C_{3b} by C_3 convertase. The C_{3b} fragment then acts to opsonize target particles. The C_{3a} fragment, as well as the product of C^5 convertase, C_{5a}, serves to attract and activate leukocytes to the site of inflammation (chemotaxis) as well as to promote vasodilatation. The final product of the three pathways of the complement cascade is the membrane attack complex (MAC), comprised of C_{5b6789}, which lyses various pathogens by incorporating itself into their cell membrane, forming a transmembrane channel by which ion displacement results in membrane disruption.

Both C_{3a} and C_{5a}, as well as C_{4a}, act as anaphylatoxins, promoting the release of histamine and other vasoactive substances from mast cells and basophils. Studies in which these products were injected into live subjects recreated the bronchoconstriction and circulatory collapse seen in anaphylaxis.

BIBLIOGRAPHY

Kumar V, Abbas AK, Fausto N, Aster JC, Perkins JA. Acute and chronic inflammation. In Kumar V, Abbas AK, Aster JC (eds.), *Robbins and Cotran Pathologic Basis of Disease, Professional Edition*, 8th ed. Maryland Heights, MO: W. B. Saunders; 2010: Chapter 2.

Levinson W. Complement. In: Levinson W (ed.), *Review of Medical Microbiology & Immunology*, 12th ed. New York, NY: McGraw-Hill; 2012:Chapter 63.

Phelan HA, Eastman AL, Frotan A, Gonzalez RP. Shock and hypoperfusion states. In: O'Leary JP (ed.), *The Physiologic Basis of Surgery*, 4th ed. Philadelphia, PA: Lippincott. Williams & Wilkins, 2008, 87–111.

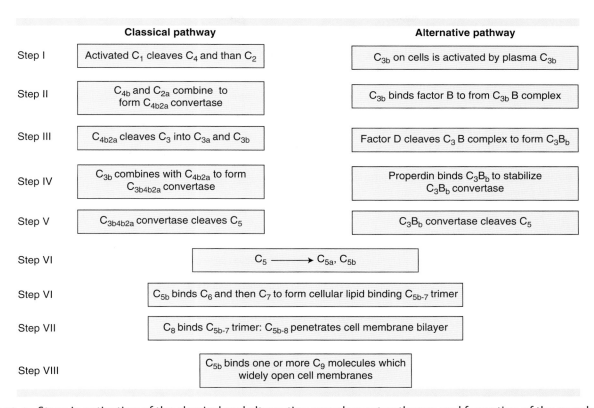

Classical pathway

Step I	Activated C_1 cleaves C_4 and than C_2
Step II	C_{4b} and C_{2a} combine to form C_{4b2a} convertase
Step III	C_{4b2a} cleaves C_3 into C_{3a} and C_{3b}
Step IV	C_{3b} combines with C_{4b2a} to form C_{3b4b2a} convertase
Step V	C_{3b4b2a} convertase cleaves C_5

Alternative pathway

Step I	C_{3b} on cells is activated by plasma C_{3b}
Step II	C_{3b} binds factor B to from C_{3b} B complex
Step III	Factor D cleaves C_3 B complex to form C_3B_b
Step IV	Properdin binds C_3B_b to stabilize C_3B_b convertase
Step V	C_3B_b convertase cleaves C_5

Step VI — $C_5 \longrightarrow C_{5a}, C_{5b}$

Step VI — C_{5b} binds C_6 and then C_7 to form cellular lipid binding C_{5b-7} trimer

Step VII — C_8 binds C_{5b-7} trimer: C_{5b-8} penetrates cell membrane bilayer

Step VIII — C_{5b} binds one or more C_9 molecules which widely open cell membranes

FIGURE 10-2. Steps in activation of the classical and alternative complement pathways and formation of the membrane attack complex, C_{5b-9}. Adapted with permission from Walport MJ: Complement. NEJM 2001; 344:1058; and Plumb ME, Sadetz JM: Proteins of the membrane attack complex, in Volkankis JE, Frank ME (eds): *The Human Complement System in Health and Disease.* New York, Marcel Dekker, 1998, p 119.

5. **(A)** Localized inflammation, as with trauma, is normally accompanied by a systemic acute phase response, a common feature of which is fever. Approximately 12–24 hours following the initiation of an acute phase response, the inflammatory mediators IL-1, IL-6, and TNF-α are found in elevated levels in the blood. These three endogenous pyrogens act on the hypothalamus, raising its set point for body temperature and resulting in a fever (see Fig. 10-3). The effects of both IL-1 and TNF-α depend on central IL-6 activity. Central IL-6 increases production of prostaglandin E_2, which directly activates the thermoregulatory center of the anterior hypothalamus raising the temperature set point; additionally, this prostaglandin induces peripheral vasoconstriction, giving an impression of "the chills," while simultaneously triggering the shiver response, again leading to the generation of body heat. Along with IL-6, neuronal afferents are believed to play a role in fever. Following a subdiaphragmatic vagotomy, animals have exhibited an attenuated fever response. This process increases body temperature through a combination of heat production, via mechanical (shivering) and chemical (uncoupled oxidative phosphorylation) thermogenesis, and heat conservation, via vasoconstriction, which redirects blood from the

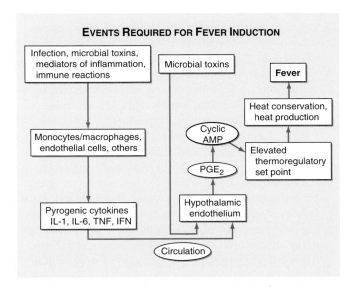

FIGURE 10-3. Fever induction events. AMP, adenosine monophosphate; PGE_2, prostaglandin E_2. From Longo DL, Fauci AS, Kasper DL, Hauser SL, Jameson J, Loscalzo J (eds.), *Harrison's Principles of Internal Medicine*, 18th ed. New York, NY: McGraw-Hill; 2012:Fig. 16-1.

periphery to the internal organs. Fever has been cited as directly inhibiting pathogen proliferation, with various bacteria and viruses growing more slowly at higher temperatures. In addition, fever enhances chemotaxis and leukocyte function; however, an elevated body temperature also elevates oxygen consumption, gluconeogenesis, and protein catabolism. IFN-α, produced by leukocytes, induces the expression of class I major histocompatibility antigens on somatic cells, activates macrophages and natural killer cells, and has antiviral effects. It has no role in fever. Both IL-4 and IL-10 act as anti-inflammatory cytokines. IL-2 promotes T-cell proliferation.

BIBLIOGRAPHY

Dinarello CA, Porat R. Fever and hyperthermia. In: Longo DL, Fauci AS, Kasper DL, Hauser SL, Jameson J, Loscalzo J (eds.), *Harrison's Principles of Internal Medicine*, 18th ed. New York, NY: McGraw-Hill; 2012:Chapter 16.

Kumar V, Abbas AK, Fausto N, Aster JC, Perkins JA. Acute and chronic inflammation. In Kumar V, Abbas AK, Aster JC (eds.), *Robbins and Cotran Pathologic Basis of Disease, Professional Edition*, 8th ed. Maryland Heights, MO: W. B. Saunders; 2010:Chapter 2.

Levinson W. Immunity. In: Levinson W (ed.), *Review of Medical Microbiology & Immunology*, 12th ed. New York, NY: McGraw-Hill; 2012:Chapter 57.

Martindale RG, Zhou M. Nutrition and metabolism. In: O'Leary JP (ed.), *The Physiologic Basis of Surgery*, 4th ed. Philadelphia, PA: Lippincott. Williams & Wilkins; 2008:112–149.

6. **(B)** Nitric oxide has been shown to have a potent antimicrobial effect. This reactive free radical gas is produced by activated neutrophils and macrophages via the enzyme inducible nitric oxide synthase (iNOS), one of three nitric oxide synthase (NOS) isoforms. Production of this inducible enzyme is stimulated by endotoxins as well as by cytokines such as IFN-γ and IL-1. The precursor molecule, L-arginine, in combination with oxygen, is converted by iNOS into nitric oxide and L-citrulline (see Fig. 10-4). The cofactors participating in this reaction include flavin mononucleotide (FMN), NADPH, tetrahydrobiopterin (H_4B), and calmodulin. The production of nitric oxide is preceded by a respiratory burst from the neutrophil or macrophage, representing a transient, prominent consumption of oxygen. This metabolic burst follows phagocytosis and may last for 3 hours, highlighting the importance of nitric oxide and oxidative killing in the antimicrobial arsenal of these phagocytes. Nitric oxide diffuses into target cells infected by intracellular pathogens, where it inhibits a number of enzymes vital to cell function.

Nitric oxide is also produced directly by the endothelium. Prior to the discovery of its chemical identity, the molecule was described as endothelium-derived relaxing factor for its potent vasodilatory effects. After

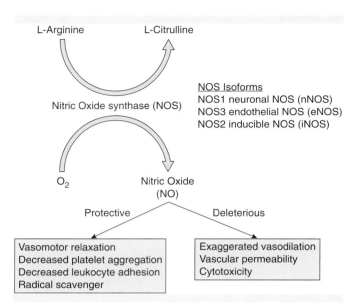

FIGURE 10-4. Production of nitric oxide via the enzyme inducible nitric oxide synthase (iNOS). From Brunicardi FC, Andersen DK, Billiar TR, et al. (eds.), *Schwartz's Principles of Surgery*, 9th ed. New York, NY: McGraw-Hill Professional; 2009:Fig. 31-11.

its synthesis in the endothelium by NOS, it diffuses into vascular smooth muscle, activating guanylyl cyclase, which produces cGMP—the vasodilatory end product.

BIBLIOGRAPHY

Barrett KE, Boitano S, Barman SM, Brooks HL. Cardiovascular regulatory mechanisms. In: Barrett KE, Boitano S, Barman SM, Brooks HL (eds.), *Ganong's Review of Medical Physiology*, 24th ed. New York, NY: McGraw-Hill; 2012:Chapter 32.

Cothren CC, Biffl WL, Moore EE. Trauma. In: Brunicardi FC, Andersen DK, Billiar TR, et al. (eds.), *Schwartz's Principles of Surgery*, 9th ed. New York, NY: McGraw-Hill Professional; 2009.

Kumar V, Abbas AK, Fausto N, Aster JC, Perkins JA. Acute and chronic inflammation. In Kumar V, Abbas AK, Aster JC (eds.), *Robbins and Cotran Pathologic Basis of Disease, Professional Edition*, 8th ed. Maryland Heights, MO: W. B. Saunders; 2010:Chapter 2.

Levinson W. Immunity. In: Levinson W (ed.), *Review of Medical Microbiology & Immunology*, 12th ed. New York, NY: McGraw-Hill; 2012:Chapter 57.

7. **(C)** The shock state is characterized by decreased perfusion such that the supply of oxygenated blood to the peripheral tissues is unable to maintain aerobic metabolism. Shock is categorized into hypovolemic, cardiogenic, neurogenic, cardiac compressive, and septic. Despite its different manifestations, shock is typified by end-organ dysfunction secondary to a deficiency of oxygen and, consequently, to a paucity of adenosine triphosphate

(ATP) in cells. On the cellular level, oxidative phosphorylation by mitochondria produces ATP, which generates the energy necessary for metabolism. Without this energy, cells become disrupted, followed by the death of the organism as a whole.

In the absence of oxygen, cells rely solely on anaerobic metabolism to produce ATP. Cells convert to an anaerobic metabolism on reaching their anaerobic threshold, the primary determinant of which is oxygen availability. As with aerobic glycolysis, pyruvate is generated from glucose; however, in anaerobic glycolysis, pyruvate then is reduced to lactate via lactate dehydrogenase (see Fig. 10-5).

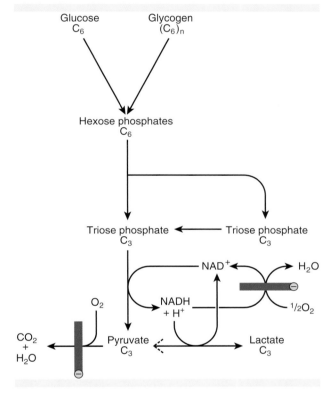

FIGURE 10-5. Aerobic and anaerobic metabolism of glucose. From Murray RK, Bender DA, Botham KM, Kennelly PJ, Rodwell VW, Weil PA (eds.), *Harper's Illustrated Biochemistry*, 29th ed. New York, NY: McGraw-Hill; 2012:Fig. 18-1.

In the presence of plentiful hydrogen ions, lactic acid results from lactate. Ultimately, 2 moles of ATP are created from 1 mole of glucose. Thus, the energy available for cellular work is severely curtailed in comparison to aerobic metabolism. The energy deficit leads to cell disruption secondary to the loss of transmembrane potential and death.

The amount of lactate produced in the course of anaerobic metabolism reflects the oxygen deficit resulting from the hypoperfused state (type A lactic acidosis). Accordingly, lactic acid serves as an indicator

of the severity of shock. Numerous studies have suggested that levels of lactic acid predict survival in shock patients, despite the etiology (see Fig. 10-6). Conversely, the success of resuscitation is signaled by a decline in the lactate level.

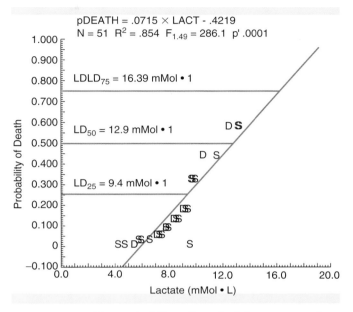

FIGURE 10-6. The probability of survival decreases as the initial arterial lactate of intensive care unit patients increases. Reproduced with permission from Dunham CM, Siegel JH, Weireter L, et al. Oxygen debt and metabolic acidemia or quantitative predictors of mortality and the severity of the ischemic insult in hemorrhagic shock. *Crit Care Med.* 1991;19:231.

BIBLIOGRAPHY

Champe PC, Harvey RA. *Lippincott's Illustrated Reviews: Biochemistry*, 5th ed. Philadelphia, PA: JB Lippincott; 2011:69–136.

Maier RV. Approach to the patient with shock. In: Longo DL, Fauci AS, Kasper DL, Hauser SL, Jameson J, Loscalzo J (eds.), *Harrison's Principles of Internal Medicine*, 18th ed. New York, NY: McGraw-Hill; 2012:Chapter 270.

Zuckerbraun BS, Peitzman AB, Billiar TR. Shock. In: Brunicardi F, Andersen DK, Billiar TR, et al. (eds.), *Schwartz's Principles of Surgery*, 9th ed. New York, NY: McGraw-Hill; 2010:Chapter 5.

8. **(D)**

9. **(B)**

Explanation for questions 8 and 9

Hypovolemic shock arises from the depletion of the circulating blood volume. Trauma patients most commonly present with this category of shock. Among the many causes of hypovolemic shock are hemorrhage, emesis, diarrhea, excessive diuresis, dehydration, gastrointestinal fistula, burn injury, and anaphylaxis. The volume losses involved in hypovolemic shock emanate from any of the three fluid compartments in the body: intracellular, extracellular, and intravascular. Hemorrhage exemplifies a loss from the intravascular space, whereas dehydration features depletion from both the intracellular and extracellular spaces. A pure extracellular fluid hypovolemia is typified by burns, diarrhea, and a gastrointestinal fistula. Despite these differences, in general, hypovolemic shock is characterized by a decrease in preload and in cardiac filling pressures, which ultimately results in a diminished cardiac output and a compromised peripheral perfusion. The severity of hypovolemic shock depends on the rate and the extent of the volume loss. The premorbid condition of the patient determines the ability of compensatory mechanisms to counteract the shock state. Hypovolemic shock is categorized into mild, moderate, and severe based on the symptoms and signs, volume of fluid losses, and organ systems affected (Table 10-1).

TABLE 10-1 The Pathophysiology and Clinical Features of the Categories of Hypovolemia

	Pathophysiology	Clinical Features
Mild (deficit <20% of blood volume)	Decreased perfusion of organs that are able to tolerate ischemia (skin, fat, skeletal muscle, bone). Redistribution of blood flow to critical organs.	Subjective complaints of feeling cold. Postural changes in blood pressure and pulse. Pale, cool, clammy skin. Flat neck veins. Concentrated urine.
Moderate (deficit = 20–40% of blood volume)	Decreased perfusion of organs that withstand ischemia poorly (pancreas, spleen, kidneys).	Subjective complaint of thirst. Blood pressure is lower than normal in the supine position. Oliguria.
Severe (deficit >40% of blood volume)	Decreased perfusion of brain and heart.	Patient is restless, agitated, confused, and often obtunded. Low blood pressure with a weak and often thready pulse. Tachypnea may be present. If allowed to progress, cardiac arrest results.

With mild hypovolemia, a loss of less than 20% of the circulating blood volume, perfusion to organs such as the skin, skeletal muscle, and bone is decreased. These organs are able to sustain a relative ischemia for short periods of time, allowing blood to be shunted to organs intolerant of ischemia. The decrease in intravascular volume lessens the stimulation of baroreceptors located in the aortic arch, atria, and carotid bodies, resulting in a decreased parasympathetic but an elevated sympathetic outflow; norepinephrine is released from the postsynaptic sympathetic nerves and adrenal medulla, whereas epinephrine is discharged from the adrenal medulla. This adrenergic discharge achieves an increase in myocardial contractility and heart rate as well as the constriction of the vascular smooth muscle, augmenting blood pressure. Vasoconstriction of the vessels produces the pale, cold, and clammy skin characteristic of shock. Constriction of the large veins and venules—which normally contain 60% of the total blood volume—permits an increase in preload to the heart, as the blood from these capacitance vessels is redistributed to the circulation. Accordingly, the collapse of the cutaneous veins comprises another sign of hypovolemic shock. The skin manifestations of hypovolemic shock are most pronounced in the lower extremities, especially the plantar surfaces of the feet. More subtle signs of mild hypovolemia include minimal oliguria (urine output <0.5 mL/kg/h in adults), postural hypotension (a sustained decrease in systolic blood pressure of >10 mmHg with an alteration in position), and a subjective feeling of cold. Overall, heart rate, blood pressure, and respiratory rate are unchanged. In the absence of continued intravascular losses, the compensatory mechanisms to mild hypovolemic shock assure survival without further treatment. Moderate hypovolemia is classified as the depletion of 20–40% of the blood volume. Perfusion of organs such as the kidney, spleen, pancreas, and gastrointestinal tract—less tolerant of ischemia—is sacrificed in order to supply the heart and brain with blood. In particular, the kidney reacts to the vasoconstriction of its afferent vessels to the cortex, induced by norepinephrine and epinephrine, by decreasing the glomerular filtration pressure below that required to maintain filtration into Bowman's capsule; as a result, oliguria ensues. The fall in renal perfusion also provokes the release of renin from the juxtaglomerular apparatus (see Fig. 10-7).

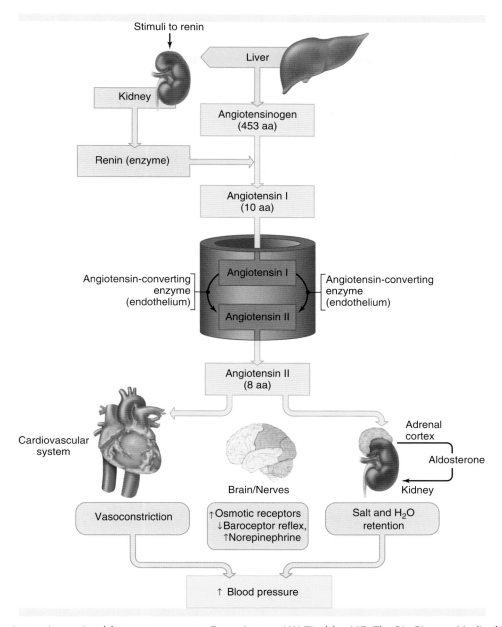

FIGURE 10-7. Renin-angiotensin-aldosterone system. From Janson LW, Tischler ME. *The Big Picture: Medical Biochemistry*. New York, NY: McGraw-Hill; 2012:Fig. 18-4.

Renin promotes the conversion of angiotensinogen to angiotensin I in the liver, ultimately resulting in the production of angiotensin II, a potent vasoconstrictor and catalyst for the issuance of aldosterone from the adrenal zona glomerulosa. Aldosterone participates in the compensatory mechanisms to hypovolemic shock by promoting the reabsorption of sodium in the distal convoluted tubules of the kidney and, therefore, by conserving the free water that contributes to intravascular volume. Also, in response to a decrease in intravascular volume of greater than 5% or a plasma osmolality higher than 285 mOsm, vasopressin is released from the posterior pituitary (neurohypophysis). Vasopressin, like angiotensin II, acts as a peripheral vasoconstrictor. Moreover, vasopressin promotes the reabsorption of free water in the collecting ducts of the kidney. The intravascular volume is further enhanced by fluid shifts between the extracellular and intravascular compartments, potentiated by a decrease in the hydrostatic pressure within the capillary bed. The adrenergic discharge promotes a greater degree of constriction in the precapillary than the postcapillary sphincter, resulting in a pressure differential between the extracellular and intravascular spaces: fluid and electrolytes are consequently transferred into the intravascular compartment until the oncotic pressure of the interstitium surpasses that of the intravascular space, at which point the fluid shift reverses. In sum, moderate hypovolemic shock is characterized by a normal blood pressure in conjunction with tachycardia, pronounced oliguria, incipient mental status changes, and thirst.

In severe hypovolemic shock, greater than 40% of the blood volume is depleted. Without intervention, perfusion of the heart and brain is compromised, resulting in ischemic injury and, ultimately, death, often by cardiac arrest. In particular, the blood supply to the brain remains intact until a pressure below 70 mmHg is reached. The poor perfusion exacerbates the manifestations of the shock state. The characteristic appearance of a patient in severe hypovolemic shock includes agitation, confusion, hypotension, tachycardia, tachypnea, oliguria, and a narrowed pulse pressure. Continuation of the volume depletion heightens and then eventually overwhelms the compensatory mechanisms.

BIBLIOGRAPHY

Cothren CC, Biffl WL, Moore EE. Trauma. In: Brunicardi FC, Andersen DK, Billiar TR, et al. (eds.), *Schwartz's Principles of Surgery*, 9th ed. New York, NY: McGraw-Hill Professional; 2009.

Holcroft JW, Anderson JT, Sena MJ. Shock and acute pulmonary failure in surgical patients. In: Doherty GM (ed.), *Current Diagnosis & Treatment: Surgery*, 13th ed. New York, NY: McGraw-Hill; 2010:Chapter 12.

Maier RV. Approach to the patient with shock. In: Longo DL, Fauci AS, Kasper DL, Hauser SL, Jameson J, Loscalzo J (eds.), *Harrison's Principles of Internal Medicine*, 18th ed. New York, NY: McGraw-Hill; 2012:Chapter 270.

Phelan HA, Eastman AL, Frotan A, Gonzalez RP. Shock and hypoperfusion states. In: O'Leary JP (ed.), *The Physiologic Basis of Surgery*, 4th ed. Philadelphia, PA: Lippincott. Williams & Wilkins; 2008:87–111.

10. **(A)** Fluid resuscitation plays an integral role in the treatment of patients in hypovolemic shock. Crystalloid solutions are currently advocated as the best initial fluid selection. The typical crystalloid is 0.9% sodium chloride, attractive for a sodium concentration (154 mM) similar to that of plasma. This isotonic fluid is also expected to distribute in the extravascular and intravascular compartments in proportions equivalent to that of plasma: 75 and 25%, respectively; however, only 20% of the administered fluid will remain in the intravascular space after 2 hours, leading to "third spacing." In addition, the equivalent chloride concentration of 154 mM in normal saline, significantly greater than that of plasma, induces a hyperchloremic metabolic acidemia;

such a mild acidemia may serve to enhance myocardial contractility. However, in the presence of a preexisting hyperchloremic metabolic acidosis, lactated or acetated Ringer's solution acts to buffer the acidemia, transforming the lactate or acetate to an organic acid that is then converted to carbon dioxide and water in the liver via the Kreb's cycle. Fluids containing dextrose, such as 5% dextrose in 0.45% sodium chloride, should be avoided because of the osmotic diuretic effect of glucose.

Colloids expand the intravascular space to an equivalent degree but in smaller volumes than crystalloids through an increase in the oncotic pressure within vessels: 1 g of albumin will draw 18 mL of fluid into the intravascular space. It is thought, however, that colloids ultimately travel to the interstitium via blood vessels made permeable by inflammation, leading to an intractable edema. Albumin, the most commonly administered colloid, has been associated with pulmonary dysfunction when given in large volumes as well as coagulopathy, hypocalcemia, and myocardial dysfunction. The colloid dextran has not been adequately studied in the setting of acute fluid resuscitation. Additionally, administration of this solution has been complicated by renal failure, anaphylaxis, and bleeding.

BIBLIOGRAPHY

Alderson P, Schierhout G, Roberts I, Bunn F. Colloids versus crystalloids for fluid resuscitation in critically ill patients. *Cochrane Database Syst Rev* 2002;4:1–36.

Annane D, Siami S, Jaber S, et al. Effects of fluid resuscitation with colloids vs crystalloids on mortality in critically ill patients presenting with hypovolemic shock: the CRISTAL randomized trial. *JAMA* 2013;310(17):1809–1817.

Cothren CC, Biffl WL, Moore EE. Trauma. In: Brunicardi FC, Andersen DK, Billiar TR, et al. (eds.), *Schwartz's Principles of Surgery*, 9th ed. New York, NY: McGraw-Hill Professional; 2009.

11. **(C)** Death due to trauma with hemorrhagic shock is arranged in a trimodal distribution: immediate (at the scene), within the first 24 hours, and 1 week or more following the injury. In the acute period after trauma, mortality is attributable to massive hemorrhage or neurologic injury. Direct injury to an organ contributes to a primary multiple organ dysfunction in this early period. In contrast, late deaths, occurring at least 1 week subsequent to the trauma, generally arise from secondary multiple organ dysfunction syndrome (MODS). This condition develops in 30–60% of these trauma patients and is associated with up to an 80% mortality rate, depending on the number of organ systems affected.

MODS is defined as the failure of multiple organs in a critically ill patient in whom the maintenance of homeostasis requires intervention. This syndrome appears as

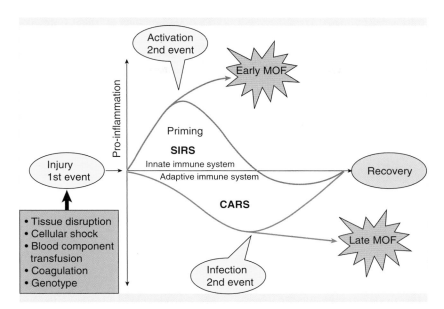

FIGURE 10-8. CARS, compensatory anti-inflammatory response system; MOF, multiple organ failure; SIRS, systemic inflammatory response syndrome. From Mattox KL, Moore EE, Feliciano DV (eds.), *Trauma*, 7th ed. New York, NY: McGraw-Hill; 2013.

the end point in a variety of conditions, not isolated to trauma and hemorrhagic shock. In the case of trauma, the prevalence of MODS is ascribed to a two-hit phenomenon, suggesting that trauma represents an initial insult that predisposes the immune system to react later to a lesser injury with a massive response, mediated primarily by neutrophils, resulting in great collateral damage (see Fig. 10-8). The primed neutrophils mediate further tissue injury by means of proteolytic enzymes, reactive oxygen species, and vasoactive substances. Following traumatic hemorrhagic shock, the patient is resuscitated into not only a local but also a systemic inflammatory response syndrome (SIRS), with generalized inflammation generated within 1 hour of injury.

Neutrophils and monocytes are first activated, releasing inflammatory mediators. TNF-α, IL-1, and IL-6 are particularly implicated in the evolution of MODS, found in studies to induce this syndrome and to be present in elevated levels. Additionally, the coagulation and alternative complement cascades are initiated. In the absence of further injury, SIRS is beneficial to recovery from the trauma. The second, often trivial, insult, however, results in an enhanced immune response from the already primed immune cells, notably neutrophils. This second hit may arise from a mild infection, pulmonary aspiration, or blood transfusion (Table 10-2). Ultimately, organs not involved in the original trauma experience an alteration in function. Usually, the lung is affected first, with kidneys, liver, and gastrointestinal tract dysfunction occurring later. The compensatory anti-inflammatory response system (CARS) results from

TABLE 10-2 Risk Factors Associated with the Development of Multiple Organ Dysfunction Following Trauma

First insult
    Severity of tissue injury
    Shock-ischemia/reperfusion
    Severity of the systemic inflammatory response

Second insult
    Infection
    Transfusion
    Secondary operative procedures

Host factors
    Age
    Preexisting conditions

persistent anti-inflammation and leaves patients susceptible to infection. The anti-inflammation creates a preconditioned state where the patient is protected against a second hit. However, this state delays the healing process, increases apoptosis, and depresses adaptive immune responses. Immunoparalysis ensues, leading to impaired wound healing, recurrent nosocomial infections, and late multiple organ failure.

BIBLIOGRAPHY

Gentile LF, Cuenca AG, Efron PA, et al. Persistent inflammation and immunosuppression: a common syndrome and new horizon for surgical intensive care. *J Trauma Acute Care Surg* 2012;72(6):1491–1501.

Sauaia A, Moore FA, Moore EE. Multiple organ failure. In: Mattox KL, Moore EE, Feliciano DV (eds.), *Trauma*, 7th ed. New York, NY: McGraw-Hill; 2013:Chapter 61.

Walley KR. Shock. In: Hall JB, Schmidt GA, Wood LH (eds.), *Principles of Critical Care*, 3rd ed. New York, NY: McGraw-Hill; 2005:Chapter 21.

12. **(C)**

13. **(C)**

Explanation for questions 12 and 13

Neurogenic shock is a form of vasogenic shock in which spinal cord injury (or spinal anesthesia) causes vasodilatation. Among the causes of neurogenic shock are certain neurologic disorders, high spinal anesthesia, fainting, and medications that antagonize the adrenergic system; however, the most common cause of this phenomenon is traumatic spinal cord injury. A spinal cord injury usually results from damage to the cervical, lower thoracic, or upper lumbar regions. The most common mechanism of the injury is an impact with persistent compression, often associated with burst fractures, fracture-dislocation, missile injury, and ruptured discs (Table 10-3). Neurogenic shock arises from the loss of autonomic innervation to the vasculature below the affected level. The magnitude of neurogenic shock depends on the severity and level of the injury, with actual shock developing only following damage above the midthoracic level. Its manifestations emanate from the pronounced sympathetic discharge produced above the level of the denervation. Sympathetic activation results in the loss of arteriolar tone and, thus, massive

TABLE 10-3 Mechanisms of Spinal Cord Injury

Mechanical Force	Mechanism of Injury
Impact plus persisting compression	Burst fracture Fracture-dislocation Disc rupture
Impact alone (temporary compression)	Hyperextension
Distraction	Hyperflexion
Laceration, transection	Burst fracture Laminar fracture Fracture-dislocation Missile

Reproduced with permission from Tator CH. Pathophysiology and pathology of spinal cord injury. In: Wilkins RH, Rengachary SS (eds.), *Neurosurgery*, 2nd ed., vol. II. New York, NY: McGraw-Hill; 1996:2847.

vasodilatation. The venules are similarly affected: blood pools in these capacitance vessels within the denervated areas of the body. The accumulation of blood in the venous system is aggravated by the inability of the muscles of the extremities to assist in returning the blood to the heart. While the total blood volume is unchanged, the circulating blood volume—the preload—is lessened. In sum, neurogenic shock presents as central hypotension (a low systemic vascular resistance) with a decreased cardiac output, PCWP, and central venous pressure. The effect of spinal cord injury on heart rate is variable, depending on the level of denervation: bradycardia ensues from a lesion above the midthoracic sympathetic outflow tract, whereas lower lesions present with tachycardia. Above the midthoracic level, myocardial contractility is also depressed. The loss of autonomic reflexes to the spinal cord below the lesion is accompanied by immediate flaccid paralysis, an absence of sensation, and tendon areflexia. The condition of spinal shock has a duration of 1–6 weeks, but in a minority of patients, it is permanent. In contradistinction to hypovolemic shock, neurogenic shock features warm, pink skin in the denervated areas secondary to the cutaneous vasodilatation. Mentation is often intact. Urine output remains normal or elevated.

Treatment of neurogenic shock centers on the usual trauma protocols, with the establishment of an airway and intravenous access being of highest priority. Stabilization of the cervical spine must be ensured with a cervical collar. The diagnosis of hypovolemic shock should be entertained despite a lesion that solely suggests neurogenic shock. Resuscitation is started with intravenous fluids, which function to increase the circulating blood volume and, thus, the preload. Often, this intervention is sufficient to elevate the blood pressure. A failure of intravenous fluids to improve hypotension may point to occult bleeding. In the absence of such bleeding, vasoactive agents may be used if fluid resuscitation is insufficient to elevate the preload. Commonly, α-adrenergic agents such as phenylephrine or norepinephrine are relied on for this treatment, especially in the case of tachycardia; refractory hypotension with bradycardia usually requires dopamine and, often, atropine. These vasoactive medications are generally given in low doses and weaned off rapidly. An elevation in the blood pressure serves to obviate progressive spinal cord ischemia. Once the acute resuscitation phase is completed, a radiographic survey may be performed and definitive treatment of the injury pursued. For instance, an unstable spine requires surgical fixation.

Head trauma itself is never a cause of hypotension. Via the Cushing reflex, the increased intracranial pressure (ICP) seen with head trauma generally results in hypertension and bradycardia. Moreover, intracranial bleeding cannot alone be responsible for hypovolemic shock, as the rigid adult skull is unable to accommodate large volumes of blood; an acute increase in intracranial volume affects a large increase in the ICP, with shifting of the brain or herniation the result.

BIBLIOGRAPHY

Alarcon LH, Puyana J, Peitzman AB. Management of shock. In: Mattox KL, Moore EE, Feliciano DV (eds.), *Trauma*, 7th ed. New York, NY: McGraw-Hill; 2013:Chapter 12.

Carlson GD, Gorden CD, Nakazawa S, et al. Sustained spinal cord compression. Part II. Effect of methylprednisolone on regional blood flow and recovery of somatosensory evoked potentials. *J Bone Joint Surg* 2003;85-A(1):95–101.

Cothren CC, Biffl WL, Moore EE. Trauma. In: Brunicardi FC, Andersen DK, Billiar TR, et al. (eds.), *Schwartz's Principles of Surgery*, 9th ed. New York, NY: McGraw-Hill Professional; 2009.

Fenves AZ, Rao A, Emmett M. Shock and hypoperfusion states. In: O'Leary JP (ed.), *The Physiologic Basis of Surgery*, 4th ed. Philadelphia, PA: Lippincott Williams & Wilkins; 2008:87–111.

14. **(B)** The Trendelenburg position, if it does not complicate other aspects of care, is useful in the treatment of neurogenic shock. The Trendelenburg position allows for the translocation of venous blood from the extremities to the heart by gravity. This method, developed in the late nineteenth century by the surgeon Friedrich Trendelenburg, became popular during World War I as an anti-shock position; however, this technique is of value only in neurogenic shock, where the massive dilatation of the venous system results in pooling of blood in the capacitance vessels of the extremities. The increased return of blood to the heart from these expanded vessels improves the cardiac preload and reduces the degree of hypotension. This maneuver has no application in hypovolemic shock, where the blood volume is low and the vessels are severely constricted. In this hypovolemic situation, no additional blood is transferred to the heart from the already-depleted vessels. The heart, in fact, is required to expend more energy to deliver blood to the viscera and elevated lower extremities.

BIBLIOGRAPHY

Holcroft JW, Anderson JT, Sena MJ. Shock & acute pulmonary failure in surgical patients. In: Doherty GM (eds.), *Current Diagnosis & Treatment: Surgery*, 13th ed. New York, NY: McGraw-Hill; 2010:Chapter 12.

15. **(D)**

16. **(A)**

17. **(B)**

Explanation for questions 15 through 17

Cardiogenic shock represents a failure of the mechanical pump function of the heart. This condition may arise from valvular heart disease (insufficiency or stenosis), arrhythmia, obstructive myocardial hypertrophy, papillary muscle rupture, or myocardial contusion; however, the most prevalent cause of cardiogenic shock is an acute MI, especially left ventricular pump dysfunction. Seventy-five percent of patients who have cardiogenic shock complicating acute MIs develop signs of cardiogenic shock within 24 hours after onset of infarction. Pulmonary rales and S3 gallop are audible in most patients with left ventricular pump dysfunction.

Treatment of MI associated with cardiogenic shock depends on early revascularization. In the SHOCK study, a significant improvement in the survival rate was reported with the early revascularization strategy as opposed to the initial medical stabilization with delayed revascularization group at 6 months and 1 year; however, the 13.2% reduction in mortality was not observed in subjects over the age of 75 years old. The initial goal of therapy is the avoidance of sustained end-organ damage by maintaining an adequate blood pressure, usually with vasopressor agents. An IABP provides additional hemodynamic support by reducing systolic afterload. The result is increased cardiac output and coronary blood flow without an increase in myocardial oxygen demand. Close monitoring of respiratory and cardiovascular parameters is required in an intensive care setting. Both aspirin and heparin should be administered.

The successful treatment of MI complicated by cardiogenic shock rests on identifying the condition and then intervening with a revascularization procedure. Despite the advances in therapies offered for MI and cardiogenic shock, the mortality remains high. Studies investigating novel therapies such as nitric oxide inhibitors continue.

BIBLIOGRAPHY

Hochman JS, Sleeper LA, Webb JG, et al. Early revascularization in acute myocardial infarction complicated by cardiogenic shock. *N Engl J Med* 1999;341:625–634.

Jaffrey SR. Nitric oxide. In: Katzung BG, Masters SB, Trevor AJ (eds.), *Basic & Clinical Pharmacology*, 12th ed. New York, NY: McGraw-Hill; 2012:Chapter 19.

Walley KR. Shock. In: Hall JB, Schmidt GA, Wood LH (eds.), *Principles of Critical Care*, 3rd ed. New York, NY: McGraw-Hill; 2003:Chapter 21.

18. **(A)**

19. **(B)**

Explanation for 18 and 19

Infarction of the right ventricle appears in one-third of acute inferior wall MIs; however, most right-sided MIs are recognized only at autopsy. This condition is suggested by the combination of an inferior wall MI and hypotension. Cardiogenic shock complicates a right ventricular MI in approximately 32% of cases. Dysfunction of the right ventricle restricts the delivery of blood to the lungs and left ventricle, causing peripheral venous congestion. In addition, the sudden dilatation of the right ventricle that accompanies a right ventricular MI produces a leftward shift in the intraventricular septum, compromising left ventricular filling. The characteristic findings on physical examination include jugular venous distension, no rales, and a positive Kussmaul sign (increased distension of the jugular veins with inspiration). A chest radiograph reveals clear lung fields. On an ECG, ST elevation of the right chest leads, V3 and V4, is found; however, this classic sign disappears several hours following the onset of the MI.

Echocardiography remains the most reliable diagnostic tool for a right ventricular MI. An echocardiogram demonstrates right ventricular dilatation and hypokinesis. Tricuspid regurgitation may be evident because of the acute increase in right ventricular dimensions and, consequently, in the diameter of the tricuspid annulus. Right heart catheterization displays a high central venous pressure (>12 mmHg), low to normal PCWP, and low to normal cardiac index. The initial intervention in treating a right ventricular MI is to administer fluids, with the goal of a PCWP greater than 18 mmHg, in order to improve the preload to the left ventricle. Systemic vasodilators and diuretics are avoided to prevent further hypotension. Inotropic support with dopamine or dobutamine is initiated for hypotension resistant to fluid resuscitation. Revascularization by thrombolysis or percutaneous transluminal coronary angioplasty is the definitive therapy for right ventricular MI. The mortality of an acute MI is worsened by the involvement of the right ventricle. The right ventricle often requires 3 days to recover its function; however, intact left ventricular function in the face of a right ventricular MI improves survival.

BIBLIOGRAPHY

Antman EM, Braunwald E. Acute myocardial infarction. In: Braunwald E, Fauci AS, Kasper DL, et al. (eds.), *Principles of Internal Medicine*, 15th ed., vol. 1. New York, NY: McGraw Hill; 2001:1386–1398.

Saltzberg MT, Sable JS, Parrillo JE. Acute heart failure and shock. In: Crawford MH, Dimarco JP, Asplund K, et al. (eds.), *Cardiology*. London, United Kingdom: Mosby; 2001:5.3.1–5.3.12.

20. **(C)**

21. **(A)**

Explanation for questions 20 and 21

In the setting of cardiogenic shock, the IABP enhances hemodynamic parameters. Although surgical placement was once widely practiced, this mechanical device is now usually inserted percutaneously via the femoral artery using a modified Seldinger technique and directed into the thoracic aorta. Within the aorta, the balloon inflates in early diastole, augmenting coronary arterial perfusion, and rapidly deflates in early systole, reducing the afterload against which the left ventricle must contract (see Fig. 10-9). The decrease in afterload allows the aortic valve to open at a lower systolic pressure, reducing myocardial oxygen consumption.

In relation to the ECG, balloon inflation occurs on the T wave, whereas deflation is coincident with the R wave (see Fig. 10-10). The timing of counterpulsation may also be guided by the arterial waveform, with inflation commencing at the dicrotic notch and deflation at the upstroke of the waveform. Among the physiologic effects

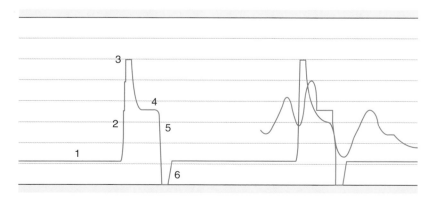

FIGURE 10-9. A normal balloon pressure waveform. 1—fill pressure, 2—rapid inflation, 3—peak inflation artifact, 4—inflation plateau pressure, 5—rapid deflation, 6—peak deflation pressure. Reproduced with permission from Daily EK, Schroeder JS. *Techniques of Bedside Hemodynamic Monitoring*, 5th ed. St. Louis, MO: Mosby; 1994:250.

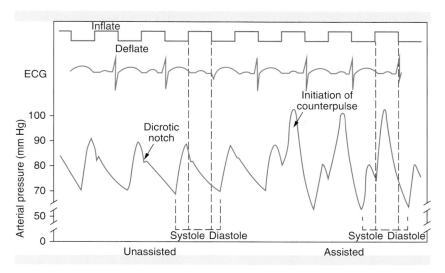

FIGURE 10-10. Counterpulsation in relation to electrocardiography (ECG) and the arterial waveform. Reproduced with permission from Daily EK, Schroeder JS. *Techniques of Bedside Hemodynamic Monitoring*, 5th ed. St. Louis, MO: Mosby; 1994:253.

of intra-aortic balloon pumping are a rise in diastolic pressure of 90% and an increase in cardiac output of 20–50%.

Counterpulsation is applied to candidates for aggressive revascularization who remain hypotensive despite maximal treatment with vasopressors. Also, IABP placement is recommended prior to transfer of a cardiogenic shock patient to a tertiary care center. This device is not a replacement for revascularization, serving only as a temporary measure to improve hemodynamic parameters.

Despite its advantages, IABP is complicated by bleeding and vascular damage in 5–20% of cases, with injuries such as groin hematoma, aortic dissection or perforation, systemic emboli, and limb ischemia because of thromboembolism. Percutaneous insertion of the IABP is associated with a higher rate of complications than is surgical placement (20% vs. 5%). Vascular complications are more common in elderly women and diabetics. Contraindications for placement include aortic incompetence, severe peripheral vascular disease, and aortic aneurysm or dissection. In general, other indications for placement of an IABP include recurrent intractable ventricular arrhythmias complicated by hypotension; severe angina post-MI as a temporizing measure prior to revascularization; acute mitral regurgitation or ventricular septal defect coincident with an MI; and patients with large areas of myocardium at risk for ischemia secondary to pronounced coronary artery disease.

BIBLIOGRAPHY

Antman EM, Braunwald E. Acute myocardial infarction. In: Braunwald E, Fauci AS, Kasper DL, et al. (eds.), *Principles of Internal Medicine*, 15th ed., vol. 1. New York, NY: McGraw Hill; 2001:1386–1398.

Schwartz CF, Crooke GA, Grossi EA, Galloway AC. Acquired heart disease. In: Brunicardi F, Andersen DK, Billiar TR, et al. (eds.), *Schwartz's Principles of Surgery*, 9th ed. New York, NY: McGraw-Hill; 2010:Chapter 21.

22. **(B)**

23. **(C)**

Explanation for questions 22 and 23

This patient has developed cardiac tamponade as a result of penetrating trauma to his chest. Cardiac tamponade exemplifies compressive cardiogenic shock, in which the pump mechanism of the heart fails because of extrinsic factors acting on the heart or the great vessels. Impingement on these cardiovascular structures compromises diastolic filling and, consequently, cardiac output. Among the causes of compressive cardiogenic shock are air embolism, tension pneumothorax, diaphragmatic rupture, and intestinal distention.

Cardiac tamponade is a life-threatening disorder commonly resulting from penetrating chest trauma, although it is also frequently encountered with blunt injuries. Nontraumatic etiologies of cardiac tamponade include malignancy, idiopathic pericarditis, cardiac surgery, tuberculosis, and uremia. Beck's triad refers to the characteristic signs of cardiac tamponade: hypotension, muffled heart sounds, and jugular venous distension. However, these "typical" findings are discovered infrequently. Pulsus paradoxus, a reduction in the systolic blood pressure of 10 mmHg or more with inspiration, may be noted. An

ECG may reveal a decrease in the amplitude of the QRS complex or electrical alternans. A globular cardiac silhouette is the distinctive radiographic finding in cardiac tamponade, rarely seen clinically. Because these signs and typical study results are seldom present, a high index of suspicion must be maintained. The diagnosis may be suggested if a hypotensive patient exhibits a transient improvement in blood pressure following a fluid bolus.

The pathophysiology of cardiac tamponade has been well understood since the nineteenth century. At its most basic, cardiac tamponade is defined as impingement on the heart by the accumulation of pericardial effluents, including blood, pus, and air. The pericardium is an inelastic tissue that poorly tolerates increases in its volume. The intrapericardial volume is shared by the heart as well as the pericardial fluid, which normally amounts to 15–30 mL of fluid. The pericardial fluid first occupies the small pericardial reserve volume, slightly distending the pericardium.

As seen in Fig. 10-12, further increases in this volume exceed the distensibility of the pericardium, manifest by the steep pressure–volume curve. The heart and the pericardial fluid are thus forced to compete for space within the unyielding pericardium. The cardiac chambers become compressed, compromising their diastolic filling and, ultimately, cardiac output. The mean diastolic pressures among the four cardiac chambers equalize, with the relatively thinner right atrium and ventricle the first to be affected. The cardiac index and pulmonary wedge pressures are reduced. Pulsus paradoxus occurs secondary to an increase in right ventricular filling during inspiration, at the expense of the left ventricle, with a shift of the intraventricular septum to the left; this pattern is reversed in expiration.

Confirmation of the diagnosis rests on the FAST examination, the subxiphoid pericardial window, or transesophageal and transthoracic echocardiography. Several studies have advocated the FAST examination as the preferred manner of diagnosis of cardiac tamponade, because it is inexpensive, readily available, reliable, and quickly learned. The definitive treatment of cardiac tamponade involves the release of the pericardial fluid and repair of any cardiac or great vessel injury via an emergent thoracotomy or median sternotomy. Emergent resuscitative thoracotomy in the emergency department is the appropriate course of action for a patient who loses vital signs in the trauma bay with ultrasound-confirmed tamponade.

BIBLIOGRAPHY

Alarcon LH, Puyana J, Peitzman AB. Management of shock. In: Mattox KL, Moore EE, Feliciano DV (eds.), *Trauma*, 7th ed. New York, NY: McGraw-Hill; 2013:Chapter 12.

Belenkie I. Pericardial disease. In: Hall JB, Schmidt GA, Wood LH (eds.), *Principles of Critical Care*, 3rd ed. New York, NY: McGraw-Hill; 2005:Chapter 28.

24. **(C)**

25. **(B)**

Explanation for questions 24 and 25

Anaphylactic shock represents an acute, systemic allergic reaction. This immunologically mediated phenomenon is described as an immediate hypersensitivity reaction. This condition is an anamnestic response to an antigen through the release of preformed inflammatory mediators from mast cells. Agents that are responsible for anaphylactic shock include drugs (penicillins, sulfonamides), food (nuts, shellfish, chocolate), and insect venom (fire ants, Hymenoptera) (Table 10-4). Anaphylactic shock because of penicillin is associated with 400–800 deaths per year in the United States. Only minute quantities of the antigen are required to instigate this potentially life-threatening reaction. IgE antibodies are formed to these various antigens. In a sensitized individual, these antibodies are bound to high affinity Fc-ε receptors (Fc-εRI) on the surface of mast cells. Although basophils possess similar receptors, their contribution to anaphylaxis is minimal. Anaphylaxis occurs when an antigen binds to the IgE antibody-Fc-εRI complex. Following cross-linking of two or more of these complexes, a series of reactions occurs such that the mast cell releases a variety of mediators from its cytoplasmic granules. In the immediate phase of anaphylaxis, preformed mediators such as histamine as well as the arachidonic acid derivatives are liberated. The late phase features TNF-α, IL-4, and platelet-activating factor, formed following the degranulation of the mast cells. The late phase occurs approximately 6 hours after antigen contact.

This condition is characterized by vascular collapse and airway obstruction. The preformed mediators released in the immediate phase provoke a generalized vasodilatation of the arterioles, giving rise to a profound hypotension. An increase in vascular permeability further contributes to hypotension by the depletion of intravascular fluid. Accordingly, the hematocrit and blood viscosity increase. The cardiac output and, consequently, coronary artery perfusion decline secondary to the diminished preload. The coronary artery perfusion is worsened by the low systemic vascular resistance as well as by coronary artery spasm, precipitated by the stimulation of cardiac histamine H_1 receptors. The enhanced vascular permeability also promotes the development of laryngeal edema and, thus, airway obstruction. Pulmonary compromise is increased by the bronchoconstriction instigated by histamine and the leukotrienes. In the skin, the increased vascular permeability presents as angioedema.

TABLE 10-4 Etiologic Agents for Anaphylactic Shock

Haptens
β-Lactam antibiotics
Sulfonamides
Nitrofurantoin
Demeclocycline
Streptomycin
Vancomycin
Local anesthetics
Others
Serum products
Gamma globulin
Immunotherapy for allergic diseases
Heterologous serum
Foods
Nuts
Shellfish
Buckwheat
Egg white
Cottonseed
Milk
Corn
Potato
Rice
Legumes
Citrus fruits
Chocolate
Others
Venoms
Stinging insects, especially Hymenoptera, fire ants
Hormones
Insulin
Adrenocorticotropic hormone
Thyroid-stimulating hormone
Enzymes
Chymopapain
L-Asparaginase
Miscellaneous
Seminal fluid
Others

Reproduced with permission from Bongard FS. Shock and resuscitation. In: Bongard FS, Sue DY (eds.), *Current Critical Care: Diagnosis and Treatment.* Stamford, CT: Appleton & Lange; 1994:29.

Following exposure to an antigen, anaphylactic shock may manifest within seconds up to 1 hour. Initially, patients note pruritus and anxiety. Palpitations and weakness precede cardiovascular signs such as tachycardia, hypotension, arrhythmias, and myocardial ischemia.

The reduction in coronary artery perfusion may precipitate an MI. Respiratory symptoms commence with a feeling of a "lump in the throat," progressing to dyspnea, hoarseness, and a cough. The patient may exhibit rhinorrhea and nasal congestion. Additional complaints involve crampy abdominal pain, bloating, and nausea, with emesis and diarrhea developing later. The characteristic cutaneous manifestations are urticaria and angioedema. Urticaria is typified by swelling, erythema, and itching (see Fig. 10-11).

Conjunctival injection, diaphoresis, and lacrimation may also become apparent. Neurologic disturbances of syncope and seizures may occur. On laboratory evaluation, an elevated histamine and mast cell tryptase are often found. The blood eosinophil level is generally normal. Activation of the coagulation cascade may precipitate disseminated intravascular coagulation.

The treatment of anaphylactic shock relies on ventilatory and circulatory support. Intubation is performed prior to the development of laryngeal edema, ensuring a secure airway. Hypotension is counteracted with epinephrine. Epinephrine halts the production of the mediators of anaphylactic shock by increasing the intracellular concentration of cyclic adenosine monophosphate. This drug is given subcutaneously (0.3–0.5 mL) or intravenously (5–10 mL) every 5 minutes as needed. A patient who normally receives β-blocking medications may not respond to sympathomimetic drugs such

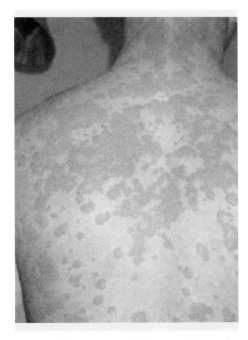

FIGURE 10-11. Diffuse urticarial lesions. Reproduced with permission from Roitt I, Brostoff J, Male D. *Immunology,* 6th ed. Edinburgh, United Kingdom: Mosby; 2001:324.

as epinephrine. The alternative medication is glucagon. Bronchoconstriction is reversed with inhaled racemic epinephrine or β-adrenergic nebulizers. Antihistamine agents treat the skin and gastrointestinal manifestations of anaphylactic shock. The preferred histamine antagonists are intravenous diphenhydramine (1 mg/kg) and ranitidine (50 mg over 5 minutes). Vasopressor agents may be initiated for refractory hypotension. Steroids attenuate the late phase of anaphylactic shock. Prognosis depends on the premorbid condition of the patient and the severity of the symptoms.

BIBLIOGRAPHY

Moss J, Mertes P. Anaphylactic and anaphylactoid reactions. In: Hall JB, Schmidt GA, Wood LH (eds.), *Principles of Critical Care*, 3rd ed. New York, NY: McGraw-Hill; 2005:Chapter 106.

Terr AI. Anaphylaxis and urticaria. In: Parslow TG, Stites DP, Terr AI, Imboden JB (eds.), *Medical Immunology*, 10th ed. New York, NY: McGraw-Hill; 2001:370–379.

26. **(D)** Cytokines function in mediating the inflammatory response. These small proteins, produced by diverse cells, possess a myriad of important biological effects, acting locally in an autocrine or paracrine manner. A cytokine is categorized as pro- or anti-inflammatory, based on the T-helper subset from which it originates. A naive CD4$^+$ T cell (Th0) ultimately develops into a helper T cell of the Th1 or Th2 lineage following stimulation from IL-12 and IFN-γ–inducing factor or IL-4, respectively (see Fig. 10-12).

Additional stimuli that influence the lineage of the helper T cell include the type of pathogen, the site of the infection, and the size of the inoculum. The Th1 cells are associated with cell-mediated immunity, protecting the host from intracellular pathogens via the cytotoxic T cell (CD8$^+$), as well as with type IV delayed hypersensitivity. In addition, this subset of helper T cells activates macrophages and promotes antibody production. The cytokines released by the Th1 cells, including IL-2, IFN-γ, and LT-α, are regarded as proinflammatory mediators. While promoting the differentiation of Th0 cells to the Th1 lineage, IFN-γ also downregulates Th2 production. In contrast, Th2 is responsible for humoral immunity, enhancing B-cell maturation. The cytokines created by the Th2 subset include IL-4, IL-5, IL-6, IL-9, IL-10, and IL-13. In particular, IL-4, IL-10, and IL-13 play a prominent anti-inflammatory role in immune function. IL-4, generated from mast cells, eosinophils, and basophils as well as the Th2 cells, interferes with proinflammatory mediators such as IL-1 and IL-8 and inhibits the conversion of Th0 cells to the Th1 subtype. This anti-inflammatory cytokine also promotes B-cell differentiation and inhibits the translocation of NF-κB to the nucleus. Cytokines such as IL-3, TNF-α, and granulocyte-macrophage colony-stimulating factor (GM-CSF) are generated by both cell types. The balance achieved between the proinflammatory Th1 and the anti-inflammatory Th2 cells determines the progression of the inflammatory process.

Traditionally, sepsis has been described as an uncontrolled inflammatory response. Studies have demonstrated that the proinflammatory cytokines IL-1 and TNF-α feature prominently in early sepsis; however, more recent studies suggest that the cells of the Th2 lineage as well as their anti-inflammatory cytokines become more prevalent as the septic process continues.

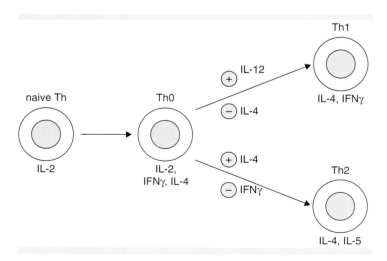

FIGURE 10-12. Differentiation of Th0 cells into the Th1 or Th2 lineage. Reproduced with permission from Imboden JB, Seaman WE. T lymphocytes and natural killer cells. In: Parslow TG, Stites DP, Terr AI, Imboden JB (eds.), *Medical Immunology*, 10th ed. New York, NY: Lange; 2001:141.

BIBLIOGRAPHY

Alarcon LH, Fink MP. Mediators of the inflammatory response. In: Townsend CM (ed.), *Textbook of Surgery: The Biological Basis of Modern Surgical Practice*, 18th ed. Philadelphia, PA: W.B. Saunders; 2008:44–68.

Hotchkiss RS, Karl IE. Medical progress: the pathophysiology and treatment of sepsis. *N Engl J Med* 2003;348(2):138–150.

Munford RS. Severe sepsis and septic shock. In: Longo DL, Fauci AS, Kasper DL, Hauser SL, Jameson J, Loscalzo J (eds.), *Harrison's Principles of Internal Medicine*, 18th ed. New York, NY: McGraw-Hill; 2012:Chapter 271.

27. **(A)** TNF-α is a major cytokine that, in conjunction with IL-1, has a prominent role in the acute inflammatory response. This proinflammatory cytokine is released primarily by macrophages and monocytes, but is also derived from nucleated cells such as natural killer cells and neutrophils, after proper stimulation. Mediators responsible for production of TNF-α include IL-1, IFN-γ, IFN-α, GM-CSF, IL-2, and TGF-β (Table 10-5). Other factors that induce TNF-α formation are LPS, ultraviolet light, protozoa, and viral infection. Following the initial impetus for TNF-α release, a variety of cytokines act to regulate its output.

TNF-α has a myriad of biological functions in inflammation (Table 10-6). Among these are neutrophil

TABLE 10-5 Factors Inducing TNF-α Release

Endogenous Factors
Cytokines (TNF-α, IL-1, IFN-γ, GM-CSF, IL-2)
Platelet-activating factor
Myelin P2 protein
Microbe-Derived Factors
Lipopolysaccharide
Zymosan
Peptidoglycan
Streptococcal pyrogenic exotoxin A
Streptolysin O
Lipoteichoic acid
Staphylococcal enterotoxin B
Staphylococcal toxic shock syndrome toxin-1
Lipoarabinomannan

Reproduced with permission from Fink MP. The role of cytokines as mediators of the inflammatory response. In: Townsend CM (ed.), *Textbook of Surgery: The Biological Basis of Modern Surgical Practice*, 16th ed. Philadelphia, PA: W. B. Saunders; 2001:34.

recruitment, augmentation of superoxide production by neutrophils, angiogenesis, and initiation of the coagulation cascade. Moreover, TNF-α is able to trigger apoptosis, cell death, via the intracellular "death domain" of its receptor, TNF-R1.

BIBLIOGRAPHY

Alarcon LH. Fink MP. Mediators of the inflammatory response. In: Townsend CM (ed.), *Textbook of Surgery: The Biological Basis of Modern Surgical Practice*, 18th ed. Philadelphia, PA: W.B. Saunders; 2008:44–68.

Jan BV, Lowry SF. Systemic response to injury and metabolic support. In: Brunicardi F, Andersen DK, Billiar TR, et al. (eds.), *Schwartz's Principles of Surgery*, 9th ed. New York, NY: McGraw-Hill; 2010:Chapter 2.

Levinson W. Host defenses. In: Levinson W (ed.), *Review of Medical Microbiology and Immunology*, 13th ed. New York, NY: McGraw-Hill; 2014.

Levinson W. Immunity. In: Levinson W (ed.), *Review of Medical Microbiology and Immunology*, 12th ed. New York, NY: McGraw-Hill; 2012:Chapter 57.

Reinhart K, Karzai W. Anti-tumor necrosis factor therapy in sepsis: update on clinical trials and lessons learned. *Crit Care Med* 2001;29(7):S121–S125.

28. **(A)** Septic shock is characterized by a derangement of systemic oxygen metabolism: although oxygen delivery is elevated, its extraction at the periphery is reduced. As a result, the arterial-venous oxygen difference is reduced, and mixed venous oxygenation is increased. A typical patient with septic shock demonstrates adequate oxygen delivery but exhibits signs of refractory hypoxia, notably a persistent lactic acidosis. Systemic oxygen delivery (DO_2) is determined by arterial oxygen content (CaO_2) and cardiac output (CO): $CaO_2 \times CO \times 10$. Despite the improved cardiac index and oxygen delivery, these patients did not experience better outcomes. Instead, the treatment group had an in-unit mortality of 50% as compared to the 30% mortality of the control group. In general, oxygen extraction was equivalent between the two groups, because the treatment group developed a decline in oxygen consumption, although the supply of oxygen increased. An insufficient supply of oxygen was thus discounted as being responsible for the persistent lactic acidosis of sepsis. In response to this scenario, an arterial-to-venous cutaneous shunt was proposed to be the cause of the poor peripheral oxygen extraction.

BIBLIOGRAPHY

Ely E, Goyette RE. Sepsis with acute organ dysfunction. In: Hall JB, Schmidt GA, Wood LH (eds.), *Principles of Critical Care*, 3rd ed. New York, NY: McGraw-Hill; 2005:Chapter 46.

TABLE 10-6 Physiologic Effects of the Infusion of TNF-α and IL-1 on Human Subjects

Effect	IL-1	TNF
Fever	+	+
Headache	+	+
Anorexia	+	+
Increased plasma ACTH level	+	+
Hypercortisolemia	+	+
Increased plasma nitrite/nitrate levels	+	+
Systemic arterial hypotension	+	+
Neutrophilia	+	+
Transient neutropenia	+	+
Increased plasma acute phase protein levels	+	+
Hypoferremia	+	+
Hypozincemia	+	+
Increased plasma level of IL-1RA	+	+
Increased plasma level of TNF-R1 and TNF-R2	+	+
Increased plasma level of IL-6	+	+
Increased plasma level of IL-8	+	+
Activation of coagulation cascades	−	+
Increased platelet count	+	−
Pulmonary edema	−	+
Hepatocellular injury	−	+

Reproduced with permission from Fink MP. The role of cytokines as mediators of the inflammatory response. In: Townsend CM (ed.), *Textbook of Surgery: The Biological Basis of Modern Surgical Practice*, 16th ed. Philadelphia, PA: W.B. Saunders; 2001:31.

Ra JH, Pascual JL, Schwab CW. The septic response. In: Cameron JL (ed.), *Current Surgical Therapy*, 10th ed. St. Louis, MO: Mosby; 2011:1143–1148.

Ronco JJ. Tissue dysoxia in sepsis: getting to know the mitochondrion. *Crit Care Med* 2002;30(2):483–484.

29. **(A)** The proinflammatory cytokines TNF-α, IL-1, and IL-6 independently trigger the hypothalamic-pituitary-adrenal (HPA) axis but act synergistically. Glucocorticoids potentiate vasoconstrictor systems while counteracting the various vasodilatory mediators; also, volume expansion is achieved via the mineralocorticoid properties of glucocorticoids (see Fig. 10-13). In addition to an occult adrenal insufficiency, sepsis is also accompanied by a peripheral resistance to glucocorticoids with the cytokines IL-2 and IL-4 promoting alterations in the affinity of the glucocorticoid receptor via the transcription factor NF-κB.

Cortisol has many effects in modulating inflammation. This endogenous substance acts by binding to glucocorticoid receptors located in the cytoplasm or nucleus. The association of cortisol and the receptor exposes the DNA binding site, previously camouflaged by heat shock proteins, on the receptor. The cortisol-receptor complex travels to the nucleus and binds to certain DNA sequences, glucocorticoid response elements, in the promoter region of various genes. By attaching to these elements, the transcription of specific genes is either promoted or inhibited. For instance, cortisol enhances the production of IκB, the inhibitor of the transcription factor NF-κB; the increased IκB allows NF-κB to be relocated to the cytoplasm, where it has no effect. Consequently, by restricting the synthesis of chemokines, cortisol reduces the accumulation of inflammatory cells in the tissues. In addition, cortisol reduces levels of IL-1, IL-2, IL-3, IL-6, IFN-γ, GM-CSF, and TNF-α. The inflammatory process is also interrupted

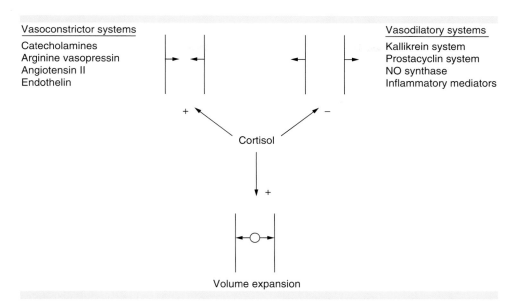

FIGURE 10-13. Effect of cortisol on arterial blood pressure. NO, nitric oxide. Reproduced with permission from Meduri GU. Rationale for glucocorticoid treatment in septic shock and unresolving ARDS. In: Baue AE, Faist E, Fry DE (eds.), *Multiple Organ Failure: Pathophysiology, Prevention, and Therapy.* New York, NY: Springer, 2000, 516.

by suppressing the expression of COX-2 and inducible nitric oxide synthase.

Corticosteroids were the first medications applied as immunotherapeutic agents in septic shock. These early studies of corticosteroids, given for short durations at high doses, demonstrated no survival benefit; however, interest in corticosteroids was renewed by two small randomized studies in which treatment with low doses of hydrocortisone for long durations (>5 days) was associated with a more rapid weaning of vasopressor agents. Similarly, healthy volunteers administered hydrocortisone prior to a local endotoxin challenge did not develop vasoplegia to norepinephrine.

BIBLIOGRAPHY

Annane D. Corticosteroids for septic shock. *Crit Care Med* 2001;29(7):S117–S120.

Hotchkiss RS, Karl IE. Medical progress: the pathophysiology and treatment of sepsis. *N Engl J Med* 2003;348(2):138–150.

Levinson W. Immunity. In: Levinson W (ed.), *Review of Medical Microbiology & Immunology*, 12th ed. New York, NY: McGraw-Hill; 2012:Chapter 57.

Ra JH, Pascual JL, Schwab CW. The septic response. In: Cameron JL (ed.), *Current Surgical Therapy*, 10th ed. St. Louis, MO: Mosby; 2011:1143–1148.

30. **(A)**

31. **(D)**

Explanation for questions 30 and 31

A significant proportion of the mortality of septic shock is attributable to the subsequent MODS. The lung appears as the first target of dysfunction, followed by the kidneys, gastrointestinal tract, and liver. A series of 154 septic patients from a study by Herbert and colleagues determined that acute lung injury (ALI) and acute respiratory distress syndrome (ARDS) were the most common manifestations of MODS. The classification of the lung damage as ALI or ARDS depends on its severity. An ALI arises in a setting of inflammation and pronounced capillary permeability and is defined as an acute-onset injury characterized by a PaO_2/FiO_2 <300 and a pulmonary artery wedge pressure of <18 mmHg with bilateral infiltrates evident on a chest radiograph. ARDS represents a more severe form of ALI, with a PaO_2/FiO_2 <200. Lung injury occurs in 30–80% of the cases of septic shock, most of which present as ARDS. In a 1996 meta-analysis, Garber and colleagues identified sepsis as the most common inciting factor for ARDS.

The lung dysfunction of ARDS emanates from the exaggerated immune response to the infecting pathogen. Neutrophils appear as the primary mediator of this damage, being the predominant cell type in biopsy specimens from ARDS-afflicted lungs. The presence of neutrophils is coincident with an increase in oxidant activity. Oxygen free radicals serve to inhibit surfactant activity by damage to its lipid components and to type II pneumocytes, the source of surfactant. Moreover, the cytotoxic products of neutrophils promote endothelial damage, resulting in protein-rich pulmonary edema, accumulating in both the alveoli and interstitium. Immune agents such as platelet-activating factor, prostaglandins, and the leukotrienes further contribute to this enhanced vascular permeability, which is accompanied by an increase in pulmonary vascular resistance. Activation of the coagulation cascade produces numerous microthrombi within the pulmonary circulation; hypoperfusion of the lung and right-to-left shunting thus arise. Autopsy studies of the lung reveal interstitial and alveolar edema, atelectasis, microthrombi, and hyaline membrane formation. Clinically, this is manifest as hypoxemia because of a ventilation-perfusion mismatch, decreased functional residual capacity, elevated airway resistance, and a pronounced reduction in lung compliance.

Treatment of ARDS rests on the support of pulmonary function while limiting additional lung injury. A majority of patients with ARDS require mechanical ventilation, with the goal of keeping the PaO_2 greater than 60 mmHg or the oxygen saturation higher than 90%. The ventilation-perfusion mismatch may prevent an increase in PaO_2 despite the administration of supplemental oxygen; however, an FiO_2 of less than 50% is recommended to avoid further lung injury from oxygen toxicity. The application of PEEP is essential in maximizing oxygen exchange and, thus, PaO_2. Alveoli are predisposed to collapse at end expiration because of low lung volumes, pulmonary edema, and the deficiency of surfactant. The application of PEEP prevents this collapse, making more alveoli available for gas exchange (see Fig. 10-14).

Additionally, studies have suggested that PEEP may redirect pulmonary artery circulation to better ventilated areas of the lung, lessening the ventilation-perfusion mismatch. Yet, PEEP may contribute to lung injury by inducing barotrauma through alveolar overdistention. Also, cardiac output may be compromised by the addition of PEEP; consequently, the systemic delivery of oxygen is reduced. Other strategies for the management of ARDS include inverse ratio ventilation, high-frequency jet ventilation, and prone positioning.

BIBLIOGRAPHY

Abraham E, Matthay MA, Dinarello CA, et al. Consensus conference definitions for sepsis, septic shock, acute lung injury, and acute respiratory distress syndrome: time for a reevaluation. *Crit Care Med* 2000;28(1):232–235.

Acute Respiratory Distress Syndrome Network. Ventilation with lower tidal volumes as compared with traditional tidal volumes for acute lung injury and the acute respiratory distress syndrome. *N Engl J Med* 2000;342(18):1301–1308.

Buchman TG. Multiple organ dysfunction and failure. In: Cameron JL (ed.), *Current Surgical Therapy*, 10th ed. St. Louis, MO: Mosby; 2011:1149–1153.

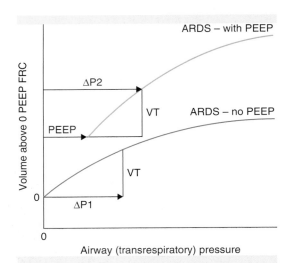

FIGURE 10-14. Relationship between airway pressure and volume in a patient with adult respiratory distress syndrome (ARDS). By adding positive end-expiratory pressure (PEEP) to the mechanical ventilation, the pressure-volume curve demonstrates greater lung compliance. FRC, functional residual capacity; VT, dead space. Reproduced with permission from Sue DY. Respiratory failure. In: Bongard FS, Sue DY (eds.), *Current Critical Care Diagnosis and Treatment*. Stamford, CT: Appleton & Lange; 1994.

Girard TD, Bernard GR. Mechanical ventilation in ARDSA state-of-the-art review. *Chest J* 2007;131:921–929.

Sauaia A, Moore FA, Moore EE. Multiple organ failure. In: Mattox KL, Moore EE, Feliciano DV (eds.), *Trauma*, 7th ed. New York, NY: McGraw-Hill; 2013:Chapter 61.

32. **(B)**

33. **(A)**

Explanation for questions 32 and 33

A prominent feature of septic shock is vasopressor-resistant hypotension, attributable to a pronounced systemic vasodilatation. This massive vasodilatation has been ascribed to nitric oxide, a free radical gas derived from the three isomers of the enzyme nitric oxide synthase. Under normal physiologic conditions, nitric oxide, produced from the constitutive enzyme endothelial nitric oxide synthase (eNOS), maintains a baseline of vasodilatation, regulating tissue perfusion. Inhibition of eNOS with guanidine-substituted L-arginine analogs promotes severe systemic and pulmonary hypertension. In the presence of inflammatory agents such as TNF-α, IL-1, and endotoxin, inducible nitric oxide synthase (iNOS) is generated from macrophages and vascular smooth muscle, following the tyrosine kinase–induced activation of the transcription factor NF-κB. As part of a normal inflammatory response, nitric oxide and its free radical derivatives contribute to the eradication of the invading pathogens. In addition, the nitric oxide created by iNOS promotes the dilatation of neighboring blood vessels via the intracellular messenger cGMP. Nitric oxide activates the enzyme soluble guanylate cyclase, which catalyzes the conversion of guanosine triphosphate (GTP) to cGMP by binding to its iron-heme component. This intracellular messenger induces a cGMP-dependent protein kinase within the cells of vascular smooth muscle to open calcium and potassium channels, thereby achieving vasodilatation.

With septic shock, the amount of nitric oxide generated becomes exuberant. In an *in vitro* model of sepsis, in which endothelial cells and endotoxin were placed in culture, nitrite, the stable end product of nitric oxide, was revealed in a concentration that far exceeded that associated with the baseline production of nitric oxide (millimoles vs. micromoles). Similar studies in adults with severe sepsis produced equivalent results, albeit in amounts smaller than in rodent models. However, the initial release of nitric oxide, within the first 2 hours of the onset of septic shock, is ascribed to eNOS, because iNOS is not yet present. Yet, the contribution of eNOS to the abundant output of nitric oxide is transient. Ochoa and colleagues measured elevated levels of nitrite in patients suffering from septic shock, correlating this finding with hypotension and an increased cardiac output. Inhibition of nitric oxide synthase in septic patients has resulted in an improved responsiveness to vasopressors. Moreover, iNOS knock-out mice afflicted with septic shock exhibit a diminished degree of hypotension, culminating in a survival advantage. Further benefits associated with the inhibition of iNOS include diminished peroxynitrite generation and attenuation of the suppression of mitochondrial respiration.

Despite its adverse effects, nitric oxide appears to play a physiologic role in maintaining tissue perfusion in the presence of septic shock. It is likely that this action is directed by the constitutive isomers of NOS, eNOS, and neuronal NOS (nNOS). Septic shock is associated with a localized vasoconstriction within various organs, including the mesenteric, pulmonary, and renal circulations. This is counteracted by the vasodilatory action of nitric oxide. In a canine model of septic shock, nonselective inhibition of NOS led to a diminished splanchnic perfusion, with gastrointestinal and liver injury the result. Nitric oxide provides further benefits in septic shock, among which are a reduction in neutrophil adhesion and decreased platelet aggregation. In sum, the search for an inhibitor of nitric oxide synthesis or action must consider the detrimental as well as beneficial contributions of nitric oxide to septic shock.

BIBLIOGRAPHY

Alarcon LH, Fink MP. Mediators of the inflammatory response. In: Townsend CM (ed.), *Textbook of Surgery: The Biological Basis of Modern Surgical Practice*, 18th ed. Philadelphia, PA: W.B. Saunders; 2008:44–68.

Jaffrey SR. Nitric oxide. In: Katzung BG, Masters SB, Trevor AJ (eds.), *Basic & Clinical Pharmacology*, 12th ed. New York, NY: McGraw-Hill; 2012:Chapter 19.

Levinson W. Immunity. In: Levinson W (eds.), *Review of Medical Microbiology & Immunology*, 12th ed. New York, NY: McGraw-Hill; 2012:Chapter 57.

Sheehan M, Wong HR. Yet another potential role for nitric oxide in the pathophysiology of septic shock. *Crit Care Med* 2002;30(6):1393–1394.

34. **(C)** Since its development in 1970, the pulmonary artery catheter, or the Swan-Ganz catheter, has remained an essential tool in the management of critically ill patients. This flexible, balloon-tipped, flow-directed catheter is inserted via a central vein (internal jugular or subclavian vein) and directed through the right heart to a branch of the pulmonary artery. As the catheter is advanced, its location is signaled by variations in the waveform and pressures (see Fig. 10-15).

At a catheter length of 50–55 cm, a pulmonary capillary wedge tracing is obtained. A more accurate PCWP is generated when the distal tip of the catheter lies in zone III of the lung, where the column of blood between the pulmonary artery and the left atrium remains uninterrupted (see Fig. 10-16).

In zones I and II, intermittent vascular collapse from surrounding high airway pressures interferes with the continuity of this column of blood. The pulmonary artery catheter directly measures cardiac output, pulmonary artery pressures, and the mixed venous oxygen saturation. The PCWP, obtained when the balloon is inflated, approximates left atrial pressure and, therefore, left ventricular end-diastolic pressure (LVEDP) and volume (LVEDV). The correlation of the PCWP and left atrial pressure is best at a pressure less than 25 mmHg; at a pressure greater than 25 mmHg, the LVEDP is overestimated. The PCWP serves as a reliable indication of cardiac preload, based on the assumptions that the mitral valve is normal; no pulmonary vascular disease exists; the column of blood between the distal tip of the catheter in the pulmonary artery and the left atrium is intact; and the LVEDP and LVEDV are directly related. In the absence of a left-to-right or a right-to-left shunt, cardiac output is accurately determined by a thermodilution technique. The oxygen saturation of blood within the pulmonary artery represents the mixed venous oxygen saturation (SvO_2), measured by reflectance spectrophotometry. The systemic utilization of oxygen—the difference between oxygen delivery and its consumption in the periphery—is reflected by the SvO_2. In the case

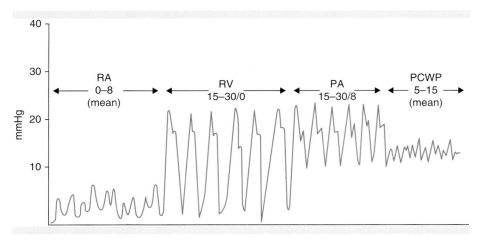

FIGURE 10-15. Evolution of the pulmonary artery catheter waveform during the advancement from the right atrium to the pulmonary arterial branch (wedge position). The pressure of each chamber is also shown. PA, pulmonary artery; PCWP, pulmonary capillary wedge pressure; RA, right atrium; RV, right ventricle. Reproduced with permission from Bongard FS, Sue DY. Critical care monitoring. In: Bongard FS, Sue DY (eds.), *Current Critical Care Diagnosis and Treatment.* Stamford, CT: Appleton & Lange; 1994:179.

of a low SvO_2, the supply of oxygen may be deficient or, alternatively, the use of oxygen by the tissues may be increased. A septic patient, however, demonstrates an elevated SvO_2, resulting from a decrease in consumption of oxygen by the peripheral tissues.

No absolute indications for pulmonary artery catheter placement exist. Among the situations in which the catheter has been recommended for use include shock refractory to fluid resuscitation, oliguria despite adequate volume replacement, multiple organ failure, cardiac or major vascular surgery, multisystem trauma, and complicated MI. Pulmonary artery catheter–related complications occur during either its placement or utilization (Table 10-7). The most common complication

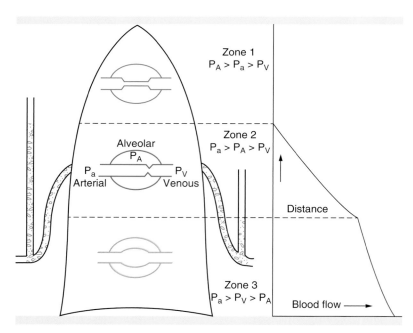

FIGURE 10-16. Pulmonary zones. In zone III of the lung, the column of blood between the pulmonary artery catheter tip and the left atrium is uninterrupted by collapse of the surrounding airways, allowing for a more accurate estimation of left ventricular end-diastolic volume and pressure. P_a, arterial pressure; P_A, alveolar pressure; P_v, venous pressure. Reproduced with permission from Bongard FS, Sue DY. Critical care monitoring. In: Bongard FS, Sue DY (eds.), *Current Critical Care Diagnosis and Treatment.* Stamford, CT: Appleton & Lange; 1994:180.

TABLE 10-7 Complications of Pulmonary Artery Catheterization (PAC)

Complications related to central vein cannulation
Complications related to insertion and use of the PAC
Tachyarrhythmias
Right bundle branch block
Complete heart block (preexisting left bundle branch block)
Cardiac perforation
Thrombosis and embolism
Pulmonary infarction due to persistent wedging
Catheter-related sepsis
Pulmonary artery rupture and pseudoaneurysm
Knotting of the catheter
Endocarditis, bland and infective
Pulmonic valve insufficiency
Balloon fragmentation and embolization

(From Hall JB, Schmidt GA, Wood LH (eds.). *Principles of Critical Care*, 3rd ed. New York, NY: McGraw-Hill; 2005:Table 13-2).

(50%) is a self-limited arrhythmia, evident on insertion of the catheter through the tricuspid and pulmonary valves. Other complications linked to catheter placement include pneumothorax, catheter knotting, right bundle branch block, tracheal laceration, innominate artery injury, pulmonary artery rupture, and bleeding. The routine use of the catheter is affiliated with air emboli, thromboemboli, infective endocarditis, sepsis, aseptic thrombotic endocarditis, and rupture of the chordae tendineae. These more serious complications transpire in less than 1 in 1000 insertions. Sandham and colleagues (2003) undertook a randomized trial comparing goal-directed therapy guided by a pulmonary artery catheter with standard treatment not employing this tool. No significant difference was demonstrated in the mortality or 10-month survival rates among the two groups. The pulmonary artery catheter cohort did exhibit an increased incidence of pulmonary embolus (8 vs. 0%). In sum, the authors detected no benefit to therapy directed by a pulmonary artery catheter; however, the decision to use a pulmonary artery catheter must be tailored to the individual patient.

BIBLIOGRAPHY

Manikon M, Grounds M, Rhodes A. The pulmonary artery catheter. *Clin Med* 2002;2(2):101–104.

Sandham JD, Hull RD, Brant RF, et al. A randomized, controlled trial of the use of pulmonary-artery catheters in high-risk surgical patients. *N Engl J Med* 2003;348(1):5–14.

Walley KR. Shock. In: Hall JB, Schmidt GA, Wood LH (eds.), *Principles of Critical Care*, 3rd ed. New York, NY: McGraw-Hill; 2005:Chapter 21.

West JB. *Respiratory Physiology: The Essentials*. Philadelphia, PA: Lippincott Williams & Wilkins; 2012.

35. **(B)** The gastrointestinal tract has been studied extensively as a portal by which occult hypoperfusion may be detected. Gastric tonometry is one of the few methods for direct measurement of splanchnic perfusion. This minimally invasive technique, using a balloon-tipped nasogastric tube, directly measures the partial pressure of carbon dioxide (PCO_2) in the mucosa of the stomach. Gastric tonometry relies on the principle that, at equilibrium, the PCO_2 of the mucosa and lumen of a hollow organ is equivalent. Following placement of a saline-filled silicone balloon, permeable to carbon dioxide, the saline equilibrates with the carbon dioxide of the mucosa, a process with a duration of approximately 60 minutes. Ultimately, the PCO_2 of the saline solution approximates that of the mucosa. The mucosal pH is then calculated using the Henderson-Hasselbalch equation, with the bicarbonate level provided by an arterial blood gas. The normal mucosal pH ranges from 7.35 to 7.41. The PCO_2 obtained by tonometry correlates well with values determined directly, especially after including a correction factor for incomplete equilibration; however, the mucosal pH, under conditions of ischemia, varies depending on the method of measurement, direct or tonometric. Air tonometry also serves as an adequate substitute for saline. The determination of gastric mucosal PCO_2 and pH is also limited by gastric acid secretion and intragastric feeding, both of which have unpredictable effects on these values. Sources of error include the contamination of the saline solution with residual fluids or bacteria, temperature fluctuations, blood gas analyzer bias, inadequate correction factors, and catheter dead space. Gastric tonometry has not demonstrated a clear advantage compared with conventional resuscitation end points and its use has not been widely adopted.

BIBLIOGRAPHY

Coimbra R, Doucet J, Bansal V. Principles of critical care. In: Mattox KL, Moore EE, Feliciano DV (eds.), *Trauma*, 7th ed. New York, NY: McGraw-Hill; 2013:Chapter 55.

Lee CC, Marill KA, Carter WA, Crupi RS. A current concept of trauma-induced multiorgan failure. *Ann Emerg Med* 2001;38(2):170–176.

Zuckerbraun BS, Peitzman AB, Billiar TR. Shock. In: Brunicardi F, Andersen DK, Billiar TR, et al. (eds.), *Schwartz's Principles of Surgery*, 9th ed. New York, NY: McGraw-Hill; 2010:Chapter 5.

CHAPTER 11

HEAD AND NECK

ERYNNE A. FAUCETT AND AUDREY B. ERMAN

QUESTIONS

1. Which intraoperative technique during parotidectomy is used to locate the main trunk of the extracranial facial nerve?
   (A) Identification of posterior aspect of the sternocleidomastoid muscle
   (B) Identification of the anterior belly of the digastric muscle
   (C) Retrograde tracking of the marginal mandibular nerve
   (D) Retrograde tracking of the greater auricular nerve
   (E) Identification of the tympanosquamousal suture line

2. Which of the following is part of the oral cavity?
   (A) Tonsillar fossa
   (B) Soft palate
   (C) Base of tongue
   (D) Uvula
   (E) Retromolar trigone

3. A newborn has respiratory distress with evidence of cyanosis immediately following delivery. During laryngoscopy for intubation, the anesthesiologist notes a pedunculated mass emanating from somewhere in the posterior naso- or oropharynx. The mass does not interfere with intubation, but on further examination it appears to have hair on its ventral surface. Figure 11-1 shows the magnetic resonance imaging (MRI) obtained to evaluate the mass. The most likely diagnosis is
   (A) Glioma
   (B) Craniopharyngioma
   (C) Teratoma
   (D) Hemangioma
   (E) Lymphangioma

4. A 7-year-old presents to your office with a right-sided neck mass. The mother states that the mass seems to fluctuate in size and drains clear fluid every time the child eats. On examination, you find a small pore anterior to the right sternocleidomastoid (SCM) muscle (see Fig. 11-2). The most likely diagnosis is
   (A) First branchial cleft cyst
   (B) First branchial cleft fistula
   (C) Second branchial cleft cyst
   (D) Second branchial cleft fistula
   (E) Third branchial cleft cyst

5. A 58-year-old man undergoes a left-sided modified radical neck dissection (MRND) for an unknown primary. While dissecting inferior and lateral to the carotid sheath, the operative field is suddenly inundated with a milky fluid. What structure was injured?
   (A) Cisterna chyli
   (B) Thoracic duct
   (C) Left internal jugular vein
   (D) A cystic left thyroid lobe
   (E) Trachea

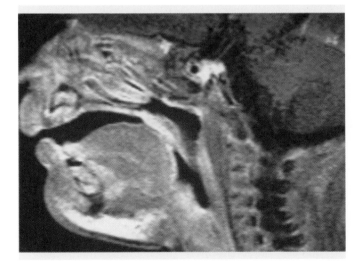

FIGURE 11-1. T1-weighted sagittal magnetic resonance image of head and neck with mass in oral cavity and nasopharynx.

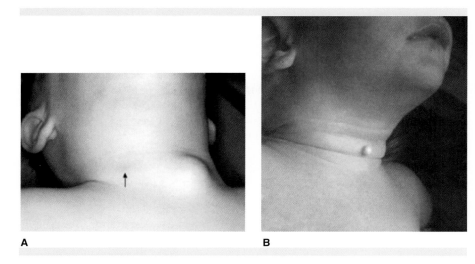

FIGURE 11-2. Arrow pointing to small pore anterior to sternocleidomastoid muscle. From *Azizkhan RG. Head and Neck Lesions.* In: Ziegler MM, Azizkhan RG, Allmen D, Weber TR. eds. Operative Pediatric Surgery, Second Edition. New York, NY: McGraw-Hill; 2014.

6. A 60-year-old man has a squamous cell carcinoma (SCC) involving the middle of the left true vocal cord. There is 3-mm supraglottic extension on the left and no reduction in cord mobility. The treatment that will best preserve voice quality is
   (A) Laser excision
   (B) Cordectomy
   (C) Primary radiation
   (D) Chemotherapy
   (E) Hemilaryngectomy

7. A 2-year-old child swallows a short straight pin and is brought to the emergency department (ED) by his parents. On examination, he is alert and able to control his secretions. He has been in no respiratory distress and remains afebrile. What is the appropriate course of action?
   (A) Follow up in the clinic in 10 days
   (B) Perform endoscopy if the pin is found in the stomach or esophagus on x-ray
   (C) Perform endoscopy whether or not a pin is seen on x-ray
   (D) Admit the child for observation and daily abdominal plain films until the pin is passed in the stool
   (E) Counsel the parents to strain the child's stool and feed him a high-roughage diet if the pin is radiographically identified in the stomach

8. A 14-year-old boy is involved in a dirt bike crash sustaining a "clothesline" injury. On examination, a 7-cm laceration over the anterior neck, subcutaneous emphysema, and a nonexpanding hematoma are noted. He is unable to lay flat and has a muffled voice. On flexible laryngoscopy, mild edema of the supraglottis and glottis, reduced vocal cord abduction, and bloody secretions in the subglottis are seen. Initial management of this patient would involve

   (A) Nasal intubation, laryngeal and cervical spine computed tomography (CT), and exploration and repair with intraoperative tracheotomy
   (B) An awake tracheostomy under local anesthesia, laryngeal and cervical CT endoscopy, and exploration and repair
   (C) Percutaneous tracheostomy, cervical spine series, and exploration and repair with stenting
   (D) Oral intubation, laryngeal and cervical spine CT, endoscopy, and exploration and repair
   (E) Nasal intubation, laryngeal and cervical CT, endoscopy, and exploration and repair

9. A 40-year-old man presents 8 days after trauma to the face with a midfacial wound and swelling of the cheek. The laceration was repaired by another physician who noted transection of the parotid duct but did not repair it. His facial nerve function is normal on examination. Your next step in management is
   (A) Perform a sialogram
   (B) Irradiate the parotid gland
   (C) Empiric antibiotics for infection
   (D) Explore the wound from an intraoral approach
   (E) Place a pressure dressing over gland to prevent sialocele development

10. A 19-year-old woman presents to the ED with a few days' history of fever and pain in the submandibular region. Over the last several hours, she has been having more trouble speaking with pain in her tongue and is afraid to lie down because she has trouble breathing. On oral examination, the floor of mouth is indurated, swollen, and very tender. The patient has very poor dentition, but there is no evidence of an abscess. Her submandibular and submental regions are also tender

and indurated. What diagnosis are you most concerned about?

(A) Vincent angina
(B) Periodontal abscess
(C) Ludwig angina
(D) Retropharyngeal abscess
(E) Submandibular and sublingual gland sialadenitis

11. Which of the following tumors is most likely to occur bilaterally?

(A) Pleomorphic adenoma
(B) Monomorphic adenoma
(C) Papillary cystadenoma lymphomatosum
(D) Cystadenoma
(E) Mucoepidermoid carcinoma

12. A 20-year-old man involved in an altercation presents to the ED with epistaxis and nasal airway obstruction. When inspecting his nose externally, you feel crepitus when moving the nasal bones and mild flattening of the dorsum. You note no active bleeding. On anterior rhinoscopy, you see an ecchymotic, swollen area on both sides of the caudal septum (see Fig. 11-3). What is the next step in management?

(A) Perform a closed reduction of nasal bones.
(B) Place internal nasal splints to stabilize the fracture.
(C) Drain the septal hematoma.
(D) Place anterior nasal packing to treat the epistaxis.
(E) Obtain facial x-rays if they were not already performed.

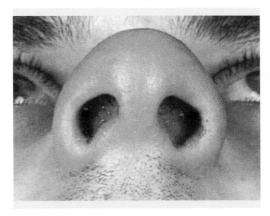

FIGURE 11-3. Anterior nares.

13. A 50-year-old man has a 2-day history of headaches and proptosis with limited vision of the right eye. Vision has been reduced to light perception only, and the globe is displaced inferior and laterally. Rhinoscopy shows swelling in the middle meatus with some purulent drainage. What is the next step in management?

(A) Obtain a CT scan of the orbits and sinuses, and then perform an ethmoidectomy.
(B) Give intravenous (IV) aqueous penicillin G 2 million U every 4 hours.

(C) Give IV levofloxacin 500 mg every 24 hours.
(D) Perform immediate exploration of the orbits.
(E) Give oral dexamethasone 4 mg daily for 1 week.

14. A 24-year-old woman sustained a zone 1 stab injury to the neck during an assault by her boyfriend. She reports several episodes of bright red emesis but denies hoarseness. On examination, she has a midline nonexpanding moderate-sized neck hematoma and is hemodynamically normal. An angiogram was performed, which was negative for any major vascular injury. Intraoperatively, an anterior tracheal laceration across the first and second tracheal rings was noted. The next step in evaluation would include inspection of the

(A) Course of both recurrent nerves
(B) Cricothyroid membrane and external branch of the superior laryngeal nerve
(C) Posterior tracheal wall
(D) Innominate artery
(E) Brachiocephalic vein

15. A 46-year-old man was struck by a train and suffered a nonpenetrating temporal bone fracture. Immediately after the injury, his facial nerve function seems intact; however, the next day, he developed some facial nerve weakness that evolved into complete paralysis by the fourth day (see Figs. 11-4 and 11-5). What is the next step?

(A) Obtain a high-resolution temporal bone CT to see if bony fragments are impinging on the facial nerve.
(B) Obtain electroneuronography (ENOG) to determine the need for surgical intervention.
(C) Proceed with immediate exploration of the facial nerve for decompression.
(D) Obtain a facial electromyogram (EMG) to determine the need for surgical intervention.
(E) Give oral steroids and continue to observe the patient because the prognosis for recovery is good.

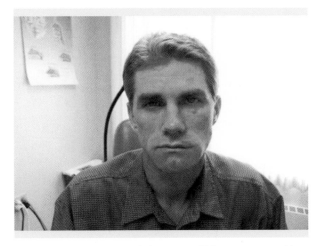

FIGURE 11-4. Patient with history of blunt temporal bone trauma at rest.

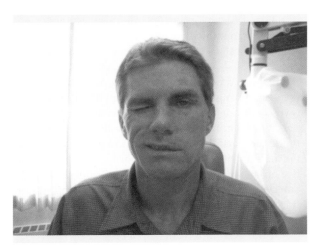

FIGURE 11-5. Patient with gross facial asymmetry on maximum effort.

16. A 6-year-old boy on a bike collides into a fence. A CT scan of the head/face is obtained (see Fig. 11-6). What would make this a LeFort III fracture?
    (A) Presence of pyramidal fractures
    (B) Presence of naso-orbito-ethmoid fractures (NOE complex)
    (C) Presence of a unilateral horizontal maxillary fracture
    (D) Presence of a bilateral horizontal maxillary fracture
    (E) Craniofacial dysjunction

17. A 60-year-old man with a history of hypertension and coronary artery disease presents to the ED with bleeding from the right nare. He is on aspirin 325 mg daily as well as Plavix for a percutaneous transluminal coronary angioplasty with stent placed 5 years ago. You place an anterior nasal pack, and he has no bleeding until 20 minutes later. He then bleeds through your pack and is bleeding from his mouth. Your next step in management is
    (A) Place a new anterior pack and admit him for observation
    (B) Place a posterior nasal pack and admit him for observation
    (C) Place a posterior nasal pack and admit him to a monitored floor
    (D) Schedule him for an internal maxillary artery ligation
    (E) Schedule embolization with interventional radiology

18. A 46-year-old patient developed acute respiratory distress syndrome (ARDS) and ultimately underwent a tracheostomy. Two weeks following his tracheostomy, you are called to see him about bright red pulsatile blood from around his tracheostomy site. Which of the following reduces the likelihood of this complication?
    (A) Use of a rigid tracheostomy
    (B) Tracheostomy placement between the third and fourth tracheal rings

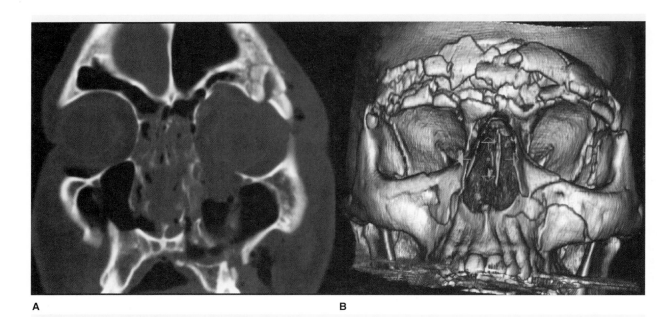

A   B

FIGURE 11-6. Coronal computed tomography scan of facial fractures. From From Mattox K, Moore E, Feliciano D (eds.). *Trauma*, 7th ed. New York, NY: McGraw-Hill; 2012:Fig. 21-15.

(C) Tracheostomy placement between the second and third tracheal rings

(D) Tracheostomy placement between the fourth tracheal rings

(E) Use of sharply angulated tracheostomy tubes

19. A 75-year-old farmer presents with a 3.0-cm ulcerated lesion of his lower lip. On examination, you find that it involves the central portion of the lower lip. A biopsy confirms squamous cell carcinoma. The optimal treatment for this patient would be
(A) Primary full-thickness excision
(B) Vermilionectomy and bilateral supraomohyoid neck dissections
(C) Radiation therapy
(D) Mohs micrographic surgery
(E) Full-thickness excision and bilateral supraomohyoid neck dissections

20. A 67-year-old patient presents with an ulcerating lesion of the cervical esophagus that does not directly involve the wall between the esophagus and larynx. It does, however, extend into the thoracic esophagus for 2 cm. The patient is consented for a total laryngopharyngoesophagectomy. The best reconstructive option is
(A) Gastric pull-up
(B) Radial forearm free flap
(C) Pectoralis major myocutaneous tubed flap
(D) Jejunal free flap/transfer
(E) Cervical skin flaps

21. An 80-year-old woman who is a nursing home patient is brought to the hospital with a gastrointestinal (GI) bleed. She ultimately undergoes a left hemicolectomy for diverticulosis and has a lengthy postoperative ileus. On postoperative day 5, she complains of a sour taste in her mouth and her right cheek feeling warm and very tender. She is febrile, and you notice a swelling inferomedial to her ear. What is the most likely bacterial cause of these symptoms?
(A) *Staphylococcus aureus*
(B) *Pseudomonas*
(C) *Burkholderia pseudomallei*
(D) *Streptococcus viridians*
(E) *Streptococcus pneumoniae*

22. A 47-year-old man undergoes resection of a right lateral tongue and retromolar trigone SCC with a wide local resection with hemiglossectomy and modified neck dissection. There is a significant soft tissue deficit, and you decide to use a pectoralis myocutaneous flap for reconstruction. What is the arterial supply to this flap?
(A) The deep epigastric artery
(B) The external carotid artery
(C) The supraclavicular artery

(D) The thoracoacromial artery
(E) The thoracodorsal artery

23. The most likely pathogen to be involved with supraglottitis (epiglottitis) is
(A) *S pneumoniae*
(B) *Haemophilus influenzae*
(C) Influenza virus
(D) Parainfluenza virus
(E) *S aureus*

24. What structure passes through the foramen ovale?
(A) Infraorbital nerve
(B) Crania nerve V_3
(C) Meningeal artery
(D) Sphenopalatine artery
(E) Cranial nerve V_2

25. What study is used to monitor response to therapy for necrotizing otitis externa?
(A) Technetium-99 scan
(B) Gallium-67 scan
(C) CT scan
(D) MRI
(E) Culture

26. Nasopharyngeal carcinoma is strongly associated with which virus?
(A) Cytomegalovirus (CMV)
(B) Varicella-zoster virus
(C) Herpes simplex virus (HSV)
(D) Epstein-Barr virus (EBV)
(E) Human papillomavirus (HPV)

27. What type of flap is raised and pivoted into a defect along an arc in a curvilinear fashion?
(A) Rotation
(B) Island
(C) Transposition
(D) Hinge
(E) Random

28. Pott puffy tumor is seen most commonly with which of these conditions?
(A) Otitis media
(B) Frontal sinus fracture
(C) Ethmoid sinusitis
(D) Bacterial pharyngitis
(E) Cervical spinal infection

ANSWERS AND EXPLANATIONS

1. **(C)** The facial nerve begins as the fascioacoustic primordium during the third week of gestation, and by

the eleventh week, most of its branching is complete. The facial nerve is the most superficial structure to pass through the parotid gland, dividing it into superficial and deep lobes. The nerve first exits the skull base at the stylomastoid foramen and then courses anteriorly and somewhat inferiorly toward the posterior surface of the parotid gland. The pes anserinus is the point at which the facial nerve divides into its temporozygomatic (upper) and cervicofacial (lower) divisions within the parotid gland (see Fig. 11-7). Once the anterior border of the parotid is reached, the nerve will have divided into its five branches: temporal, zygomatic, buccal, marginal mandibular, and cervical (see Fig. 11-8). In children under age 3, the mastoid bone is poorly developed, and the facial nerve courses much more superficially and caudally.

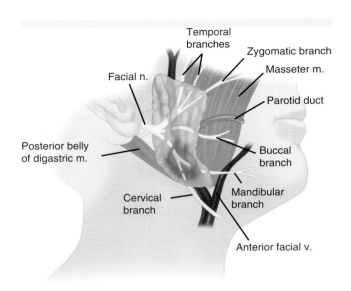

FIGURE 11-8. Identification of the main trunk of the facial nerve and Stensen's duct. From Brunicardi F, Andersen DK, Billiar TR, et al. (eds.), *Schwartz's Principles of Surgery*, 10th ed. New York, NY: McGraw-Hill; 2014:Fig. 18-44.

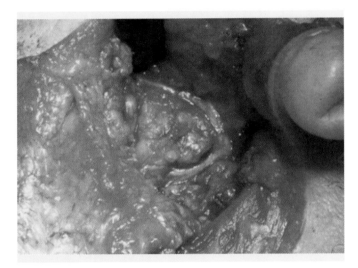

FIGURE 11-7. Intraoperative photograph of the pes anserinus in the parotid gland.

A superficial parotidectomy begins with a preauricular incision that curves around the lobule of the ear to the mastoid extending into the neck past the angle of the mandible in a natural skin crease. Anterior and posterior skin flaps are developed to ensure exposure of the entire gland. The mastoid and anterior border of the sternocleidomastoid (SCM) are located. The posterior belly of the digastric is then located, which marks the level of the nerve from a superficial to deep plane. The gland is then separated by blunt dissection from the cartilage of the external auditory canal, and the tragal pointer (the medial-most aspect of the cartilaginous portion of the external auditory canal [EAC]) is exposed. The main trunk of the facial nerve is identified approximately 1 cm medial and anterior the tragal pointer, exiting the stylomastoid foramen immediately

posterior to the styloid process entering the parotid gland immediately anterior to the insertion of the digastric muscle into the mastoid tip.

The tympanomastoid suture line is used as another landmark: the main trunk can be found 6–8 mm deep to this suture line. Any of the branches if identified first peripherally can be followed retrograde to the main trunk or "pes." The marginal mandibular branch is often used for this and can be found following the posterior facial vein superiorly. The greater auricular nerve is derived from cervical roots C2 and C3 and supplies sensation to the inferior part of the auricle as well as the neck and the area between the mastoid and angle of the mandible. Although it is one of the early structures encountered during parotidectomy, it is not used specifically as a landmark for the main trunk. A deep lobe or total parotidectomy would involve taking the portion of the parotid gland deep to the facial nerve requiring complete skeletonization of the nerve branches.

BIBLIOGRAPHY

Carrasco VN, Zdanski CJ, Logan TC, et al. Facial nerve paralysis. In: Lee KJ (ed.), *Essential Otolaryngology Head and Neck Surgery*, 8th ed. New York, NY: McGraw Hill; 2003:169–191.

Sunwoo J, Lewis JS, McJunkin J, et al. Malignant neoplasms of the salivary glands. In: Cummings CW, Fredrickson JM, Harker LA, et al. (eds.), *Otolaryngology Head & Neck Surgery: Pediatric*, 5th ed. St. Louis, MO: Mosby; 2010:1178–1199.

2. **(E)** The oral cavity extends from the cutaneous vermilion border of the lips to the anterior tonsillar pillars (the mucosa-covered palatoglossus muscle). The posterior border of the oral cavity also includes the circumvallate papillae inferiorly and the junction of the hard and soft palate superiorly. The oral cavity has eight subunits: lips, buccal mucosa, floor of mouth, anterior two-thirds of the tongue (i.e., oral tongue), upper and lower alveolar ridges, hard palate, and retromolar trigone (RMT). The lips represent a transition from external skin to internal mucous membrane that occurs at the vermillion border.

The salivary ducts traverse the mucosa to drain into the oral cavity. These include Stensen's duct of the parotid gland, the papilla of which is located lateral to the second molars; Wharton's duct of the submandibular gland, which is found in the midline floor of mouth adjacent to the frenulum of the tongue; and ducts of Rivinius of the sublingual gland, which drain into the floor of mouth or into Wharton's duct itself.

The vascular supply of the oral cavity is derived from several branches of the external carotid artery. These include the lingual artery, which supplies the oral tongue and tongue base. It is found deep to the hypoglossus muscle. The internal maxillary artery branches into the descending palatine artery, ultimately dividing into the greater and lesser palatine arteries to supply the hard and soft palate, respectively, and the posterior, middle, and anterior superior alveolar arteries and nasopalatine artery, which supply the upper alveolar ridge. The lesser palatine artery anastomoses posteriorly with a branch of the facial artery, the ascending palatine artery. The mandibular teeth and gingiva are vascularized by the inferior alveolar artery. Venous drainage of the palate is via the pterygoid plexus (hard palate) and pharyngeal plexus (soft palate) and tongue and floor of mouth via the lingual vein. Lymphatic drainage occurs via submandibular (hard palate, lateral tongue), deep jugular (most subunits), lateral pharyngeal, parotid, and submental nodes (tip of tongue).

BIBLIOGRAPHY

Deschler DG, Erman AB. Oral cavity cancer. In: Bailey BJ, Johnson JT, Newlands SD (eds.), *Head & Neck Surgery Otolaryngology*, 5th ed., vol. 2. Philadelphia, PA: Lippincott Williams & Wilkins; 2014:1849–1874.

Farrior JB, Lee KJ. Embryology of clefts and pouches. In: Lee KJ (ed.), *Essential Otolaryngology Head and Neck Surgery*, 10th ed. New York, NY: McGraw-Hill; 2012:269–284.

Robbins KT, Malone J. Carcinoma of the oral cavity, pharynx and esophagus. In: Lee KJ (ed.), *Essential Otolaryngology Head and Neck Surgery*, 10th ed. New York, NY: McGraw-Hill; 2012:695–723.

3. **(C)** The differential diagnosis for airway obstruction in the neonate is broad and includes congenital anatomic anomalies, nasal masses, neoplastic lesions, and teratomas. The first group of disorders involves congenital anatomic anomalies. These may involve the nose, nasopharynx, and oropharynx and include etiologies such as choanal atresia, pyriform aperture stenosis, and craniofacial anomalies such as the micrognathia and glossoptosis found in the Pierre-Robin sequence. Choanal atresia can be diagnosed at birth by the inability to pass an 8-French catheter into the oropharynx. Other congenital anomalies in the nasopharynx would include nasopharyngeal cysts, which can be intra- or extra-adenoidal or branchial cleft in origin.

An important group of nasal masses are those of neuroectodermal origin. These include gliomas, encephaloceles, and dermoids. Only the encephalocele is characterized by an ependyma-lined tract that communicates with the ventricles of the brain. The encephalocele can be characterized by a positive Furstenberg test. The Furstenberg test is performed by compression of the jugular veins, which causes increased cerebrospinal fluid (CSF) pressure, leading to enlargement of the encephalocele. Anomalies of the larynx would include laryngomalacia, laryngeal webs, cysts, laryngoceles, subglottic stenosis, laryngeal atresia, or laryngeal clefts.

Neoplastic lesions include hemangiomas, lymphangiomas, and craniopharyngiomas. Hemangiomas can be located anywhere in the upper aerodigestive tract; however, there is a propensity for the anterior subglottic region. Hemangiomas of the subglottis do not produce symptoms of stridor or airway obstruction at birth because they are small initially; however, they begin to proliferate several weeks after birth. Lymphangiomas are caused by failure of lymph spaces to link to the rest of the lymphatic system. They range in size from lymphangioma simplex to the large multicystic cystic hygroma. The craniopharyngioma is a tumor of the nasopharynx derived from Rathke's pouch elements. Rathke's pouch contains the ectoderm that becomes the anterior pituitary gland, and the tumor itself contains well-differentiated epithelial elements.

Teratomas are benign masses originating from pleuripotential cells. Most are located sacrococcygeal, with the head and neck region being the second most common site for teratomas in infants. Teratomas in the head and neck region occur in the nasopharynx, oral cavity, orbit, neck, and thyroid. After birth, teratomas can present as large neck masses that cause airway obstruction. The teratoma is part of a spectrum of masses, which includes the dermoid cyst, the teratoid cyst, and epignathi. The dermoid is the most common and has both epidermal and mesodermal elements and can have hair. The teratoid cyst and teratoma contain all three germ layers, but the teratoma has much more cellular differentiation (and can exhibit hair growth as well). Epignathi also contain all three germ layers and are the most differentiated with complete organs and/or body parts.

BIBLIOGRAPHY

Alper CM, Robison JG. Head and neck masses in children. In: Bailey BJ, Johnson JT, Newlands SD (eds.), *Head & Neck Surgery Otolaryngology*, 5th ed., vol. 1. Philadelphia, PA: Lippincott Williams & Wilkins; 2014:1589–1606.
Chan Y, Das S, Scannell R. Highlights and pearls. In: Lee KJ (ed.), *Essential Otolaryngology Head and Neck Surgery*, 10th ed. New York, NY: McGraw-Hill; 2012:949–1056.
Wetmore RF, Potsic WP. Differential diagnosis of neck masses. In: Cummings CW, Fredrickson JM, Harker LA, et al. (eds.), *Otolaryngology Head & Neck Surgery: Pediatric*, 5th ed. St. Louis, MO: Mosby; 2010:2812–2821.

4. **(D)** The structures of the head and neck are derived from the branchial arches, grooves (clefts), or pharyngeal pouches. The arches are mesodermal, the grooves are ectodermal, and the pouches endodermal in origin. Much of the development of the arches occurs in the first 8 weeks of embryonic life. Each of the arches is associated with a nerve, artery, and bar of cartilage, whereas the pouches become glandular or are associated with the digestive tract. A cervical sinus develops where structures of each arch develop. Eventually the sinus is obliterated by the growth of the arch derivatives. When the sinus does not obliterate, a branchial arch anomaly exists. These anomalies come in three forms: a sinus, cyst, or fistula. The sinus has an opening in the mucosa of the foregut or skin and ends in the soft tissue of the neck. The fistula is a complete tract with an internal and external opening indicating persistence of both a groove and a pouch. The fistula can present as intermittent swelling or with drainage. The cyst is formed from remnants of the grooves or sinuses.

The path of the first arch anomaly starts at the external auditory canal and is divided into two types as described by Work. Type I is a duplication of the membranous canal alone and contains only ectodermal elements without cartilage or adnexa. It is found medial to the concha and may extend to the postauricular area, running superior to the facial nerve, the nerve for the second branchial arch. Type II is the more common type and involves duplication of both the membranous and cartilaginous external auditory canal and can be intimately associated with the facial nerve and have a tract at the level of the mandible. These first arch anomalies should be differentiated from the preauricular pits or cysts,

which are inclusion cysts from fusion of the auricular hillocks (which are derivatives of the first and second arch) during development of the pinna. Surgical excision is the treatment of choice, and if the parotid gland is involved with the tract, a superficial parotidectomy with facial nerve dissection may be required for complete removal.

The second branchial arch anomaly, which is the most common type of branchial arch defect, has a pathway that begins at the tonsillar bed and, if a complete fistulous tract, will open just anterior to the ipsilateral SCM (see Fig. 11-9). The tract passes between the internal and external carotid arteries and lies superficial to derivatives of the third arch. Second arch derivatives include all facial muscles, posterior belly of the digastric muscle, styloid muscle, and lesser cornu and body of the hyoid bone. These anomalies can be identified by ultrasound or contrast-enhanced CT or MRI. Surgical excision, usually via two stair step incisions, is the treatment of choice.

The third branchial arch anomaly has a tract that extends from the pyriform sinus, runs deep to the bifurcation of the carotid and cranial nerve IX but superficial to cranial nerve XII, and opens (if a fistula) in the skin of the lower neck anterior to the SCM. The fourth arch anomaly has a similar course but loops around the subclavian on the right and around the arch of the aorta on the left.

BIBLIOGRAPHY

Farrior JB, Lee KJ. Embryology of clefts and pouches. In: Lee KJ (ed.), *Essential Otolaryngology Head and Neck Surgery*, 10th ed. New York, NY: McGraw-Hill; 2012:269–284.
Graney DO, Sie KCY. Anatomy and developmental embryology of the neck. In: Cummings CW, Fredrickson JM, Harker LA, et al. (eds.), *Otolaryngology Head & Neck Surgery: Pediatric*, 5th ed. St. Louis, MO: Mosby; 2010:2577–2586.
Pincus RL. Congenital cysts and sinuses of the head and neck. In: Bailey BJ, Johnson JT, Newlands SD (eds.), *Head & Neck Surgery Otolaryngology*, 5th ed., vol. 1. Philadelphia, PA: Lippincott Williams & Wilkins; 2012:1607–1616.

5. **(B)** Patients with unknown primary carcinomas frequently present with an asymmetric neck mass, and up to two-thirds of the primaries are discovered on the initial examination. If the first examination fails to reveal a primary site, the examination should be repeated to concentrate on less visible areas of the upper aerodigestive tract. CT or T2-weighted MRI scans, direct laryngoscopy, and fine-needle aspiration (FNA) should also be considered. In cases where no primary is found, broad treatment of the neck with radiation, including possible neck dissection is the recommended treatment option (see Fig. 11-10).

There are several complications associated with neck dissections including infection, bleeding, chylous fistula, seroma, facial/cerebral edema, blindness, and carotid artery rupture.

The incidence of chyle leak as a complication in neck dissection is 1–2% of cases. The thoracic duct is located medial and inferior to a left common carotid artery and the vagus nerve. At this point, it arches upward, forward, and laterally, passing behind the internal jugular vein and in front of the anterior scalene muscle and the phrenic nerve. It then opens into the internal jugular vein at the level IV lymph node region.

To test for possible injury of the duct during surgery, positive airway pressure is required for greater than 30 seconds or more, and the operative field should be examined for milky or oily fluid in the region just lateral to the carotid sheath and internal jugular vein low in the neck (inferior aspect of level IV).

In the postoperative period, drains should be observed for any high-output or milky drainage. The presence of chylomicrons may not necessarily indicate a chylous fistula (or chyle leak). Normal triglyceride content of neck drainage is approximately 100 mg/dL. If the drain content is less than 600 mL/d, then conservative management should be started. Conservative treatment starts with continuous suction drainage, fluid replacement, head of bed elevation, and a low- or nonfat diet. If an oral diet does not decrease chylous output, further nutrition recommendations include medium-chain triglycerides, which are directly absorbed into the portal system and bypass the lymphatic system. This alone may obviate the need for total parenteral nutrition (TPN). Indications for surgical exploration would include output >600 mL/d because these fistulas do not respond to conservative measures. If a chyle leak progresses to the mediastinum, then it may cause a chylothorax that must be treated with a thoracotomy.

BIBLIOGRAPHY

Medina JE, Vasan NR. Neck dissection. In: Bailey BJ, Johnson JT, Newlands SD (eds.), *Head & Neck Surgery Otolaryngology*, 5th ed., vol. 2. Philadelphia, PA: Lippincott Williams & Wilkins; 2014:1807–1838.

Robbins KT, Samant S, Romen O. Neck dissection. In: Cummings CW, Fredrickson JM, Harker LA, et al. (eds.), *Otolaryngology Head & Neck Surgery*, 5th ed., vol. 2. St. Louis, MO: Mosby; 2010:1702–1725.

6. **(C)** Cancer of the larynx typically originates on the true vocal cord itself (in 75% of cases), and it is this location where it has the best prognosis. This particular cancer is staged as a T2 and we can assume N0

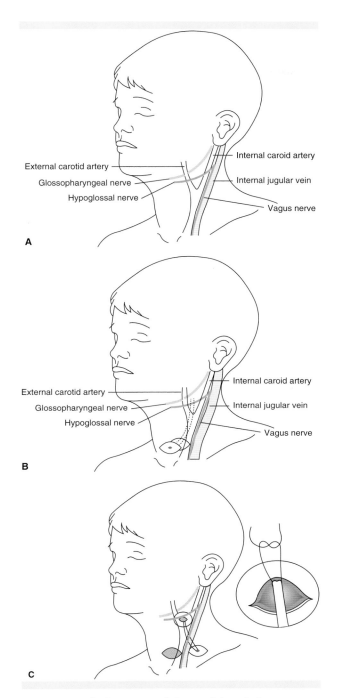

FIGURE 11-9. A. Anatomy of the neck in relation to a second branchial cleft fistula. **B.** The fistula opening is circumscribed by an incision. The tract is carefully dissected away from surrounding neck structures by staying on the fistula wall. The tract courses cephalad between the external and internal carotid arteries. A counter incision (*dotted line*) may be required to complete the dissection. **C.** The tract is ligated as it enters the pharynx (*inset*), and the incisions are closed in layers with absorbable sutures. From Azizkhan RG. *Head and Neck Lesions*. In: Ziegler MM, Azizkhan RG, Allmen D, Weber TR. eds. Operative Pediatric Surgery, Second Edition. New York, NY: McGraw-Hill; 2014.

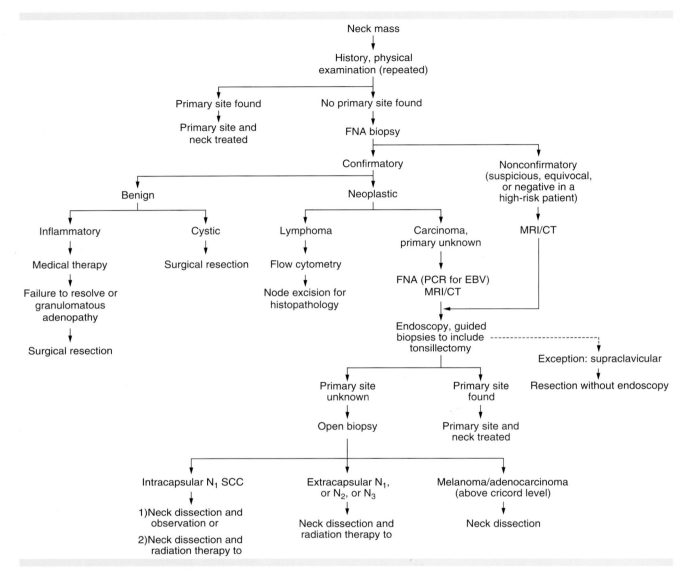

FIGURE 11-10. Algorithm for workup of an unknown primary. CT, computed tomography; EBV, Epstein-Barr virus; FNA, fine-needle aspiration; MRI, magnetic resonance imaging; PCR, polymerase chain reaction; SCC, squamous cell carcinoma. Reprinted from Cummings CW, Fredrickson JM, Harker LA, et al. *Otolaryngology–Head and Neck Surgery*, 3rd ed. St. Louis, MO: CV Mosby; 1998:1686–1699, copyright 1998, with permission from Elsevier.

(see Table 11-1). Early laryngeal carcinoma is usually treated with one modality, including radiation, transoral/endoscopic laser excision, or cold knife excision. Partial laryngectomies can also be considered; however, they are thought to be high in morbidity. Current treatment options include radiation, transoral/endoscopic laser excision or cold knife excision, or partial laryngeal surgeries. Historically, radiation therapy has been the treatment of choice for early glottic carcinoma because of the advantages of avoiding surgery and hospitalization and good voice quality; however, the voice never

returns completely to normal. Endoscopic laser excision/cordectomy as it has been refined is now showing evidence of equivalent cure rates and nearly equivalent voice preservation. Single modality cure with radiation is approximately 85% with radiation and 90–95% with surgical salvage. If a cancer recurs after radiation therapy, then radiation cannot be used again because the patient has likely been treated with the maximal lifetime dose of radiation.

Early glottic carcinoma is diagnosed by the physical symptoms and signs. The patient typically complains

TABLE 11-1 Staging for Malignant Laryngeal Disorders

Supraglottis	
T1	Tumor limited to one subsite of supraglottis
T2	Tumor involving more than one adjacent subsite of supraglottis, glottis, or region outside the supraglottis (vallecula, tongue base, medial wall of pyriform sinus)
T3	Tumor causes vocal cord fixation and/or invades preepiglottic space, postcricoid area Moderately advanced local disease
T4a	Tumor invades through thyroid cartilage, and/or invades tissues beyond the larynx Very advanced local disease
T4b	Tumor invades prevertebral space, encases carotid artery or invades mediastinal structures
Glottis	
T1	Tumor limited to vocal cord; may involve anterior or posterior commissure
T2	Tumor extends to supraglottis, glottis, and/or impaired vocal cord mobility
T3	Vocal cord fixation Moderately advanced local disease
T4a	Tumor invades through thyroid cartilage, and/or invades tissues beyond the larynx Very advanced local disease
T4b	Tumor invades prevertebral space, encases carotid artery or invades mediastinal structures
Subglottis	
T1	Tumor limited to the subglottis
T2	Tumor extends to vocal cord with normal or impaired mobility
T3	Vocal cord fixation Moderately advanced local disease
T4a	Tumor invades through cricoid or thyroid cartilage, and/or invades tissues beyond the larynx Very advanced local disease
T4b	Tumor invades prevertebral space, encases carotid artery or invades mediastinal structures
N0	No cervical lymph nodes positive
N1	Single ipsilateral lymph node ≤3 cm
N2a	Single ipsilateral lymph node >3 cm and ≤6 cm
N2b	Multiple ipsilateral lymph nodes, each ≤6 cm
N2c	Bilateral or contralateral lymph nodes, each ≤6 cm
N3	Single or multiple lymph nodes >6 cm
M0	No distant metastases
M1	Distant metastases present

Concus AP, Tran TN, Sanfilippo NJ, DeLacure MD. Chapter 31. Malignant Laryngeal Lesions. In: Lalwani AK. eds. CURRENT Diagnosis & Treatment in Otolaryngology—Head & Neck Surgery, 3e. New York, NY: McGraw-Hill; 2012.

of hoarseness and "globus" or a "lump in the throat" sensation. Some may even present with dysphagia. The history should be carefully sought for alcohol and tobacco abuse. The initial examination should involve careful listening of the acoustical features of the voice, assessment of swallowing and respiration during the examination, palpation, and careful inspection of the oral cavity, oropharynx, and hypopharynx by means of fiberoptic laryngoscopy. Careful palpation of the neck to rule out neck metastases is crucial. CT scan

Stage	Tumor	Nodes	Metastases
I	T1	N0	M0
II	T2	N0	M0
III	T3	N0	M0
	T1–3	N1	M0
IVA	T4a	N0–2	M0
	T1–4a	N0	M0
IVB	T4b	any N	M0
	any T	N3	M0
IVC	any T	any N	M1

is important to check for any soft tissue infiltration, although this is less of an issue with early glottic carcinoma. The final stage is direct laryngoscopy with biopsies and mapping of the lesion.

The anatomy of the glottis lends early glottic carcinomas a good prognosis. This is chiefly because the glottis proper has very few lymphatics, and cancers confined to the true vocal cords present with neck metastases in 5% of cases. When the mobility of the cord is affected, this implies invasion of the thyroarytenoid muscle and probable involvement of the paraglottic space; the tumor then has wide access to other subsets of the larynx (see Fig. 11-11).

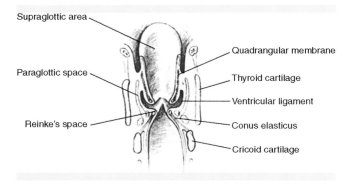

FIGURE 11-11. Coronal view of larynx demonstrating natural barriers to tumor spread, the quadrangular membrane, and conus elasticus. Reprinted from Lee KJ. *Essential Otolaryngology: Head and Neck Surgery*, 8th ed. New York, NY: McGraw-Hill; 2001; copyright 2003, with permission from McGraw-Hill.

BIBLIOGRAPHY

Beasley NJP, Gullane PJ. Cancer of the larynx, paranasal sinuses and temporal bone. In: Lee KJ (ed.), *Essential Otolaryngology*

Head and Neck Surgery, 8th ed. New York, NY: McGraw-Hill; 2010:596–616.

Sinha P, Okuyemi O, Haughey B. Early laryngeal cancer. In: Bailey BJ, Johnson JT, Newlands SD (eds.), *Head & Neck Surgery Otolaryngology*, 5th ed., vol. 2. Philadelphia, PA: Lippincott Williams & Wilkins; 2014:1940–1960.

Wippold FJ. Malignant tumors of the larynx. In: Cummings CW, Fredrickson JM, Harker LA, et al. (eds.), *Otolaryngology Head & Neck Surgery: Pediatric*, 5th ed. St. Louis, MO: Mosby; 2010:1462–1511.

7. **(E)** Young children make up the majority of patients suffering from foreign body aspiration: children under 3 account for between 70 and 80% of all foreign body aspirations.

The signs and symptoms of esophageal foreign body aspiration are dyspnea or airway distress, drooling, and dysphagia. The posterior wall between the anterior esophagus and posterior trachea is very compliant, and if a large foreign body is engaged here, it can compress the airway from behind. Any evidence of fever, tachycardia, tachypnea, and increasing pain should raise concern for esophageal perforation and possible mediastinal emphysema or retropharyngeal abscess. The most common area for an esophageal foreign body to lodge is at the level of the cricopharyngeus or at C6. If it lodges elsewhere, investigation for another anatomical disorder of the esophagus is warranted.

When an esophageal foreign body is suspected, it is important to obtain a radiologic evaluation (posterior to anterior [PA] and lateral chest x-rays) to assess location, size, and object. It is imperative to obtain a lateral airway and chest film to look for possible battery ingestion. Typically, small sharp objects pass spontaneously, and thus, this type of ingestion can be treated conservatively. An observation period of 8–16 hours is considered in an asymptomatic healthy child. Objects that require immediate removal include disc batteries or a patient presenting with airway symptoms. Disc batteries can cause esophageal perforation within 8–12 hours of ingestion, but if imaging reveals that it has passed into the stomach, these ingestions can be treated more conservatively. Coins less than 20 mm in diameter (dimes, pennies) can pass spontaneously. Other objects that are high risk for causing perforation are long straight pins, chicken and fish bones, and toothpicks.

BIBLIOGRAPHY

Friedman EM, Yunker WK. Ingestion injuries and foreign bodies in the aerodigestive tract. In: Bailey BJ, Johnson JT, Newlands SD (eds.), *Head & Neck Surgery Otolaryngology*, 5th ed., vol. 1. Philadelphia, PA: Lippincott Williams & Wilkins; 2014:1399–1408.

Holinger LD, Poznanovic, SA. Foreign bodies of the airway and esophagus. In: Cummings CW, Fredrickson JM, Harker LA, et al.

(eds.), *Otolaryngology Head & Neck Surgery: Pediatric*, 5th ed. St. Louis, MO: Mosby; 2010:2935–2943.

Robbins KT, Malone J. Carcinoma of the oral cavity, pharynx and esophagus. In: Lee KJ (ed.), *Essential Otolaryngology Head and Neck Surgery*, 10th ed. New York, NY: McGraw-Hill; 2012:695–723.

8. **(B)** External laryngeal trauma is diagnosed on the basis of history and physical findings. A patient who presents with evidence of anterior neck trauma should be assumed to have upper airway trauma. This compounded with subcutaneous emphysema, voice changes, and orthopnea should arouse suspicion for disruption of the larynx or trachea. As in any trauma situation, the "ABCs" come first: airway, breathing, and circulation. Although on fiberoptic examination, this patient had "mild edema," it is presumably early after the trauma and the entire injury may have not evolved. There is potential for worsening of the edema and bleeding in the next 8–12 hours. Therefore, an awake tracheostomy is the best option. The addition of general anesthesia in this situation may cause laryngospasm during induction and may cause complete airway obstruction. In addition, "clothesline" injuries are high risk for being associated with laryngotracheal separation. Any situation in which this is considered precludes oral or nasal intubation because intubation may worsen the existing damage or convert a partial laryngotracheal or cricotracheal separation into a complete separation.

Some external laryngeal trauma can be treated conservatively with medical management. Conditions include minor edema or hematomas with intact mucosa, single nondisplaced thyroid cartilage fractures, and small lacerations without exposed cartilage. Medical management would include elevation of the head of bed with bed rest to reduce edema. Corticosteroids are probably only beneficial in the early postinjury period, and antibiotics are used in the event of lacerations or mucosal tears as prophylaxis. Cool humidified air is important to prevent crust formation with tracheostomies and with mucosal tears. Voice rest is sometimes recommended to reduce edema or hematoma progression. Gastroesophageal reflux prevention is also important with either H2 blockers or proton pump inhibitors. Any patient not meeting the criteria for conservative management should proceed to surgery.

BIBLIOGRAPHY

Jordan JR, Norris BK, Stringer SP. Laryngeal trauma. In: Bailey BJ, Johnson JT, Newlands SD (eds.), *Head & Neck Surgery Otolaryngology*, 5th ed., vol. 1. Philadelphia, PA: Lippincott Williams & Wilkins; 2012:1141–1152.

Sandhu GS, Nouraei RS. Laryngeal and esophageal trauma. In: Cummings CW, Fredrickson JM, Harker LA, et al. (eds.), *Otolaryngology Head & Neck Surgery: Pediatric*, 5th ed. St. Louis, MO: Mosby; 2010:933–942.

9. **(D)** Penetrating parotid gland injuries have the potential to involve both Stensen's duct (parotid duct) and the facial nerve. Wounds occurring posterior to the anterior masseter muscle may injure the duct. These injuries can carry with them several sequelae including sialoceles, fistulas, and infections.

Parotid duct injuries should be considered in any deep laceration or penetrating injury of the cheek. They can be assessed by cannulating the papilla intraorally. It is also important to thoroughly examine the gland both visually and with palpation. Lacrimal probes and angiocatheters can be used to further manipulate the duct. If the duct is not readily found, the gland can be massaged to expel saliva and uncover the duct orifice. Inspection ideally should be done in the operating room.

Parenchymal injury can be treated conservatively by closing the capsule of the gland after thorough debridement. Pressure dressings may be applied to prevent saliva accumulation. If a swelling develops after injury, it can be aspirated and tested for amylase to prove parenchymal origin. A sialogram may be used in this instance as well. Persistent sialoceles or fistulas to the skin can be treated with tympanic neurectomy, total parotidectomy, atropine or repeated aspiration, Botox injection, or pressure dressings.

If the duct itself is transected, then it should be debrided at the ends and repaired under magnification with 7-0 or 8-0 monofilament suture over a 20- or 22-gauge silastic catheter or stent to prevent placing backwall sutures and to prevent stricture formation when left in place for up to 14 days. The catheter is either sutured to the orifice intraorally or brought out through the parenchyma externally. If the distal duct is injured significantly and there is adequate length of the proximal portion, this portion can be diverted to the buccal mucosa. Some surgeons have also employed vein grafts in this instance.

If an injury goes unnoticed and overlying tissue is repaired, significant inflammation within the wound can result in dehiscence, abscess formation, or parotitis. An injury should be considered with any increasing pain, erythema, or edema after a soft tissue repair.

BIBLIOGRAPHY

Hill JD, Hamilton GS. Facial trauma: soft tissue lacerations and burns. In: Cummings CW, Fredrickson JM, Harker LA, et al. (eds.), *Otolaryngology Head & Neck Surgery: Pediatric*, 5th ed. St. Louis, MO: Mosby; 2010:302–317.

Shemen LJ. Salivary glands: benign and malignant diseases. In: Lee KJ (ed.), *Essential Otolaryngology Head and Neck Surgery*, 10th ed. New York, NY: McGraw-Hill; 2010:535–565.

10. **(C)** This scenario describes a neck space infection with abscess. Most adult neck space infections are caused by odontogenic or salivary gland infections, although tonsillar and pharyngeal infections still account for the majority of pediatric neck space infections. Other etiologies include preexisting congenital anomalies (i.e., branchial cleft sinuses), trauma, upper respiratory tract infections, iatrogenic causes, or spread from a superficial infection.

    The patient in this question is exhibiting signs of a submandibular space infection that has progressed. Ludwig angina usually originates in the submandibular and sublingual space and then disseminates to the entire floor of mouth spaces by way of the posterior border of the mylohyoid to both bilateral submandibular and sublingual spaces and the submental space (see Fig. 11-12). The infections have the potential to spread quickly from one space to another and, if not treated appropriately, can rapidly progress to a gangrenous cellulitis with brawny induration involving bilateral sublingual,

submental (between anterior bellies of the digastric muscles and between the mylohyoid muscle and skin), and submandibular spaces. This infection does not spread through lymphatics, but rather direct involvement of fascial planes. The clinical presentation is marked by drooling, severe pain, trismus, dysphagia, and tongue swelling. Respiratory distress is a late finding and signals impending airway compromise. Airway obstruction happens quickly in these patients, and preemptive tracheostomy should be considered in all patients presenting with floor of mouth swelling.

The typical microorganisms involved are consistent with oral flora, such as *Peptostreptococcus*, *Streptococcus pyogenes*, *Fusobacterium*, as well as *Bacteroides melaninogenicus* and *S aureus*. Penicillin remains the drug of choice, but any antibiotic with a similar spectrum (i.e., clindamycin, first-generation cephalosporins) is usually adequate. Most neck space infections in the abscess stage require surgical drainage and antibiotics.

Vincent angina, also known as trench mouth, is an acute necrotizing ulcerative gingivitis secondary to a *Spirochaeta denticulate* and *Borrelia vincentii*. Patients present with high fevers, headaches, malodorous breath, drooling, and gingival bleeding.

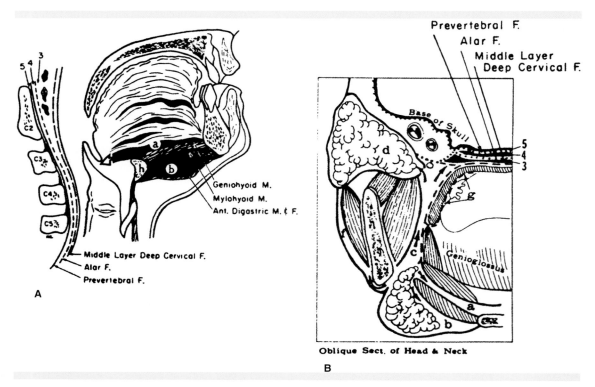

FIGURE 11-12. Anatomic relationships in Ludwig angina. Sagittal **A.** and oblique **B.** sections of head and neck: a, sublingual space; b, submylohyoid space; c, lateral pharyngeal space; d, parotid gland; e, masticator space; f, peritonsillar space; g, hyoid bone; 3, retropharyngeal space; 4, danger space; 5, prevertebral space. Reproduced with permission from Blomquist IK, Bayer AS: Life-threatening deep fascial space infections of the head and neck. *Infect Dis Clin North Am* 2:237, 1988.

A retropharyngeal abscess can also present with symptoms of dysphagia and odynophagia, snoring, noisy breathing, and cervical adenopathy, but airway obstruction is less common. Retropharyngeal infections are more common in children because lymph nodes (which are the typical source) regress or atrophy by the age of 4 or 5.

BIBLIOGRAPHY

Doerr TD. Odontogenic infections. In: Bailey BJ, Johnson JT, Newlands SD (eds.), *Head & Neck Surgery Otolaryngology*, 5th ed., vol. 1. Philadelphia, PA: Lippincott Williams & Wilkins; 2014:770–781.

Gillespie B. Neck spaces and fascial planes. In: Lee KJ (ed.), *Essential Otolaryngology*, 10th ed. New York, NY: McGraw-Hill; 2010:557–575.

11. **(C)** This characteristic is that of a Warthin tumor (aka, papillary cystadenoma lymphomatosum), the second most common type of benign neoplasm of the parotid gland. This tumor rarely is found in the other major or minor salivary glands. It represents approximately 6–10% of parotid gland tumors, and in 10% of cases, tumors are bilateral. Several epidemiologic characteristics are singular to a Warthin tumor. It is commonly found in men between the fourth and seventh decades of life; however, the incidence has increased in women. It is more common in smokers and can be multifocal. The tumor may arise from either heterotopic salivary duct tissue or from glandular inclusions within lymph nodes. This is thought to be because the parotid, although the first salivary gland to develop, is the last to be encapsulated and incorporates lymphoid tissue. Papillary fronds with a double layer of oncocytic cells are seen, with the inner layer of cells having nuclei that face the basement membrane. These cells have a high density of mitochondria. Copious lymphoid tissue is associated with the tumor, and is at the center of the papillary fronds. There are usually multiple cystic components as well that contain a brown mucinous material. On occasion, metaplastic squamous epithelium may be found, which could lead to a misdiagnosis of squamous cell carcinoma (SCC) on fine needle aspiration (FNA). The treatment of choice for Warthin tumors is surgical excision.

The most common benign neoplasm of the salivary glands is the pleomorphic adenoma, also known as benign mixed tumor, which arises from the intercalated duct cells and myoepithelial cells. This lesion contains both connective tissue and epithelial elements. These tumors are most commonly found in the parotid gland, followed by the submandibular gland and the minor salivary glands. When found in the parotid gland, 90% are superficial to the facial nerve. Microscopically, spindle and stellate cells in a myxoid stroma are seen, and frequently these tumors have fine

extensions throughout the capsule of the gland; recurrence is common if only an enucleation rather than a complete superficial parotidectomy is performed. These can degenerate into the carcinoma ex pleomorphic adenoma in up to 25% of cases if the tumor has been present for several years.

BIBLIOGRAPHY

Calzada GG, Hanna EY. Benign neoplasms of the salivary glands. In: Cummings CW, Fredrickson JM, Harker LA, et al. (eds.), *Otolaryngology Head & Neck Surgery: Pediatric*, 5th ed. St. Louis, MO: Mosby; 2010:1163–1177.

Witt R. Salivary glands diseases. In: Lee KJ (ed.), *Essential Otolaryngology Head and Neck Surgery*, 10th ed. New York, NY: McGraw-Hill; 2012:488–505.

12. **(C)** The nasal bone is the most frequently fractured facial bone. A history of trauma to the nose with epistaxis should raise concern for a nasal fracture. Diagnosis relies heavily on the physical examination, and signs of crepitus of the nasal cartilaginous and bony framework and obvious external deformity are pathognomic. X-rays have not been shown to be helpful in adding to diagnostic accuracy. In nearly 50% of cases, nasal x-rays may not reveal a fracture when one is actually present. A careful rhinoscopic examination should be performed because there are few injuries and/or complications associated with nasal trauma to the nose that require immediate repair or attention. A septal hematoma presents with nasal airway obstruction, usually bilaterally. Less often do patients with a septal hematoma present with epistaxis. Septal hematoma is one of the most severe early complication of trauma to the nose (see Fig. 11-13).

The hematoma develops in the plane between the perichondrium of the septal cartilage and the cartilage itself. As the cartilage receives its blood supply from the perichondrium, the hematoma causes ischemic injury and eventually degeneration of the cartilaginous septum. A devastating cosmetic and functional consequence of this is the "saddle nose" deformity. Another complication is a septal abscess, usually caused by *S aureus* 6–7 days after trauma. This can lead to cavernous sinus thrombosis because of valveless veins of the so-called "danger triangle" of the face (bounded by the superior most aspect of the nasal dorsum and the lateral edges of the lips). If septal hematoma is found early, then it can be aspirated with a 25-gauge needle. If left for longer, then bilateral incisions called Killian incisions can be done. These are performed at the 1-cm caudal end of the septum. These should be staggered to prevent septal perforation. Nasal packing or splints are placed to avoid reaccumulation of blood.

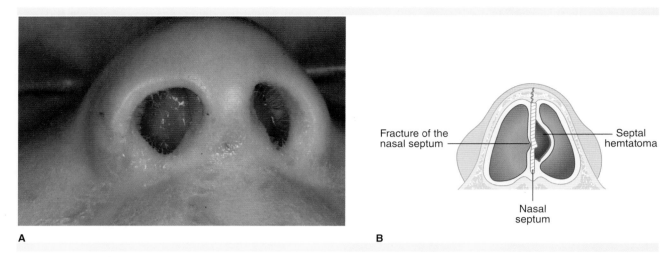

FIGURE 11-13. **A and B.** Septal hematoma. **A.** From Knoop KJ, Stack LB, Storrow AB, Thurman RJ. *The Atlas of Emergency Medicine*, 3rd ed. New York, NY: McGraw-Hill; 2009:Fig. 5-40. **B.** From Knoop KJ, Stack LB, Storrow AB, Thurman RJ. *The Atlas of Emergency Medicine*, 3rd ed. New York, NY: McGraw-Hill; 2009.

BIBLIOGRAPHY

Chan Y. The nose, acute and chronic sinusitis. In: Lee KJ (ed.), *Essential Otolaryngology Head and Neck Surgery*, 10th ed. New York, NY: McGraw-Hill; 2012:397–415.

Chegar BE, Tatum SA. Nasal fractures. In: Cummings CW, Fredrickson JM, Harker LA, et al. (eds.), *Otolaryngology Head & Neck Surgery: Pediatric*, 5th ed. St. Louis, MO: Mosby; 2010:496–507.

13. **(A)** About 3% of patients with acute rhinosinusitis have orbital manifestations, and complicated rhinosinusitis is the most common cause of orbital infection. Infections spread by direct extension and thrombophlebitis of ethmoidal veins. The ethmoid is the most commonly involved sinus because of its proximity to the eye. Patients with changes in visual acuity require immediate operative intervention, because complications can lead to blindness. Other complications may include neurologic infections: subdural and epidural abscesses and meningitis. In cases of ethmoid sinusitis, decompressing the infection or abscess if present, can be performed via the lamina papyracea, the medial wall of the orbit (see Fig. 11-14).

Orbital complications are classified by the Chandler classification system. Stage I is simply inflammatory edema or preseptal cellulitis (orbital septum of the eyelid) of the lids. Extraocular muscles are not involved. Stage II indicates orbital cellulitis with edema of the contents of the orbit. The first two stages should be aggressively treated with intravenous antibiotics against *S pneumoniae* and *H influenzae* to prevent progression to stage III. Stage III is a subperiosteal abscess that is beneath the periosteum of the lamina papyracea; the globe is displaced inferolaterally, and vision is affected. Stage IV is an orbital abscess that is accompanied by ptosis, chemosis, and ophthalmoplegia with visual loss. Stage V, cavernous sinus thrombosis, is the most severe. This stage can be fatal if not treated aggressively and is seen with bilateral eye findings and meningitis. Aside from intravenous antibiotics and drainage of the abscess, some physicians choose to heparinize to minimize thrombosis, although there is conflicting evidence of benefit. Later stages (III–V) are associated with

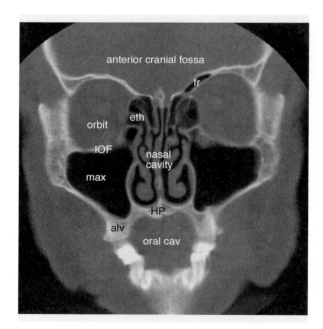

FIGURE 11-14. Coronal computed tomography of face. From Lalwani A. *Current Diagnosis & Treatment Otolaryngology–Head and Neck Surgery*, 3rd ed. New York, NY: McGraw-Hill; 2011:Fig. 3-96.

polymicrobial infections including streptococci, staphylococci, *H influenzae*, and the anaerobes *Bacteroides*, *Peptostreptococcus*, and/or *Fusobacterium*.

Orbital complications are typically treated with an external approach rather than an endoscopic approach, although the trend is changing. Because the ethmoid sinuses are the most frequently involved, at minimum, an endoscopic sinus surgery to remove a portion of the lamina papyracea to allow for abscess drainage is performed.

BIBLIOGRAPHY

Giannoni CM. Complications of rhinosinusitis. In: Cummings CW, Fredrickson JM, Harker LA, et al. (eds.), *Otolaryngology Head & Neck Surgery: Pediatric*, 5th ed. St. Louis, MO: Mosby; 2010:573–585.

14. **(C)** There are three horizontal zones in the neck that are used to describe penetrating neck injuries. Zone I comprises the root of the neck to the inferior border of the cricoid cartilage. This represents a dangerous area due to the vascular structures in close proximity to the thorax. This zone has a mortality rate of 12%. Zone II is the most exposed and the largest zone in surface area, extending from the inferior cricoid border to the angle of the mandible. It is the most common zone to be injured; however, mandatory exploration is not usually recommended, because angiography is suggested to ensure integrity of great vessels. Zone III begins at the angle of the mandible and extends to the base of the skull.

Signs of significant vascular injury include shock, hematoma or hemorrhage, pulse and neurologic deficits, and bruits or thrills in the neck. Arterial injury most often involves the carotid artery, followed by the subclavian artery. The patient in this case study has had a negative angiography, ruling out vascular injury.

Signs of laryngotracheal injury include hemoptysis, subcutaneous emphysema, dyspnea, stridor, and hoarseness depending on the exact location of the injury. Esophageal or pharyngeal injury is associated with dysphagia or odynophagia, subcutaneous emphysema, and possibly hematemesis.

A posterior tracheal wall injury should be sought because delay in diagnosis could result in a tracheoesophageal (TEP) fistula. Other complications of penetrating neck trauma include airway obstruction, neck abscess, mediastinitis, vocal cord paresis or paralysis, and cervical spine osteomyelitis.

BIBLIOGRAPHY

Hom DM, Maisel RH. Penetrating and blunt trauma to the neck. In: Cummings CW, Fredrickson JM, Harker LA, et al. (eds.), *Otolaryngology Head & Neck Surgery*, 3rd ed., vol. 2. St. Louis, MO: Mosby; 2010:1625–1635.

Stewart M. Penetrating face and neck trauma. In: Bailey BJ, Johnson JT, Newlands SD (eds.), *Head & Neck Surgery Otolaryngology*, 5th ed., vol. 1. Philadelphia, PA: Lippincott Williams & Wilkins; 2014:1131–1152.

15. **(E)** Temporal bone fractures are usually associated with blunt or closed head injury. Motor vehicle accidents rank first in causes, whereas smaller numbers are caused by falls and sports-related injury. These fractures are diagnosed by physical findings, but fine-cut (1-mm) CT scans and/or MRIs are essential to evaluate for facial nerve involvement.

Temporal bone fractures are divided into three types (see Fig. 11-15). Seventy to 90% are longitudinal fractures, named according to their plane relative to the petrous apex. These extend to the region of the foramina lacerum and ovale and pass through the external auditory canal. Longitudinal fractures are frequently associated with conductive hearing loss, either because of tympanic membrane trauma, hemotympanum, or direct

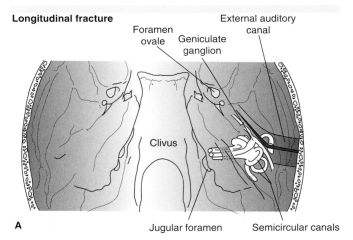

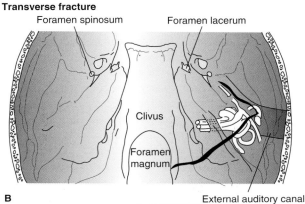

FIGURE 11-15. Temporal bone fracture types. From Lalwani A. *Current Diagnosis & Treatment Otolaryngology–Head and Neck Surgery*, 3rd ed. New York, NY: McGraw-Hill; 2011:Fig. 59-1.

ossicular disruption. Bleeding is also seen from the ear canal. CSF otorrhea is possible if a fracture involves the tegmen tympani, which is the roof of the middle ear and mastoid. Facial paralysis is seen in 10–20% of cases due to the proximity of the fracture line to the perigeniculate region of the facial nerve.

Transverse temporal bone fractures are most commonly due to severe occipital injuries. Because of their perpendicular course relative to the petrous apex, these fractures involve the bony labyrinth and can cause profound sensorineural hearing loss with vertigo. Transverse fractures are associated with facial nerve injury in 50% of cases, as the labyrinthine segment of the facial nerve can be injured. CSF otorrhea and meningitis are frequently seen in patients with these fractures.

Patients with delayed paralysis following normal function at the time of injury have the best prognosis. These patients can be observed, and function should return in 6 months to a year. Proper eye care is important with artificial tears or moisture chambers. Steroids may be helpful in the acute situation. Patients with obvious bony disruption of the facial canal on CT scan (defined as a diastasis in the facial canal of 1 mm or greater or a spicule of bone in the canal) with immediate paralysis and facial nerve injuries associated with CSF otorrhea are at greatest risk for permanent nerve paralysis.

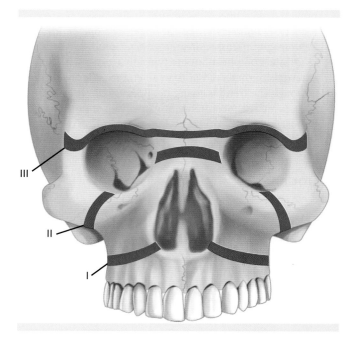

FIGURE 11-16. LeFort classification system. From Brunicardi F, Andersen DK, Billiar TR, et al. (eds.). *Schwartz's Principles of Surgery*, 10th ed. New York, NY: McGraw-Hill; 2014.

BIBLIOGRAPHY

Brodie HA. Management of temporal bone trauma. In: Cummings CW, Fredrickson JM, Harker LA, et al. (eds.), *Otolaryngology Head & Neck Surgery: Pediatric*, 5th ed. St. Louis, MO: Mosby; 2010:2036–2048.

Diaz RC, Kamal SM, Brodie HA. Middle ear and temporal bone trauma. In: Bailey BJ, Johnson JT, Newlands SD (eds.), *Head & Neck Surgery Otolaryngology*, 5th ed., vol. 2. Philadelphia, PA: Lippincott Williams & Wilkins; 2014:2410–2432.

16. **(E)** Midface fractures in adults and children can be classified by the LeFort system (see Fig. 11-16). The vertical buttresses of the face are the nasomaxillary, zygomaticomaxillary, and pterygomaxillary bony buttresses. These are important in maintenance of the vertical height of the face and must withstand the strong vertical masticatory forces. The horizontal buttresses of the face are important in facial width maintenance and bridging the vertical buttresses together but are weaker than the vertical buttresses. These components include the inferior orbital rims, greater wing of sphenoid, medial and lateral pterygoid plates, zygomatic process of the temporal bone, and the maxillary alveolus and palate. In most cases, LeFort and midface fractures in general are caused by anterior impact forces.

A LeFort I fracture (horizontal maxillary fracture) indicates separation of the palate from the rest of the maxilla. The fracture line extends through the pterygoid plates, maxillary sinus, and floor of the nose/pyriform aperture. A floating or mobile palate is a sign of this fracture and is demonstrated by being able to pull the entire palate forward while stabilizing the forehead with the other hand. A LeFort II fracture (pyramidal dysjunction) occurs when the palate and nose are separated from the cranium and the fracture line extends through the pterygoid plates, lateral and anterior maxillary walls, inferior orbital rims, medial orbital wall (lamina papyracea), nasofrontal suture, and bony septum. The palate-nose complex is then mobile with respect to the rest of the face. A LeFort III fracture (complete craniofacial dysjunction) occurs at the level of the skull base, separating the zygomas from the temporal bones and frontal bones, crossing the lateral orbits and medial orbits, and reaching the midline at the nasofrontal junction. This fracture also violates the nasal septum and pterygoid plates.

BIBLIOGRAPHY

Kellman RM. Maxillofacial trauma. In: Cummings CW, Fredrickson JM, Harker LA, et al. (eds.), *Otolaryngology Head & Neck Surgery: Pediatric*, 5th ed. St. Louis, MO: Mosby; 2010:318–341.

17. **(C)** Epistaxis, or nosebleed, is one of the most common ear, nose, and throat emergencies, affecting up to

60% of individuals in their lifetimes, with 6% requiring medical care. Terminal branches of the external and internal carotid arteries supply nasal cavity mucosa. Epistaxis more commonly occurs in older individuals because of vessel wall aging with fibrosis and slower vasoconstriction and in the winter months because of cold, dry air exposure. Other risk factors include trauma (nose picking, most common in children), nasal sprays intranasal or sinus tumors, allergies, medications such as antiplatelet agents and anticoagulants, and anatomic deformities such as septal deviation. Systemic factors and diseases putting patients at epistaxis risk include hypertension, hereditary hemorrhagic telangiectasia (Osler-Weber-Rendu disease, an autosomal dominant disease with associated mucosal telangiectasias and pulmonary arteriovenous malformations), von Willebrand disease, hemophilia, nutritional deficiencies, alcohol abuse with associated hepatic disease, and lymphoreticular disorders or malignancies.

The initial assessment of a patient with epistaxis should focus on the amount of blood loss over what period of time should be assessed. Special attention should be given to the patient with coronary ischemia history and a low hematocrit. One must then determine from which side the bleeding originates and whether the bleeding is anterior or posterior (see Fig. 11-17). Endoscopy is the procedure of choice, but visualization is difficult with profuse bleeding.

There are different treatment options for epistaxis including topical treatment, cautery, nasal packing, maxillary artery ligation, endoscopic sphenopalatine artery ligation, ligation of the external carotid artery, and ligation of the anterior ethmoidal artery, and embolization.

An anterior bleed is treated with an anterior pack, which traditionally is a 6-foot piece of Vaseline-impregnated strip gauze, which is the most secure. An antibacterial ointment is used to cover the gauze, and if this controls the bleeding, the patient is discharged with pain medication and antibiotic prophylaxis against *S aureus* and sinus pathogens, with instructions to return in 3–5 days for pack removal. Other methods of anterior packing are with expandable sponges, microfibrillar collagen slurries, or absorbable cellulose fiber packings. Small-volume bleeds with obvious focal sources can be treated with silver nitrate chemical cauterization. The two reasons an anterior pack fails are inadequate packing and a posterior bleed.

Posterior nasal packing can result in significant morbidity when compared to anterior nasal packing. The traditional pack employed a Foley balloon catheter to tamponade posterior bleeding with an anterior gauze pack. There are now double balloon devices to serve the same purpose. These packs are left in place for days as well; however, patients must be admitted, typically to a

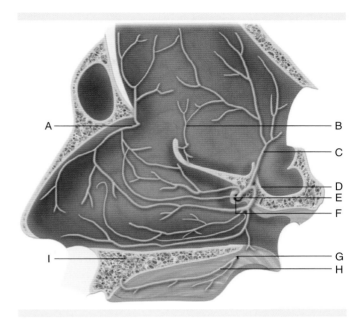

FIGURE 11-17. Nasal blood supply. Major nasal blood vessels and their relative positions are depicted. Note that the nasal septum has been reflected superiorly. A, anterior ethmoidal artery; B, posterior ethmoidal artery; C, posterior septal nasal artery; D, lateral nasal artery; E, sphenopalatine artery; F, sphenopalatine foramen; G, greater palatine foramen; H, greater palatine artery; I, incisive canal. Reprinted from Gates GA. *Current therapy in Otolaryngology—Head and Neck Surgery*, 6th ed. St. Louis, MO: Mosby; 1998; copyright 1998, with permission from Elsevier.

monitored floor, for observation. Pain control is crucial to avoid blood pressure fluctuations. Pack insertion complications include nasovagal reflexes (reflex bradycardia), hypovolemic shock, topical anesthetic, and vasoconstrictor complications.

Surgical management of nosebleeds is usually reserved for patients whose bleeding is refractory to conservative modalities, who have chronic epistaxis, or who have sustained a life-threatening amount of blood loss. The goal of surgical intervention is to ligate the offending arterial source while not disturbing surrounding structures and to preserve nasal function. Transnasal endoscopic sphenopalatine artery ligation has become an immediate surgical option for refractory posterior nosebleeds and may be considered an alternative therapy to packing.

BIBLIOGRAPHY

Bleier BS, Schlosser RJ. Epistaxis. In: Bailey BJ, Johnson JT, Newlands SD (eds.), *Head & Neck Surgery Otolaryngology*, 5th ed., vol. 2. Philadelphia, PA: Lippincott Williams & Wilkins; 2014:501–508.

Randall DA. The nose and paranasal sinuses. In: Lee KJ (ed.), *Essential Otolaryngology Head and Neck Surgery*, 8th ed. New York, NY: McGraw-Hill; 2003:682–723.

Simmen DB, Jones NS. Epistaxis. In: Cummings CW, Frederickson JM, Harker LA, et al. (eds.), *Otolaryngology Head & Neck Surgery: Pediatric*, 5th ed. St. Louis, MO: Mosby; 2010:682–693.

18. **(C)** Tracheotomies are performed to provide temporary openings in the trachea for longer term ventilation. Tracheostomies, on the other hand, are the permanent counterpart to the tracheotomy, because of the creation of a skin-lined tract to the trachea. Indications for tracheostomy include relief of upper airway obstruction (acute and chronic), prolonged mechanical ventilation, and enabling for more tracheobronchial toilet.

Elective tracheotomies are performed in the operating room, and the patient's head is hyperextended with use of a shoulder roll (if there are no contraindications to hyperextension). A horizontal incision is made approximately 3–5 cm long midway between the cricoid and the sternal notch through the platysma. When strap muscles are seen, they are divided in the midline vertically, and the thyroid isthmus is

encountered and either retracted upward or divided sharply via electrocautery. A cricoid hook is used to retract the entire framework of the inferior cricoid upward while the pretracheal fascia is bluntly dissected away. At this point, there are variations. Some surgeons remove a cartilage window at the second or third cartilage ring, but a large proportion still use the Bjork flap described first in 1960. The Bjork flap is an inferiorly based flap of the anterior portion of a single ring sutured to the inferior skin margin. It is designed for ease of tube insertion especially in the event the patient is accidentally decannulated so that no false passages are created.

Complications are divided into intraoperative, immediate postoperative, and late postoperative. Intraoperative complications include hemorrhage, pneumothorax, pneumomediastinum, fire, intraoperative tracheoesophageal fistula, and postobstructive pulmonary edema. Immediate postoperative complications include tube obstruction, displaced tracheostomy tube, postoperative hemorrhage, wound infection, and subcutaneous emphysema. Late postoperative complications include granulation tissue, tracheoesophageal fistula, tracheoinnominate

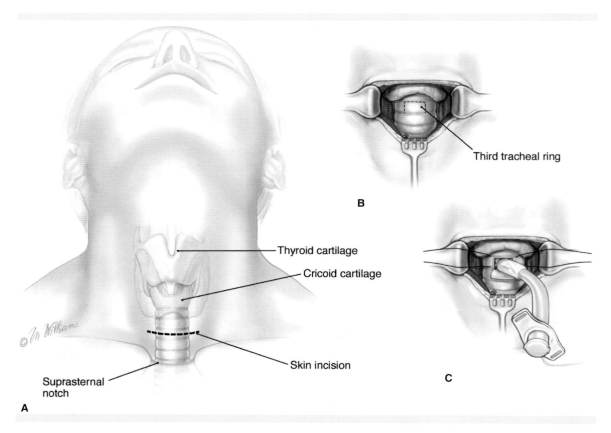

FIGURE 11-18. Tracheostomy. From Sugarbaker D, Bueno R, Krasna M, Mentzer S. *Adult Chest Surgery*. New York, NY: McGraw-Hill; 2009:Fig. 45-1.

fistula, tracheal stenosis, tracheomalacia, tracheocutaneous fistula, and depressed scar.

Tracheoinnominate fistula is most often seen 2–3 weeks after tracheostomy, and results from either low placement of the tracheostomy (below the fourth tracheal ring) or hyperinflation of the tracheal cuff. It can also occur in the setting of an aberrant or abnormally high innominate artery, use of an excessive long or curved tube that can erode through the trachea into the vessel wall, prolonged pressure on the tracheal wall by an inflated cuff, or a tracheal infection.

A tracheoinnominate fistula should be considered if a patient with a tracheostomy tube is having bright red pulsatile blood from the tracheostomy site. Patients commonly experience a minor "sentinel" bleed prior to the massive hemorrhage that occurs if the diagnosis is delayed. Diagnosis of tracheoinnominate fistula is best done by bronchoscopy through the mouth, CT scan of the neck, or direct examination in the operating room.

There are several methods of temporizing an actively bleeding tracheoinnominate fistula (see Fig. 11-19). If the fistula is secondary to cuff erosion, hyperinflation of the tracheal cuff will occlude the arterial injury. If the fistula is the result of cannula erosion, orotracheal intubation followed by removal of the tracheal cannula and insertion of a digit into the stoma to apply manual pressure against the sternum will tamponade the arterial injury. In some cases, the tracheostomy may require further opening to allow for passage of a finger. In either case, operative repair of the tracheoinnominate fistula is required immediately and is most commonly accomplished by resection of the involved segment of the innominate artery, with or without reconstruction. Endovascular stenting of the innominate artery has also been described.

BIBLIOGRAPHY

Kost KM. Advanced airway management—intubation and tracheotomy. In: Bailey BJ, Johnson JT, Newlands SD (eds.), *Head & Neck Surgery Otolaryngology*, 5th ed., vol. 3. Philadelphia, PA: Lippincott Williams & Wilkins; 2014:908–944.

19. **(E)** Lip cancer is one of the most common malignant tumors of the head and neck, with an incidence of approximately 2 per 100,000. It is disproportionately found in the lower lip as compared to the upper lip because the upper lip tends to be shaded from actinic exposure. The most common histologic subtype involving the lower lip is squamous cell carcinoma (SCC), whereas in the skin of the upper lip, basal cell carcinoma (BCC) is the most common type. The typical patient with lip cancer is a male who is 50–70 years of age. Risk factors include fair complexion, immunosuppression, tobacco use, and exposure to sunlight. These patients usually present with an ulcerated lesion on the vermillion or cutaneous surface, or least likely on the mucosal surface. Differential diagnosis for a lip lesion includes keratoacanthoma, minor salivary gland tumors, malignant melanoma, and tumors of the mesenchymal origin.

For early-stage lesions (small T2 and T1), both surgery and radiation are equally effective; however, surgical excision with negative margins is the preferred treatment. Five-year survival rates are about 90%. Advantages of surgery are rapidity of treatment, histologic evaluation, better overall cure in advanced lesions, and avoidance of radiation-induced morbidity to surrounding structures. The disadvantage is that surgery is invasive as compared to radiation, and cosmesis can be an issue with certain excisions. Radiation is delivered by brachytherapy implants or external-beam radiation via orthovoltage photon or electron beams. Radiation is low risk and is appropriate in patients who are poor surgical candidates. However, it takes an extended period of time to complete, and surrounding tissues are subjected to radiation damage.

Surgical options include full-thickness excision in the shape of a V, W, or rectangle to help with closure. Superficial carcinomas can be excised with Mohs micrographic excision. An 8- to 10-mm minimum normal tissue margin should be taken with the lesion. Marginal mandibulectomy (single cortex) may need to be incorporated in lesions encroaching the alveolar ridge or outer mandibular cortex, and segmental mandibulectomy is needed for tumors invading the mandible. Elective neck dissection is only recommended in recurrent or advanced-stage tumors or high-grade tumors. Lymph node basins that require removal are the intraparotid, submandibular, and submental lymph nodes for cancer of the upper lip. Submental and bilateral submandibular lymph nodes in those with carcinoma of the lower lip involving the central one-third of the lip as well as the upper jugular group of lymph nodes should be removed (see Fig. 11-20). There is controversy as to whether modified or selective neck dissections should be performed. Combined surgery and adjuvant radiation are required in advance local disease as in the case of T4 lesions or those with positive lymph nodes after neck dissection.

BIBLIOGRAPHY

Puscas L, Fritz MA, Esclamado RM. Lip cancer. In: Bailey BJ, Johnson JT, Newlands SD (eds.), *Head & Neck Surgery Otolaryngology*, 5th ed., vol. 2. Philadelphia, PA: Lippincott Williams & Wilkins; 2014:1788–1805.

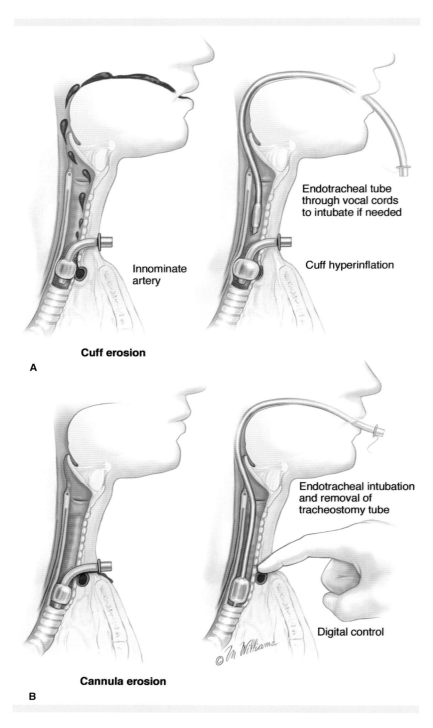

Endotracheal tube
through vocal cords
to intubate if needed

Cuff hyperinflation

Innominate
artery

Cuff erosion

A

Endotracheal intubation
and removal of
tracheostomy tube

Digital control

Cannula erosion

B

FIGURE 11-19. Interventions for tracheoinomminate fistula. From Sugarbaker D, Bueno R, Krasna M, Mentzer S. *Adult Chest Surgery*. New York, NY: McGraw-Hill; 2009:Fig. 54-2.

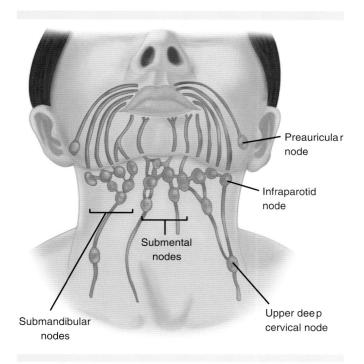

FIGURE 11-20. Lymphatics of the lip. From Brunicardi F, Andersen DK, Billiar TR, et al. (eds.), *Schwartz's Principles of Surgery*, 10th ed. New York, NY: McGraw-Hill; 2014:Fig. 18-20.

Wein RO, Malone JP, Weber RS. Malignant neoplasms of the oral cavity. In: Cummings CW, Fredrickson JM, Harker LA, et al. (eds.), *Otolaryngology Head & Neck Surgery: Pediatric*, 5th ed. St. Louis, MO: Mosby; 2010:1291–1318.

20. **(A)** There are several reconstructive options for a pharyngolaryngectomy defect, but the appropriate choice depends on the size of the defect and tissues involved. The options available are free tissue transfer with a jejunal autograft, colon interposition, anterolateral thigh flap (ALT), a radial forearm fasciocutaneous flap, a pectoralis major myocutaneous flap, and a gastric pull-up procedure. In this patient, the gastric pull-up would be the procedure of choice because the defect and lesion involve the thoracic esophagus. It is also a useful procedure if a total esophagectomy is required for skip lesions in the esophagus (see Figs. 11-21 and 11-22).

The chief advantage of the gastric pull-up is the need for a single anastomosis as opposed to multiple anastomoses. With a single anastomosis, there is less opportunity for stricture or fistula formation. The stomach is elevated up through the posterior mediastinum without the need for a thoracotomy by using blunt dissection. The stomach relies then on vascularity from the right

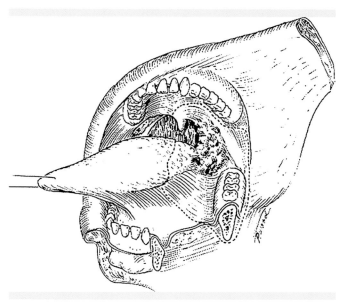

FIGURE 11-21. Gastric pull-up. From Cummings CW, Fredrickson JM, Harker LA, et al. *Otolaryngology–Head and Neck Surgery*, 3rd ed. St. Louis, MO: CV Mosby; 1998; copyright 1998, with permission from Elsevier.

gastric and gastroepiploic vessels, while the left gastric, short gastrics, and left gastroepiploic origins are divided. A Kocher maneuver is used to mobilize the duodenum, which allows for anastomosis as high as the nasopharynx if needed, and vagotomy and pyloroplasty are performed to help with gastric emptying. A jejunostomy tube is used for postoperative decompression. The gastric fundus is opened for the pharyngeal anastomosis. There is

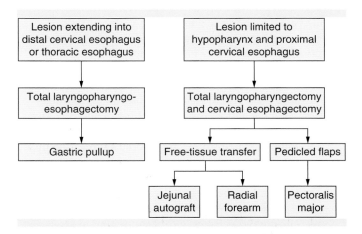

FIGURE 11-22. Reconstructive options for cervical esophagectomy and laryngopharyngectomy defects. Cummings CW, Fredrickson JM, Harker LA, et al. *Otolaryngology–Head and Neck Surgery*, 3rd ed. St. Louis, MO: CV Mosby; 1998; copyright 1998, with permission from Elsevier.

a 5–15% mortality rate with gastric pull-up. The most likely complication of this procedure is pneumothorax or hemothorax because of the mediastinal dissection. This can be treated with a chest tube. There are several potential long-term GI side effects, including emesis, early satiety, and dumping and regurgitation of bile and/or food.

BIBLIOGRAPHY

Bhayani MK, Weber RS. Hypopharyngeal and cervical esophageal cancer. In: Bailey BJ, Johnson JT, Newlands SD (eds.), *Head & Neck Surgery Otolaryngology*, 5th ed., vol. 2. Philadelphia, PA: Lippincott Williams & Wilkins; 2014:1917–1939.

Chepeha DB. Reconstruction of the hypopharynx and cervical esophagus. In: Cummings CW, Fredrickson JM, Harker LA, et al. (eds.), *Otolaryngology Head & Neck Surgery: Pediatric*, 5th ed. St. Louis, MO: Mosby; 2010:1448–1461.

21. **(A)** This case is typical of acute bacterial parotitis or sialadenitis. This usually occurs in individuals with dehydration from any cause. *S aureus* is the most common cultured organism responsible for these infections, which is seen in up to 90% of cases. *S pyogenes*, *S viridans*, *S pneumoniae*, and *H influenzae* can be seen in community-acquired cases. The anaerobic bacteria most commonly cultured were *Peptostreptococcus*, *Bacteroides* species, *Prevotella* species, and *Fusobacterium*. *B pseudomallei* is a common cause in Southeast Asia.

The pathophysiology of acute parotitis is retrograde bacterial infection through Stensen's duct. Mucoid saliva, which has a high-molecular-weight glycoprotein and sialic acid, has superior bacteriostatic activity because of the ability to trap bacteria. Mucoid saliva also has a higher lysozyme and IgA concentration. because the parotid expresses predominantly serous saliva, it is at a relative disadvantage compared to the other salivary glands. Salivary stasis can occur with decreased production, ductal stricture, or calculi (stones). Poor oral hygiene also contributes to infection. When a patient is NPO (nothing by mouth), stimulation of salivary flow by mastication is not possible, and food itself helps prevent bacterial aggregation by a detergent-like action.

The treatment of parotitis is both local and systemic. The patient must be adequately hydrated, and if applicable, good oral hygiene measures should be observed. Warm compresses are used for comfort and to assist with drainage of pus from the duct. Sialagogues (lemon drops or lemons) can be used to assist in stimulation of salivary flow. The most important arm of treatment is intravenous antibiotics preferably with antipenicillinase properties. An improvement should be seen within 24–48 hours, and if not, then imaging with CT scan or ultrasound should be considered to look for an abscess. An algorithm for evaluation and treatment of salivary gland inflammation is given in Fig. 11-23.

BIBLIOGRAPHY

Rogers J, McCaffrey TV. Inflammatory disorders of the salivary glands. In: Cummings CW, Fredrickson JM, Harker LA, et al. (eds.), *Otolaryngology Head & Neck Surgery: Pediatric*, 5th ed. St. Louis, MO: Mosby; 2010:1151–1161.

Walvekar RR, Bowen MA. Nonneoplastic diseases of the salivary glands. In: Bailey BJ, Johnson JT, Newlands SD (eds.), *Head & Neck Surgery Otolaryngology*, 5th ed., vol. 1. Philadelphia, PA: Lippincott Williams & Wilkins; 2014:703–715.

22. **(D)** The pectoralis major myocutaneous flap is the most frequently used axial flap used in head and neck reconstruction. It is very well vascularized by perforating branches of the thoracoacromial artery, which originates from the second part of the axillary artery. It gives off the lateral thoracic artery, which can contribute to blood supply of the flap. The thoracodorsal artery supplies the latissimus dorsi muscle and flap. The pectoralis muscle origin is at the medial clavicle, costal cartilage and sternum, and the external oblique aponeurosis, and it inserts into the intertubercular sulcus of the humerus. The flap is used as an island or pedicle flap but more frequently as an island flap. It can also be used as an osteomyocutaneous flap with a rib in some cases. Other options for oral tongue reconstruction include a radial forearm free flap and a submental artery pedicled flap.

BIBLIOGRAPHY

Taylor SM, Haughey BH. Reconstruction of the oropharynx. In: Cummings CW, Fredrickson JM, Harker LA, et al. (eds.), *Otolaryngology Head & Neck Surgery: Pediatric*, 5th ed. St. Louis, MO: Mosby; 2010:1375–1392.

23. **(B)** Despite the advent and widespread use of the *H influenzae* type b (HIB) vaccine, *H influenzae* type b still remains the most common cause of epiglottitis. Historically, the disease was more common in children between ages 2 and 6; however, with vaccine use, the incidence in children has dropped significantly. Other bacteria that are found commonly include other types of *H influenzae*, β-hemolytic streptococci, *Staphylococcus*, *Klebsiella pneumoniae*, *Bacteroides melaninogenicus*, and *Mycobacterium tuberculosis*. The presentation in children is fever, difficulty breathing, and irritability. Other symptoms include shallow respiration, retractions, drooling, muffled speech, and

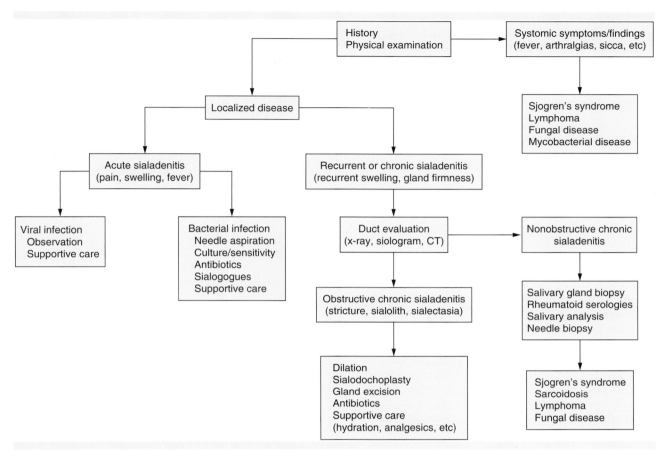

FIGURE 11-23. Algorithm for management of acute and chronic sialadenitis. Cummings CW, Frederickson JM, Harker LA, et al. *Otolaryngology–Head and Neck Surgery*, 3rd ed. St. Louis, MO: CV Mosby; 1998; copyright 1998, with permission from Elsevier.

dysphagia. There is a rapid onset of pain. Stridor occurs later when airway obstruction is nearly complete. Patients sit forward and upright in a "sniffing" position to relieve some of the respiratory obstruction.

BIBLIOGRAPHY

Duncan NO. Infections of the airway in children. In: Cummings CW, Fredrickson JM, Harker LA, et al. (eds.), *Otolaryngology Head & Neck Surgery: Pediatric*, 5th ed. St. Louis, MO: Mosby; 2010:2803–2810.

24. **(B)** The cranial skull base is a complex anatomical region that houses multiple vital structures. Any disease process in this region has the potential to affect the function of the various contents of the skull base foramina. The skull base can be simplified by separating it into an anterior, middle, and posterior cranial fossa.

The anterior cranial fossa (ACF) is formed by three bones: frontal, ethmoid, and sphenoid. The main component is the frontal bone, and the floor is chiefly composed of the orbital plates of the frontal bone and ends at the anterior border of the greater wing of sphenoid. The fovea ethmoidalis is the portion of the ethmoid sinuses that forms part of the ACF floor. The foramina of the ACF include the cribriform plate, which transmits the olfactory nerve (cranial nerve [CN] I), and the foramen cecum, which transmits the emissary vein and is the place of origin of the sagittal sinus.

The middle cranial fossa is formed by the greater wing and body of the sphenoid bone, the squamous part of the temporal bone, and a portion of the petrous temporal bone. The foramina from anterior to posterior are:

Optic canal (transmits optic nerve [CN II] and the ophthalmic artery)

Superior orbital fissure (transmits CN III, IV, ophthalmic division of the trigeminal nerve [CN V1], and superior and inferior divisions of the ophthalmic vein)

Inferior orbital fissure (transmits the maxillary division of the trigeminal nerve [CN V2], zygomatic branch of the maxillary nerve, and the ascending branches from the pterygopalatine ganglion, infraorbital vessels, and the anastomosis between inferior ophthalmic vein and pterygoid venous plexus)

Foramen rotundum (transmits maxillary division of trigeminal nerve [CN V2])

Foramen ovale (transmits mandibular division of trigeminal nerve [CN V3])

Foramen spinosum (transmits the middle meningeal artery)

Foramen lacerum (carries the artery of pterygoid canal, the nerve of the pterygoid canal, and some its accompanying venous plexi)

The posterior cranial fossa can be examined posterior, inferior, and medial to the temporal bone. There are five foramina of the posterior cranial fossa. The foramen magnum carries the medulla oblongata, spinal accessory nerve roots (CN XI), vertebral arteries, anterior and posterior spinal arteries, and occipitoaxial ligament. The jugular foramen transmits the beginning of the internal jugular vein and CNs IX, X, and XI. The hypoglossal canal carries CN XII. The internal acoustic meatus transmits the facial nerve (CN VII) and the vestibuloacoustic nerve (CN VIII). The stylomastoid foramen transmits the facial nerve (CN VII) and the stylomastoid artery.

BIBLIOGRAPHY

Pincheiro-Neto CD, Synderman CH, Gardner PA. Cranial base surgery. In: Cummings CW, Fredrickson JM, Harker LA, et al. (eds.), *Otolaryngology Head & Neck Surgery: Pediatric*, 5th ed. St. Louis, MO: Mosby; 2010:2081–2096.

25. **(B)** Necrotizing otitis externa is frequently referred to as malignant otitis externa, although this is a misnomer as the condition is not a neoplastic process but rather a potentially life-threatening external ear infection. It is a rare process that is usually seen in the elderly, diabetics, and the immunocompromised. Patients usually present with a long history of severe otalgia and otorrhea. Granulation tissue through the floor of the external ear canal at the bony cartilaginous junction is pathognomonic for this disease process.

   Pseudomonas aeruginosa is the causative organism in a majority of cases, although cases of *S aureus*, have been reported. *Aspergillus* species are the most common fungal pathogens. CT scan of the temporal bone with IV contrast is the usual first imaging modality. It provides excellent bony detail and can outline extension of disease and specific location. It is very poor at monitoring response to therapy, however, because remineralization of the osteomyelitic bone must occur for

changes to be detected by CT, and sometimes this may not take place. A technetium-99m bone scan is performed when clinical suspicion is high but the CT scan is negative for disease. The bone scan highlights areas of increased osteoblastic activity whether it is because of bone destruction or bone repair. The gallium-67 scan is important in monitoring necrotizing otitis externa and its resolution. Gallium-67 citrate and indium 111-labeled leukocyte scans reveal areas of high inflammatory cell activity. They indicate an active infection but are not as accurate in locating the entire extent of the osteomyelitis. The gallium-67 scan reverts to normal, however, when resolution progresses. Sequential scanning is recommended.

BIBLIOGRAPHY

Guss J, Ruckenstein MJ. Infections of the external ear. In: Cummings CW, Fredrickson JM, Harker LA, et al. (eds.), *Otolaryngology Head & Neck Surgery: Pediatric*, 5th ed. St. Louis, MO: Mosby; 2010:1944–1949.

Melvin TN, Rramanathan M. Microbiology, infections, and antibiotic therapy. In: Bailey BJ, Johnson JT, Newlands SD (eds.), *Head & Neck Surgery Otolaryngology*, 5th ed., vol. 1. Philadelphia, PA: Lippincott Williams & Wilkins; 2014:131–140.

26. **(D)** Nasopharyngeal carcinomas (NPC) and lymphomas are the two most common malignant neoplasms of the nasopharynx with NPC accounting for approximately 90% of the total. In children, a group in which NPC is rare, the differential of a nasopharyngeal mass should include embryonal rhabdomyosarcoma, neuroblastoma, non-Hodgkin lymphoma, and juvenile nasopharyngeal angiofibroma. Although uncommon in the United States, it makes up nearly 20% of cancers in China. The etiology of NPC has been linked to genetic susceptibility at the HLA-A2, HLA-B-SIN 2, HLA Bw46, and B17 loci. In addition, the Epstein-Barr virus (EBV) has shown a close association with NPC. EBV antibodies are acquired earlier in life in tropical countries, when compared to industrialized countries; however, by adulthood, 90–95% of people have EBV antibodies. EBV is a herpes virus, with a central core of DNA and an envelope causing a persistent and chronic infection especially in B lymphocytes, and the latent membrane protein of the virus may be the inciting agent in carcinogenesis. IgA antibodies to the EBV viral capsid antigen and early antigen diffuse component help in the diagnosis of occult disease or identification of recurrence; however, they are less helpful with the detection of recurrent or persistent disease. Clonal EBV DNA has been found in premalignant lesions. EBV antigens and Epstein-Barr–encoded ribonucleic acids (EBERs) are expressed on NPC cells. Both of these are not present on normal nasopharynx cells.

The majority of people infected with EBV do not develop NPC. Also, the expression of EBNA-1 and LMP-1 is not seen in normal nasopharynx cells suggesting that EBV is not the inciting event in NPC. Its role in development is a result of latent infection of the transformed epithelial cells of the nasopharynx.

BIBLIOGRAPHY

Robbins KT, Malone J. Carcinoma of the oral cavity and pharynx. In: Lee KJ (ed.), *Essential Otolaryngology Head and Neck Surgery*, 10th ed. New York, NY: McGraw-Hill; 2012:695–723.

Tan L, Loh T. Benign and malignant tumors of the nasopharynx. In: Cummings CW, Fredrickson JM, Harker LA, et al. (eds.), *Otolaryngology Head & Neck Surgery: Pediatric*, 5th ed. St. Louis, MO: Mosby; 2010:1348–1357.

27. **(A)** Local flaps are designed immediately next to or near the location of a cutaneous defect. There are several ways to classify local flaps: blood supply, shape, location, or method of transfer. Most local flaps are based on a random pattern blood supply from unnamed arteries in the subdermal plexus. In contrast, larger regional flaps use axial pattern blood supply dependent on larger named arteries. Two general types of local skin flaps in terms of the method of transfer are those that rotate around a fixed point to reach a defect and those that are advanced into a defect. The first group can be referred to as pivotal flaps, which include rotation, transposition, and interpolated (island) flaps. The second group are advancement flaps, which are shaped linearly and are stretched into the defect after appropriate relaxing incisions are made. These include unipedicle, bipedicle, V-Y, hinged flaps, rectangular monopedicled or bipedicled flaps, and the V-Y advancement flap.

The rotation flap has a curvilinear shape and is best designed for triangular defects. It rotates in an arc, and a back cut or Z-plasty may be done to address redundant tissue at the base. Vascularity is dependable because of the broad base. The flap should be based inferiorly to restrict flap edema and assist with lymphatic drainage. A special type of rotation flap is the rhomboid flap, which is used frequently in the head and neck. The rotation flap is helpful in repairing medial cheek defects, and large rotational flaps are helpful in repairing large posterior and upper neck defects (see Figs. 11-24 and 11-25). The transposition flap is a pivotal flap that has a linear axis but can be designed like a rotational flap in that one border is a border of the defect. It has the advantage of the ability to be designed further away from the defect with an axis independent of the linear axis. Optimum skin for closure can be selected this way. The interpolated flap has a base located away from the defect and is also based on a linear axis. It is passed either over or under a complete bridge of skin.

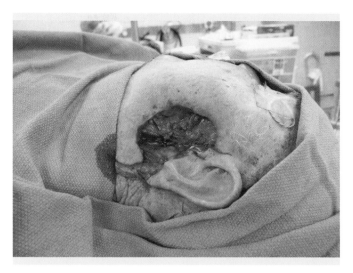

FIGURE 11-24. Defect after removal of preauricular squamous cell carcinoma and superficial parotidectomy.

The advancement flap is based on sliding of donor tissue in a straight line without any lateral movement. Bipedicled advancement flaps are useful in lip and forehead defects. Burow's triangles are excised from the base to avoid a standing cutaneous cone (dog-ear deformity) at the base of the donor site. The V-Y advancement involves pushing the donor skin into the defect by a primary straight line closure of the donor site. It is useful in treating contracted scars that distort critical aesthetic areas such as the vermilion border or eyelid. It is widely used in the repair of cleft lip–nasal deformities to lengthen the columella. A hinge flap is designed either linearly or curvilinearly, and the pedicle is based on one

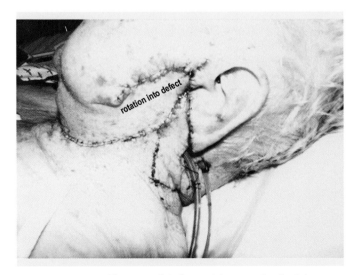

FIGURE 11-25. Closure of defect with a cervicofacial rotation flap.

margin of the defect. The flap is turned on to the defect like a page in a book, but a second graft is required for the exposed deep surface that is now external. It is used primarily in full-thickness nasal defects and in replacing internal nasal lining.

BIBLIOGRAPHY

Baker SR. Reconstruction of facial defects. In: Cummings CW, Fredrickson JM, Harker LA, et al. (eds.), *Otolaryngology Head & Neck Surgery: Pediatric*, 5th ed. St. Louis, MO: Mosby; 2010:343–372.

Jewett B. Local cutaneous flaps and grafts. In: Bailey BJ, Johnson JT, Newlands SD (eds.), *Head & Neck Surgery Otolaryngology*, 5th ed., vol. 3. Philadelphia, PA: Lippincott Williams & Wilkins; 2014:2797–2823.

28. **(B)** Pott puffy tumor is a term used to describe a soft tissue swelling caused by a subperiosteal abscess over the region of the frontal sinus. This occurs when the anterior table of the frontal sinus is involved in an osteomyelitic process, which can be caused by sinusitis or by as result of a mucocele that has developed after a fracture. The offending organism in many cases is *S aureus*.

A malignancy of the frontal sinus, though exceedingly rare, should be considered in the differential. The pathophysiologic of development of a mucocele with subsequent osteomyelitis is an obstructed frontal sinus outflow tract. These can develop several years after the initial fracture, with the average being 7.5 years.

BIBLIOGRAPHY

Strong EB. Frontal sinus fractures. In: Bailey BJ, Johnson JT, Newlands SD (eds.), *Head & Neck Surgery Otolaryngology*, 5th ed., vol. 2. Philadelphia, PA: Lippincott Williams & Wilkins; 2014:1255–1271.

CHAPTER 12

THYROID AND PARATHYROID

AMIT D. TEVAR AND DINESH P. TEVAR

QUESTIONS

1. A 34-year-old woman presents with a large right-sided thyroid nodule seen on ultrasound. What information in her history and workup would make her at higher risk for a differentiated thyroid cancer?
   (A) She underwent radiation treatment after resection of a left lower extremity sarcoma 2 years ago.
   (B) Her thyroid-stimulating hormone (TSH) level is suppressed.
   (C) She grew up in an iodine-deficient area.
   (D) She had acne as a teenager that was treated with radiation.
   (E) She had scoliosis as a teenager requiring frequent spinal x-rays.

2. The patient in Question 2 was found to be hyperthyroid on laboratory evaluation. In which situation would anti-thyroid medication followed by radioactive iodine (RAI) be appropriate?
   (A) Graves disease
   (B) Cold nodule on iodine uptake scan, correlating with the ultrasound finding, with increased uptake in the surrounding parenchyma
   (C) Hot nodule on iodine uptake scan, correlating with ultrasound finding, with suppressed background
   (D) Hashimoto thyroiditis
   (E) If thyroglobulin levels are within normal limits

3. Which of the following ultrasound findings is most suggestive of malignancy?
   (A) Complete halo
   (B) Hypoechogenicity
   (C) Hyperechogenicity
   (D) Wider than tall
   (E) Anechogenicity

4. A recommendation of repeat fine-needle aspiration (FNA) in 3 months would be appropriate for which Bethesda category?
   (A) Atypia of undetermined significance or follicular lesion of undetermined significance
   (B) Benign
   (C) Follicular neoplasm or suspicious for follicular neoplasm
   (D) Suspicious for malignancy

5. Which of the following is the *most accurate* statement with regard to FNA of thyroid nodules?
   (A) The false-positive rate is ~2%.
   (B) The false-negative rate is ~15%.
   (C) Ultrasound must be used for a reliable result.
   (D) FNA findings classified as atypia of undetermined significance have a malignancy rate of 15–30%.
   (E) FNA diagnosis of follicular neoplasm has a malignancy rate of 1–4%.

6. A 35-year-old woman presents with a painless midline mass above the hyoid bone for the past 4 months. She denies any history of neck radiation or previous surgery. The mass is 2 × 2 cm on physical examination and elevates with tongue protrusion. What is the most common malignancy associated with this condition?
   (A) Follicular
   (B) Hürthle cell
   (C) Papillary
   (D) Medullary
   (E) Anaplastic

7. A professional singer has a left thyroid lobectomy for a large thyroid nodule with compression symptoms. Post-operatively, she notices she is having trouble hitting some notes and projecting her voice. The ligation of which vessel resulted in this nerve injury?
   (A) Inferior thyroid artery
   (B) Superior thyroid artery
   (C) Inferior thyroid vein
   (D) Middle thyroid vein
   (E) Thyrocervical trunk

8. Which of the following is the most common postoperative complication seen in thyroid surgery?
   (A) Recurrent laryngeal nerve injury
   (B) Superior laryngeal nerve injury
   (C) Transient hypoparathyroidism
   (D) Permanent hypoparathyroidism
   (E) Hematoma

9. A 42-year-old woman presents with bulging eyes and symptoms of hyperthyroidism including palpitations, heat intolerance, and anxiety. What will an iodine uptake scan show?
   (A) No uptake in the thyroid gland
   (B) High uniform uptake throughout both lobes of the thyroid
   (C) High multifocal uptake within both lobes of the thyroid
   (D) High unifocal uptake in the right upper lobe
   (E) Low uniform uptake in a single lobe

10. The patient in Question 9 undergoes treatment with methimazole for 18 months, after which therapy was discontinued. What is her chance of having a durable cure?
    (A) 1–10%
    (B) 15–25%
    (C) 20–30%
    (D) 40–50%
    (E) 65–75%

11. A 42-year-old woman underwent thyroid lobectomy for a large nodule causing compressive symptoms. FNA preoperatively showed a benign colloid nodule. On final pathology, a 5-mm focus of papillary thyroid cancer is noted. What is the next step in treatment?
    (A) Completion thyroidectomy followed by radioactive iodine ablation
    (B) Completion thyroidectomy without radioactive iodine ablation
    (C) Completion thyroidectomy with ipsilateral central neck dissection
    (D) TSH suppressive therapy
    (E) No further treatment needed

12. A 45-year-old woman presents with a 3.1-cm nodule in the lower pole of the left thyroid lobe. There are no palpable lymph nodes, and no other lesions are found during ultrasound evaluation. FNA shows a well-differentiated papillary carcinoma. What is the most appropriate treatment?
    (A) Total thyroidectomy
    (B) Total thyroidectomy with postoperative iodine-131 (^{131}I) therapy
    (C) Lobectomy with 1-cm margins
    (D) Lobectomy with postoperative ^{131}I therapy
    (E) Observation with interval ultrasound examination and thyroglobulin measurement

13. A 35-year-old woman is found to have a solitary, painless 2-cm thyroid lesion. FNA indicates a follicular lesion. What is the most appropriate management of this patient?
    (A) Total thyroidectomy with ^{131}I therapy
    (B) Magnetic resonance imaging (MRI) of the lesion
    (C) Thyroid lobectomy
    (D) Open excisional biopsy with permanent section pathology
    (E) Measure carcinoembryonic antigen (CEA) and calcitonin levels

14. A 78-year-old woman presents with a rapidly enlarging right-sided neck mass, voice changes, and some worsening compressive symptoms. She has right vocal cord paralysis on fiber-optic laryngoscopy. FNA shows anaplastic thyroid cancer. What is the most appropriate next step in her treatment?
    (A) Chemotherapy followed by total thyroidectomy, central neck dissection and right-sided lateral neck dissection
    (B) Chemotherapy and external-beam radiation, followed by surgical debulking and tracheostomy placement
    (C) Ultrasound of the neck, computed tomography (CT) of neck and chest, and fluorodeoxyglucose (FDG) positron emission tomography (PET) to assess extent of disease
    (D) Biopsy of any distant metastasis
    (E) External-beam radiation followed by total thyroidectomy

15. A 40-year-old woman presents with a 1-cm left-sided thyroid nodule that demonstrates medullary thyroid carcinoma on FNA. What is the next step in the treatment of this patient?
    (A) Measure calcitonin and CEA to determine extent of disease
    (B) Total thyroidectomy with central neck dissection and postoperative ^{131}I treatment

(C) Total thyroidectomy with central neck dissection

(D) Total thyroidectomy with postoperative chemora-diation therapy

(E) Measure calcium and plasma fractionated metanephrines

16. Which of the following is the most common site of origin for isolated metastatic lesions to the thyroid?
    (A) Kidney
    (B) Breast
    (C) Colon
    (D) Soft tissue
    (E) Lung

17. A 31-year-old woman develops sudden onset of neck pain radiating to the jaw with a temperature of 40°C 4 days after being treated for "strep throat." Thyroid function tests are normal, and the white blood cell count is 24,000. The thyroid is tender, but there are no obvious areas of fluctuance found on physical examination. What is the most appropriate form of treatment?
    (A) Total thyroidectomy
    (B) Operative incision and drainage
    (C) Intravenous antibiotics
    (D) High-dose immunosuppression
    (E) FNA

18. A 42-year-old woman presents with symptoms of hypothyroidism with a painless, enlarged, firm, rubbery thyroid gland on exam. Which diagnosis is most consistent with her condition?
    (A) Hashimoto thyroiditis
    (B) Acute suppurative thyroiditis
    (C) Riedel thyroiditis
    (D) Painless thyroiditis
    (E) Subacute de Quervain thyroiditis

19. A 27-year-old woman with a history of lupus develops symptoms of hyperthyroidism 2 months after delivery of her first child. Three months later, she develops symptoms of hypothyroidism that persist. A small, nontender goiter is present. What is the best method of treatment for her disease?
    (A) ^{131}I treatment
    (B) Total thyroidectomy
    (C) FNA
    (D) Thyroid hormone replacement
    (E) High-dose steroids

20. Which of the following statements is *true* regarding the origin of the parathyroids?
    (A) The two inferior glands are usually found near the posterior aspect of the thyroid capsule.

(B) The two superior glands are usually found near the posterior aspect of the thyroid capsule.

(C) Thirty-five percent of normal people have a fifth parathyroid gland.

(D) The parathyroid glands arise from the fourth and fifth branchial pouches.

(E) The inferior glands arise from the fourth branchial pouch.

21. Parathyroid hormone (PTH) acts indirectly on which organ to increase calcium levels?
    (A) Small bowel
    (B) Kidney
    (C) Bone
    (D) Liver
    (E) Skin

22. A 58-year-old woman without any significant past medical history presents to her primary care physician for her routine yearly physical. She has had some vague complaints of fatigue, but has otherwise been in good health. Her calcium level was noted to be elevated on her blood work. Which of the following is the most likely etiology of her disease?
    (A) Vitamin D toxicity
    (B) Malignancy
    (C) Primary hyperparathyroidism
    (D) Sarcoidosis
    (E) Secondary hyperparathyroidism

23. In patients with primary hyperparathyroidism, which of the following will cause worsening hypercalcemia?
    (A) Amiodarone
    (B) Furosemide
    (C) Hydrochlorothiazide
    (D) Bisphosphonate
    (E) Calcitonin

24. A 33-year-old woman has had elevated serum calcium levels since birth. Further evaluation demonstrates a normal PTH and hypocalciuria. She denies any symptoms. What is the most appropriate treatment?
    (A) Subtotal parathyroidectomy
    (B) Technetium-99m (^{99m}Tc)-sestamibi
    (C) Bisphosphonates
    (D) Observation
    (E) Minimally invasive parathyroidectomy

25. A 47-year-old woman develops symptomatic hypercalcemia, and further workup demonstrates primary hyperparathyroidism. Surgical treatment shows the following gross and permanent histologic sections (see Fig. 12-1).

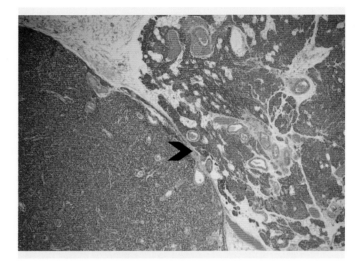

FIGURE 12-1. Hematoxylin and eosin stain of parathyroid tissue. From Kemp W, Burns D, Brown T. *Pathology: The Big Picture*. New York, NY: McGraw-Hill; 2007.

What is the most likely etiology of her disease?
(A) Single adenoma
(B) Familial hypocalciuric hypercalcemia
(C) Hyperplasia
(D) Carcinoma
(E) Exogenous calcium intake

26. A 48-year-old woman with primary hyperparathyroidism has a T score of less than –1.8 at the left distal radius on her dual-energy x-ray absorptiometry (DEXA) scan but is otherwise asymptomatic. What is the next step in her management?
(A) Cystoscopy
(B) Serum oxalate measurement
(C) Parathyroid localization studies
(D) Bilateral neck exploration
(E) Observation

27. A patient with primary hyperparathyroidism undergoes surgical exploration. A single irregularly enlarged parathyroid gland is found that invades into surrounding tissue. The specimen histology is shown in Fig. 12-2. What is the most appropriate surgical resection?
(A) Single parathyroidectomy, with visual inspection of the other three glands
(B) Subtotal parathyroidectomy

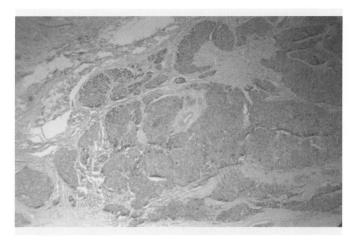

FIGURE 12-2. Frozen section of parathyroid tissue.

(C) En bloc gland resection, with ipsilateral thyroid lobectomy and cervical thymus and central neck dissection
(D) Total parathyroidectomy with reimplantation
(E) En bloc gland resection, with ipsilateral thyroid lobectomy and cervical thymus and central and lateral neck dissections

28. Surgical exploration for a patient with primary hyperparathyroidism reveals all four glands to be enlarged. What is the most appropriate treatment?
(A) Closure with localization study
(B) Biopsy of all glands
(C) Subtotal parathyroidectomy
(D) Excision of the largest gland
(E) Selective venous PTH sampling

29. In a 65-year-old woman with primary hyperparathyroidism, which of the following is a contraindication to minimally invasive parathyroidectomy?
(A) Calcium >12 μg/dL
(B) Large parathyroid adenoma noted in the right paraesophageal space
(C) History of ionizing radiation exposure to the neck
(D) Amiodarone-induced hyperparathyroidism
(E) Inability to acquire preoperative imaging

ANSWERS AND EXPLANATIONS

1. **(D)** Although thyroid nodules are common within the general population, thyroid malignancy overall is still relatively rare. Approximately 5% of thyroid nodules are eventually found to harbor malignancy; the overwhelming majority of these will be differentiated thyroid cancer (papillary, follicular). Therapeutic doses of radiation to

the head/neck region have been shown to increase the risk of thyroid malignancy. Prior to knowing its potential harmful effects, radiation was used for treatment of benign conditions such as acne, recurrent tonsillitis, tinea capitis, and external otitis; therefore, it is important to elicit this information from the patient. Other patients at increased risk of thyroid-related disease secondary to radiation exposure include those exposed to high levels of radiation related to nuclear disasters (e.g., Chernobyl) and patients who have received therapeutic radiation for the treatment of lymphoma or head/neck malignancies. There seems to be a dose-dependent relationship between the amount of radiation and the risk for thyroid malignancy.

BIBLIOGRAPHY

Miller BS, Gauger PG. Thyroid gland. In: Mulholland MW, Lillemoe KD, Doherty GM, et al. (eds.), *Greenfield's Surgery: Scientific Principles and Practice*, 5th ed. Philadelphia, PA: Lippincott Williams & Wilkins; 2010:Chapter 75.

Procopiou M, Meier CA. Evaluation of thyroid nodules. In: Oertli D, Udelsman R (eds.), *Surgery of the Thyroid and Parathyroid Glands*. New York, NY: Springer; 2012:197–205.

2. **(C)** The algorithm for evaluation of thyroid nodules includes early measurement of serum TSH (see Fig. 12-3).

   If the TSH is suppressed, the patient should undergo a thyroid uptake scan to determine if the nodule is hyperfunctioning ("hot"). If so, the likelihood of malignancy is minimal and treatment focuses on medical control

of hyperthyroidism (antithyroid medication followed by RAI). In patients with Graves disease, total thyroidectomy is indicated to both treat the Graves disease and resect the nodule. If the nodule is nonfunctioning ("cold"), then further workup with FNA is required. Thyroglobulin levels are not helpful in the setting of a patient with an *in situ* thyroid gland.

BIBLIOGRAPHY

Lee GA, Masharani U. Disorders of the thyroid gland. In: Lalwani AK (ed.), *Current Diagnosis & Treatment in Otolaryngology–Head & Neck Surgery*, 3rd ed. New York, NY: McGraw-Hill; 2012:Chapter 42.

Miller BS, Gauger PG. Thyroid gland. In: Mulholland MW, Lillemoe KD, Doherty GM, et al. (eds.), *Greenfield's Surgery: Scientific Principles and Practice*, 5th ed. Philadelphia, PA: Lippincott Williams & Wilkins; 2010:Chapter 75.

Procopiou M, Meier CA. Evaluation of thyroid nodules. In: Oertli D, Udelsman R (eds.), *Surgery of the Thyroid and Parathyroid Glands*. New York, NY: Springer; 2012:197–205.

3. **(B)** Ultrasound is a commonly used modality that employs sound waves to image thyroid nodules. It is a simple noninvasive test that can reliably visualize thyroid lesions and can be performed in the office setting, although results are operator-dependent. It can reliably differentiate solid from cystic lesions, but it lacks the ability to definitively distinguish malignant from benign lesions, although certain characteristics are associated with higher rates of malignancy (see Fig. 12-4).

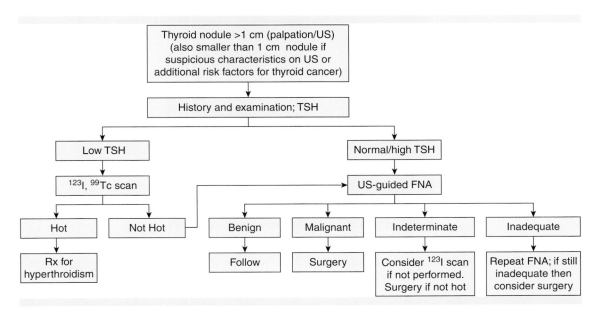

FIGURE 12-3. Algorithm for the management of thyroid nodules. FNA, fine-needle aspiration; TSH, thyroid-stimulating hormone; US, ultrasound. From Lalwani AK (ed). *Current Diagnosis & Treatment in Otolaryngology–Head & Neck Surgery*, 3rd ed. New York, NY: McGraw-Hill; 2012.

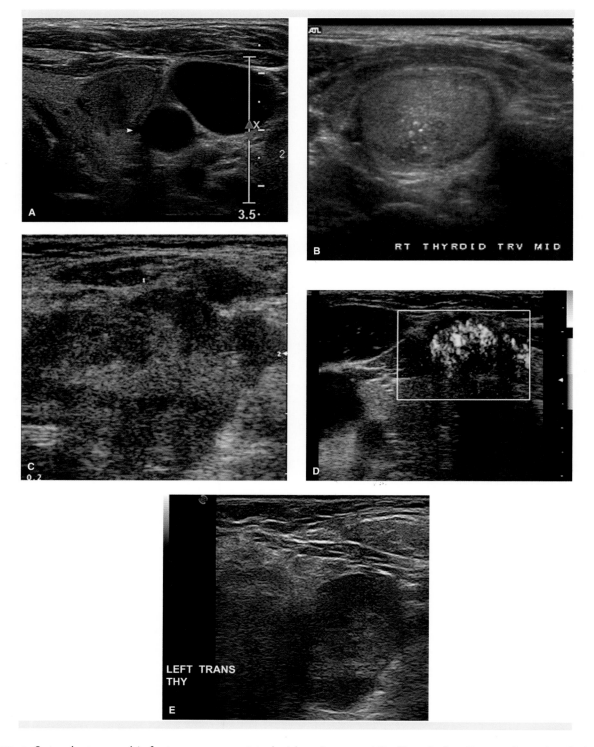

FIGURE 12-4. Several sonographic features are associated with an increased likelihood of malignant thyroid pathology. **A.** Hypoechoic nodule medial to the carotid artery; *arrow* denotes interface between nodule and artery. **B.** Microcalcifications within a nodule. **C.** Irregular margins. **D.** Increased intranodular vascularity as seen on duplex imaging. **E.** "Taller than wide" appearance on transverse view. **(A)** From Braakman HM, Knippenberg SA, de Bondt BJ, Lodder J. An unusual cause of transient neurologic deficits: compression of the carotid artery by a thyroid cystic nodule. *J Stroke Cerebrovasc Dis* 2010;19(1):73–74. **(B)** From Jin J, McHenry C. Thyroid incidentaloma. *Best Pract Res Clin Endocrinol Metab* 2012;26(1):83–96. **(C–E)** From Kangelaris G, Kim TB, Orloff LA. Role of ultrasound in thyroid disorders. *Otolaryngol Clin North Am* 2012;7(2):197–210, with permission from Elsevier.

Suspicious features include hypoechogenicity in comparison to thyroid parenchyma, microcalcifications, increased vascularity, irregular borders, absent halo, and a nodule that is taller than wide. Malignant lesions are found to be hypoechogenic on ultrasound in almost 80% of cases. When the finding of a hypoechogenic lesion is combined with microcalcifications, irregular borders, and taller than wide shape, the sensitivity for malignancy increases. Simple cysts, hyperechogenic solid nodules, and spongiform architecture are all associated with benign lesions. Ultrasound may aid in localization and examination of nodules, but FNA or excisional biopsy is necessary to definitively determine presence of malignancy.

TABLE 12-1 Bethesda System

Bethesda Category	Rate of Malignancy
Nondiagnostic or unsatisfactory	1–4%
Benign	0–3%
Atypia of undetermined significance or follicular lesion	5–15%
Follicular neoplasm or suspicious for a follicular neoplasm	15–30%
Suspicious for malignancy	60–75%
Malignant	97–99%

BIBLIOGRAPHY

Cooper DS, Doherty GM, Haugen BR, et al. Revised American Thyroid Association management guidelines for patients with thyroid nodules and differentiated thyroid cancer. *Thyroid* 2009;19(11):1–48.

Miller BS, Gauger PG. Thyroid gland. In: Mulholland MW, Lillemoe KD, Doherty GM, et al. (eds.), *Greenfield's Surgery: Scientific Principles and Practice*, 5th ed. Philadelphia, PA: Lippincott Williams & Wilkins; 2010:Chapter 75.

Wiesner W, Engel H, Steinbrich W, et al. Diagnostic imaging of the thyroid and radioiodine therapy. In: Oertli D, Udelsman R (eds.), *Surgery of the Thyroid and Parathyroid Glands*. New York, NY: Springer; 2012:35–57.

4. **(A)**

5. **(A)**

Explanation for 4 and 5

FNA has become the mainstay for the diagnosis of thyroid nodules. It remains a technically simple procedure with a high yield of information and minimal complications. It is a cost-effective tool that can be performed in the office setting. Using aseptic technique, a 25-gauge needle is inserted into the nodule, approaching it from a medial to lateral direction either by palpation or under ultrasound guidance. Some use the aspiration technique, whereas others favor the nonaspiration technique to acquire the specimen. Once the mass is entered, the needle is moved in and out rapidly within the nodule to gather as much cellular material within the needle as possible. The aspirate is immediately placed on a cytology specimen slide and fixed with the pathologist's choice of fixative. Three to five specimens are usually obtained for a single nodule. Several results can be obtained.

In 2009, the Bethesda system for cytopathology was introduced. There are six designations that were made to standardize how thyroid cytology specimens are categorized (see Table 12-1).

Each of these categories has very specific findings, and the creation of this system has allowed reliable communication between different facilities, specialists, and other members of the care team. These diagnostic criteria have also given us the capability to estimate the chance of malignancy within each of these subsets. A benign result will be malignant 0–3% of the time, whereas a malignant result will be a cancer 97–99% of the time. With patients who are found to have atypia of undetermined significance or follicular lesion of undetermined significance, a repeat FNA will give a more definitive result in most cases (80%).

The false-negative rates of FNA range from 0–3% for a benign reading. Diagnosis of follicular malignancy is particularly difficult. It requires tissue architecture showing vascular and/or capsular invasion for unequivocal identification, which cannot be determined by FNA; therefore, lobectomy is generally required for definitive diagnosis.

Studies have reported decreased rates of both nondiagnostic and false-negative cytology results when FNA is performed using ultrasound guidance, but the palpation method can be used when appropriate. If a patient has a nondiagnostic FNA result, then repeat FNA with ultrasound guidance should be considered in 3 months from initial FNA.

BIBLIOGRAPHY

Cibas E, Syed A. The Bethesda system for reporting thyroid cytopathology. *Am J Clin Pathol* 2009;132:658–665.

Cooper DS, Doherty GM, Haugen BR, et al. Revised American Thyroid Association management guidelines for patients with thyroid nodules and differentiated thyroid cancer. *Thyroid* 2009;19(11):1–48.

Karakla DW, Bak MJ. The management of thyroid nodules. In: Cameron JL (ed.), *Current Surgical Therapy*, 11th ed. Philadelphia, PA: Elsevier; 2014:642–645.

6. **(C)** The patient described in the question has the classic findings of a thyroglossal duct cyst (see Fig. 12-5). This lesion results from an incomplete involution of

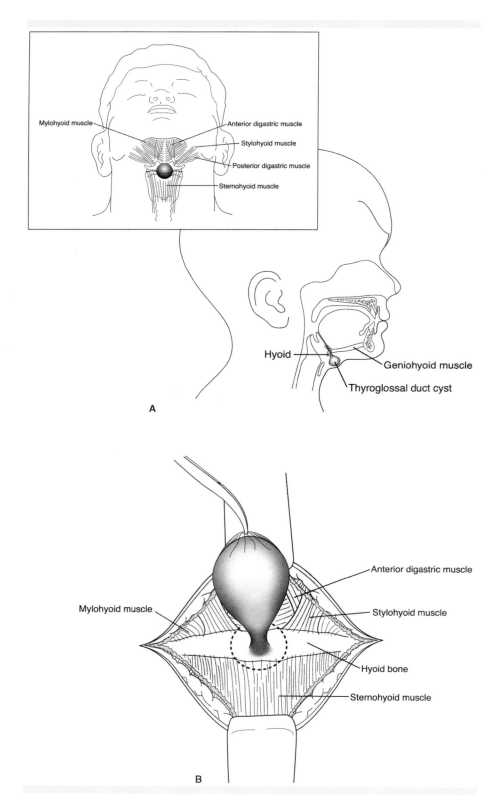

FIGURE 12-5. Thyroglossal duct cyst. **A.** Anterior neck anatomy and a thyroglossal duct cyst extending through the hyoid bone. Lateral view and anterior frontal view (*inset*). The incision is represented by the *dotted line*. **B.** The platysma has been opened and the cyst dissected free, exposing the hyoid and deep anterior cervical muscles. The *dotted line* marks the area that will be incised with electrocautery.

embryonic elements during the path of descent of the thyroid from the floor of the mouth (foramen cecum) to the low anterior neck. The cyst is generally lined with stratified squamous or pseudostratified columnar epithelium with mucus-secreting glands. A majority of thyroglossal duct cysts present in early childhood as a painless midline neck mass, with infection or drainage from a fistula. Often the mass will elevate with tongue protrusion.

There is a small chance of developing a carcinoma within a thyroglossal duct cyst, with the most common cell type being papillary carcinoma. Papillary carcinoma is diagnosed in up to 10% of patients undergoing thyroglossal duct cyst excision in adulthood.

The Sistrunk procedure, which was first described in 1920, is still the recommended procedure. It involves complete cyst excision in continuity with the involved portion of the hyoid bone. The procedure has proved to have minimal morbidity. Recurrence occurs up to 10% of the time and is associated with inadequate excision of the tract.

BIBLIOGRAPHY

Miller BS, Gauger PG. Thyroid gland. In: Mulholland MW, Lillemoe KD, Doherty GM, et al. (eds.), *Greenfield's Surgery: Scientific Principles and Practice*, 5th ed. Philadelphia, PA: Lippincott Williams & Wilkins; 2010:Chapter 75.

Oldham KT, Aiken JJ. Pediatric head and neck. In: Mulholland MW, Lillemoe KD, Doherty GM, et al. (eds.), *Greenfield's Surgery: Scientific Principles and Practice*, 5th ed. Philadelphia, PA: Lippincott Williams & Wilkins; 2010:Chapter 105.

7. **(B)** The symptoms described in the question occur after injury to the external branch of the superior laryngeal nerve. This is most commonly injured during the mobilization of the superior pedicle (see Fig. 12-6).

Understanding the relationship of the nerves associated with the thyroid gland is important in avoiding injuries during thyroidectomy. The recurrent laryngeal nerve originates from the vagus and provides motor function to all muscles of the larynx, except the cricothyroid muscle. On the right, the nerve loops under the subclavian artery, and on the left, it passes under the arch of the aorta and then continues to travel cephalad in the tracheal esophageal groove on each side to the insertion site at the cricothyroid joint (see Fig. 12-7).

The recurrent laryngeal nerve is intimately associated with the inferior thyroid artery, whereas the external branch of the superior laryngeal nerve is most commonly in proximity to the superior thyroid artery and vein (see Fig. 12-8). It is during the mobilization of the superior pedicle that most injuries to the external

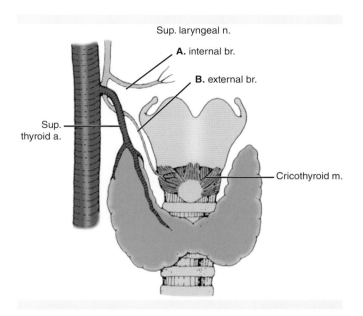

FIGURE 12-6. Relationship between the **A.** internal and **B.** external branches of the superior laryngeal nerve with the superior thyroid artery and the upper pole of the thyroid gland. Modified from Droulias C, Tzinas S, Harlaftis N, Akin JT Jr, Gray SW, Skandalakis JE. The superior laryngeal nerve. *Am Surg* 1976;42:635–638; with permission.

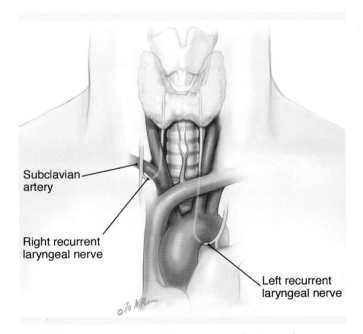

FIGURE 12-7. Anatomy of the recurrent laryngeal nerve. Modified from Droulias C, Tzinas S, Harlaftis N, Akin JT Jr, Gray SW, Skandalakis JE. The superior laryngeal nerve. *Am Surg* 1976;42:635–638; with permission.

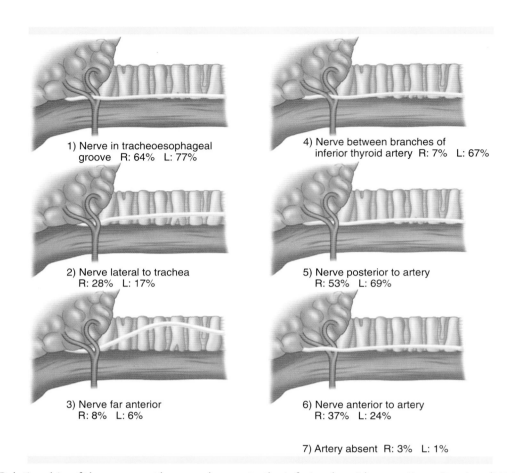

1) Nerve in tracheoesophageal groove R: 64% L: 77%

2) Nerve lateral to trachea R: 28% L: 17%

3) Nerve far anterior R: 8% L: 6%

4) Nerve between branches of inferior thyroid artery R: 7% L: 67%

5) Nerve posterior to artery R: 53% L: 69%

6) Nerve anterior to artery R: 37% L: 24%

7) Artery absent R: 3% L: 1%

FIGURE 12-8. Relationship of the recurrent laryngeal nerve to the inferior thyroid artery. From Brunicardi F, Andersen DK, Billiar TR, et al. (eds.), *Schwartz's Principles of Surgery*, 10th ed. New York, NY: McGraw-Hill; 2014.

branch of the superior laryngeal nerve occur, which is why these vessels must be ligated as close to the thyroid as possible. Injury to the external branch of the superior laryngeal nerve results in the inability to attain and sustain high-pitched notes and the loss of ability to project one's voice.

The superior laryngeal nerve also originates from the vagus nerve and divides into internal and external branches. The internal superior laryngeal nerve provides mostly sensory function, whereas the external superior laryngeal nerve provides motor function to the cricothyroid muscle.

BIBLIOGRAPHY

Duke WS, Terris DJ. Hyperthyroidism. In: Cameron JL, Cameron AM (eds.), *Current Surgical Therapy*, 11th ed. Philadelphia, PA: Elsevier; 2014:666–658.

Miller BS, Gauger PG. Thyroid gland. In: Mulholland MW, Lillemoe KD, Doherty GM, et al. (eds.), *Greenfield's Surgery: Scientific Principles and Practice*, 5th ed. Philadelphia, PA: Lippincott Williams & Wilkins; 2010:Chapter 75.

8. **(C)** Thyroid surgery is routinely performed at high-volume centers with minimal morbidity and mortality. Nerve injuries are uncommon, yet frequently discussed due to the serious morbidity that can result. Unilateral injuries, associated with ipsilateral vocal cord paralysis, result in hoarseness, whereas bilateral cord injuries may lead to airway obstruction. Postoperatively, patients with bilateral nerve injury may present with stridor requiring immediate intubation or surgical airway.

Temporary recurrent laryngeal nerve injury has been reported in 1.4–5.9% of patients undergoing thyroid surgery, although the true risk is difficult to determine due to different methods of identification and lack of standardized reporting. Recurrent laryngeal stretch or crush injuries generally improve within 4–6 weeks, but may take several months to a year to fully recover. Injuries present after 1 year are considered permanent. Permanent recurrent laryngeal nerve injury occurs in 1–3% of all thyroidectomy patients.

Suspected recurrent laryngeal injuries are best diagnosed with fiber-optic examination or indirect laryngoscopy. Unilateral injuries may benefit from medialization of the cord to improve voice quality. Superior laryngeal nerve injuries are more difficult to diagnose. The best method of diagnosis is laryngeal videostroboscopy and spectrographic analysis. This permits early diagnosis and treatment with speech rehabilitation.

Hematoma occurs secondary to hemorrhage deep to the strap muscles, and patients present with stridor followed by complete loss of the airway. This diagnosis should be made at the bedside and warrants immediate treatment. The incision should be emergently opened at the bedside to evacuate the hematoma and reestablish the airway. Simultaneously, an operative suite should be prepared for further exploration, ligation of bleeding sites, and wound closure.

The most common complication of thyroid surgery is transient hypoparathyroidism, occurring in up to 40% of patients. Hypoparathyroidism is considered transient if it resolves less than 6 months from time of surgery. Mild asymptomatic hypocalcemia does not require calcium supplementation, although patients with severe disturbances may require intravenous supplementation, which should be transitioned to oral calcium, with or without calcitriol, and tapered as appropriate. In 2% of patients, permanent hypoparathyroidism, lasting >6 months postoperatively, may require lifelong calcium and vitamin D supplementation to treat persistent hypocalcemia.

BIBLIOGRAPHY

Frilling A, Weber F, Kornasiewitcz O. Complications in thyroid and parathyroid surgery. In: Oertli D, Udelsman R (eds.), *Surgery of the Thyroid and Parathyroid Glands*. New York, NY: Springer; 2012:197–205.
Miller BS, Gauger PG. Thyroid gland. In: Mulholland MW, Lillemoe KD, Doherty GM, et al. (eds.), *Greenfield's Surgery: Scientific Principles and Practice*, 5th ed. Philadelphia, PA: Lippincott Williams & Wilkins; 2010:Chapter 75.

9. **(B)** This patient has Graves disease, which is an autoimmune disease characterized by thyroid-stimulating antibodies (TSAb), also known as thyroid-stimulating immunoglobulin (TSI), that result in activation of TSH receptors, leading to unregulated hyperthyroidism. Graves disease is the most common autoimmune disease in the United States. The peak age of incidence is between 40 and 60 years. Patients will most often present with symptoms of hyperthyroidism, though in rare cases Graves disease can initially present with exophthalmos alone. Other clinical manifestations specific to Graves disease include diffuse goiter, dermopathy, and lymphoid hyperplasia. Common diseases associated with Graves are diabetes mellitus, Addison disease, vitiligo, pernicious anemia, myasthenia gravis, alopecia, and other autoimmune diseases.

Laboratory evaluation of Graves disease shows hyperthyroidism with elevated T_3/T_4 levels and a low serum TSH, along with elevated TSI/TSAb. The differential diagnosis of hyperthyroidism includes Graves disease, toxic nodular goiter, toxic nodule, thyroiditis, and iatrogenic hyperthyroidism, which can be distinguished on thyroid scintigraphy.

Thyroid scintigraphy gives a picture of the functional status of the thyroid. It is based on the idea that active thyroid cells take up iodine. Thyroid scintigraphy uses ^{99m}Tc to allow us to see the rate of isotope uptake within the thyroid. Graves affects the whole thyroid and therefore projects a picture of high uptake throughout both lobes on thyroid scintigraphy.

BIBLIOGRAPHY

Miller BS, Gauger PG. Thyroid gland. In: Mulholland MW, Lillemoe KD, Doherty GM, et al. (eds.), *Greenfield's Surgery: Scientific Principles and Practice*, 5th ed. Philadelphia, PA: Lippincott Williams & Wilkins; 2010:Chapter 75.
Wiesner W, Engel H, Steinbrich W, et al. Diagnostic imaging of the thyroid and radioiodine therapy. In: Oertli D, Udelsman R (eds.), *Surgery of the Thyroid and Parathyroid Glands*. New York, NY: Springer; 2012:25–33.

10. **(D)** Treatment of Graves disease can be accomplished through antithyroid drugs, radioactive iodine, or thyroidectomy. The two antithyroid medications most commonly used are methimazole and propylthiouracil (PTU; may be used in pregnancy). These medications may take 2–4 weeks before improvement of symptoms is noted. After discontinuation of the antithyroid medications, 50–60% of patients will have recurrence of disease.

Radioactive iodine is the most common treatment in the United States. It takes 4–8 weeks before results are seen in most patients. This treatment is not ideal in patients with severe disease who need more immediate resolution of their hyperthyroidism, and it is also contraindicated in pregnancy and in patients with severe ophthalmopathy. The main side effect of radioactive iodine treatment is hypothyroidism.

Thyroidectomy is the preferred method of treatment of patients with a large goiter or with nodules. Euthyroid state should be obtained prior to surgery with the use of antithyroid medications and β-blockade for control of symptoms. Potassium iodide (Lugol's) solution can be given 7–10 days prior to surgery to decrease vascularity of the thyroid gland to facilitate thyroidectomy.

BIBLIOGRAPHY

Christ-Crain M, Morgenthaler NG, Mueller B. Evaluation of hyper-
    thyroidism and hyperthyroid goiter. In: Oertli D, Udelsman R
    (eds.), *Surgery of the Thyroid and Parathyroid Glands*. New York,
    NY: Springer; 2012:25–33.
Miller BS, Gauger PG. Thyroid gland. In: Mulholland MW, Lillemoe
    KD, Doherty GM, et al. (eds.), *Greenfield's Surgery: Scientific
    Principles and Practice*, 5th ed. Philadelphia, PA: Lippincott
    Williams & Wilkins; 2010:Chapter 75.

11. **(E)** Microcarcinomas are defined as papillary thyroid
cancers that are less than 1 cm in size. They are generally asymptomatic and usually found when thyroidectomy is done for other indications. Although strictly
speaking they are still carcinomas, generally they do
not necessitate further treatment. Prognosis is excep-
tional, with a 0.4% cause-specific mortality rate. If a
microcarcinoma is found after lobectomy, adequate
treatment has already been performed. In these cases,
completion thyroidectomy and radioiodine scanning
are not necessary.

BIBLIOGRAPHY

Miller BS, Gauger PG. Thyroid gland. In: Mulholland MW, Lillemoe
    KD, Doherty GM, et al. (eds.), *Greenfield's Surgery: Scientific
    Principles and Practice*, 5th ed. Philadelphia, PA: Lippincott
    Williams & Wilkins; 2010:Chapter 75.

12. **(B)** Papillary thyroid carcinoma (PTC) constitutes
approximately 80–85% of all thyroid cancers. It is
found more commonly in iodine-sufficient areas and
occurs more often in women, with a peak incidence
between 20 and 30 years of age. On ultrasound, PTC is
generally solid or predominantly solid and hypoechogenic, often with infiltrative irregular margins and
increased nodular vascularity. Microcalcifications, if
present, are suggestive of PTC, but may be difficult to
distinguish from colloid.

   PTCs arise from follicular cells and are characterized
by distinct architecture, often associated with calcifications, psammoma bodies, squamous metaplasia, and
fibrosis. Nuclear features allow for FNA diagnosis of
PTC, and findings include large, overlapping nuclei
that are clear (Orphan Annie nuclei) and intranuclear
grooves.

   The management algorithm for PTC is shown in
Fig. 12-9.

   As a whole, the prognosis is excellent, despite that
>30% of PTCs are multifocal, with cervical lymph node
involvement being present in approximately 30–40% of
people, and distant metastases occurring in 2–14%. At
least 70% of PTCs are iodine avid, and thus, radioactive

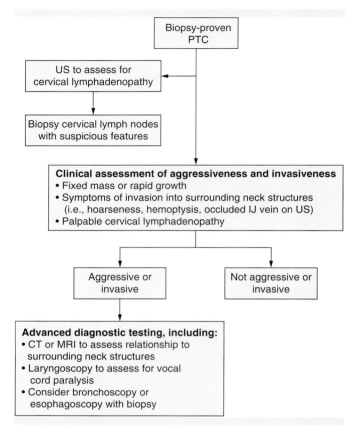

FIGURE 12-9. Management algorithm for papillary thyroid
cancer (PTC). CT, computed tomography; IJ, internal jugular; MRI, magnetic resonance imaging; US, ultrasound.
From Morita S, Dackiw A, Zeiger M. *McGraw-Hill Manual:
Endocrine Surgery.* New York, NY: McGraw-Hill; 2009.

iodine (RAI) scanning and ablation are important
adjuncts in treatment of PTC. Papillary lesions have
classic histologic findings of overlapping nuclei with
ground-glass appearance and longitudinal grooves
(see Fig. 12-10).

   Cancer spread is generally through lymphatic channels. Survival is >90% at 10 years with well-differentiated
lesions appropriately treated.

BIBLIOGRAPHY

Cooper DS, Doherty GM, Haugen BR, et al. Revised American
    Thyroid Association management guidelines for patients with
    thyroid nodules and differentiated thyroid cancer. *Thyroid*
    2009;19(11):1–48.
Miller BS, Gauger PG. Thyroid gland. In: Mulholland MW, Lillemoe
    KD, Doherty GM, et al. (eds.), *Greenfield's Surgery: Scientific
    Principles and Practice*, 5th ed. Philadelphia, PA: Lippincott
    Williams & Wilkins; 2010:Chapter 75.

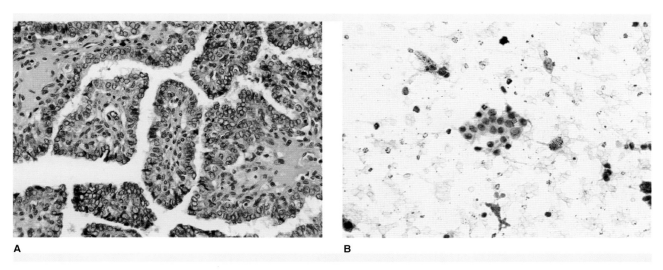

A   **B**

FIGURE 12-10. Papillary thyroid cancer. **A.** Hematoxylin-eosin stain. **B.** Fine-needle aspiration biopsy specimen from a papillary thyroid cancer showing typical intranuclear cytoplasmic inclusions in the center of the slide. From Brunicardi F, Andersen DK, Billiar TR, et al. (eds.), *Schwartz's Principles of Surgery*, 10th ed. New York, NY: McGraw-Hill; 2014.

Wu LS, Roman S. Surgery for solitary thyroid nodule including differentiated thyroid cancer. In: Oertli D, Udelsman R (eds.), *Surgery of the Thyroid and Parathyroid Glands*. New York, NY: Springer; 2012:207–214.

13. **(C)** The diagnostic dilemma of differentiating follicular cancer from benign follicular adenoma is not one that can be solved with FNA. The diagnosis of follicular cancer is made on permanent section with evidence of capsular and/or vascular invasion; therefore, if FNA shows a follicular lesion, thyroid lobectomy is generally recommended for definitive diagnosis (see Fig. 12-11).

   Approximately 15–30% of these lesions are found to harbor malignancy on final pathologic examination. Frozen section is unreliable in definitively ruling out follicular carcinoma intraoperatively. Those who are found to have invasive follicular carcinoma should have a completion thyroidectomy, followed by ^{131}I therapy when indicated.

   Follicular thyroid cancer (FTC) makes up about 10–20% of all thyroid cancers. It occurs more often in females, with a peak incidence in the fifth decade of life. Compared to papillary thyroid cancer, FTC tends to present as a solitary lesion and is more often found to have extrathyroidal extension. About 30% patients with FTC have distant metastases at the time of diagnosis. Follicular cancer more commonly spreads hematogenously, with lung and bone frequently involved, yet 10% of patients will also have nodal involvement. About 80% of FTC will be iodine avid, making ^{131}I an important adjunct to treatment. The classic histologic findings seen with these lesions are follicular changes, without the nuclear changes seen with papillary cancer.

BIBLIOGRAPHY

Cooper DS, Doherty GM, Haugen BR, et al. Revised American Thyroid Association management guidelines for patients with thyroid nodules and differentiated thyroid cancer. *Thyroid* 2009;19(11):1–48.

Miller BS, Gauger PG. Thyroid gland. In: Mulholland MW, Lillemoe KD, Doherty GM, et al. (eds.), *Greenfield's Surgery: Scientific Principles and Practice*, 5th ed. Philadelphia, PA: Lippincott Williams & Wilkins; 2010:Chapter 75.

14. **(C)** Anaplastic cancer accounts for 1–2% of thyroid cancers. It is most common in elderly patients with a long-standing history of a goiter. There is evidence that anaplastic cancers may arise from dedifferentiation of papillary or follicular thyroid carcinomas. Anaplastic thyroid carcinoma is rapidly lethal, and essentially all are too advanced at presentation to be successfully treated. Diagnosis is often made by FNA but may require surgical excision for definitive diagnosis. A multidisciplinary approach with medical oncology, surgery, radiation oncology, and palliative care should be implemented immediately upon diagnosis. For evidence of airway compromise, surgical debulking and tracheostomy should be performed. The tumor should be evaluated on imaging, and comprehensive workup for metastatic disease should be performed. If imaging indicates

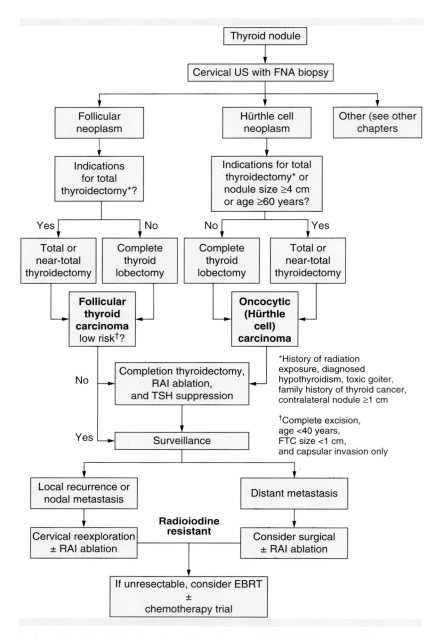

FIGURE 12-11. Diagnostic algorithm for follicular thyroid carcinoma (FTC). EBRT, external-beam radiotherapy; FNA, fine-needle aspiration; RAI, radioactive iodine; TSH, thyroid-stimulating hormone; US, ultrasound. From Morita S, Dackiw A, Zeiger M. *McGraw-Hill Manual: Endocrine Surgery.* New York, NY: McGraw-Hill; 2009.

unresectability of the primary disease, then external-beam radiation with or without chemotherapy should be initiated neoadjuvently. Prognosis is uniformly poor, with a median survival of 5–6 months.

BIBLIOGRAPHY

Miller BS, Gauger PG. Thyroid gland. In: Mulholland MW, Lillemoe KD, Doherty GM, et al. (eds.), *Greenfield's Surgery: Scientific Principles and Practice,* 5th ed. Philadelphia, PA: Lippincott Williams & Wilkins; 2010:Chapter 75.

Smallridge RC, Ain KB, Asa SL, et al. American Thyroid Association guidelines for the management of anaplastic thyroid cancer. *Thyroid* 2012;22(11):1104–1134.

15. **(E)** Approximately 75% of patients with medullary thyroid carcinoma (MTC) are found to have sporadic disease, whereas 20–25% are found to have a familial syndrome. Compared to the differentiated thyroid

cancers, MTC is a more aggressive malignancy with a 10-year survival of 69–89%. Patients have evidence of lymph node involvement at presentation in 50–75% of cases. Exclusion of pheochromocytoma and parathyroid disease must be performed before proceeding to surgery.

The treatment of choice for sporadic and inherited disease is based on surgical resection, in that adjuvant treatment is not indicated in the treatment of MTC. There is no role for postoperative ^{131}I therapy, as C cells are not iodine avid. Chemotherapy is not indicated, but external-beam radiation therapy decreases local recurrence in high-risk patients. Serum calcitonin and carcinoembryonic antigen (CEA) levels are used as markers for recurrence and also to gauge progression of disease.

In patients without evidence of distant metastasis on imaging (most commonly bone, liver, and lung involvement) or with small-volume metastatic disease, surgical resection should include total thyroidectomy with central lymph node dissection. There are varying opinions in regard to prophylactic lateral neck dissection. The majority do not favor prophylactic lateral neck dissection and believe that compartment-oriented lymph node dissection should only be done when metastatic nodes are identified. In patients with distant metastasis, less aggressive neck surgery should be done to avoid morbidity (maintain swallowing and speech) while gaining locoregional control, especially in light of inability to achieve curative resection.

BIBLIOGRAPHY

Kloos RT, Eng C, Evans DB, et al. Medullary thyroid cancer management guidelines of the American Thyroid Association. *Thyroid* 2009;19(6):565–612.
Miller BS, Gauger PG. Thyroid gland. In: Mulholland MW, Lillemoe KD, Doherty GM, et al. (eds.), *Greenfield's Surgery: Scientific Principles and Practice*, 5th ed. Philadelphia, PA: Lippincott Williams & Wilkins; 2010:Chapter 75.

16. **(A)** Rarely, isolated spread from other primary cancers can occur to the thyroid. The most common type of tumor that will result in thyroid metastases is renal cell carcinoma, although breast, lung, gastrointestinal carcinomas, melanoma, and sarcoma have also been reported. The treatment for patients with isolated metastatic lesions should take into account the prognosis of the primary lesion. If the thyroid is the only site of metastasis, resection may have some benefit.

BIBLIOGRAPHY

Miller BS, Gauger PG. Thyroid gland. In: Mulholland MW, Lillemoe KD, Doherty GM, et al. (eds.), *Greenfield's Surgery: Scientific Principles and Practice*, 5th ed. Philadelphia, PA: Lippincott Williams & Wilkins; 2010:Chapter 75.
Sipple RS, Chen H. Thyroid lymphoma and other metastatic lesions. In: Oertli D, Udelsman R (eds.), *Surgery of the Thyroid and Parathyroid Glands*. New York, NY: Springer; 2012:259–267.

17. **(C)** Acute suppurative thyroiditis is a rare finding due to the thyroid's excellent blood supply and ample lymphatic drainage. It is most often caused by gram-positive organisms, with *Staphylococcus aureus* being the most common, although *Streptococcus pyogenes*, *Streptococcus pneumoniae*, and *Haemophilus influenzae* are also frequently found on culture. Fungal infection can also be seen in the immunosuppressed host.

In general, the thyroid is secondarily infected from tonsils, pharynx, thyroglossal duct cyst, trauma to the neck, or recent surgery. Patients usually present with anterior neck pain and tenderness with fever, pharyngitis, and erythema over the affected area. Pain is usually worsened with swallowing and can radiate to the jaw and ear. It is paramount that the examining physician carefully searches for evidence of abscess cavities, which can be present.

Thyroid function tests are typically normal. Ultrasound is the best method for examining the thyroid gland for abscess collections. Further studies are generally unnecessary, although FNA/aspiration with culture can be used to guide antibiotic management. Once the diagnosis is confirmed and the organism is identified, the treatment is appropriate antibiotic therapy. If an abscess is present, incision and drainage are necessary.

BIBLIOGRAPHY

Heizmann O, Oertli D. Thyroiditis. In: Oertli D, Udelsman R (eds.), *Surgery of the Thyroid and Parathyroid Glands*. New York, NY: Springer; 2012:153–164.
Miller BS, Gauger PG. Thyroid gland. In: Mulholland MW, Lillemoe KD, Doherty GM, et al. (eds.), *Greenfield's Surgery: Scientific Principles and Practice*, 5th ed. Philadelphia, PA: Lippincott Williams & Wilkins; 2010:Chapter 75.

18. **(A)** The patient in the question has classic findings of Hashimoto thyroiditis, also referred to as chronic lymphocytic thyroiditis or autoimmune thyroiditis. Common presenting symptoms are painless goiter and hypothyroidism with an enlarged, firm, rubbery thyroid gland on examination. This disease is the most common cause of hypothyroidism in the United States and occurs more often in areas of adequate iodine intake. It predominantly affects women (9:1), peak incidence is between the ages of 30 and 60 years, and there is some degree of genetic predisposition.

A small subset of patient may present with hyperthyroidism, referred to as Hashitoxicosis. Patients may

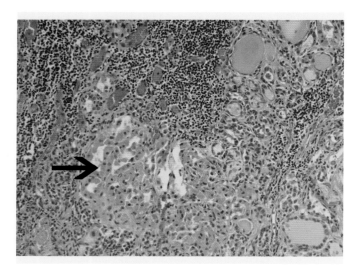

FIGURE 12-12. Hashimoto thyroiditis. From Kemp W, Burns D, Brown T. *Pathology: The Big Picture.* New York, NY: McGraw-Hill; 2007.

also be euthyroid on presentation yet generally progress to be hypothyroid over time at a rate of approximately 5% per year. On laboratory evaluation, thyroperoxidase (TPO) antibodies are elevated in 70–90% of patients with Hashimoto thyroiditis, whereas thyroglobulin antibodies are elevated 40–70%. Imaging studies are not necessary in the diagnosis of Hashimoto thyroiditis, but ultrasound is used to evaluate for nodules. FNA should be performed on any nodules that meet criteria to exclude the presence of PTC or lymphoma, which has a slightly higher incidence in patients with this disease.

The histologic findings seen in Hashimoto thyroiditis are diffuse plasma cell and lymphocytic infiltration, extensive fibrosis, and gland destruction (see Fig. 12-12).

Management of Hashimoto thyroiditis includes thyroid hormone replacement for hypothyroidism and appropriate treatment of any nodules noted. Thyroidectomy is indicated for suspicion of malignancy, cosmetically unsightly goiters, and compressive symptoms.

BIBLIOGRAPHY

Heizmann O, Oertli D. Thyroiditis. In: Oertli D, Udelsman R (eds.), *Surgery of the Thyroid and Parathyroid Glands.* New York, NY: Springer; 2012:153–164.

Miller BS, Gauger PG. Thyroid gland. In: Mulholland MW, Lillemoe KD, Doherty GM, et al. (eds.), *Greenfield's Surgery: Scientific Principles and Practice,* 5th ed. Philadelphia, PA: Lippincott Williams & Wilkins; 2010:Chapter 75.

Parker C, Sterward D. The management of thyroiditis. In: Cameron JL, Cameron AM (eds.), *Current Surgical Therapy,* 11th ed. Philadelphia, PA: Elsevier; 2014:649–652.

19. **(D)** The patient described in the question has the classic findings of postpartum painless thyroiditis. This disease is characterized by lymphocytic inflammation of the thyroid after pregnancy. It occurs within 1 year of delivery in 2–16% of women and is more prevalent in women with known history of autoimmune disorders. It can cause transient or permanent thyroid dysfunction. The classic pattern begins with thyrotoxicosis. This usually is first seen 1–6 months after delivery and lasts for up to 2 months. This is followed by a hypothyroid phase that lasts between 4 and 6 months. A majority of women (80%) will return to a euthyroid state within a year of delivery. A small fraction of women develop persistent hypothyroidism.

On physical examination, patients will have a firm, nontender goiter. Thyroid peroxidase antibodies and thyroglobulin antibodies are elevated in 85% of these patients. If Graves is suspected, iodine uptake scan may be useful to distinguish painless postpartum thyroiditis (low uptake) from Graves disease (high uptake).

Treatment is usually not necessary for either the thyrotoxicosis or hypothyroid phases of the disease. If the patient does have a persistent hypothyroid state, replacement therapy is indicated. An attempt to discontinue thyroid hormone at 6–9 months should be done to determine if the patient has returned to a euthyroid state.

BIBLIOGRAPHY

Heizmann O, Oertli D. Thyroiditis. In: Oertli D, Udelsman R (eds.), *Surgery of the Thyroid and Parathyroid Glands.* New York, NY: Springer; 2012:153–164.

Parker C, Sterward D. The management of thyroiditis. In: Cameron JL, Cameron AM (eds.), *Current Surgical Therapy,* 11th ed. Philadelphia, PA: Elsevier; 2014:649–652.

20. **(B)** The anatomy of the parathyroid gland is variable, and a thorough understanding of the embryologic and adult anatomy is essential in locating the glands during difficult preservations or resections (see Fig. 12-13).

The usual pattern for parathyroid glands is two superior parathyroid glands and two inferior thyroid glands, with each gland weighing 30–50 mg. The glands are normally oval and flat but change into a more globular state when abnormal. The superior glands arise from the fourth pharyngeal pouch with the lateral thyroid. Their location tends to be more uniform; they are located on the posterior surface of the capsule of the upper pole of the thyroid in proximity to where the recurrent laryngeal nerve enters the larynx. The inferior glands arise from the third pharyngeal pouch. These glands are more variable and can be found from the pharynx to the

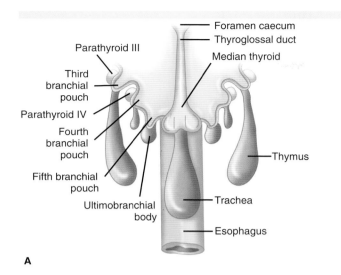

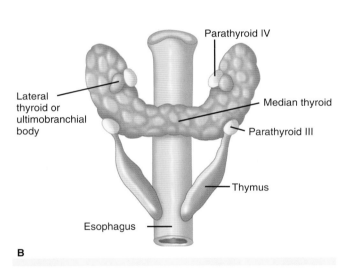

FIGURE 12-13. Parathyroid embryology. Reproduced with permission from Henry J. Applied embryology of the thyroid and parathyroid glands. In: Randolph G, ed. *Surgery of the Thyroid and Parathyroid Glands*. Philadelphia: W. B. Saunders Company; 2003. Copyright Elsevier.

mediastinum but are most often located near the inferior thyroid margin. Occasionally, the parathyroid gland will be found completely embedded in the body of the thyroid.

BIBLIOGRAPHY

Doherty GM. Parathyroid glands. In: Mulholland MW, Lillemoe KD, Doherty GM, et al. (eds.), *Greenfield's Surgery: Scientific Principles and Practice*, 5th ed. Philadelphia, PA: Lippincott Williams & Wilkins; 2010:Chapter 76.

Stewart WB, Rizzolo LJ. Embryology and surgical anatomy of the thyroid and parathyroid glands. In: Oertli D, Udelsman R (eds.), *Surgery of the Thyroid and Parathyroid Glands*. New York, NY: Springer; 2012:15-24.

21. **(A)** Parathyroid hormone (PTH), calcitonin, and vitamin D, in concert, regulate calcium homeostasis (see Fig. 12-14).

Under normal physiologic circumstances, PTH is released in response to hypocalcemia. The main physiologic response elicited by PTH is to increase plasma calcium levels. PTH has its primary physiologic effects on kidney and bone. In the kidney, PTH increases calcium

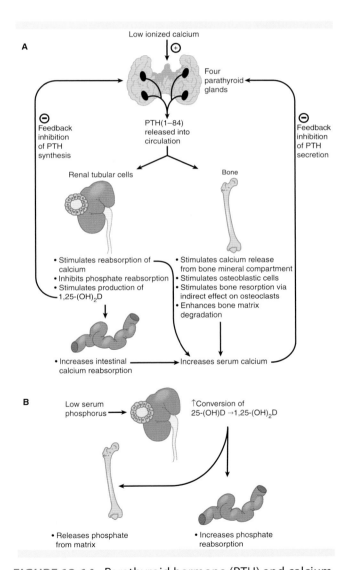

FIGURE 12-14. Parathyroid hormone (PTH) and calcium homeostasis. From McPhee S, Papadakis M. *Current Medical Diagnosis and Treatment 2011*. New York, NY: McGraw-Hill; 2010.

absorption and phosphate excretion. It also increases the activity of 1α-hydroxylase, the enzyme responsible for formation of the active form of vitamin D [1,25(OH)$_2$D]. The site of PTH regulation of Ca^{2+} reabsorption is the distal tubules.

In the bone, PTH binds osteoclast receptors and increases their function while inhibiting osteoblast function, resulting in rapid calcium release from bone matrix into the extracellular compartment.

In the intestine, PTH increases the absorption of calcium indirectly via vitamin D$_3$ activation. Cholecalciferol (vitamin D$_3$) is produced by the effect of sunlight on 7-dehydrocholesterol in the skin. Cholecalciferol is then hydroxylated to calcifediol (25-hydroxyvitamin D), and further hydroxylated to its active form of calcitriol (1,25-dihydroxyvitamin D). This activated form results in a greater absorption of calcium and phosphate from the intestine. PTH directly increases the hydroxylation of calcifediol to calcitriol.

BIBLIOGRAPHY

Brown EM, Arnold A. In: Oertli D, Udelsman R. *Surgery of the Thyroid and Parathyroid Glands*. New York, NY: Springer; 2012:413–432.

Doherty GM. Parathyroid glands. In: Mulholland MW, Lillemoe KD, Doherty GM, et al. (eds.), *Greenfield's Surgery: Scientific Principles and Practice*, 5th ed. Philadelphia, PA: Lippincott Williams & Wilkins; 2010:Chapter 76.

22. **(C)** Hypercalcemia occurs in 0.1–0.5% of the population, with the most common etiology in the outpatient setting being primary hyperparathyroidism (PHPT), present in approximately 1% of the population (incidence increases to 2% over the age of 55).

Hyperparathyroidism and resulting hypercalcemia affect several organ systems in the body. Renal symptoms develop because hypercalcemia leads to an increase in urinary calcium excretion and PTH increases the excretion of phosphate and produces urinary alkalosis. This combination increases risk of stone formation. Bone disease is a direct effect of PTH, causing bone resorption and resulting in osteopenia/osteoporosis. Gastrointestinal manifestations are general nonspecific complaints of nausea, constipation, and abdominal pain. In addition, although nonspecific, neurocognitive symptoms include fatigue, lethargy, confusion, memory loss, concentration issues, and depression. Cardiac effects can be seen on electrocardiogram showing shortened QT interval and widening of the T wave. When calcium levels are extremely elevated, bradycardia and complete heart block can be seen.

The only definitive treatment of primary hyperparathyroidism is surgical resection of the affected gland(s).

BIBLIOGRAPHY

Doherty GM. Parathyroid glands. In: Mulholland MW, Lillemoe KD, Doherty GM, et al. (eds.), *Greenfield's Surgery: Scientific Principles and Practice*, 5th ed. Philadelphia, PA: Lippincott Williams & Wilkins; 2010:Chapter 76.

Patel ND, Zeiger MA. Primary hyperparathyroidism. In: Cameron JL, Cameron AM (eds.), *Current Surgical Therapy*, 11th ed. Philadelphia, PA: Elsevier; 2014:666–673.

Stewart WB, Rizzolo LJ. Embryology and surgical anatomy of the thyroid and parathyroid glands. In: Oertli D, Udelsman R (eds.), *Surgery of the Thyroid and Parathyroid Glands*. New York, NY: Springer; 2012:15–24.

23. **(C)** In patients with primary hyperparathyroidism, medications that can cause increased calcium levels should be discontinued. Although certain diuretics (furosemide) can be used to decrease calcium levels, thiazides decrease the excretion of calcium, causing increased blood levels.

Intravenous hydration and furosemide will generally correct symptoms of hypercalcemia and decrease calcium levels in patients with hyperparathyroidism. Malignant hypercalcemia may be more difficult to manage and may require the use of bisphosphonates, which inhibit the action of osteoclasts and/or calcitonin. Calcitonin is a fairly poor hypercalcemic treatment agent but has a short time to onset of action and minimal adverse effects. Hemodialysis may also be used in refractory cases of hypercalcemia.

BIBLIOGRAPHY

Doherty GM. Parathyroid glands. In: Mulholland MW, Lillemoe KD, Doherty GM, et al. (eds.), *Greenfield's Surgery: Scientific Principles and Practice*, 5th ed. Philadelphia, PA: Lippincott Williams & Wilkins; 2010:Chapter 76.

24. **(D)** The patient described in the question has familial hypocalciuric hypercalcemia (FHH) disease. This is an autosomal dominant disease that expresses itself as an error in the calcium-sensing receptor (CASR). This will cause the baseline serum calcium level to be higher than normal. These patients are generally asymptomatic. Key laboratory findings include hypercalcemia, hypocalciuria, and normal to slightly elevated PTH levels.

The diagnosis of FHH is suspected when 24-hour urinary calcium is low despite the elevated blood levels of calcium. A calcium and creatinine ratio is then determined using the following equation:

$$(\text{Urinary calcium/PLASMA calcium}) \times (\text{Plasma creatinine/Urinary creatinine}) = \text{Ca/Cr clearance ratio}$$

If this ratio is 0.02 or less, then genetic counseling is warranted and genetic testing for mutations in the CASR gene may be recommended. Genetic testing is especially helpful in patients with a ratio between 0.01 and 0.02 where differentiating FHH from PHPT is not possible. It is important to identify patients with FHH, because they do not benefit from surgery.

BIBLIOGRAPHY

Doherty GM. Parathyroid glands. In: Mulholland MW, Lillemoe KD, Doherty GM, et al. (eds.), *Greenfield's Surgery: Scientific Principles and Practice*, 5th ed. Philadelphia, PA: Lippincott Williams & Wilkins; 2010:Chapter 76.

Patel ND, Zeiger MA. Primary hyperparathyroidism. In: Cameron JL, Cameron AM (eds.), *Current Surgical Therapy*, 11th ed. Philadelphia, PA: Elsevier; 2014:666–673.

25. **(A)** Primary hyperparathyroidism (PHPT) is defined as the autonomous secretion of PTH, resulting in hypercalcemia. This is the most common cause of hypercalcemia in the outpatient population. Women are two-thirds more likely to have PHPT.

The systemic manifestations of PHPT are due to hypercalcemia. Bone pain, fragility fractures, nephrolithiasis, proximal muscle weakness, depression, nausea, vomiting, concentration issues, irritability, and gastrointestinal symptoms can all result from elevated levels of calcium (see Fig. 12-15).

Laboratory tests will be able to reliably diagnose primary hyperparathyroidism. Elevated calcium levels along with elevated or inappropriately normal PTH levels confirm the diagnosis. Ionized calcium levels are useful in determining an accurate calcium level in patients with albumin fluctuations. Creatinine and vitamin D levels should be evaluated to exclude secondary hyperparathyroidism. All patients with hypercalcemia should have a 24-hour urinary calcium/creatinine ratio measured to rule out familial hypocalciuric hypercalcemia (FHH). This distinction is essential in making sure patients with FHH do *not* undergo parathyroidectomy, because surgery is not indicated.

The most common etiology of primary hyperparathyroidism is a single adenoma, which is found in 80–85% of patients.

BIBLIOGRAPHY

Doherty GM. Parathyroid glands. In: Mulholland MW, Lillemoe KD, Doherty GM, et al. (eds.), *Greenfield's Surgery: Scientific Principles and Practice*, 5th ed. Philadelphia, PA: Lippincott Williams & Wilkins; 2010:Chapter 76.

Patel ND, Zeiger MA. Primary hyperparathyroidism. In: Cameron JL, Cameron AM (eds.), *Current Surgical Therapy*, 11th ed. Philadelphia, PA: Elsevier; 2014:666–673.

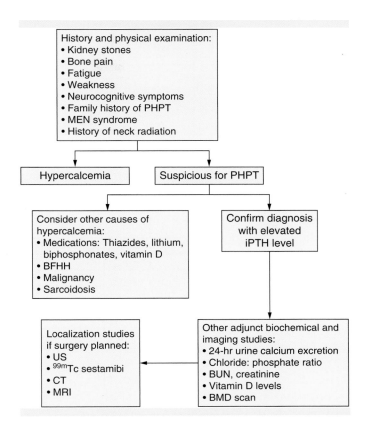

FIGURE 12-15. Diagnostic evaluation for patients with primary hyperparathyroidism (PHPT). BFHH, benign familial hypocalciuric hypercalcemia; BMD, bone mineral density; BUN, blood urea nitrogen; CT, computed tomography; iPTH, intact parathyroid hormone; MEN, multiple endocrine neoplasia; MRI, magnetic resonance imaging; PTH, parathyroid hormone; ^{99m}Tc, technetium pertechnetate; US, ultrasonography. From Morita S, Dackiw A, Zeiger M. *McGraw-Hill Manual: Endocrine Surgery.* New York, NY: McGraw-Hill; 2009.

26. **(C)** The approach to a patient with primary hyperparathyroidism is shown in Fig. 12-16.

In patients with otherwise asymptomatic primary hyperparathyroidism, indications for surgery include:

1. Age <50 years old

2. Calcium >1 mg/dL above normal

3. DEXA scan T-score <–2.5 indicating osteoporosis

4. Glomerular filtration rate <60 mL/min

5. Vertebral fractures on imaging (x-ray, CT, MRI)

6. 24-Hour urinary calcium >400 mg/d

7. Nephrolithiasis, nephrocalcinosis on imaging (ultrasound, x-ray, CT)

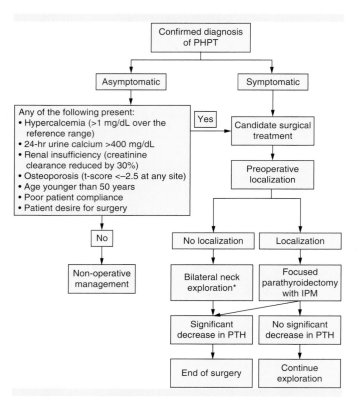

FIGURE 12-16. Management of patients with primary hyperparathyroidism (PHPT). *Jugular venous sampling. IPM, intraoperative parathyroid hormone monitoring; PTH, parathyroid hormone. From Morita S, Dackiw A, Zeiger M. *McGraw-Hill Manual: Endocrine Surgery.* New York, NY: McGraw-Hill; 2009.

Once the decision for surgical management has been made, localization studies aid in planning surgery. Given that 80–85% of patients have a single adenoma, minimally invasive parathyroidectomy can be performed using intra-operative PTH levels to verify biochemical cure.

A combination of studies gives the best chance of localizing the affected parathyroid. The most commonly used imaging studies are ultrasound, ^{99m}Tc-sestamibi scan, and CT. Sestamibi with single photon emission computed tomography (SPECT) can pick up abnormal parathyroid tissue in 80–90% of patients. It is limited in patients with smaller adenomas or in patients with thyroid nodules. Ultrasound is heavily operator- and equipment-dependent. When high-resolution equipment is used, sensitivity is 70–90% with a specificity of 90–98%. Ultrasound also has the benefit of giving more detailed anatomic information and being able to evaluate any possible thyroid nodules that may be present. If there is thyroid pathology that requires surgical intervention, it can be addressed concurrently with the parathyroid disease. When sestamibi and ultrasound are concordant, localization improves to 94–99%. Utilization of CT has

also increased, especially in the reoperative setting. A four-dimensional CT, consisting of precontrast, postcontrast, and delayed images, is particularly useful in identifying parathyroid adenomas. Reported sensitivity can be up to 88%, with a specificity of 92%.

BIBLIOGRAPHY

Patel ND, Zeiger MA. Primary hyperparathyroidism. In: Cameron JL, Cameron AM (eds.), *Current Surgical Therapy*, 11th ed. Philadelphia, PA: Elsevier; 2014:666–673.

Udelsman R, Akerstrom G, Biagini C, et al. The surgical management of asymptomatic primary hyperparathyroidism: proceedings of the Fourth International Workshop. *J Clin Endocrinol Metab* 2014;99:1–12.

27. **(C)** The figure presented in the question demonstrates parathyroid carcinoma, which is a rare cause of primary hyperparathyroidism (<1%). The diagnosis is made with evidence of invasion into surrounding structures. Parathyroid carcinoma is resistant to chemotherapy or radiation therapy; therefore, complete surgical resection is the only option for long-term cure.

Appropriate surgery includes en bloc resection of the affected parathyroid gland, thyroid lobe, cervical thymus, and central neck dissection. Lateral neck lymphadenectomy is generally not indicated unless grossly involved. Meticulous technique must be used to avoid rupture of the capsule to prevent tumor spillage, because it increases the risk of recurrence.

BIBLIOGRAPHY

Pasieka, JL, Khalil M. Parathyroid carcinoma. In: Oertli D, Udelsman R (eds.), *Surgery of the Thyroid and Parathyroid Glands.* New York, NY: Springer; 2012:537–554.

28. **(C)** Surgical exploration for primary hyperparathyroidism starts with a Kocher incision. The thyroid lobes are carefully rotated in a medial fashion, and the inferior thyroid artery and the recurrent laryngeal nerve are identified. The superior glands remain more constant and are usually found along the dorsal surface of the upper portion of the thyroid. The inferior glands are more variable in location. If the inferior glands are not visualized after initial exploration, the thymus must be pulled up and inspected (see Fig. 12-17).

The operation for a single adenoma is resection of the affected gland. Primary hyperparathyroidism caused by four-gland hyperplasia can be treated by subtotal parathyroidectomy (3.5 glands) or total parathyroidectomy with autotransplantation into brachioradialis of the nondominant arm. It is vital to leave approximately 40 mg of tissue. In the event that three normal glands are identified, but the

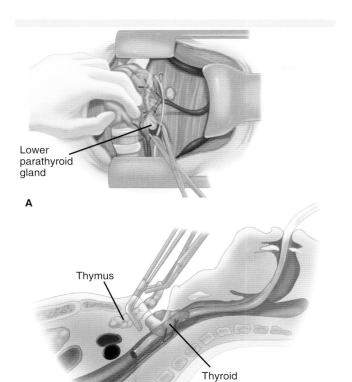

A

B

C

FIGURE 12-17. Exposure for parathyroidectomy. From Brunicardi F, Andersen DK, Billiar TR, et al. (eds.), *Schwartz's Principles of Surgery*, 10th ed. New York, NY: McGraw-Hill; 2014.

fourth parathyroid cannot be found, the upper pole should be mobilized and the entire dorsal surface must be palpated, as well as the retrolaryngeal, retrotracheal, and posterior mediastinal spaces. The most common locations of ectopic parathyroid glands are shown in Fig. 12-18.

If it is a lower parathyroid that is not found, transcervical thymectomy can be performed and thyroid lobectomy can be considered.

Sternotomy is not recommended at this point. Instead, the visualized glands are biopsied, the wound is closed, localization studies are obtained, and the patient is reexplored at a later date.

BIBLIOGRAPHY

Doherty GM. Parathyroid glands. In: Mulholland MW, Lillemoe KD, Doherty GM, et al. (eds.), *Greenfield's Surgery: Scientific Principles and Practice*, 5th ed. Philadelphia, PA: Lippincott Williams & Wilkins; 2010:Chapter 76.

Wu LS, Roman S. Conventional surgical management of primary hyperparathyroidism. In: Oertli D, Udelsman R (eds.), *Surgery of the Thyroid and Parathyroid Glands*. New York, NY: Springer; 2012:463–473.

29. **(E)** Bilateral cervical exploration is the gold standard in the treatment of primary hyperparathyroidism, though minimally invasive parathyroidectomy has gained widespread acceptance. If preoperative imaging is not possible or does not localize a parathyroid adenoma, a bilateral exploration should be performed. Although a history of ionizing radiation to the head/neck region does increase the incidence of multigland disease, a minimally invasive parathyroidectomy is acceptable if imaging successfully localizes the enlarged gland and intraoperative PTH confirms biochemical cure. Amiodarone does not induce hyperparathyroidism but may cause thyroiditis.

BIBLIOGRAPHY

Doherty GM. Parathyroid glands. In: Mulholland MW, Lillemoe KD, Doherty GM, et al. (eds.), *Greenfield's Surgery: Scientific Principles and Practice*, 5th ed. Philadelphia, PA: Lippincott Williams & Wilkins; 2010:Chapter 76.

Siperstein AE, Milas M. Comprehensive parathyroidectomy for the treatment of PHPT. Fischer JE, Jones DB, Pomposelli FB, et al. *Fischer's Master of Surgery*, 6th ed. Philadelphia, PA: Lippincott Williams & Wilkins; 2011:Chapter 39.

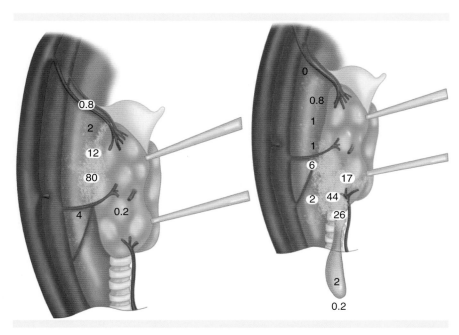

FIGURE 12-18. Location of ectopic upper and lower parathyroid glands. Reproduced with permission from Akerström G, et al. Surgical anatomy of human parathyroid glands. *Surgery*.1984;95:15. Copyright Elsevier.

CHAPTER 13

MULTIPLE ENDOCRINE NEOPLASIA

RACHEL MORRIS AND LILAH F. MORRIS

QUESTIONS

1. The gene involved in the pathogenesis of multiple endocrine neoplasia (MEN) type 2 syndromes is
   (A) *MEN1*
   (B) *RET*
   (C) *APC*
   (D) *P53*
   (E) None of the above

2. The chromosome carrying the gene associated with MEN1 is
   (A) Chromosome 14
   (B) Chromosome 13
   (C) Chromosome 12
   (D) Chromosome 11
   (E) Chromosome 10

3. What percentage of MEN1 patients develop hyperparathyroidism?
   (A) 10%
   (B) 30%
   (C) 60%
   (D) 75%
   (E) 95%

4. What is the most common presentation in MEN1 patients?
   (A) Pituitary adenoma
   (B) Primary hyperparathyroidism
   (C) Gastrinoma
   (D) Papillary thyroid cancer
   (E) Pheochromocytoma

5. A 35-year-old patient with recently diagnosed hyperparathyroidism (HPT) also gives a history of poorly controlled gastroesophageal reflux disease and chronic diarrhea. Fasting serum gastrin is 650 pg/mL. What is the expected response to a secretin test?
   (A) Increase in gastrin
   (B) No change in gastrin
   (C) Decreased gastrin
   (D) Secretin testing would not be relevant

6. MEN-associated gastrinomas are most frequently found in what anatomic location?
   (A) Head of the pancreas
   (B) Tail of the pancreas
   (C) Gastric antrum
   (D) Duodenum
   (E) Jejunum

7. A 40-year-old man has recently been diagnosed with sporadic HPT. Compared to MEN1-associated HPT, this patient's disease is most likely to involve
   (A) A single parathyroid gland
   (B) All four parathyroid glands
   (C) The thyroid gland
   (D) The pituitary gland
   (E) None of the above

8. A 50-year-old man with a recently diagnosed gastrinoma is noted to have a serum calcium of 12.5 mg/dL. A serum PTH level is drawn and found to be elevated. Although proton pump inhibitors have been prescribed, the patient has persistent reflux symptoms. The next most appropriate step in managing this patient's reflux symptoms would be
   (A) Total parathyroidectomy with autotransplantation
   (B) Sestamibi scan
   (C) Addition of an H2 blocker
   (D) Distal pancreatectomy
   (E) Highly selective vagotomy

9. Which patient should undergo genetic testing for MEN1?
   (A) A 58-year-old woman with newly diagnosed hyperparathyroidism
   (B) A 60-year-old man with metastatic pancreatic adenocarcinoma
   (C) A 12-year-old girl with medullary thyroid cancer
   (D) A 21-year-old woman with a calcium level of 11.8 mg/dL
   (E) None of the above

10. In MEN1, the most common pancreaticoduodenal tumors are
    (A) Gastrinomas
    (B) Nonfunctioning tumors
    (C) Insulinomas
    (D) Somatostatinomas
    (E) VIPomas

11. A male patient with a pituitary neoplasm in the setting MEN1 would be most likely to present with which of the following clinical findings?
    (A) Galactorrhea
    (B) Hypogonadism
    (C) Abdominal striae
    (D) Hyperthyroidism
    (E) Acral enlargement

12. Medullary thyroid cancer associated with MEN2 syndromes
    (A) Is more aggressive in MEN2B than MEN2A and most often unilateral
    (B) Is more aggressive in MEN2B than MEN2A and most often bilateral
    (C) Is more aggressive in MEN2A than MEN2B and most often unilateral
    (D) Is more aggressive in MEN2A than MEN2B and most often bilateral
    (E) None of the above

13. Medullary thyroid cancer accounts for what percentage of all thyroid malignancies?
    (A) 5–10%
    (B) 15–20%
    (C) 25–30%
    (D) 35–40%
    (E) 45–50%

14. What percentage of Medullary thyroid cancers are familial?
    (A) 10%
    (B) 25%
    (C) 40%
    (D) 65%
    (E) 80%

15. A 22-year-old woman is being evaluated for a multinodular thyroid noted on physical examination by her primary physician. She also gives a recent history of "terrible headaches" and anxiety. She is noted to have a serum calcitonin level of 1400 pg/mL. Which of the following is the most important laboratory test to perform prior to any surgical intervention?
    (A) Serum calcium
    (B) Serum parathyroid hormone level
    (C) 24-hour urine catecholamines
    (D) Serum thyroid-stimulating hormone (TSH) and free T_4 levels
    (E) Serum phosphorous

16. A 17-year-old woman is diagnosed with medullary thyroid cancer (MTC) in a 2-cm nodule in the right thyroid lobe. She has no evidence of lymphadenopathy on preoperative imaging. Preoperative *RET* testing is positive for MEN2A. What operation should be performed?
    (A) There is no effective surgical therapy for MTC
    (B) Right thyroid lobectomy
    (C) Total thyroidectomy
    (D) Total thyroidectomy with bilateral central lymph node dissection
    (E) Total thyroidectomy with central lymph node dissection and right-sided modified radical neck dissection

17. Which of the following is most likely to be associated with MEN2B?
    (A) Hyperparathyroidism
    (B) Ganglioneuromas
    (C) Obesity
    (D) Pituitary adenoma
    (E) Retinoblastoma

18. A 45-year-old man presents to your office with a history of MTC. He underwent total thyroidectomy 4 years ago. He now presents with poorly controlled hypertension, severe paroxysmal headaches, and palpitations. Urinary catecholamines are elevated, and magnetic resonance imaging of the abdomen is performed as shown in Fig. 13-1.
    Which of the following medications should be initiated on this visit?
    (A) Esmolol
    (B) Sodium nitroprusside
    (C) Isoproterenol
    (D) Phenoxybenzamine
    (E) Calcium gluconate

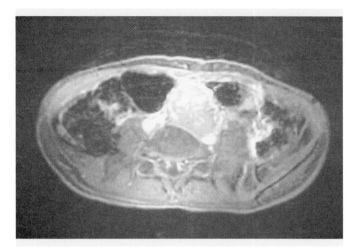

FIGURE 13-1. Magnetic resonance imaging of the abdomen.

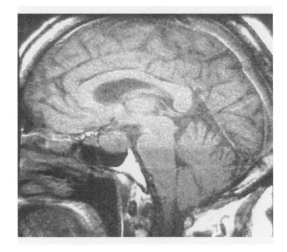

FIGURE 13-2. Magnetic resonance image of the brain.

19. A 24-year-old woman presents to her physician complaining of intermittent fatigue, confusion, and diaphoresis. She states that these symptoms are especially prominent on waking in the morning but seem to get better after she has her usual glass of orange juice. Routine laboratory workup reveals hypercalcemia, an elevated parathyroid hormone (PTH) level, and no other abnormalities. A monitored 24-hour fast reproduces her symptoms. Laboratory analysis while she is symptomatic reveals an inappropriately elevated serum insulin level and a corresponding blood glucose of 48 mg/dL. A 1.7-cm tumor in the head of the pancreas is found on computed tomography (CT) scan. What is the most appropriate surgical management?
    (A) Pancreaticoduodenectomy
    (B) Total pancreatectomy
    (C) Distal pancreatectomy with enucleation of grossly visible tumor in the head of the pancreas
    (D) Simple enucleation of grossly visible tumor
    (E) No surgery is indicated

20. A 37-year-old nonlactating woman presents to her primary care physician complaining of milky discharge from both breasts. Initial workup reveals an elevated prolactin level as well as elevated serum calcium and serum parathyroid hormone levels. The patient is currently asymptomatic with regard to her hypercalcemia. Magnetic resonance imaging (MRI) of the brain is shown in Fig. 13-2.
    The most appropriate initial therapy for this problem is
    (A) Bromocriptine therapy
    (B) Transsphenoidal resection
    (C) Carbidopa/levodopa therapy
    (D) Octreotide therapy
    (E) Radiation therapy

21. A 31-year-old pregnant woman who has undergone total thyroidectomy for medullary thyroid cancer with a history of a MEN2B mutation presents to your office inquiring about prophylactic treatment for her baby. The most appropriate recommendation is
    (A) Total thyroidectomy in the first 6 months of life
    (B) Total thyroidectomy before age 5
    (C) Total thyroidectomy by age 20
    (D) No surgical treatment is necessary
    (E) Yearly serum calcitonin measurement starting at age 2

ANSWERS AND EXPLANATIONS

1. **(B)** MEN2 syndromes are characterized by the presence of medullary thyroid cancer (MTC) and pheochromocytomas. The MEN2A variant is further characterized by primary hyperparathyroidism (HPT). MEN2B, on the other hand, is notable for mucosal and musculoskeletal abnormalities, which include neuromas of the mouth and lips, "marfanoid" habitus, and ganglioneuromatosis of the bowel myenteric and submucosal plexus. Additional abnormalities associated with MEN2B include congenital hip dislocation, pes cavus, pectus excavatum, and kyphosis. Both MEN2 syndromes are inherited in an autosomal dominant fashion with nearly 100% penetrance but varying degrees of expressivity. Mutations in the *RET* (*re*arranged *during transfection*) proto-oncogene, which maps to chromosome 10, have been identified in individuals with MEN2 syndromes. This gene encodes a receptor tyrosine kinase important in transmembrane signal transduction.

MEN2A variants are characterized by mutations in one of five codons, which specify highly conserved cysteine residues in the extracellular domain (see Fig. 13-3).

In the nonmutated *RET* gene, two cysteine residues are juxtaposed and a resultant disulfide bond is formed. When the *RET* gene is mutated such that one of these cysteine residue is replaced, the free remaining cysteine residue is available to form a disulfide bond with a cysteine residue of a neighboring receptor. When this aberrant disulfide bond is formed, dimerizing the two receptors, the result is a constitutively activated tyrosine kinase and unopposed signal transduction (see Fig. 13-4).

In contrast to MEN2A, MEN2B variants are characterized by a single point mutation in the catalytic domain of the *RET* gene product. This mutation, specifying

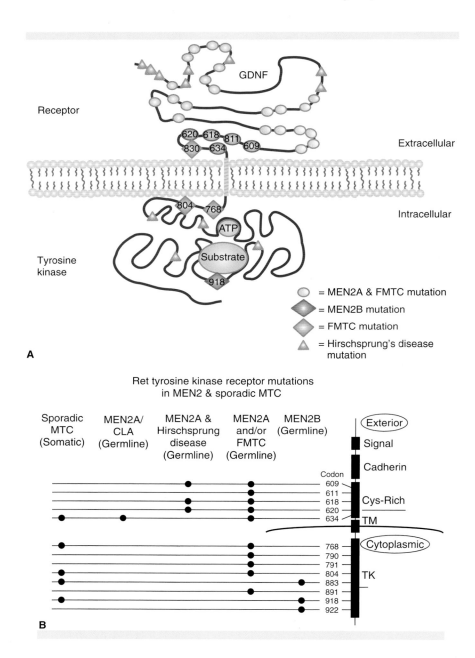

FIGURE 13-3. Structure of the RET tyrosine kinase receptor. *RET* mutations in multiple endocrine neoplasia (MEN) type 2 **(A)** and sporadic medullary thyroid cancer (MTC) **(B)**. CLA, cutaneous lichen amyloidosis; FMTC, familial medullary thyroid cancer. **A** Reproduced with permission from Wells S and Franz C: Medullary carcinoma of the thyroid. *World J Surg* 24:954, 2000, Springer-Verlag.

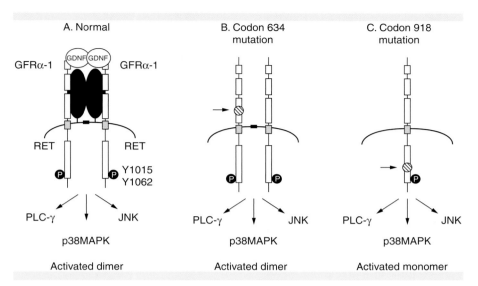

FIGURE 13-4. *RET* mutations in the cysteine-rich extracellular domain lead to dimerization and constitutive activation, whereas mutations in the intracellular domain result in changed substrate specificity.

replacement of a methionine with a threonine residue at the tyrosine kinase domain, occurs most frequently at codon 918 and results in changed substrate specificity.

In both MEN2 syndromes, there seems to be a strong correlation between disease phenotype and mutation at a specific codon. This seems to be especially true with regard to prediction of pheochromocytomas and HPT and may offer clinicians valuable information in disease treatment and surveillance among kindred of MEN2 patients.

BIBLIOGRAPHY

Carling T, Roman SA. Multiple endocrine neoplasia type 2. In: Morita SY, Dackiw AB, Zeiger MA (eds.), *McGraw-Hill Manual: Endocrine Surgery*. New York, NY: McGraw-Hill; 2010:Chapter 22.

Gagel RF, Marx SJ. Multiple endocrine neoplasia. In: Larsen PR, Kronenberg HM, Shlomo M, Polonsky KS (eds.), *Williams Textbook of Endocrinology*, 10th ed. Philadelphia, PA: W. B. Saunders; 2003:1741.

Larsen PR, Kronenberg HM, Melmed S, Polonsky KS (eds.). *Williams Textbook of Endocrinology*, 10th ed. Philadelphia, PA: W. B. Saunders; 2003:51–52, 1741–1742.

Lal G, Clark OH. Thyroid, parathyroid, and adrenal. In: Brunicardi F, Andersen DK, Billiar TR, et al. (eds.), *Schwartz's Principles of Surgery*, 9th ed. New York, NY: McGraw-Hill; 2010:Chapter 38.

Yip L, Cote GJ, Shapiro SE, et al. Multiple endocrine neoplasia type 2: evaluation of the genotype-phenotype relationship. *Arch Surg* 2003;138(4):409–416.

2. **(D)** MEN1 is characterized by the presence of HPT, adenomas of the anterior pituitary, and neuroendocrine tumors (NETs) of the pancreas and duodenum.

Clinically overt disease is usually recognized between the third and fifth decades; however, laboratory abnormalities are frequently apparent much earlier. Like MEN2 syndromes, MEN1 is inherited in an autosomal dominant fashion. The gene responsible for MEN1 has been mapped to chromosome 11 and codes for a 610–amino acid protein called menin, which consists of 10 exons, only nine of which are translated during creation of an mRNA transcript. The gene product is ubiquitously expressed in many tissues, most notably thymus, thyroid, and pancreas. Although recognized for its importance in the pathogenesis of MEN1, the precise function of the menin protein is not well understood and is an area of active research.

In contrast to *RET*, which requires only a single mutated gene in order to produce MEN2 syndromes, *MEN1* follows the so-called "two-hit" hypothesis of tumorigenesis, requiring both an inherited faulty copy of the gene as well as a second somatic mutation in order to produce disease. *MEN1* is a tumor-suppressor gene, coding for a nuclear protein. The second hit in approximately 90% of MEN patients involves chromosomal deletions at the 11q13 locus; however, some studies have shown other somatic mutations in the remaining MEN1 patients, even in the absence of 11q13 deletions.

BIBLIOGRAPHY

Norton JA, Bollinger RR, Chang AE, et al. (eds.), *Surgery: Basic Science and Clinical Evidence*. New York, NY: Springer-Verlag; 2000:955–966.

Pannett AA, Thakker RV. Somatic mutations in MEN type 1 tumors, consistent with the Knudsen "two-hit" hypothesis. *J Clin Endocrinol Metab* 2001;86(9):4371–4374.

Skogseid B. Multiple endocrine neoplasia type 1. *Br J Surg* 2003;90(4):383–385.

3. **(E)** Primary hyperparathyroidism is the first and most common clinical manifestation of MEN1. Approximately 95% of MEN1 patients are affected by primary hyperparathyroidism. Sporadic primary hyperparathyroidism is most common in women in the fifth to seventh decades of life, with 85% of patients having a single adenoma. MEN1-associated primary hyperparathyroidism occurs equally in men and women, typically presents in the teens, is a multiglandular disease with nodular hyperplasia, is associated with ectopic and supernumerary glands, and frequently recurs. Indications for parathyroidectomy are the same in sporadic and MEN1-associated disease.

BIBLIOGRAPHY

Brandi ML, Gagel RF, Angeli A, et al. Guidelines for diagnosis and therapy of MEN type 1 and type 2. *J Clin Endocrinol Metab* 2001;86(12):5658–5671.

Lal G, Clark OH. Thyroid, parathyroid, and adrenal. In: Brunicardi F, Andersen DK, Billiar TR, et al. (eds.), *Schwartz's Principles of Surgery*, 9th ed. New York, NY: McGraw-Hill; 2010:Chapter 38.

Thakker RV, Newey PJ, Walls GV, et al. Clinical practice guidelines for MEN1. *J Clin Endocrinol Metab* 2012;97:2990–3011.

4. **(B)** MEN1 most commonly presents between 20 and 40 years of age, but mutations are highly penetrant; 50% of carriers are symptomatic by 20 years of age, and >95% are symptomatic by 50 years of age. The disease equally affects men and women and individuals of different ethnic and racial backgrounds. Incidence ranges from 1/10,000 to 1/100,000. As mentioned earlier, among those with MEN1, nearly 95% are diagnosed with HPT by 50 years of age, making this the most common manifestation of MEN1.

MEN1 neoplasias affect an entire tissue type. Thus, although 85% of patients with sporadic primary hyperparathyroidism have a single hyperfunctioning adenoma, all patients with MEN1-associated primary hyperparathyroidism have multigland hyperplastic disease (see Fig. 13-5), frequently associated with supernumerary glands. These patients require a standard bilateral neck exploration in order to visualize all parathyroid glands. The surgical procedure of choice is a matter of controversy. Some surgeons advocate subtotal parathyroidectomy, leaving behind a remnant of parathyroid tissue. Others prefer total parathyroidectomy with autotransplantation of a

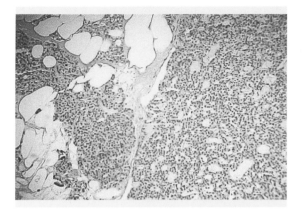

FIGURE 13-5. Histologic representation of parathyroid hyperplasia.

portion of parathyroid tissue to the forearm. The latter procedure may preclude the morbidity associated with reexploration of the neck should the patient manifest persistent or recurrent HPT requiring surgical intervention, but leaves the patient at risk for permanent aparathyroidism. In both procedures, a bilateral cervical thymectomy is also performed to remove any potential ectopic parathyroid tissue. Additionally, because both of the previously mentioned procedures carry a risk of postoperative hypoparathyroidism, some advocate cryopreservation of resected parathyroid tissue in anticipation of a future need for autotransplantation.

BIBLIOGRAPHY

Brandi ML, Gagel RF, Angeli A, et al. Guidelines for diagnosis and therapy of MEN type 1 and type 2. *J Clin Endocrinol Metab* 2001;86(12):5658–5671.

Goldman L, Bennett JC (eds.). *Cecil Textbook of Medicine*, 21st ed. Philadelphia, PA: W. B. Saunders; 2000:1402–1403.

Lambert LA, Shapiro SE, Lee JE, et al. Surgical treatment of hyperparathyroidism in patients with multiple endocrine neoplasia type 1. *Arch Surg* 2005;140:374–382.

Larsen PR, Kronenberg HM, Melmed S, Polonsky KS (eds.). *Williams Textbook of Endocrinology*, 10th ed. Philadelphia, PA: W. B. Saunders; 2003:1292–1294.

5. **(A)** Developing in 30–80% of MEN1 patients, neuroendocrine tumors (NETs) of the pancreas and duodenum constitute the second most common manifestation of MEN1 after HPT. The majority of these tumors are nonfunctioning. Among functional tumors, the two most common are gastrinoma and insulinoma. Among MEN1 patients with functional neuroendocrine pancreaticoduodenal tumors, approximately 47% have gastrinomas and 12% have insulinomas. Other rare functional NETs

include VIPomas and somatostatinomas. One-fourth of patients with gastrinoma will have MEN1. Patients with gastrinoma typically present with Zollinger-Ellison syndrome (ZES). The most common manifestations include epigastric pain and reflux esophagitis because of increased gastric acid secretion. Also noteworthy is the presence of a secretory diarrhea in many patients with gastrinoma, and in some patients, this may be the only symptom.

Patients with suspected gastrinoma should have a serum gastrin level drawn. Fasting serum gastrin levels greater than 100 pg/mL are concerning for gastrinoma and should prompt a secretin test to confirm the diagnosis. Serum gastrin levels >1000 pg/mL with a gastric pH <2 are virtually diagnostic of ZES. The secretin test is performed by measuring serum gastrin levels after administration of 2 U/kg of secretin intravenously (IV). Infusion of secretin normally diminishes serum gastrin levels. A positive secretin test is confirmed by an increase in serum gastrin to at least 200 pg/mL above the basal value.

MEN1-associated gastrinomas are malignant in a majority of cases with a tendency to metastasize to liver, lymphatics, and bone. Liver metastases may ultimately lead to death in a subset of this patient population with aggressive tumor growth. Initial therapy in all gastrinomas is directed toward control of gastric acid hypersecretion.

Unfortunately, gastrinomas are rarely amenable to curative resection because they are typically multifocal. Extrapancreatic tumors are found most frequently within the duodenal wall with more than 90% of duodenal gastrinomas occurring in the first or second portions of the duodenum. MEN-associated gastrinomas may also be found within peripancreatic lymph nodes. The multifocal nature of MEN1-associated gastrinomas stands in contrast to sporadic gastrinomas, which are more likely to be solitary tumors. For these reasons, curative surgical resection is most frequently undertaken in sporadic ZES. Surgical management of gastrinomas in MEN1 patients with a goal of cure is more controversial. Some advocate resection for cure, whereas others argue for wide local excision only as a palliative debulking procedure or in an attempt to limit ongoing metastatic spread.

BIBLIOGRAPHY

Dickson PV, Rich TA, Xing Y, et al. Achieving eugastrinemia in MEN1 patients: both duodenal inspection and formal lymph node dissection are important. *Surgery* 2011;150(6):1143–1152.

Fathia G, Venzon DJ, Ojeaburu JV, et al. Prospective study of the natural history of gastrinoma in patients with MEN1: definition of an aggressive and a nonaggressive form. *J Clin Endocrinol Metab* 2001;86(11):5282–5293.

Feldman M, Tschumy WO, Friedman LS, Sleisinger MH (eds.). *Sleisinger and Fordtran's Gastrointestinal and Liver Disease: Pathophysiology, Diagnosis, Management*, 7th ed. Philadelphia, PA: W. B. Saunders; 2002:782–792.

6. **(D)** The majority of gastrinomas occur within the so-called gastrinoma triangle. This space is bounded by the confluence of the cystic and common hepatic ducts superiorly, the junction of the head and neck of the pancreas medially, and the junction of the second and third portions of the duodenum inferiorly (see Fig. 13-6).

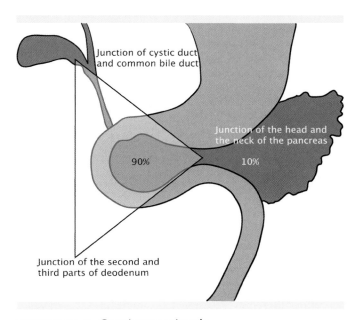

FIGURE 13-6. Gastrinoma triangle.

Both sporadic and MEN-associated gastrinomas occur most frequently within the pancreas and duodenum. Although there seems to be an equal number occurring in each of these two locales when all gastrinomas are considered, evidence suggests MEN-associated disease has a predilection for the duodenum, with upward of 80% being found in the duodenal wall. When occurring within the duodenal wall, gastrinomas are found most frequently within the first and second portions of the duodenum. Gastrinomas have also been found in the peripancreatic lymph nodes as well as in ectopic locations such as ovary, liver, common bile duct, and gastric pylorus. As noted in previous discussions, MEN-associated gastrinomas tend to be multifocal, making curative resection difficult.

BIBLIOGRAPHY

Feldman M, Tschumy WO, Friedman LS, Sleisenger MH (eds.). *Sleisenger and Fordtran's Gastrointestinal and Liver Disease: Pathophysiology, Diagnosis, Management*, 7th ed. Philadelphia, PA: W. B. Saunders; 2002:782–792.

Harvey A, Berber E. Gastrinoma. In: Morita SY, Dackiw AB, Zeiger MA (eds.), *McGraw-Hill Manual: Endocrine Surgery*. New York, NY: McGraw-Hill; 2010:Chapter 18.

7. **(A)** Sporadic primary HPT is clinically distinct from its MEN-associated counterpart. One of the ways in which these two entities differ is in the number of glands involved. Whereas MEN-associated disease affects all parathyroid tissue causing multiglandular parathyroid hyperplasia, sporadic primary HPT tends to involve only a single gland.

The difference in number of glands involved in sporadic versus MEN-associated disease has important implications for surgical management of patients with primary HPT. In MEN-associated HPT, most surgeons advocate subtotal or total parathyroidectomy. The specifics of which procedure to perform in MEN-associated disease, however, are controversial. Some surgeons advocate total parathyroidectomy with autotransplantation, while others prefer subtotal or 3½ gland parathyroidectomy.

MEN1 is a disease of all parathyroid tissue, requiring a subtotal or total parathyroidectomy with concomitant bilateral cervical thymectomy. In contrast, surgical therapy for sporadic adenomas may be directed at removal of the single adenomatous gland. A more targeted operation is directed by sestamibi scanning and/or CT scanning. Sestamibi scanning using technetium-99m (^{99m}Tc) sestamibi, which is taken up by parathyroid tissue, will localize 70–80% of enlarged and hyperfunctional parathyroid glands. Such localization may then allow dissection of a limited area of the neck. Decrease of intraoperative PTH by 50% or more at 10 minutes following resection of all abnormal parathyroid tissue may be used to confirm surgical cure. Failure of intraoperative PTH test levels to fall both into the normal range and also to levels less than one-half of preoperative levels may suggest the need for further neck exploration.

BIBLIOGRAPHY

Augustine MM, Bravo PE, Zeiger MA. Surgical treatment of primary hyperparathyroidism. *Endocr Pract* 2011;17(Suppl 1):75–82.

Katai M. Primary hyperparathyroidism in patients with multiple endocrine neoplasia type 1: comparison with sporadic hyperparathyroidism. *Horm Metab Res* 2001;33(8):499–503.

8. **(A)** The majority of gastrinomas are sporadic and account for approximately 75% of all patients with Zollinger-Ellison syndrome. However, nearly one-fourth of patients with gastrinomas have a genetic syndrome.

HPT is the most common abnormality in patients with MEN1. Present in virtually all MEN1 patients by 50 years of age, this endocrinopathy leads to elevated serum calcium in the setting of an inappropriately elevated parathyroid hormone level. NETs of the pancreas and duodenum, with gastrinomas being the most common, develop in 30–80% of MEN1 patients. The third type of endocrinopathy associated with MEN1 is anterior pituitary adenoma, developing in 15–50% of MEN1 patients. Prolactinomas constitute the most frequent type of pituitary neoplasm in this setting.

This patient has both a gastrinoma and a laboratory diagnosis of HPT, strongly suggesting a diagnosis of MEN1. When these two endocrinopathies coexist, the hypercalcemia of HPT actually can lead to increased gastrin secretion. This, in turn, may make management of symptoms associated with gastrinoma more difficult. For this reason, surgical treatment of HPT is advocated as part of the initial treatment of gastrinoma. If normocalcemia can be achieved, gastrin secretion decreases, basal acid output diminishes, and the symptoms of marginally controlled reflux frequently improve.

Although there is some controversy among parathyroid surgeons regarding which procedure to perform for MEN-associated HPT, the most appropriate option listed earlier would be total parathyroidectomy with autotransplantation. This procedure is performed through a cervical neck incision. A bilateral neck exploration is done with identification and removal of all four parathyroid glands. A transcervical thymectomy is also performed.

BIBLIOGRAPHY

Brandi ML, Gagel RF, Angeli A, et al. Guidelines for diagnosis and therapy of MEN type 1 and type 2. *J Clin Endocrinol Metab* 2001;86(12):5658–5671.

Norton JA, Bollinger RR, Chang AE, et al. (eds.). *Surgery: Basic Science and Clinical Evidence*. New York, NY: Springer-Verlag; 2000:955–966.

9. **(D)** As noted previously, the gene responsible for MEN1 is located on chromosome 11q13 and codes for a protein called menin. Although the precise function of menin is poorly understood, this 610–amino acid protein is thought to play a role in cell growth and proliferation via interaction with the transcription factor JunD, nuclear factor-κB, and other proteins.

Since identification of the gene associated with MEN1, attention has been directed toward genetic testing and screening, which might allow earlier identification and treatment of patients with the disease. Identification has been made possible through direct DNA sequencing techniques and haplotype analysis in connection with biochemical and imaging tests. Genetic testing should be considered in patients with a suspicious family history, multiple MEN1-associated disease processes, or young age of presentation with primary hyperparathyroidism.

When genetic testing reveals definite or probable MEN1 mutations, more frequent biochemical testing for malignant tumors should be undertaken, although no formal protocol has been developed. Close observation has been shown to increase detection of biochemical abnormalities associated with neoplasias. When genetic testing is inconclusive or there is a high clinical suspicion, patients should also have increased surveillance performed.

BIBLIOGRAPHY

Brandi ML, Gagel RF, Angeli A, et al. Guidelines for diagnosis and therapy of MEN type 1 and type 2. *J Clin Endocrinol Metab* 2001:86(12);5658–5671.

Lal G, Clark OH. Thyroid, parathyroid, and adrenal. In: Brunicardi F, Andersen DK, Billiar TR, et al. (eds.), *Schwartz's Principles of Surgery*, 9th ed. New York, NY: McGraw-Hill; 2010:Chapter 38.

Thakkar RV, Newey PJ, Walls GV, et al. Clinical practice guidelines for MEN1. *J Clin Endocrinol Metab* 2012;97:2990–3011.

Townsend CM (ed.). *Sabiston Textbook of Surgery: The Biological Basis of Modern Surgical Practice*, 16th ed. Philadelphia, PA: W. B. Saunders; 2001:697–707.

Whaley J, Lairmore TC. Multiple endocrine neoplasia type 1. In: Morita SY, Dackiw AB, Zeiger MA (eds.), *McGraw-Hill Manual: Endocrine Surgery*. New York, NY: McGraw-Hill; 2010:Chapter 21.

10. **(B)** NETs of the pancreas and duodenum are the second most common endocrinopathy associated with MEN1, occurring in anywhere from 30–80% of all patients with this syndrome. Gastrinomas, accounting for 47% of MEN-associated, functional pancreaticoduodenal tumors, lead to hypergastrinemia and Zollinger-Ellison syndrome; however, the most common type of NET is nonfunctional. These nonfunctional tumors produce symptoms by exerting mass effect on surrounding structures.

Other common types of NETs of the pancreas and duodenum in MEN include gastrinoma and insulinoma. These two tumor types account for the majority of functional enteropancreatic NETs in MEN1, comprising 47% and 12% of functional tumors, respectively. MEN1-associated pancreatic tumors produce a field defect; they affect all pancreatic tissue, so resection is reserved for symptom control. MEN1-associated gastrinomas tend to be aggressive, with up to 50% presenting with metastases to the liver. Functional NETs secreting vasoactive intestinal peptide (VIP), glucagon, or somatostatin are decidedly less common.

BIBLIOGRAPHY

Akerström G, Stålberg P. Surgical management of MEN-1 and -2: state of the art. *Surg Clin North Am* 2009;89(5):1047–1068.

Norton JA, Bollinger RR, Chang AE, et al. (eds.). *Surgery: Basic Science and Clinical Evidence*. New York, NY: Springer-Verlag; 2000:955–966.

Townsend CM (ed.). *Sabiston Textbook of Surgery: The Biological Basis of Modern Surgical Practice*, 16th ed. Philadelphia, PA: W. B. Saunders; 2001:629–645, 697–707.

11. **(B)** Pituitary neoplasms are the third most frequent type of tumor associated with MEN1, affecting approximately 50% of patients with the disease. The most common type of functional pituitary adenoma is a prolactinoma, accounting for approximately 62% of MEN1-associated pituitary adenomas. The next most common type of pituitary adenoma is growth hormone–secreting adenomas, accounting for 10% pituitary adenomas. Other functional pituitary tumor types include adrenocorticotropic hormone (ACTH)–producing tumors and "cosecreting" adenomas, which release multiple substances. Pituitary adenomas may also become symptomatic due to mass effect, including compression of the optic chiasm, which may cause visual field defects. Finally, in rare cases, an enlarging pituitary adenoma may cause hypopituitarism by compression of the adjacent normal gland.

According to one multicenter study, the mean age of patients diagnosed with MEN1-associated pituitary disease was 38 years old, with 25% of patients diagnosed by age 26. There was a near 2:1 female predominance. The vast majority (85%) are macroadenomas. MEN1-associated pituitary adenomas are associated with mutation of a tumor-suppressor protein called menin located at chromosome location 11q13. This is in contradistinction to sporadic pituitary adenomas, which do not appear to share the same mechanism of tumorigenesis.

Males and females with prolactinomas may present in very different ways despite a common pathology. Women who have prolactinomas typically present with amenorrhea or galactorrhea. In contrast, men with prolactin-secreting tumors typically present with hypogonadism.

BIBLIOGRAPHY

Goldman L, Bennett JC (eds.). *Cecil Textbook of Medicine*, 21st ed. Philadelphia, PA: W. B. Saunders; 2000:1210–1212.

Larsen PR, Kronenberg HM, Melmed S, Polonsky KS (eds.). *Williams Textbook of Endocrinology*, 10th ed. Philadelphia, PA: W. B. Saunders; 2003:184–185.

Thakker RV, Newey PJ, Walls GV, et al. Clinical practice guidelines for multiple endocrine neoplasia type 1 (MEN1). *J Clin Endocrinol Metab* 2012;97(9):2990–3011.

Townsend CM (ed.). *Sabiston Textbook of Surgery: The Biological Basis of Modern Surgical Practice*, 16th ed. Philadelphia, PA: W. B. Saunders; 2001:629–645, 697–707.

Verges B, Boureille F, Goudet P, et al. Pituitary disease in MEN type 1: data from the France-Belgium MEN1 multicenter study. *J Clin Endocrinol Metab* 2002;87(2):457–465.

12. **(B)** MTC is a tumor of the parafollicular cells of the thyroid gland, which secrete calcitonin. Accounting for 10% of all thyroid malignancies, MTC is a feature common to both MEN2 syndromes with a penetrance of greater than 90%. Although, sporadic MTC accounts for 75% of all MTC cases, familial forms are a significant source of morbidity and mortality among this patient population. All patients diagnosed with medullary thyroid cancer should undergo genetic (*RET*) testing. MTC is generally the first manifestation of MEN2 and the major cause of death of those with these syndromes.

In contrast to sporadic MTC, where the tumors tend to be unilateral and unifocal, MEN2-associated MTC tends to be bilateral and multifocal. Furthermore, whereas onset of sporadic disease tends to occur in the fifth and sixth decades of life, hereditary MTC tends to occur much earlier. This seems to be especially true in MEN2B where disease may be diagnosed as early as 2 years of age, with metastasis already having occurred in upward of 70% of patients at the time of diagnosis.

This difference in clinical behavior, with MEN2B being far more aggressive, can likely be attributed to differing mutations in the RET protein, a tyrosine kinase that regulates cell growth. In fact, although MEN2 syndromes, as well as the closely related familial medullary thyroid cancer (FMTC), all share a mutated *RET* proto-oncogene in their pathogenesis, the location of this mutation within the protein can vary from syndrome to syndrome. For example, in MEN2A, mutations most often affect one of five cysteine residues at codons 609, 611, 618, 620, or 634. These codons correlate to portions of the extracellular domain of the *RET* proto-oncogene, and mutations likely alter ligand binding. In MEN2B, however, mutations involving a methionine residue at codon 918, which corresponds to a portion of the intracellular domain, have been most commonly implicated.

Total thyroidectomy is recommended for all patients with any hereditary MTC in light of its propensity for multifocality and bilateral gland involvement. Furthermore, early, elective total thyroidectomy is advocated in the treatment of MEN2 patients diagnosed by genetic screening before gross disease is evident. Surgery between the ages of 5 and 10 years is recommended in patients carrying MEN2A mutations. Earlier surgery is advocated for patients found to have the MEN2B mutation due to its more aggressive nature. Among patients found to have mutations consistent with MEN2B, surgery is advocated during the first year of life. Total thyroidectomy should also include a central compartment node dissection for patients with MTC. Prophylactic surgery should include total thyroidectomy alone.

In cases of recurrent or inoperable disease, external-beam radiation therapy has been used in an attempt to control local disease. Doxorubicin-based chemotherapy has also been employed in treating more widespread disease; however, neither radiation nor chemotherapy has yielded very promising results. Research on other treatment modalities is ongoing. Early detection and complete surgical excision of tumor tissue remain the best hope for long-term survival.

BIBLIOGRAPHY

Townsend CM (ed.). *Sabiston Textbook of Surgery: The Biological Basis of Modern Surgical Practice*, 16th ed. Philadelphia, PA: W. B. Saunders; 2001:697–707.

Wella SA Jr, Franz C. Medullary carcinoma of the thyroid. *World J Surg* 2000;24(8):952–956.

Yip L, Cote GJ, Shapiro SE, et al. Multiple endocrine neoplasia type 2: evaluation of the genotype and phenotype relationship. *Arch Surg* 2003;138(4):409–416.

13. **(A)** Thyroid cancer is relatively rare, accounting for only 1% of all newly diagnosed cancers yearly in the United States; however, thyroid malignancy accounts for over 90% of all endocrine tumors. Papillary thyroid cancers account for approximately 80% of all thyroid malignancies, with its incidence peaking in the third or fourth decades. Follicular thyroid cancer accounts for approximately 10% of all thyroid malignancies and has a slightly older age of onset. MTC accounts for an additional 5% of all thyroid malignancies, has a slight female predominance, and is familial 20% of the time, as in MEN2 syndromes and FMTC (see Fig. 13-7).

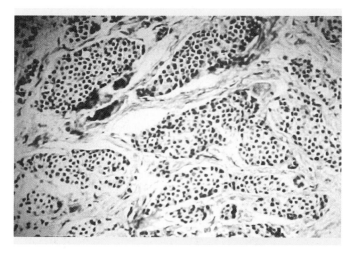

FIGURE 13-7. Histologic representation of medullary thyroid carcinoma.

MTC involves calcitonin-producing parafollicular or C cells. In sporadic cases, it tends to be unilateral with a later age of onset. It is most commonly located in uppermost third of the thyroid lobes (see Fig. 13-8). Approximately 15% of patients have evidence of locally advanced disease at the time of diagnosis in sporadic cases. In a familial setting, multiglandular involvement and multifocality are the rule. Overt malignancy is preceded by C-cell hyperplasia, which may be detectable histopathologically in the absence of gross or palpable disease. Unfortunately, these tumors have a tendency toward early metastasis.

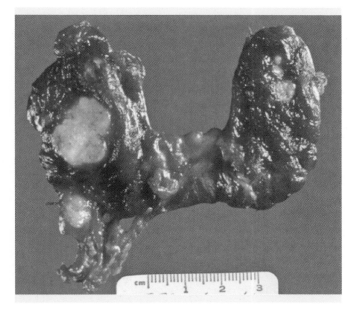

FIGURE 13-8. Resected thyroid showing medullary thyroid cancer (MTC). From Morita SY, Dackiw APB, Zeiger MA. *McGraw-Hill Manual: Endocrine Surgery.* New York, NY: McGraw-Hill; 2009:Fig. 6-1.

MTCs may secrete a variety of substances, including calcitonin, serotonin, ACTH, carcinoembryonic antigen (CEA), histaminase, and VIP. The most common of these is calcitonin. With the advent of genetic screening for *RET* gene mutations, the role of serum calcitonin measurements has largely been relegated to one of monitoring patients for recurrent disease. Every patient with MTC should undergo testing for the *RET* proto-oncogene mutation.

BIBLIOGRAPHY

American Thyroid Association Guidelines Task Force. Medullary thyroid cancer: management guidelines of the American Thyroid Association. *Thyroid* 2009;19(6):565–612.

Callender GG, Hu MI, Evans DB, Perrier ND. Medullary thyroid carcinoma. In: Morita SY, Dackiw AB, Zeiger MA (eds.), *McGraw-Hill Manual: Endocrine Surgery.* New York, NY: McGraw-Hill; 2010:Chapter 6.

Engelbach M, Gîrges R, Forst T, Pfâtzner A, et al. Improved diagnostic methods in the follow-up of medullary thyroid carcinoma by highly specific calcitonin measurements. *J Clin Endocrinol Metab* 2000;85(5):1890–1894.

14. **(B)** MTC accounts for about 5% of all thyroid malignancies. Although sporadic in 80% of cases, MTC may be inherited in as many as 20% of those affected. Inherited cases include those associated with MEN2A and MEN2B, which have been described earlier, as well as familial medullary thyroid cancer (FMTC). MEN2A is the most common setting in which inherited MTC occurs. FMTC is least common when considering inherited MTCs.

FMTC is defined by the presence of kindreds with at least four members having MTC but not having any of the other classic findings associated with the MEN2 syndromes. Like MEN2 syndromes, FMTC is associated with germline mutations in the *RET* proto-oncogene. FMTC behaves more like MEN2A than MEN2B, having a more indolent course. This is likely attributable to the similarities in the causative mutations, which typically involve the cysteine-rich extracellular domain. Additional mutations at codon 768, which codes for a portion of the intracellular domain, have also been observed in patients with FMTC; however, like MTC in both of the MEN2 syndromes, diagnosis of the disease requires early, elective total thyroidectomy with central compartment node dissection. Although the specific timing of surgery is a matter of debate among surgeons, the general consensus seems to be elective removal at the age of 5 years in FMTC. The same recommendation applies to MEN2A as noted previously. Diagnosis of FMTC should be made cautiously, because incorrect diagnosis may lead clinicians to miss the additional diagnoses of hyperparathyroidism and pheochromocytoma.

Because MTC is the most frequent cause of death among patients with MEN2 syndromes or FMTC, early diagnosis and treatment are paramount. This is accomplished most easily in inherited MTC by genetic screening of the family members of patients confirmed to have MTC. When predisposing germline mutations in the *RET* gene are detected, total thyroidectomy is recommended.

When MEN2 syndromes are suspected, it is essential to rule out the simultaneous presence of a pheochromocytoma by assessing urine catecholamines. Pheochromocytoma may be present in up to 24% of MEN2 patients at the time their thyroid disease is diagnosed. If pheochromocytoma is discovered, adrenalectomy should be performed first, followed by thyroidectomy.

BIBLIOGRAPHY

American Thyroid Association Guidelines Task Force. Medullary thyroid cancer: management guidelines of the American Thyroid Association. *Thyroid* 2009;19(6):565–612.

Callender GG, Hu MI, Evans DB, Perrier ND. Medullary thyroid carcinoma. In: Morita SY, Dackiw AB, Zeiger MA (eds.), *McGraw-Hill Manual: Endocrine Surgery*. New York, NY: McGraw-Hill; 2010:Chapter 6.

Yip L, Cote GJ, Shapiro SE, Ayers GD, et al. Multiple endocrine neoplasia type 2: evaluation of the genotype and phenotype relationship. *Arch Surg* 2003;138(4):409–416.

15. **(C)** The presence of severe headaches and anxiety occurring with MTC should arouse suspicion that there may be a synchronous pheochromocytoma. Pheochromocytoma may be present in up to 24% of MEN2 patients at the time their thyroid disease is diagnosed. Undiagnosed pheochromocytomas present significant difficulties for the anesthesiologist, and patients will require α-blockade, preferably phenoxybenzamine, in the weeks leading up to surgery to minimize anesthetic risks and facilitate intraoperative blood pressure control. For this reason, 24-hour urine catecholamines must be checked prior to surgery so that an occult pheochromocytoma is not missed. If catecholamine values are abnormally elevated, computed tomography (CT) scan or magnetic resonance imaging (MRI) is usually confirmatory.

    If a pheochromocytoma is identified in this patient, removal of the pheochromocytoma is the operative priority with subsequent total thyroidectomy. Pheochromocytomas in MEN2 syndromes may be unilateral or bilateral and are characterized by hyperplastic chromaffin tissue. Although chromaffin cells frequently invade the adrenal capsule, metastasis is rare.

    In terms of treatment, unilateral laparoscopic adrenalectomy is performed in cases where the contralateral gland is radiographically normal in sporadic cases. This approach allows preservation of adrenal function from the contralateral gland, thus minimizing the risk of postoperative adrenal insufficiency. Although this approach is most reasonable in patients with unilateral, sporadic disease, MEN2 syndromes frequently go on to develop disease in the contralateral gland. In fact, upward of 50% of MEN patients presenting with unilateral tumors eventually develop bilateral disease. Therefore, in an attempt to preserve cortical function in MEN patients who either do have or may go on to have bilateral disease, some endocrine surgeons advocate cortical-sparing adrenalectomy. This approach allows for the possibility of cortical preservation even when bilateral pheochromocytomas are resected.

BIBLIOGRAPHY

Brandi ML, Gagel RF, Angeli A, et al. Guidelines for diagnosis and therapy of MEN type 1 and type 2. *J Clin Endocrinol Metab* 2001;86(12):5658–5671.

Larsen PR, Kronenberg HM, Melmed S, Polonsky KS (eds.). *Williams Textbook of Endocrinology*, 10th ed. Philadelphia, PA: W. B. Saunders; 2003:1733–1737.

Morita SY, Dackiw AB, Zeiger MA. Pheochromocytoma and paraganglioma. In: Morita SY, Dackiw AB, Zeiger MA (eds.), *McGraw-Hill Manual: Endocrine Surgery*. New York, NY: McGraw-Hill; 2010:Chapter 15.

Townsend CM (ed.). *Sabiston Textbook of Surgery: The Biological Basis of Modern Surgical Practice*, 16th ed. Philadelphia, PA: W. B. Saunders; 2001:697–707.

16. **(D)** As has been noted in previous discussions, MTC accounts for about 5% of all thyroid malignancies and is inherited in as many as 20% of those affected. Inherited cases include those associated with MEN2 syndromes and FMTC. MEN2A and FMTC have a more indolent course than MEN2B, which often affects the very young and is frequently diagnosed at an advanced stage except in cases where rigorous familial screening is undertaken. Since chemotherapeutic regimens and external-beam radiation have proved disappointing, efforts have been redoubled to screen for inherited MTC among kindred of those diagnosed with these tumors. Although monitoring serum calcitonin and radionuclide scanning have been used in the past for surveillance among kindred with MTC, especially in confirmed cases of inherited disease, these modalities have largely been supplanted by genetic screening for mutations in the *RET* proto-oncogene. This technique is now considered the most sensitive means of screening for MTC in kindred of patients diagnosed with inherited MTC.

    In terms of surgical management, total thyroidectomy is the primary management for both the treatment of proven MTC and prevention of MTC in MEN2 carriers. The management of the cervical lymph nodes is more complex. Cervical lymph node dissection is not necessary in patients with MEN2A undergoing prophylactic thyroidectomy. Patients with proven cancer (sporadic or hereditary) should undergo total extracapsular thyroidectomy with bilateral central neck dissection. The lateral compartments are dissected only if there is fine-needle aspiration cytologic evidence of disease spread.

BIBLIOGRAPHY

Callender GG, Hu MI, Evans DB, Perrier ND. Medullary thyroid carcinoma. In: Morita SY, Dackiw AB, Zeiger MA (eds.), *McGraw-Hill Manual: Endocrine Surgery*. New York, NY: McGraw-Hill; 2010:Chapter 6.

Clayman GL, El-Baradie TS. Medullary thyroid cancer. *Otolaryngol Clin North Am* 2003;36(1):91–105.

Townsend CM (ed.). *Sabiston Textbook of Surgery: The Biological Basis of Modern Surgical Practice*, 16th ed. Philadelphia, PA: W. B. Saunders; 2001:697–707.

17. **(B)** The MEN2 syndromes, as discussed previously, are notable for the presence of MTC and pheochromocytomas. In addition to these endocrinopathies, MEN2B is further distinguished by nonendocrine features including marfanoid body habitus, mucosal neuromas, ganglioneuromas, and skeletal abnormalities (see Fig. 13-9). Although MEN2B is an autosomal dominant trait, many cases appear to represent new mutations.

The mucosal neuromas most often occur on the oral mucosa, lips, and tongue. These neuromas are almost invariably present by 10 years of age and occasionally at birth. These neuromas may also involve the corneal nerves. Notable for an increase in both size and number of nerves, these corneal neuromas are visible by slit lamp ophthalmologic examination. Ganglioneuromatoses of the gastrointestinal (GI) tract are also frequent, affecting predominantly the large and small bowel. Occasionally, the esophagus may also be involved. These GI ganglioneuromas often lead to GI dysmotility, problems with chronic constipation, and even megacolon. In some instances, bowel obstruction may also result. The skeletal abnormalities associated with MEN2B are multiple and include a tall, slender Marfanoid habitus, pectus excavatum, kyphosis, pes planus or cavus, and congenital hip dislocation. In contrast to true Marfanoids, MEN2B patients do not typically develop aortic arch disease or ectopia lentis.

Because mucosal neuromas and habitus may be the first clinical presentation of MEN2B, physicians need to be alert to these traits. This is important because these characteristic phenotypic features may presage the discovery of MTC, which, in MEN2B in particular, is very aggressive. Because MTC is the most frequent cause of death among MEN2 patients and because early diagnosis and surgical removal provide the only hope of cure, recognition of mucosal neuromas should prompt a workup for MTC including measurement of serum calcitonin and genetic screening for the *RET* mutation.

BIBLIOGRAPHY

American Thyroid Association Guidelines Task Force. Medullary thyroid cancer: management guidelines of the American Thyroid Association. *Thyroid* 2009;19(6):565–612.

Goldman L, Bennet JC (eds.). *Cecil Textbook of Medicine*, 21st ed. Philadelphia, PA: W. B. Saunders; 2000:1407.

Lal G, Clark OH. Thyroid, parathyroid, and adrenal. In: Brunicardi F, Andersen DK, Billiar TR, et al. (eds.), *Schwartz's Principles of Surgery*, 9th ed. New York, NY: McGraw-Hill; 2010:Chapter 38.

Larsen PR, Kronenberg HM, Melmed S, Polonsky KS (eds.). *Williams Textbook of Endocrinology*, 10th ed. Philadelphia, PA: W. B. Saunders; 2003:1739.

18. **(D)** Anyone undergoing surgery for MTC should undergo screening for pheochromocytoma. This clinical scenario does not specify whether such an evaluation was undertaken. Nevertheless, this patient presents with complaints and findings that suggest he has a pheochromocytoma, especially in light of his history of MTC. Resection of the mass is now needed.

Pheochromocytomas are rare catecholamine-secreting tumors that most frequently occur in the adrenal medulla; however, they also may arise in any sympathetic ganglia. In this case, the patient's mass occurs in the pelvis,

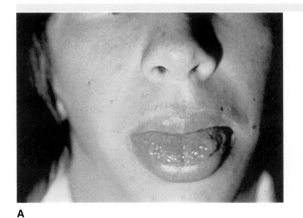 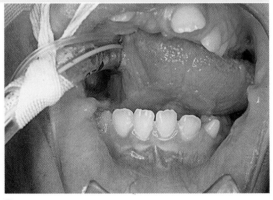

A   **B**

FIGURE 13-9. Features of multiple endocrine neoplasia (MEN) type 2B: thickened lips **A.** and mucosal neuromas **B.** From Brunicardi F, Andersen D, Timothy Billiar T, et al. *Schwartz's Principles of Surgery*, 9th ed. New York, NY: McGraw-Hill; 2009: Fig. 38-20.

abutting a lumbar vertebra. Pheochromocytomas have also been noted in such diverse places as the right atrium, spleen, broad ligament of the ovary, and the organ of Zuckerkandl. The organ of Zuckerkandl, located at the aortic bifurcation, is the most common extra-adrenal site. Extra-adrenal tumors secrete norepinephrine only because they lack the enzyme ethanolamine-*N*-methyl transferase. This is in contradistinction to adrenal tumors, which secrete both norepinephrine and epinephrine.

Although rare in the general population, these tumors are found with greater frequency in patients who have predisposing conditions, such as MEN2 syndromes, von Recklinghausen disease, and von Hippel-Lindau disease. Inherited pheochromocytoma syndromes account for 10% of all pheochromocytomas and are frequently bilateral.

Typical symptoms include hypertension, profuse sweating, headaches, and palpitations. Although the most common clinical finding is hypertension, when all pheochromocytomas are considered, severe hypertension may not be a prominent finding in MEN2 patients because these patients are diagnosed earlier in the course of their disease are a result of screening. When suspected clinically, 24-hour urine catecholamines should be measured. The normal value for total urine catecholamines is 100 mg/24 h. Values two to three times greater are typical of patients who have a pheochromocytoma. CT scanning and MRI are most often used for tumor localization, although 3-iodobenzylguanidine (MIBG) scanning and octreotide scanning may also be used.

Patients with pheochromocytomas are particularly subject to intraoperative hypertension resulting from tumor manipulation and the subsequent release of excessive catecholamines. In severe cases, this hypertension may lead to stroke or death. Therefore, every effort should be made to optimize these patients prior to surgery. This optimization includes α-adrenergic blockade with either prazosin or phenozybenzamine as well as volume resuscitation to compensate for the vasodilatory effects of α-blockade. Effective therapy is achieved with good blood pressure control and mild postural hypotension. Patients using phenozybenzamine usually require doses in the range of 60–250 mg/d. When patients experience persistent tachycardia on this α-blockade regimen, β-blockade with propranolol is recommended. Preoperative α-blockade is generally required for a minimum of 10–14 days prior to surgery. When intraoperative hypertension occurs, nitroprusside is generally the agent of choice for blood pressure control.

BIBLIOGRAPHY

American Thyroid Association Guidelines Task Force. Medullary thyroid cancer: management guidelines of the American Thyroid Association. *Thyroid* 2009;19(6):565–612.

Larsen PR, Kronenberg HM, Melmed S, Polonsky KS (eds.). *Williams Textbook of Endocrinology*, 10th ed. Philadelphia, PA: W. B. Saunders; 2003:1739.

Miller RD (ed.). *Anesthesia*, 5th ed. Philadelphia, PA: Churchill Livingstone; 2000:924–925.

19. **(C)** As noted in previous discussions, NETs of the pancreas and duodenum constitute the second most common endocrine abnormality associated with MEN1. Although gastrinomas are the most common type of functional pancreaticoduodenal tumor, accounting for anywhere from 50 to 70% of functional, MEN-associated NETs, insulinomas constitute the second most common type of functional tumor. When present, these tumors produce symptoms of neuroglycopenia during fasting. These symptoms include anxiety, tremor, confusion, sweating, seizure, and syncope and are frequently most prominent in the morning. Also significant in making the diagnosis is a remarkable improvement or resolution of the symptoms after administration of glucose. Because these tumors are rare, exogenous insulin administration should be excluded as an alternative diagnosis. This can be done by careful history as well as measurement of serum C-peptide and proinsulin levels. Proinsulin is a natural precursor to endogenous insulin and should be elevated when oversecretion of endogenous insulin occurs. C-peptide, a cleavage product of endogenous insulin production, should be elevated as well. If proinsulin and C-peptide levels are normal, this finding may suggest exogenous administration of insulin. Some also advocate measurement of serum sulfonylureas to rule out oral hypoglycemic abuse.

Initial management of insulinomas is directed at controlling hypoglycemia. This is first attempted with diet and medications. Frequent meals are advocated with small snacks between normal meals and at bedtime. Additionally, complex carbohydrates, such as those found in potatoes, bread, and rice, are preferable to simple carbohydrates because the former are digested more slowly, leading to more consistent blood glucose levels. Medical therapy with diazoxide or octreotide has also been used with some success in managing hypoglycemia. Diazoxide works by both inhibiting insulin release from pancreatic β cells and enhancing glycogenolysis. Octreotide works by interactions with somatostatin receptors on the tumor, decreasing insulin secretion. Although medical therapy has been used with some success over the long term in small numbers of patients, its primary role is in controlling hypoglycemia in anticipation of a definitive surgical procedure.

Surgical removal of insulinomas is frequently challenging because these tumors are notoriously difficult to localize. This is in part because of their small size. Ninety percent of MEN1-associated insulinomas are also multifocal, in contrast to sporadic insulinomas, which are multifocal only 10% of the time. In fact, historically as many as 20–60% of insulinomas could not be visualized preoperatively and as many as 20% could not be visualized during exploration, even when excellent exposure of the pancreas was achieved. Standard preoperative imaging modalities, such as CT, MRI, and ultrasound, though frequently used, are often inadequate, correctly localizing only 10–30%. Among more invasive imaging techniques, abdominal angiography is perhaps most sensitive, localizing up to 60% of tumors. When intraoperative imaging is an option, intraoperative ultrasound (IOUS) is the most effective modality, identifying anywhere from 80–90% of tumors. This modality is widely advocated now as a standard part of any abdominal exploration for insulinoma.

Surgical exploration is typically performed through either a midline laparotomy or bilateral subcostal incisions depending on surgeon's preference. An extensive Kocher maneuver is performed, and the pancreas is mobilized by dividing the gastrocolic ligament and opening the posterior peritoneal lining of the lesser sac. Although sporadic insulinomas are frequently benign and amenable to simple enucleation, this is not the case for MEN1-associated tumors, which are often multifocal, involving all parts of the pancreas. Therefore, a more extensive procedure is warranted in treating MEN1-associated disease. Most surgeons now favor enucleation of gross disease in the head of the pancreas combined with distal subtotal pancreatectomy.

BIBLIOGRAPHY

Brandi ML, Gagel RF, Angeli A, et al. Guidelines for diagnosis and therapy of MEN type 1 and type 2. *J Clin Endocrinol Metab* 2001;86(12):5658–5671.

Feldman M, Friedman LS, Sleisenger MH (eds.). *Sleisenger and Fordtrans Gastrointestinal and Liver Disease: Pathophysiology, Diagnosis, Management*, 7th ed. Philadelphia, PA: W. B. Saunders; 2002:993–994, 1005.

Norton JA, Bollinger RR, Chang AE, et al. *Surgery: Basic Science and Clinical Evidence*. New York, NY: Springer-Verlag; 2000:956–958.

Townsend CM (ed.). *Sabiston Textbook of Surgery: The Biological Basis of Modern Surgical Practice*, 16th ed. Philadelphia, PA: W. B. Saunders; 2001:652–653, 697–707.

Vanderveen K, Grant C. Insulinoma. In: Morita SY, Dackiw AB, Zeiger MA (eds.), *McGraw-Hill Manual: Endocrine Surgery*. New York, NY: McGraw-Hill; 2010:Chapter 17.

20. **(A)** Pituitary adenomas occur in anywhere from 15–50% of MEN1 patients, with a significantly higher frequency in women than men by nearly 2:1 in some studies. The mean age of onset is approximately 38 =years with 25% diagnosed by 26 years of age and as many as 75% diagnosed by the fifth decade. The most common type of functional pituitary adenoma among both MEN and non-MEN patients is prolactinoma. Among MEN1 patients, prolactinomas account for upward of 62% of all functional pituitary adenomas. The next most common tumors are growth hormone–secreting adenomas (9%), followed by ACTH-secreting tumors (4%). Additionally, a small percentage of pituitary adenomas may secrete multiple substances.

In terms of tumor size, approximately 85% of pituitary tumors occurring in MEN1 patients are macroadenomas, defined as tumors measuring at least 1 cm in diameter. This stands in contrast to non-MEN tumors where macroadenomas occur in approximately 42% of patients. This is clinically significant because macroadenomas are far more likely to cause symptoms from compression of surrounding structures than microadenomas, which measure less than 1 cm. When prolactinoma is the diagnosis, the oversecretion of prolactin most often results in hypogonadism in men and amenorrhea or galactorrhea in women. Galactorrhea was the presenting complaint of the patient in this particular clinical vignette.

Treatment of prolactinomas has generally involved medical treatment with dopamine agonists, such as bromocriptine, and/or transsphenoidal surgical resection. Clinical research has shown that microadenomas typically respond well to transsphenoidal resection, as measured by normalization of serum prolactin levels; however, treatment with a dopamine agonist has also been shown to induce normalization of prolactin levels and tumor shrinkage in many of these patients, as well. Therefore, patients with microadenomas are frequently offered either surgery or medical treatment.

When patients have macroadenomas, most surgeons and endocrinologists recommend medical management with a dopamine agonist such as bromocriptine as first-line treatment. This recommendation is based on lower observed rates of prolactin normalization following surgery for macroadenomas compared to microadenomas (32 vs 71%). Furthermore, transsphenoidal or craniotomy resection of macroadenomas is associated with increased morbidity and is currently deemed to pose more risk to the patient than is justified by the anticipated rate of postoperative hormone normalization. Therefore, for this patient who has galactorrhea and a pituitary macroadenoma by MRI, bromocriptine is the preferred initial treatment. If this line of treatment fails, surgical resection does remain an option with or without external-beam radiation for any residual disease.

BIBLIOGRAPHY

Abeloff MD, Armitage JO, Lichter AS, et al. (eds.). *Clinical Oncology*, 2nd ed. Philadelphia, PA: Churchill Livingstone; 2000:1171–1174.

Townsend CM (ed.). *Sabiston Textbook of Surgery: The Biological Basis of Modern Surgical Practice*, 16th ed. Philadelphia, PA: W. B. Saunders; 2001:697–707, 1527–1528.

Verges B, Boureille F, Goudet P, et al. Pituitary disease in MEN type 1: data from the France-Belgium MEN1 multicenter study. *J Clin Endocrinol Metab* 2002;87(2):457–465.

Whaley J, Lairmore TC. Multiple endocrine neoplasia type 1. In: Morita SY, Dackiw AB, Zeiger MA (eds.), *McGraw-Hill Manual: Endocrine Surgery*. New York, NY: McGraw-Hill; 2010:Chapter 21.

21. **(A)** When a patient is diagnosed with MTC, genetic screening for a mutant *RET* gene should be undertaken. If the patient does, in fact, have a defective gene, *RET* screening in all first-degree relatives is then recommended. Germline mutations affecting codon 634 are most often associated with MEN2A syndromes. Codons 768 and 891 are aberrant in FMTC. Codon 918 is the culprit most often in MEN2B.

All family members with *RET* mutations predisposing them to MTC should undergo total thyroidectomy as soon as they are able to tolerate the procedure. Infants born to families known to have the predisposing *RET* mutation should undergo screening at birth. When the MEN2B *RET* mutation is identified, total thyroidectomy should be done as soon as possible and is generally advocated within the first 6 months of life. If the MEN2A or FMTC *RET* mutations are identified, surgery may generally be deferred until the child is 5 years old.

BIBLIOGRAPHY

American Thyroid Association Guidelines Task Force. Medullary thyroid cancer: management guidelines of the American Thyroid Association. *Thyroid* 2009;19(6):565–612.

Brandi ML, Gagel RF, Angeli A, et al. Guidelines for diagnosis and therapy of MEN type 1 and type 2. *J Clin Endocrinol Metab* 2001;86(12):5658–5671.

Carling T, Roman SA. Multiple endocrine neoplasia type 2. In: Morita SY, Dackiw AB, Zeiger MA (eds.), *McGraw-Hill Manual: Endocrine Surgery*. New York, NY: McGraw-Hill; 2010:Chapter 22.

CHAPTER 14

PITUITARY

JONNAE Y. BARRY AND ALEXANDER G. CHIU

QUESTIONS

1. Which statement about pituitary microadenomas is true?
   (A) By definition, they are less than 1.0 cm in size.
   (B) They are best seen on coronal T2 gadolinium-enhanced magnetic resonance scans.
   (C) They are rarely found at autopsy in asymptomatic individuals.
   (D) Fifteen percent will enlarge to macroadenomas.

2. A 19-year-old woman has had amenorrhea and galactorrhea for 13 months. Her prolactin level is 100 ng/mL (normal 4–23 ng/mL for nonpregnant women). She brought a recent magnetic resonance image (MRI) with her (see Fig. 14-1). After other causes of hyperprolactinemia have been ruled out, she should
   (A) Begin medical therapy with dopamine agonists
   (B) Begin medical therapy with oral contraceptives
   (C) Begin calcium supplementation
   (D) Undergo transsphenoidal resection of the lesion

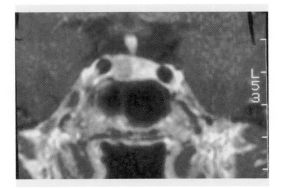

FIGURE 14-1. Coronal magnetic resonance scan (T1 with contrast).

3. A 45-year-old truck driver presents to your office reporting painless loss of vision. On exam, you discover bitemporal hemianopsia and decreased visual acuity. He also states that he has put on "a lot of weight," feels tired, and has decreased libido. An MRI scan is obtained as shown in Fig. 14-2. The most important diagnostic test in this situation is
   (A) Serum cortisol level
   (B) Thyroid function tests
   (C) Prolactin level
   (D) Computed tomography (CT) scan

4. A 30-year-old woman presents with signs of fulminant Cushing syndrome that have developed over the past 4 months. She does not take any medications. Which of the following would be a fairly specific finding in her case?
   (A) Hypotension
   (B) Peripheral neuropathy
   (C) Striae
   (D) Anemia

5. If the patient from Question 4 had a negative MRI for pituitary abnormality, with and without contrast, what is the most likely etiology of her Cushing syndrome?
   (A) Adrenal tumor
   (B) Adenocarcinoma of the lung
   (C) Exogenous steroid use
   (D) Pituitary tumor

6. After excluding exogenous glucocorticoid use, what diagnostic test should be ordered if you suspect Cushing syndrome?
   (A) Insulin tolerance test
   (B) Early morning salivary cortisol
   (C) 48-hour dexamethasone suppression test
   (D) Random serum cortisol or plasma adrenocorticotropic hormone (ACTH) level

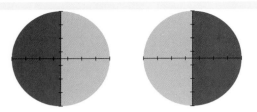

Bitemporal Hemianopia

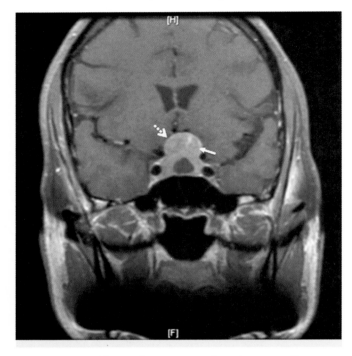

FIGURE 14-2. Magnetic resonance imaging scan. From McKean SC, Ross JJ, Dressler DD, Brotman DJ, Ginsberg JS. *Principles and Practice of Hospital Medicine.* New York, NY: McGraw-Hill; 2012:Fig. 152-2.

7. A corticotropin-releasing hormone (CRH) stimulation test is conducted in a patient with Cushing syndrome who had an intermediate ACTH level. The results show no response of ACTH to CRH. This result is most consistent with
   (A) ACTH-dependent Cushing
   (B) ACTH-independent Cushing
   (C) A normal result
   (D) Cushing disease

8. The best test to distinguish between pituitary and ectopic secretion of corticotropin is
   (A) High-dose dexamethasone suppression test
   (B) High-resolution CT of the head
   (C) CRH stimulation test
   (D) Selective inferior petrosal sinus sampling

9. A 46-year-old man with Cushing syndrome and history of low back pain presents to the emergency department with progressive lower extremity weakness in all muscle groups and new-onset radicular symptoms. What is the most likely diagnosis?
   (A) Vertebral body compression fracture with cord injury
   (B) Thoracic disk herniation
   (C) Epidural lipomatosis
   (D) Spinal stenosis

10. The treatment for compression fracture of the thoracic spine, when associated with the osteoporosis that accompanies Cushing disease, is
    (A) Prolonged bed rest and narcotics
    (B) Polymethyl methacrylate injection
    (C) Endoscopic transthoracic stabilization
    (D) Bracing and medical therapy for osteoporosis

11. The best test to confirm suspected acromegaly is
    (A) Growth hormone (GH) level >5 ng/mL
    (B) GH level >25 ng/mL
    (C) Failure of GH to suppress with 75 mg of glucose
    (D) Elevated insulin-like growth factor (IGF)-1 level

12. Patients with acromegaly are at increased risk of
    (A) Atrophy of the thyroid gland
    (B) Carcinoma of the colon
    (C) Coronary artery disease
    (D) Hypotension

13. A 60-year-old man presents with acromegaly. An MRI demonstrates a mass in the pituitary with superior extension above the sella (see Fig. 14-3). The patient's GH, prolactin, and IGF-1 are grossly elevated. He is

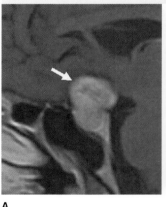 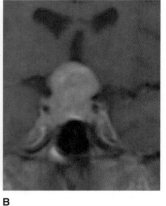

A　　　　B

FIGURE 14-3. Magnetic resonance imaging scan. From Doherty GM (ed.). *Current Diagnosis & Treatment: Surgery,* 13th ed. New York, NY: McGraw-Hill; 2010:Fig. 36-17.

not currently having visual deficits. The best immediate treatment option would be
(A) Transsphenoidal excision
(B) Radiosurgery
(C) Long-acting octreotide
(D) Bromocriptine

14. Your patient with acromegaly must have a cholecystectomy. The safest method for intubating this patient for his surgery is
(A) Awake fiberoptic intubation
(B) Rigid laryngoscope
(C) Nasal intubation
(D) Extra-large endotracheal tube

15. A 40-year-old women is admitted for deep vein thrombosis (DVT). The following morning, she begins to experience retro-orbital headache, visual field deficits and vomiting. She has no medical conditions but is currently in her second cycle of *in vitro* fertilization (IVF) treatments. On exam, she has ptosis of the left eyelid and is unable to move her left eye up, down, or inward. She is most likely suffering from
(A) Subarachnoid hemorrhage
(B) Pituitary apoplexy
(C) Horner syndrome
(D) Medication-related oculomotor neuropathy

ANSWERS AND EXPLANATIONS

1. **(A)** The "gold standard" for classifying pituitary adenomas is based on immunohistochemistry and electron microscopy. However, from a surgical standpoint, they can be classified by size and growth characteristics. In the simplest form, adenomas are divided into two groups: microadenomas (<10 mm in diameter) and macroadenomas (≥10 mm in diameter). To further classify macroadenomas, it can be useful to use a system that takes into account grade, degree, and direction of extrasellar extension (stage). Microadenomas of the pituitary are best visualized with a coronal T1 MRI. Eighty to 95% of such studies will show a focal hypointense lesion within an otherwise homogenous adenohypophysis. The excellent sensitivity of unenhanced T1-weighted spin echo (SE) MRI for microadenomas has made it the primary sequence for imaging the pituitary gland. Contrast is reserved for those cases in which there is good clinical or biochemical evidence of a pituitary adenoma with a negative or equivocal plain MRI. In most cases, the best imaging routine is to perform a plain scan followed by a repeat T1-weighted coronal sequence immediately after intravenous injection of contrast (gadolinium). Autopsy studies have repeatedly shown that 20–25% of the general population harbor small pituitary microadenomas. Microadenomas are usually clinically silent and occur in patients without apparent endocrine symptoms. Whereas very few microadenomas will show interval growth, more than one-third of macroadenomas will increase in size.

BIBLIOGRAPHY

Atlas S. *Magnetic Resonance Imaging of the Brain and Spine*, 4th ed. Philadelphia, PA: Lippincott Williams & Wilkins; 2009.

Jane J, Thapar K, Laws E. Pituitary tumors. In: Winn HR (ed.), *Youmans Neurological Surgery*, 6th ed. Philadelphia, PA: W. B. Saunders; 2011:1476–1510.

2. **(A)** The MRI shown in Fig. 14-1 shows a microadenoma on the right side of the sella. Regardless of cause, the classic features of prolactin excess in women are galactorrhea and amenorrhea. In men, decreased libido and impotence are common. The elevated prolactin level, combined with the findings on MRI, makes prolactinoma a likely diagnosis. However, pituitary incidentalomas are very common, and other possible etiologies must be excluded. Other common causes of increased prolactin secretion include pregnancy, hypothalamic-pituitary disorders, primary hypothyroidism, and drug ingestion (estrogen therapy, oral contraceptives, dopamine antagonists, monoamine oxidase inhibitors [MAOIs], intravenous cimetidine, and verapamil). Other causes can include nipple stimulation, chest wall lesions, spinal cord lesions, chronic renal failure, or severe liver disease. Prolactin secretion from the pituitary is primarily under inhibitory control by dopamine, which is secreted by the hypothalamus. Increased production of prolactin will suppress luteinizing hormone (LH) and follicle-stimulating hormone (FSH) production, leading to decreased estrogen production. In the short term, these abnormalities can lead to galactorrhea and hypogonadism. In the long term, osteoporosis can become a concern. Although most microadenomas do not progress, control of prolactin hypersecretion is recommended for cessation of galactorrhea and return to normal gonadal function. This can usually be achieved with dopamine agonists such as cabergoline or bromocriptine. Of these, cabergoline is the usual therapy of choice due to its more favorable side effect profile and success rate of 90% in treating microadenomas. Once prolactin levels have been restored to normal levels, fertility will also be restored. Therefore, women not wishing to become pregnant should be counseled about use of birth control. The risk of major expansion of an existing adenoma during pregnancy is less than 2%, and although no late toxicity from dopamine agonists taken during pregnancy has been reported, studies are limited at this time. Women are advised to discontinue their medication and obtain a pregnancy test if they miss a period. Transsphenoidal resection is an option for patients who do not respond to medical therapy.

BIBLIOGRAPHY

Javorsky BR, Aron DC, Findling JW, Tyrrell J. Hypothalamus and pituitary gland. In: Gardner DG, Shoback D (eds.), *Greenspan's Basic & Clinical Endocrinology*, 9th ed. New York, NY: McGraw-Hill; 2011.

3. **(C)** The image shown in Fig. 14-2 is a coronal MRI demonstrating a pituitary macroadenoma (*solid arrow*) with superior extension and compression of the optic chiasm (*dashed arrow*). Superior extension of such an adenoma can compress the optic chiasm, leading to visual disturbances, as seen in this patient. A classic finding is bitemporal hemianopsia. In addition, the mass effect on native pituitary tissue can lead to hypopituitarism. Extension of such tumors into the cavernous sinus may result in diplopia, ophthalmoplegia, and involvement of the cranial nerves, especially the third nerve. Prolactinomas compose 30–40% of all pituitary tumors; therefore, a prolactin level should be drawn for diagnostic purposes. Given this patient's severe visual deficits, urgent medical therapy should be initiated including dopamine agonist therapy and steroids; this therapy should not be delayed while waiting for lab tests to return. Dopamine agonists will suppress prolactin secretion and cause the adenoma to shrink, which should improve or restore visual and neurologic deficits. In addition, steroids reduce tumor edema and treat a potential adrenal crisis. If the patient had presented with more severe vision loss, had more sudden onset of symptoms, or had headache and change in mental status, a CT scan would be useful to differentiate subarachnoid hemorrhage from pituitary apoplexy.

BIBLIOGRAPHY

Jain SH, Katznelson L. Pituitary disease. In: McKean SC, Ross JJ, Dressler DD, Brotman DJ, Ginsberg JS (eds.), *Principles and Practice of Hospital Medicine*. New York, NY: McGraw-Hill; 2012.

Nelson BK. Pituitary apoplexy. In: Adams JG (ed.), *Emergency Medicine*, 2nd ed. Philadelphia, PA: W. B. Saunders; 2013:1439–1441.e1.

Parker KL, Schimmer BP. Introduction to endocrinology: the hypothalamic-pituitary axis. In: Brunton LL, Chabner BA, Knollmann BC (eds.), *Goodman & Gilman's The Pharmacological Basis of Therapeutics*, 12th ed. New York, NY: McGraw-Hill; 2011.

4. **(C)** The term Cushing syndrome encompasses a constellation of clinical features. Truncal obesity and thin frail skin resulting in reddish purple striae across the abdomen can be common findings (see Fig. 14-4).

In addition, hirsutism, balding, ecchymosis, hypertension, glucose intolerance, development of a supraclavicular fat pad, rounding of the facies, proximal muscle weakness, and thin extremities may also be present. Cushing syndrome is a term used to describe the clinical abnormalities associated with excess glucocorticoid

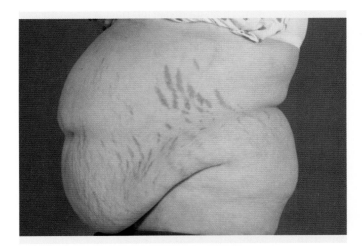

FIGURE 14-4. Truncal obesity and reddish purple striae across the abdomen in Cushing syndrome. From Kantarjian HM, Wolff RA, Koller CA. *The MD Anderson Manual of Medical Oncology*, 2nd ed. New York, NY: McGraw-Hill; 2011: Fig. 38-21.

circulation when the etiology is identified outside the pituitary gland. Cushing disease is the term reserved for clinical findings caused by pituitary adrenocorticotropic hormone (ACTH) excess from a tumor within the pituitary itself. In Cushing disease, there is hyperplasia of pituitary cells that produce ACTH, which stimulates the adrenal glands, resulting in the common clinical findings listed earlier. In patients with clinical features suggesting Cushing syndrome, the initial screening test is the overnight dexamethasone suppression test. If Cushing disease is suspected after initial screening, an MRI of the pituitary gland is useful for localization. Treatment of an ACTH-secreting pituitary adenoma usually requires transsphenoidal resection of the lesion, with a cure rate approaching 80%. After surgery, roughly 10% of patients will experience complications such as cerebrospinal fluid (CSF) leak, transient diabetes insipidus, visual abnormalities, or meningitis. Twenty percent of patients will have incomplete excision of the lesion and experience recurrence or persistence of symptoms.

BIBLIOGRAPHY

Ferri FF. Cushing's disease and syndrome. In: Ferri FF (ed.), *Ferri's Clinical Advisor 2014*. Maryland Heights, MO: Mosby; 2014:308–308.

Ropper AH, Samuels MA. The hypothalamus and neuroendocrine disorders. In: Ropper AH, Samuels MA (eds.), *Adams and Victor's Principles of Neurology*, 9th ed. New York, NY: McGraw-Hill; 2009.

5. **(D)** Even with negative imaging, the most likely etiology of this patient's Cushing syndrome is a pituitary tumor. In fact, only 70% of microadenomas, some as small as 3 mm in diameter, can be detected with high-resolution, gadolinium-enhanced MRI. Although iatrogenic causes account for most cases of Cushing syndrome due to widespread use of therapeutic high-dose glucocorticoids, the question stem clearly states she is not taking any medications. Of the spontaneous causes of Cushing syndrome, Cushing disease is the most common cause in adults, accounting for 70% of cases. Cushing syndrome can be divided into two groups: ACTH dependent and ACTH independent. The ACTH-dependent forms include pituitary-dependent Cushing syndrome (Cushing disease), ectopic tumor source, ectopic CRH production (rarely), and exogenous ACTH administration. ACTH-independent causes include adrenal adenoma, adrenal carcinoma, and primary pigmented nodular adrenal disease (PPNAD). Of these other causes of Cushing syndrome, adrenal adenomas account for 8–19%, adrenal carcinomas account for 6–7%, and ectopic ACTH syndrome accounts for 6–15% of cases.

BIBLIOGRAPHY

Bertagna X, Guignat L, Raux-Demay MC, Guilhaume B, Girard F. Cushing's disease. In: Melmed S (ed.), *The Pituitary*, 3rd ed. Philadelphia, PA: Elsevier; 2011:533–617.

Morris DG, Grossman A, Nieman LK. Cushing's syndrome. In: Jameson JL, De Groot LJ (eds.), *Endocrinology*, 6th ed. Philadelphia, PA: W. B. Saunders; 2010:282–311.

Winn HR. Pituitary tumors. In: Winn HR (ed.), *Youmans Neurological Surgery*, 3rd ed. Philadelphia, PA: W. B. Saunders; 2011:1476–1510.

6. **(C)** The current guidelines released by the Endocrine Society in 2008 state that patients with multiple and progressive features compatible with Cushing syndrome should undergo one test with high diagnostic accuracy to aid in diagnosis. Acceptable tests include a urine free cortisol (UFC; at least two measurements), late-night salivary cortisol (two measurements), 1-mg overnight dexamethasone suppression test (DST), or longer low-dose DST (2 mg/d for 48 hours). The test chosen depends on the individual patient's preference. The guidelines specifically recommend against using a random serum cortisol, plasma ACTH level, urinary 17-ketosteroid, insulin tolerance test, loperamide test, or tests designed to determine etiology of Cushing syndrome (e.g., pituitary or adrenal imaging). In individuals with an abnormal test, referral to an endocrinologist is warranted.

BIBLIOGRAPHY

Nieman LK, Biller BMK, Findling JW, et al. The diagnosis of Cushing's syndrome: an Endocrine Society clinical practice guideline. *J Clin Endocrinol Metab* 2008;93(5):1526–1540.

7. **(B)** Normally CRH is released from the hypothalamus in response to stress. It is secreted at the median eminence into the hypothalamo-hypophyseal portal system where it travels to the anterior lobe of the pituitary to stimulate the release of ACTH. ACTH, in turn, acts to stimulate the adrenal glands to produce cortisol, glucocorticoids, mineralocorticoids, and dehydroepiandrosterone (DHEA). Therefore, a normal physiologic response to a bolus of CRH, whether from the hypothalamus or given exogenously, as in this test, would be to increase ACTH release from the pituitary. In ACTH-dependent Cushing (i.e., Cushing disease or an ectopic tumor), excess CRH will also stimulate increased release of ACTH. A patient with an ACTH-independent cause of Cushing (i.e., adrenal tumor) would be expected to have low levels of ACTH at baseline due to the negative feedback of cortisol on the pituitary and hypothalamus. This can be useful in diagnosing these patients without conducting a CRH stimulation test. However, if a patient with ACTH-independent Cushing initially had an intermediate ACTH level and a CRH stimulation test were conducted, there would be little or no effect on the level of ACTH measured because the pituitary is already suppressed.

BIBLIOGRAPHY

Molina PE. Chapter 6. Adrenal Gland. In: Molina PE. eds. *Endocrine Physiology, 4e.* New York, NY: McGraw-Hill; 2013. http://accessmedicine.mhmedical.com.ezproxy2.library.arizona.edu/content.aspx?bookid=507&Sectionid=42540506.

Javorsky BR, Aron DC, Findling JW, Tyrrell J. Chapter 4. Hypothalamus and Pituitary Gland. In: Gardner DG, Shoback D. eds. *Greenspan's Basic & Clinical Endocrinology, 9e.* New York, NY: McGraw-Hill; 2011. http://accessmedicine.mhmedical.com.ezproxy2.library.arizona.edu/content.aspx?bookid=380&Sectionid=39744044.

8. **(D)** Dexamethasone suppresses ACTH through feedback inhibition in both pituitary and ectopic sources, but pituitary tumors are much more responsive, with ACTH levels dropping much lower in a high-dose dexamethasone test. However, a more sensitive and specific method for distinguishing between the two is the use of inferior petrosal sinus sampling (IPSS). This is done by simultaneous sampling of the peripheral blood and the inferior petrosal sinuses bilaterally after a dose of CRH is given. A significant rise in ACTH in

the petrosal blood, but not the peripheral, is consistent with a pituitary source. The bilateral sampling can be helpful for lateralization of the tumor as well, especially if not visualized on MRI. In several studies, IPSS has been demonstrated to have 95% sensitivity and 93% specificity.

BIBLIOGRAPHY

Invitti C, Pecori Giraldi F, de Martin M, Cavagnini F. Diagnosis and management of Cushing's syndrome: results of an Italian multicentre study. Study Group of the Italian Society of Endocrinology on the Pathophysiology of the Hypothalamic-Pituitary-Adrenal Axis. *J Clin Endocrinol Metab* 1999;84(2):440–448.
Kaltsas GA, Giannulis MG, Newell-Price JD, et al. A critical analysis of the value of simultaneous inferior petrosal sinus sampling in Cushing's disease and the occult ectopic adrenocorticotropin syndrome. *J Clin Endocrinol Metab* 1999;84(2):487–492.

9. **(C)** Epidural lipomatosis is nonneoplastic accumulation of fatty tissue in the epidural space of the thoracic or lumbar spine. It is most commonly associated with chronic corticosteroid excess, obesity, or hypothyroidism. Seventy-five percent of cases are associated with exogenous steroid use. Patients typically have been on corticosteroids for greater than 6 months, are obese, and cushingoid. With removal of corticosteroids, the fatty tissue can regress, but severe neurologic symptoms warrant laminectomy. A spinal MRI will be highly suggestive of the diagnosis with findings of epidural fat thickness greater than 7 mm (see Fig. 14-5).

This patient's presentation is classic, with low back pain being present long before other symptoms. Vertebral body compression is not a common cause of radicular symptoms but can be a source of back pain. Disk herniation could explain this patient's symptoms; however, he has involvement of multiple spinal cord levels, which argues against disk herniation as a cause. Although spinal stenosis is associated with back and leg pain, this type of pain is often worse with movement and relieved with sitting or spine flexion. Spinal stenosis is also more prevalent in the sixth or seventh decades of life.

BIBLIOGRAPHY

Fenton DS. Epidural lipomatosis. In: Czervionke LF, Fenton DS (eds.), *Imaging Painful Spine Disorders*. Philadelphia, PA: W. B. Saunders; 2011:222–227.
Rosenbaum RB, Kula RW. Disorders of bones, joints, ligaments, and meninges. In: Daroff RB, Fenichel GM, Jankovic J, Mazziotta JC (eds.), *Bradley's Neurology in Clinical Practice*, 6th ed. Philadelphia, PA: W. B. Saunders; 2012:1824–1854.e2

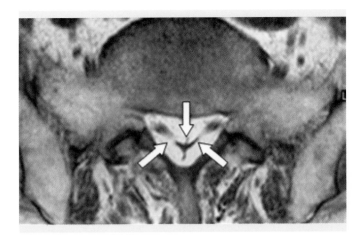

FIGURE 14-5. T1-weighted magnetic resonance imaging axial view of L5-S1. Hyperintense tissue (indicated by *arrows*), consistent with adipose tissue, is circumferentially compressing the spinal cord.

10. **(B)** Percutaneous treatment of painful osteoporotic vertebral compression fractures can be accomplished with injection with polymethyl methacrylate (PMMA), bone cement used in orthopedic surgeries. This is a minimally invasive, radiologically guided procedure that can serve to decrease pain and increase function for symptomatic patients. In retrospective case studies, immediate pain relief was achieved in 70–90% of cases, with complications occurring less than 1% of the time (see Fig. 14-6).

BIBLIOGRAPHY

Lin W, Cheng T, Lee Y, et al. New vertebral osteoporotic compression fractures after percutaneous vertebroplasty: retrospective analysis of risk factors. *J Vasc Interv Radiol* 2008;19:225–232.
Rowland L. *Merritt's Neurology*, 12th ed. Philadelphia, PA: Lippincott Williams & Wilkins; 2010.

11. **(C)** Growth hormone is secreted in a pulsatile manner; therefore, a random level would not be helpful in the diagnosis of acromegaly. The gold standard for diagnosis is measurement of GH after 75 g of oral glucose. Suppression to less than 0.4 ng/mL excludes the diagnosis. Lack of suppression establishes the diagnosis. Other situations that can lead to decreased suppression are pregnancy, puberty, oral contraceptive pill use, poorly controlled diabetes, and hepatic or renal insufficiency. IGF-1 levels are reflective of the 24-hour GH concentration and correlate well with clinical activity of the hormone.

BIBLIOGRAPHY

Bope ET, Kellerman RD. Section 11. In: Bope ET, Kellerman RD (eds.), *Conn's Current Therapy*. Philadelphia, PA: W. B. Saunders; 2014:687–774.

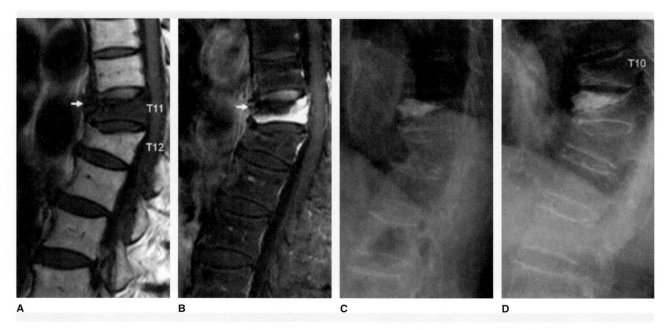

FIGURE 14-6. Images obtained in a 78-year-old woman with a history of T12 fracture. **A.** Sagittal fast spin echo T1-weighted magnetic resonance image (MRI) shows low signal intensity in the bone marrow and a loss of vertebral body height at the T11 vertebra. A fluid-filled vacuum cleft was noted (*arrow*). **B.** Sagittal MRI obtained with fat saturation shows high signal intensity within the T11 vertebra. A fluid-filled vacuum cleft was noted (*arrow*). **C.** Lateral radiograph obtained after vertebroplasty shows restoration of the vertebral height and correction of spinal kyphosis. **D.** Radiograph obtained 3 months after vertebroplasty, after the patient returned with a new onset of back pain, shows a new deformity of the T10 vertebra. From Lin W, Cheng T, Lee Y, et al. New vertebral osteoporotic compression fractures after percutaneous vertebroplasty: retrospective analysis of risk factors. *J Vasc Interv Radiol* 2008;19:225–232.

12. **(B)** Overgrowth of bone is the classic feature associated with acromegaly, particularly of the face and skull. Long term, this increases the risk for disabling degenerative arthritis. Hypersecretion of GH leads to excessive IGF-1 production by the liver, which is the mediator of many other systemic effects. GH excess leads to generalized organ hypertrophy, clinically evident as thyromegaly and enlargement of the submandibular glands. Cardiomyopathy, hypertension, and cardiomegaly are a significant cause of morbidity and mortality in acromegaly. Obstructive and central sleep apnea are also common. In addition, glucose intolerance occurs in 50–70% of patients. Patients with acromegaly are also at increased risk for development of colon polyps and colon cancer, with recent estimates suggesting they are at double the risk of the general population.

BIBLIOGRAPHY

Javorsky BR, Aron DC, Findling JW, Tyrrell J. Hypothalamus and pituitary gland. In: Gardner DG, Shoback D (eds.), *Greenspan's Basic & Clinical Endocrinology*, 9th ed. New York, NY: McGraw-Hill; 2011.

Melmed S. Acromegaly. In: Jameson J, De Groot L (eds.), *Endocrinology*, 6th ed. Philadelphia, PA: W. B. Saunders; 2010:262–281.

13. **(C)** This patient has a macroadenoma with extrasellar extension, which is not causing compressive symptoms. Therefore, there is no need for urgent surgical decompression. In fact, 40–60% of macroadenomas are unlikely to be controlled with surgery alone. Transsphenoidal surgery is the treatment of choice for intrasellar microadenomas (<10 mm), noninvasive macroadenomas, and tumors causing compressive symptoms. For other situations, including this patient, there are currently three drug classes available to treat acromegaly: dopamine agonists, somatostatin receptor ligands, and GH receptor antagonists. Of these, serotonin receptor ligands are most appropriate for first-line therapy in tumors that have low probability for surgical cure. Radiosurgery should be considered a third-line therapy, usually reserved for patients who cannot achieve tumor growth control or normalization of hormone levels with surgery or medical therapy.

BIBLIOGRAPHY

Melmed S, Colao A, Barkan A, et al. Guidelines for acromegaly management: an update. *J Clin Endocrinol Metab* 2009;94(5):1509–1517.

14. **(A)** Patients with acromegaly characteristically will have difficult airways. This is due to a number of factors. First, the increased size of facial bones, particularly the mandible, makes face mask sealing difficult. This can become particularly dangerous with attempted ventilation after the induction of anesthesia. Enlargement of the tongue and other soft tissues of the pharynx not only makes laryngoscopy difficult, but these changes also predispose to sleep apnea and further complicate ventilation. In addition, tracheal intubation may be challenging because the glottis can be narrowed due to enlargement of the vocal cords. Second, enlargement of the thyroid can compress the trachea, further complicating intubation. As with obese patients and those with obstructive sleep apnea, the safest technique for intubation is with the awake fiberoptic technique. Additionally, the use of a small endotracheal tube can facilitate easier passage through the cords. Patients with acromegaly may also have enlarged nasal turbinates, making nasal intubation a less viable option.

BIBLIOGRAPHY

Flint PW, Haughey BH, Lund VJ, et al. Surgical management of the difficult adult airway. In: Bhatti NI (ed.), *Cummings Otolaryngology Head & Neck Surgery*. New York, NY: Elsevier; 2010:121–129.
Walters TL. Acromegaly. In: Bready LL, Dillman D, Noorily SH (eds.), *Decision Making in Anesthesiology*, 4th ed. Philadelphia, PA: Elsevier; 2007:200–202.

15. **(B)** The patient has findings consistent with pituitary apoplexy (see Fig. 14-7), which is due to hemorrhage or infarct within the pituitary gland. Although pituitary tumors are common, apoplexy is a rare but serious complication. Factors that may precipitate this complication include endocrine stimulation (in the form of diagnostic studies), head trauma, pregnancy (Sheehan syndrome), anticoagulation, hypertension, recent cardiac surgery, diabetic ketoacidosis, and ovarian stimulation medications. The combination of anticoagulation and ovarian stimulation medications in this patient likely triggered a hemorrhage into an undiagnosed pituitary macroadenoma. The visual disturbances she is experiencing are

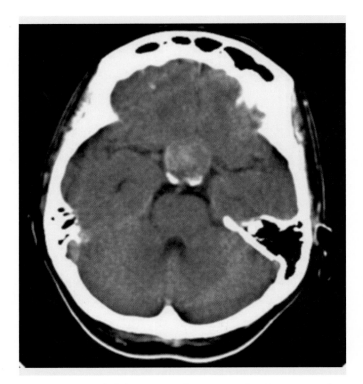

FIGURE 14-7. Axial computed tomography demonstrating evidence of hemorrhage within the pituitary gland, seen as areas of patchy enhancement.

likely due to the tumor's proximity to the optic chiasm. Additionally, nerves passing through the cavernous sinus can also be affected (CN III, IV, V1, and V2). Acute hypopituitarism is a major concern in these patients who may develop adrenal crisis. In addition, delay in diagnosis and treatment can lead to permanent blindness, nerve palsies, or death. She should be treated with parenteral corticosteroids immediately. There is currently controversy regarding surgical intervention rather than conservative medical management. However, definitive therapy involves transsphenoidal decompression of the pituitary.

BIBLIOGRAPHY

Nelson BK. Pituitary apoplexy. In: Adams JG (ed.), *Emergency Medicine*, 2nd ed. Philadelphia, PA: Saunders; 2013:1439–1441.e1431.
Tan T, Caputo C, Mehta A, Hatfield E, Martin N, Meeran K. Pituitary macroadenomas: are combination antiplatelet and anticoagulant therapy contraindicated? A case report. *J Med Case Rep.* 2007;1:74.

CHAPTER 15

BREAST SURGERY

GREGORY LARRIEUX AND RACHEL A. GREENUP

QUESTIONS

1. The long thoracic nerve
   (A) Innervates the latissimus dorsi muscle
   (B) Arises from the posterior cord of the brachial plexus
   (C) Is located deep to the axillary artery and vein and then travels superficial to the deep fascia of the serratus anterior muscle
   (D) Is also called the internal respiratory nerve of Bell
   (E) Has minimal significant sequelae if damaged during axillary dissection

2. Axillary lymph nodes are classified according to the relationship with the
   (A) Axillary vein
   (B) Pectoralis major muscle
   (C) Pectoralis minor muscle
   (D) Axillary nerve
   (E) Serratus anterior muscle

3. All of the following are important features of a patient's initial assessment and are known risk factors for breast cancer *except*
   (A) Family history of breast cancer
   (B) Age of menarche
   (C) History of atypical hyperplasia
   (D) Radiation exposure as a teenager
   (E) History of ductal adenosis

4. All of the following are part of the Gail model calculation of 5-year and lifetime breast cancer risk *except*
   (A) Race
   (B) Age of first menses
   (C) Age of first live birth/full-term pregnancy
   (D) Age at menopause
   (E) Number of first-degree relatives with breast cancer

5. Epidermal growth factor receptors (EGFR)
   (A) Are autocrine factors
   (B) Have no known mitogenic activity
   (C) Are related to acquired tamoxifen resistance
   (D) Have not been shown to have any response to estrogen
   (E) Have no known role in apoptosis

6. Which of the following is true regarding *BRCA2*?
   (A) The incidence of breast cancer among *BRCA2* carriers is approximately 30%.
   (B) It is not associated with an increased risk of male breast cancer.
   (C) It plays a role in DNA damage response pathways.
   (D) It is a cystosolic protein.
   (E) It is associated with a 40% lifetime risk of ovarian cancer.

7. Which of the following is true regarding Li-Fraumeni syndrome?
   (A) It accounts for 10% of hereditary breast cancers.
   (B) It occurs as a result of proto-oncogene mutation.
   (C) Criteria include leukemia in a first-degree relative.
   (D) It is rarely associated with breast cancer in males.
   (E) It has autosomal recessive inheritance.

8. A 35-year-old woman arrives at your office stating that she has a 1-month history of a palpable right breast lump. On physical examination, you are able to palpate a 1-cm solid, mobile, firm nodule at the 2 o' clock position. Your diagnostic evaluation for this newly found breast mass includes
   (A) Mammogram
   (B) Ultrasound
   (C) Core-needle biopsy
   (D) Short-term follow-up
   (E) All of the above

9. Characteristics of a malignant lesion on an ultrasound include all of the following *except*
   (A) Irregular borders
   (B) Asymmetry
   (C) Posterior enhancement
   (D) Poorly circumscribed
   (E) High acoustic attenuation

10. Breast magnetic resonance imaging (MRI)
    (A) Is a valuable screening tool among high-risk women (i.e., *BRCA* mutation carriers)
    (B) Has high specificity but low sensitivity
    (C) Should be added to annual diagnostic mammogram for routine surveillance in average-risk women previously treated for breast cancer
    (D) Should not be used if the patient has a breast implant
    (E) Cannot differentiate between scar tissue and cancer recurrence

11. Breast cellulitis found in a lactating patient
    (A) Is best treated with incision and drainage in the operating room
    (B) Is reason for the infant to stop breast-feeding
    (C) That develops into an abscess is diagnosed by fever, leukocytosis, and a fluctuant mass
    (D) Is treated by antibiotics, warm packs, and emptying the breast
    (E) Involves multiple organisms

12. The most common cause of nipple discharge is
    (A) Carcinoma
    (B) Fibrocystic disease
    (C) Intraductal papilloma
    (D) Ductal ectasia
    (E) Trauma

13. Which of the following is true regarding phyllodes tumor?
    (A) Present in older women when compared to fibroadenomas
    (B) Are rarely malignant
    (C) Require wide local excision
    (D) Are at a high risk of recurrence approximating 20%
    (E) All of the above

14. A 22-year-old college senior presents to your clinic stating that she has recently found a new breast mass. She reports that this initially caused discomfort but has since resolved. She has no nipple discharge or other complaints. You do an ultrasound in the office and find the following (see Fig. 15-1):
    Your recommendations to her are
    (A) Partial mastectomy with sentinel node biopsy
    (B) Total mastectomy with sentinel node biopsy followed by immediate reconstruction
    (C) Core needle biopsy (CNB)
    (D) Needle localized excisional biopsy
    (E) Close follow-up

15. Which of the following is true regarding gynecomastia?
    (A) Mastectomy is first-line treatment.
    (B) It is pathologic in neonates.

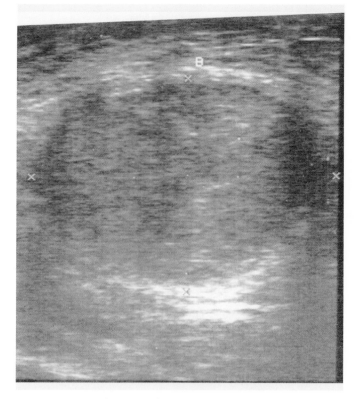

FIGURE 15-1. Ultrasound in 22-year-old woman.

    (C) It increases the risk of subsequent breast cancer.
    (D) It most commonly due to idiopathic causes.
    (E) It rarely warrants psychotherapy in affected patients.

16. A 67-year-old man arrives at your office with a 1-month history of right breast pain, greatest in the subareolar area. He now is able to palpate a mass. He denies any nipple discharge or skin changes. Your next step is
    (A) Clinical breast examination and office ultrasound
    (B) Mammogram
    (C) Measure estrogen and testosterone levels
    (D) Ask the patient to stop all medications
    (E) Give reassurance that this is not cancer and see him back in 6 months to 1 year for a repeat examination

17. A 34-year-old woman is referred to your office for evaluation of breast pain. She describes the pain as burning that is occasionally sharp in nature. It is mostly located in the subareolar area and seems to be fairly well localized. When asked when the pain occurs, she states that it is always present and is very troublesome to her. On physical examination, she has dense glandular tissue throughout both breasts, but no discrete nodules. Your working diagnosis at this point is
    (A) Cyclical breast pain
    (B) Noncyclical breast pain

(C) Cancer
(D) Psychosomatic pain
(E) Tietze syndrome

18. Your next step in management of the patient in Question 17 is
    (A) Reassurance
    (B) Start a diuretic
    (C) Refer her to a psychologist
    (D) Give a steroid injection
    (E) Perform a surgical excision of the painful area

19. Tamoxifen
    (A) Is an estrogen receptor (ER) agonist
    (B) Is an ER antagonist
    (C) Has been shown to decrease the incidence of recurrent breast cancer by 47%
    (D) Has been shown to decrease the risk of future breast cancer by 49% in high-risk patients
    (E) All of the above

20. Following a needle localized excisional biopsy for microcalcifications, pathology demonstrates fibrocystic changes associated with sclerosing adenosis and ductal hyperplasia with lobular carcinoma *in situ* (LCIS) at the margin. There is no atypia or evidence of malignancy. In reviewing the pathology with your patient, your recommendations include
    (A) Reexcision of the lumpectomy cavity due to positive margins followed by radiation therapy
    (B) A contralateral "mirror" breast biopsy in the same region because this disease is bilateral
    (C) Close follow-up due to her future cancer risk of 1% per year
    (D) Bilateral mastectomy with sentinel lymph node biopsy on the affected side
    (E) Consideration of hormone replacement therapy

21. With respect to inherited breast cancer, which of the following statements is *true*?
    (A) Most newly diagnosed breast cancers in women are related to either *BRCA1* or *BRCA2* positivity.
    (B) Early age of onset, multiple primary tumors, and bilateral cancers are typical in inherited breast cancer.
    (C) The lifetime risk of developing breast cancer if carrying a *BRCA1* or *BRCA2* gene mutation is approximately 50%.
    (D) Patients carrying the *BRCA1* or *BRCA2* gene should have a prophylactic bilateral mastectomy before the age of 25 if possible.
    (E) Careful surveillance with monthly breast self-examination, annual physician physical examination, and total breast ultrasound will minimize risk

associated with a strong pedigree of inherited breast cancers.

22. A 40-year-old woman presents with a 2-cm mass in her right breast first detected by mammography (see Fig. 15-2).

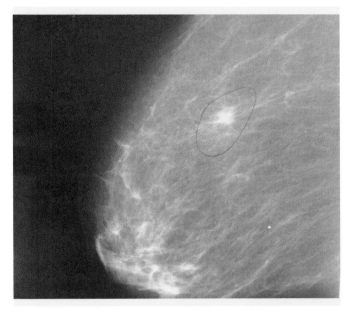

FIGURE 15-2. Mammogram showing an irregular, speculated mass in the right breast. Core biopsy reveals invasive ductal carcinoma.

Radiographic core biopsy of the lesion is selected for diagnosis and reveals infiltrating ductal carcinoma. She has no palpable axillary lymph nodes. Appropriate therapy for the patient would include
    (A) Modified radical mastectomy
    (B) Partial mastectomy (lumpectomy) with sentinel lymph node biopsy
    (C) Neoadjuvant chemotherapy followed by lumpectomy
    (D) Lumpectomy with axillary node dissection
    (E) Lumpectomy followed by axillary radiation

23. A sentinel lymph node biopsy in the patient described in Question 22 reveals metastatic carcinoma. There is no evidence of distant metastases on further investigation. Her stage by the American Joint Committee on Cancer (AJCC) TNM staging system is
    (A) I
    (B) II
    (C) III
    (D) IV
    (E) V

24. A 65-year-old woman presents with a large (5-cm) mass in her right breast. On physical exam, there is overlying ulceration of the skin and concern for fixation to the underlying pectoralis muscle. She is noted to have several enlarged, matted axillary lymph nodes on examination. Core biopsy reveals ER-negative, progesterone receptor (PR)-negative, human epidermal growth factor receptor 2 (HER2)-negative invasive ductal carcinoma of the breast. After staging scans demonstrate no evidence of distant metastatic disease, her management should begin with
    (A) Mastectomy with sentinel lymph node biopsy
    (B) Neoadjuvant chemotherapy
    (C) Radiation therapy
    (D) Aromatase inhibitors

25. Which of the following is *true* with respect to sentinel lymph node biopsy?
    (A) Localization of the sentinel node is successful in only approximately 75% of cases.
    (B) It misses isolated micrometastases in nonsentinel nodes in 20% of cases.
    (C) It is unnecessary in patients with primary tumors less than 1 cm (T1a), because the rate of metastases is less than 1%.
    (D) The time from injection to accumulation of dye in the sentinel node is longer for the radioactive tracer than isosulfan (Lymphazurin) dye.
    (E) When properly performed, it should yield a single sentinel lymph node.

26. Which of the following statements is *incorrect* regarding ductal carcinoma *in situ*?
    (A) Breast-conservation therapy should be done for localized disease, particularly of the noncomedo variety.
    (B) Axillary lymph node dissection is not necessary.
    (C) The most common clinical presentation is a palpable mass.
    (D) After breast-conserving surgery, radiotherapy is administered in tangential fields to the whole breast.
    (E) There is no role for chemotherapy in the treatment of ductal carcinoma *in situ* (DCIS).

27. A 45-year-old man presents with a 2-cm, painless subareolar mass of his left breast, with nipple retraction. Physical examination reveals no lymph node involvement. A fine-needle biopsy of the mass is performed and reveals infiltrating ductal carcinoma with positive hormone receptors. Further workup reveals no evidence of metastatic disease. What is the most appropriate treatment plan?
    (A) Hormone therapy with tamoxifen
    (B) Wide local excision with sentinel lymph node biopsy
    (C) Segmental mastectomy
    (D) Modified radical mastectomy
    (E) Radical mastectomy

28. A 29-year-old woman in her second trimester of pregnancy presents with stage II invasive ductal carcinoma. The lesion is visualized on ultrasound, and there is no evidence of metastatic or lymph node disease. Which of the following is the most appropriate treatment option?
    (A) Routine ultrasound examination, followed by postpartum lumpectomy, axillary dissection, chemotherapy, and irradiation
    (B) Lumpectomy and axillary dissection, followed by postpartum chemotherapy and irradiation
    (C) Lumpectomy and axillary dissection, followed by immediate chemotherapy and postpartum irradiation
    (D) Lumpectomy and axillary dissection, followed by immediate chemotherapy and irradiation
    (E) Termination of pregnancy, lumpectomy, axillary dissection, chemotherapy, and irradiation

29. A 22-year-old woman in her ninth week of pregnancy presents with a painless lump in her left breast. Physical examination reveals both breasts to be fibrous and dense. A 2-cm lesion is palpated in the left breast. No nipple discharge is noted, and there are no palpable lymph nodes of either axilla. Which of the following imaging studies should be used first to evaluate the lesion?
    (A) Ultrasound
    (B) Single-view mammogram
    (C) Two-view mammogram
    (D) MRI

30. Criteria for consideration of genetic testing for hereditary breast cancer syndromes include
    (A) Personal history of breast cancer diagnosed at ≤40 years old
    (B) Personal history of epithelial ovarian cancer at any age
    (C) Any male breast cancer
    (D) Triple-negative breast cancer phenotype diagnosed at ≤60 years old
    (E) All of the above

ANSWERS AND EXPLANATIONS

1. **(C)** The anatomy of the axilla is shown in Fig. 15-3. The long thoracic nerve, or the external respiratory nerve of Bell, arises from the fifth, sixth, and seventh cervical nerves and passes deep to the axillary artery and vein, staying close to the chest wall. It innervates the serratus anterior muscle. This muscle is important in stabilizing the scapula on the thorax. Injury to the long thoracic nerve results in a winged scapula. This can lead to significant morbidity.

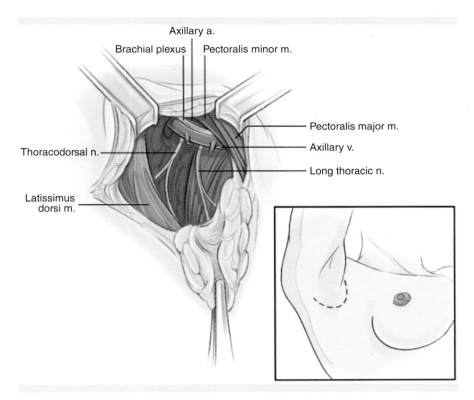

FIGURE 15-3. Axillary nerves. Reproduced with permission from Petrek JA, Blackwood MM. Axillary dissection: current practice and technique. *Curr Prob Surg.* 1995;32:285.

The thoracodorsal nerve arises from the posterior cord of the brachial plexus and passes beneath the axillary vein. It runs in the posterior axilla and through the areolar tissue containing the lymph nodes. It innervates the latissimus dorsi muscle. Loss or injury of the thoracodorsal nerve results in weakness of extension, internal rotation, and adduction of the humerus. This can be well tolerated by most patients.

BIBLIOGRAPHY

Osbourne M. Breast anatomy and development. In: Harris JR, Lippman ME, Morrow M, et al. (eds.), *Diseases of the Breast*, 2nd ed. Philadelphia, PA: Lippincott Williams & Wilkins; 2000:6–9.

Spratt J, Donegan W, Tobin G. Gross anatomy of the breast. In: Donegan W, Spratt J (eds.), *Cancer of the Breast*, 5th ed. St. Louis, MO: W.B. Saunders; 2002:32–37.

2. **(C)** The axillary lymph nodes are classified according to their relationship with the pectoralis minor muscle (see Fig. 15-4).

   Level I: lateral to the lateral border of the pectoralis minor

   Level II: posterior to the pectoralis minor

   Level III: medial to the medial border of the pectoralis minor

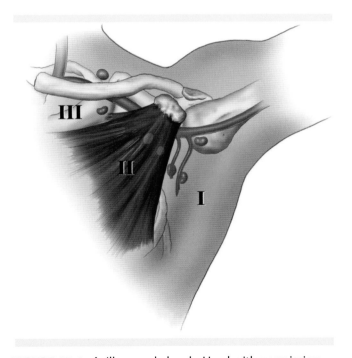

FIGURE 15-4. Axillary node levels. Used with permission from Visual Art © 2012. The University of Texas MD Anderson Cancer Center.

Rotter's nodes, or interpectoral nodes, are anterior to the pectoralis minor muscle. The pathway of metastasis follows the direction of lymph flow to the lymph nodes (I, then to II and III).

Axillary lymph node status is one of the most important prognostic indicators for breast cancer. The likelihood of node-positive disease is directly related to the size of the tumor, not other tumor markers (estrogen/progesterone receptors, Her2/neu status) (Table 15-1).

TABLE 15-1 Axillary Nodes and Tumor Size

Tumor Size (cm)	Chance of Node-Positive Disease (%)
0.1–0.5	11
0.6–1.0	15
1.1–1.3	25
1.4–1.6	34
1.7–2.0	43

Lymph node status also gives an indication about overall survival.

Subsequent therapy is often based on the status of the lymph nodes. If the patient has lymph node–positive disease, then chemotherapy should be strongly considered.

BIBLIOGRAPHY

Osbourne M. Breast anatomy and development. In: Harris JR, Lippman ME, Morrow M, et al. (eds.), *Diseases of the Breast*, 2nd ed. Philadelphia, PA: Lippincott Williams & Wilkins; 2000:4–6.
Spratt J, Donegan W, Tobin G. Gross anatomy of the breast. In: Donegan W, Spratt J (eds.), *Cancer of the Breast*, 5th ed. St. Louis, MO: W.B. Saunders; 2002:39–43.

3. **(E)** There are many known risk factors for breast cancer. The most important risk factor is being female. There is a 100:1 ratio of female breast cancers as compared to male breast cancers.

Increased estrogen exposure also increases the risk of breast cancer, and factors that increase the number of menstrual cycles, such as early menarche, nulliparity, and late menopause, are associated with increased risk. Obesity is also associated with breast cancer risk, because the major source of estrogen in postmenopausal women is the conversion of androstenedione to estrone by adipose tissue. Alcohol consumption and a high-fat diet are also implicated, as are radiation exposure when younger than 30 years old (i.e., as treatment for Hodgkin lymphoma) and a prior history of breast cancer (0.5–1% risk per year).

Also, some forms of benign breast disease place the patient at increased risk for developing breast cancer in the future. This includes atypical hyperplasia (four to five times the risk) and lobular carcinoma *in situ* (LCIS) (8–10 times the risk). Benign papillomas, adenomas, ductal ectasia, cysts, and the like do not increase a patient's risk significantly.

BRCA1 and *BRCA2* are tumor-suppressor genes that play a significant role in breast cancer development. *BRCA1* is located on chromosome 17 and is also linked to ovarian, prostate, and colon cancer. *BRCA2* is located on chromosome 13 and is linked to male breast cancer, a lesser rate of ovarian cancer, and prostate and colon cancer. Having one of the genes confers a 60–80% lifetime risk of developing breast cancer; however, only 5–10% of all breast cancer cases are genetically driven.

BIBLIOGRAPHY

Hunt KK, Robertson JR, Bland KI. The breast. In: Brunicardi F, Andersen DK, Billiar TR, et al. (eds.), *Schwartz's Principles of Surgery*, 10th ed. New York, NY: McGraw-Hill; 2014.
Shahid T, Soroka J, Kong EH, et al. Structure and mechanism of action of the BRCA2 breast cancer tumor suppressor. *Nat Struct Mol Biol* 2014;21(11):962–968.

4. **(D)** The Gail model is a statistical model based on data from the Breast Cancer Detection Demonstration Project, a mammography screening program conducted in the 1970s. The model incorporates race, age, age at first menses, age at first live birth, number of first-degree relatives with breast cancer, and number of previous biopsies, including benign results and those with atypical hyperplasia. The program derives 5-year and lifetime risks for breast cancer by multiplying relative risks from several categories (Table 15-2).

A risk greater than 1.7% at 5 years deserves further addressing, and the patient should be appropriately counseled regarding her increased risk. Tamoxifen has now been shown to decrease the 5-year and lifetime risks in these patients by almost 50%. This is based on the NSABP-P1 study data. Further studies are ongoing to examine the role of other estrogen-blocking drugs, such as raloxifene (Evista; STAR trial).

BIBLIOGRAPHY

Hunt KK, Robertson JR, Bland KI. The breast. In: Brunicardi F, Andersen DK, Billiar TR, et al. (eds.), *Schwartz's Principles of Surgery*, 10th ed. New York, NY: McGraw-Hill; 2014.
Armstrong K, Eisen A, and Barbara Weber B. Assessing the risk of breast cancer. *N Engl J Med* 2000;342:564–571.

5. **(C)** Epidermal growth factor receptor (EGFR) is a family of transmembrane tyrosine kinase receptors. The family

TABLE 15-2 Relative Risk Estimates for the Gail Model

Variable	Relative Risk
Age at menarche (years)	
≥14	1.00
12–13	1.10
<12	1.21
Number of biopsy specimens/history of benign breast disease, age <50 y	
0	1.00
1	1.70
≥2	2.88
Number of biopsy specimens/history of benign breast disease, age ≥50 y	
0	1.02
1	1.27
≥2	1.62
Age at first live birth (years)	
<20 y	
Number of first-degree relatives with history of breast cancer	
0	1.00
1	2.61
≥2	6.80
20–24 y	
Number of first-degree relatives with history of breast cancer	
0	1.24
1	2.68
≥2	5.78
25–29 y	
Number of first-degree relatives with history of breast cancer	
0	1.55
1	2.76
≥2	4.91
≥30 y	
Number of first-degree relatives with history of breast cancer	
0	1.93
1	2.83
≥2	4.17

From Brunicardi F, Andersen DK, Billiar TR, et al. (eds.), *Schwartz's Principles of Surgery*, 10th ed. New York, NY: McGraw-Hill; 2014:Table 17-6.

includes HER1 (EGFR), HER2, HER3, and HER4. This group of growth factor receptors is also known as c-erb-b2, c-erb-b3, and c-erb-b4. When EGFR is activated, tyrosine kinase activity is induced, leading to autophosphorylation and subsequent activation of nuclear transcription factors.

Overexpression of EGFR in breast cancer correlates with estrogen receptor–negative status and with overexpression of p53 and Ki-67. *HER2/neu* (c-erb-b2) is overexpressed in 20–30% of breast cancer cases and is both an important prognostic factor and a predictive factor in breast cancer. When overexpressed in breast cancer, *HER2/neu* promotes enhanced growth and proliferation and increases invasive and metastatic capabilities, resulting in poorly differentiated tumors with high proliferation rates, positive lymph nodes, decreased hormone receptor expression, and an increased risk of recurrence and death due to breast cancer.

Routine testing of the primary tumor specimen for *HER2/neu* expression should be performed on all invasive breast cancers. This can be done with immunohistochemical analysis to evaluate for overexpression of the cell-surface receptor at the protein level or by using fluorescence in situ hybridization (FISH) to evaluate for gene amplification. In patients whose tumors overexpress *HER2/neu*, treatment with trastuzumab (Herceptin) is warranted. Trastuzumab is a recombinant humanized monoclonal antibody directed against *HER2/neu* and is first-line treatment of women with *HER2/neu*-overexpressing metastatic breast cancer as well as women with early-stage breast cancer when used in combination with chemotherapy. Patients who receive trastuzumab in combination with chemotherapy have a 40–50% reduction in the risk of breast cancer recurrence and approximately a one-third reduction in breast cancer mortality compared with chemotherapy alone.

BIBLIOGRAPHY

Hunt KK, Robertson JR, Bland KI. The breast. In: Brunicardi F, Andersen DK, Billiar TR, et al. (eds.), *Schwartz's Principles of Surgery*, 10th ed. New York, NY: McGraw-Hill; 2014.

van Diest PJ, Buerger H, Kuijper A, van der Wall E. Breast carcinogenesis. In: Kuerer HM (ed.), *Kuerer's Breast Surgical Oncology*. New York, NY: McGraw-Hill; 2010:Chapter 1.

6. **(C)** *BRCA2* is located on chromosome 13q. It is a tumor-suppressor gene that plays a role in the DNA damage response pathways. *BRCA2* is associated with an approximately 85% lifetime risk of breast cancer and 20% risk of ovarian cancer in female carriers. Males that carry the *BRCA2* gene have a 6% lifetime risk of developing breast cancer, nearly 100 times the general population risk. *BRCA2* mutations are also associated with an increased risk of

melanoma, colon, prostate, pancreatic, biliary, and stomach cancers. Patients who develop breast cancer tend to be slightly older than those patients with *BRCA1*. The tumors also tend to be less aggressive than those associated with *BRCA1*. *BRCA2* tumors are more like sporadic tumors, yet the inheritance is autosomal dominant, with approximately half of children of carriers inheriting the trait.

BRCA1 is located on chromosome 17q11. It is also a nuclear protein that plays a role in transcription, cell-cycle control, and DNA damage response pathways. It is thought to affect transcription factors and can enhance p53 transactivation. Germline mutations in *BRCA1* are implicated in up to 45% of hereditary breast cancers and 80% of hereditary ovarian cancers. Female mutation carriers have an approximate 85% lifetime risk of developing breast cancer and up to a 40% lifetime risk of developing ovarian cancer. The breast cancers linked to *BRCA1* tend to be poorly differentiated invasive ductal carcinomas. In addition, *BRCA1* is also a factor in prostate cancer and possible colon cancer.

BIBLIOGRAPHY

Hunt KK, Robertson JR, Bland KI. The breast. In: Brunicardi F, Andersen DK, Billiar TR, et al. (eds.), *Schwartz's Principles of Surgery*, 10th ed. New York, NY: McGraw-Hill; 2014.

Krontiras H, Awonuga O, Bland K. Molecular targets in breast cancer. In: Cameron J (ed.), *Current Surgical Therapy*, 11th ed. Philadelphia, PA: Elsevier; 2014:579–583.

Robinson L. Genetic predisposition syndromes. In: Kuerer HM (ed.), *Kuerer's Breast Surgical Oncology*. New York, NY: McGraw-Hill; 2010:Chapter 8.

Shahid T, Soroka J, Kong EH, et al. Structure and mechanism of action of the BRCA2 breast cancer tumor suppressor. *Nat Struct Mol Biol* 2014;21(11):962–968.

7. **(D)** Li-Fraumeni syndrome (LFS) is an autosomal dominant disease that was first documented in families whose children had sarcomas. Criteria for classic LFS in an individual (the proband) include: (1) a bone or soft tissue sarcoma when younger than 45 years, (2) a first-degree relative with cancer before age 45 years, and (3) another first- or second-degree relative with either a sarcoma diagnosed at any age or any cancer diagnosed before age 45 years. LFS is due to germline mutations in the *TP53* tumor suppressor gene located on chromosome 17p, which codes for the p53 protein.

TP53 is a tumor suppressor gene located on chromosome 17q13. This gene is responsible for a multifunctional DNA damage response protein. When *TP53* undergoes mutation, it functions as an inhibitor of p53. Unmutated p53 is a nuclear protein that affects DNA damage response proteins as well. p53 normally acts to block the cell cycle at the G_1-S phase, to induce apoptosis, and to allow induction of differentiation. This all in turn slows cellular growth and allows for DNA repair. Inhibition or loss of p53 function may lead to cellular instability.

LFS is characterized by early-onset breast cancer, bone and soft tissue sarcomas, brain tumors, acute leukemia, lymphoma, and adrenal cortical carcinoma. It is estimated that over 75% of these women develop breast cancer between the ages of 22 and 45 years, and 45% of women with this mutation will develop breast cancer before the age of 60, but overall, LFS accounts for only 1% of hereditary breast cancer. Interestingly, male breast cancer has rarely been reported in families with LFS.

The current recommendations for patients with LFS include:

1. Children and adults should undergo comprehensive annual physical examination.

2. Children and adults should be encouraged see a physician promptly for evaluation of lingering symptoms and illnesses.

3. Women should undergo breast cancer monitoring, with annual breast MRI and twice annual clinical breast examination beginning at age 20–25 years. The use of mammograms has been controversial because of radiation exposure and limited sensitivity. When included, annual mammograms should alternate with breast MRI, with one modality every 6 months.

4. Adults should consider routine screening for colorectal cancer with colonoscopy every 2–3 years beginning no later than age 25 years.

5. Individuals should consider organ-targeted surveillance based on the pattern of cancer observed in their family. Intensified surveillance with whole-body MRI protocols for adults and children who carry a germline *TP53* mutation are being evaluated in investigational settings.

BIBLIOGRAPHY

Meric-Bernstam F, Pollock RE. Oncology. In: Brunicardi F, Andersen DK, Billiar TR, et al. (eds.), *Schwartz's Principles of Surgery*, 10th ed. New York, NY: McGraw-Hill; 2014.

Robinson L. Genetic predisposition syndromes. In: Kuerer HM (ed.), *Kuerer's Breast Surgical Oncology*. New York, NY: McGraw-Hill; 2010:Chapter 8.

Schneider K, Zelley K, Nichols KE, et al. Li-Fraumeni syndrome. 1999 Jan 19 [Updated April 11, 2013]. In: Pagon RA, Adam MP, Ardinger HH, et al. (ed.), *GeneReviews®* [Internet]. Seattle (WA): University of Washington, Seattle; 1993-2014. http://www.ncbi.nlm.nih.gov/books/NBK1311/. Accessed November 15, 2015.

8. **(E)** The initial evaluation for a palpable breast mass in a 40-year-woman should include a diagnostic

mammogram and ultrasound. Cystic masses that are amenable to aspiration with complete resolution can be followed closely with a 6-week follow-up ultrasound. Without complete resolution, cystic masses should undergo core biopsy or be excised to rule out a cystic cancer.

If the mass is solid, a core biopsy should be performed regardless of appearance on imaging. Benign findings on core biopsy can be followed with close surveillance, but any atypia or abnormality should warrant surgical excision. Appropriate treatment can then be initiated.

Core needle biopsy is preferred over a fine-needle aspirate when evaluating breast masses by providing a definitive histologic diagnosis, including tumor receptors (i.e., estrogen receptor status and *in situ* versus invasive cancer). Fine-needle aspiration only gives a cytologic diagnosis.

Although only 5% of breast masses among women under 40 are malignant, it is important that a thorough evaluation including diagnostic mammogram, ultrasound, and core biopsy be performed and the lesion closely followed.

BIBLIOGRAPHY

Bleicher M. In: Harris J, Lippman M, Morrow M, Osborne C (eds.), *Diseases of the Breast*, 4th ed. Philadelphia, PA: Lippincott Williams & Wilkins; 2010:32–41.

Giuliano AE. Breast disorders. In: Doherty GM (ed.), *Current Diagnosis & Treatment: Surgery*, 13th ed. New York, NY: McGraw-Hill; 2010:Chapter 17.

Hunt KK, Robertson JR, Bland KI. The breast. In: Brunicardi F, Andersen DK, Billiar TR, et al. (eds.), *Schwartz's Principles of Surgery*, 10th ed. New York, NY: McGraw-Hill; 2014.

Kern K. Diagnostic options in symptomatic breast disease. In: Cameron J (ed.), *Current Surgical Therapy*, 7th ed. St. Louis, MO: Mosby; 2001:680–681.

Kopans D. Imaging analysis of breast lesions. In: Harris JR, Lippman ME, Morrow M, et al. (eds.), *Diseases of the Breast*, 2nd ed. Philadelphia, PA: Lippincott Williams & Wilkins; 2000:135–137.

9. **(C)** Malignant lesions seen on ultrasound tend to have irregular or spiculated borders and are poorly circumscribed, asymmetric, and hypoechoic. They have a high acoustic attenuation that leads to posterior shadowing. The accuracy of characterizing a malignant lesion on ultrasound is 80% for T1 lesions, 93% for T2 lesions, and 100% for T3 lesions. This gives an overall accuracy of 88.9%.

Benign lesions tend to have smooth borders and are well circumscribed, symmetric, and hypo-/iso-/anechoic. They may have posterior enhancement with apparent bilateral shadowing; this is especially true of cysts (see Fig. 15-6).

Solid benign lesions tend to have smooth borders, are well circumscribed, and are hypoechoic. They tend to be wider than taller (see Fig. 15-7).

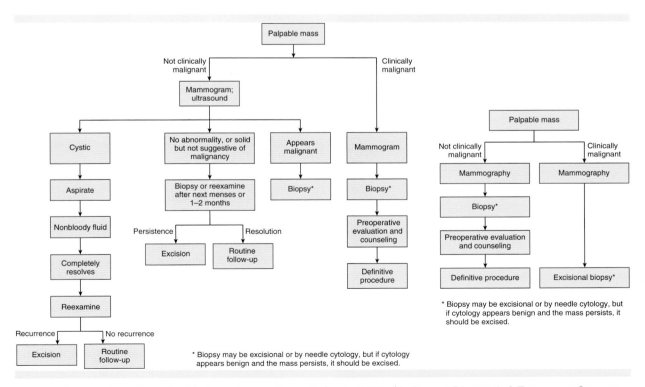

FIGURE 15-5. Approach to the palpable breast mass. From Doherty GM (ed.). *Current Diagnosis & Treatment: Surgery*, 13th ed. New York, NY: McGraw-Hill; 2010:Figs. 17-4 and 17-5.

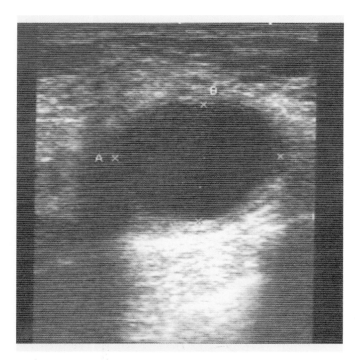

FIGURE 15-6. Benign cystic lesion.

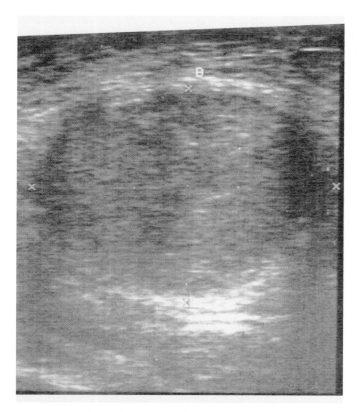

FIGURE 15-7. Benign solid lesion.

BIBLIOGRAPHY

Gadd M. Screening for breast cancer. In: Cameron J (ed.), *Current Surgical Therapy*, 11th ed. Philadelphia, PA: Elsevier; 2014:568–570.

Hunt KK, Robertson JR, Bland KI. The breast. In: Brunicardi F, Andersen DK, Billiar TR, et al. (eds.), *Schwartz's Principles of Surgery*, 10th ed. New York, NY: McGraw-Hill; 2014.

Mackey A, Ananthakrishnan P. Breast ultrasound. In: Schrope B (ed.), *Surgical and Interventional Ultrasound*. New York, NY: McGraw-Hill; 2014:Chapter 5.

10. **(A)** Breast MRI is a very sensitive, but not specific, imaging test. Some studies have shown specificity to be as low as 30%. MRI provides further diagnostic evaluation in women with known cancers and is also a valuable screening tool among high-risk women. Gadolinium is used to aid enhancement. Dedicated breast coils are used, and both breasts are imaged at the same time. Most examinations can be completed within 30 minutes. Invasive cancers do demonstrate enhancement; however, *in situ* cancers may not enhance. Current approved indications for breast MRI are (1) tumor staging to determine extent of diseases, (2) differentiating scar tissue from cancer recurrence, and (3) evaluating axillary metastasis of unknown origin. MRI is the best way to evaluate implant rupture and is safe to use in women with breast implants.

BIBLIOGRAPHY

Behrendt CE, Tumyan L, Gonser L, et al. Evaluation of expert criteria for preoperative magnetic resonance imaging of newly diagnosed breast cancer. *Breast* 2014;23(4):341–345.

Mahoney M. Breast imaging: mammography, sonography, and emerging technologies. In: Donegan W, Spratt J (eds.), *Cancer of the Breast*, 5th ed. St. Louis, MO: W.B. Saunders; 2002:305–306.

Morris E, Port E. Breast magnetic resonance imaging. In: Kuerer HM (ed.), *Kuerer's Breast Surgical Oncology*. New York, NY: McGraw-Hill; 2010:Chapter 35.

Roth S. Imaging analysis: magnetic resonance imaging. In: Harris JR, Lippman ME, Morrow M, et al. (eds.), *Diseases of the Breast*, 4th ed. Philadelphia, PA: Lippincott Williams & Wilkins; 2010:152–169.

11. **(D)** Mastitis is a parenchymal infection of the mammary glands. Symptoms most commonly appear during the third to fourth week postpartum, with unilateral breast engorgement preceding local inflammation characterized by a firm erythematous and painful breast. Cellulitis associated with lactation is caused by gram-positive cocci (most commonly staphylococci) from the infant's nose and throat. It is best treated by oral antibiotics, warm packs, and keeping the breast emptied. The infant does not need to be weaned and can continue to breastfeed without any ill effect.

Approximately 10% of women with mastitis develop a breast abscess. An abscess should be suspected based on failure of improvement with mastitis treatment, as well as fever, leukocytosis, or point tenderness. A fluctuant mass does not usually develop because of the diffuse fibrous septa. Sonographic-guided needle aspiration using local anesthesia has a success rate of 80–90%. If an abscess does form, it should be drained in the operating room, usually under a general anesthetic. At this point, the infant should be weaned.

Breast infections found in the nonlactating patient are usually caused by multiple organisms. They are often recurrent and are associated with periductal mastitis or ductal ectasia. Acutely, the infections should be treated with antibiotics and drainage. If the infection is chronic and relapsing, the acute infection needs to be treated with antibiotics, and the subareolar duct system should be excised.

BIBLIOGRAPHY

Cunningham F, Leveno KJ, Bloom SL, Hauth JC, Rouse DJ, Spong CY. The puerperium. In: Cunningham F, Leveno KJ, Bloom SL, Hauth JC, Rouse DJ, Spong CY (eds.), *Williams Obstetrics*, 23rd ed. New York, NY: McGraw-Hill; 2010:Chapter 30.

Hunt KK, Robertson JR, Bland KI. The breast. In: Brunicardi F, Andersen DK, Billiar TR, et al. (eds.), *Schwartz's Principles of Surgery*, 10th ed. New York, NY: McGraw-Hill; 2014.

12. **(C)** The most common cause of nipple discharge in a nonlactating breast is duct ectasia, followed by intraductal papilloma and carcinoma. Mammary duct ectasia is a dilation of the subareolar duct in peri- and postmenopausal women, which results in a viscous white or green discharge. Duct excision is recommended when nipple discharge is persistent and troublesome.

Intraductal papilloma is a benign condition occurring in the major lactiferous ducts, usually of premenopausal women. Patients may present with serous or bloody nipple discharge. Multiple papillomas do appear to have an increased risk of future cancer. These occur in younger women and are less frequently associated with nipple discharge.

Pathologic nipple discharge is characterized as a spontaneous, persistent bloody or clear fluid arising from a single duct without signs of mastitis. Twenty percent of nipple discharge in older women is associated with ductal carcinoma *in situ* (DCIS). The chance of an underlying cancer rises as the patient's age increases.

Fibrocystic disease may also cause nipple discharge; however, this is usually green or yellow/brown in color.

Galactorrhea manifests as bilateral milky discharge not associated with pregnancy or lactation. Numerous drugs can cause milky nipple discharge, including psychotropic agents. Prolactin levels should be obtained, and if elevated, evaluation for a pituitary tumor should be done.

BIBLIOGRAPHY

Giuliano AE. Breast disorders. In: Doherty GM (ed.), *Current Diagnosis & Treatment: Surgery*, 13th ed. New York, NY: McGraw-Hill; 2010:Chapter 17.

Hunt KK, Robertson JR, Bland KI. The breast. In: Brunicardi F, Andersen DK, Billiar TR, et al. (eds.), *Schwartz's Principles of Surgery*, 10th ed. New York, NY: McGraw-Hill; 2014.

Osborne MP, Boolbol SK, Asad J. Benign conditions of the breast. In: Kuerer HM (ed.), *Kuerer's Breast Surgical Oncology*. New York, NY: McGraw-Hill; 2010:Chapter 16.

13. **(E)** Phyllodes tumors, also known as cystosarcoma phyllodes, are stromal tumors. They are well circumscribed and do not have a true capsule. The cut surface of one of these tumors tends to be mucoid.

Phyllodes tend to occur in an older population when compared to fibroadenomas (FAs). FAs are also stromal tumors, and it is thought that phyllodes may arise from these benign tumors. Phyllodes tend to occur in the fourth decade of life and most commonly present as painless mobile masses. On mammogram and ultrasound, they are similar in appearance to fibroadenomas—smooth, solid, and with multilobulated margins. There may also be fluid within the mass on ultrasound, suggesting phyllodes over FA.

Seventy-five percent of phyllodes tumors are benign. Similar to other stromal tumors, malignancy is difficult to establish and is based on histologic appearance. Stromal overgrowth is now considered the most important predictor of aggressive behavior. Other characteristics that are considered are cellular atypia, mitotic activity, and tumor margins.

Phyllodes tend to recur regardless of benign or malignant status (Table 15-3). The reported

TABLE 15-3 Characteristics of Phyllodes Tumors

Benign	<2 mitoses per 10 high-power fields No more than mild atypia No stromal overgrowth Well-circumscribed tumor
Borderline	2–5 mitoses per 10 high-power fields Moderate atypia No stromal overgrowth Tumor margins infiltrative
Malignant	>10 mitoses per 10 high-power fields Marked atypia Stromal overgrowth present Tumor margins infiltrative

incidence is 20–25% of recurrence. Current recommendations for initial surgical treatment of these tumors are wide local excision with at least a 1-cm margin. This can usually be done without requiring a mastectomy and is based on tumor–to–breast mass ratio. Regional lymph node metastases are rare and axillary evaluation is not warranted. Radiation therapy is also not indicated because this is not a multifocal disease like ductal breast cancer. The tumors are only weakly radiosensitive; however, radiation therapy may offer some palliation for malignant or recurrent disease.

BIBLIOGRAPHY

Calhoun K, Lawton T, Kim J, Lehman C, Anderson B. In: Harris J, Lippman M, Morrow M, Osborne C (eds.), *Diseases of the Breast*, 4th ed. Philadelphia, PA: Lippincott Williams & Wilkins; 2010:781–792.

Hunt KK, Robertson JR, Bland KI. The breast. In: Brunicardi F, Andersen DK, Billiar TR, et al. (eds.), *Schwartz's Principles of Surgery*, 10th ed. New York, NY: McGraw-Hill; 2014.

Jacobs L, Hardin R. The management of benign breast disease. In: Cameron J (ed.), *Current Surgical Therapy*, 11th ed. Philadelphia, PA: Elsevier; 2014:565–567.

Osborne MP, Boolbol SK, Asad J. Benign conditions of the breast. In: Kuerer HM (ed.), *Kuerer's Breast Surgical Oncology*. New York, NY: McGraw-Hill; 2010:Chapter 16.

14. **(C)** Given her age and the mass's typical appearance on ultrasound, this is most likely a fibroadenoma (FA).

FAs can present at any age but are most common in adolescent and young women. The masses are most commonly painless and found incidentally by the patient. On exam, they are typically described as well circumscribed, rubbery, and mobile. On ultrasound, they have benign features: elliptical, iso- or hypoechoic, "wider than tall" solid masses with smooth margins. Most FAs are <3 cm, and those >6 cm are termed "giant fibroadenomas."

Any new breast mass deserves serious evaluation and workup to exclude malignancy. FAs can be reliably diagnosed by either fine-needle aspiration or core needle biopsy, usually under ultrasound guidance. Conservative management with short-term follow-up rather than surgical excision can be offered provided there is no associated atypia. Proceeding with mastectomy, either partial or total, is not appropriate without tissue diagnosis first. A needle localized excisional biopsy is not required because this is a palpable mass.

Transformation of an FA to invasive cancer is a rare event; however, recent studies show that a subgroup of women may be a higher risk of future cancer. This group includes women with a "complex fibroadenoma," such as those with sclerosing adenosis, papillary apocrine hyperplasia, cysts, or epithelial calcifications, as well as women with a family history of breast cancer and women who displayed parenchymal proliferation adjacent to the FA.

BIBLIOGRAPHY

Donegan W. Common benign conditions of the breast. In: Donegan W, Spratt J (eds.), *Cancer of the Breast*, 5th ed. St. Louis, MO: W.B. Saunders; 2002:71–73.

Hunt KK, Robertson JR, Bland KI. The breast. In: Brunicardi F, Andersen DK, Billiar TR, et al. (eds.), *Schwartz's Principles of Surgery*, 10th ed. New York, NY: McGraw-Hill; 2014.

Jacobs L, Hardin R. The management of benign breast disease. In: Cameron J (ed.), *Current Surgical Therapy*, 11th ed. Philadelphia, PA: Elsevier; 2014:565–567.

Osborne MP, Boolbol SK, Asad J. Benign conditions of the breast. In: Kuerer HM (ed.), *Kuerer's Breast Surgical Oncology*. New York, NY: McGraw-Hill; 2010:Chapter 16.

15. **(D)** Gynecomastia is enlargement of the male breast due to benign proliferation of glandular tissue. This tends to occur in infancy, at puberty, and in old age, with the highest prevalence in men 50–80 years old. The prevalence of gynecomastia also increases body mass index (BMI), likely due to the increased aromatase activity in adipose tissue.

Gynecomastia results from an imbalance of the normal hormonal milieu or a change in breast tissue sensitivity to estrogen. The testes secrete 95% of the total body testosterone and only 15% of the circulating estradiol. The vast majority of circulating estradiol is from the peripheral conversion of testosterone and adrenal steroids via the aromatase enzyme (see Fig. 15-8).

The potential causes of gynecomastia are numerous. Any cause of androgen deficiency can lead to gynecomastia, reflecting an increased estrogen/androgen ratio, as estrogen synthesis still occurs by aromatization of residual adrenal and gonadal androgens. Clinical evaluation for gynecomastia includes a thorough review of prescription and over-the-counter medications, drug and alcohol history, testicular exam, and blood tests (Table 15-4).

Increased human chorionic gonadotropin (hCG) level or increased estradiol with a normal/decreased luteinizing hormone (LH) level would be an indication for referral and additional imaging evaluation, including testicular ultrasound. In the neonate, the etiology is often a response to circulating material estrogens. In young men, a testicular lesion must be excluded (see Fig. 15-9). Despite the long list, about three-fourths of patients have idiopathic gynecomastia.

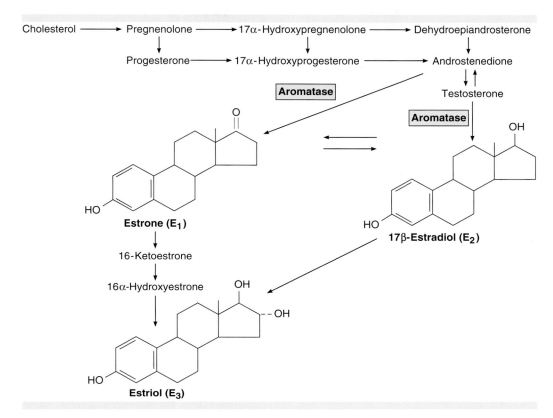

FIGURE 15-8. Biosynthesis and metabolism of estrogen. From Barrett KE, Barman SM, Boitano S, Brooks H. *Ganong's Review of Medical Physiology*, 24th ed. New York, NY: McGraw-Hill; 2012:Fig. 22-16.

TABLE 15-4 Gynecomastia: Drug-Induced Causes

Increased Estrogen	Decreased Testosterone	Unknown
Steroids	Cimetidine	Lasix
Heroin	Diazepam	Isoniazid
Digoxin	Ketoconazole	Theophylline
Cannabis	Phenytoin	Tricyclics
	Spironolactone	Verapamil
	Chemotherapy	Amiodarone
		Clonidine
		Captopril
		Nifedipine
		Amiloride
		Phenothiazine
		Reglan
		Omeprazole

BIBLIOGRAPHY

Bhasin S, Jameson J. Disorders of the testes and male reproductive system. In: Longo DL, Fauci AS, Kasper DL, Hauser SL, Jameson J, Loscalzo J (eds.), *Harrison's Principles of Internal Medicine*, 18th ed. New York, NY: McGraw-Hill; 2012:Chapter 346.

Hunt KK, Robertson JR, Bland KI. The breast. In: Brunicardi F, Andersen DK, Billiar TR, et al. (eds.), *Schwartz's Principles of Surgery*, 10th ed. New York, NY: McGraw-Hill; 2014.

Laronga C, Tollin S, Turaga K. History, physical examination, and staging. In: Kuerer HM (ed.), *Kuerer's Breast Surgical Oncology*. New York, NY: McGraw-Hill; 2010:Chapter 12.

16. **(A)** As with any new breast mass, a serious evaluation and workup are indicated. Breast cancer represents less than 1% of all cancers in men with an annual incidence of about 1 case in 100,000 men; the male-to-female ratio is 1:100. The median age of diagnosis is 65–71 years, and risk factors are similar to women, with hormonal factors, particularly estrogen exposure, and family history playing predominant roles. Klinefelter syndrome, although rare, confers a 58-fold higher risk of breast cancer.

A clinical breast examination can be very helpful in differentiating a clinical cancer from gynecomastia. Gynecomastia most commonly presents as tender diffuse

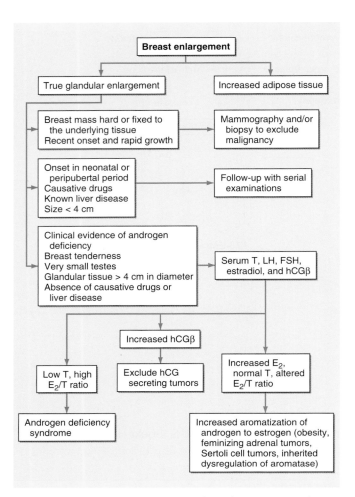

FIGURE 15-9. Diagnostic approach to the patient with gynecomastia. FSH, follicle-stimulating hormone; hCG, human chorionic gonadotropin; LH, luteinizing hormone; T, testosterone. From Longo DL, Fauci AS, Kasper DL, Hauser SL, Jameson J, Loscalzo J (eds.). *Harrison's Principles of Internal Medicine*, 18th ed. New York, NY: McGraw-Hill; 2012:Fig. 346-5.

enlargement of both breasts. Cancers, on the other hand, tend to be unilateral and hard. Nipple discharge in men is also considered pathologic, as are masses associated with ulceration.

Mammography is the preferred mode of diagnosis of male breast cancer, although false-negatives occur in 10–20% of men. Ultrasound is a useful adjunct and can also quickly distinguish cystic from solid lesions. Fine-needle aspiration (FNA) and core biopsy are used for pathologic evaluation.

Invasive ductal carcinoma accounts for 85% of the cancers. Treatment is a modified radical mastectomy. Survival statistics are similar stage for stage when compared to their female counterparts. Men, in general, are diagnosed at a later stage, and this accounts for the apparent increased mortality rates.

BIBLIOGRAPHY

El-Tamer M, Pocock B. Male breast cancer. In: Kuerer HM (ed.), *Kuerer's Breast Surgical Oncology*. New York, NY: McGraw-Hill; 2010:Chapter 21.

Hardin R, Tsangaris T. Male breast cancer. In: Cameron J (ed.), *Current Surgical Therapy*, 11th ed. Philadelphia, PA: Elsevier; 2041:618–620.

17. **(B)**

18. **(A)**

Explanations for 17 and 18

Mastalgia, or breast pain, is a common complaint and a common reason for referral to a breast center. Evaluation of breast pain should include a thorough history and examination. Typical types of mastalgia can be described as cyclical pronounced, noncyclical, trauma, musculoskeletal/chest wall, and miscellaneous uncommon causes.

Cyclical pronounced mastalgia is the most common. It is related to the menstrual cycle, especially ovulation. Patients complain of "heaviness" and "tenderness." Nodularity is common, especially in the upper outer quadrants, and also tends to fluctuate with the menstrual cycle. The pain is often in the upper outer quadrant, may be bilateral, and can radiate down the arm.

Noncyclical mastalgia is not related to the menstrual cycle. The pain is different from cyclical pain in that it is more localized and described as a "burning" or "pulling." Nodularity is typically less pronounced, but it is present in greater than 50% of the patients.

Musculoskeletal pain is usually unilateral. It is often either lateral chest wall pain or costochondral junction pain (Tietze syndrome). Pain can be generally reproduced. Treatment includes local injection of anesthetic and steroids.

Trauma can often be localized to a previous biopsy site. The etiology of this pain is uncertain but may be related to postsurgical/procedural infection or hematoma or to placing the incision across Langer's lines.

An uncommon cause of mastalgia is cancer. Literature reports a 7–24% frequency of breast pain as a symptom of operable breast cancer. The pain associated with a cancer is generally unilateral, persistent, and stable in its position.

The idea that mastalgia is psychosomatic can be traced back to Sir Astley Cooper in 1829; however, recent studies have shown no greater tendency toward mental illness in this population over other patients.

Treatment of mastalgia begins with excluding cancer and giving reassurance. For refractory cyclical pain, evening primrose oil is a safe first option. This contains essential fatty acids and is believed to correct a deficiency that may lead to mastalgia. Side effects are rare. Second-line therapy is danazol. This drug is limited by its side effects (weight gain, acne, hirsutism, and amenorrhea). Third-line treatment is bromocriptine and is also limited by its side effects, especially nausea and vomiting. The most efficacious of these medications is danazol. Noncyclical breast pain is less responsive to medications. Efficacy in descending order is danazol, bromocriptine, and evening primrose oil. In select instances, steroid and local anesthetic injections have proven beneficial. Musculoskeletal pain and Tietze syndrome can be treated with steroid/local anesthetic injections.

Surgery is a last-resort option, and in most cases, segmental resection of the breast is not sufficient. Mastectomy is required. Even with complete removal of the offending breast tissue, pain is persistent in 50% of the patients. In addition, complications may occur with the mastectomy and/or reconstruction that may result in additional pain.

BIBLIOGRAPHY

Hoffman BL, Schorge JO, Schaffer JI, et al. Breast disease. In: Hoffman BL, Schorge JO, Schaffer JI, et al. (eds.), *Williams Gynecology*, 2nd ed. New York, NY: McGraw-Hill; 2012: Chapter 12.

Laronga C, Tollin S, Turaga K. History, physical examination, and staging. In: Kuerer HM (ed.), *Kuerer's Breast Surgical Oncology*. New York, NY: McGraw-Hill; 2010:Chapter 12.

19. **(E)** Tamoxifen, a selective estrogen receptor (ER) agonist antagonist, first came into the market in the 1970s. It is a well-studied drug. The antagonist effects of tamoxifen are related to its competitive binding of the estrogen receptor, especially in breast tissue. This results in a reduced transcription of estrogen-related proteins and effective blockade of cell cycle in G_1. This in turn then translates to ineffective tumor growth. The National Surgical Adjuvant Breast and Bowel Project (NSABP) has performed a series of studies investigating the role of tamoxifen in breast cancer care. Tamoxifen has been shown to reduce breast cancer mortality by nearly one-third when given as adjuvant treatment, as well as reduce the risk of contralateral breast cancer by nearly 40%.

Current guidelines recommend 5 years of tamoxifen as adjuvant therapy for premenopausal women with tumors expressing ER or progesterone receptor (PR) hormone receptors, regardless of age or nodal status. Tamoxifen is also an effective adjuvant therapy for postmenopausal women, with aromatase inhibitors used as an adjunct endocrine therapy either concurrently or following tamoxifen.

Tamoxifen has apparent estrogen agonist effects on the endometrial lining, as shown by the increase in endometrial cancer found in women being treated with the drug. This risk is about 1%. In addition, there is an increased risk of venous embolic phenomena that is related to the estrogen agonist effects. Tamoxifen also increases bone density and improves lipid profiles—both related to ER agonist activity. The major side effects that women complain about while taking tamoxifen are hot flashes and sleep disturbances—similar to menopausal symptoms attributed to decreased estrogen.

BIBLIOGRAPHY

Fisher B, Kignam J, Bryant J, Wolmark N. Five versus more than five years of tamoxifen for lymph node-negative breast cancer: updated findings of the National Surgical Adjuvant Breast and Bowel Project B-14 randomized trial. *J Natl Cancer Inst* 2001;93:684–690.

Francis PA. Endocrine therapy. In: Kuerer HM (ed.), *Kuerer's Breast Surgical Oncology*. New York, NY: McGraw-Hill; 2010:Chapter 86.

Mamounas EP, Wickerham D, Fisher B, Geyer CE, Julian TB, Wolmark N. The NSABP experience. In: Kuerer HM (ed.), *Kuerer's Breast Surgical Oncology*. New York, NY: McGraw-Hill; 2010:Chapter 42.

20. **(C)** Lobular carcinoma *in situ* (LCIS) is a noninvasive disease in the lobules or terminal ducts first described it in 1941. The true incidence of LCIS in unknown, because it is not typically detected on routine screening measures (i.e., mammography or clinical breast examination). More commonly, it is an incidental pathologic finding discovered on core biopsy or surgical pathology. LCIS is not seen macroscopically. Microscopically, it is often a solid proliferation of small cells with distinct borders and uniform, small nuclei. The cells often distend the lobules and terminal ducts (see Fig. 15-10).

LCIS is felt to be a risk factor for the future development of breast cancer. The majority of women with LCIS do not go on to develop cancer, but when they do, it is most commonly invasive ductal cancer. The risk is bilateral. The risk of future cancer is 1% per year indefinitely.

Therapy for LCIS is tamoxifen. Tamoxifen can decrease the risk of breast cancer by almost 50%. Hormone replacement therapy is not recommended among women at high risk for breast cancer. If there are contraindications to tamoxifen therapy or if the patient is unable or unwilling to comply with close follow-up, bilateral prophylactic mastectomy with or without reconstruction is also an option.

There is no indication for reexcision, sentinel lymph node biopsy, standard chemotherapy, radiation therapy, or mirror biopsies.

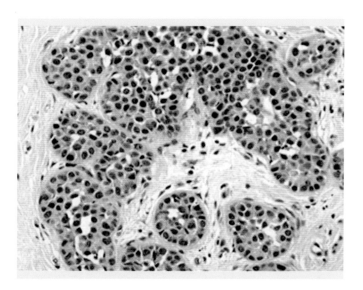

FIGURE 15-10. Lobular carcinoma *in situ*. From Kuerer H. *Kuerer's Breast Surgical Oncology.* New York, NY: McGraw-Hill; 2010:Fig. 17-1B.

BIBLIOGRAPHY

Smart CE, Smart CE, Furnival CM, Furnival CM, Lakhani SR, Lakhani SR. High-risk lesions: ALH/LCIS/ADH. In: Kuerer HM (ed.), *Kuerer's Breast Surgical Oncology.* New York, NY: McGraw-Hill; 2010:Chapter 17.

Wang T, Urist M. Ductal and lobular in situ carcinoma of the breast. In: Cameron J (ed.), *Current Surgical Therapy*, 11th ed. Philadelphia, PA: Elsevier; 2014:602–606.

21. **(B)** The overwhelming majority of newly diagnosed breast cancers are sporadic. Approximately 5% are felt related to *BRCA1* or *BRCA2* mutations. Hereditary breast cancers are more likely to occur at younger age, involve both sides, or include multiple organs (especially ovary) compared with sporadic cases. Inheritance pattern is autosomal dominant with variable penetrance. Lifetime breast cancer risk associated with *BRCA1* or *BRCA2* is estimated to be 85%. Management options thus include screening with self-examination, mammography, and even breast magnetic resonance imaging (MRI) beginning at age 25. Although controversial, bilateral prophylactic mastectomy, chemoprevention with tamoxifen or aromatase inhibitors, and contralateral prophylactic mastectomy when managing ipsilateral breast cancer should be considered.

BIBLIOGRAPHY

Kriege M, Brekelmans C, Boetes C, et al. Efficacy of MRI and mammography for breast cancer screening in women with a familial or genetic predisposition. *N Engl J Med* 2004;351:427–436.

Lynch HT, Marcus JM, Lynch JF, et al. Breast cancer genetics. In: *The Breast: Comprehensive Management of Benign and Malignant Disorders*, 3rd ed. St. Louis, MO: W.B. Saunders; 2004:380–392.

Scheuer L. Outcome of preventive surgery and screening for breast and ovarian cancer in BRCA mutation carriers. *J Clin Oncol* 2002;20:1260.

Shahid T, Soroka J, Kong EH, et al. Structure and mechanism of action of the BRCA2 breast cancer tumor suppressor. *Nat Struct Mol Biol* 2014;21(11):962–968.

22. **(B)** The initial surgical management of clinically localized breast cancer must address the primary cancer in the breast and sample axillary lymph nodes for staging. This may be accomplished by partial mastectomy with sentinel lymph node biopsy, partial mastectomy with axillary lymph node dissection, or modified radical mastectomy. For early-stage (I and II) breast cancer, mastectomy with axillary staging and breast-conserving surgery with axillary staging and radiation therapy are considered equivalent treatments. Relative contraindications to breast-conservation therapy include (1) prior radiation therapy to the breast or chest wall, (2) persistently positive surgical margins after reexcision, (3) multicentric disease, and (4) scleroderma or lupus erythematosus. Alternative means of primary tumor therapy, including laser, radiofrequency, or cryoablation, are under investigation but not clinically applicable at present.

Adjuvant chemotherapy for patients with early-stage invasive breast cancer is considered for patients with node-positive cancers, patients with cancers that are >1 cm, and patients with node-negative cancers of >0.5 cm when adverse prognostic features are present. Adverse prognostic factors include blood vessel or lymph vessel invasion, high nuclear grade, high histologic grade, *HER2/neu* overexpression or amplification, and negative hormone receptor status. Adjuvant endocrine therapy is considered for women with hormone receptor–positive cancers, and use of an aromatase inhibitor is recommended if the patient is postmenopausal.

BIBLIOGRAPHY

Fisher B, Anderson S, Bryant J, et al. Twenty year follow up of a randomized trial comparing total mastectomy, lumpectomy, and lumpectomy plus irradiation for the treatment of invasive breast cancer. *N Engl J Med* 2002;347:1233–1240.

23. **(B)** Currently, the most widely used description of breast cancer staging is the TNM system. This has been popularized by the AJCC, sponsored by the American Cancer Society and the American College of Surgeons.

The system demands an assessment of the primary tumor, regional lymph nodes, and any distant metastasis.

TABLE 15-5 AJCC Staging for Breast Cancer

1. Primary tumor (T)
   - Tx: primary tumor cannot be assessed
   - T0: no primary tumor
   - Tis: carcinoma *in situ*
   - T1: tumor ≤2 cm
   - T2: tumor >2 cm but ≤5 cm
   - T3: tumor >5 cm
   - T4: tumor with extension to chest wall, skin edema or ulceration, or inflammatory carcinoma

2. Regional lymph nodes (N)
   - Nx: regional lymph nodes cannot be assessed
   - N0: no regional lymph node metastasis
   - N1: metastases to mobile axillary lymph nodes
   - N2: metastases to fixed, matted, or clinically apparent axillary lymph nodes or internal mammary nodes
   - N3: metastases to axillary and infraclavicular lymph nodes, clinically apparent internal mammary nodes or supraclavicular lymph nodes

3. Distant metastasis (B)
   - Mx: distant metastasis cannot be assessed
   - M0: no distant metastasis
   - M1: distant metastasis

4. Stage grouping

Stage	T	N	M
Stage 0	TIS	N0	M0
Stage IA	T1[a]	N0	M0
Stage IB	T0	N1mi	M0
	T1[a]	N1mi	M0
Stage IIA	T0	N1[b]	M0
	T1[a]	N1[b]	M0
	T2	N0	M0
Stage IIB	T2	N1	M0
	T3	N0	M0
Stage IIIA	T0	N2	M0
	T1[a]	N2	M0
	T2	N2	M0
	T3	N1	M0
	T3	N2	M0
Stage IIIB	T4	N0	M0
	T4	N1	M0
	T4	N2	M0
Stage IIIC	Any T	N3	M0
Stage IV	Any T	Any N	M1

Defining various groups of TNM stages with similar prognoses allows appropriate consensus treatment recommendations. Further, the system aids the design, conduct, and analysis of clinical trials. The AJCC TNM clinical staging system can be found at AJCC 7th Edition Staging for Breast Cancer: https://cancerstaging.org/references-tools/quickreferences/Documents/BreastMedium.pdf:

BIBLIOGRAPHY

American Joint Committee on Cancer. Breast. In: Edge SB, Byrd DR, Compton CC, et al. (eds.), *AJCC Cancer Staging Manual*, 7th ed. New York, NY: Springer; 2010:347–376.

Hunt KK, Robertson JR, Bland KI. The breast. In: Brunicardi F, Andersen DK, Billiar TR, et al. (eds.), *Schwartz's Principles of Surgery*, 10th ed. New York, NY: McGraw-Hill; 2014.

24. **(B)** Advanced breast cancer poses a serious threat to life by means of systemic disease. Even if micrometastases are undetectable by diagnostic testing, the high rate of distant treatment failure suggests their presence. Therefore, after staging scans are performed, neoadjuvant chemotherapy is usually initiated with systemic treatment. Chemotherapy followed by surgery has been demonstrated to yield improved local control and survival. Thus, initial treatment of stage III and stage IV breast cancer, including inflammatory cancer, is by systemic chemotherapy. Surgical treatment of locally advanced cancers should be reserved for the rare cases of palliation or poor response to or growth during chemotherapy (see Fig. 15-11).

BIBLIOGRAPHY

Hortobagyi G, Singletary SE, Strom E. Locally advanced breast cancer. In: Harris JR, Lippman ME, Morrow M (eds.), *Diseases of the Breast*, 4th ed. Philadelphia, PA: Lippincott Williams & Wilkins; 2010:745–761.

Hunt KK, Robertson JR, Bland KI. The breast. In: Brunicardi F, Andersen DK, Billiar TR, et al. (eds.), *Schwartz's Principles of Surgery*, 10th ed. New York, NY: McGraw-Hill; 2014.

25. **(D)** Sentinel lymph node biopsy has emerged as a safe and accurate approach to assessing axillary lymph nodes for metastases from breast cancer (see Fig. 15-12). The successful identification of one or more sentinel lymph nodes is reported to be between 85 and 100%. Sensitivity and specificity rates for the procedure are 90–100%, as compared to completion axillary lymph node dissection. A serious reservation has been the possibility of skip metastases involving nonsentinel lymph nodes (or false-negative sentinel node), but this has been demonstrated to occur in less than 10% of patients. Several series have

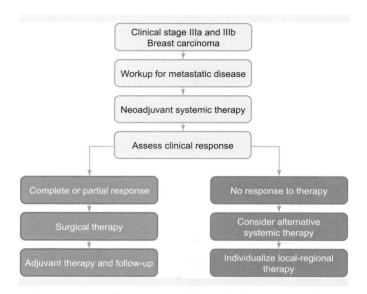

FIGURE 15-11. Treatment pathways for local-regional breast cancer. From Brunicardi F, Andersen DK, Billiar TR, et al. (eds.). *Schwartz's Principles of Surgery*, 10th ed. New York, NY: McGraw-Hill; 2014:Fig. 17-31.

revealed positive sentinel nodes in T1 tumors (<2 cm), ranging from 5 to 44%. Multiple sentinel lymph nodes are common, with an average yield of two to three nodes. The technique of sentinel node biopsy involves injection of dye in either a subareolar or peritumoral location. The dye used is either radiocolloid or 1% isosulfan blue. The optimal interval from injection to identification of the sentinel node in surgery is approximately 2 hours for the radioisotope, as opposed to 5 minutes for the isosulfan blue.

BIBLIOGRAPHY

Garreau JR, Giuliano AE. Sentinel lymph node biopsy. In: Kuerer HM (ed.), *Kuerer's Breast Surgical Oncology*. New York, NY: McGraw-Hill; 2010:Chapter 62.

Tuttle TM, Zogakis TG, Dunst CM, et al. A review of technical aspects of sentinel lymph node identification for breast cancer. *J Am Coll Surg* 2002;195:261–267.

Veronesi U, Pahanelli G, Viale G, et al. A randomized comparison of sentinel node biopsy with routine axillary dissection in breast cancer. *N Engl J Med* 2003;349:546–553.

26. **(C)** Ductal carcinoma *in situ* (DCIS) of the breast consists of the clonal proliferation of cells that appear malignant and that accumulate within the lumens of the mammary duct. There is no evidence of invasion beyond the epithelial basement membrane into the adjacent breast stroma. This lesion, which is a precursor to invasive ductal carcinoma, is frequently diagnosed on screening mammography. The incidence of DCIS is increasing,

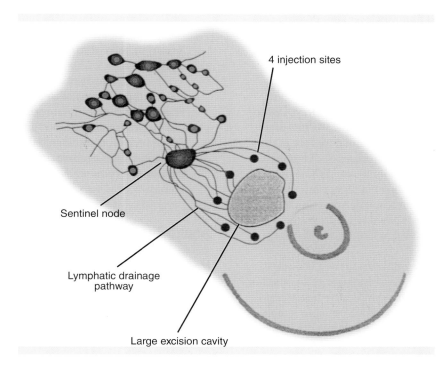

4 injection sites

Sentinel node

Lymphatic drainage
pathway

Large excision cavity

FIGURE 15-12. Sentinel lymph node biopsy. Modified from Feldman SM, Krag DN, McNally RK, Moor BB, Weaver DL, Klein P. Limitation in gamma probe localization of the sentinel node in breast cancer patients with large excisional biopsy. *J Am Coll Surg* 188:248–254, 1999; with permission.

and, because of screening mammography, the disease is diagnosed in an increasing proportion of asymptomatic patients. The most common clinical presentation is that of calcifications on mammography. Approximately 47,000 cases of DCIS will be diagnosed this year. DCIS accounts for nearly 20% of all breast cancers detected by screening (one case of DCIS detected per 1300 screening mammograms) in North America. DCIS will evolve into an invasive ductal carcinoma in approximately 30–50% of patients over 10 years.

The options for surgical treatment include simple mastectomy or breast-conserving surgery. After breast-conserving surgery, radiotherapy is administered in tangential fields to the whole breast. According to the results of NSABP-B17, breast-conserving therapy is an effective option in the management of DCIS. The use of radiotherapy after lumpectomy significantly decreases the rate of recurrence. The presence of comedo necrosis and surgical margin involvement are the most commonly used predictors of the likelihood of recurrence. If relapse occurs after breast-conserving therapy, the chance of an invasive component is approximately 50%. The risk for in-breast recurrence at 5 years after breast-conserving therapy is approximately 8%.

There is no role for chemotherapy in the treatment of DCIS. Neither dissection of axillary lymph nodes nor mapping of sentinel lymph nodes is routinely warranted in patients with DCIS, owing to the very low incidence of axillary metastases. Intense surveillance needs to be maintained for a patient's lifetime.

BIBLIOGRAPHY

Burstein HJ, Polyak K, Wong JS, Lester SC, Kaelin CM. Ductal carcinoma in situ of the breast. *N Engl J Med* 2004;350(14):1430–1441.

Meric F, Robinson EK, Hunt KK. Noninvasive breast cancer. In: Feig BW, Berger DH, Fuhrman GM (eds.), *The M.D. Anderson Surgical Oncology Handbook*, 3rd ed. Philadelphia, PA: Lippincott Williams & Wilkins; 2003:1–13.

Wang T, Urist M. Ductal and lobular in situ carcinoma of the breast. In: Cameron J (ed.), *Current Surgical Therapy*, 11th ed. Philadelphia, PA: Elsevier; 2014:602–606.

27. **(D)** Male breast carcinoma remains a rare cause of cancer in men, accounting for less than 1% of cases of cancer in men. The incidence of this disease has remained stable, at approximately 1400–2000 new cases per year over the past several decades. The average age at diagnosis is 68 years, which is older than the age of diagnosis seen in women.

At 10%, the proportion of noninvasive carcinomas in men is much higher than that of women. This is likely due to the ease of detection of smaller breast lesions in the comparatively smaller quantity of tissue seen in the male breast. The most common histologic subtype of invasive carcinomas remains invasive ductal carcinoma. This accounts for more than 80% of all invasive breast lesions in men. All subtypes of invasive carcinoma found in women have been reported in men. Nearly all of the noninvasive lesions in men are DCIS, but unlike females, DCIS in males is almost always low to intermediate grade, and in more than 75%, it is of the papillary subtype. The lack of terminal lobules in the male breast results in minimal incidence of lobular carcinoma *in situ* and invasive lobular carcinoma. Review of reported literature has shown a higher incidence of hormone receptors than in women. Approximately 74% of male breast lesions are shown to be progesterone receptor positive, and 81% are found to be estrogen receptor positive.

Significant prognostic indicators in men include lymph node status, tumor size, histologic grade, and hormone receptor status. The most indicative negative prognostic indicator in male breast cancer remains lymph node status. Staging and survival outcomes are similar to those found in women.

The most common presenting sign in men with breast lesions is a painless subareolar mass (50–97%). Other common presenting signs and symptoms include nipple retraction (10–51%), local pain (4–20%), and nipple ulceration (4–17%). Male patients who present with a breast lesion should undergo a thorough physical examination to evaluate for multiple lesions, contralateral disease, and lymph node involvement. Carcinomas can be differentiated on mammogram by their irregular boarder and spiculated margins, but the diagnostic use of mammograms remains limited in men because of the paucity of tissue in the male breast. All lesions should have a fine-needle aspiration performed to evaluate tumor histology and hormone status.

Treatment of patients with nonmetastatic disease involves removal of all breast tissue and lymph node dissection. The local recurrence and survival rates are similar between radical mastectomy and modified radical mastectomy; as such, the recommended treatment is the less morbid modified radical mastectomy. The small quantity of male breast tissue and the need for lymph node dissection in invasive disease limit the use of breast-conservation therapy.

The role of adjuvant chemotherapy and radiation therapy in male invasive breast cancer remains unclear. The low incidence of the disease makes it difficult to determine which patients would have increased risk of recurrence and would benefit from adjuvant therapy. Most centers use the same guidelines in men as they do for women and recommend adjuvant chemotherapy if lymph nodes are involved or if the tumor is greater than 1 cm and radiation therapy for tumors that are T3

or T4 or if more than four lymph nodes are involved. All male patients with hormone receptor–positive lesions benefit from adjuvant tamoxifen treatment for 5 years.

For metastatic disease of hormone receptor–positive lesions, the mainstay of treatment is hormonal therapy. First-line treatment is tamoxifen. If there is evidence of disease progression, second-line hormonal agents can be added including aminoglutethimide, progestins, antiandrogens, GnRH agonists, steroids, or androgens. Chemotherapy is recommended for receptor-negative metastatic lesions.

BIBLIOGRAPHY

Dickerson R, Lippman ME. Pathogenesis of breast cancer. In: Harris J, Lippman ME, Morrow M, et al. (eds.), *Disease of the Breast*, 2nd ed., vol. 200. Philadelphia, PA: Lippincott Williams & Wilkins; 2014:281–302.

Giordano SH, Buzdar AU, Hortobagyi GN. Breast cancer in men. *Ann Intern Med* 2002;137:678–687.

Hardin R, Tsangaris T. Male breast cancer. In: Cameron J (ed.), *Current Surgical Therapy*, 11th ed. Philadelphia, PA: Elsevier; 2041:618–620.

28. **(C)**

29. **(A)**

Explanations for questions 28 and 29

After cervical cancer, breast cancer remains the second most common malignancy encountered in pregnancy. During pregnancy, breast cancer most commonly presents as a painless mass in up to 95% of patients. The differential diagnosis of breast lesions during pregnancy includes cancer, lactating adenoma, fibroadenoma, cystic disease, lobular hyperplasia, galactocele, abscess, and lipoma. Eighty percent of all breast masses found during pregnancy are benign.

The interpretation of diagnostic tests and physical examination becomes difficult during pregnancy as breast weight and firmness increase. Ultrasound remains the best first imaging choice of the pregnancy patient and can differentiate between cystic and solid masses. Mammographic evaluation during pregnancy is a comparatively benign radiographic test, exposing the fetus to only 0.0004 Gy. Interpretation is often difficult with the density changes of the pregnant breast; as a result, there is a high-false negative rate. MRI may prove to be a useful imaging tool in the pregnant patient, but currently, the risks and benefits are undetermined. Radiographs and bone scan imaging searching for metastatic disease in pregnant patients without symptoms or laboratory abnormalities remains low yield.

Biopsy is essential in the evaluation of breast lesions in the pregnant patient. It can be done by core needle or fine-needle aspiration, as most patients present with palpable, painless masses. The pathologist must be made aware of the patient's pregnancy and trimester to avoid misdiagnosis secondary to breast changes. Lactation must be stopped prior to the biopsy to avoid milk fistulas. This can be done with ice packs and breast bindings.

The histology of breast cancer in pregnancy parallels that of the nonpregnant female. There is a higher incidence of lymph node metastases and lower incidence of positive hormone receptor status. The cause of this is multifactorial and may include delay in diagnosis, breast cancer at a younger age, breast hypervascularity, and physiologic changes associated with pregnancy (hormone level, downregulation of hormone receptors, and immunosuppressed state).

Treatment of breast cancer in the pregnant patients involves a thorough understanding of the risks involved with each treatment modality in each trimester of pregnancy. The clinician must also comprehend the consequences of delaying treatment. Surgery remains the mainstay of treatment. The risks of surgery involve preterm labor, spontaneous abortion, and congenital abnormalities. Surgery can be performed safely at any stage of pregnancy. Adjuvant therapy with irradiation and chemotherapy are conclusively linked to birth defects. The teratogenicity and increased likelihood of newborn malignancy with irradiation is cumulative dose dependent, and irradiation is contraindicated during any part of the pregnancy. Chemotherapy has the greatest teratogenic risk during the first trimester and is recommended for use only after 12 weeks.

Stage I and II lesions during the first trimester should be treated with modified radical mastectomy, because it eliminates the need for postoperative chemotherapy or irradiation, neither of which should be offered in the first trimester.

Patients with stage I and II lesions presenting in the second and third trimester can again be offered modified radical mastectomy. Another option would be to offer breast-conservation therapy, followed immediately by chemotherapy and postpartum radiation therapy. There is no benefit survival or recurrence difference between modified radical mastectomy and breast-conservation therapy in the pregnant patient.

Prognosis of breast cancer in pregnant patients in early stages (I and II) is similar to age-matched nonpregnant patients. Decreased survival is noted in pregnant patients in later stages. Patients should be advised to avoid pregnancy for 2 years following treatment for stage I and II cancers and for 5 years for stage III cancers and to avoid childbearing after stage IV cancers. Women should also avoid breast-feeding during chemotherapy.

Termination of pregnancy has not been shown to increase maternal survival.

BIBLIOGRAPHY

Cunningham F, Leveno KJ, Bloom SL, Hauth JC, Rouse DJ, Spong CY. Neoplastic diseases. In: Cunningham F, Leveno KJ, Bloom SL, Hauth JC, Rouse DJ, Spong CY (eds.), *Williams Obstetrics*, 23rd ed. New York, NY: McGraw-Hill; 2010:Chapter 57.

Woo JC, Yu T, Hurd TC. Breast cancer in pregnancy. *Arch Surg* 2003;138:91–98.

30. **(E)** Review of family history is an important component of the history of any new breast cancer diagnosis. Although many women have family history of breast cancer, a strong family history of breast and ovarian cancer should prompt referral for consideration of genetic testing. A strong family history of multiple affected family members with breast, ovarian, or pancreas cancer or glioblastoma should prompt referral for consideration of genetic testing for a *BRCA1* mutation.

Criteria for consideration of genetic testing include personal history of breast cancer in women less than or equal to 40 years old, personal history of epithelial ovarian cancers at any age, any male breast cancer, and more recently, any triple-negative breast cancer diagnosed in women age 60 years or less.

BIBLIOGRAPHY

Isaacs C, Peshkin B, Schwartz M. Genetic testing and management of patients with hereditary breast cancer. *Diseases of the Breast*, 4th ed. Philadelphia, PA: Lippincott Williams & Wilkins; 2010:225–247.

National Comprehensive Cancer Network. NCCN Guidelines for Genetic/Familial High-Risk Assessment: Breast and Ovarian. www.nccn.org/physician_gls. Accessed November 15, 2015.

CHAPTER 16

GASTROINTESTINAL PHYSIOLOGY

RACHEL RUSSO, ELEANOR CURTIS, AND AARON CARR

QUESTIONS

1. Which of the following statements regarding innervation of the gastrointestinal (GI) tract is true?
   - (A) Sympathetic innervation has a primarily excitatory effect on the GI tract.
   - (B) Parasympathetic innervation is supplied solely by the vagus nerve and its branches.
   - (C) The enteric nervous system is composed of a serosal plexus and submucosal plexus.
   - (D) Local reflex activity occurs in the enteric nervous system in the absence of any sympathetic or parasympathetic innervation.
   - (E) Most sympathetic fibers terminate in the mucosa.

2. Which of the following is a component of the normal swallowing mechanism?
   - (A) Depression of the soft palate
   - (B) Posteriosuperior movement of the hyoid bone
   - (C) Initiation of a peristaltic wave down the esophageal body
   - (D) Vagally mediated contraction of the smooth muscle of the upper esophageal sphincter (UES)
   - (E) Coordination of the swallowing mechanism by the swallowing center in the cortex

3. Regarding the esophageal phase of swallowing, which is correct?
   - (A) The vagus nerve innervates both skeletal and smooth muscle.
   - (B) There is a clear line of demarcation between the skeletal muscle of the upper one-third of the esophagus and the smooth muscle of the lower two-thirds.
   - (C) Atropine stimulates esophageal motility.

   - (D) The force of esophageal peristalsis is greater than esophageal occlusion pressure.
   - (E) Relaxation of the lower esophageal sphincter coincides with passage of the food bolus into the distal esophagus.

4. The lower esophageal sphincter (LES)
   - (A) Is defined anatomically
   - (B) Is a zone of continuous high pressure
   - (C) Relaxes when the stomach is distended
   - (D) Cannot be detected with manometry
   - (E) Has no relationship to the angle of His

5. Which of the following has been shown to increase LES pressure?
   - (A) Cholecystokinin (CCK)
   - (B) Ethanol
   - (C) Estrogen
   - (D) Theophylline
   - (E) Motilin

6. Vomiting is a reflex behavior best characterized by which of the following?
   - (A) It is caused by relatively few stimuli.
   - (B) The vomiting center, located in the pons, acts to coordinate the vomiting reflex.
   - (C) Vomiting is accompanied by reverse peristalsis of the esophagus.
   - (D) The chemoreceptor trigger zone is located on the floor of the fourth ventricle and can elicit vomiting following exposure to certain substances.
   - (E) Failure of the LES to relax is the most notable motor difference between retching and vomiting.

7. Which of the following best characterizes the electrolyte and acid/base disturbances seen with protracted (>24 h) vomiting?

	Plasma pH	Urine pH	Plasma Chloride	Plasma Potassium
(A)	Alkalosis	Alkauria	Hypochloremia	Hypokalemia
(B)	Alkalosis	Aciduria	Hypochloremia	Hypokalemia
(C)	Alkalosis	Aciduria	Hyperchloremia	Hypokalemia
(D)	Alkalosis	Aciduria	Hyperchloremia	Hyperkalemia
(E)	Alkalosis	Alkauria	Hyperchloremia	Hyperkalemia

8. Gastric protein digestion is notable for
   (A) Secretion of pepsinogen by parietal cells
   (B) Leading to malnutrition if impaired
   (C) Conversion of pepsinogen to pepsin by pepsinogenase
   (D) Cessation of pepsin activity when it encounters the alkaline environment of the duodenum
   (E) Cleavage of terminal peptide bonds by pepsin

9. Which of the following increases gastrin release?
   (A) Antral acidification
   (B) Fatty acids in the antrum
   (C) Carbohydrates in the antrum
   (D) Gastric distension
   (E) Somatostatin release

10. A patient has been prescribed famotidine to treat a peptic ulcer. At which location in the parietal cell does famotidine act?
    (A) Histamine receptors
    (B) Acetylcholine receptors
    (C) CCK2 receptors
    (D) H-K ATPase
    (E) Mucosal layer

11. Truncal vagotomy causes an increased rate of gastric emptying of liquids by
    (A) Increasing the rate of the gastric "pacemaker"
    (B) Destroying the receptive relaxation reflex in the proximal stomach
    (C) Decreasing resting pyloric tone
    (D) Increasing the amplitude of gastric contractions
    (E) Eliminating the potentiating effect of cholinergic input on somatostatin release

12. Carbohydrate digestion and absorption is characterized by
    (A) Digestion of starch by brush border enzymes
    (B) Transportation of glucose, galactose, and fructose across the luminal membrane by an active transport system

    (C) Increased activity of brush border enzymes in the jejunum relative to the ileum
    (D) Initiation of digestion in the duodenum by amylase secreted from the pancreas
    (E) Decreased osmotic effect as starch is digested into oligosaccharides

13. Lingual lipase and pancreatic lipase
    (A) Are inactivated in an acidic environment
    (B) Cleave triglycerides primarily into monoglycerides and fatty acids
    (C) Make use of a coenzyme
    (D) Are secreted in active form
    (E) Are activated by trypsin

14. Cholecystokinin
    (A) Relaxes the sphincter of Oddi
    (B) Inhibits gastric acid secretion
    (C) Inhibits gallbladder contractions
    (D) Causes mesenteric vasodilation
    (E) Inhibits pancreatic exocrine secretions

15. The intestines play an important role in calcium metabolism. Which of the following patients might be expected to have impaired calcium absorption?
    (A) A patient taking penicillin for otitis media
    (B) A patient with gastric hypersecretion
    (C) A patient with colon cancer
    (D) A patient taking cholestyramine
    (E) A patient with hyperparathyroidism

16. A patient has undergone an ileal resection. Which of the following conditions would the patient be least likely to develop?
    (A) Alopecia
    (B) Megaloblastic anemia
    (C) Nephrolithiasis
    (D) Steatorrhea
    (E) Cholelithiasis

17. Which of the following dietary adjustments is appropriate for a patient with a chylothorax?
    (A) Removal of all galactose from the diet.
    (B) Use of medium-chain triglycerides (MCTs) as the only source of fat
    (C) Intake of long-chain triglycerides as the only source of fat
    (D) Consumption of aromatic amino acids as the only source of protein
    (E) A gluten-free diet

18. Which of the following peptides is matched to its correct effect?
    (A) Secretin acts to increase pancreatic endocrine secretions.

(B) Motilin plays an important role in digestion by increasing enteric motility during a meal.

(C) Somatostatin works in concert with CCK to increase pancreatic exocrine secretions.

(D) Gastric inhibitory peptide (GIP) inhibits acid production and insulin release.

(E) Bombesin acts to stimulate GI motility.

19. Small intestinal motility is characterized by which of the following?

(A) A "pacemaker potential" that is responsible for initiating peristaltic contractions

(B) Both peristaltic and segmental contractions

(C) Mean transit time through the small intestine of 24 h

(D) Increasing motility more distally in the bowel

(E) A migrating motor complex (MMC) that serves to facilitate the digestion of consumed protein

20. Host defense mechanisms in the gut include both immunologic and nonimmunologic components. One important agent is immunoglobulin (Ig) A. Which of the following statements regarding IgA in the intestines is correct?

(A) It is produced in quantities second only to IgG.

(B) B cells in the follicle of Peyer's patches are responsible for its release.

(C) It is secreted as a monomer bound to a glycoprotein, which facilitates transepithelial migration.

(D) Antigen-specific IgA production to antigens first encountered in the gut can be found in other secretory tissues and can even be transferred via breast milk.

(E) IgA incapacitates bacteria by binding them and promoting phagocytosis.

21. What is the primary fuel source of enterocytes?

(A) Glucose

(B) Glutamine

(C) Ketones

(D) Medium-chain triglycerides

(E) Arginine

22. What portion of the colon absorbs the majority of fluid?

(A) Ascending colon

(B) Transverse colon

(C) Descending colon

(D) Sigmoid colon

(E) Rectum

23. Which of the following is the primary energy source for colonocytes?

(A) Glutamine

(B) Short-chain fatty acids

(C) Glucose

(D) Medium-chain triglycerides

(E) Alanine

24. Which of the following statements regarding the defecatory mechanism is correct?

(A) There is voluntary control of the internal anal sphincter.

(B) Passage of feces into the rectal vault results in reflex contraction of the internal anal sphincter.

(C) Squatting aids in defecation by straightening the anorectal angle.

(D) The external anal sphincter is composed of smooth muscle.

(E) In the setting of normal innervation and musculature, incontinence is rare even with rectal volumes greater than 600 mL.

25. The concentration of which electrolyte in pancreatic secretions increases as the rate of secretion increases?

(A) Sodium

(B) Potassium

(C) Chloride

(D) Bicarbonate

(E) Calcium

26. Islets of Langerhans

(A) Account for 30% of pancreatic mass

(B) Are composed chiefly of alpha cells

(C) Secret bicarbonate into the duodenum via the pancreatic duct

(D) Have varying cellular compositions depending on their location within the pancreas

(E) Are found in lesser numbers in the liver

27. Regarding normal human bile,

(A) Cholesterol is the most prevalent lipid

(B) Deoxycholic acid is the most prevalent bile acid

(C) Lethicin is the most prevalent phospholipid

(D) Micelles with a higher bile acid concentration are able to solubilize more cholesterol

(E) Lecithin-rich micelles form a spherical shape

28. With regard to the enterohepatic circulation, which of the following is a true statement?

(A) The primary means of replenishing the bile acid pool is by enteric absorption from dietary sources.

(B) The level of bile acids in the serum undergoes a postprandial increase.

(C) The highest concentration of bile acids in the body is found in hepatic bile.

(D) Most of the bile acids that leave the body do so in the urine.

(E) Chenodeoxycholic acid is metabolized to ursodeoxycholic acid in the liver before being secreted.

29. Which of the following would you expect following a cholecystectomy?
    (A) Fasting levels of bile acids in the serum are lower.
    (B) The proportion of bile acids extracted by the liver is increased.
    (C) Bile acids are predominantly stored in the liver.
    (D) There is a relative increase in the number of secondary bile acids.
    (E) An elevation of serum bilirubin level exists.

30. Which of the following statements concerning the hepatic acinus is correct?
    (A) Zone 1 hepatocytes are the first to regenerate.
    (B) Bilirubin is mainly absorbed in zone 1.
    (C) Zone 3 hepatocytes are furthest from the hepatic venules.
    (D) Solutes that enter hepatocytes by simple diffusion are absorbed mainly in zone 3.
    (E) The sinusoidal endothelium is characterized by tight junctions with numerous carrier proteins for facilitated diffusion.

31. Which of the following statements regarding hepatic carbohydrate metabolism is correct?
    (A) Insulin facilitates gluconeogenesis.
    (B) Insulin promotes glucose uptake by hepatocytes.
    (C) Glucose storage as fat is more energy efficient than as glycogen.

    (D) Alanine is converted to glucose by deamination to ribose, which is then phosphorylated and enters the phosphogluconate pathway.
    (E) Glucose is the primary fuel source of hepatocytes.

ANSWERS AND EXPLANATIONS

1. **(D)** Innervation of the GI tract can be broadly divided into three categories: sympathetic, parasympathetic, and enteric. Sympathetic innervation is chiefly inhibitory, decreasing motility and secretions; however, sympathetic fibers stimulate contraction of the muscularis mucosa and of certain sphincters. These nerve fibers are typically adrenergic fibers arising from prevertebral and paravertebral plexuses. Few fibers terminate on muscle itself, instead exercising an inhibitory effect by terminating in the submucosal and myenteric plexuses and inhibiting synaptic transmission. Sympathetic fibers also cause vasoconstriction of blood vessels and provide innervation to glandular structures.

   Parasympathetic innervation to the preponderance of the GI tract is conveyed through the vagus nerve and its branches. The distal colon, however, receives parasympathetic innervation from the hypogastric plexus. Like sympathetic fibers, parasympathetic fibers mainly terminate in the submucosal and myenteric plexuses. Unlike sympathetic fibers, they have a stimulatory effect on GI motility and secretions.

   The enteric nervous system is composed primarily of the submucosal plexus (Meissner's plexus) and the myenteric plexus (Auerbach's plexus). These plexuses consist of ganglia connected by unmyelinated fibers (Fig. 16-1).

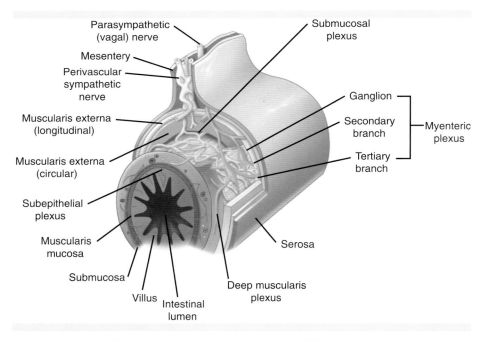

FIGURE 16-1. Enteric nervous system (from Brunicardi FC, Andersen DK, Billiar TR, et al., eds. *Schwartz's Principles of Surgery.* 9th ed. New York, NY: McGraw-Hill; 2009: Fig. 26-16. Copyright © The McGraw-Hill Companies, Inc. All rights reserved).

Other, less-well-defined, plexuses also contribute to the enteric nervous system. The enteric nervous system is influenced by sympathetic and parasympathetic innervation but consists of a rich pathway of afferent and efferent nerves such that much of the activity of the gut, including local reflex activity, continues even in the absence of any extrinsic input.

BIBLIOGRAPHY

Silbernagl S, Despopoulos A. *Color Atlas of Physiology*. 6th ed. Stuttgart, Germany: Thieme; 2008:236–237.

2. **(C)** Swallowing is a complex activity with distinct phases. The pharyngeal phase of swallowing begins when food is pushed posteriorly from the oral cavity into the oropharynx and hypopharynx by the tongue. At the same time, the soft palate elevates, pulled by the levator levi palatini and tensor veli palatini muscles, to prevent passage of the food bolus into the nasopharynx and to allow for the creation of positive pressure in the oropharynx. The hyoid bone moves upward and anteriorly, bringing the epiglottis under the tongue and elevating the larynx, allowing for opening of the retrolaryngeal space. As well, the larynx closes at the level of the epiglottis.

As the tongue moves back and the posterior pharyngeal constrictors contract, hypopharyngeal pressure rises to 60 mmHg. As the cricopharyngeus relaxes, this pressure gradient between the hypopharynx and the thoracic esophagus serves, in conjunction with the peristaltic contractions of the pharyngeal constrictors, to propel the food bolus into the esophagus. The UES then closes to prevent retrograde passage of food. Initially, the pressure of the UES will reach twice the resting pressure but will return to normal with further progression of the food bolus. The muscles of the UES and upper third of the esophagus are striated muscles and receive innervation from the vagus nerve and its recurrent laryngeal branches. The whole act of swallowing is coordinated by the swallowing center, located in the medulla, which acts through cranial nerves V, VII, X, XI, and XII, as well as motor nerves C1–C3 to control the swallowing mechanism. It works in conjunction with areas of the brainstem devoted to respiration to smoothly transform the pharynx from a respiratory to a gustatory conduit (Fig. 16-2).

BIBLIOGRAPHY

Chung DH, Evers MB. The digestive system. In: O'Leary JP, ed. *The Physiologic Basis of Surgery*. 4th ed. Philadelphia, PA: Lippincott Williams & Wilkins; 2008:475–507.
Peters JH, Little VR, Watson TJ. Esophageal anatomy and physiology and gastroesophageal reflux disease. In: Mulholland MW, Lillemoe KD, Doherty GM, et al., eds. *Greenfield's Surgery: Scientific Principles and Practice*. 5th ed. Philadelphia, PA: Lippincott Williams & Wilkins; 2011: Chapter 41.
Waters PF, Demeester TR. Foregut motor disorders and their surgical management. *Med Clin North Am* 1981;65:1235–1241.

3. **(A)** The esophageal phase of swallowing is initiated by the pharyngeal phase, as the UES relaxes in a reflex mediated by the swallowing center of the brainstem. The rapid closing of the UES creates an increase in intraluminal pressure to 60 mmHg, twice the resting level. The peristaltic wave then continues from the pharynx through the esophagus, traveling 2–4 cm/s. Despite high occlusive pressures, the propulsive force of the esophagus is weak, aided by the negative pressure gradient in the thorax. Once food reaches the LES, the bolus must overcome the increased pressure of the abdomen to enter the stomach. The LES, which is tonically contracted, relaxes with the pharyngeal phase of swallowing, which allows for passage of the food bolus on the initiation of the next swallow. Tonicity of the LES is increased by alpha-adrenergic neurotransmitters, beta-blockers, or increased vagal tone and is decreased by caffeine, alcohol, and calcium channel blockers, which can contribute to gastric reflux.

Anatomically, the striated muscles of the upper third of the esophagus receive innervation from the vagus and its recurrent laryngeal branches. There is a gradual transition from striated to smooth muscle that occurs over the middle third of the esophagus. The smooth muscle derives innervation from the vagus via cholinergic fibers synapsing on the myenteric plexus—therefore, atropine impairs esophageal motility.

BIBLIOGRAPHY

Chung DH, Evers MB. The digestive system. In: O'Leary JP, ed. *The Physiologic Basis of Surgery*. 4th ed. Philadelphia, PA: Lippincott Williams & Wilkins; 2008:475–507.
Peters JH, Little VR, Watson TJ. Esophageal anatomy and physiology and gastroesophageal reflux disease. In: Mulholland MW, Lillemoe KD, Doherty GM, et al., eds. *Greenfield's Surgery: Scientific Principles and Practice*. 5th ed. Philadelphia, PA: Lippincott Williams & Wilkins; 2011: Chapter 41.
Waters PF, Demeester TR. Foregut motor disorders and their surgical management. *Med Clin North Am* 1981;65:1235–1241.

4. **(C)** The LES cannot be defined anatomically but can be detected manometrically by an increase in pressure above the gastric baseline as the probe is withdrawn into the esophagus. There are two situations in a normal subject when this high-pressure zone is absent: (1) when the stomach is distended to allow for a belch and (2) during

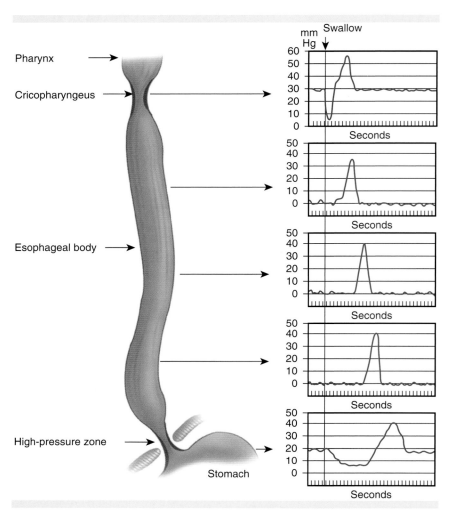

FIGURE 16-2. Demonstration of manometry in response to swallowing. Reproduced with permission from Waters PF, DeMeester TR: Foregut motor disorders and their surgical management. *Med Clin North Am* 65:1238, 1981. Copyright Elsevier.

swallowing. The three most important characteristics for determining the efficacy of the LES in preventing reflux are its resting pressure, overall length, and length exposed to intra-abdominal pressure. The resting pressure and overall length act in concert. A shorter zone of high pressure requires a higher resting pressure to prevent reflux and vice versa. The length of sphincter in the abdomen is also important, as high intra-abdominal pressure can overcome the resting pressure of the LES if this pressure is applied only to the stomach and not also to a significant portion of the LES. As mentioned previously, the LES relaxes with gastric distension to allow belching. Even without this reflex, gastric distension works to lower the resistance of the LES by pulling on the terminal esophagus, in effect incorporating it into the fundus. This then shortens the length of the LES, particularly

the component exposed to intra-abdominal pressure. Patients with a normal angle of His are more resistant to this process, as measured by a higher intragastric pressure required to overcome the sphincter, than are patients with a hiatal hernia.

BIBLIOGRAPHY

Peters JH, Little VR, Watson TJ. Esophageal anatomy and physiology and gastroesophageal reflux disease. In: Mulholland MW, Lillemoe KD, Doherty GM, et al., eds. *Greenfield's Surgery: Scientific Principles and Practice.* 5th ed. Philadelphia, PA: Lippincott Williams & Wilkins; 2011: Chapter 41.

5. **(E)** A wide array of substances has been demonstrated to affect the resting pressure of the LES. Alpha-adrenergic

innervation increases the LES pressure, and beta-adrenergic stimulation decreases it. Hormones that have been shown to increase LES pressure include gastrin, motilin, bombesin, beta-enkephalins, and substance P. Medications that increase LES pressure are antacids, cholinergics, alpha-adrenergic agonists, and metoclopramide. Those that have been shown to decrease LES pressure include CCK, estrogen, glucagons, progesterone, somatostatin, secretin, and vasoactive intestinal peptide (VIP). Medications that lower LES pressure include anticholinergics, barbiturates, calcium channel blockers, caffeine, diazepam, dopamine, meperidine, and theophylline. Dietary factors can also decrease LES tone and include peppermint, chocolate, ethanol, caffeine, and fat.

BIBLIOGRAPHY

Peters JH, Little VR, Watson TJ. Esophageal anatomy and physiology and gastroesophageal reflux disease. In: Mulholland MW, Lillemoe KD, Doherty GM, et al., eds. *Greenfield's Surgery: Scientific Principles and Practice*. 5th ed. Philadelphia, PA: Lippincott Williams & Wilkins; 2011: Chapter 41.

6. **(D)** Vomiting is defined as expulsion of gastric and sometimes enteric contents via the oral cavity. There are a large number of stimuli that may precipitate vomiting. Once initiated, however, the reflex is the same. Retrograde peristalsis occurs in the small intestines. Retrograde peristalsis combined with pyloric and gastric relaxation results in the enteric contents being pushed into the stomach. The pylorus then contracts as gastric distension acts via a reflex mechanism to cause relaxation of the LES. The abdominal wall muscles then contract, causing an increase in the intra-abdominal pressure, which forces the gastric contents into the esophagus. The UES relaxes, allowing continued passage of the vomitus out through the oral cavity. Occurring concomitantly with the GI events, inspiration against a closed glottis occurs, which decreases the intrathoracic pressure and aids the passage of gastric contents into the esophagus. Closure of the glottis, along with approximation of the vocal cords and anterior movement of the larynx, serves to prevent aspiration. The chief difference between retching and vomiting is that in the case of retching, the UES does not relax, preventing passage of gastric contents into the pharynx. The reflex of vomiting is controlled by the vomiting center, which is located in the medulla. A wide variety of stimuli can elicit vomiting, including gastric or duodenal distension, dizziness, pharyngeal stimulation, injury to the genitourinary system, and exposure to emetics, which may act by stimulating gastric or duodenal receptors or may act directly on the central nervous system by stimulating the chemoreceptor trigger zones located in the floor of the fourth ventricle.

BIBLIOGRAPHY

Silbernagl S, Despopoulos A. *Color Atlas of Physiology*. 6th ed. Stuttgart, Germany: Thieme; 2008:236–237.

7. **(B)** Gastric secretions are rich in hydrogen ions, potassium, and chloride. As these ions are lost to the body with vomiting, a resultant hypokalemic, hypochloremic, metabolic alkalosis results. The body compensates by decreasing the respiratory rate and increasing renal bicarbonate secretion in an attempt to normalize the acid/base balance. With protracted vomiting, however, a paradoxical aciduria occurs. The patient becomes dehydrated secondary to sodium and fluid losses in the vomitus, stimulating the renin-angiotensin-aldosterone axis to preserve sodium. This results in sodium retention in the kidney with a reciprocal loss of potassium and hydrogen ions.

BIBLIOGRAPHY

Kellum JA, Puyana JC, Gomez H. Acid base disorders. In: Ashley SW, Cance WG, Jurkovich GJ, et al., eds. *ACS Surgery—Scientific American Surgery*. Hamilton, ON: Decker Intellectual Properties; 2014: Chapter 812.

8. **(D)** Unlike carbohydrates, digestion of proteins does not begin until the food bolus reaches the stomach. Pepsin is the end product of the proenzyme pepsinogen, which is secreted by chief cells and converted to pepsin by hydrochloric acid. Pepsinogen production is stimulated by food in the stomach and low gastric pH. Once converted into the active form of pepsin, the enzyme works as an endopeptidase by disrupting peptide bonds involving aromatic amino acids. Pepsin is inactivated by the alkaline milieu of the duodenum. At this point, proteases produced by the pancreas continue protein digestion. Because of the presence of pancreatic proteases, pepsin is not a necessary component of protein digestion in the normal state, becoming essential only if pancreatic function is abnormal. Pancreatic proteases may be endopeptidases, such as trypsin or chymotrypsin, or exopeptidases, such as carboxypeptidases A and B. They are secreted as proenzymes, and trypsinogen is activated by enterokinase, with trypsin then activating the other proteases. Proteases cleave proteins into tripeptides, dipeptides, or amino acids, all of which can be absorbed by enterocytes, usually involving sodium-mediated transport. Once in

the cytosol, further enzymes digest tri- and dipeptides to single amino acids before they are released into the portal blood.

BIBLIOGRAPHY

Chung DH, Evers MB. The digestive system. In: O'Leary JP, ed. *The Physiologic Basis of Surgery.* 4th ed. Philadelphia, PA: Lippincott Williams & Wilkins; 2008:475–507.

9. **(D)** The primary factors stimulating gastrin release are vagal stimulation, food in the antrum, and gastric distension. Both polypeptides and amino acids result in increased gastrin release—fats and carbohydrates have no effect. Gastric distension increases gastrin release via cholinergic pathways. Prolonged alkalinization (>8 h) will increase gastrin release, while acute alkalinization does not directly cause release of gastrin but does potentiate the release by other stimuli. The primary inhibitor of gastrin release is antral acidification (pH < 2.5). Increased acid in the antrum results in somatostatin release from antral D cells, which then inhibits gastrin release. Indeed, a reciprocal inhibitory relationship exists between gastrin and somatostatin, such that the release of one inhibits the release of the other.

BIBLIOGRAPHY

Barrett KE, Boitano S, Barman SM, Brooks HL. Overview of gastrointestinal function and regulation. In: Barrett KE, Boitano S, Barman SM, Brooks HL, eds. *Ganong's Review of Medical Physiology.* 24th ed. New York, NY: McGraw-Hill; 2012: Chapter 25.
Chung DH, Evers MB. The digestive system. In: O'Leary JP, ed. *The Physiologic Basis of Surgery.* 4th ed. Philadelphia, PA: Lippincott Williams & Wilkins; 2008:475–507.

10. **(A)** The three main stimulants to acid production by the parietal cells are histamine, gastrin, and acetylcholine. The main inhibitors are somatostatin and prostaglandins.

    Adrenergic stimulation acts indirectly to upregulate somatostatin production and downregulate gastrin production. Histamine is released by mast cells located in the lamina propria and diffuses to the mucosa. Histamine receptors are located on the basal membrane of the parietal cell and are classified as H_2 receptors. When stimulated by the binding of histamine, they activate adenylate cyclase, which catalyzes the conversion of adenosine triphosphate (ATP) to cyclic adenosine monophosphate (cAMP). This, in turn, leads to activation of protein kinase C, which causes further protein phosphorylation, ultimately

leading to stimulation of the proton pump. H_2 blockers, such as famotidine, act to impede gastric acid secretion by competitively binding to the receptors, which provides reversible inhibition of histamine-mediated gastric acid production.

Cholinergic stimulation and gastrin act through a similar pathway to increase acid production. Whether they act through identical pathways is unknown. What is known is that both rely on increases in intracellular calcium. This is accomplished by catalyzing the conversion of phosphatidylinositol-4,5-bisphosphate (PIP_2) into inositol triphosphate (IP_3) and diacylglycerol (DAG). IP_3 causes release of intracellular calcium stores from the endoplasmic reticulum, leading to stimulation of a protein kinase (not protein kinase C) with subsequent protein phosphorylation and proton pump activation. The proton pump is a membrane-bound H^+-K^+ ATPase that exchanges cytoplasmic H^+ for luminal K^+. To maintain a ready supply of K^+ on the luminal side of the plasma membrane, luminal K^+ is repleted from intracellular stores. With activation of the H^+-K^+ ATPase, OH^- is produced, which is then converted to HCO_3^- by carbonic anhydrase. HCO_3^- is in turn exchanged for Cl^- at the basal membrane. Chloride ions then diffuse across the canalicular membrane into the lumen. In sum, then, the proton pump results in net movement of H^+ and Cl^- into the lumen and HCO_3^- into the interstitial space (Fig. 16-3).

BIBLIOGRAPHY

Barrett KE, Boitano S, Barman SM, Brooks HL. Overview of gastrointestinal function and regulation. In: Barrett KE, Boitano S, Barman SM, Brooks HL, eds. *Ganong's Review of Medical Physiology.* 24th ed. New York, NY: McGraw-Hill; 2012: Chapter 25.
Peters JH, Little VR, Watson TJ. Esophageal anatomy and physiology and gastroesophageal reflux disease. In: Mulholland MW, Lillemoe KD, Doherty GM, et al., eds. *Greenfield's Surgery: Scientific Principles and Practice.* 5th ed. Philadelphia, PA: Lippincott Williams & Wilkins; 2011: Chapter 41.

11. **(B)** When considering gastric motility, the stomach can be broken down into two regions—the proximal one-third and distal two-thirds. These regions do not correspond to any gross anatomic distinctions but serve differing roles in the gastric handling of a food bolus. The proximal one-third of the stomach has no pacemaker potential or action potentials. Because of this, there is no peristaltic contraction, only prolonged, tonic contractions that serve to increase the intraluminal pressure of the proximal stomach. By contrast, the distal two-thirds of the stomach has a pacemaker located approximately one-third of the way along the greater

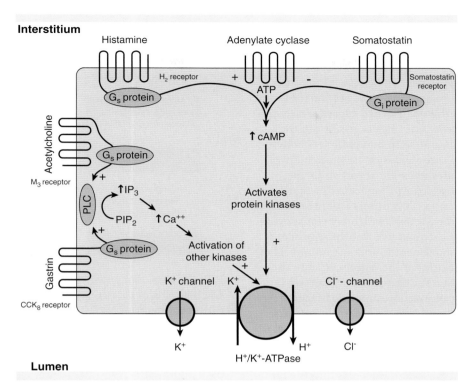

FIGURE 16-3. The parietal cell and stimulants of gastric acid secretion. Reproduced with permission from Mercer DW, Liu TH, Castaneda A: Anatomy and physiology of the stomach, in Zuidema GD, Yeo CJ (eds): *Shackelford's Surgery of the Alimentary Tract,* 5th ed., Vol. II. Philadelphia: Saunders, 2002, p 3. Copyright Elsevier.

curvature. Pacesetter potentials, or electrical control activity (ECA), cause partial depolarizations that occur at a rate of 3/min. By themselves, they do not stimulate a contraction but must be coupled with an action potential to cause smooth muscle contractions. When contractions occur, they spread more rapidly along the greater curvature so that the peristaltic wave reaches the pylorus in a coordinated fashion from all parts of the stomach. The pylorus typically tightens before the peristaltic wave arrives, resulting in a backwash of gastric contents. The repeated churning aids in the digestion of foodstuffs and causes solid food particles to be broken down into smaller particles until they are small enough to pass through the pylorus, typically less than 1 mm. For liquids, however, the rate-determining factor in gastric emptying is the pressure gradient between the stomach and the duodenum. Vagotomy, either truncal or proximal, causes a loss of receptive relaxation. This causes an increase in intragastric pressure and leads to an increased emptying rate of liquids. However, it does not change the tone of the pylorus, the strength of contractions, or the rate of the gastric pacemaker. Pyloroplasty is often done in conjunction with vagotomy to prevent delayed gastric emptying.

BIBLIOGRAPHY

Chung DH, Evers MB. The digestive system. In: O'Leary JP, ed. *The Physiologic Basis of Surgery.* 4th ed. Philadelphia, PA: Lippincott Williams & Wilkins; 2008:475–507.

Peters JH, Little VR, Watson TJ. Esophageal anatomy and physiology and gastroesophageal reflux disease. In: Mulholland MW, Lillemoe KD, Doherty GM, et al., eds. *Greenfield's Surgery: Scientific Principles and Practice.* 5th ed. Philadelphia, PA: Lippincott Williams & Wilkins; 2011: Chapter 41.

12. **(C)** Ingested carbohydrates can be broadly thought of as simple sugars, such as glucose or fructose; disaccharides, such as sucrose or lactose; starches, such as amylose; and undigestible fibers, such as cellulose. Digestion of carbohydrates is initiated in the mouth by salivary amylase. Salivary amylase is inactivated in the stomach when the gastric pH is reduced to less than 4.0. Before inactivation, however, amylase hydrolyzes starch into maltose, maltotriose, and alpha-limit dextrins by cleaving internal alpha-glycosidic bonds. Fibers such as cellulose are indigestible because their beta-glycosidic bonds are not hydrolyzed by amylase or any other human enteric enzyme. Amylase secreted by the pancreas completes the hydrolysis of starch, usually by the time the proximal

jejunum is reached. These oligosaccharides, along with such dietary disaccharides as lactose, are digested by the brush border enzymes to form glucose, galactose, and fructose. Deficiency of brush border enzymes, as seen with lactase deficiency in lactose intolerance, can result in cramping and diarrhea secondary to the osmotic burden of the unabsorbed sugars. The activity of the brush border enzymes is greatest in the duodenum and jejunum, with markedly less activity in the ileum. Once carbohydrates are broken down into monosaccharides, they are absorbed by the enterocytes. Fructose absorption occurs primarily via facilitated diffusion. This differs from the transport of glucose and galactose, which are transported into the enterocyte via an active transport system that couples their movement to that of sodium. They are then transported out of the enterocyte into the interstitial space via a sodium-independent carrier. The osmotic value of one molecule of starch is equal to that of one molecule of maltose or glucose. Therefore, as starch is digested, the osmotic effect is increased; however, under normal circumstances, the absorptive mechanisms along the brush border work rapidly, preventing massive fluid shifts into the luminal space.

BIBLIOGRAPHY

Chung DH, Evers MB. The digestive system. In: O'Leary JP, ed. *The Physiologic Basis of Surgery*. 4th ed. Philadelphia, PA: Lippincott Williams & Wilkins; 2008:475–507.

McKenzie S, Evers BM. Small intestine. In: Townsend CM, Beauchamp RD, Evers BM, Mattox KL, eds. *Sabiston Textbook of Surgery: The Biological Basis of Modern Surgical Practice*. 19th ed. Philadelphia, PA: Saunders Elsevier; 2012: Chapter 50.

13. **(D)** The initial step in lipid metabolism is the breakdown of triglycerides, which are the main component of dietary fat (Fig. 16-4). Two of the enzymes involved in this process are lingual and pancreatic lipase. Both enzymes are secreted in active form and remain active even in an acidic environment. Lingual lipase is active from a pH of 2.2 to 6.0, and while pancreatic lipase is most active at an alkaline pH of 8.0, it is not inactivated until the pH is less than 3.0. Lingual lipase acts to hydrolyze the ester linkages in the 1 and 3 positions of the triglyceride molecule, and its actions result in free fatty acids and diglycerides. Pancreatic lipase acts to hydrolyze triglycerides primarily into free fatty acids and monoglycerides. Pancreatic lipase must first, however, gain access to the glyceride moiety of the triglyceride. This is accomplished through the actions of colipase, a coenzyme secreted by the pancreas as the proenzyme

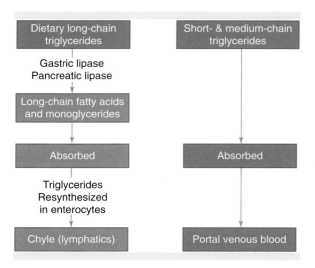

FIGURE 16-4. Fat digestion (from Brunicardi FC, Andersen DK, Billiar TR, et al., eds. *Schwartz's Principles of Surgery*. 10th ed. New York, NY: McGraw-Hill; 2014: Fig. 28-9. Copyright © The McGraw-Hill Companies, Inc. All rights reserved).

procolipase before being activated by trypsin. Colipase binds to lipase and causes a structural transformation that enables lipase to successfully compete with bile salts for access to the glyceride moiety. Lingual lipase does not use a coenzyme.

Other enzymes important to lipid digestion are also secreted by the pancreas. Phospholipase A_2 acts to catalyze phospholipids into lysophospholipids and free fatty acids. Both bile salts and calcium are required for this hydrolysis, and phospholipase A_2 acts on both dietary and biliary phospholipids. It is secreted as a proenzyme and requires activation by trypsin. Another pancreatic enzyme important for lipid digestion is cholesterol esterase. This enzyme acts to hydrolyze a variety of lipid ester linkages, including cholesterol; vitamins A, D, C, and E; as well as the ester linkages found in triglycerides. Like phospholipase A_2, its activity is dependent on bile salts. On the completion of enzymatic digestion, dietary lipids have been metabolized into free fatty acids, 2-monoglycerides, and phospholipids.

Enzymatic digestion can be impaired by a number of conditions, leading to fat malabsorption and resultant diarrhea. These include pancreatic insufficiency, although only 10–15% of normal pancreatic exocrine function is needed for adequate lipid digestion; hypersecretion of gastric hydrochloric acid to the point that lipase is persistently inactivated; and failure of enterohepatic circulation such that enzymatic activity is impaired by the resulting bile salt deficiency.

BIBLIOGRAPHY

Barrett KE, Boitano S, Barman SM, Brooks HL. Digestion, absorption, and nutritional principles. In: Barrett KE, Boitano S, Barman SM, Brooks HL, eds. *Ganong's Review of Medical Physiology.* 24th ed. New York, NY: McGraw-Hill; 2012: Chapter 26.

14. **(A)** A variety of peptides serve to act in an endocrine, paracrine, or autocrine manner to regulate the complex interrelationships between the stomach, small bowel, gallbladder, and pancreas. One such peptide is CCK, which is found in the central nervous system, as well as in the GI tract. In the gut, CCK is found in I cells of the duodenum and jejunum. Its release is stimulated by fatty acids and peptides in the duodenal lumen. When released, it acts to upregulate small intestinal digestion. It aids in micelle formation by stimulating the gallbladder to contract, while at the same time relaxing the sphincter of Oddi, leading to increased bile secretion. Along with secretin, it acts to increase pancreatic bicarbonate and exocrine secretions, neutralizing gastric acid in the duodenum and assisting with protein digestion. Finally, while CCK increases small intestinal motility, it acts to inhibit gastric emptying, ensuring that the small intestinal digestive mechanisms do not become overwhelmed. CCK is not known to affect gastric acid secretion or mesenteric vasodilation directly.

BIBLIOGRAPHY

Chung DH, Evers MB. The digestive system. In: O'Leary JP, ed. *The Physiologic Basis of Surgery.* 4th ed. Philadelphia, PA: Lippincott Williams & Wilkins; 2008:475–507.

15. **(D)** The recommended daily intake of calcium is 1000 mg. Calcium must be ionized as a soluble salt to be absorbed. Calcium is primarily absorbed in the duodenum and, to a lesser extent, in the proximal jejunum. To absorb ionized calcium, a number of hormonal, enteric, and physiologic factors must work in concert. Vitamin D acts to facilitate calcium absorption by upregulating various calcium-specific transport proteins. Parathyroid hormone acts indirectly to increase calcium absorption by stimulating the hydroxylation of 25-OH vitamin D in the kidney, resulting in the metabolically active $1,25\text{-}(OH)_2$ vitamin D. This active transport is necessary when low intraluminal concentrations of calcium are present, but passive absorption can be observed if the intraluminal concentration rises to high levels.

Intraluminal factors that enhance calcium absorption include bile acids, amino acids, and certain medications, such as penicillin and chloramphenicol, which create soluble calcium salts. Sugars also act to enhance calcium absorption by altering fluid transport. Gastric acid should theoretically enhance calcium absorption by causing the dissociation of calcium compounds and dissolving insoluble compounds. In practice, however, gastric acid has been demonstrated to have no significant effect. Other factors such as fatty acids and cholestyramine bind to calcium to form relatively insoluble complexes that impair absorption.

A healthy mucosal surface is necessary for adequate calcium absorption. Conditions such as Crohn's disease and celiac sprue inhibit calcium absorption. Similarly, patients experience malabsorption of calcium after intestinal bypass if food is redirected past the duodenum or proximal jejunum. Primary biliary cirrhosis has also been implicated in decreased calcium absorption, as have a variety of other factors, including glucocorticoids, thyroxine, thiazides, and aging, either by direct effects on the intestine or secondary to alterations in vitamin D metabolism. Conversely, growth hormone, estrogens, prolactin, and sarcoidosis increase calcium absorption through multifactorial mechanisms.

BIBLIOGRAPHY

Barrett KE, Boitano S, Barman SM, Brooks HL. Digestion, absorption, and nutritional principles. In: Barrett KE, Boitano S, Barman SM, Brooks HL, eds. *Ganong's Review of Medical Physiology.* 24th ed. New York, NY: McGraw-Hill; 2012: Chapter 26.

16. **(A)** Up to 50% of the small bowel may be resected with expectation of normal GI function; however, because of specialized absorptive or secretory properties, the duodenum, proximal jejunum, and distal ileum must be spared. Because it is the sole or primary absorptive site for a range of substances found in the gut, resection of the distal ileum can result in an array of deficiency states. Loss of the distal ileum results in decreased bile salt absorption, and the losses often exceed the capacity of the liver to produce new bile salts, reducing the total bile salt pool. This has two adverse effects. First, it results in lithogenic bile and formation of cholesterol gallstones. Second, there is a decreased ability to form micelles, and fat absorption is therefore impeded, resulting in steatorrhea, which is then worsened by the osmotic diarrhea caused by excessive bile salts in the colon. This dearth of bile salts also results in impaired absorption of the fat-soluble vitamins A, D, E, and K. Fat malabsorption results in the formation of insoluble calcium salts from the binding of calcium to fatty acids. This serves to decrease the intraluminal calcium concentration such that oxalate, which normally precipitates as an insoluble calcium salt, is free to pass into the colon in soluble form, where it is then absorbed. Increased oxalate absorption leads to hyperoxaluria and the formation of kidney stones. Finally, vitamin B_{12} is absorbed in the distal ileum, and the deficiency thereof results in megaloblastic anemia.

BIBLIOGRAPHY

Chung DH, Evers MB. The digestive system. In: O'Leary JP, ed. *The Physiologic Basis of Surgery*. 4th ed. Philadelphia, PA: Lippincott Williams & Wilkins; 2008:475–507.

17. **(B)** Following digestion into monoglycerides and fatty acids in the intestinal lumen, lipid breakdown products are absorbed, and the process is reversed in the enterocyte, resulting in reformation of triglycerides. The triglycerides are then formed into chylomicrons, which are large spheres consisting of a hydrophobic core covered by phospholipids and apolipoproteins. The chylomicron then exits the enterocyte across the basolateral membrane and is taken up by the intestinal lymphatic system, as chylomicrons are too large to fit through the capillary junctions and enter the portal venous system. Chylomicrons travel through the lymphatics to the cisterna chyle and thoracic duct before entering the systemic circulation. Medium-chain fatty acids, however, secondary to their increased polarity, are to some degree water soluble and can therefore be directly absorbed without the need for bile salt–facilitated solubilization into micelles. Similarly, once in the enterocyte, they can be transported into the portal venous system as fatty acids without undergoing reassembly into triglycerides. They are thus able to bypass the lymphatic system and decrease the effluent seen in cases of chylothorax. Sugars such as galactose or proteins such as gluten do not have a significant effect on chyle formation.

BIBLIOGRAPHY

Barrett KE, Boitano S, Barman SM, Brooks HL. Digestion, absorption, and nutritional principles. In: Barrett KE, Boitano S, Barman SM, Brooks HL, eds. *Ganong's Review of Medical Physiology*. 24th ed. New York, NY: McGraw-Hill; 2012: Chapter 26.

18. **(E)** A variety of peptides serve to act in an endocrine, paracrine, or autocrine manner to regulate the complex interrelationships between the stomach, small bowel, gallbladder, and pancreas. These include secretin, which is found in the S cells of the duodenum and jejunum and is released in response to duodenal fat, acid, or bile salts. It acts with CCK to increase pancreatic secretions rich in bicarbonate. It has a feedback mechanism such that its release is inhibited when the duodenal pH rises above 4.5. Secretin is notable for causing an unexpected increase in gastrin release and gastric acid production when applied exogenously to a patient with Zollinger-Ellison's syndrome.

Somatostatin is a widely distributed peptide, found in both the central and peripheral nervous systems, as well as in the GI tract. Somatostatin acts like a global brake on the GI system, decreasing motility, as well as gastric, enteric, and pancreatic secretions.

GIP is found in the K cells of the duodenum. It acts as a true hormone to inhibit gastric acid secretion and stimulate insulin release. Its own release is stimulated by intraluminal amino acids, glucose, and fatty acids.

Motilin is found throughout the small intestine but is present in higher concentrations more proximally. It is released during fasting and has an important role in gut motility, serving some role in the initiation of migrating motor complexes. Its release is inhibited by somatostatin, secretin, pancreatic polypeptides, and intraluminal fat. Neurotensin is another peptide found in the central nervous system as well as the gut. In the GI tract, it is located predominantly in the ileum. It is released in response to luminal fatty acids and acts to inhibit gastric acid secretion and intestinal motility while stimulating pancreatic exocrine secretions and causing mesenteric vasodilation. Other peptides of note include peptide YY, which is found in the distal ileum and colon, released in response to intraluminal fat, and acts to inhibit gastric emptying and acid production, as well as pancreatic exocrine secretions; and bombesin, which stimulates GI motility and secretions and can be used as a tumor marker for small bowel cancers.

BIBLIOGRAPHY

Chung DH, Evers MB. The digestive system. In: O'Leary JP, ed. *The Physiologic Basis of Surgery*. 4th ed. Philadelphia, PA: Lippincott Williams & Wilkins; 2008:475–507.

19. **(B)** The normal resting potential of human enterocytes is −50 to −70 mV. Depolarizations called pacemaker potentials occur at regular intervals but do not cause muscular contractions. Instead, additional neural or chemical stimuli are needed to exceed the excitation threshold and cause an action potential. Thus, while the pacemaker potential is necessary for a contraction to occur, and is thus able to regulate the rate of contractions, it does not itself initiate peristaltic contractions. In the duodenum, these depolarizations occur 11–13 times/min, while they slow to 8–10 times/min in the ileum. Once a contraction occurs, it can be either a peristaltic contraction or a segmental one. Segmental contractions occur as circular muscle acts to churn intestinal contents and causes mixing of the food bolus and exposure to the luminal mucosa. Peristaltic contractions, however, are the result of contractions of longitudinal muscle and serve to propel intestinal contents distally by a combination of proximal contraction and distal relaxation. These contractions serve to propel the intestinal contents fairly briskly, with a mean transit time through the intestines of just under

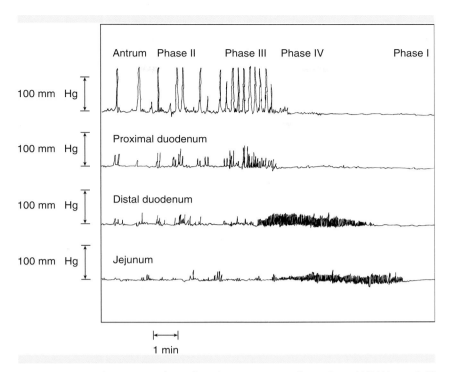

FIGURE 16-5. Migrating motor complex. Reproduced with permission from Rees WDW, et al: Human interdigestive and postprandial gastrointestinal motor and gastrointestinal hormone patterns. *Dig Dis Sci.* 27(4):321, 1982. Copyright 1982, with kind permission of Springer Science + Business Media.

4 h. This transit time is shortened by meals high in glucose and lengthened by meals high in fat. The MMC is mediated by motilin. It occurs during the fasting state and serves to clear the intestines of residual material (Fig. 16-5). When present, it cycles every 9–12 min, beginning in the proximal bowel and progressing distally to the terminal ileum. There are four phases. Phase I is a quiescent phase. During phase II, irregular, intermittent contractions occur. In phase III, the intestines exhibit regular, high-amplitude contractions before progressing to phase IV, which, like phase II, has irregular, intermittent contractions. The MMC moves at a rate of 4–6 cm/min in the proximal small bowel and 1–2 cm/min more distally. Control for the MMC rests in the enteric nervous system and is destroyed with enteric resection. While extrinsic innervation can modulate the MMC, it continues to occur even after total extrinsic denervation.

BIBLIOGRAPHY

Chung DH, Evers MB. The digestive system. In: O'Leary JP, ed. *The Physiologic Basis of Surgery.* 4th ed. Philadelphia, PA: Lippincott Williams & Wilkins; 2008:475–507.

McKenzie S, Evers BM. Small intestine. In: Townsend CM, Beauchamp RD, Evers BM, Mattox KL, eds. *Sabiston Textbook of Surgery: The Biological Basis of Modern Surgical Practice.* 19th ed. Philadelphia, PA: Saunders Elsevier; 2012: Chapter 50.

20. **(D)** Host defense mechanisms in the gut include both immunologic and nonimmunologic components. Some of the nonimmunologic processes include hydrochloric acid secretion by the stomach and mucus production, which serves to entrap bacteria. Peristalsis acts to clear the gut of harmful agents, while various enzymes lyse bacteria and toxins. The rapid turnover of epithelial cells seen in the intestines serves to slough infected cells and prevent deeper penetration of harmful organisms, and competition from endogenous, nonpathogenic organisms prevents harmful bacteria from colonizing the gut. Peyer's patches are large collections of lymphoid follicles with intervening interfollicular areas that are rich in T cells. A specialized epithelium composed of membrane cells (M cells) covers the Peyer's patch and acts as an antigen presenter by transporting particles from the intestinal lumen and delivering them to the underlying immune cells.

    B cells mature in the germinal centers of the follicles in response to antigen under the regulation of T cells in the interfollicular areas. But, while B cell maturation occurs in Peyer's patches, immunoglobulin secretion does not occur until they migrate to the lamina propria. The vast majority of B cells (80–90%) here produce IgA. Unlike in the serum, IgA in mucosal tissue exists as a dimer, connected by a J chain and linked to a transmembrane glycoprotein secretory component that facilitates transmembrane migration. Unlike other antibodies that act via the complement cascade, IgA inhibits bacterial activity by binding to the offending agent and promoting entrapment within the mucin layer, as well as by directly impeding bacterial activity by binding to external bacterial effector mechanisms such as fimbriae. Exposure to antigens in the gut will lead to antigen-specific IgA secretion in other mucosal tissues as well. Following stimulation in the Peyer's patch, mature B cells migrate to mesenteric lymph nodes before eventually entering the systemic circulation via the thoracic duct. From there, they localize to other mucosa-associated lymphoid tissue. In this way, IgA can be secreted into breast milk and impart antigen-specific immunity to the GI tract of an infant. IgA is the third most abundant antibody, behind IgG and IgM.

BIBLIOGRAPHY

McKenzie S, Evers BM. Small intestine. In: Townsend CM, Beauchamp RD, Evers BM, Mattox KL, eds. *Sabiston Textbook of Surgery: The Biological Basis of Modern Surgical Practice*. 19th ed. Philadelphia, PA: Saunders Elsevier; 2012: Chapter 50.

21. **(B)** Glutamine is the chief fuel source of enterocytes. It is absorbed either from the gut lumen or from the arterial circulation. Glutamine is formed in peripheral tissues from glutamate and ammonia by the actions of glutamine synthetase. In the enterocyte, glutamine is broken down into glutamate and ammonia. Glutamate enters the tricarboxylic acid cycle, while the ammonia is taken up in the portal circulation and delivered to the liver where it is used to form urea. About 50% of the ammonia in the portal circulation comes from glutamine metabolism, with the remainder coming as a result of bacterial metabolism.

BIBLIOGRAPHY

Rodwell VW. Biosynthesis of the nutritionally nonessential amino acids. In: Murray RK, Bender DA, Botham KM, Kennelly PJ, Rodwell VW, Weil P, eds. *Harper's Illustrated Biochemistry*. 29th ed. New York, NY: McGraw-Hill; 2012: Chapter 27.
Shelton AA, Chang G, Welton ML. Small intestine. In: Doherty GM, ed. *Current Diagnosis and Treatment: Surgery*. 13th ed. New York, NY: McGraw-Hill; 2010: Chapter 29.

22. **(A)** Water comprises approximately 90% of small intestinal contents that pass into the colon. The colon will absorb roughly 90% of this water before passing the remainder in the stool. The majority of water absorption occurs in the right colon as a passive response to an osmotic gradient established via the active transport of sodium, powered by the Na^+-K^+ ATPase on the basolateral membrane of colonic epithelial cells. The electrochemical gradient thus created also allows for passive passage of K^+ into the colonic lumen. The colon is also a site of chloride absorption with reciprocal excretion of bicarbonate.

BIBLIOGRAPHY

Sweeney JF. Colonic anatomy and physiology. In: Greenfield L, ed. *Surgery: Scientific Principles and Practice*. 3rd ed. Philadelphia, PA: Lippincott Williams & Wilkins; 2001:1066–1067.

23. **(B)** Colonocytes are unable to actively absorb glucose or amino acids; however, bacteria in the colonic lumen metabolize carbohydrates and proteins into short-chain fatty acids, principally acetate, propionate, and butyrate. In fact, these short-chain fatty acids are the predominant anions in the colon. Short-chain fatty acids appear to be absorbed both by passive means and by carrier-mediated transport. Short-chain fatty acids account for 7–10% of all the calories absorbed and serve as the primary fuel source for colonocytes.

BIBLIOGRAPHY

Fry RD, Mahmoud NN, Maron DJ, Bleier JIS. Colon and rectum. In: Townsend CM, Beauchamp RD, Evers BM, Mattox KL, eds. *Sabiston Textbook of Surgery: The Biological Basis of Modern Surgical Practice*. 19th ed. Philadelphia, PA: Saunders Elsevier; 2012:1294–1380.
McKenzie S, Evers BM. Small intestine. In: Townsend CM, Beauchamp RD, Evers BM, Mattox KL, eds. *Sabiston Textbook of Surgery: The Biological Basis of Modern Surgical Practice*. 19th ed. Philadelphia, PA: Saunders Elsevier; 2012: Chapter 50.

24. **(C)** The defecatory mechanism begins with the passage of a fecal bolus into the rectum. Rectal distension is transmitted via parasympathetic mechanoreceptors; however, the rectosphincteric reflex is mediated by the myenteric plexus and results in relaxation of the internal anal sphincter as the rectum contracts. At this time, voluntary contraction of the striated muscle of the external anal sphincter can forestall defecation; however, at rectal volumes exceeding 400 mL, incontinence can commonly occur, even in the setting of normal innervation and musculature. There

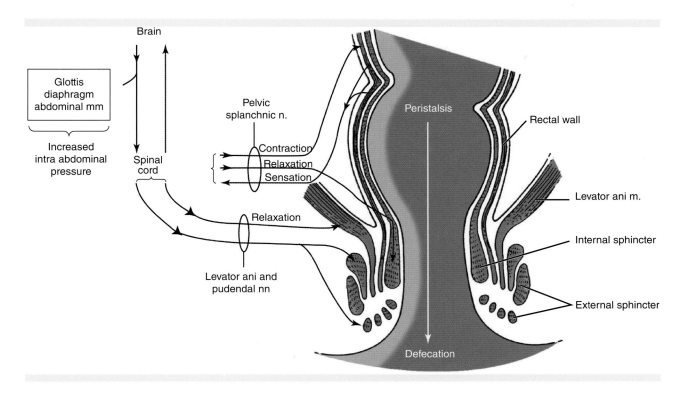

FIGURE 16-6. Neural pathways in the defecatory mechanism (from Skandalakis JE, Colborn GL, Weidman TA, et al. *Skandalakis' Surgical Anatomy.* New York, NY: McGraw-Hill; 2004: Fig. 18-50. Copyright © The McGraw-Hill Companies, Inc. All rights reserved).

is no voluntary control over the relaxation of the internal sphincter. Once a socially acceptable situation is reached, a squatting position is assumed, which serves to straighten the anorectal junction, facilitating the passage of fecal material. The anorectal junction is further straightened by relaxation of the pelvic musculature, particularly the puborectalis muscle. A Valsalva maneuver is performed as the external anal sphincter relaxes, allowing passage of the stool out through the anus.

BIBLIOGRAPHY

Chung DH, Evers MB. The digestive system. In: O'Leary JP, ed. *The Physiologic Basis of Surgery.* 4th ed. Philadelphia, PA: Lippincott Williams & Wilkins; 2008:475–507.

Fry RD, Mahmoud NN, Maron DJ, Bleier JIS. Colon and rectum. In: Townsend CM, Beauchamp RD, Evers BM, Mattox KL, eds. *Sabiston Textbook of Surgery: The Biological Basis of Modern Surgical Practice.* 19th ed. Philadelphia, PA: Saunders Elsevier; 2012:1294–1380.

25. **(D)** Pancreatic secretions consist of water and electrolytes secreted by centroacinar and intercalated duct cells and digestive enzymes from acinar cells. The secretions are alkalotic, and the concentration of bicarbonate increases from 20 mmol/L in the resting state to 150 mmol/L under conditions of maximal secretion. As bicarbonate concentration increases, there is a concomitant decrease in the chloride concentration such that the total concentration of the two anions remains constant and equal to their combined concentration in the plasma. The acinar cells secrete three main categories of enzymes: lipases, amylases, and proteases. The lipases secreted by the pancreas include pancreatic lipase, phospholipases A and B, and cholesterol esterase, which act to hydrolyze lipids. Amylase hydrolyzes carbohydrates into monosaccharides and disaccharides and alpha-limit dextrins. Proteases act to digest protein and are notable for being secreted into the intestinal lumen in inactive, proenzyme form. One of these proenzymes, trypsinogen, is activated either by an acidic environment or by the enteric enzyme enterokinase into its active form, trypsin. Trypsin then activates the other proteases. Pancreatic secretion can be increased by a variety of stimuli. Vagal stimulation increases both bicarbonate and enzymatic secretion. Secretin results in an increase in bicarbonate and fluid secretion but has little effect on enzyme secretion. VIP has similar effects but with less potency. CCK, as well as bombesin

TABLE 16-1 Factors Affecting Pancreatic Secretion*

Stimulus	Enzyme Production	Bicarbonate/ Volume Production
Vagus	↑	↑
Secretin	–	↑
VIP	–	↑
CCK	↑	–
Gastrin	↑	–
Bombesin	↑	–
Pancreatic polypeptide	↓	↓
Somatostatin	↓	↓
Glucagon	↓	↓
Sham feeding	↑	↓
Duodenal acid	–	↑
Fatty acids	↑	↑
Amino acids	↑	–

*Bicarbonate and total volume show concomitant increases or decreases. Production of enzymes may be independent from that of bicarbonate.

and gastrin to a lesser degree, is a strong stimulator of enzyme secretion, while having little effect on bicarbonate or fluid secretion (Table 16-1).

BIBLIOGRAPHY

Jensen EH, Borja-Cacho D, Al-Refaie WB, Vickers SM. Exocrine pancreas. In: Townsend CM, Beauchamp RD, Evers BM, Mattox KL, eds. *Sabiston Textbook of Surgery: The Biological Basis of Modern Surgical Practice.* 19th ed. Philadelphia, PA: Saunders Elsevier; 2012: Chapter 56.

26. **(D)** The pancreas can functionally be divided into the exocrine and endocrine pancreas. Structurally, this correlates with the acinar cells and ductal network for the exocrine pancreas and the islets of Langerhans for the endocrine pancreas. The islets of Langerhans contribute little to pancreatic mass, accounting for only 2% of its weight. Within the islets of Langerhans can be found alpha cells, which secrete glucagon; beta cells, which produce insulin; delta cells, which manufacture somatostatin; and pancreatic polypeptide cells, which, not surprisingly, produce pancreatic polypeptide. Beta cells are the most predominant cell type; they are located centrally within the islet and account for 70% of the mass

of the endocrine pancreas. The other cell types account for a smaller percentage of the endocrine pancreas mass, with pancreatic polypeptide cells accounting for 15%, alpha cells for 10%, and delta cells for 5%.

Islets have varying compositions depending on their location within the pancreas. While beta and delta cells are relatively uniform in their distribution, alpha cells are found in greater predominance in the body and tail, while pancreatic polypeptide cells are more plentiful in the uncinate process. The acinar cells and ducts account for 80% of pancreatic mass. Acinar cells produce the enzymes necessary for digestion. Centroacinar cells secrete fluid and bicarbonate. Together, these cells form a structural unit called an acinus. The cells in an acinus secrete their products into an acinar lumen, which drains into intercalated ducts, which in turn drain into interlobular ducts. The interlobular ducts eventually coalesce into the main pancreatic duct. which carries the products of pancreatic exocrine production into the duodenum (Fig. 16-7, Table 16-2).

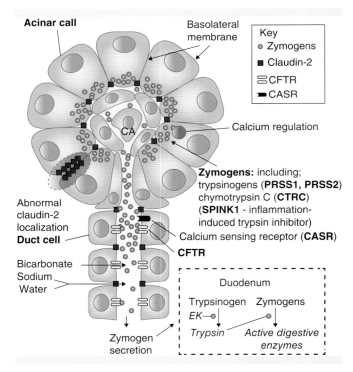

FIGURE 16-7. Pancreatic acinus. Acinar cells secrete enzymes and centroacinar cells secrete water and bicarbonate into the acinar lumen. The acinar lumen in turn drains into intercalated ducts and eventually into the main pancreatic duct. Reproduced with permission from Bell RH Jr: Atlas of pancreatic surgery. In: Bell RH Jr, Rikkers LF, Mulholland MW (eds): *Digestive Tract Surgery: A Text and Atlas.* Philadelphia: Lippincott-Raven, 1996, p 969.

TABLE 16-2 Comparison of the Various Cells Comprising the Islets of Langerhans

Cell	Endocrine Product	% of Pancreatic Endocrine Mass	Location in Pancreas
α-Cells	Glucagon	10	Body and tail
β-Cells	Insulin	70	Uniform
δ-Cells	Somatostatin	5	Uniform
Pancreatic polypeptide cells	Pancreatic polypeptide	15	Uncinate process

BIBLIOGRAPHY

Jensen EH, Borja-Cacho D, Al-Refaie WB, Vickers SM. Exocrine pancreas. In: Townsend CM, Beauchamp RD, Evers BM, Mattox KL, eds. *Sabiston Textbook of Surgery: The Biological Basis of Modern Surgical Practice*. 19th ed. Philadelphia, PA: Saunders Elsevier; 2012: Chapter 56.

27. **(C)** Bile is a solution composed chiefly of water, which accounts for about 85% of its volume. Because cholesterol is nonpolar and insoluble in water, and because bile acids and phospholipids are amphipathic, these lipids form micelles in solution. Cholesterol aggregates centrally in association with the nonpolar aspects of the bile acids and phospholipids. The polar, hydrophilic aspects of these molecules are found on the periphery, in contact with the aqueous environment. When rich in bile salts, the micelles form into a spherical shape, but when rich in lecithin, they form disk-shaped micelles, which tend to be larger and are capable of solubilizing more cholesterol. The main lipid component in bile is the bile acids, with the two main primary bile acids, cholic acid and chenodeoxycholic acid, accounting for about 80% of all bile acids. Phospholipids, of which lecithin is the most prevalent, account for about 20% of all lipids. Cholesterol is the least-prevalent lipid, accounting for less than 10%. In addition to lipids, bile contains smaller amounts of proteins, chiefly albumin, and various electrolytes. The concentration of the main electrolytes approximates that of plasma. Of course, bilirubin is also present in bile, almost exclusively in conjugated form.

BIBLIOGRAPHY

Barrett KE, Boitano S, Barman SM, Brooks HL. Transport and metabolic functions of the liver. In: Barrett KE, Boitano S, Barman SM, Brooks HL, eds. *Ganong's Review of Medical Physiology*. 24th ed. New York, NY: McGraw-Hill; 2012: Chapter 28.

Mulvihill, SJ. Liver, biliary tract, and pancreas. In: O'Leary JP, ed. *The Physiologic Basis of Surgery*. 4th ed. Philadelphia, PA: Lippincott Williams & Wilkins; 2008:508–532.

28. **(B)** Understanding of the enterohepatic circulation of bile acids began with Moritz Schiff in 1855, who observed an increased rate of bile secretion in dogs in proportion to the amount of exogenous bile instilled into their small intestines. New bile acids are typically added to the pool by conversion of cholesterol to one of the two primary bile acids, either chenodeoxycholic acid or cholic acid. The concentration of bile acids in hepatocytes is low (<50 µmol), as active secretion prevents the accumulation of bile acids. Hepatic bile, on the other hand, is quite concentrated (20,000–40,000 µmol). This bile either flows freely into the duodenum or, if the sphincter of Oddi is contracted, will flow into the gallbladder. Once in the gallbladder, water is absorbed from the bile across the mucosa, resulting in the highest concentration of bile acids (50,000–200,000 µmol).

With the release of CCK in response to a meal, the gallbladder contracts and the sphincter of Oddi relaxes, causing flow of the bile into the small intestine. A small amount of bile acids will be passively absorbed in the proximal intestine, but most will proceed distally. Chenodeoxycholic acid and cholic acid may undergo transformation into ursodeoxycholic acid and deoxycholic acid, respectively, by enteric bacteria. Most of these bile acids, both primary and secondary, will be actively absorbed in the terminal ileum. A small percentage of bile acids will pass into the colon. Some of these will be reabsorbed, and the rest will be lost to the body in the feces. This accounts for almost all of the loss of bile acids. The bile acids absorbed by the terminal ileum will pass back to the liver bound to albumin in portal blood, where they will be extracted by hepatocytes. The percentage of bile acids extracted remains relatively constant, as the capacity for bile acid extraction greatly exceeds the typical bile acid load seen by the liver.

Thus, as enterohepatic circulation of bile acids is increased by a meal, a greater absolute number of bile acids will bypass the liver and enter the systemic circulation, resulting in a postprandial increase in the serum bile acid level. Bile acids in the systemic circulation can be excreted in the urine, but urine losses are negligible for three main reasons. First, the hepatic extraction of bile acids from portal venous blood is extremely efficient. Second, most bile acids in the blood are protein bound, and third, bile acids are reabsorbed by the renal tubules (Fig. 16-8).

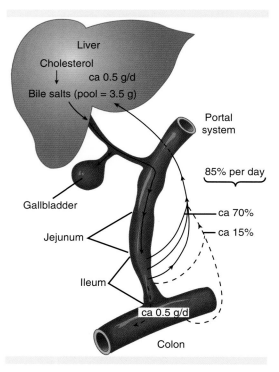

FIGURE 16-8. Enterohepatic circulation (from Doherty GM, ed. *Current Diagnosis and Treatment: Surgery.* 13th ed. New York, NY: McGraw-Hill; 2010: Fig. 25-5).

BIBLIOGRAPHY

Barrett KE, Boitano S, Barman SM, Brooks HL. Transport and metabolic functions of the liver. In: Barrett KE, Boitano S, Barman SM, Brooks HL, eds. *Ganong's Review of Medical Physiology.* 24th ed. New York, NY: McGraw-Hill; 2012: Chapter 28.

29. **(D)** For patients with a normal gallbladder in the fasting state, over half of the bile acid pool will be stored in the gallbladder. Alterations in function or surgical removal of the gallbladder therefore cause changes in characteristics of the bile acid pool. After cholecystectomy, bile passes directly into the intestines, which essentially serves as the storage reservoir for bile salts; however, this is not a static process, and distal passage of the bile acids results in absorption in the terminal ileum and an increase in enterohepatic cycling. This, in turn, results in slight elevations in the fasting serum bile acid levels, as the percentage of bile acids extracted by the liver remains constant. Because a greater proportion of bile acids is located enterically, the bile acids are more exposed to bacterial biotransformation and a relative increase in secondary bile acids is seen, although patients who have undergone cholecystectomy have a smaller total pool of bile acids. In patients with celiac sprue, conversely, CCK release is impaired, and the gallbladder does not

effectively contract in response to a meal. This results in a large number of bile acids being sequestered in the gallbladder and leads to a greatly enlarged bile acid pool.

BIBLIOGRAPHY

Barrett KE, Boitano S, Barman SM, Brooks HL. Transport and metabolic functions of the liver. In: Barrett KE, Boitano S, Barman SM, Brooks HL, eds. *Ganong's Review of Medical Physiology.* 24th ed. New York, NY: McGraw-Hill; 2012: Chapter 28.

30. **(A)** The acinus is a diamond-shaped mass that composes the smallest functional unit of the liver. Its apices are the hepatic venules, and its axis is defined by the terminal braches of the portal vein and hepatic artery, in conjunction with the bile ductules. The hepatocytes within the acinus are further subdivided based on their proximity to the portal venules. Those hepatocytes closest to the venules are in zone 1, those at an intermediate distance in zone 2, and those hepatocytes furthest from the portal venules, and thus closest to the hepatic venules, are termed zone 3 hepatocytes. Obviously, zone 1 hepatocytes, being closest to the terminal portal venule, receive the best blood supply and are therefore the last cells to die and the first to regenerate and are in general more resistant to toxic insults than zone 3 hepatocytes. They are also the first cells exposed to solutes that are taken up by simple diffusion and therefore most such solutes enter zone 1 hepatocytes. Zones 1 and 2 are also the sites of uptake of most solutes that require receptor-mediated endocystosis, while albumin-bound solutes, such as bilirubin, are taken up in all three zones. The endothelium of the hepatic sinusoids is characterized by large fenestrations, which allow for the passage of relatively large particles into contact with the hepatocytes.

BIBLIOGRAPHY

Sicklick JK, D'Angelica M, Fonng Y. The liver. In: Townsend CM, Beauchamp RD, Evers BM, Mattox KL, eds. *Sabiston Textbook of Surgery: The Biological Basis of Modern Surgical Practice.* 19th ed. Philadelphia, PA: Saunders Elsevier; 2012: Chapter 54.

31. **(B)** One of the chief functions of the liver is maintaining a steady concentration of glucose in the blood. Glucose, fructose, and galactose are the three monosaccharides that are the endpoint of intestinal carbohydrate digestion. Both fructose and galactose are capable of enzymatic conversion to glucose. These hexoses are carried in portal blood to the liver. The rate of glucose uptake by the hepatocyte is greatly increased by insulin. Phosphorylated glucose does not leave the hepatocyte,

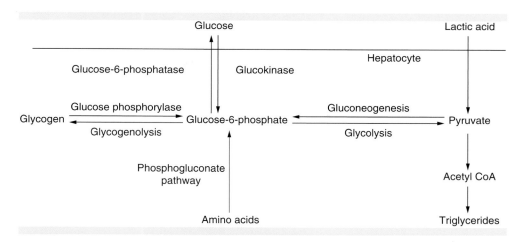

FIGURE 16-9. A schematic of the hepatic metabolism of carbohydrates.

and the cleavage of the phosphate group by glucose-6-phosphatase is necessary for glucose release. Glycogenesis is favored after feeding, as insulin reduces cAMP levels. Glucokinase facilitates the phosphorylation of glucose to glucose-6-phosphate (G6P). G6P will then be converted to glucose-1-phosphate and ultimately to glycogen. As the hepatic glycogen capacity is reached, excess glucose is converted to fat by the glycolytic pathway. Phosphofructokinase, induced by insulin, facilitates the conversion of fructose-6-phosphate to fructose-1,6-bisphosphate, the rate-limiting step of glycolysis. One molecule of glucose will yield two molecules of pyruvate, which will then undergo conversion to acetyl–coenzyme A (CoA), which then acts as the building block for triglyceride synthesis. The conversion of glucose into triglycerides is fairly efficient, with about 85% of the energy retained. The efficiency of glucose storage as glycogen, however, is a remarkable 97%. In the fasting state, when blood glucose levels fall, glucagon is released, and insulin secretion diminishes. This favors glycogenolysis and gluconeogenesis. Glucagon acts to increase intracellular levels of cAMP, which activates phosphorylase A, the enzyme responsible for liberating glucose molecules from glycogen. Glucose can then be released from the hepatocyte into the systemic circulation after cleavage of

the phosphate group by glucose-6-phosphatase. When hepatic glycogen stores are exhausted, some amino acids, glycerol, or lactate can serve as substrates for glucose production. This process is simplest for alanine, which can be converted to pyruvic acid by deamination and then undergoes conversion to glucose by a reversal of the glycolytic pathway. Other amino acids are converted to three to five carbon sugars and undergo subsequent conversion to glucose via the phosphogluconate pathway. About 40% of amino acids in the body cannot be converted into glucose. Interestingly, while the liver is central to glucose metabolism, it derives most of its energy from ketoacid oxidation (Fig. 16-9).

BIBLIOGRAPHY

Barrett KE, Boitano S, Barman SM, Brooks HL. Digestion, absorption, and nutritional principles. In: Barrett KE, Boitano S, Barman SM, Brooks HL, eds. *Ganong's Review of Medical Physiology*. 24th ed. New York, NY: McGraw-Hill; 2012: Chapter 26.

Sicklick JK, D'Angelica M, Fonng Y. The liver. In: Townsend CM, Beauchamp RD, Evers BM, Mattox KL, eds. *Sabiston Textbook of Surgery: The Biological Basis of Modern Surgical Practice*. 19th ed. Philadelphia, PA: Saunders Elsevier; 2012: Chapter 54.

CHAPTER 17

ESOPHAGUS

SHAKIRAT OYETUNJI AND LEAH BACKHUS

1. A 33-year-old female arrives at the emergency department following a suspected suicide attempt in which she swallowed an unknown cleaning solution. The patient is obtunded and unable to provide any history. Vital signs are as follows: temperature 98.6°F, blood pressure (BP) 136/88 mmHg, heart rate (HR) 114 bpm, and respiratory rate (RR) 36 breaths/min. On examination, she is drooling from the mouth, and there are visible burns in the oropharynx and crepitus in the neck and upper chest. Which of the following is the most immediate next appropriate step in management?
   (A) Endotracheal intubation
   (B) Administer broad-spectrum intravenous antibiotics
   (C) Perform endoscopy
   (D) Administer intravenous corticosteroids
   (E) Placement of nasogastric tube with continuous gastric lavage

2. For the surgical treatment of gastroesophageal reflux disease (GERD), which of the following antireflux procedures is *not* associated with an appropriate indication?
   (A) Nissen fundoplication for scleroderma
   (B) Toupet fundoplication for peptic stricture
   (C) Belsey Mark IV fundoplication for low-amplitude peristalsis
   (D) Collis gastroplasty with Nissen fundoplication for short esophagus
   (E) Heller myotomy and Dor fundoplication for achalasia

3. Which of the following statements is true?
   (A) The esophageal mucosal epithelium normally consists of columnar cells.
   (B) The right vagus nerve is located anterior to the esophagus, whereas the left vagus nerve is posterior to the esophagus.
   (C) The lower third of the esophagus consists of striated muscle, and the upper two-thirds consists of smooth muscle.
   (D) The esophageal muscle is made of an outer longitudinal muscle layer overlying an inner circular muscle layer.
   (E) The embryonic esophagus forms from the primitive midgut.

4. A 76-year-old White male complains of a 6-month history of hypersalivation, intermittent dysphagia, and a 15-lb weight loss. His primary care physician suspects esophageal carcinoma and refers the patient to you. The barium esophagogram obtained is shown in Fig. 17-1. What treatment should you recommend to this patient?
   (A) Pneumatic dilation
   (B) Bougienage
   (C) Diverticulectomy or diverticulopexy alone
   (E) Esophagectomy

5. A 46-year-old female complains of epigastric burning pain that has been worsening in recent months. She has been self-medicating with over-the-counter agents with only mild relief in symptoms. She undergoes esophagoscopy, which reveals moderate-to-severe esophagitis. Which of the following medications is most effective for healing the esophagus?
   (A) Drug A binds the proton pump in gastric parietal cells and inhibits gastric acid production.
   (B) Drug B antagonizes histamine 2 (H_2) receptors to inhibit stimulation of acid secretion.
   (C) Drug C is a dopamine antagonist that promotes motility.
   (D) Drug D neutralizes gastric acidity and stimulates prostaglandin activity.
   (E) Drug E anticholinergic agent that decreases esophageal contractions and saliva production

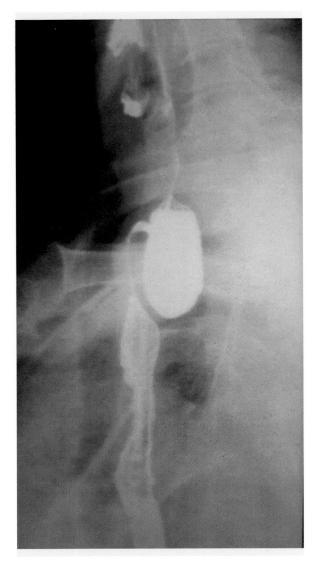

FIGURE 17-1. Barium esophagogram (from Gerald M Doherty: *Current Diagnosis and Treatment: Surgery.* 14th ed. New York, NY: McGraw-Hill; 2015: Fig. 20-6).

6. A 48-year-old male with achalasia is treated with pneumatic dilatation. There was mild improvement in symptoms during the first several months, but he now complains of regurgitation and weight loss. What is the preferred treatment for this patient?
   (A) Fundoplication
   (B) Botulinum toxin injection
   (C) Esophagectomy
   (D) Heller myotomy and fundoplication
   (E) None of the above

7. Approximately 24 h after an uneventful transhiatal esophagectomy with a cervical esophagogastric anastomosis for esophageal carcinoma, the patient develops

respiratory distress requiring emergent intubation. The postintubation chest radiograph shows an infiltrate in the right middle lobe. What is the likely etiology of this complication?
   (A) Phrenic nerve injury
   (B) Tracheal laceration
   (C) Gastric outlet obstruction
   (D) Esophagogastric anastomotic leak
   (E) Recurrent laryngeal nerve injury

8. A 76-year-old female with a 12-month history of dysphagia is admitted to the hospital for pneumonia. A barium esophagogram shows a tracheoesophageal fistula (TEF). Endoscopic biopsies at this site reveal squamous cell carcinoma. What is the preferred treatment?
   (A) Esophagectomy
   (B) Cervical esophagostomy and gastric tube placement
   (C) Esophageal stent placement
   (D) Radiation therapy
   (E) Chemoradiation followed by esophagectomy

9. The gastroesophageal junction is located above the diaphragmatic hiatus in which type(s) of hiatal hernia?
   (A) Type II only
   (B) Types I, II, and III
   (C) Types I, III, and IV
   (D) Types II and III
   (E) Types I, II, III, and IV

10. A 49-year-old female with Barrett's esophagus undergoes routine surveillance esophagoscopy. Random biopsies reveal low-grade dysplasia. Which of the following recommendations should you make to this patient?
    (A) No change in treatment required with continued routine endoscopic surveillance in 2–3 years
    (B) Nissen fundoplication to eliminate the need for future endoscopic surveillance
    (C) Repeat endoscopic surveillance in several months' time regardless of choice of therapy
    (D) Increased dose of proton pump inhibitors (PPIs) to allow regression of the dysplastic epithelium
    (E) Esophagectomy because of the risk of invasive adenocarcinoma

11. A 42-year-old business executive presents with occasional symptoms of intense chest pain during swallowing. An electrocardiogram was unremarkable; however, a barium swallow was obtained during these symptoms and is shown in Fig. 17-2. Which of the following regarding this abnormality is true?
    (A) The incidence of psychiatric disorders is increased in patients with this condition.
    (B) Surgical management should be the first line of therapy.
    (C) Manometry is usually nondiagnostic.

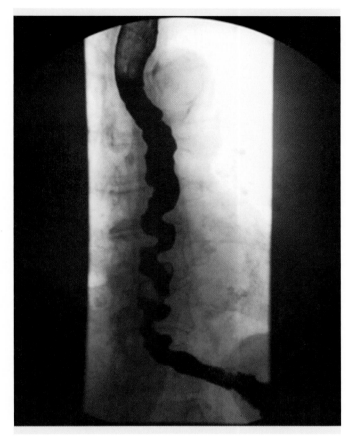

FIGURE 17-2. Barium esophagogram. (Courtesy of John M. Braver, MD).

(D) A normal barium esophagogram excludes this diagnosis.
(E) Esophagectomy is the surgical procedure of choice.

12. Which of the following studies is the most accurate method for evaluating regional lymph node involvement in esophageal cancer?
(A) Barium esophagogram
(B) Endoscopic ultrasound (EUS)
(C) Computed tomography (CT)
(D) Positron emission tomography (PET)
(E) Magnetic resonance imaging (MRI)

13. A 40-year-old female complains of a 3-month history of dysphagia. The EUS and CT scan obtained are shown in Figs. 17-3A and 17-3B, respectively. What is the likely etiology of the patient's symptoms?
(A) Squamous cell carcinoma
(B) Congenital duplication cyst

(C) Fibrovascular polyp
(D) Leiomyoma
(E) Benign stricture

14. Which of the following statements is true?
(A) The majority of esophageal carcinomas in the United States are squamous cell carcinomas.
(B) There are no identified risk factors for esophageal carcinoma.
(C) The incidence of squamous cell carcinoma of the esophagus has risen dramatically as a result of gastroesophageal reflux and Barrett's metaplasia.
(D) Esophageal adenocarcinoma occurs more frequently in females than in males.
(E) Black males have an increased risk of developing squamous cell carcinoma of the esophagus.

15. A 54-year-old male complains of dysphagia and a sticking sensation in his chest after meals. He also experiences regurgitation of undigested food and has lost 10 lb in the last 2 months. A barium esophagogram is obtained and is shown in Fig. 17-4. Which of the following should be considered in the differential diagnosis?
(A) Malignancy
(B) Achalasia
(C) Chagas disease
(D) Stricture
(E) All of the above

16. Which of the following tests are used to guide management of GERD?
(A) Endoscopy
(B) Upper gastrointestinal series
(C) Manometry
(D) Esophageal pH monitor
(E) All of the above

17. Starting with the innermost structure, what is the correct order of the layers of the esophageal wall?
(A) Epithelium, muscularis propria, muscularis mucosa, submucosa, periesophageal tissue
(B) Epithelium, submucosa, muscularis propria, muscularis mucosa, lamina propria
(C) Epithelium, lamina propria, muscularis mucosa, submucosa, muscularis propria
(D) Mucosa, submucosa, muscularis mucosa, muscularis propria, periesophageal tissue
(E) Mucosa, muscularis propria, lamina propria, submucosa, muscularis mucosa

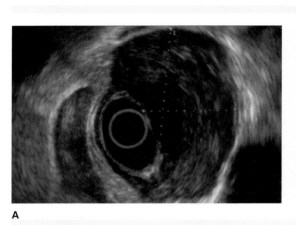
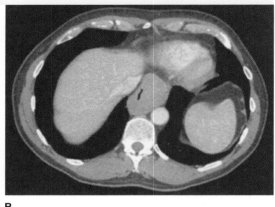

A   B

FIGURE 17-3. (A) Endoscopic esophageal ultrasound; (B) CT scan. Image provided by Dr. Irving Waxman and Dr. Mariano Gonzalez-Haba Ruiz, University of Chicago, Department of Gastroenterology.

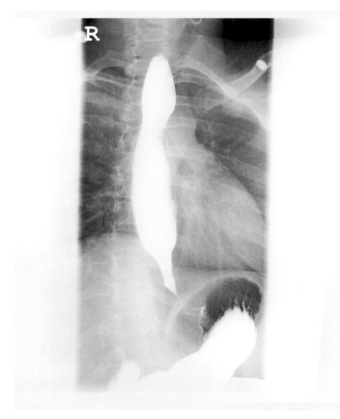

FIGURE 17-4. Barium esophagogram. Courtesy of John M. Braver, MD.

18. Which of the following statements regarding GERD is true?
    (A) The LES must be permanently defective for GERD to occur.
    (B) The presence of pepsin in refluxed gastric juice potentiates the injurious effects of gastric acid on esophageal mucosa.
    (C) The reflux of duodenal juice tends to neutralize acidic gastric juice and therefore causes less injury to the esophageal mucosa than gastric content reflux alone.
    (D) Patients with normal LES pressures will not develop clinically significant reflux.
    (E) The presence of *Helicobacter pylori* is associated with GERD.

19. A 59-year-old male with a several-month history of dysphagia is diagnosed with adenocarcinoma of the distal esophagus. An EUS shows the tumor to invade peri-esophageal tissue but not adjacent structures. CT scans of the chest and abdomen show no distant metastasis. The patient is otherwise healthy. Which of the following treatments provide the best chance for long-term survival?
    (A) Chemotherapy followed by surgery
    (B) Chemoradiation alone
    (C) Chemoradiation followed by surgery
    (D) Surgery alone
    (E) Chemoradiation after surgery

20. A 68-year-old female reports a 3-year history of dyspha-gia and epigastric pain. She has been hospitalized twice in the last year for aspiration pneumonia. Her primary physician orders the barium esophagogram shown in Fig. 17-5. What treatment will provide the best long-term improvement in this patient's symptoms?

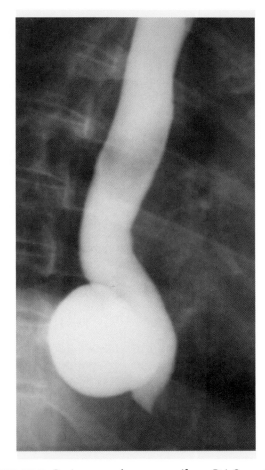

FIGURE 17-5. Barium esophagogram (from D.J. Sugarbaker, R. Bueno, Y. L. Colson, M. T. Jaklitsch, M. J. Krasna, S. J. Mentzer, M. Williams, A. Adams: *Adult Chest Surgery*. 2nd ed. New York, NY: McGraw Hill; 2013: Fig. 30-2. Copyright © The McGraw-Hill Companies, Inc. All rights reserved).

   (A) Pneumatic esophageal dilation
   (B) Hiatal hernia repair and fundoplication
   (C) Diverticulopexy or diverticulectomy
   (D) Diverticulectomy and myotomy
   (E) Esophagectomy

21. Which of the following inhibits LES relaxation?
   (A) Atropine
   (B) Nitric oxide (NO)

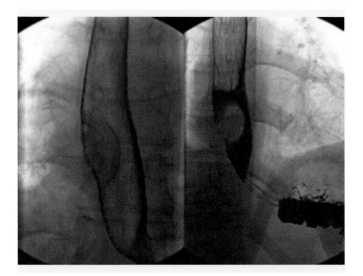

FIGURE 17-6. Barium esophagogram. Image provided by The Human Imaging Research Office at The University of Chicago.

   (C) Cholecystokinin (CCK)
   (D) Gastric distention
   (E) Pharyngeal stimulation

22. A 38-year-old male complains of dysphagia and regur-gitation. A barium esophagogram is obtained (see Fig. 17-6). An endoscopic esophageal ultrasound is sub-sequently performed, which demonstrates a submucosal cystic mass with normal overlying mucosa. Which of the following is true?
   (A) Endoscopic biopsy is usually indicated.
   (B) Occurs most frequently in geriatric patients.
   (C) The lining consists of squamous epithelium.
   (D) Potential complications include compression of adjacent structures, ulceration, hemorrhage, and infection.
   (E) Surgical resection is not indicated in most cases.

23. Which of the following is *not* an advantage of a transhia-tal esophagectomy compared to a transthoracic approach with an intrathoracic anastomosis?
   (A) Avoiding a thoracotomy incision
   (B) Decreased operative mortality
   (C) Decreased mortality with an anastomotic leak
   (D) Decreased incidence of postoperative gastroesopha-geal reflux
   (E) Decreased risk of pulmonary complications

24. Which of the following patients is expected to have the *least* benefit from antireflux surgery?
    (A) A 36-year-old male with no improvement in reflux symptoms after a 6-week course of H_2 receptor antagonist therapy
    (B) A 52-year-old female with a 10-year history of GERD and Barrett's metaplasia
    (C) A 44-year-old male taking PPIs for 5 years with linear ulceration in the distal esophagus
    (D) A 41-year-old female whose reflux symptoms are well controlled on escalating doses of PPIs
    (E) A 49-year-old male with asthma and a 10-year history of reflux whose symptoms are well controlled with PPIs

25. A 24-year-old female swallowed drain cleaning solution containing concentrated lye. Which of the following complications is she *most* likely to experience several weeks after the injury?
    (A) Tracheoesophageal fistula
    (B) Esophageal stricture
    (C) Esophageal carcinoma
    (D) Hiatal hernia
    (E) Esophageal perforation

26. Which of the following protects esophageal mucosa against acid-induced injury?
    (A) High-pressure zone in the distal esophagus
    (B) Esophageal peristalsis and gravity
    (C) Swallowed saliva
    (D) Submucosal gland secretions
    (E) All of the above

27. A 74-year-old male complains of postprandial fullness and bloating over the past 9 months. He presents to the emergency department with epigastric pain and dry retching. Attempts to pass a nasogastric tube are unsuccessful (Fig. 17-7). Which of the following regarding this abnormality is true?
    (A) Surgery is indicated because of the risk of obstruction, bleeding, and particularly strangulation.
    (B) Open repair is safer and more effective compared to laparoscopic repair.
    (C) Fundoplication is not necessary once the primary abnormality is repaired.
    (D) Gastroesophageal reflux is not commonly associated with this disorder.
    (E) This abnormality is secondary to a congenital defect.

28. Which of the following arteries does not supply blood to the esophagus:
    (A) Inferior thyroid artery
    (B) Left gastric artery
    (C) Bronchial arteries
    (D) Inferior phrenic artery
    (E) Internal thoracic artery

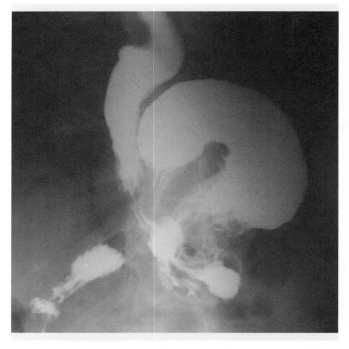

FIGURE 17-7. Barium esophagogram (from Brunicardi FC, Andersen DK, Billiar TR, et al., eds. *Schwartz's Principles of Surgery.* 10th ed. New York, NY: McGraw-Hill; 2014: Fig. 25-18. Copyright © The McGraw-Hill Companies, Inc. All rights reserved).

29. A 79-year-old male with dysphagia and 30-lb weight loss over the last 6 months is diagnosed with adenocarcinoma of the distal esophagus. Chest and abdominal CT scans demonstrate multiple hepatic and pulmonary nodules. Which of the following is *least* likely to benefit this patient?
    (A) Radiation therapy
    (B) Endoscopic stenting
    (C) Gastrostomy tube placement
    (D) Photodynamic therapy
    (E) Esophagectomy

30. A 58-year-old male with a history of GERD undergoes routine esophagogastroscopy. The endoscopist notes salmon-pink mucosa extending 2 cm above the gastroesophageal junction. Biopsies of this area reveal columnar epithelium-containing goblet cells. Which of the following is true regarding this patient?
    (A) Because the abnormality extends only 2 cm above the gastroesophageal junction, the risk of adenocarcinoma is not increased.
    (B) Reflux of duodenal contents (i.e., bile) into the esophagus is protective against the development of this abnormality.
    (C) This is a benign condition that does not require further studies or treatment.

(D) The presence of *H. pylori* gastritis increases the risk of developing this abnormality.

(E) The presence of goblet cells increases the risk of dysplasia and subsequent adenocarcinoma.

31. A 58 year-old female with a history of Raynaud's syndrome presents with a 2-year history of heartburn and a "sensation of food getting stuck." A barium esophagogram is obtained (Fig. 17-8). Which of the following statements regarding this condition is *false*?

(A) Decreased LES pressures may play a role.

(B) Complications include Barrett's esophagus, esophagitis, and stricture.

(C) Prokinetic drugs provide no benefit.

(D) PPIs are used in first-line therapy in the early stages of this condition.

(E) The primary abnormality is a motility disorder.

Directions (Questions 32 and 33): For each of these two questions, choose the *best answer* from the following lettered set:

(A) Nothing by mouth, intravenous antibiotics only

(B) Primary repair with local tissue reinforcement

(C) Esophagectomy with immediate reconstruction

(D) Proximal and distal diversion, jejunostomy feeding tube

(E) Esophageal stent placement with thoracostomy tube placement

32. A 65-year-old male with a history of GERD underwent a routine esophagoduodenoscopy 24 h ago. He now has subcutaneous emphysema in the neck and upper chest; a barium esophagram is shown in Fig. 17-9. He is afebrile and hemodynamically stable. What is the appropriate treatment?

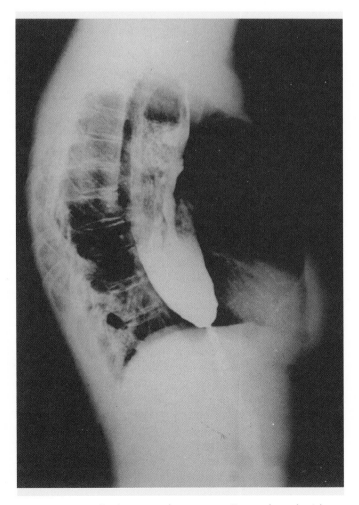

FIGURE 17-8. Barium esophagogram. Reproduced with permission from Waters PF, DeMeester TR: Foregut motor disorders and their surgical management. *Med Clin North Am.* 65:1253, 1981. Copyright Elsevier.

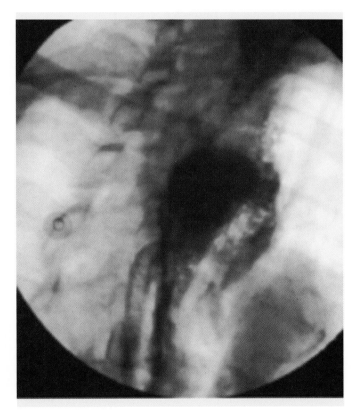

FIGURE 17-9. Barium esophagram (from D.J. Sugarbaker, R. Bueno, Y. L. Colson, M. T. Jaklitsch, M. J. Krasna, S. J. Mentzer, M. Williams, A. Adams: *Adult Chest Surgery.* 2nd ed. New York, NY: McGraw Hill; 2013: Fig. 48-3. Copyright © The McGraw-Hill Companies, Inc. All rights reserved).

33. A 19-year-old male presents to the emergency department with acute onset of substernal chest pain and hematemesis. His medical history is significant for bulimia, and he admits to retching after a large meal prior to the onset of symptoms. A chest x-ray shows a right-sided pleural effusion, and a barium esophagram shows a small, contained leak in the midthoracic esophagus. What is the appropriate management?

ANSWERS AND EXPLANATIONS

1. **(A)** The presentation of the patient described should raise suspicion for ingestion of a caustic substance. Household agents capable of producing caustic injuries include detergents, bleaches, drain cleaners, and ammonia products. Lye substances, which cause liquefactive necrosis, generally result in deeper penetration and tissue injury than acid agents, which cause coagulative necrosis. It is helpful to ascertain the nature of the product ingested, as this may determine the distribution and severity of injury. However, it will rarely affect subsequent management.

Following ingestion of a caustic agent, destruction of the superficial epithelium occurs, and necrosis may extend into mucosa and muscularis. The injured tissue is invaded by bacteria and leukocytes. Between the second and fifth days, the necrotic tissue forms a cast and sloughs. Following this phase, granulation tissue forms at the periphery of injury as tissue repair begins. Collagen deposition continues for several months. Scar contraction begins following the second week and frequently results in esophageal shortening and stricture formation.

The acute clinical course is marked by oral and substernal pain, odynophagia, dysphagia, drooling, and hematemesis. Pulmonary symptoms may occur with aspiration of caustic material. With severe injuries, visceral perforation may occur along with septicemia, mediastinitis, hemorrhage, and possibly death. Initial treatment should follow the usual guidelines for managing trauma patients. The airway should be assessed with the recognition that laryngeal inflammation and edema may progress rapidly to airway obstruction; in this scenario, the patient's drooling and obtunded state require oropharyngeal intubation in anticipation of this event. The circulatory status should also be addressed and resuscitation with intravenous fluids begun. Broad-spectrum antibiotics are warranted if perforation is suspected. A nasogastric tube may be placed under fluoroscopy to drain gastric contents.

Any evidence of perforation as demonstrated by physical examination or radiographic studies mandates surgical exploration. Subcutaneous emphysema, fever, hypotension, and peritonitis may be signs of perforation. Esophagography with water-soluble contrast may be performed when perforation is suspected. Endoscopy provides the best means of assessing the severity of injury in the absence of perforation. Patients with gastric injuries or linear esophageal burns require hospital observation for possible transmural extension of these injuries. Patients in whom endoscopy demonstrates near-circumferential esophageal burns are at risk for strictures, which may occur any time after the second week. Corticosteroids have been used in the past as prophylactic therapy against stricture formation, but clinical trials have shown no benefit from steroid administration.

BIBLIOGRAPHY

Hugh TB, Kelly MD. Corrosive ingestion and the surgeon. *J Am Coll Surg* 1999;189:508–522.
Maish SM. Esophagus. In: Townsend CM, Beauchamp DR, Evers MB, et al., eds. *Sabiston Textbook of Surgery: The Biological Basis of Modern Surgical Practice*. 19th ed. Philadelphia, PA: Saunders; 2012:1040–1043.

2. **(A)** The surgical treatment of GERD has evolved greatly since Rudolf Nissen in 1956 first described the 360-degree fundoplication that bears his name. The principle behind surgical treatment is the restoration of the mechanical barrier between the stomach and distal esophagus. In this regard, the original Nissen fundoplication successfully created an anatomic flap valve and increased LES pressure to prevent reflux; however, side effects were frequent and included bloating, dysphagia, early satiety, and inability to vomit. Partial fundoplications were then suggested as alternatives to Nissen's procedure. These procedures left a portion of esophagus uncovered to decrease LES pressures and provide less outflow resistance. Examples of partial fundoplications include the original Toupet (180-degree posterior wrap), Thal (90-degree anterior patch), and Dor (180-degree anterior wrap). Although these procedures decreased the incidence of dysphagia and bloating, the resistance to reflux was also reduced; as such, these partial fundoplications are only performed for GERD in patients with esophageal dysmotility (Fig. 17-10).

As surgical treatment of gastroesophageal reflux became more common, several special situations deserved recognition. The most common postoperative complaint following antireflux surgery is dysphagia, particularly in patients with motility abnormalities who undergo a 360-degree fundoplication. Therefore, manometry should be performed prior to antireflux surgery to identify patients with motility disorders who would likely benefit from a partial fundoplication. When peristalsis is absent, impaired, or of low magnitude, partial fundoplications performed using laparoscopic

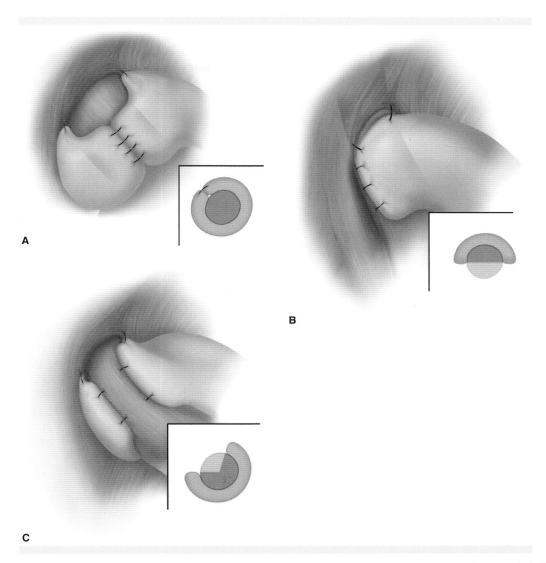

FIGURE 17-10. Different fundoplication wraps. A. Complete; B. anterior (Dor); C. posterior (Toupet). From Oelschlager B, Eubanks T, Pellegrini C. *Sabiston Textbook of Surgery,* 18th ed, Chapter 42. Copyright Elsevier/Saunders.

techniques should be considered. In the setting of achalasia, a Heller myotomy in conjunction with a partial fundoplication, such as the Dor 180-degree anterior wrap, is appropriate.

A basic principle in antireflux surgery is to create a tension-free fundoplication below the diaphragm crus. A fundoplication is destined to fail if esophageal length is insufficient to allow a tension-free repair. This is most common in long-standing reflux disease in which chronic inflammation results in fibrotic shortening of the esophagus. Other conditions associated with short esophagus include caustic ingestion, paraesophageal hernia, scleroderma, and Crohn's disease. In these situations, mobilization of the mediastinal esophagus may provide sufficient length for the fundoplication. Occasionally, a Collis gastroplasty, in which neoesophagus is formed from stapled division of the gastric fundus, is required to provide additional esophageal length.

Of the choices discussed, the Nissen procedure performed for GERD associated with scleroderma is most likely to result in obstructive symptoms because of absence of contractility in the distal esophagus. A partial fundoplication would surgically treat the reflux disease while minimizing the incidence of postoperative dysphagia as compared to a complete fundoplication in these cases. In addition, esophageal shortening is frequently found in patients with scleroderma, which may necessitate a gastroplasty procedure.

BIBLIOGRAPHY

Cai W, Watson DI, Lally CJ, et al. Ten-year clinical outcome of a prospective randomized clinical trial of laparoscopic Nissen versus anterior 180 (degrees) partial fundoplication. *Br J Surg* 2008;95:1501–1505.

Gee DW, Andreoli MT, Rattner DW. Measuring the effectiveness of laparoscopic antireflux surgery: Long term results. *Arch Surg* 2008;143:482–487.

Horvath KD, Swanstrom LL, Jobe BA. The short esophagus: pathophysiology, incidence, presentation, and treatment in the era of laparoscopic antireflux surgery. *Ann Surg* 2000;232:630–640.

Smith CD. Antireflux surgery. *Surg Clin North Am.* 2008 Oct; 88(5):943–58, v.

Soper NJ, Hungness ES. Laparoscopic antireflux surgery. In: Fischer JE, Jones DB, Pomposelli FB, et al., eds. *Fischer's Mastery of Surgery.* 6th ed. Philadelphia, PA: Lippincott Williams & Wilkins, 2011: Chapter 71.

3. **(D)** At approximately 3 weeks' gestation, fusion of septa arising from the primitive foregut results in formation of the esophagus and upper trachea. The esophagus elongates and is structurally formed by 5–6 weeks' gestation, but the epithelial lining continues to develop. The initial epithelium is stratified columnar in type, which is covered by ciliated columnar cells at 8 weeks' gestation. At 5 months' gestation, stratified squamous epithelium replaces the ciliated columnar layer. The muscular layers develop along a similar timeline as the epithelium. The inner circular muscle layer develops at 6 weeks' gestation, and the outer longitudinal layer forms by 9 weeks' gestation. The muscularis propria consists entirely of smooth muscle initially, with striated muscle gradually developing in the upper third. By 5 months' gestation, the upper third of the esophagus is striated muscle and the lower two-thirds smooth muscle, which is the normal ratio at birth. The position of the vagus nerves on the esophagus results from unequal growth of the greater curve of the stomach relative to the lesser curve, so that the left vagus nerve is positioned anterior to the esophagus and the right nerve posteriorly.

BIBLIOGRAPHY

Lerut T, Coosemans W, Decaluwé H, et al. Anatomy of the esophagus. In: Fischer JE, Jones DB et al., eds. *Mastery of Surgery.* 6th ed. Philadelphia, PA: Lippincott Williams & Wilkins; 2011:664.

Maish SM. Esophagus. In: Townsend CM, Beauchamp DR, Evers MB, et al., eds. *Sabiston Textbook of Surgery: The Biological Basis of Modern Surgical Practice.* 19th ed. Philadelphia, PA: Saunders; 2012:1013–1015.

Patti MG, Gantert W, Way LW. Surgery of the esophagus, anatomy and physiology. *Surg Clin North Am* 1997;77:959–970.

4. **(D)** The barium esophagogram is diagnostic for a pharyngoesophageal, or Zenker's, diverticulum. This is a false diverticulum that occurs at the transition between the oblique fibers of the thyropharyngeus muscle and the horizontal fibers of the cricopharyngeus muscle. Zenker and von Zeimssen first summarized 27 cases of pharyngoesophageal diverticula in 1877 and suggested that these pouches resulted from forces acting within the esophageal lumen against an area of resistance. Killian in 1907 identified this area of weakness as the space between the inferior pharyngeal constrictor muscles and the cricopharyngeus muscle. Zenker's diverticulum occurs predominantly in the seventh and eighth decades of life and more often in men than women. The etiology of pharyngoesophageal diverticula is thought to be related to incoordination in the swallowing mechanism and upper esophageal sphincter dysfunction. These abnormalities raise the intraluminal pressure and cause herniation of mucosa and submucosa through the area of potential weakness near the junction of pharynx and esophagus.

Symptoms are highly characteristic and include dysphagia, regurgitation of undigested food, gurgling noises with swallowing, retrosternal pain, and respiratory obstruction. The most serious complication is respiratory infection as a result of aspiration. A history of dysphagia and weight loss may raise suspicion of malignancy, but a barium esophagogram, which is diagnostic for a Zenker's diverticulum with no other abnormalities, essentially excludes this possibility. A concomitant sliding hiatal hernia is not an uncommon finding on esophagogram. Upper gastrointestinal endoscopy, while possible if performed carefully, is usually not necessary to confirm the diagnosis and may risk perforation at the diverticulum site.

There is no effective medical therapy other than observation of small, asymptomatic diverticula. Surgical therapy is indicated in symptomatic patients as untreated diverticula will continue to progress in size and potentially result in pulmonary morbidity. Simple resection of the pouch with primary closure was one of the early approaches to pharyngoesophageal diverticula; however, the underlying motor dysfunction was not addressed with this technique, and the persistent functional obstruction resulted in suture line disruptions. The most important component of surgical therapy is an esophagomyotomy. This involves dissection to the base of the diverticulum and division of the cricopharyngeus muscle fibers in a vertical direction. Because most pouches are directed posteriorly or to the left, the procedure is usually performed through a left cervical incision and may include resection of the pouch, especially those larger than 3–4 cm. Diverticulopexy, which involves anchoring the pouch to the posterior pharyngeal wall or prevertebral fascia, performed concurrently with myotomy is another option. Endoscopic stapling of the wall separating the diverticular and esophageal lumens has been used with some success. To date, however, endoscopic techniques have been shown to be less effective at providing symptomatic relief compared to open myotomy. Esophagectomy is not indicated for Zenker's diverticulum without evidence of malignancy.

BIBLIOGRAPHY

Gutschow CA, Hamoir M, Rombaux P, et al. Management of pharyngoesophageal (Zenker's) diverticulum: which technique? *Ann Thorac Surg* 2002;74:1677–1683.

Jacobs IN, Rabkin D, DelGaudio JM, Skandalakis JE. Pharynx. In: Skandalakis JE, Colburn GL, Weidman TA, et al., eds. *Skandalakis' Surgical Anatomy.* New York, NY: McGraw-Hill; 2004; Chapter 13.

Maish SM. Esophagus. In: Townsend CM, Beauchamp DR, Evers MB, et al., eds. *Sabiston Textbook of Surgery: The Biological Basis of Modern Surgical Practice.* 19th ed. Philadelphia, PA: Saunders; 2012:1023–1025.

5. **(A)** The initial treatment of gastroesophageal reflux disease is nonoperative and includes behavioral modification as well as pharmacotherapy. Behavior modification includes avoiding fatty foods, alcohol, and cigarette smoking; substituting frequent smaller meals for large meals; and avoiding eating for several hours before lying down. The mainstay of medical therapy is with antisecretory drugs that help reduce symptoms of GERD, promote healing of esophageal epithelium, and prevent recurrence and complications of GERD.

   Many patients initiate therapy on their own early in the course of disease with over-the-counter medications such as antacids or H_2 receptor antagonists. Antacids work by neutralizing acidic gastric juices, thus increasing intragastric pH. This results in a more neutral pH when gastric reflux does occur, and the conversion of pepsinogen to pepsin, which has been demonstrated to intensify the severity of esophageal injury, is reduced at a pH greater than 4.0. Antacids also stimulate the release of gastrin and prostaglandins, which protect esophageal mucosa. Antacids provide quick relief of symptoms, but their duration of action is short, and they must be administered several times a day. Moreover, antacids do not affect acid secretion. Adverse reactions of antacids are usually mild and consist of gastrointestinal disturbances. Calcium- and aluminum-containing antacids can cause constipation, while magnesium salts can cause diarrhea. Antacids may also interact with many other drugs, altering their rate or extent of absorption, and therefore should be taken at least 2 h before or after other medications. The H_2 receptor antagonists competitively inhibit histamine at H_2 receptors, resulting in reduced gastric acid secretion. They also reduce gastrin-induced acid and pepsin release. H_2 receptor antagonists have relatively few and minor side effects, including headache, dizziness, diarrhea, and rash. Drug interactions are most common with cimetidine, which inhibits cytochrome P-450 enzymes involved with drug metabolism. Metabolism of drugs such as warfarin, tricyclic antidepressants, and theophylline are inhibited by cimetidine.

   Proton pump inhibitors are the agent of choice with severe GERD or the presence of esophageal mucosal damage. PPIs such as omeprazole bind irreversibly and noncompetitively to the H^+/K^+-ATP pump, thereby inhibiting acid secretion. These drugs are the most effective inhibitors of acid secretion because they block the final pathway for acid release. The maximal effect occurs after approximately 4 days of therapy, and the effects linger for the life of the parietal cell. Thus, the acid suppression will persist for 4 to 5 days after therapy has ended, so the patient needs to be off therapy for 1 week before being evaluated with pH monitoring. They are longer acting than alternative medications and usually only require once-a-day dosing. PPIs have been demonstrated to be more effective than H_2 receptor antagonists at providing symptomatic relief and allowing healing of reflux-induced esophagitis. The most common side effects reported with PPIs include nausea, diarrhea, constipation, abdominal pain, headache, and dizziness.

BIBLIOGRAPHY

Peters JH, Little VR, Watson, TJ. Esophageal anatomy and physiology and gastroesophageal reflux disease. In: Mulholland MW, Lillemoe KD, Doherty GM, et al., eds. *Greenfield's Surgery: Scientific Principles and Practice.* 5th ed. Philadelphia, PA: Lippincott Williams & Wilkins; 2011:647–648.

Petersen RY, Pellegrini CA, Oelschlager BK. Hiatal hernia and gastroesophageal reflux disease. In: Townsend CM, Beauchamp DR, Evers MB, et al., eds. *Sabiston Textbook of Surgery: The Biological Basis of Modern Surgical Practice.* 19th ed. Philadelphia, PA: Saunders; 2012:1073.

Smith CD. Antireflux surgery. *Surg Clin North Am* 2008 Oct; 88(5):943–958, v.

Vivian EM, Thompson MA. Pharmacologic strategies for treating gastroesophageal reflux disease. *Clin Ther* 2000;22:654–672.

Wang Y-K, Hsu W-H, Wang SSW, et al., Current pharmacological management of gastroesophageal reflux disease. *Gastroenterol Res Pract* 2013; Article ID 983653.

6. **(D)** The initial treatment of achalasia is usually nonoperative and may include pharmacologic therapy, esophageal dilation, or botulinum toxin injections into the LES. Nitrates and calcium channel blockers have been shown to decrease LES pressure, but adverse effects of these medications and the development of tolerance lead to ultimate failure of pharmacologic management. Botulinum toxin injections into the LES and esophageal dilation can improve dysphagia in some patients, but the duration of relief is variable, and repeated treatments are often required.

Esophageal myotomy remains the gold standard of therapy for achalasia and is indicated when conservative management fails or in younger patients who are more likely to benefit from the long-term effects of surgical treatment. Heller originally described myotomy of the LES. This approach has been modified and can now be performed laparoscopically. Myotomy involves division of the circular and longitudinal muscles of the lower esophagus. Extension of the myotomy to the muscle of the cardia is recommended based on literature by Oelschlager et al. (2003); they reported higher efficacy of Heller myotomy when it included a 3-cm cardiomyotomy. In their study, the LES pressure was significantly lower after extended gastric myotomy and a Toupet fundoplication versus standard myotomy and a Dor fundoplication (9.5 vs. 15.8 mmHg). Dysphagia was both less frequent and less severe after extended gastric myotomy and Toupet fundoplication.

The procedure can be performed through transthoracic and transabdominal approaches. The length of myotomy and the need for a concomitant antireflux procedure remain controversial. Some studies have shown transabdominal myotomy with fundoplication to have the lowest incidence of postoperative gastroesophageal reflux. If a fundoplication is performed, a subtotal wrap is recommended to minimize postoperative dysphagia in these patients who have an underlying motility disorder. Per oral endoscopic myotomy (POEM), an incisionless submucosal myotomy, has been described as a less-invasive surgical treatment. A submucosal injection is used to expand the submucosal space at a point 10–15 cm proximal to the LES, followed by a 2-cm long mucosal incision using an electrical knife. The endoscope is inserted into the submucosal space, and with sequential submucosal injection and submucosal dissection using an electrical knife, a dilation balloon, or a combination thereof. A long submucosal tunnel is created along the right wall of the esophagus and is extended beyond the LES approximately 2–4 cm into the submucosa of the cardia along the lesser curvature. The endoscope is then withdrawn to approximately 2–3 cm distal to the mucosal incision site where the start of the myotomy will take place, thus offsetting the mucosal defect and the muscle defect, which is the ingenious and critical feature of this technique that allows secure closure. At the starting point of the myotomy, the muscle is dissected until the plane between the inner circular and outer longitudinal layer is exposed. At that point, the circular muscle myotomy is initiated by hooking the circular fibers with the knife and cutting them, proceeding distally until the myotomy is extended about 2 cm into the cardia (cardiomyotomy).

Swanstrom et al. reported 6-month physiological and symptomatic outcomes after POEM for achalasia in a prospective series of 18 patients; all patients had dysphagia relief, 83% having relief of noncardiac chest pain. There was significant, though mild, gastroesophageal reflux postoperatively in 46% of patients in 6-month pH studies.

Esophagectomy is reserved for end-stage achalasia, which is identified by progressive dilatation and marked tortuosity of the esophagus. Resection of the diseased esophagus is the only treatment for this irreversible condition. Reconstruction can be with gastric transposition or a colonic conduit.

BIBLIOGRAPHY

Adler DG, Romero Y. Primary esophageal motility disorders. *Mayo Clin Proc* 2001;76:195–200.

Banbury MK, Rice TW, Goldblum JR, et al. Esophagectomy with gastric reconstruction for achalasia. *J Thorac Cardiovasc Surg* 1999:117:1077–1085.

Oelschlager BK, Chang L, Pellegrini CA. Improved outcome after extended gastric myotomy for achalasia. *Arch Surg* 2003 May;138(5):490–495.

Swanstrom LL, Kurian A, Dunst CM, Sharata A, Bhayani N, Rieder E. Long-term outcomes of an endoscopic myotomy for achalasia: the POEM procedure. *Ann Surg* 2012 Oct;256(4):659-667.

Tatum RP, Pellegrini CA. How I do it: laparoscopic Heller myotomy with Toupet fundoplication for achalasia. *J Gastrointest Surg* 2009;13(6):1120–1124.

7. (**E**) Dissection in the left tracheoesophageal groove may result in recurrent laryngeal nerve neuropraxia or even permanent paresis. Accordingly, caution should be undertaken to avoid retraction injury to prevent neuropraxia during this dissection and cervical esophagogastric anastomosis. Injury to the recurrent nerve results in vocal cord incompetence and a propensity to aspirate. Patients who manifest postoperative hoarseness should be evaluated with laryngoscopy. If recurrent nerve injury is suspected, either vocal cord injection or phonoplastic surgery is indicated to minimize the risk of aspiration prior to beginning oral feeding.

A tracheal laceration is a rare complication and is usually identified intraoperatively when large amounts of air begin escaping through the operative field or when the anesthesiologist notices a sharp decrease in ventilatory pressure. If tracheal injury is not recognized intraoperatively, it may present in the early postoperative period with persistent air leak through chest tubes or subcutaneous emphysema in the face and neck. Bronchoscopic examination will reveal the injury.

Gastric atony or gastric outlet obstruction can contribute to postoperative aspiration following esophagectomy; however, with vocal cord competence it is less likely to cause aspiration. Phrenic nerve injury is extremely rare after esophagectomy and is identified by an elevated hemidiaphram on chest radiograph. A cervical esophagogastric anastomotic leak may present with fevers and leukocytosis. It is usually noticed several days postoperatively, however, and should be well controlled through drains placed at the time of surgery and therefore not affect the lungs.

Vascular injury during transhiatal esophagectomy is a rare but life-threatening complication. As the esophagus is in close vicinity to the aorta, pulmonary vessels, and the azygous vein, these blood vessels can be injured during its resection. There may be a higher risk in tumors located in the midesophagus. Management involves prompt identification and control via a dilated hiatus or a thoracotomy. Javed et al. (2011) reported intrathoracic vascular injury in 1.4% of patients in a series of 710 transhiatal esophagectomies.

BIBLIOGRAPHY

Gandhi SK, Naunheim KS. Complications of transhiatal esophagectomy. *Chest Surg Clin North Am* 1997;7:601–610.

Hulscher JBF, ter Hofstede E, Kloek J, et al. Injury to the major airways during subtotal esophagectomy: incidence, management, and sequelae. *J Thorac Cardiovasc Surg* 2000;120:1093–1096.

Javed A, Pal S, Chaubal GN, Sahni P, Chattopadhyay TK. Management and outcome of intrathoracic bleeding due to vascular injury during transhiatal esophagectomy. *J Gastrointest Surg* 2011 Feb;15(2):262–626.

Katariya K, Harvey JC, Pina E, et al. Complications of transhiatal esophagectomy. *J Surg Oncol* 1994;57:157–163.

Orringer MB, Marshall B, Iannettoni MD. Transhiatal esophagectomy: clinical experience and refinements. *Ann Surg* 1999;230:392–400.

8. **(C)** The prognosis of malignant TEF secondary to esophageal carcinoma is extremely poor. Most patients die within 3 months from pulmonary complications. The disease is typically inoperable because of extensive mediastinal invasion. When surgical resection is possible, esophagectomy with enteric interposition for palliation restores swallowing ability; however, there is little justification for performing a noncurative procedure with relatively high associated morbidity and mortality. Esophageal intubation, especially with self-expanding metallic stents, provides the best means of palliation by preventing recurrent aspiration and restoring swallowing ability. Esophageal stents are preferred over alternative palliative therapies because they provide immediate relief of dysphagia. The stents are placed by endoscopy under fluoroscopic guidance and occlude the esophageal side of the fistula so that oral intake can be resumed without the risk of aspiration.

Self-expanding stents maintain luminal patency when subsequent therapies, such as radiation or chemotherapy, result in tumor shrinkage. Potential complications of stent placement include infection, tumor ingrowth at the ends, and stent migration.

Radiation with or without chemotherapy offers little curative potential in unresectable esophageal cancer. It may provide some symptomatic relief of dysphagia but usually requires 1–2 months before this effect is appreciated. Neither radiation nor chemotherapy contributes to closure of TEFs, which will continue to cause significant morbidity and mortality. The therapies themselves can cause life-threatening complications as well as increase the risks of concurrent stent placement by compromising tissue viability in proximity of the tumor. Cervical esophagostomy with gastric tube placement would divert secretions away from the TEF and decrease the risk of aspiration but would not allow the patient to eat normally and therefore is not optimal palliation.

BIBLIOGRAPHY

Madhusudhan C, Saluja SS, Pal S, et al. Palliative stenting for relief of dysphagia in patients with inoperable esophageal cancer: impact on quality of life. *Dis Esophagus* 2009;22(4):331–336.

Peters JH, Little VR, Watson, TJ. Esophageal anatomy and physiology and gastroesophageal reflux disease. In: Mulholland MW, Lillemoe KD, Doherty GM, et al., eds. *Greenfield's Surgery: Scientific Principles and Practice.* 5th ed. Philadelphia, PA: Lippincott Williams & Wilkins; 2011:647–648.

Weigel TL, Frumiento C, Gaumintz E. Endoluminal palliation for dysphagia secondary to esophageal carcinoma. *Surg Clin North Am* 2002;82:747–761.

Xinopoulos D, Dimitroulopoulos D, Moschandrea J, et al. Natural course of inoperable esophageal cancer treated with metallic expandable stents: quality of life and cost-effectiveness analysis. *J Gastroenterol Hepatol* 2004;19(12):1397–1402.

9. **(C)** There are four types of hiatal hernias. In type I hernias, the gastroesophageal junction is displaced superior to the hiatus. This is also known as a sliding hiatal hernia because the gastric cardia migrates back and forth between the posterior mediastinum and the peritoneal cavity. Type I hernias are the most common and are often associated with gastroesophageal reflux. Type II hernias, also termed paraesophageal hernias, are characterized by an upward displacement of the gastric fundus with a normally positioned gastroesophageal junction. Type III hernias have both sliding and paraesophageal components and with the gastroesophageal junction displaced above the diaphragm along with all or part of the stomach. Type IV hernias are simply type III hernias that involve displacement of additional organs into the chest. The exact cause of paraesophageal hernias

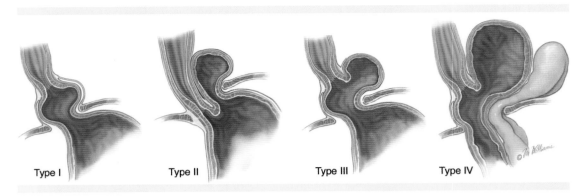

FIGURE 17-11. Four types of hiatal (paraesophageal) hernias. (from D.J. Sugarbaker, R. Bueno, Y. L. Colson, M. T. Jaklitsch, M. J. Krasna, S. J. Mentzer, M. Williams, A. Adams: *Adult Chest Surgery*. 2nd ed. New York, NY: McGraw Hill; 2013: Fig. 37-3. Copyright © The McGraw-Hill Companies, Inc. All rights reserved).

is unknown, but it is thought to be related to the structural deterioration of the phrenoesophageal membrane and becomes more prevalent with advancing age. The phrenoesophageal membrane is stretched over time with repeated movement of the esophagus during swallowing and as intra-abdominal pressures are exerted against the membrane (Fig. 17-11).

BIBLIOGRAPHY

Burakoff R, Chan WW. Overview of esophageal motility disorders. In: Sugarbaker DJ, Bueno R, Colson YL, et al., eds. *Adult Chest Surgery*. 2nd edition. New York, NY: McGraw-Hill; 2013:267.

Hashemi M, Sillin LF, Peters JH. Current concepts in the management of paraesophageal hiatal hernia. *J Clin Gastroenterol* 1999;29:8–13.

Landreneau RJ, Del Pino M, Santos R. Management of paraesophageal hernias. *Surg Clin North Am* 2005 Jun;85(3):411–432.

Petersen RY, Pellegrini CA, Oelschlager BK. Hiatal hernia and gastroesophageal reflux disease. In: Townsend CM, Beauchamp DR, Evers MB, et al., eds. *Sabiston Textbook of Surgery: The Biological Basis of Modern Surgical Practice*. 19th ed. Philadelphia, PA: Saunders; 2012:1067–1069.

10. **(C)** Barrett's esophagus is the most serious complication of GERD. Approximately 10% of patients with GERD will have Barrett's metaplasia, which is defined as the presence of columnar metaplasia extending 3 cm or greater into the esophagus or specialized intestinal-type metaplasia of any length. Nondysplastic Barrett's epithelium has been estimated to progress to dysplasia at a rate of 5–10% per year, with adenocarcinoma developing in 1% of cases per year. If there is no dysplasia present, medical therapy with PPIs should be continued with routine endoscopic surveillance every 2–3 years. Although PPIs reduce the volume of gastric acid reflux, it does not entirely eliminate gastric and duodenal reflux. Columnar metaplasia may continue to occur. Some authors advocate the use of surgical antireflux procedures to restore LES function.

Despite effective antireflux surgery, the incidence of adenocarcinoma in patients with Barrett's esophagus has not decreased. As a result, routine endoscopic surveillance is required in all patients with Barrett's esophagus. Once dysplasia is identified on histology specimens, management should be tailored according to the severity of dysplasia. If the specimens are indeterminate for dysplasia, high-dose PPIs should be instituted to resolve any inflammation, and a repeat biopsy should be performed in 3–6 months. If repeat biopsy is still indeterminate for dysplasia, then the patient should be treated as if low-grade dysplasia were present. The presence of low-grade dysplasia should raise concern because it represents progression of a disease process that eventually leads to adenocarcinoma. Low-grade dysplasia may be treated with aggressive medical therapy or antireflux surgery and repeat biopsy every 6 months. Most authors agree that the presence of high-grade dysplasia is an indication to perform resection via either endoscopic mucosal resection or esophagectomy. Studies have shown that 30–40% of patients with high-grade dysplasia who undergo esophagectomy pathologically demonstrate invasive adenocarcinoma in the resected specimens despite negative findings on repeat endoscopy and EUS.

BIBLIOGRAPHY

Milind R, Attwood SE. Natural history of Barrett's esophagus. *World J Gastroenterol* 2012 Jul 21;18(27):3483–3491.

Peters JH, Little VR, Watson, TJ. Esophageal anatomy and physiology and gastroesophageal reflux disease. In: Mulholland MW, Lillemoe KD, Doherty GM, et al., eds. *Greenfield's Surgery: Scientific Principles and Practice*. 5th ed. Philadelphia, PA: Lippincott Williams & Wilkins; 2011:647–648.

Smith CD. Antireflux surgery. *Surg Clin North Am* 2008 Oct; 88(5):943–958, v.

Spechler SJ, Souza RF. Barrett's esophagus. *N Engl J Med* 2014 Aug 28;371(9):836–845.

11. **(A)** The barium esophagogram shows disruption of peristalsis with tertiary activity producing segmentation of the esophagus, typical of diffuse esophageal spasm (DES) (Fig. 17-12). DES is characterized by normal peristalsis intermittently interrupted by simultaneous contractions. The disorder is uncommon and its cause unknown. Some evidence suggests a defect in neural inhibition along the esophageal body. Esophageal spasm has been linked to GERD and stressful events. Chest pain and dysphagia, the most common presenting symptoms, are usually intermittent, which may make establishing a diagnosis of DES challenging.

The classic finding of the "corkscrew" or "rosary-bead" appearance of the esophageal body may be seen during a barium swallow study; however, the absence of these findings on barium swallow does not eliminate the possibility of DES, particularly if the patient is asymptomatic during the study. Conversely, symptoms of chest pain do not always correlate with spastic activity. Esophageal manometry is usually diagnostic for DES and helps distinguish it from other esophageal motility disorders. Diagnostic criteria include simultaneous contractions in the esophageal body in greater than 30% (but less than 100%) of wet swallows and mean simultaneous

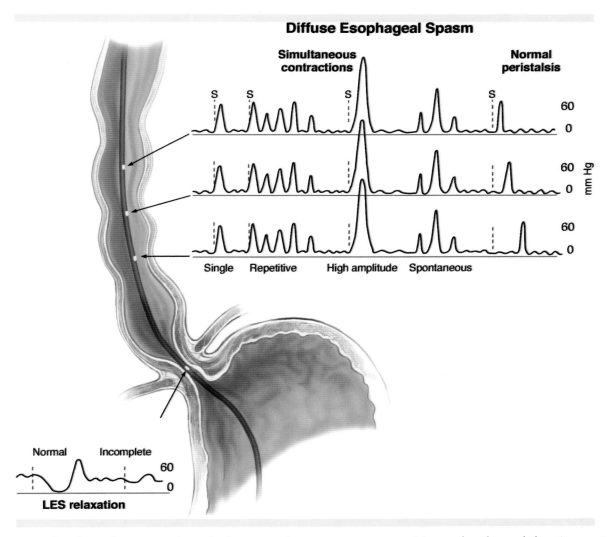

FIGURE 17-12. Esophageal manometric study demonstrating spontaneous, repetitive, and prolonged-duration contractions in diffuse esophageal spasm (LES, lower esophageal sphincter; S, swallow).(from D.J. Sugarbaker, R. Bueno, Y. L. Colson, M. T. Jaklitsch, M. J. Krasna, S. J. Mentzer, M. Williams, A. Adams: Adult Chest Surgery. 2nd ed. New York, NY: McGraw Hill; 2013: Fig. 33-5. Copyright © The McGraw-Hill Companies, Inc. All rights reserved).

contraction amplitude greater than 30 mmHg. Other criteria less consistently found include repetitive contractions (greater than three peaks), prolonged duration (greater than 6 s) of contractions, and abnormalities of LES relaxation. If manometry shows all contractions to be simultaneous, with associated impaired LES relaxation, then the diagnosis of achalasia should be considered.

Initial treatment of DES should be medical. Reassurance that the patient's symptoms are not cardiac related is often beneficial. Nitrates and calcium channel blockers can decrease high-amplitude contractions, thereby relieving symptoms of chest pain, but results are variable, and long-term efficacy has not been adequately assessed. The incidence of psychiatric disorders such as anxiety, depression, and somatization is increased in patients with spastic disorders of the esophagus. Accordingly, psychotropic drugs such as trazodone and imipramine have shown some success in symptom relief. Botulinum toxin injections and pneumatic dilation have also shown some clinical response, but the duration of effect is variable.

Esophageal myotomy should be reserved for patients in whom medical therapy has failed. The results of surgery are not as predictable with DES compared to achalasia. Myotomy decreases the intensity of esophageal contractions, but the frequency of contractions is often unaffected, and symptoms occasionally persist despite surgery. Myotomy may also result in a hypocontractile esophagus, which can result in dysphagia. When surgery is contemplated, a long myotomy from the aortic arch to the LES is the procedure of choice.

BIBLIOGRAPHY

Adler DG, Romero Y. Primary esophageal motility disorders. *Mayo Clin Proc* 2001;76:195–200.

Khandelwal S, Oelschlager BK. Benign esophageal disorders. In: Zinner MJ, Ashley SW. *Maingot's Abdominal Operations*. 12th ed. New York, NY: McGraw-Hill; 2013: Chapter 14.

Prakash C, Clouse RE. Esophageal motor disorders. *Curr Opin Gastroenterol* 2002;18:454–463.

Richter JE. Oesophageal motility disorders. *Lancet* 2001;358:823–828.

Spechler SJ, Castell DO. Classification of oesophageal motility abnormalities. *Gut* 2001;49:145–151.

12. **(B)** Endoscopic ultrasound is the procedure of choice for evaluating primary tumor depth, regional nodal disease, and involvement of adjacent structures. The accuracy of lymph node staging ranges from 50 to 88% based on EUS characteristics, such as lymph node size, shape, border characteristics, and central echogenicity. EUS can also accurately identify suspicious lymph nodes in the celiac axis and disease in the left liver lobe, both

of which are considered distant metastases. EUS with fine-needle aspiration (FNA) under real-time guidance is usually recommended to cytologically document the presence of metastatic disease in suspicious-appearing lymph nodes, particularly when the presence of distant metastases will change therapy. CT scanning of the chest and abdomen may also detect regional and nonregional lymph node metastases, but assessment of T and N stage with CT is not as accurate as EUS. Invasion of surrounding mediastinal structures may also be suggested by CT scan; however, operative exploration is not infrequently required to confirm unresectability. CT scanning is relied on to determine the presence of metastatic disease with 85–90% accuracy.

Positron emission tomography is also used in the evaluation of esophageal cancer. Although lacking complete specificity, PET is sensitive in identifying sites of tumor activity and is useful in the evaluation of metastatic disease. Flamen et al. (2000) reported 95% sensitivity of PET in identifying primary tumor in esophageal cancer and 82% accuracy of identifying stage IV disease. Unfortunately, PET is not as sensitive in assessing lymph node involvement. Flamen et al. (2000) reported a significantly lower sensitivity compared to EUS, 33% versus 81%, respectively, which is attributed to the inability of separating 18-fluorodeoxyglucose uptake in the primary tumor from uptake in surrounding lymph nodes. PET is also not reliable for predicting primary tumor depth (T stage). Other disadvantages include high cost and lack of availability compared to conventional staging modalities. The routine use of PET for staging esophageal cancer requires further evaluation.

Magnetic resonance imaging is not routinely used for staging esophageal carcinoma. In select cases, MRI can accurately detect T4 disease with direct tumor extension into adjacent organs, such as the aorta or trachea, but the relatively high cost and lack of significant imaging improvement compared to conventional CT scans limit its use for this disease. Video-assisted thoracoscopy (VATS) and laparoscopy are highly accurate methods of evaluating nodal disease in esophageal carcinoma. The disadvantages of these procedures include the need for general anesthesia, the costs and risks associated with surgery, and recovery, which may delay neoadjuvant chemoradiation therapy. As a result, VATS and laparoscopy are infrequently used in the initial evaluation of esophageal cancer.

BIBLIOGRAPHY

Kucharczuk JC, Kaiser LR. Esophageal injury, diverticula, and neoplasms. In: Mulholland MW, Lillemoe KD, Doherty GM, et al., eds. *Greenfield's Surgery: Scientific Principles and Practice*. 5th ed. Philadelphia, PA: Lippincott Williams & Wilkins; 2011:629–648.

Lada MJ, Peters JH. The management of esophageal carcinoma. In: Cameron JL, ed. *Current Surgical Therapy*. 10th ed. St. Louis, MO: Mosby; 2011:47–49.

Maish SM. Esophagus. In: Townsend CM, Beauchamp DR, Evers MB, et al., eds. *Sabiston Textbook of Surgery: The Biological Basis of Modern Surgical Practice*. 19th ed. Philadelphia, PA: Saunders; 2012:1052–1053.

13. **(D)** An extrinsic mass with a smooth surface on barium esophagogram combined with a hypoechoic mass with smooth margins in the muscularis propria on EUS is consistent with leiomyoma. Leiomyomas are smooth muscle tumors of the muscularis propria and account for 70% of benign esophageal tumors. They typically occur in patients between 20 and 50 years of age and occur with equal frequency in males and females. Most leiomyomas are located in the middle or distal thirds of the esophagus. Tumors less than 5 cm are rarely symptomatic and are usually found incidentally during endoscopy or contrast studies obtained for nonrelated symptoms. Symptomatic leiomyomas may present with dysphagia or retrosternal pain. Leiomyomas have a characteristic appearance on barium esophagogram, typically showing a concave submucosal defect with sharp borders. Esophagoscopy is indicated to exclude malignancy or other occult pathology, but attempts at direct biopsy are typically not diagnostic as these tumors are located beneath the submucosal layer. Cells for cytologic analysis can be obtained with FNA under EUS guidance if the diagnosis based on contrast studies and EUS findings is in question.

Asymptomatic leiomyomas can be managed conservatively; leiomyomas larger than 5 cm should be resected. The conventional approach is through a thoracotomy incision or upper midline laparotomy for distal tumors. After splitting of the overlying muscle layers, a plane can be found between tumor and mucosa. The leiomyoma is an encapsulated mass that is relatively avascular and can be easily enucleated while preserving the submucosal layer. The split muscle edges should then be reapproximated. The procedure has been performed successfully with VATS, which has the advantage of reduced postoperative pain.

BIBLIOGRAPHY

Kucharczuk JC, Kaiser LR. Esophageal injury, diverticula, and neoplasms. In: Mulholland MW, Lillemoe KD, Doherty GM, et al., eds. *Greenfield's Surgery: Scientific Principles and Practice*. 5th ed. Philadelphia, PA: Lippincott Williams & Wilkins; 2011:629–648.

Lee LS, Singhal S, Brinster CJ, et al. Current management of esophageal leiomyoma. *J Am Coll Surg*. 2004 Jan;198(1):136–146.

Maish SM. Esophagus. In: Townsend CM, Beauchamp DR, Evers MB, et al., eds. *Sabiston Textbook of Surgery: The Biological Basis*

of Modern Surgical Practice. 19th ed. Philadelphia, PA: Saunders; 2012:1047–1049.

Punpale A, Rangole A, Bhambhani N, et al. Leiomyoma of esophagus. *Ann Thorac Cardiovasc Surg* 2007;13:78–81.

14. **(E)** Esophageal cancer represents 4% of newly diagnosed cancers in the United States. It occurs most commonly in the seventh decade of life and is 1.5–3 times more common in men than in women. The cause of esophageal carcinoma is unknown but is thought to be related to mucosal injury from prolonged exposure to noxious stimuli. Alcohol consumption and cigarette smoking have been shown to be risk factors for squamous cell carcinoma. The histology of esophageal carcinoma can be seen as a progression from dysplastic cells to carcinoma *in situ,* which is limited to the mucosa. Once carcinoma extends beyond the basement membrane, early invasive carcinoma is present.

Worldwide, squamous cell carcinoma accounts for approximately 95% of esophageal cancer. Squamous cell carcinoma had been the predominant form of esophageal cancer in the United States until recently, when the incidence of adenocarcinoma doubled in the 1990s. Adenocarcinoma is now the most common type of esophageal carcinoma in the United States. This shift has been attributed to gastroesophageal reflux and secondary columnar metaplasia seen with Barrett's disease. In the United States, black males have a greater risk of developing squamous cell carcinoma, whereas white males have a greater risk of adenocarcinoma.

BIBLIOGRAPHY

Lepage C, Drouillard A, Jouve JL, Faivre J. Epidemiology and risk factors for oesophageal adenocarcinoma. *Dig Liver Dis* 2013 Aug;45(8):625–629.

Maish SM. Esophagus. In: Townsend CM, Beauchamp DR, Evers MB, et al., eds. *Sabiston Textbook of Surgery: The Biological Basis of Modern Surgical Practice*. 19th ed. Philadelphia, PA: Saunders; 2012:1049–1052.

Peters JH, Little VR, Watson, TJ. Esophageal anatomy and physiology and gastroesophageal reflux disease. In: Mulholland MW, Lillemoe KD, Doherty GM, et al., eds. *Greenfield's Surgery: Scientific Principles and Practice*. 5th ed. Philadelphia, PA: Lippincott Williams & Wilkins; 2011:647–648.

15. **(E)** A dilated proximal esophagus with bird-beak tapering on barium esophagogram is suggestive of achalasia or an achalasia-like motility disorder. Achalasia is an esophageal motility disorder characterized by inadequate LES relaxation and aperistalsis of the esophageal body (Fig. 17-13). The etiology is unknown but is theorized to be related to the degeneration of inhibitory neurons that affect relaxation of esophageal smooth muscle. These parasympathetic ganglion cells reside in the myenteric

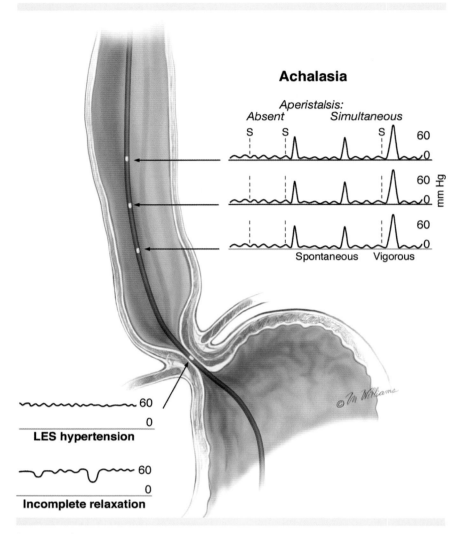

FIGURE 17-13. Classic features of achalasia revealed on esophageal manometry (LES, lower esophageal sphincter; S, swallow) (from D.J. Sugarbaker, R. Bueno, Y. L. Colson, M. T. Jaklitsch, M. J. Krasna, S. J. Mentzer, M. Williams, A. Adams: *Adult Chest Surgery*. 2nd ed. New York, NY: McGraw Hill; 2013: Fig. 33-3. Copyright © The McGraw-Hill Companies, Inc. All rights reserved).

plexus between the longitudinal and circular muscle layers of the esophagus. The smooth muscle of the LES is normally contracted at rest and relaxes when stimulated by inhibitory neurons, as occurs with swallowing. In achalasia, resting LES pressures may be increased, and diminished relaxation of the LES is seen with swallowing. Loss of inhibitory neurons also affects normal peristalsis in the esophageal body.

Although the etiology of achalasia is unknown, infection with the parasite *Trypanosoma cruzi* (Chagas disease) seen in Central and South America causes loss of intramural ganglion cells and results in aperistalsis with inadequate LES relaxation, producing a motor abnormality identical to primary achalasia. Malignancies at the

gastroesophageal junction can cause a pseudoachalasia that has the same radiographic and manometric findings as primary achalasia. In addition, strictures of the distal esophagus can cause proximal esophageal dilatation but would be differentiated from achalasia on the basis of endoscopic and manometric findings.

As with other esophageal motility disorders, achalasia typically produces symptoms of chest pain and dysphagia. Patients may complain of a sticking sensation in the chest after swallowing and may drink large volumes of water to force food into the stomach. As the disease progresses, regurgitation of undigested food may occur, and the risk of aspiration increases. Weight loss may also be seen and may raise the concern of malignancy.

Manometry is required for diagnosis. Classic manometric findings include an elevated resting LES pressure, lack of peristalsis, and incomplete relaxation of the LES with swallows. These findings are highly reproducible, unlike other esophageal motility disorders. Radiographic studies typically include a barium esophagogram, which shows a dilated proximal esophagus with tapering "bird-beak" appearance in the distal esophagus. Retained food may be seen in portions of the esophagus as well as air-fluid levels in the distal esophagus. Endoscopy with biopsy is useful for ruling out malignancy as well as benign conditions such as strictures or stromal tumors that can mimic achalasia.

BIBLIOGRAPHY

Maish SM. Esophagus. In: Townsend CM, Beauchamp DR, Evers MB, et al., eds. *Sabiston Textbook of Surgery: The Biological Basis of Modern Surgical Practice*. 19th ed. Philadelphia, PA: Saunders; 2012:1049–1058.

Patti MG, Herbella FA. Achalasia and other esophageal motility disorders. *J Gastrointest Surg* 2011 May;15(5):703–707. doi:10.1007/s11605-011-1478-x. Epub 2011 Mar 11.

Spechler SJ, Castell DO. Classification of oesophageal motility abnormalities. *Gut* 2001;49:145–151.

16. **(E)** Diagnostic testing is essential in planning the management of GERD. The gold standard for diagnosing reflux is the 24-h pH probe. Electrodes that measure fluctuation in pH are placed in the esophagus. Over the course of 24 h, the patient notes specific times that he or she experiences reflux symptoms. Reflux is calculated as the total percentage of time the pH is below 4. Abnormal reflux occurs when the pH is less than 4 more than 1% of the time in the proximal esophagus and more than 4% of the time in the distal esophagus. Correlation between the patient's symptoms and drops in pH are also taken into account when interpreting the study.

Barium esophagram is an integral part of the assessment and management of patients with GERD before, and especially after, antireflux procedures. It is useful in the definition of the morphology and function of the esophagus and the detection of esophageal motility disturbances and abnormal clearance that may accompany reflux esophagitis. Fluoroscopic observation during the barium esophagram using multiple barium swallows reliably evaluates primary esophageal peristalsis.

Manometry evaluates the function of the esophageal body and LES. Esophageal body function is evaluated by placing several channels along the esophageal body, and peristaltic activity is measured at each channel with swallowing. Patients should normally have greater than 80% of peristaltic activity transmitted to each channel with swallows. The amplitude of the peristaltic wave can also be measured, with normal values greater than 30 mmHg. Patients demonstrating compromised peristalsis by manometry are likely to experience dysphagia following a 360-degree fundoplication. A partial fundoplication should be considered in these cases.

Endoscopy is important in the workup of gastroesophageal reflux because it excludes other pathology and evaluates the severity of esophageal injury. Mucosal changes can be directly visualized and biopsies obtained to evaluate for metaplasia or dysplasia; however, endoscopy is not sensitive for diagnosing gastroesophageal reflux because many patients may not have obvious mucosal changes. Gastric scintigraphy helps identify patients with delayed gastric emptying, which may contribute to gastroesophageal reflux. A gastric-emptying procedure may benefit these patients.

BIBLIOGRAPHY

Eubanks TR, Pellegrini CA. Hiatal hernia and gastroesophageal reflux disease. In: Townsend CM, Beauchamp DR, Evers MB, et al., eds. *Sabiston Textbook of Surgery: The Biological Basis of Modern Surgical Practice*. 16th ed. Philadelphia, PA: Saunders; 2001:757–759.

Patti MG, Diener U, Tamburini A, et al. Role of esophageal function tests in the diagnosis of gastroesophageal reflux disease. *Dig Dis Sci* 2001;46:597–602.

Telem DA, Rattner DW. Gastroesophageal reflux disease. In: Cameron JL, ed. *Current Surgical Therapy*. 10th ed. St. Louis, MO: Mosby; 2011:10–11.

17. **(C)** The esophagus consists of three layers: the mucosa, submucosa, and muscularis propria. The mucosa consists of a squamous epithelium, lamina propria, and muscularis mucosa. The epithelium, the innermost layer, is made of nonkeratinizing squamous cells. The squamous epithelium ends abruptly in the distal 1–2 cm of esophagus, where the junctional columnar epithelium of the gastric cardia begins. This transition point, known as the "Z line," is readily apparent on endoscopy as small projections of red gastric epithelium extend upward into the pink-white squamous epithelium. Beneath the epithelium lies the lamina propria, which is a loose matrix of collagen and elastic fibers and contains lymphatics. Surrounding the lamina propria is the muscularis mucosa, which contains mainly longitudinal muscle fibers (Fig. 17-14).

The submucosa consists of loose connective tissue containing blood vessels; nerve fibers, including Meissner's plexus; lymphatics; and submucosal glands. The submucosa contains elastic and fibrous tissue and is the strongest layer of the esophageal wall. The muscularis

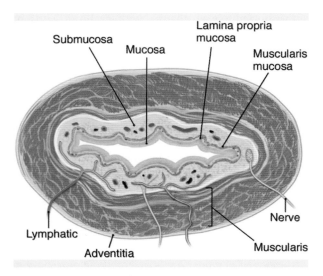

FIGURE 17-14. Layers of the esophagus. Courtesy of John M. Braver, MD.

propria consists of an inner circular layer and an outer longitudinal layer. This muscle layer provides the propulsive force for swallowing. The myenteric, or Auerbach's, plexus is located between the circular and longitudinal muscle layers. On EUS, four distinct layers (superficial mucosa, deep mucosa, submucosa, and muscularis propria) can be visualized. The periesophageal tissue can be seen as a fifth layer on EUS.

BIBLIOGRAPHY

Lerut T, Coosemans W, Decaluwé H, et al. Anatomy of the esophagus. In: Fischer JE, Jones DB, et al., eds. *Mastery of Surgery*. 6th ed. Philadelphia, PA: Lippincott Williams & Wilkins; 2011:670.

Linden PA. Overview: anatomy and pathophysiology of esophageal reflux disease. In: Sugarbaker DJ, Bueno R, Colson YL, et al., eds. *Adult Chest Surgery*. 2nd ed. New York, NY: McGraw-Hill; 2013: Chapter 37.

Telem DA, Rattner DW. Gastroesophageal reflux disease. In: Cameron JL, ed. *Current Surgical Therapy*. 10th ed. St. Louis, MO: Mosby; 2011:10–11.

18. **(B)** Everyone experiences some degree of symptomatology from transient reflux of gastric contents into the esophagus. Yet, not everyone develops clinically significant GERD because of defense mechanisms, which protect the esophageal mucosa from acid-induced injury; these defenses include esophageal motor activity, gravity, and buffering secretions from saliva and submucosal glands. Reflux develops when these defense mechanisms are impaired, such as in esophageal motility disorders. The most common cause of GERD, however, is a defective LES. LES competence depends on baseline sphincter pressure, overall length, and length exposed to intra-abdominal positive pressure. The LES does not have to be permanently defective for GERD to occur. Transient relaxation of the LES may be the cause of early gastroesophageal reflux. The sequelae of esophageal mucosal injury include esophagitis, stricture, and Barrett's metaplasia. The development of these complications is usually related to a defective LES.

The components of refluxed gastric juice include gastric acid and pepsin as well as biliary and pancreatic secretions from duodenal contents. Gastric acid alone causes minimal damage to the esophageal mucosa. The presence of pepsin in the acidic environment of refluxed gastric juice appears to be the major injurious agent. The addition of duodenal contents in refluxed juice results in a more alkaline environment. In this setting, bile acids and the pancreatic enzyme trypsin play a significant role in mucosal injury.

The significance of *H. pylori* in the development of peptic ulcer disease has been well documented. *Helicobacter pylori* does not potentiate the development of GERD and in fact may have a protective effect in esophageal disease. The presence of *H. pylori* strains with the cytotoxin-associated gene A (cagA+) has an inverse association with esophagitis, Barrett's epithelium, and adenocarcinoma of the distal esophagus.

BIBLIOGRAPHY

Buttar NS, Falk GW. Pathogenesis of gastroesophageal reflux and Barrett esophagus. *Mayo Clin Proc* 2001;76:226–234.

Mittal RK, Balaban DH. Mechanisms of disease: the esophagogastric junction. *N Engl J Med* 1997;336:924–932.

Peters JH, Little VR, Watson, TJ. Esophageal anatomy and physiology and gastroesophageal reflux disease. In: Mulholland MW, Lillemoe KD, Doherty GM, et al., eds. *Greenfield's Surgery: Scientific Principles and Practice*. 5th ed. Philadelphia, PA: Lippincott Williams & Wilkins; 2011:647–648.

Warburton-Timms VJ, Charlett A, Valori RM, et al. The significance of cagA+ *H. pylori* in reflux oesophagitis. *Gut* 2001;49:341–346.

19. **(C)** Despite advances in surgical techniques and adjuvant therapies, esophageal cancer remains an aggressive disease with poor prognosis. Surgery has been the mainstay of treatment; however, 5-year survival following surgery alone for locally advanced disease ranges between 20 and 25%. The unacceptably poor outcomes with surgery alone prompted investigation into additional therapies.

Neoadjuvant chemotherapy alone has not conclusively shown any survival advantages. A large multicenter phase III study in the United States randomizing patients to chemotherapy followed by surgery compared to surgery alone (Kelsen et al. 1998) demonstrated no survival advantage to preoperative chemotherapy: 14.9 months for the patients who received preoperative chemotherapy and 16.1 months for those who underwent immediate surgery ($p = 0.53$). At 1 year, the survival rate was 59% for those who received chemotherapy and 60% for those who had surgery alone; at 2 years, survival was 35% and 37%, respectively. A similar phase III study completed in Europe (Clark 2001), however, demonstrated survival advantage to preoperative chemotherapy, with median survival of 16.8 months in the preoperative chemotherapy group compared with 13.3 months in the surgery-only group. The 2-year survival rates were 43% in the preoperative chemotherapy group compared with 34% in the surgery-only group.

Some oncologists and radiation therapists believe that definitive chemoradiation therapy without surgery is optimal; however, this is based on data from earlier studies on patients with mainly squamous cell carcinoma histology. Postoperative chemotherapy or radiation therapy is difficult to administer; moreover, it has never been shown to improve survival.

To date, the most promising treatment regimen consists of preoperative chemotherapy and radiation therapy followed by surgery. The premise behind induction chemoradiation is that the tumor may be downstaged with chemoradiation, increasing the likelihood of a complete resection with tumor-free margins. In addition, micrometastases would be treated with preoperative chemoradiation. Unfortunately, there have been no large-scale prospective, randomized trials comparing induction chemoradiation followed by surgery versus surgery alone. Single-institution studies have demonstrated mixed results regarding the benefit of preoperative chemoradiation therapy. It is believed, however, that the subset of patients, estimated to range between 20 and 30%, who demonstrate a complete pathologic response following neoadjuvant chemoradiation therapy have a superior prognosis over patients who do not demonstrate a complete response. Moreover, neoadjuvant chemoradiation therapy in otherwise-healthy patients has not been shown to significantly increase operative risks. In this regard, patients with good performance status probably should be offered preoperative chemoradiation therapy prior to esophagectomy.

BIBLIOGRAPHY

Clark P. Surgical resection with or without pre-operative chemotherapy in oesophageal cancer: an updated analysis of a randomised controlled trial conducted by the UK medical research council upper GI tract cancer group. *Proc Am Soc Clin Oncol* 2001; abstract 502:126a.

Kelsen DP, Ginsberg R, Pajak T, et al. Preoperative chemotherapy followed by operation versus operation alone for patients with localized esophageal cancers: a U.S. national intergroup study. *N Engl J Med* 1998;339:1979–1984.

Maish SM. Esophagus. In: Townsend CM, Beauchamp DR, Evers MB, et al., eds. *Sabiston Textbook of Surgery: The Biological Basis of Modern Surgical Practice*. 19th ed. Philadelphia, PA: Saunders; 2012:1058–1063.

Urba SG, Orringer MB, Turrisi A, et al. Randomized trial of preoperative chemoradiation versus surgery alone in patients with locoregional esophageal carcinoma. *J Clin Oncol* 2001;19:305–313.

Urschel JD, Vasan HB, Blewett CJ. A meta-analysis of randomized controlled trials that compared neoadjuvant chemotherapy and surgery to surgery alone for respectable esophageal cancer. *Am J Surg* 2002;183:274–279.

20. **(D)** The barium esophagogram shows an epiphrenic, or lower, esophageal diverticulum. Epiphrenic diverticula, which occur in the distal 10 cm of the esophagus, are the most common type of esophageal diverticula (Fig. 17-15). They are usually false diverticula that result from pulsion forces leading to mucosal herniation at an area of focal weakness in the esophageal wall.

There is an increasing amount of evidence to suggest a link between esophageal diverticula and motility disorders. In fact, findings of epiphrenic diverticula should raise suspicion of an underlying motility disorder, and manometry should be performed. Achalasia is the most common esophageal motility disorder; however, diverticula occur in less than 5% of patients with achalasia. DES is less prevalent than achalasia, but pulsion diverticula occur more frequently in these patients.

Small and asymptomatic diverticula may be observed. Symptomatic or large diverticula warrant operative intervention. Symptoms of dysphagia, regurgitation of undigested food, and even aspiration are primarily felt to be a result of the underlying motility disorder, with a lesser contribution from the diverticulum itself. The most important component of any surgical treatment is therefore esophagomyotomy. Myotomy treats the underlying motor disorder and prevents recurrence or suture line disruption following diverticulectomy. Addition of an antireflux procedure is controversial but should be included when myotomy is performed transabdominally.

BIBLIOGRAPHY

Grant KS, DeMeester SR. Resection of esophageal diverticula. In: Sugarbaker DJ, Bueno R, Colson YL, et al., eds. *Adult Chest Surgery*. 2nd ed. New York, NY: McGraw-Hill; 2013: Chapter 30.

Nehra D, Lord RV, DeMeester TR, et al. Physiologic basis for the treatment of epiphrenic diverticulum. *Ann Surg* 2002;235:346–354.

Thomas ML, Anthony AA, Fosh BG, et al. Oesophageal diverticula. *Br J Surg* 2001;88:629–642.

21. **(A)** The LES has been the focus of intense research because of its role in gastroesophageal reflux and esophageal motility disorders. The LES is a zone of high pressure in the area of the diaphragmatic hiatus that extends

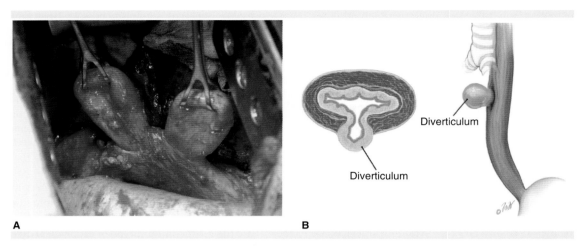

FIGURE 17-15. A. The epiphrenic esophageal diverticulum depicted in the intraoperative photograph is of the pulsion variety. Pulsion diverticula (B) are not covered by the muscle layers of the esophageal wall and thus are considered false diverticula. (from D.J. Sugarbaker, R. Bueno ,Y. L. Colson, M. T. Jaklitsch, M. J. Krasna ,S. J. Mentzer, M. Williams, A. Adams: *Adult Chest Surgery*. 2nd ed. New York, NY: McGraw Hill; 2013: Fig. 30-1. Copyright © The McGraw-Hill Companies, Inc. All rights reserved).

over an axial distance of 2–3 cm. This zone maintains a pressure higher than intragastric pressure with inspiration and expiration, but the pressure drops significantly in response to swallow-induced peristalsis. LES tone and relaxation are controlled by central and peripheral mechanisms. Neural control of the LES involves cholinergic and noncholinergic inhibitory pathways. Contraction of the crural diaphragm increases LES pressure, whereas gastric distention, esophageal distention, and pharyngeal and laryngeal inhibitory reflexes stimulate pathways resulting in LES relaxation.

Nitric oxide plays an important role in the relaxation of the LES. Studies in animals and humans have shown that blocking NO production with a NO synthase inhibitor reduces LES relaxation. CCK has also been shown to increase the rate of LES relaxation. Intravenous infusion of a CCK antagonist into healthy human volunteers resulted in a significant reduction in LES relaxation following oral feeding. Atropine, on the other hand, inhibits LES relaxation, as demonstrated by esophageal manometry. Atropine has been shown to reduce the incidence of gastroesophageal reflux when assessed by esophageal pH monitoring in patients receiving postprandial atropine infusions.

BIBLIOGRAPHY

Gawrieh S, Shaker R. Peripheral mechanisms affecting the lower esophageal sphincter tone. *Gastroenterol Clin North Am* 2002;31:S21–S33.
Mittal RK, Balaban DH. Mechanisms of disease: the esophagogastric junction. *N Engl J Med* 1997;336:924–932.
Peters JH, Little VR, Watson, TJ. Esophageal anatomy and physiology and gastroesophageal reflux disease. In: Mulholland MW, Lillemoe KD, Doherty GM, et al., eds. *Greenfield's Surgery: Scientific Principles and Practice*. 5th ed. Philadelphia, PA: Lippincott Williams & Wilkins; 2011:647–648.

22. **(D)** Esophageal duplication cysts are rare congenital anomalies of the foregut, accounting for 0.5–2.5% of all esophageal tumors. Most duplications are discovered in infants and children, although 25–30% are found in the adult population. Duplication cysts result from developmental errors in the fifth to eighth weeks of embryonic life. During this time, the primitive foregut divides into dorsal and ventral segments. The dorsal segment elongates to form the esophagus and the ventral portion develops into the tracheobronchial tree. Vacuoles that form in the foregut during the solid-tube stage of development normally coalesce to form the esophageal lumen. It is theorized that failure of the vacuoles to coalesce results in formation of a duplication cyst. Esophageal cysts are lined by ciliated epithelium that may be columnar, squamous, or pseudostratified. Bronchogenic cysts are similarly lined by ciliated columnar epithelium and may contain cartilage. It is often difficult to differentiate bronchogenic cysts from esophageal cysts because of their close embryologic relationship. Many authors thus refer to these lesions collectively as foregut cysts.

Most duplication cysts are asymptomatic and are discovered incidentally while evaluating the esophagus for other pathology. When symptoms do occur, they typically include dysphagia, regurgitation, anorexia, chest pain, wheezing, and cough. Chest radiography may show a posterior mediastinal mass. Barium esophagogram frequently demonstrates a filling defect with smooth edges in the esophagus. Endoscopic examination reveals a submucosal lesion with normal overlying mucosa, which may suggest a diagnosis of the more common leiomyoma. Biopsy should not be performed because it will not penetrate the submucosal location of the mass and may complicate future surgical intervention. Evaluation of duplication cysts with CT provides useful information about the size, location, and relationship to adjacent structures. The most accurate diagnostic modality, however, is EUS. EUS can distinguish cystic lesions from solid masses and shows the relationship to the esophageal wall. Moreover, EUS can differentiate bronchogenic from esophageal duplication cysts, which may not be apparent by CT imaging and can, therefore, be helpful with surgical planning.

Once the diagnosis of esophageal duplication cyst is established, surgical resection is usually indicated because of the potential for serious complications. These complications include compression of surrounding structures, ulceration with subsequent hemorrhage, suppurative infection, and rupture. Early attempts at treatment included marsupialization of the cyst and needle aspiration, but recurrences have been reported following incomplete surgical removal. Because most cysts are located in the right posterior mediastinum, cyst excision is conventionally performed through a posterolateral thoracotomy. Both vagus nerves should be identified and preserved. Similar to surgery for esophageal leiomyomas, extramucosal dissection can usually be performed with the mucosa left intact. The muscle edges should be reapproximated following cyst excision to prevent formation of a pseudodiverticulum. Thoracoscopic resection has recently been demonstrated to be as safe and effective as open surgery in select cases.

BIBLIOGRAPHY

Cioffi U, Bonavina L, Matilde D, et al. Presentation and surgical management of bronchogenic and esophageal duplication cysts in adults. *Chest* 1998;113:1492–1496.

Whitaker JA, Deffenbaugh LD, Cooke AR. Esophageal duplication cyst. *Am J Gastroenterol* 1980;73:329–332.

Ziesat M, Paruch J, Ferguson MK. Overview: anatomy and pathophysiology of benign esophageal disease. In: Sugarbaker DJ, Bueno R, Colson YL, et al., eds. *Adult Chest Surgery*. 2nd ed. New York, NY: McGraw-Hill; 2013: Chapter 28.

23. **(B)** Surgical resection provides the best means of palliation and provides a potential for cure for localized esophageal carcinoma. There are several options for surgical resection; these can be broadly divided into transthoracic and transhiatal approaches. The transthoracic approach can be performed through a single thoracoabdominal incision or separate thoracic and abdominal incisions. The tumor-containing portion of the esophagus and the proximal stomach and regional lymph nodes are resected, and an intrathoracic esophagogastric anastomosis is usually performed. With the transhiatal approach, the entire intrathoracic esophagus is bluntly dissected through upper midline abdominal and neck incisions, thus avoiding a thoracotomy. The stomach is anastomosed to the cervical esophagus above the level of the clavicles.

Both transhiatal and transthoracic approaches have advantages and disadvantages. The most feared complication of a transthoracic procedure with an intrathoracic anastomosis is anastomotic leak. Although this complication is rare in most series, when leak does occur, it is associated with higher morbidity and mortality than leaks that occur in the neck. A leak in a cervical anastomosis can usually be managed conservatively with open drainage to establish a controlled fistula. On the other hand, intrathoracic leaks often require operative intervention, which may include takedown of the anastomosis and diversion through an esophagostomy. The risk of intrathoracic leak can be minimized for transthoracic approaches that involve initial right thoracotomy followed by abdominal and neck incisions by performing a cervical esophagogastric anastomosis or the so-called three-port approach. This approach is mandatory for cancers that involve the mid-to-upper esophagus that are adjacent to the membranous wall of the trachea.

Another disadvantage of the transthoracic approach is the need for both thoracic and abdominal incisions, which may increase postoperative pain and therefore result in more respiratory complications. In addition, the incidence of gastroesophageal reflux may be increased, particularly when performed through a single left thoracoabdominal incision. The disadvantage of the transhiatal approach is limited exposure through the diaphragmatic hiatus, resulting in potential life-threatening injuries to mediastinal structures. In addition, lack of a mediastinal lymph node dissection may result in an incomplete resection of gross disease and early recurrence.

A recent randomized trial comparing extended transthoracic to transhiatal resections for adenocarcinoma in the mid-to-distal esophagus found lower morbidity in transhiatal esophagectomy as compared to transthoracic resection, but there was no significant difference in operative mortality. As both approaches have potential limitations and neither has conclusively been demonstrated superior, the specific approach used should be based on tumor location, tumor extent, and finally surgeon preference.

BIBLIOGRAPHY

Bousamra M, Haasler GB, Parviz M. A decade of experience with transthoracic and transhiatal esophagectomy. *Am J Surg* 2002;183:162–167.

Boyle MJ, Franceschi D, Livingstone AS. Transhiatal versus transthoracic esophagectomy: complication and survival rates. *Am Surg* 1999;65:1137–1141.

Hulscher JBF, van Sandick JW, de Boer AGEM, et al. Extended transthoracic resection compared with limited transhiatal resection for adenocarcinoma of the esophagus. *N Engl J Med* 2002;347:1662–1669.

Maish SM. Esophagus. In: Townsend CM, Beauchamp DR, Evers MB, et al., eds. *Sabiston Textbook of Surgery: The Biological Basis of Modern Surgical Practice.* 19th ed. Philadelphia, PA: Saunders; 2012:1058–1063.

24. **(A)** Ideal candidates for an antireflux operation are patients who show a response to medical therapy but are either unwilling or unable to take daily medications. Antireflux surgery is indicated when medical therapy has failed (usually determined by several months of high-dose PPIs or escalating doses of PPIs), with objectively documented severe reflux, when complications of GERD occur, and in patients who favor a single intervention rather than long-term pharmacologic therapy (e.g., young patients or those with financial considerations). Severe reflux can be objectively documented with a 24-h esophageal pH study, LES incompetence by manometry, or with mucosal changes on endoscopic examination. Complications of GERD include erosive esophagitis, stricture, and Barrett's esophagus. Patients with these abnormalities should undergo fundoplication. In general, patients whose remaining life expectancy exceeds 10 years may avoid costly long-term drug therapy by undergoing antireflux surgery.

The development of a stricture represents failure of medical therapy and is an indication for antireflux surgery. A malignant etiology must be excluded prior to surgery, and dilation may be appropriate. Manometry is especially important in this setting as impaired peristalsis necessitates consideration of a partial fundoplication. With Barrett's metaplasia, antireflux surgery can arrest progression of disease and allow healing of ulceration, although it does not prevent subsequent development of adenocarcinoma. If biopsies show high-grade dysplasia or *in situ* carcinoma, resection should be performed.

A significant proportion of patients with GERD have concomitant respiratory disease, such as asthma. The etiology of respiratory symptoms may be related to aspiration of gastric contents or bronchoconstriction in response to acid in the esophagus. Medical therapy of GERD in patients with asthma improves respiratory symptoms in 25–50% of patients, but fewer than 15% have an objective improvement in pulmonary function. Antireflux surgery, on the other hand, improves respiratory symptoms in nearly 90% of children and 70% of adults and is thus the preferred therapy for patients with asthma and GERD.

BIBLIOGRAPHY

Bowrey DJ, Peters JH, DeMeester TR. Gastroesophageal reflux disease in asthma: effects of medical and surgical antireflux therapy on asthma control. *Ann Surg* 2000;231:161–172.

Peters JH, Little VR, Watson, TJ. Esophageal anatomy and physiology and gastroesophageal reflux disease. In: Mulholland MW, Lillemoe KD, Doherty GM, et al., eds. *Greenfield's Surgery: Scientific Principles and Practice.* 5th ed. Philadelphia, PA: Lippincott Williams & Wilkins; 2011:647–648.

Telem DA, Rattner DW. Gastroesophageal reflux disease. In: Cameron JL, ed. *Current Surgical Therapy.* 10th ed. St. Louis, MO: Mosby; 2011:10–11.

25. **(B)** Ingestion of caustic substances has both immediate and long-term effects on the gastrointestinal tract. Caustic injuries occur most commonly in young children who accidentally swallow these substances and adults who attempt suicide. Corrosive agents include acids, alkalis, bleach, and detergents. Of these, alkalis are most damaging because they produce a liquefactive necrosis that results in deeper tissue penetration. Acids, on the other hand, cause a coagulative necrosis that limits tissue penetration. Hydrofluoric acid is an exception because it produces liquefactive injury similar to alkalis.

Following the ingestion of either acid or alkali, there is reflex pyloric spasm, which prevents passage of the corrosive agent into the duodenum; however, gastric contraction also occurs, which results in regurgitation of the substance back into the esophagus. Meanwhile, the esophagus is vigorously contracting against a closed cricopharyngeus to propel the substance into the stomach. This seesaw activity lasts approximately 3–5 min, after which esophagogastric atony occurs, and the substance passes into the duodenum.

Esophageal injury continues for 24–48 h following exposure to caustic agents. It is during this time that esophageal wall necrosis and subsequent perforation may occur. Inflammatory cells infiltrate the submucosa in the first few days after injury. Granulation tissue forms over sloughing necrotic tissue approximately 10 days postinjury. By the third week, fibroblastic proliferation is present. The fibrosis that occurs results in stricture formation, which represents the most common complication following caustic injury to the esophagus. The amount of fibrosis that occurs is related to the severity of the initial injury. Full-thickness burns or circumferential ulcerations of the esophagus, accordingly, have the highest potential for stricture formation.

Because of the high incidence of stricture formation following severe caustic esophageal injury, prophylactic measures have been attempted. Unfortunately, most, if not all, of these therapies have little proven benefit in preventing strictures. Corticosteroids, esophageal stenting, prophylactic bougienage, and esophageal rest using nasoenteric feeding or parental nutrition have been previously used to prevent stricture formation, but there is little evidence to suggest any benefits. Vigilant anticipation, including patient counseling regarding the possibility of stricture development and reporting any symptoms of dysphagia for early intervention with dilatation is perhaps the best means of managing this late complication.

Another potential consequence of esophageal caustic injury is TEF formation. TEFs usually present within the first few weeks after injury; however, they are less common than simple stricture formation. Symptoms include progressive pneumonia, choking, coughing with feedings, or aspiration of bile-stained mucus from the airway. Hiatal hernia is a late complication that usually occurs many years after caustic injury as a presumed result of esophageal foreshortening. Another long-term complication of esophageal scarring because of caustic injury is malignant degeneration. The incidence of esophageal carcinoma is 1000-fold greater after caustic injury than in the general population.

BIBLIOGRAPHY

Hugh TB, Kelly MD. Corrosive injection and the surgeon. *J Am Coll Surg* 1999;189:508–522.

Kikendall JW. Caustic ingestion injuries. *Gastroenterol Clin North Am* 1991;20:847–857.

Maish SM. Esophagus. In: Townsend CM, Beauchamp DR, Evers MB, et al., eds. *Sabiston Textbook of Surgery: The Biological Basis of Modern Surgical Practice.* 19th ed. Philadelphia, PA: Saunders; 2012:1058–1063.

26. **(E)** The main barrier to reflux of gastric contents into the esophagus is the LES. The sphincter mechanism is not an anatomically distinct structure but is formed from the intrinsic smooth muscle of the distal esophagus and the skeletal muscle of the crural diaphragm. The LES normally has a resting baseline pressure greater than the baseline pressure of the stomach. When this high-pressure zone is compromised, reflux of gastric contents occurs. The tonic resistance of the LES is a function of both its pressure and the overall length over which this pressure is exerted. The shorter the length, the higher the pressure must be to maintain sufficient resistance for the sphincter to be competent.

Thus, an abnormally short length of high-pressure zone can lead to significant reflux even with normal LES pressures. For example, gastric distention causes the sphincter length to shorten, thus decreasing the pressure threshold for reflux to occur. This accounts for postprandial symptoms seen early in the course of disease. Transient increases in intra-abdominal pressure may also overcome LES pressure and result in reflux.

Transient relaxation of the LES occurs in everyone, but not everyone develops clinically significant reflux because of the existence of other defense mechanisms. Gravity and esophageal peristalsis play a large role in limiting the contact time between gastric contents and the esophageal mucosa. Salivary gland secretions help buffer the acidic contents of gastric reflux, and secretions from esophageal submucosal glands also provide additional buffering to restore neutral pH in the esophageal lumen. Esophageal submucosal glands secrete mucus that contains a high concentration of bicarbonate, and secretory activity occurs in response to acidification of the esophageal lumen.

BIBLIOGRAPHY

Long JD, Orlando RC. Esophageal submucosal glands: structure and function. *Am J Gastroenterol* 1999;94:2818–2824.

Mittal RK, Balaban DH. Mechanisms of disease: the esophagogastric junction. *N Engl J Med* 1997;336:924–932.

Peters JH, Little VR, Watson, TJ. Esophageal anatomy and physiology and gastroesophageal reflux disease. In: Mulholland MW, Lillemoe KD, Doherty GM, et al., eds. *Greenfield's Surgery: Scientific Principles and Practice.* 5th ed. Philadelphia, PA: Lippincott Williams & Wilkins; 2011:647–648.

27. **(A)** The barium esophagogram demonstrates a type III paraesophageal hernia, where both gastric cardia and the gastroesophageal junction are displaced above the diaphragmatic hiatus. As a paraesophageal hernia develops, the stomach commonly rotates around its longitudinal axis so that the anterior and posterior walls of the gastric body are transposed. A volvulus may develop with upward displacement of the cardia.

Many patients with paraesophageal hernia may be asymptomatic or complain of mild symptoms, such as postprandial fullness, bloating, epigastric or substernal discomfort, and nausea. Symptoms of gastroesophageal reflux are commonly associated with paraesophageal hernia. Complications may result from gastric incarceration, pulmonary compromise from decreased lung expansion or aspiration, and bleeding from mechanical or ischemic gastric ulcerations. The risk of complications justifies surgical repair in most cases of paraesophageal hernia. Certainly, if gastric incarceration is suspected, then emergent surgery is indicated. Barium swallow is diagnostic, and chest roentgenogram occasionally shows an air-fluid level behind the cardiac silhouette.

Once identified, paraesophageal hernias should be surgically repaired. This can be performed through a transabdominal or transthoracic approach, and laparoscopic repair has recently been shown to be equally effective and safe compared to open repair. Surgical repair consists of hernia reduction, crural closure, and fundoplication. The need for fundoplication is controversial, but many authors advocate its inclusion for several reasons. Of patients with paraesophageal hernia, 60 to 70% have increased esophageal exposure to gastric acid based on 24-h pH monitoring. It is also difficult to adequately assess the presence of GERD in all patients with paraesophageal hernia, especially those presenting on an emergent basis. Finally, dissection at the gastroesophageal junction may lead to postoperative reflux.

BIBLIOGRAPHY

Landreneau RJ, Del Pino M, Santos R. Management of paraesophageal hernias. *Surg Clin North Am* 2005 Jun;85(3):411–432.
Maish SM. Esophagus. In: Townsend CM, Beauchamp DR, Evers MB, et al., eds. *Sabiston Textbook of Surgery: The Biological Basis of Modern Surgical Practice.* 19th ed. Philadelphia, PA: Saunders; 2012:1058–1063.

28. **(E)** The distribution of arterial blood supply to the esophagus is segmental based on embryologic development. The cervical esophagus receives its blood supply from branches of the inferior thyroid artery. The bronchial arteries supply the upper portion of the thoracic esophagus, and the midthoracic esophagus is supplied by vessels directly originating from the descending thoracic aorta. The lower thoracic and intra-abdominal esophagus is nourished by branches of the left gastric and inferior phrenic arteries. There is often a communicating vessel between the inferior phrenic and left gastric arteries, commonly referred to as Belsey's artery. Branches from these arteries run within the muscularis propria and give rise to branches that course within the submucosa. There are extensive anastomoses, which account for the rarity of esophageal infarction. Mobilization of the distal esophagus must be approached with extreme caution to avoid injury to the arterial branches originating from the left gastric and inferior phrenic systems. This is especially important with left thoracotomy approaches as these vessels may retract beneath the diaphragm before they are adequately controlled (Fig. 17-16).

Venous drainage of the esophagus occurs through an extensive submucosal venous plexus. The submucosal plexus communicates through perforating branches with longitudinally oriented veins on the outer esophageal surface. Branches from the upper two-thirds of the esophagus lead into the inferior thyroid vein and azygous system, with eventual drainage into the superior vena cava. The lower esophagus drains into the left gastric veins and short gastric veins, which are part of the portal venous system. The caval and portal systems thus communicate through the submucosal veins. Portal hypertension may lead to dilations of the submucosal plexus, which are commonly referred to as esophageal varices.

BIBLIOGRAPHY

Ebright MI, Krasna MJ. Overview of esophageal and proximal stomach malignancy. In: Sugarbaker DJ, Bueno R, Colson YL, et al., eds. *Adult Chest Surgery.* 2nd ed. New York, NY: McGraw-Hill; 2013; Chapter 10.
Lerut T, Coosemans W, Decaluwé H, et al. Anatomy of the esophagus. In: Fischer JE, Jones DB, et al., eds. *Mastery of Surgery.* 6th ed. Philadelphia, PA: Lippincott Williams & Wilkins; 2011:670.
Peters JH, Little VR, Watson, TJ. Esophageal anatomy and physiology and gastroesophageal reflux disease. In: Mulholland MW, Lillemoe KD, Doherty GM, et al., eds. *Greenfield's Surgery: Scientific Principles and Practice.* 5th ed. Philadelphia, PA: Lippincott Williams & Wilkins; 2011:647–648.

29. **(E)** Esophageal cancer exhibits aggressive behavior, initially spreading along the extensive submucosal lymphatic channels and then frequently involving regional lymph nodes. More distant lymph node involvement, such as of cervical or celiac nodes, is currently considered metastatic disease. The primary tumor may directly extend into adjacent structures, such as the aorta, trachea, diaphragm, and lung. The most common sites for distant metastases are the liver, lung, and pleura.

Esophageal cancer with evidence of metastatic disease equates to unresectable stage IVb disease, and any treatment will be palliative, with an expected survival of only 3–6 months. Although surgical resection can be used for palliation of malignant dysphagia, the morbidity and mortality associated with surgery make it a less-than-ideal option. Radiation therapy can be administered externally or via an endoluminal catheter (brachytherapy) and may provide some relief of dysphagia. One to two months may be required for appreciable symptom improvement, and potential complications include radiation-induced esophagitis with persistent dysphagia. Of note, chemoradiation therapy usually provides the better long-term palliation as compared to radiation therapy alone but would be poorly tolerated in a patient nearly 80 years of age with significant weight loss.

Endoscopic intubation and stenting provide excellent relief of dysphagia. Plastic stents were commonly used

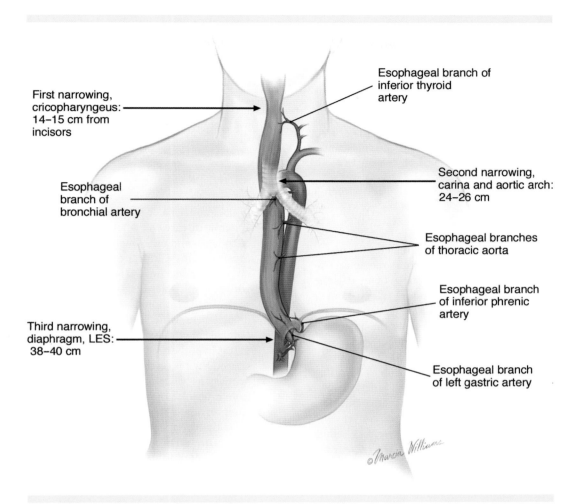

First narrowing,
cricopharyngeus:
14–15 cm from
incisors

Esophageal branch of
inferior thyroid
artery

Esophageal
branch of
bronchial artery

Second narrowing,
carina and aortic arch:
24–26 cm

Esophageal branches
of thoracic aorta

Esophageal branch
of inferior phrenic
artery

Third narrowing,
diaphragm, LES:
38–40 cm

Esophageal branch
of left gastric artery

FIGURE 17-16. Arterial blood supply of the esophagus (from D.J. Sugarbaker, R. Bueno, Y. L. Colson, M. T. Jaklitsch, M. J. Krasna, S. J. Mentzer, M. Williams, A. Adams: Adult Chest Surgery. 2nd ed. New York, NY: McGraw Hill; 2013: Fig. 10-2. Copyright © The McGraw-Hill Companies, Inc. All rights reserved).

prior to 1990, with mixed results. The internal diameters were usually less than 12 mm, and they required initial dilation of the malignant stricture to accommodate the large external diameters. Over the past decade, self-expanding metallic stents have become available for palliation of unresectable esophageal tumors. They are easier to insert, have larger internal diameters, and are less likely to cause perforation than the older plastic stents. They can expand as the tumor shrinks with concurrent use of other therapies, and silicone coatings prevent tumor ingrowth. Self-expanding metal stents provide excellent relief of malignant dysphagia and are the treatment of choice for malignant TEF. Complications include bleeding, perforation, and distal migration. Care must be taken to avoid placement of stents across the gastroesophageal junction as this may lead to gastroesophageal reflux.

Photodynamic therapy is a recent development that uses a photosensitive compound that is activated by laser energy at a specific wavelength, thus generating cytotoxic singlet oxygen, causing cell death. Malignant cells selectively retain the photosensitive agent hematoporphyrin, which is given intravenously 48–72 h prior to endoscopic application of laser energy. Once activated, the singlet oxygen generated kills neoplastic cells, resulting in tumor slough. The depth of tissue injury is usually between 2 and 5 mm, and multiple sessions may be required to achieve an adequate clinical response. The most common complication is photosensitizer-induced skin injury, which occurs when patients are exposed to radiant heat, such as sunlight or strong fluorescent lighting, within 30 days of treatment.

BIBLIOGRAPHY

Lada MJ, Peters JH. The management of esophageal carcinoma. In: Cameron JL, ed. *Current Surgical Therapy.* 10th ed. St. Louis, MO: Mosby; 2011:47–54.

Kucharczuk JC, Kaiser LR. Esophageal injury, diverticula, and neoplasms. In: Mulholland MW, Lillemoe KD, Doherty GM, et al., eds. *Greenfield's Surgery: Scientific Principles and Practice.* 5th ed. Philadelphia, PA: Lippincott Williams & Wilkins; 2011:629–648.

Schuchert MJ, Go C, Luketich JD. Esophageal stents. In: Cameron JL, ed. *Current Surgical Therapy,* 10th ed. St. Louis, MO: Mosby; 2011:58–64.

Weigel TL, Frumiento C, Gaumintz E. Endoluminal palliation for dysphagia secondary to esophageal carcinoma. *Surg Clin North Am* 2002;82:747–761.

30. **(E)** It has been estimated that approximately 10% of patients with GERD will develop Barrett's metaplasia. Barrett's esophagus has traditionally been defined as the presence of columnar mucosa extending at least 3 cm into the esophagus. Recent studies have shown that specialized intestinal-type epithelium has the potential to degenerate into dysplasia and subsequently adenocarcinoma, which may occur in segments of columnar mucosa shorter than 3 cm. The progression to Barrett's esophagus begins at the gastroesophageal junction, where repetitive exposure of distal esophageal squamous mucosa to gastric acid results in metaplasic conversion to gastric-type epithelium. As the severity of reflux increases, the length of columnar metaplasia increases, and intestinal metaplasia may develop. Current evidence supports the role of duodenal contents in the pathogenesis of Barrett's metaplasia. Studies have shown that esophageal bile acid exposure is increased in patients with Barrett's esophagus, and bile acid gastritis is associated with an increased incidence of Barrett's metaplasia.

The diagnosis of Barrett's esophagus is made on endoscopy and biopsy. Endoscopically, columnar mucosa has a salmon-pink appearance, in contrast to the pearly white appearance of squamous epithelium. Barrett's is suspected when this salmon-pink columnar mucosa extends, often with flame-shaped projections, into the white squamous epithelium, above the gastroesophageal junction. Histologic examination may show gastric fundic-type epithelium, gastric junctional-type epithelium, or specialized columnar epithelium that has a villiform surface and contains goblet cells. The presence of goblet cells differentiates specialized columnar cells from normal columnar cells and is the hallmark of intestinal metaplasia.

The role of *H. pylori* in gastritis and peptic ulcer disease has been well documented. Several authors reported an inverse relationship of *H. pylori* with the development of reflux esophagitis, Barrett's esophagus, dysplasia, and adenocarcinoma. In particular, they speculated that the cagA+ strain of *H. pylori* is associated with a lower incidence of esophageal mucosal disease.

BIBLIOGRAPHY

Oksanen A, Sipponen P, Karttunen R, et al. Inflammation and intestinal metaplasia at the squamocolumnar junction in young patients with or without *Helicobacter pylori* infection. *Gut* 2003;52:194–198.

Spechler SJ, Souza RF. Barrett's esophagus. *N Engl J Med* 2014 Aug 28;371(9):836-845.

31. **(C)** Scleroderma or progressive systemic sclerosis is a systemic disease characterized by excessive deposition of collagen and other matrix elements in skin and other organ systems. Clinically significant gastrointestinal involvement occurs in approximately 50% of all patients with systemic sclerosis. In addition, many patients with scleroderma without GI symptoms have subclinical involvement, which is documented by abnormalities on esophageal motility testing.

It is hypothesized that gastrointestinal involvement by scleroderma is secondary to either vascular ischemia or primary nerve damage. Neural dysfunction may result from arteriolar changes in the vasa nervorum or by compression of nerve fibers by collagen deposition. Vascular changes mainly involve the small arteries, which demonstrate a mononuclear inflammatory response. Subsequent fibroblastic changes induce severe sclerosis of the intima of the small arteries and interstitium. The vascular and neurogenic changes result in smooth muscle atrophy, which is the basis for the clinical features of scleroderma. Muscle function is diminished but capable of responding early in the disease process, during which time treatment with prokinetic drugs may be beneficial. As the disease progresses, muscle fibrosis occurs, and muscle function is permanently lost.

The esophagus is the most frequently involved gastrointestinal organ in scleroderma. The primary manifestation of esophageal involvement in scleroderma is GERD. Several mechanisms contribute to the development of reflux. Decreased LES pressure results in an increased frequency of reflux, and impaired peristalsis prevents clearance of refluxed material back into the stomach. Furthermore, many patients with scleroderma have a coexistent sicca syndrome and therefore have reduced acid-neutralizing capacity of swallowed saliva. Current evidence suggests that disordered motility is the primary abnormality contributing to GERD in scleroderma.

In patients with scleroderma, GERD is more likely to result in complications such as erosive esophagitis, Barrett's esophagus, and strictures. Manometric findings of low LES pressures and low-amplitude peristalsis have been found to correlate with the development of esophagitis. Endoscopy should be routinely performed in patients with scleroderma with reflux to evaluate for Barrett's metaplasia. Although 24-h ambulatory pH testing is highly sensitive in the diagnosis of GERD, it is not necessary when there is documented abnormal manometry or endoscopic findings.

Treatment of GERD in patients with scleroderma is similar to treatment of patients without scleroderma. First-line therapy consists of behavioral modification and antisecretory drugs or prokinetic agents. Prokinetic agents are beneficial earlier in the disease process, prior to muscle fibrosis. If medical therapy fails, antireflux surgery may be considered. Although usually extremely effective in the treatment of GERD, results of antireflux surgery in patients with scleroderma are not as promising. The esophageal motor dysfunction makes it challenging to create a wrap that is sufficient to prevent reflux, yet not too tight to cause dysphagia. Furthermore, chronic inflammation and fibrosis often result in esophageal shortening, which may necessitate an esophageal lengthening procedure.

BIBLIOGRAPHY

Bassotti G, Battaglia E, Debernardi V, et al. Esophageal dysfunction in scleroderma: relationship with disease subsets. *Arthritis Rheum* 1997;40:2252–2259.

Ling TC, Johnston BT. Esophageal investigations in connective tissue disease: which tests are most appropriate? *J Clin Gastroenterol* 2001;32:33–36.

Rose S, Young MA, Reynolds JC. Gastrointestinal manifestations of scleroderma. *Gastroenterol Clin North Am* 1998;27:563–594.

Sjogren RW. Gastrointestinal motility disorders in scleroderma. *Arthritis Rheum* 1994;37:1265–1282.

32. **(B)**

33. **(E)** Esophageal perforation is commonly a life-threatening emergency. Successful management relies on prompt recognition and initiation of treatment. Delay in diagnosis results in increased morbidity and mortality and can affect the choice of therapy. The majority of perforations (60%) are iatrogenic following endoscopy, esophageal dilatations, difficult endotracheal intubations, and other forms of instrumentation. Trauma accounts for approximately 20% of esophageal perforations and spontaneous rupture for another 15%. Boerhaave's syndrome, emetogenic perforation of the esophagus, is caused by forceful or increased intra-abdominal pressure. Symptoms vary according to the location of perforation, size of the perforation, and time duration since injury. Cervical perforations may present with neck pain, dysphagia, and odynophagia. Palpation of the neck may reveal crepitus. Thoracic perforations may present with substernal or epigastric pain as well as dysphagia. Abdominal perforations usually present with epigastric pain radiating to the back or left shoulder with signs of peritoneal irritation. Without treatment, frank sepsis and respiratory failure may develop.

The plain chest radiograph may appear normal early after esophageal perforation. Radiographic findings suggestive of perforation, however, include pneumomediastinum, subcutaneous emphysema, pleural effusion, and hydropneumothorax. The diagnostic study of choice in any patient suspected of having an esophageal perforation is a contrast radiograph of the esophagus. A water-soluble contrast esophagogram followed by barium, if necessary, is diagnostic in 90% of patients. CT scan of the chest and upper abdomen with oral contrast is also being used with more frequency. The site of perforation can often be defined on chest CT, as well as any areas of mediastinal or pleural space fluid collections that require drainage.

Treatment of esophageal perforation should be tailored to each individual patient. Factors to consider include the location of perforation, the extent of tissue necrosis, time interval since injury, and the presence of underlying esophageal disease. If an esophageal perforation is suspected, immediate treatment should begin with cessation of all oral intake, intravenous fluid resuscitation, gastric decompression, and broad-spectrum antibiotic therapy to cover both aerobic and anaerobic organisms.

In the stable patient with mild symptoms and a well-contained leak on esophagogram, nonoperative management can be successful. Patients meeting these criteria can be managed with cessation of oral intake, total parenteral nutrition, and antibiotics. If there is evidence of pleural contamination, such as the scenario in question 33, drainage of pleural contents can be performed via placement of a chest tube or video-assisted thoracoscopic decortication. A repeat esophagogram is performed in 7–14 days. Oral intake may be resumed following resolution or stabilization of the leak. Signs of clinical deterioration with conservative management should prompt surgical intervention.

In the absence of underlying esophageal pathology such as malignancy, primary repair with drainage of the contaminated area should be initially considered. This option is best suited for patients with early presentation demonstrating hemodynamic stability and minimal contamination. Primary repair is performed by exposing the entire length of mucosal injury, debriding any nonviable tissue, and closing the defect in two layers. The submucosal layer can frequently be stapled followed by interrupted suture closure of the muscular wall. The suture line can then be reinforced with a flap of parietal pleura, intercostal muscle, or gastric fundus (Fig. 17-17). When perforation is associated with underlying esophageal disease, any pathology causing distal obstruction must

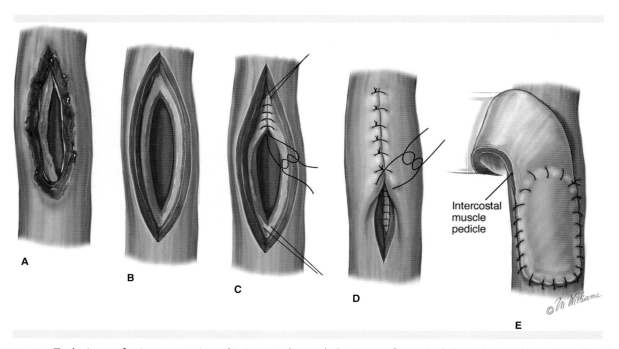

FIGURE 17-17. Technique of primary repair and intercostal muscle buttress of a typical thoracic esophageal perforation. A. The mucosa is often torn further underneath the muscle tear. B. The muscle tear is opened further to expose the limits of the mucosal tear, and both are debrided back to healthy tissue. C. The mucosa is closed with fine 4-0 absorbable sutures with knots tied on the inside. D. The muscle is closed in a second layer. E. An intercostal muscle is carefully sutured around the circumference of the repair site to provide a third layer of protection (from D.J. Sugarbaker, R. Bueno, Y. L. Colson, M. T. Jaklitsch, M. J. Krasna, S. J. Mentzer, M. Williams, A. Adams: *Adult Chest Surgery.* 2nd ed. New York, NY: McGraw Hill; 2013: Fig. 48-9. Copyright © The McGraw-Hill Companies, Inc. All rights reserved).

be addressed to prevent breakdown of a primary repair. In the setting of achalasia, a distal esophagomyotomy on the side opposite of the perforation should be performed in addition to primary repair and partial gastric fundoplication buttress of the perforation site.

Perforations accompanied by esophageal malignancy or severe contaminations are best treated with esophageal resection. Proximal drainage through a cervical esophagostomy (so-called spit fistula) and a feeding tube are appropriate in anticipation of a delayed reconstruction. In the setting of hemodynamic instability or frank sepsis, the patient may not tolerate a lengthy procedure. In this situation, esophageal stent placement should be considered. The introduction of expandable bare metal stents changed the management paradigm in this patient population. Increased experience with stents has led to expanded use in patients presenting with iatrogenic perforations, particularly after delayed presentation and in those with significant associated mediastinal/pleural contamination. Although their initial use was problematic due to difficulties associated with removal of uncovered metal stents (mucosal ingrowth), several small prospective series demonstrated the utility of stents as a

primary treatment option for these patients.
This indication has been expanded to included patients following early presentation who traditionally have reasonable outcomes with open surgical repair. The introduction of covered, removable, self-expanding stent technology that is easily deployed, restricts mucosal ingrowth, and is adjustable if migration does occur has led to widespread use by thoracic surgeons for both iatrogenic and benign esophageal perforations.

BIBLIOGRAPHY

Blasberg JD, Wright CD. Management of esophageal perforation. In: Sugarbaker DJ, Bueno R, Colson YL, et al., eds. *Adult Chest Surgery.* 2nd ed. New York, NY: McGraw-Hill; 2013:48.

Maish SM. Esophagus. In: Townsend CM, Beauchamp DR, Evers MB, et al., eds. *Sabiston Textbook of Surgery: The Biological Basis of Modern Surgical Practice.* 19th ed. Philadelphia, PA: Saunders; 2012:1058–1063.

Zumbro GL, Anstadt MP, Mawulawde K, et al. Surgical management of esophageal perforation: role of esophageal conservation in delayed perforation. *Am Surg* 2002;68:36–40.

CHAPTER 18

STOMACH

NÉHA DATTA AND O. JOE HINES

QUESTIONS

1. Which of the following statements concerning vascular anatomy of the stomach is most accurate?
   - (A) The left gastric artery mainly supplies the greater curvature of the stomach.
   - (B) Occlusion of the left gastroepiploic and left gastric arteries is likely to result in clinically significant gastric ischemia.
   - (C) Bleeding gastric ulcers are often the result of posterior erosion into the gastroduodenal artery.
   - (D) Both the short gastric arteries and the left gastro-epiploic artery arise from the splenic artery in the majority of patients.

2. Which of the following statements is correct?
   - (A) The right vagus nerve gives off a branch to the liver.
   - (B) Sensation of gastric pain occurs through both vagus nerves.
   - (C) The majority of vagal fibers are motor or secretory efferents.
   - (D) The left vagal trunk winds around the esophagus and rests along the anterior surface of the esophagus after exiting the esophageal hiatus.

3. Which of the following best describes the effects of parietal cell vagotomy, in a previously normal stomach, assuming no other procedure is performed in addition to the vagotomy?
   - (A) Both liquids and solids would empty significantly faster.
   - (B) Both liquids and solids would empty significantly slower.
   - (C) Liquids would empty significantly faster, whereas the emptying rate of solids would not change significantly.
   - (D) Solids would empty significantly faster, whereas the emptying rate of liquids would not change significantly.

4. Which of the following statements concerning gastric acid secretion is *false*?
   - (A) Truncal vagotomy eliminates the cephalic phase of gastric acid secretion.
   - (B) Gastrin is the most important mediator of gastric acid secretion during the gastric phase.
   - (C) Histamine stimulates acid secretion by parietal cells.
   - (D) Parietal cells lack receptors for somatostatin.

5. Which of the following statements concerning gastrin is most accurate?
   - (A) Gastrin in high levels induces gastric mucosal hypertrophy.
   - (B) Glucose in a meal is the most potent stimulator of gastrin release.
   - (C) Gastrin-secreting cells (G cells) are found only in the gastric antrum and pylorus.
   - (D) Regular administration of antacids suppresses gastrin release.
   - (E) Omeprazole, a proton pump inhibitor (PPI), can completely suppress gastrin secretion when taken for a minimum of 2 weeks.

6. Which of the following events is *not* an essential step for acid production by parietal cells?
   - (A) Entry of one K^+ ion into the parietal cell for every H^+ released into the stomach lumen
   - (B) Hydrolysis of adenosine triphosphate (ATP) into adenosine diphosphate (ADP) and inorganic phosphate
   - (C) Inhibition of carbonic anhydrase
   - (D) Exchange of HCO_3^- for Cl^- at the basolateral membrane

7. Which of the following statements concerning *Helicobacter pylori* is most accurate?
   (A) *Helicobacter pylori* organisms bind only to gastric-type epithelium.
   (B) The majority of persons harboring *H. pylori* in their stomachs become symptomatic.
   (C) *Helicobacter pylori* organisms directly stimulate G cells to secrete gastrin, thereby increasing acid secretion.
   (D) Recurrence of duodenal ulceration after treatment for *H. pylori* infection approaches 25%.

8. Which of the following is *not* a sucralfate mechanism of action?
   (A) The negatively charged sucralfate polyanions bind positively charged proteins exposed in mucosal lesions.
   (B) Sucralfate stimulates the production of mucus, prostaglandin E2, and bicarbonate.
   (C) Sucralfate is absorbed systemically via the gastric mucosa to counter the effects of nonsteroidal anti-inflammatory drug (NSAID) use.
   (D) Sucralfate polymerizes in an acidic environment, allowing it to bind with bile salts.

9. Choose the least-appropriate combination of diagnostic test for *H. pylori* and clinical situation:
   (A) Performing the urea breath test to detect the presence of *H. pylori* in a 28-year-old otherwise-healthy male after he undergoes 12 weeks of therapy with omeprazole, clarithromycin, and amoxicillin for biopsy-proven infection
   (B) Performing antral mucosal biopsy and subsequent histologic examination for *H. pylori* organisms in a 63-year-old female with a finding of diffuse gastritis while undergoing endoscopy for epigastric pain
   (C) Performing endoscopy and antral mucosal biopsy, with subsequent histologic examination for *H. pylori* organisms, in a 35-year-old female who had a "normal" endoscopy 2 weeks ago in which biopsies were not taken
   (D) Performing repeat endoscopy with antral mucosal biopsy, with subsequent histologic examination and bacterial culture for sensitivity, in a 28-year-old otherwise-healthy male who has persistent *H. pylori* infection as detected by urea breath test after 8 weeks of therapy with omeprazole, clarithromycin, and amoxicillin

10. A 31-year-old man presents to the emergency room with nausea, vomiting, and two bouts of hematemesis over the last 24 hours. He is currently in stable condition. His past medical history is significant for a previous admission 2 months ago for hematemesis, which resolved after endoscopic coagulation. Twice within the past 2 years, he has been diagnosed by endoscopy with a duodenal ulcer and twice has failed medical therapy because of noncompliance with triple therapy (omeprazole, clarithromycin, amoxicillin). Endoscopy at this admission reveals no active bleeding and an inability to pass the endoscope past the edematous pylorus. The most appropriate therapy for this patient is as follows:
    (A) Urgent surgical exploration of the upper abdomen with vagotomy and pyloroplasty to relieve pyloric obstruction
    (B) Seven-day trial of nasogastric suction and intravenous H_2 receptor antagonists
    (C) Supportive care, including intravenous H_2 receptor antagonists, for 24 h, then elective vagotomy and antrectomy
    (D) Gastric lavage with at least 10 L of ice-cold saline

11. Which of the following statements is most accurate concerning the three most commonly performed duodenal ulcer surgeries: parietal cell vagotomy, truncal vagotomy with pyloroplasty, and truncal vagotomy with antrectomy?
    (A) Parietal cell vagotomy has the lowest ulcer recurrence rate among the three.
    (B) Truncal vagotomy with antrectomy is technically the least demanding and is the quickest to perform in an emergency situation.
    (C) Parietal cell vagotomy is associated with the lowest occurrence of postoperative dumping syndrome.
    (D) All three procedures involve severing the celiac and hepatic divisions of the vagus nerves.

12. A 65-year-old man with past medical history significant for diet-controlled diabetes mellitus and rheumatoid arthritis, for which he takes indomethacin, presents to his primary care physician with a several-month history of slowly worsening, vague epigastric pain. Referral to an endoscopist reveals mild antral gastritis and a shallow, 2-cm ulcer at the lesser curvature. The remainder of the endoscopic examination was unremarkable. Which of the following is *least* important in the care of this patient?
    (A) Endoscopic biopsies of the ulcer margin
    (B) Medical therapy to eradicate *H. pylori* after histologic analysis of antral biopsies demonstrate the organism
    (C) Referral to a surgeon for performance of an elective parietal cell vagotomy
    (D) Cessation of indomethacin

13. The patient in question 12 is prescribed a 2-week regimen of triple-drug therapy (omeprazole, clarithromycin, and amoxicillin) after histologic analysis demonstrated infection with *H. pylori*. He is also instructed to discontinue indomethacin.

The pathologist's report concerning the two biopsies of the ulcer states "necrotic tissue with prominent lymphocytic infiltration." After completing the triple-drug therapy, the patient is pain free. Six months later, the patient is seen at follow-up and complains of the same epigastric pain. Urea breath test reveals that he is no longer infected with *H. pylori*. He is again referred for endoscopy, which reveals a shallow, 4-cm ulcer at the lesser curvature. Three biopsies are taken off the ulcer margins. The pathology report states "gastric epithelium with possibly dysplastic features—cannot rule out malignancy." The next most appropriate step is

(A) Repeat endoscopy with additional ulcer margin biopsies

(B) Distal gastrectomy, including entire ulcer with 4-cm margins

(C) Distal gastrectomy, including entire ulcer with 4-cm margins, and truncal vagotomy

(D) Parietal cell vagotomy and ulcer excision with 6-cm margins

14. Type II gastric ulcers

(A) Account for the majority of gastric ulcers and occur along the lesser curvature toward the incisura

(B) Occur in the body of the stomach concurrently with a duodenal ulcer in the setting of gastric acid oversecretion

(C) Occur along the lesser curvature near the gastroesophageal junction in the setting of normal-to-low gastric acid secretion

(D) Occur at any location and are associated with NSAID use

15. A 55-year-old female journalist presents to the local emergency room complaining of severe epigastric pain. This pain started suddenly about 2 h ago, while preparing an article due in 2 days. She states that it is the worst pain she has ever experienced, and it is not getting any better. She has no past medical history and has not seen a doctor since the birth of her youngest child at 32 years of age. She occasionally uses regular-strength Tylenol for a headache. On physical examination, she has a rigid abdomen and avoids movement. An upright chest radiograph shows a thin stripe of free air under the right hemidiaphragm. Your next step is

(A) Computed tomography (CT) of the abdomen with oral and intravenous contrast

(B) Open distal gastrectomy with Billroth II reconstruction

(C) Laparoscopic truncal vagotomy with pyloroplasty and oversewing of the perforation

(D) Laparoscopic exploration and repair of the perforation with Graham patch

16. Regardless of what step you chose in question 15, it is now 6 h later, and the patient is under general anesthesia on the operating table. You perform an abdominal exploration through a vertical upper midline abdominal incision and find a 3-mm hole in the anterior portion of the second portion of the duodenum. There is minimal inflammation and scant soiling of the peritoneum with intestinal fluid. Which of the following statements is most appropriate?

(A) This problem could not have been adequately diagnosed and treated laparoscopically.

(B) The procedure of choice is suture closure of the duodenal perforation and suturing a well-vascularized portion of omentum over the repair.

(C) Because of the small size of perforation and minimal contamination, this patient probably should have undergone observation.

(D) The procedure of choice is a suture closure of the duodenal perforation and suturing a well-vascularized portion of omentum over the repair plus parietal cell vagotomy.

17. A 44-year-old male automotive mechanic remains in the surgical intensive care unit after sustaining second- and third-degree burns to 45% of his body 4 days ago. He is sedated and on mechanical ventilation and is receiving tube feedings via a transoral duodenal feeding tube. He underwent debridement with xenograft (porcine) skin grafting over his chest yesterday. He received four units of blood during and immediately after surgery and is in stable condition. This morning, while performing a regular nasogastric check for gastric reflux of tube feedings, the nurse notices a small amount of blood in the nasogastric return. A serum hemoglobin value is checked and returns 12.5 mg/dL, similar to his posttransfusion hemoglobin value yesterday evening. Six hours later, the nurse reports copious amounts of blood from the nasogastric tube. The patient's stomach is lavaged with 6 L of warm saline via the nasogastric tube, without any return of blood afterward. Which of the following is an important step in management?

(A) Arrangement for endoscopic examination within 48 hours

(B) Transfusion of 4 units of typed and crossmatched packed red blood cells

(C) Initiation of intravenous vasopressin, continued for 48 h

(D) Laboratory evaluation of coagulation by measuring prothrombin time, activated partial thromboplastin time, and platelet count

18. Continuing with the same patient as in questions 16 and 17, within 1 h of the stomach lavage, the nasogastric tube again returns copious, bright red blood. Coagulation test results return from the lab and are within normal limits. The stomach is again lavaged with warm saline to prepare for endoscopy, which reveals multiple bleeding points from the fundus and proximal body. The bleeding is too profuse to be managed endoscopically, despite several attempts of coagulation and epinephrine injection. The patient becomes mildly hypotensive and tachycardic, and his arterial oxygen saturation has fallen somewhat. A successful attempt at resuscitation is made with transfusion of 4 units of packed red blood cells, and the patient is currently normotensive and only slightly tachycardic (110 bpm). The most appropriate next step would be

(A) Selective cannulation of the left gastric artery via interventional radiology techniques, with continuous infusion of vasopressin into the left gastric artery for 48 h

(B) Surgical gastrotomy and oversewing of the bleeding gastric ulcers

(C) Surgical devascularization of the stomach by ligating the left and right gastric and gastroepiploic arteries

(D) Tamponade of the gastric ulcers with a Sengstaken-Blakemore tube

19. A 67-year-old male patient undergoes upper endoscopy as part of a workup for fecal occult hemoglobin. The only finding is a bulge, approximately 4 cm in diameter and slightly protuberant, with a small central dimple on the anterior body of the stomach. Four biopsies are taken from different areas of this bulge. Pathologic examination of biopsy specimens reveals only normal gastric mucosa. A CT scan of the abdomen is obtained to better define this abnormality, and it reveals a discreet, 5 cm by 5 cm mass that appears to be entirely within the wall of the stomach body anteriorly (Fig. 18-1). There is no apparent lymphadenopathy. The patient undergoes elective abdominal exploration, and a distal gastrectomy with inclusion of the mass with 2-cm margins is performed with gastroduodenotomy. Pathologic histologic analysis reveals "interlacing bundles of elongated cells with spindle-shaped nuclei." Which of the following statements is true regarding this tumor?

(A) Enucleation would have been the preferred surgical therapy.

(B) Surgery would have been appropriately abandoned if abdominal exploration revealed three 0.5-cm liver metastases, proven by frozen section.

(C) Five-year survival for all presentations is greater than 30%.

(D) This tumor is relatively resistant to radiation therapy.

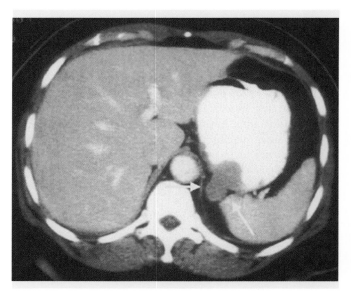

FIGURE 18-1. Computed tomographic scan of a lesion of the stomach.

20. A 55-year-old male patient who underwent truncal vagotomy and antrectomy with gastroduodenostomy (Billroth I) for recalcitrant duodenal ulcer disease 3 years ago is referred to you with worsening epigastric pain. The pain is burning and almost always present, sometimes worsening with food. He has lost an estimated 30 lb, and his primary care physician is no longer willing to prescribe narcotics for pain control until he is further evaluated. He complains of occasional vomiting, but these episodes do not relieve his pain. Of the following investigations, which should be performed first?

(A) Measurement of serum gastrin level

(B) Endoscopy with instillation of Congo red dye

(C) Trial of omeprazole (proton pump inhibitor) for 2 weeks

(D) Nuclear medicine ^{99m}Tc hepatic iminodiacetic acid (HIDA) scan

21. The patient in question 21 undergoes upper endoscopy. Findings include mucosal erythema and friability throughout the remaining stomach, three small ulcers near the gastroduodenal anastomotic line with signs of recent hemorrhage, and a small pool of bile in the dependent stomach. Biopsies are taken of several sites of the stomach. Instillation of Congo red dye and intravenous pentagastrin reveals no black color within 10 min of instillation. Histologic examination of the biopsy specimens reveals intestinal metaplasia of gastric glands, a paucity of parietal cells, and an increase in the number of mucin cells usually seen. Which one of the

following statements about this patient and his condition is *false*?

(A)   A Roux-en-Y procedure is indicated for refractory symptoms.

(B)   Consistent use of cholestyramine will improve symptoms and endoscopic findings.

(C)   A HIDA scan will not demonstrate gastric reflux.

(D)   A parietal cell vagotomy would have been less likely to result in this particular complication.

22.   A 62-year-old man undergoes upper endoscopy for a suspected duodenal ulcer. He is found not to have any duodenal or gastric ulcer disease, and the only abnormal finding is mild antral gastritis. Three biopsies are taken of the antrum. On examination of the biopsy specimens, the pathologist's report indicates "numerous spiral-shaped gram-negative organisms, presumably *H. pylori*, and multiple pockets of submucosal lymphoid tissue, cannot rule out low-grade lymphoma." The patient is referred to you for further management. The most appropriate therapy at this point is

(A)   A 2-week regimen of clarithromycin and amoxicillin, followed by repeat endoscopic evaluation with deep antral biopsies 1 month after completion

(B)   Combined chemotherapy and radiation therapy

(C)   Antrectomy with frozen section evaluation of surgical margins

(D)   Parietal cell vagotomy, followed by repeat endoscopic evaluation with deep antral biopsies 1 month later

23.   A 72-year-old man undergoes upper gastrointestinal barium study for complaints of dull epigastric pain, nausea, vomiting, and weight loss. Upper endoscopy reveals a diffusely thickened stomach lining and biopsy shows high-grade lymphoma. A CT scan of the abdomen reveals a diffusely thickened stomach (Fig. 18-2). There

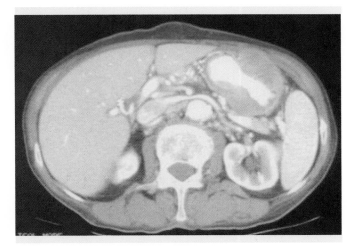

FIGURE 18-2. Computed tomographic scan of a patient with a gastric lesion.

is questionable perigastric lymph node involvement, but no apparent hepatic or splenic abnormalities. What is the next step?

(A)   Proceed with total gastrectomy and perigastric lymph node sampling

(B)   Proceed with total gastrectomy with splenectomy, including perigastric lymph nodes

(C)   After subtotal gastrectomy, a microscopically positive margin on frozen section at the duodenum warrants partial duodenectomy

(D)   Initiate chemotherapy with radiation and follow up with repeat imaging on completion

24.   A 45-year-old female patient is seen in your office for a 1-month follow-up visit after you performed omental patching, truncal vagotomy, and pyloroplasty to treat her perforated duodenal ulcer. She no longer has the burning epigastric pain that she experienced before her surgery, but complains to you of bloating and severe abdominal cramps soon after meals, followed by profuse diarrhea, sweating, and dizziness. These symptoms appeared shortly after she recovered from surgery and have not improved since surgery. She asks you for your advice about ameliorating this problem. Which of the following statements is *false*?

(A)   In most patients, these symptoms will improve significantly with minor modification of diet.

(B)   She should separate the ingestion of liquids from solids.

(C)   Octreotide can be a useful adjunct for treatment combined with diet modifications.

(D)   Regular administration of cholestyramine will likely prevent most of her symptoms.

25.   You have just begun a staging laparoscopy on a 58-year-old Asian American man with biopsy-proven gastric adenocarcinoma. Previous endoscopy revealed a diffusely thickened area of mucosa about 4 cm in diameter without ulceration in the body of the stomach. Endoscopic ultrasound (EUS) revealed a thickened body wall and perigastric lymphadenopathy. The spleen, pancreas, and liver appear normal on CT. Which of the following is true?

(A)   Given the involvement of perigastric lymph nodes, splenectomy is indicated.

(B)   A D1 lymphadenectomy with 15 lymph nodes is considered adequate for nodal sampling.

(C)   If curative gastric resection is intended, a 3-cm margin of microscopically tumor-free, normal tissue is adequate.

(D)   Extension into the gastrocolic and gastrohepatic ligaments constitutes T4 disease, and a palliative operation is indicated.

26. Which of the following statements regarding gastric adenocarcinoma is true?
    (A) Perioperative chemotherapy improves 5-year survival rates in patients with stage II or higher disease compared to surgery with curative intent alone.
    (B) Premalignant conditions include infection with *H. pylori*, hyperplastic gastric polyps, chronic gastritis, and chronic alcohol abuse.
    (C) Helical (spiral) CT scanning is superior to EUS in detecting extent of infiltration and involvement of surrounding lymph nodes.
    (D) Five-year survival rate after resection with curative intent for stage II disease is roughly 20%.

27. Which of the following lesions is likely (greater than 50% chance) to fail medical and endoscopic therapy and require surgical intervention, assuming that the patient is hemodynamically stable and has not required blood transfusion?
    (A) An exposed, 4-mm pulsating vessel visualized endoscopically on the lesser curvature of the proximal stomach in a 35-year-old man with no significant past medical history who presents with his first-ever episode of hematemesis
    (B) Two 2-cm linear tears, slowly oozing blood, seen in the mucosa of the lesser curvature approximately 1 cm distal from the gastroesophageal junction in a 45-year-old chronic alcohol abuser who presents with approximately 12 h of retching, vomiting, and hematemesis
    (C) At least 10 small, slowly oozing mucosal erosions found diffusely in the body and antrum of a 66-year-old woman who has taken sulindac for osteoarthritis for the past 10 years and presents after her first-ever bout of hematemesis
    (D) None of the above—all three patients' gastric lesions are likely to resolve after endoscopic and medical treatment

28. Which of the following medical regimens against *H. pylori* is least likely to eradicate the organism?
    (A) Omeprazole, clarithromycin, and metronidazole for 14 days
    (B) Bismuth, omeprazole, metronidazole, and tetracycline for 14 days
    (C) Ranitidine bismuth citrate, amoxicillin, and clarithromycin for 14 days
    (D) Lansoprazole and amoxicillin for 14 days

ANSWERS AND EXPLANATIONS

1. **(D)** The stomach is supplied by a rich anastomotic network of both intramural and extramural arteries. The majority of the blood supply derives from the celiac trunk via the left gastric artery (Fig. 18-3). The lesser curvature of the stomach is perfused by the left gastric artery (a branch of the celiac artery) and the right gastric artery (a branch from either the hepatic artery or the gastroduodenal artery). The greater curvature is perfused by the gastroepiploic arteries: The left gastroepiploic and short gastric arteries branch from the splenic artery, while the right gastroepiploic artery derives most often from the gastroduodenal artery with a small contribution from the superior mesenteric artery (A incorrect). In most individuals, the left gastroepiploic artery forms an anastomosis with the right gastroepiploic artery, forming an arcade along the greater curvature. Due to the extensive system of arterial anastomoses, the stomach can withstand occlusion or disruption to several supplying branches. It is routine to ligate the left gastric and the left gastroepiploic arteries when using the stomach to replace a resected esophagus, leaving the right gastroepiploic artery as the main vessel to perfuse the mobilized stomach in the chest, with a smaller contribution by the right gastric artery (B incorrect).

Erosion of a gastric ulcer into the gastroduodenal artery is uncommon. Massive hemorrhage secondary to a duodenal ulcer is often the result of erosion into the gastroduodenal artery, which is positioned immediately posterior to the first portion of the duodenum (C incorrect).

BIBLIOGRAPHY

Mahvi DM, Krantz SB. Stomach. In: Townsend CM, Beauchamp RD, Evers BM, et al., eds. *Sabiston Textbook of Surgery*. 19th ed. Philadelphia, PA: Elsevier Saunders; 2012:1182–1226.

Mulholland MW. Gastric anatomy and physiology. In: Greenfield LJ, Mulholland MW, Oldham KT, Zelenock GB, Lillemoe KD, eds. *Greenfield's Surgery: Scientific Principles and Practice*. 5th ed. Philadelphia, PA: Lippincott Williams & Wilkins; 2011: Chapter 43.

Skandalakis LJ, Colborn GL, Weidman TA, Kingsnorth AN, Skandalakis JE, Skandalakis PN. Stomach. In: Skandalakis JE, Colburn GL, Weidman TA, et al., eds. *Skandalakis' Surgical Anatomy*. New York, NY: McGraw-Hill; 2004: Chapter 15.

Zollinger RM Jr, Ellison E, Bitans M, Smith J. In: Zollinger RM Jr, Ellison E, Bitans M, Smith J, eds. *Zollinger's Atlas of Surgical Operations*. New York, NY: McGraw-Hill; 2011: Plate 1.

2. **(D)** There is both sympathetic (celiac plexus) and parasympathetic (vagus) innervation to and from the stomach (Fig. 18-4). The vagus nerve descends from the neck within the carotid sheath to enter the mediastinum. Just above the esophageal hiatus, vagal branches around the esophagus merge to form the left (anterior) and right (posterior) vagal nerves.

The *left* vagus nerve gives off a hepatic division before branching to innervate the anterior gastric wall as the

1 Celiac axis
2 Lt. gastric - 2a anterior branch
3 Lt. inf. phrenic
4 Short gastrics
5 Lt. gastroepiploic
6 Rt. gastroepiploic
7 Rt. gastric
8 Com. hepatic
9 Splenic
10 Gastroduodenal
11 Middle colic
12 Post. and ant. (sup. and inf.)
 pancreaticoduodenals
13 Sup. mesenteric
14 Sup. (dorsal)
 pancreatic
15 Inf. (transv.)
 pancreatic
16 Greater pancreatic
17 Cystic
18 Rt. hepatic
19 Lt. hepatic

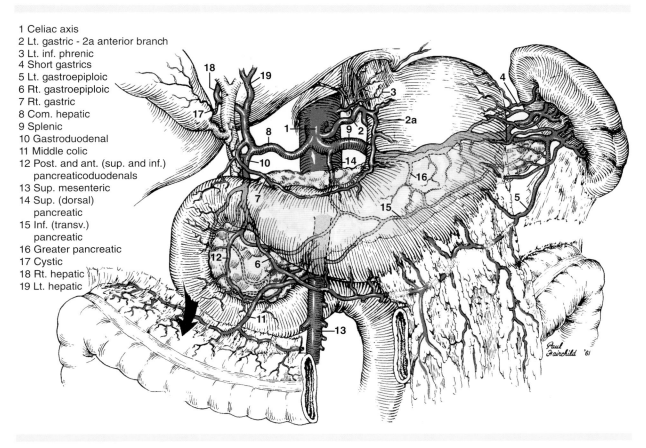

FIGURE 18-3. Arterial supply of the stomach (from Zollinger RM Jr, Ellison E, Bitans M, Smith J, eds. *Zollinger's Atlas of Surgical Operations*. New York, NY: McGraw-Hill; 2011: Plate 1, Fig. 1. Copyright © The McGraw-Hill Companies, Inc. All rights reserved).

anterior nerve of Latarjet (*A incorrect*). This hepatic division passes through the lesser omentum to provide parasympathetic innervation to the liver and biliary tract. The *right* vagus nerve gives off a celiac division, which passes into the celiac plexus and then the posterior gastric wall. The criminal nerve of Grassi is the first branch of the right vagus nerve, often incriminated in recurrent ulcers when left undivided.

Only 10% of the total vagal fibers are motor or secretory efferents. The majority of vagal fibers transmit gastrointestinal information back to the central nervous system. The sympathetic innervation is derived from spinal segments T5 through T10. Preganglionic efferent fibers from the spine synapse within the right and left celiac ganglia to postganglionic fibers, which then enter the stomach alongside the vasculature. Afferent fibers from the stomach to the central nervous system pass without synapse from the stomach wall to the dorsal spinal roots. It is within these afferent sympathetic fibers that pain stimuli are transmitted back to the central nervous system.

BIBLIOGRAPHY

Mahvi DM, Krantz SB. Stomach. In: Townsend CM, Beauchamp RD, Evers BM, et al., eds. *Sabiston Textbook of Surgery*. 19th ed. Philadelphia, PA: Elsevier Saunders; 2012:1182–1226.

3. **(C)** When a meal enters the stomach, the fundus and body undergo vagally mediated receptive relaxation. This allows the normally collapsed stomach to expand, preventing intragastric pressure from rising dangerously as it fills. Liquids in the stomach are forced to empty primarily by increased intragastric pressure, normally created by low-amplitude tonic contractions of the fundus. The increased pressure gradient between the stomach and the lower-pressure duodenum forces the liquids across the pylorus and out of the stomach. After parietal cell vagotomy, receptive relaxation is blocked, resulting in increased intragastric pressure with both liquids and solids. The relatively high intragastric pressure in this vagally denervated stomach forces liquids out at a greater rate than in the normal stomach. The emptying of solids

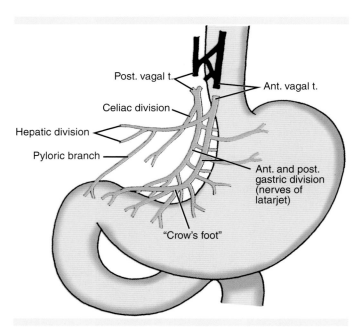

FIGURE 18-4. Innervation of the stomach (from Skandalakis LJ, Colborn GL, Weidman TA, Kingsnorth AN, Skandalakis JE, Skandalakis PN. Stomach. In: Skandalakis JE, Colburn GL, Weidman TA, et al., eds. *Skandalakis' Surgical Anatomy.* New York, NY: McGraw-Hill; 2004: Chapter 15, Fig. 15-46. Copyright © The McGraw-Hill Companies, Inc. All rights reserved).

is more dependent on the distal stomach. Strong ring contractions begin in the midbody of the stomach and proceed toward the pylorus, propelling gastric contents against a closed pylorus. The pylorus closes 2–3 s before the arrival of the antral contraction ring. Continued pulsion and retropulsion mixes the solids with the liquids, and the antral contractions grind the solids into small particles. Solid particles that are 1 mm or smaller can then pass across the pylorus, along with liquids; larger particles do not normally pass. Since a properly performed parietal cell vagotomy leaves the vagal innervation to the distal stomach intact, the emptying of solids is unaffected.

BIBLIOGRAPHY

Mahvi DM, Krantz SB. Stomach. In: Townsend CM, Beauchamp RD, Evers BM, et al., eds. *Sabiston Textbook of Surgery.* 19th ed. Philadelphia, PA: Elsevier Saunders; 2012:1182–1226.
Mulholland MW. Gastric anatomy and physiology. In: Greenfield LJ, Mulholland MW, Oldham KT, Zelenock GB, Lillemoe KD, eds. *Greenfield's Surgery: Scientific Principles and Practice.* 5th ed. Philadelphia, PA: Lippincott Williams & Wilkins; 2011: Chapter 43.

4. **(D)** The regulation of gastric acid secretion is complex and involves several mediators. The three phases of acid secretion are cephalic, gastric, and intestinal, which

occur simultaneously and not consecutively. Before food reaches the stomach, the sight, smell, or thought of food can stimulate gastric acid secretion, referred to as the cephalic phase. Vagal stimulation targets parietal and G cells. Stimulation of parietal cells via acetylcholine-muscarinic receptor interaction induces acid secretion (Fig. 18-5). Because this phase is entirely dependent on vagal nerve transmission, a truncal vagotomy will abolish the cephalic phase.

The gastric phase begins once food enters the stomach. Both the presence of partially hydrolyzed food and gastric distention stimulate the G cells of the antrum, pylorus, and duodenum to release gastrin. This response is mediated by a vasovagal reflex arc and thus is abolished by proximal gastric vagotomy. The intestinal phase is stimulated by the presence of chyme in the small intestine and accounts for only 10% of gastric acid secretion.

Gastrin is responsible for over 90% of meal-stimulated acid secretion. ECL cells and mast cells of the stomach also have receptors for gastrin (Fig. 18-5). Gastrin stimulates the release of histamine by ECL cells, which in turn stimulates parietal cell acid secretion. Parietal cells, responsible for secreting acid into the stomach lumen, are stimulated to produce acid by gastrin, histamine, and

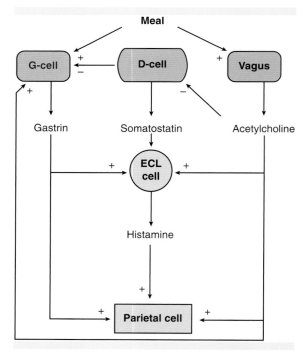

FIGURE 18-5. Gastric acid secretion; ECL = enterochromaffin-like. (Reproduced with permission from Mercer DW, Liu TH, Castaneda A: Anatomy and physiology of the stomach, in Zuidema GD, Yeo CJ (eds): *Shackelford's Surgery of the Alimentary Tract,* 5th ed., Vol. II. Philadelphia: Saunders, 2002, p 3. Copyright Elsevier.)

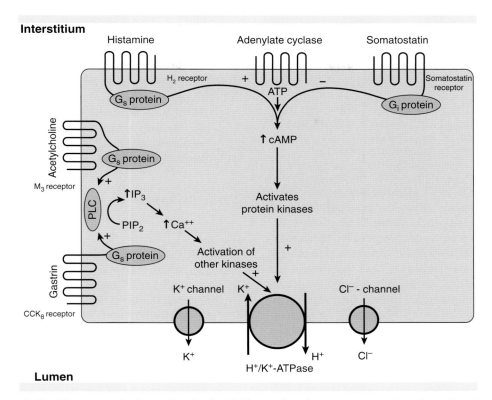

FIGURE 18-6. Control of acid secretion in the parietal cell; cAMP = cyclic adenosine monophosphate; IP_3 = inositol triphosphate; PIP_2 = phosphatidylinositol-4,5-bisphosphate. (Reproduced with permission from Mercer DW, Liu TH, Castaneda A: Anatomy and physiology of the stomach, in Zuidema GD, Yeo CJ (eds): *Shackelford's Surgery of the Alimentary Tract,* 5th ed., Vol. II. Philadelphia: Saunders, 2002, p 3. Copyright Elsevier.)

acetylcholine (Fig. 18-6). In addition to stimulation of gastric acid secretion, there are mechanisms to inhibit the parietal cell from secreting acid. In addition to stimulatory receptors for gastrin, histamine, and acetylcholine, the parietal cell expresses receptors for prostaglandin E2 and somatostatin, which inhibit acid secretion when stimulated. The most important inhibitor of acid secretion involves a negative-feedback mechanism in which gastrin-producing G cells are suppressed as the antral mucosa is exposed to acid. Gastrin production stops completely when the pH falls below 2.0, thus removing the major stimulus for parietal cells to secrete acid.

The PPIs become activated below a pH of 3 and irreversibly bind to the membrane-bound H^+K^+ ATPase of parietal cells, inhibiting proton secretion.

BIBLIOGRAPHY

Kitagawa Y, Dempsey DT. Stomach. In: Brunicardi F, Andersen DK, Billiar TR, et al., eds. *Schwartz's Principles of Surgery.* 10th ed. New York, NY: McGraw-Hill; 2014: Chapter 26.

Mahvi DM, Krantz SB. Stomach. In: Townsend CM, Beauchamp RD, Evers BM, et al., eds. *Sabiston Textbook of Surgery.* 19th ed. Philadelphia, PA: Elsevier Saunders; 2012:1182–1226.

Mulholland MW. Gastric anatomy and physiology. In: Greenfield LJ, Mulholland MW, Oldham KT, Zelenock GB, Lillemoe KD, eds. *Greenfield's Surgery: Scientific Principles and Practice.* 5th ed. Philadelphia, PA: Lippincott Williams & Wilkins; 2011: Chapter 43.

5. **(A)** Parietal cells secrete acid in response to gastrin, histamine, and acetylcholine. Gastrin is released from the G cells of the antrum, pylorus, and duodenum and reaches the fundal parietal cells by way of the systemic circulation. The presence of peptides and amino acids by the antral G cells is the primary stimulus for gastrin release. Gastric distension also stimulates gastrin release by activating cholinergic neurons that directly stimulate the G cells. Vagal cholinergic activity can also inhibit G cells, as shown by the hypergastrinemia that occurs after vagotomy.

With an intact negative-feedback system, pharmacologic acid suppression in the form of antacids or PPIs results in hypergastrinemia (*D and E incorrect*). The increased gastric pH resulting from these agents reduces somatostatin release, removing negative feedback for gastrin release, causing hypergastrinemia.

Several processes can cause hypergastrinemia. These include Zollinger-Ellison syndrome, gastric outlet obstruction, short-gut syndrome, retained antrum, antral G cell hyperplasia, pernicious anemia, atrophic gastritis, and chronic renal failure.

BIBLIOGRAPHY

Mahvi DM, Krantz SB. Stomach. In: Townsend CM, Beauchamp RD, Evers BM, et al., eds. *Sabiston Textbook of Surgery.* 19th ed. Philadelphia, PA: Elsevier Saunders; 2012:1182–1226.

Mulholland MW. Gastric anatomy and physiology. In: Greenfield LJ, Mulholland MW, Oldham KT, Zelenock GB, Lillemoe KD, eds. *Greenfield's Surgery: Scientific Principles and Practice.* 5th ed. Philadelphia, PA: Lippincott Williams & Wilkins; 2011: Chapter 43.

6. **(C)** Acid production by the parietal cell ultimately occurs via a specialized ion transport system called the proton pump. This membrane-bound protein resides in the secretory canaliculus, releasing H^+ ions into the stomach lumen. The energy to drive this exchange against a very large electrical gradient comes from the hydrolysis of ATP into ADP and phosphate. To maintain electroneutrality, K^+ ions and Cl^- ions passively diffuse across the cell membrane in a 1:1 ratio to maintain electroneutrality (*A incorrect*). The supply of chloride ions comes from an exchange of Cl^- for HCO_3^- ions at the basolateral membrane. Carbonic anhydrase catalyzes the formation of bicarbonate (HCO_3^-) from CO_2 and excess OH^- ions.

BIBLIOGRAPHY

Mulholland MW. Gastric anatomy and physiology. In: Greenfield LJ, Mulholland MW, Oldham KT, Zelenock GB, Lillemoe KD, eds. *Greenfield's Surgery: Scientific Principles and Practice.* 5th ed. Philadelphia, PA: Lippincott Williams & Wilkins; 2011: Chapter 43.

7. **(A)** *Helicobacter pylori* is a gram-negative spiral bacterium that has evolved special characteristics to survive in the hostile environment of the stomach. It utilizes flagella to burrow through the mucous layer toward the gastric epithelium, following an increasing pH gradient. It then secretes a variety of proteases and other enzymes. Urease converts urea to carbon dioxide and ammonia, which is directly toxic to gastric epithelium. *Helicobacter pylori* expresses an analogue of histamine, thereby promoting parietal cell acid secretion. (Fig. 18-7). Furthermore, parietal cell mass is increased in infected patients and has been linked to hypergastrinemia. The unchecked hypergastrinemia results in abnormally elevated acid secretion. Both basal and peak acid output are increased in ulcer patients harboring *H. pylori*, and levels return to normal after eradication by antimicrobials.

The majority of individuals harboring *H. pylori* are asymptomatic, with 10–15% developing ulceration and 1% developing adenocarcinoma. This has been attributed to expression of the CagA and VacA virulence factors by different strains: VacA promotes epithelial cell apoptosis via pore formation, while CagA disrupts infected cell shape and intracellular signaling pathways that regulate proliferation and differentiation. Several well-described mechanisms explain the relationship between *H. pylori* and enteric ulceration: (1) chronic inflammation of the gastric mucosa, (2) direct ammonia toxicity to gastric lining, (3) disruption of acid secretion homeostasis, and (4) proteases that directly degrade the mucous lining of the stomach.

BIBLIOGRAPHY

Mahvi DM, Krantz SB. Stomach. In: Townsend CM, Beauchamp RD, Evers BM, et al., eds. *Sabiston Textbook of Surgery.* 19th ed. Philadelphia, PA: Elsevier Saunders; 2012:1182–1226.

Mulholland MW. Gastric anatomy and physiology. In: Greenfield LJ, Mulholland MW, Oldham KT, Zelenock GB, Lillemoe KD, eds. *Greenfield's Surgery: Scientific Principles and Practice.* 5th ed. Philadelphia, PA: Lippincott Williams & Wilkins; 2011: Chapter 43.

8. **(C)** Sucralfate is the aluminum salt of sulfated sucrose. At a pH below 4, it polymerizes to form a viscous gel with exposed negatively charged functional groups. These exposed polyanions bind the exposed enteric mucosa, which harbors a high concentration of positively charged proteins, thereby forming a protective physical barrier in the ulcer bed. It stimulates the production of protective gastric mucus, prostaglandin E_2, and bicarbonate. Sucralfate binds bile salts and inhibits the proteolytic action of pepsin. Sucralfate stimulates the proliferation of healthy epithelium at the margin of an ulcer. There is virtually no systemic absorption of sucralfate; therefore, sucralfate is safe for use in the pregnant patient. Sucralfate is currently only approved by the Food and Drug Administration (FDA) for treatment of active duodenal ulcers without evidence of NSAID use as its effectiveness is thought to be related to countering acid oversecretion.

BIBLIOGRAPHY

Mulholland MW. Gastric anatomy and physiology. In: Greenfield LJ, Mulholland MW, Oldham KT, Zelenock GB, Lillemoe KD, eds. *Greenfield's Surgery: Scientific Principles and Practice.* 5th ed. Philadelphia, PA: Lippincott Williams & Wilkins; 2011: Chapter 43.

9. **(C)** There are many methods used commonly today to diagnose infection with *H. pylori*. The standard remains mucosal biopsy with histologic examination of the biopsy specimen for the organisms, with a reported sensitivity of 100% and specificity of 73%. There also exist rapid urease tests in which the biopsy specimen can be tested for the presence of urease activity, a characteristic of *H. pylori*. The "CLO test" (*Campylobacter*-like

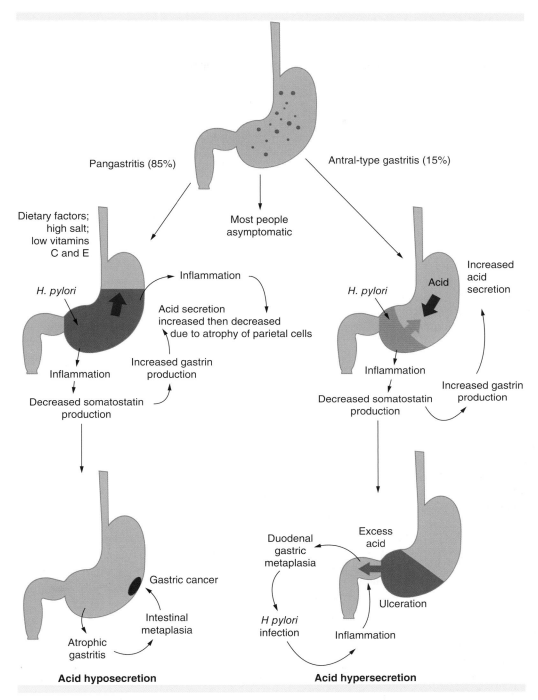

FIGURE 18-7. *Helicobacter pylori* and acid secretion. Redrawn from data in Conklin JL et al. Motor functions of the pharynx and esophagus. In: Johnson LR, ed. *Physiology of the Gastrointestinal Tract,* 3rd ed. Lippincott-Raven, 1994.

organism test) is an example of such a method. The rapid urease tests have been reported to have nearly 100% sensitivity and specificity. Culture of the biopsy specimen is not routinely performed because the organism is difficult to isolate in routine laboratories; however, if information

is needed about the organism's antimicrobial sensitivity and resistance, culture of biopsy specimens for *H. pylori* should be performed by an experienced laboratory.

Serologic testing is the method of choice as an initial screening test unless endoscopy is indicated for reasons other than diagnosis of *H. pylori*. These tests are quick, easy to perform, and relatively inexpensive, with a sensitivity of 85% and 79% specificity. Another noninvasive test is the urea breath test, in which urease activity is detected in the patient's inhaled breath after ingesting C^{14}- or C^{15}-labeled urea. This test has a reported sensitivity of 94% and 100% specificity. The breath test is the preferred method for diagnosing persistent infection after medical treatment.

In scenario A, the urea breath test is the method of choice to determine effectiveness of therapy. In scenario B, because the patient is already undergoing endoscopy for other reasons and gastritis has been observed, mucosal biopsy with either histologic examination or rapid urease test is certainly indicated. In scenario D, bacterial culture with subsequent determination of antimicrobial resistance and sensitivity are crucial to determine how to best treat this infection. In scenario C, the test of choice is the serologic test or possibly the urea breath test. The risks and cost of endoscopy are not justified to diagnose *H. pylori* when other, noninvasive tests are available.

BIBLIOGRAPHY

Mahvi DM, Krantz SB. Stomach. In: Townsend CM, Beauchamp RD, Evers BM, et al., eds. *Sabiston Textbook of Surgery*. 19th ed. Philadelphia, PA: Elsevier Saunders; 2012:1182–1226.
Mulholland MW. Gastric anatomy and physiology. In: Greenfield LJ, Mulholland MW, Oldham KT, Zelenock GB, Lillemoe KD, eds. *Greenfield's Surgery: Scientific Principles and Practice*. 5th ed. Philadelphia, PA: Lippincott Williams & Wilkins; 2011: Chapter 43.

10. **(B)** If left untreated, 10% of patients with duodenal ulcer will develop obstruction. Pyloric obstruction is indeed one of the four indications for operation on patients with duodenal ulcer: obstruction, hemorrhage, perforation, and intractability. Conservative therapy should, however, be attempted if possible . It is recommended that patients presenting with pyloric obstruction because of a swollen and inflamed pyloric channel be admitted to the hospital and treated with nasogastric suction and intravenous PPI for at least 7 days. Most patients' obstructions will clear within 1 week. If the obstruction has not cleared within 1 week with conservative therapy, then surgery is indicated. The procedure of choice in this situation is vagotomy, to definitively treat this patient's ulcer diathesis, and antrectomy. If conservative therapy is successful, there is still a chance that the patient will develop pyloric scarring and subsequent obstruction, even if the ulcer itself heals. Assuming that endoscopic biopsy excludes malignancy in this situation, the benign stricture can be dilated endoscopically in many cases, although the

majority of these patients' symptoms will recur, requiring repeat dilations or surgical correction.

BIBLIOGRAPHY

Kitagawa Y, Dempsey DT. Stomach. In: Brunicardi F, Andersen DK, Billiar TR, et al., eds. *Schwartz's Principles of Surgery*. 10th ed. New York, NY: McGraw-Hill; 2014: Chapter 26.
Mahvi DM, Krantz SB. Stomach. In: Townsend CM, Beauchamp RD, Evers BM, et al., eds. *Sabiston Textbook of Surgery*. 19th ed. Philadelphia, PA: Elsevier Saunders; 2012:1182–1226.
Mulholland MW. Gastric anatomy and physiology. In: Greenfield LJ, Mulholland MW, Oldham KT, Zelenock GB, Lillemoe KD, eds. *Greenfield's Surgery: Scientific Principles and Practice*. 5th ed. Philadelphia, PA: Lippincott, Williams & Wilkins; 2011: Chapter 43.

11. **(C)** Elective surgical intervention for gastroduodenal ulcers has become quite rare, given better understanding of the role of *H. pylori* and NSAID use in pathogenesis. However, for select patients, surgical therapy may be considered in those who are unresponsive to therapy. The goal in this setting is to reduce acid secretion. The three most common procedures performed are parietal cell vagotomy (also called proximal gastric vagotomy or highly selective vagotomy), truncal vagotomy with pyloroplasty, and truncal vagotomy with antrectomy (Figs. 18-8A and B).

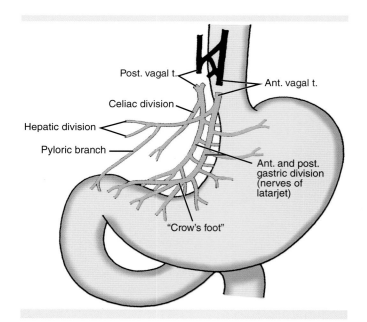

FIGURE 18-8A. (from Skandalakis LJ, Colborn GL, Weidman TA, Kingsnorth AN, Skandalakis JE, Skandalakis PN. Stomach. In: Skandalakis JE, Colburn GL, Weidman TA, et al., eds. *Skandalakis' Surgical Anatomy*. New York, NY: McGraw-Hill; 2004: Chapter 15, Fig. 15-46A. Copyright © The McGraw-Hill Companies, Inc. All rights reserved).

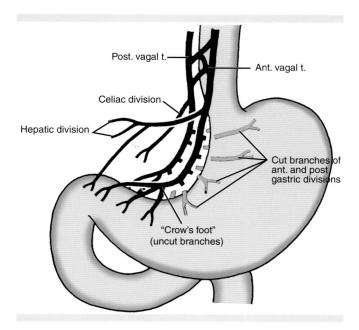

FIGURE 18-8B. Parietal cell vagotomy (from Skandalakis LJ, Colborn GL, Weidman TA, Kingsnorth AN, Skandalakis JE, Skandalakis PN. Stomach. In: Skandalakis JE, Colburn GL, Weidman TA, et al., eds. *Skandalakis' Surgical Anatomy*. New York, NY: McGraw-Hill; 2004: Chapter 15, Fig. 15-46C. Copyright © The McGraw-Hill Companies, Inc. All rights reserved).

In truncal vagotomy, the vagus nerve trunks are divided just proximal to the the hepatic and celiac branches (Fig. 18-7A). To combat the gastric atony caused by vagotomy, the pyloric mechanism must be bypassed or destroyed, allowing the stomach to drain freely. This is often achieved by pyloroplasty. The most commonly performed pyloroplasty is the Heineke-Mikulicz procedure, but the slightly more elaborate Finney and Jaboulay pyloroplasties should be available in the ulcer surgeon's armamentarium in cases of extensively scarred or otherwise deformed duodenal bulb. It is technically the least demanding of the three commonly performed procedures. A typical application of this procedure is for a patient with a bleeding duodenal ulcer who will undergo an incision across the pylorus to oversew the bleeding vessel. The rate of ulcer recurrence is 10%. The initial postoperative incidence of dumping is 10%, and this remains severe in 1%.

The addition of antrectomy is usually reserved for gastric ulcers, not duodenal ulcers. It is more effective than truncal vagotomy alone in reducing acid secretion, with an ulcer recurrence rate of 0–2%. Complications, however, include postgastrectomy syndromes in combination with postvagotomy syndromes and run as high as 20%. Reconstruction is usually gastroduodenostomy (Billroth I) or gastrojejunostomy (Billroth II). In the absence of significant duodenal scarring, a Billroth I is preferred to avoid duodenal stump leakage and afferent loop obstruction. During a Billroth II procedure, the jejunal loop is often brought up in a retrocolic fashion to minimize torsion or compression, which can promote afferent loop obstruction. Dumping syndrome occurs in 10–15% of patients postoperatively, with 1–2% of patients exhibiting severe symptoms. It is important to note, however, that these procedures are not commonly performed today with the advent of improved understanding of *H. pylori* and effective nonsurgical management.

Parietal cell vagotomy preserves vagal innervation of the antrum and therefore avoids complications associated with truncal vagotomy necessitating a drainage procedure (Fig. 18-7B). It has the lowest incidence of postoperative dumping syndrome of the three procedures. It is accomplished by transecting the nerves of Latarjet from the lesser curvature starting from a point 5 cm proximal to the gastroesophageal junction down to a point approximately 7 cm proximal to the pylorus. The hepatic and celiac divisions of the vagus trunks are preserved, while the criminal nerve of Grassi muse be sought and transected. Ulcer recurrence rates with parietal cell vagotomy are the highest among the three commonly performed procedures at 10%.

BIBLIOGRAPHY

Mahvi DM, Krantz SB. Stomach. In: Townsend CM, Beauchamp RD, Evers BM, et al., eds. *Sabiston Textbook of Surgery*. 19th ed. Philadelphia, PA: Elsevier Saunders; 2012:1182–1226.

Mulholland MW. Gastric anatomy and physiology. In: Greenfield LJ, Mulholland MW, Oldham KT, Zelenock GB, Lillemoe KD, eds. *Greenfield's Surgery: Scientific Principles and Practice*. 5th ed. Philadelphia, PA: Lippincott, Williams & Wilkins; 2011: Chapter 43.

12. **(C)**

13. **(B)**

14. **(B)**

Explanation for questions 12 through 14

This patient presented with a gastric ulcer. In the general population, gastric ulcers occur at about one-third the frequency of duodenal ulcers. Similar to duodenal ulcers, gastric ulcers are associated with *H. pylori* colonization in 85–90% of patients. A classification system based on location and acid secretion divides gastric ulcers into five groups (Fig. 18-9). Operative treatment strategy can also be generalized for each type.

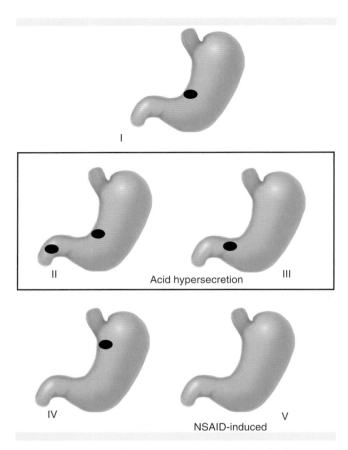

FIGURE 18-9. Gastric ulcer types. Reproduced with permission from Fisher WE, Brunicardi FC: Benign gastric ulcer, in Cameron JL (ed): *Current Surgical Therapy*, 9th ed. Philadelphia: Mosby Elsevier, 2008, p 81. Copyright Elsevier.

Type I gastric ulcers account for 60% of all cases and are not associated with gastric acid hypersecretion; in fact, many patients with this type of gastric ulcer have low acid output. Type II gastric ulcers are a combination of a gastric ulcer in the body of the stomach and another in the duodenum and are associated with acid hypersecretion.

Type III gastric ulcers occur within 3 cm of the pylorus and are often associated with acid hypersecretion. Type IV gastric ulcers occur on the lesser curvature at or near the gastroesophageal junction. Similar to type I gastric ulcers, these ulcers are not associated with acid hypersecretion. Type V gastric ulcers can occur at any location in the stomach and are associated with chronic NSAID use. These patients often initially present with hemorrhage or perforation, warranting emergency surgical treatment.

Any ulcer larger than 3 cm should be suspected of harboring malignancy and should undergo early operative excision.

In the clinical vignette, this gentleman was appropriately treated for an apparently benign type I gastric ulcer. Surgical management before a trial of medical therapy and cessation of NSAIDs is not the standard of care. At representation 6 months later, the physicians have demonstrated that he is *H. pylori* free, and he is no longer taking NSAIDs. The finding on endoscopy that the ulcer is now 4 cm in diameter is worrisome for malignancy, as is the finding of dysplasia on histologic examination of ulcer margin biopsies. At this point, surgery is indicated not only because of the increase in ulcer size after adequate medical therapy but also because malignant disease cannot be excluded. The appropriate elective operation is distal gastrectomy with inclusion of the ulcer. There is no indication for an acid-suppressing procedure in this situation.

BIBLIOGRAPHY

Mahvi DM, Krantz SB. Stomach. In: Townsend CM, Beauchamp RD, Evers BM, et al., eds. *Sabiston Textbook of Surgery*. 19th ed. Philadelphia, PA: Elsevier Saunders; 2012:1182–1226.

Mulholland MW. Gastric anatomy and physiology. In: Greenfield LJ, Mulholland MW, Oldham KT, Zelenock GB, Lillemoe KD, eds. *Greenfield's Surgery: Scientific Principles and Practice*. 5th ed. Philadelphia, PA: Lippincott, Williams & Wilkins; 2011: Chapter 43.

15. **(D)**

16. **(B)**

Explanation for questions 15 and 16

This patient has a duodenal perforation. The lifetime risk of perforation in an untreated duodenal ulcer is 10%, and perforation can occur without any preceding symptoms of duodenal ulcer (epigastric pain, bleeding). The classic presentation is an acute onset of severe pain, followed by immediate signs of peritonitis as gastric and duodenal fluids irritate the peritoneum. The classic diagnostic procedure of choice is an upright chest radiograph or left lateral decubitus radiograph, which will show free air in approximately 80% of patients with perforation. An upper gastrointestinal contrast study (performed with water-soluble contrast) may demonstrate the perforation if the diagnosis is still in question after negative chest or decubitus radiographs. Perforation of a duodenal ulcer is a strong indication for urgent surgical management. Delaying surgical treatment for more than 12 h after presentation results in increased complication rates, increased hospital stay, and increased mortality. Therefore, observation is contraindicated in the acutely perforated patient described. There are reports of nonoperative management in patients several days after perforation, with contrast radiographic evidence of perforation closure.

The surgical procedure of choice is suture oversewing of the perforation and placement of a well-vascularized portion of omentum over that suture line. The omentum can be fixed by separate sutures or by using the tails of the previously placed sutures to fix the omentum in place. The decision to add an antacid procedure depends both on the presentation of the patient and on his or her ulcer history. If the patient has no history of ulcer disease, as in the patient described, there is no indication to perform an antacid procedure. In this situation, oversewing and omental patch provide an adequate treatment of the perforation, and proper diagnosis and medical therapy of ulcer disease can be performed once the patient recovers from surgery. This is also true of the patient with NSAID-induced ulcer perforation, in which cessation of the offending agent should be adequate therapy. If the patient does have a significant history of ulcer disease, then a definitive antacid procedure should be performed, provided that three criteria are met: (1) There is no preoperative shock, (2) the perforation occurred less than 48 h previous to surgery, and (3) life-threatening medical problems do not coexist. If any of these criteria are not met, the definitive antacid procedure should be omitted.

In the hands of an experienced laparoscopist, duodenal perforation can be effectively diagnosed, sutured, and patched with omentum by laparoscopic techniques. In addition, acid-reducing procedures can be performed by surgeons with advanced laparoscopic skills.

BIBLIOGRAPHY

Mahvi DM, Krantz SB. Stomach. In: Townsend CM, Beauchamp RD, Evers BM, et al., eds. *Sabiston Textbook of Surgery*. 19th ed. Philadelphia, PA: Elsevier Saunders; 2012:1182–1226.

Mulholland MW. Gastric anatomy and physiology. In: Greenfield LJ, Mulholland MW, Oldham KT, Zelenock GB, Lillemoe KD, eds. *Greenfield's Surgery: Scientific Principles and Practice*. 5th ed. Philadelphia, PA: Lippincott, Williams & Wilkins; 2011: Chapter 43.

17. **(D)**

18. **(A)**

Explanation for questions 17 and 18

Stress gastritis occurs most often in patients who have sustained severe burns, trauma, hemorrhagic shock, sepsis, or respiratory failure. The ulcers are usually multiple and superficial, occurring most frequently in the fundus. They start to occur as soon as 12 h after the injury or insult. The exact mechanisms responsible for stress gastritis are as yet unknown, but most experts agree that mucosal ischemia is the common denominator. The diagnosis is often suspected on detection of blood from nasogastric aspirates or an otherwise-unexplained drop in hematocrit. Determination of any factors contributing to coagulopathy should be assessed and managed accordingly.

The next treatment step should be lavage of the stomach with saline. This serves to fragment blood clots, prevent gastric distension, and wash out harmful bile salts and pancreatic juices that may have refluxed into the stomach. There is disagreement on the temperature of the lavage solution. Chilled saline was traditionally used, probably in an attempt to constrict vessels, but some investigators are opposed to using cold solutions in a central body cavity for fear of lowering the temperature in an already-sick, potentially coagulopathic patient. The majority of bleeding gastritis will cease after this relatively simple management.

Regardless of whether the bleeding arrests or not, the next logical step is urgent endoscopy, both to diagnose the problem and assess severity and to definitively treat the gastric erosions with a number of techniques, including heater probe, injection of epinephrine, and laser or electrocoagulation. It would also be prudent to arrange for readily available blood products for the critically ill patient, although in this vignette there is no indication for transfusion based on laboratory parameters. Lavage of the stomach before endoscopy is an important step, serving to wash out gastric contents and blood to enable adequate visualization. Endoscopy is effective in permanent hemostasis in over 90% of patients with stress gastritis but may fail if there is profuse bleeding or many ulcerations. In this situation, endoscopy is abandoned, and the patient is taken to the interventional radiology suite. If the left gastric artery can be selectively cannulated, a continuous infusion of vasopressin for up to 72 h is likely to effectively stop the bleeding. An alternative to continuous vasopressin is embolization of the left gastric artery. If interventional radiology techniques are either unsuccessful or unavailable, then surgery is warranted to stop the bleeding.

No prospective clinical trials have been conducted that clearly define the optimal surgical procedure to perform. Long gastrotomy with oversewing of ulcers, with or without truncal vagotomy and either pyloroplasty or antrectomy, is likely the least-morbid operation, but any combination of these has a significant risk of recurrent hemorrhage. More aggressive procedures trade higher morbidity and mortality for lower recurrence rates and include subtotal gastrectomy and gastric devascularization (ligation of right and left gastric arteries plus gastroepiploic arteries). If bleeding is diffuse or a previous attempt at surgical hemostasis has failed, total gastrectomy may be the only option.

It has been shown that maintaining gastric pH above 3.5 is effective prophylaxis against gastritis. The "no acid–no ulcer" dictum has some truth in stress gastritis because it appears that acid production is necessary for its development. Antacids, intravenous H_2 receptor antagonists, and sucralfate have all shown ability with essentially equal efficacy to prevent stress gastritis in the critically ill patient. Some investigators prefer the use of sucralfate because acid-reducing agents may increase the risk of nosocomial pneumonia by favoring growth of gram-negative organisms in the more neutral stomach environment. Data supporting or rejecting this are mixed in the literature.

The Sengstaken-Blakemore tube is a transoral, dual-balloon device used to tamponade bleeding esophageal varices and has no role in the treatment of gastric ulcers.

BIBLIOGRAPHY

Mahvi DM, Krantz SB. Stomach. In: Townsend CM, Beauchamp RD, Evers BM, et al., eds. *Sabiston Textbook of Surgery*. 19th ed. Philadelphia, PA: Elsevier Saunders; 2012:1182–1226.

Mulholland MW. Gastric anatomy and physiology. In: Greenfield LJ, Mulholland MW, Oldham KT, Zelenock GB, Lillemoe KD, eds. *Greenfield's Surgery: Scientific Principles and Practice*. 5th ed. Philadelphia, PA: Lippincott, Williams & Wilkins; 2011: Chapter 43.

19. **(D)** Gastrointestinal stromal tumors (GISTs) can appear anywhere in the digestive tract, from esophagus to colon, but are most frequently found in the stomach. These were originally called leiomyoma or leiomyosarcoma, reflecting the belief that they were of smooth muscle tumor origin. More recent studies and more elaborate immunohistochemical analyses have shown that there are multiple possible origins of the cells comprising GISTs, including Schwann cells, enteric glial cells, perineural cells, and intestinal pacemaker cells. They can be asymptomatic and found incidentally or can present with symptoms such as bleeding, obstruction, nonspecific pain, or palpable mass. Bleeding occurs most frequently in larger GISTs when the overlying mucosa ulcerates.

On endoscopy, they are usually described as an extrinsic bulge, possibly with umbilication or ulceration of the overlying mucosa. Routine endoscopic biopsies are likely to reveal only normal gastric mucosa, and even intentionally deep biopsies have only a 50% diagnostic yield. Upper gastrointestinal contrast studies often show only an extrinsic mass with intact or ulcerated overlying mucosa. Abdominal CT can better define the total size of the mass and determine the presence of extragastric extension. CT-guided biopsy can often be performed but seldom contributes to the preoperative management because biopsy—whether CT guided or endoscopic—rarely is able to determine benign versus malignant disease. In fact, there is no consensus on what defines benign versus malignant GIST. One proposed method involves number of mitotic figs. per high-powered field on light microscopy, with benign being defined as fewer than 5 mitotic figs., intermediate as 6–10 mitotic figs., and malignant as more than 10 mitotic figs.

Unfortunately, there are reports of metastases occurring after complete resection of GISTs with no mitotic figs. If a gastric GIST is discovered incidentally on laparotomy, it should be excised with a margin of 2–3 cm of normal gastric tissue. This is also the procedure to be performed if the diagnosis is known or suspected preoperatively. Because of the uncertainty of malignancy, these should never be enucleated. Lymphadenectomy is not indicated as these tumors most often metastasize hematogenously. Distant metastases are discovered at presentation in less than 20% of patients. If metastases are discovered and the primary GIST can be safely removed, the primary should be excised to prevent complications of bleeding and obstruction. Radiation has not proved beneficial in these tumors, and chemotherapy, although there are some reports of response, has not shown any increase in survival. Survival is reported to be 53% at 5 years for gastric GISTs. When asymptomatic tumors are diagnosed preoperatively, they should undergo surgical excision if they are greater than 3 cm in any dimension, but it is unclear how best to treat smaller, asymptomatic GISTs.

BIBLIOGRAPHY

Greenfield LJ, Mulholland MW, Oldham KT, Zelenock GB, Lillemoe KD, eds. *Greenfield's Surgery: Scientific Principles and Practice*. 5th ed. Philadelphia, PA: Lippincott, Williams & Wilkins; 2011.

Mahvi DM, Krantz SB. Stomach. In: Townsend CM, Beauchamp RD, Evers BM, et al., eds. *Sabiston Textbook of Surgery*. 19th ed. Philadelphia, PA: Elsevier Saunders; 2012:1182–1226.

Mulholland MW. Gastric anatomy and physiology. In: Greenfield LJ, Mulholland MW, Oldham KT, Zelenock GB, Lillemoe KD, eds. *Greenfield's Surgery: Scientific Principles and Practice*. 5th ed. Philadelphia, PA: Lippincott, Williams & Wilkins; 2011: Chapter 43.

20. **(D)**

21. **(C)**

Explanation for questions 20 and 21

The approach to any patient with prior surgical intervention for ulcer disease requires detailed history taking. Included in the differential for epigastric pain after gastric surgery are gastric outlet obstruction, gastroesophageal reflux, recurrent ulcer (retained antrum or Zollinger-Ellison's syndrome), and alkaline reflux gastritis. This patient likely has alkaline reflux gastritis associated with his prior antrectomy. The combination of bile and pancreatic juices generates gastric mucosal injury. Bile acids themselves erode the protective mucosal barrier when in contact with gastric mucosa for extended times. Symptoms commonly include constant, burning epigastric pain worse with eating, nausea, and regurgitation of bitter, bilious material. Vomiting does not relieve the pain.

The diagnosis of alkaline reflux gastritis should be made after excluding all other causes. A nuclear medicine gastric-emptying study can demonstrate gastric outlet obstruction if present. Further confirmation of the diagnosis of alkaline reflux can be made with a HIDA scan. The term *HIDA* remains despite use of newer radiolabeled ^{99m}Tc molecules such as diisopropyl iminodiacetic acid DISIDA. These agents are injected intravenously and secreted in the bile. An external scintigraphic device quantifies the degree of bile refluxed into the stomach. This test is not pathognomonic, however, because even normal persons demonstrate some bile reflux; therefore, the test does not have high specificity. Serum testing for gastrin levels is usually used to rule out Zollinger-Ellison's syndrome; however, the results will be equivocal in this patient because hypergastrinemia develops postvagotomy. An additional important diagnostic tool is upper endoscopy. This can effectively diagnose gastroesophageal reflux, detect visible pathology such as recurrent ulceration, permit biopsy for *H. pylori*

colonization, and can directly visualize the enterogastric reflux of bile into the stomach. Histologic examination of damaged gastric mucosa will reveal intestinal metaplasia of gastric glands, a loss of parietal cells, and increased density of mucin cells.

Interestingly, conservative therapy for alkaline reflux gastritis is similar to treatment of acid reflux, with a few additions. Lifestyle modifications, including smoking cessation and avoidance of alcohol and other agents that promote lower esophageal sphincter relaxation are beneficial. PPIs and prokinetic agents reduce gastric irritation and increase gastric motility, respectively. Bile-absorbing agents like cholestyramine are often useful. Surgical intervention is indicated for severe or refractory symptoms. Most commonly, a Roux-en-Y diversion of the alkaline stream away from the stomach is performed. This reconstruction is inherently ulcerogenic, so if an acid-reducing procedure was not originally performed, a truncal vagotomy and antrectomy should be strongly considered in addition. An alternative procedure to the standard Roux-en-Y involves converting the original procedure to a gastroduodenostomy (Billroth I). Then, the common bile duct is disconnected from the duodenum and reanastomosed to a newly created Roux-en-Y limb, diverting the alkaline bile at least 45–60 cm from the stomach (Fig. 18-10).

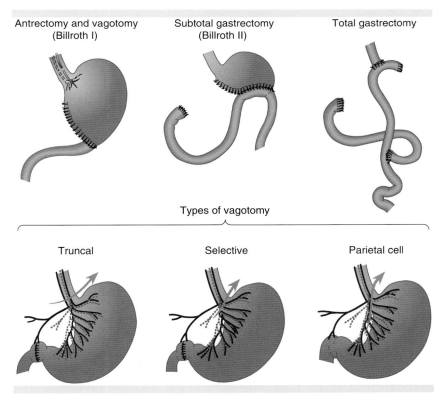

FIGURE 18-10. Alternative procedures for diverting the alkaline stream (from Doherty GM, ed. *Current Diagnosis and Treatment: Surgery*. 13th ed. New York, NY: McGraw-Hill; 2010: Fig. 23-5).

Congo red is a topical indicator dye that turns black when exposed to a pH less than 3.0. When instilled endoscopically, gastric mucosa with acid-secreting capability turns visibly black within 5 min of intravenous pentagastrin injection, thus identifying any gastric mucosa with vagal innervation intact.

Parietal cell vagotomy has almost no incidence of postoperative alkaline reflux gastritis because it does not destroy or bypass the pylorus.

BIBLIOGRAPHY

Mahvi DM, Krantz SB. Stomach. In: Townsend CM, Beauchamp RD, Evers BM, et al., eds. *Sabiston Textbook of Surgery*. 19th ed. Philadelphia, PA: Elsevier Saunders; 2012:1182–1226.

Mulholland MW. Gastric anatomy and physiology. In: Greenfield LJ, Mulholland MW, Oldham KT, Zelenock GB, Lillemoe KD, eds. *Greenfield's Surgery: Scientific Principles and Practice*. 5th ed. Philadelphia, PA: Lippincott, Williams & Wilkins; 2011: Chapter 43.

Sifrim D. Management of bile reflux. *Gastroenterol Hepatol* 2013;9(3):179–180.

22. **(A)** *Helicobacter pylori* is a carcinogen, according to the International Agency for Research on Cancer. The prevailing theory is that long-term infection and cycles of gastritis, ulceration, and atrophy cause chronic inflammation. In a subset of patients, this leads to intestinal metaplasia followed by dysplasia, then frank adenocarcinoma. *Helicobacter pylori* is also strongly associated with mucosa-associated lymphomatous tissue (MALT); infection is found in more than 90% of patients with primary gastric lymphoma. The importance of this association is demonstrated by the fact that eradication of this bacteria results in complete regression of MALT in 70–100% of cases. It is remarkable in that some early, low-grade gastric lymphomas can completely regress with antibiotic monotherapy (Fig. 18-11).

In this patient, the histological findings are suggestive of MALT, which accounts for just under 50% of all gastric lymphoma cases. Initial treatment with antibiotics targeted to eradicate *H. pylori* is indicated for stage I and II disease. In these lesions, surgical therapy is reserved for complications such as bleeding or perforation. For MALT lesions that are more advanced or do not respond to antibiotics alone, a combination of antibiotics, chemotherapy, or chemoradiation therapy is pursued. For the remainder of cases that represent high-grade lymphomas with or without a MALT component, chemoradiation is usually administered. Patients with early high-grade lesions rarely undergo surgical treatment. Stage III (locally advanced) and stage IV (disseminated) disease is treated with chemotherapy with or without radiation, with surgery reserved for any remaining disease not responsive to therapy, or for palliation. Recent case

series have demonstrated no survival benefit for primary surgical therapy in either stage I/II disease or stage III/IV disease.

BIBLIOGRAPHY

Bilimoria KY, Talamonti MS, Wayne JD. Tumors of the stomach, duodenum, and small bowel. In: Ashley SW, Cance WG, Chen H, et al. *Scientific American Surgery Online*. Hamilton, ON, Canada; Decker: Chapter 50.

Kitagawa Y, Dempsey DT. Stomach. In: Brunicardi F, Andersen DK, Billiar TR, et al., eds. *Schwartz's Principles of Surgery*. 10th ed. New York, NY: McGraw-Hill; 2014: Chapter 26.

23. **(D)** Patients with gastric lymphoma may present with nausea, vomiting, vague epigastric pain, and weight loss. Initial diagnosis is usually with endoscopy with biopsy. Additional studies for staging include basic laboratory studies, such as lactate dehydrogenase testing; imaging with CT of the chest, abdomen, and pelvis; and occasionally bone marrow biopsy.

BIBLIOGRAPHY

Bilimoria KY, Talamonti MS, Wayne JD. Tumors of the stomach, duodenum, and small bowel. In: Ashley SW, Cance WG, Chen H, et al. *Scientific American Surgery Online*. Hamilton, ON, Canada; Decker: Chapter 50.

Mulholland MW. Gastric anatomy and physiology. In: Greenfield LJ, Mulholland MW, Oldham KT, Zelenock GB, Lillemoe KD, eds. *Greenfield's Surgery: Scientific Principles and Practice*. 5th ed. Philadelphia, PA: Lippincott, Williams & Wilkins; 2011: Chapter 43.

24. **(D)** This patient's symptoms are consistent with dumping syndrome, characterized by rapid enteric transit after a high-osmotic load empties into the proximal small intestine. Gastrointestinal symptoms include fullness, nausea, vomiting, abdominal cramps, bloating, and diarrhea. Vasomotor symptoms include diaphoresis, weakness, dizziness, flushing, palpitations, blurry vision, and tachycardia. It is believed that destruction of the stomach's reservoir capacity results in the rapid delivery of hyperosmolar contents into the duodenum, and extracellular fluid shifts into the intestinal lumen to restore isotonicity. This causes an acute decrease in intravascular volume, leading to vasomotor symptoms. Humoral substances such as serotonin, neurotensin, and vasoactive intestinal peptide may also contribute to the vasomotor substances.

This syndrome may present to some degree after any gastric surgery, most often after partial gastrectomy. The Billroth II reconstruction results in a higher incidence than the Billroth I. There are two distinct forms of

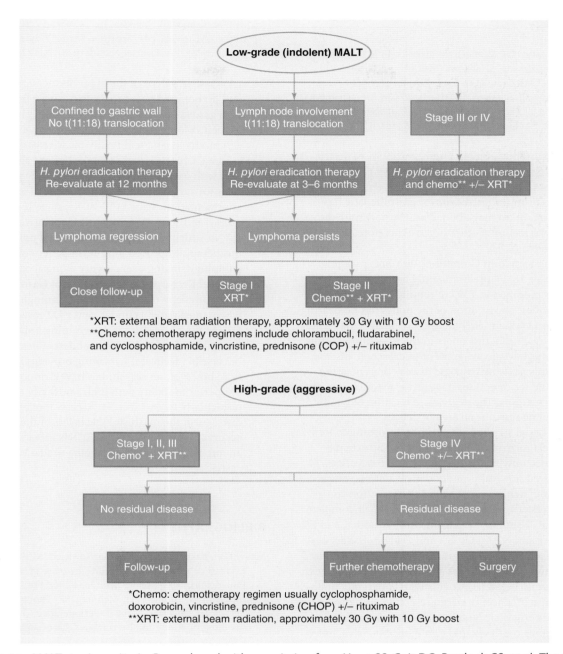

FIGURE 18-11. MALT staging criteria. Reproduced with permission from Yoon SS, Coit DG, Portlock CS, et al: *The diminishing role of surgery in the treatment of gastric lymphoma. Ann Surg* 240:28, 2004.

dumping: early and late. Early dumping usually occurs within 30 min of a meal. Late dumping occurs less frequently than early dumping. It is believed that late dumping results in excessive secretion of insulin from the pancreas. The resultant hypoglycemia is responsible for the symptoms of late dumping, intensified by the release of catecholamines.

Dietary management includes the separation of liquids and solids, decreasing liquid intake with meals, decreasing the amount of carbohydrates in meals, and avoiding extra salt. Octreotide, administered subcutaneously before meals, has been shown to improve dumping symptoms. Surgical interventions are rarely employed. The most widely used procedure is Roux-en-Y gastrojejunostomy, which takes advantage of the impaired motility of the Roux limb.

Cholestyramine, a bile acid sequestrant, has not been shown to be effective in ameliorating the symptoms of dumping syndrome.

BIBLIOGRAPHY

Kitagawa Y, Dempsey DT. Stomach. In: Brunicardi F, Andersen DK, Billiar TR, et al., eds. *Schwartz's Principles of Surgery*. 10th ed. New York, NY: McGraw-Hill; 2014: Chapter 26.

Mahvi DM, Krantz SB. Stomach. In: Townsend CM, Beauchamp RD, Evers BM, et al., eds. *Sabiston Textbook of Surgery*. 19th ed. Philadelphia, PA: Elsevier Saunders; 2012:1182–1226.

25. **(B)** Gastric adenocarcinoma represents 95% of gastric malignancies, followed by lymphomas (4%) and GISTs (1%) in the United States. Tumors that extend into the muscularis propria, gastrocolic, or gastrohepatic ligaments or omentum may not necessarily penetrate the visceral peritoneum of other organs; therefore, their classification remains T3.

    The American Joint Committee on Cancer staging system (Table 18-1), predominantly used in the United States, was modified in 1997 to require a minimum of 15 sampled nodes. The location of the nodes has no bearing in the current system. Frequently discussed is the "R status" of the resection; this refers to the resection margins. R0 resections have no evidence of microscopic disease, R1 resections have microscopic disease present at the margins, and R2 resections have gross, macroscopic disease at the margins. The degree and location of lymph node sampling remains an area of debate.

    Gastric nodal stations are grouped according to location and relation to the primary tumor. The extent of lymphadenectomy necessary for adequate resection and improved survival is under debate, with Japanese surgeons preferring a more extensive dissection compared to Western surgeons. A D0 represents incomplete resection of N1 nodes, D1 includes all N1 nodes, and D2 includes N1 and N2 nodes. D3 and D4 lymphadenectomies represent even further resections. Current standard of care in the United States is a D1 lymphadenectomy. In Western countries, most patients with apparently node-negative gastric cancer undergo resection with dissection of only the perigastric lymph nodes (D1 resection). In Japan, patients routinely undergo more extensive dissections of lymph nodes, usually D2 or D3. Japanese and German studies have shown that these more extensive node dissections improve survival. Other studies have not shown an increase in survival or have shown an increase in operative mortality with more extensive node dissections.

BIBLIOGRAPHY

Kitagawa Y, Dempsey DT. Stomach. In: Brunicardi F, Andersen DK, Billiar TR, et al., eds. *Schwartz's Principles of Surgery*. 10th ed. New York, NY: McGraw-Hill; 2014: Chapter 26.

Mahvi DM, Krantz SB. Stomach. In: Townsend CM, Beauchamp RD, Evers BM, et al., eds. *Sabiston Textbook of Surgery*. 19th ed. Philadelphia, PA: Elsevier Saunders; 2012:1182–1226.

26. **(A)** Gastric polyps of the hyperplastic type are benign and do not predispose to gastric cancer, but adenomatous gastric polyps can follow the same progression as their colonic counterparts and become dysplastic, carcinoma in situ, and finally invasive gastric adenocarcinoma. Chronic alcohol intake has not shown a correlation with gastric adenocarcinoma. The 5-year survival rates for surgery with curative intent correlates with stage at presentation: stage I (60–80%), stage II (35%), stage III (20%), and stage IV (<10%). Perioperative chemotherapy, in which patients receive pre- and postoperative chemotherapy, improved long-term patient outcomes and pathology staging over surgery along according to the Medical Research Council Adjuvant Gastric Infusional Chemotherapy (MAGIC) trial (Cunningham et al. 2006), where most patients underwent a D2 resection. While CT imaging is useful for determining bulky disease and metastasis, the sensitivity is modest at best for N1 and N2 disease. Helical CT imaging provides better resolution; however, several studies have demonstrated EUS as a superior modality with high sensitivity and specificity, particularly for N0 and N1 disease. It offers the ability to distinguish the five histologic layers of the stomach with accuracy approaching 92%. EUS is therefore considered an important adjunctive imaging modality for staging gastric cancer.

BIBLIOGRAPHY

Mahvi DM, Krantz SB. Stomach. In: Townsend CM, Beauchamp RD, Evers BM, et al., eds. *Sabiston Textbook of Surgery*. 19th ed. Philadelphia, PA: Elsevier Saunders; 2012:1182–1226.

Cunningham D, Allum WH, Stenning SP, Thompson JN, Van de Velde CJH, Nicolson M, et al. Perioperative Chemotherapy versus Surgery Alone for Resectable Gastroesophageal Cancer. N Engl J Med 2006; 6:11–20.

27. **(D)** Dieulafoy's lesion is the presence of arteries of consistently large caliber in the submucosa. These most often occur in the proximal stomach, although they have been described throughout the gastrointestinal tract. This occurs as a result of lack of the normally occurring arterial arborization once they reach the submucosa, hence the alternate name "caliber-persistent artery." These become symptomatic if the artery compresses the overlying mucosa, leading to erosion of the arterial wall and rupture. Massive hemorrhage results, and this is the usual presenting symptom. Treatment follows that of all gastric bleeding, with resuscitation of the patient

TABLE 18-1 TNM Classification of Tumors of the Stomach

T: Primary Tumor	
T0	No evidence of primary tumor
Tis	Carcinoma in situ; intraepithelial tumor without invasion of the lamina propria, high-grade dysplasia
T1	Tumor invades lamina propria, muscularis mucosae, or submucosa
T1a	Tumor invades lamina propria or muscularis mucosae
T1b	Tumor invades submucosa
T2	Tumor invades muscularis propria
T3	Tumor invades subserosa
T4	Tumor perforates serosa or invades adjacent structures
T4a	Tumor perforates serosa
T4b	Tumor invades adjacent structures

N: Regional Lymph Nodes	
N0	No regional lymph node metastasis
N1	Metastasis in 1 to 2 regional lymph nodes
N2	Metastasis in 3 to 6 regional lymph nodes
N3	Metastasis in 7 or more regional lymph nodes
N3a	Metastasis in 7 to 15 regional lymph nodes
N3b	Metastasis in 16 or more regional lymph nodes

M: Distant Metastasis	
M0	No distant metastasis
M1	Distant metastasis

Stage Grouping

Stage	T	N	M
Stage 0	Tis	N0	M0
Stage IA	T1	N0	M0
Stage IB	T2	N0	M0
	T1	N1	M0
Stage IIA	T3	N0	M0
	T2	N1	M0
	T1	N2	M0
Stage IIB	T4a	N0	M0
	T3	N1	M0
	T2	N2	M0
	T1	N3	M0
Stage IIIA	T4a	N1	M0
	T3	N2	M0
	T2	N3	M0
Stage IIIC	T4a	N3	M0
	T4b	N2, 3	M0
Stage IV	AnyT	AnyN	M1

Source: Used with permission of the American Joint Commission on Cancer (AJCC), Chicago, Illinois. The original source for this material is the AJCC Cancer Staging Manual, Seventh Edition (2010) published by Springer Science and Business Media LLC, www.springer.com.

and gastric lavage, then endoscopic examination. Many of these have stopped bleeding by the time endoscopy is performed, but if there is persistent hemorrhage, endoscopic therapy via heater probe, laser coagulator, injection, or band ligator is able to permanently stop bleeding in more than 90% of cases.

Mallory-Weiss tears are linear mucosal tears at or just below the gastroesophageal junction, usually at the lesser curvature. These were classically described as the source of profuse bleeding after a bout of retching or vomiting, but they are often found in association with other gastric pathologies, such as gastritis, ulcer, and hiatal hernia. Over 90% of bleeding tears cease after resuscitation and gastric lavage. On endoscopy, if there is active bleeding or a visible vessel, therapy is indicated via heater probe, laser coagulator, injection, or band ligator. Endoscopic therapy is highly effective even in patients with varices secondary to portal hypertension, who have a higher incidence of Mallory-Weiss tears than the general population.

Gastric ulcers secondary to chronic NSAID use, sometimes called type V gastric ulcers, almost always respond to resuscitation, withdrawal of the offending agent, and administration of acid-reducing medications such as a PPI. Endoscopic therapy may be indicated if bleeding persists after gastric lavage and supportive care. Embolization via interventional radiology techniques would be the next step in recalcitrant bleeding. Surgical therapy is occasionally needed if profuse bleeding persists or certainly if a perforation occurs.

BIBLIOGRAPHY

Mahvi DM, Krantz SB. Stomach. In: Townsend CM, Beauchamp RD, Evers BM, et al., eds. *Sabiston Textbook of Surgery*. 19th ed. Philadelphia, PA: Elsevier Saunders; 2012:1182–1226.

28.   **(D)** There are several pharmaceutical agents used in the medical treatment of ulcer disease. Some act as acid reduction agents, some as antibiotics, and some perform both functions. PPIs, such as omeprazole and lansoprazole, selectively inhibit the H^+, K^+-ATPase of parietal cells, the enzyme that is the last step in producing luminal acid. If enough drug is administered, a state of anacidity can be produced. PPIs are ineffective at eradicating *H. pylori* infections as single agents but act synergistically with antibiotics; the growth and survival of *H. pylori* is pH dependent, with slower growth rates at higher pH. H_2 receptor antagonists (famotidine, ranitidine, cimetidine, and nizatidine) reduce acid secretion by blocking activation of the histamine receptor of parietal cells. This not only prevents histamine from stimulating acid secretion but also reduces the effects of acetylcholine and gastrin on the remaining types of

receptors. H_2 receptor blockers significantly decrease acid production but will not by themselves eradicate *H. pylori*.

Bismuth compounds exhibit antimicrobial activity against several bacteria, including *H. pylori*, by an unclear mechanism. They are also synergistic with other antibiotics. Importantly, there have been no reported instances of *H. pylori* resistance to bismuth compounds. Bismuth compounds in their most commonly administered forms—bismuth subsalicylate (Pepto-Bismol) and colloidal bismuth subcitrate—are poorly absorbed and therefore must act locally against *H. pylori* in the gastric lumen. Ranitidine bismuth citrate is a compound that combines the effects of an H_2 receptor antagonist and a bismuth compound and has found an important place in the armamentarium against *H. pylori*.

The imidazoles, such as metronidazole and tinidazole, exhibit activity against *H. pylori* by damaging bacterial DNA. They are absorbed systemically and then transported to the gastric juice. Mutations can occur that allow *H. pylori* strains to prevent activation of imidazoles, rendering these strains resistant to this genre of antimicrobials.

Macrolides, like clarithromycin and erythromycin, show activity against *H. pylori* by binding to the 50S ribosomal subunit, preventing protein synthesis. Like imidazoles, they are absorbed systemically and then transported to the gastric mucosa. Macrolides show greater antimicrobial efficacy at higher pH, explaining their improved efficacy when combined with an acid reduction agent. Of all antimicrobials, clarithromycin is the most effective single agent against *H. pylori* organisms, with eradication rates of 40% when used alone. This reinforces why multiple-agent regimens are greatly preferred to single-agent regimens. Resistance to macrolides occurs when strains of *H. pylori* develop mutated ribosomal subunits that no longer strongly bind these agents.

Amoxicillin, a penicillin, is probably second only to clarithromycin in efficacy against *H. pylori*. Amoxicillin acts by preventing cell wall cross-linking. It probably acts against *H. pylori* both locally and systemically. *Helicobacter pylori* resistance to amoxicillin is rare. Like the macrolides, amoxicillin shows increased efficacy at higher pH. Tetracycline inhibits protein synthesis by binding the 30S ribosomal subunit and has shown good efficacy against *H. pylori*. Sucralfate probably exerts its antimicrobial action indirectly by promoting gastric mucus production. It is unclear if sucralfate is bactericidal or not, but it improves the minimum inhibitory concentration (MIC) of almost all antibiotics used against *H. pylori*.

In this question, all of the combinations have proven at least 90% effective and are recommended in the attempt to eradicate *H. pylori* infection except for lansoprazole plus amoxicillin. All of the currently used PPIs demonstrate comparable acid-suppressing ability, but even with the synergism between a PPI and most antibiotics, eradication rates higher than 70% have not been achieved when single antibiotics have been used. All currently recommended regimens involve some form of acid suppression and at least two antibiotics, and eradication rates have been shown to be approximately 90% or greater.

BIBLIOGRAPHY

Mahvi DM, Krantz SB. Stomach. In: Townsend CM, Beauchamp RD, Evers BM, et al., eds. *Sabiston Textbook of Surgery*. 19th ed. Philadelphia, PA: Elsevier Saunders; 2012:1182–1226.

Mulholland MW. Gastric anatomy and physiology. In: Greenfield LJ, Mulholland MW, Oldham KT, Zelenock GB, Lillemoe KD, eds. *Greenfield's Surgery: Scientific Principles and Practice*. 5th ed. Philadelphia, PA: Lippincott Williams & Wilkins; 2011: Chapter 43.

CHAPTER 19

SMALL BOWEL

MICHAEL WANDLING, MICHAEL SHAPIRO, AND MAMTA SWAROOP

QUESTIONS

1. Which of the following is true of cholecystokinin (CCK)?
   (A) Its release stimulates pancreatic acinar cell secretion, pancreatic growth, and insulin release.
   (B) It is a peptide hormone.
   (C) Its release stimulates gallbladder contraction and sphincter of Oddi relaxation.
   (D) It is released by the small bowel in response to contact with amino acids.
   (E) All of the above.

2. A 45-year-old woman presents to the emergency department with 18 h of nausea, vomiting, and cramping abdominal pain. The pain is not constant, and she denies any associated fevers. She underwent hysterectomy and bilateral oophorectomy 2 years ago. An abdominal series is consistent with a small bowel obstruction. Which of the following is true regarding the natural physiologic barrier that prevents bacterial translocation in this clinical scenario?
   (A) The gastrointestinal (GI) tract contains minimal, if any, lymphoid tissue.
   (B) The nonimmunologic defenses of the gut include epithelial tight junctions, endogenous bacteria, mucin production, gastric acid, proteolytic enzymes, and peristalsis.
   (C) Secretory immunoglobulin (Ig) A prevents colonization of bacteria in the small bowel by stimulating their adherence to the epithelial surface.
   (D) Absorption of antigens and bacterial toxins is stimulated by secretory IgA.
   (E) All of the above.

3. Which of the following is true regarding the epidemiology of Crohn's disease (CD)?
   (A) The incidence in females is equal to the incidence in males.
   (B) The incidence in American Caucasians is much greater than the incidence in individuals immigrating to the United States from Africa.

   (C) Crohn's disease affects rural dwellers more often than urban dwellers.
   (D) A family history of Crohn's is not important for first-degree relatives.
   (E) All of the above.

4. A 22-year-old woman comes to your office with complaints of daily sharp abdominal pain, a 7-lb weight loss over the last 6 weeks, and four to six bowel movements per day for the last several weeks. An upper GI endoscopy was unremarkable. Her colonoscopy was suggestive of Crohn's disease. Which of the following findings is suggestive of Crohn's disease over ulcerative colitis (UC)?
   (A) There are ulcerated lesions in the distal sigmoid colon, followed by a patch of normal colon and then more ulcers near the splenic flexure. The rectum appears to be spared.
   (B) There is an absence of perianal fistulas.
   (C) Microscopic evaluation of a lesion reveals superficial, partial-thickness inflammation.
   (D) Absence of circumferential wrapping of mesenteric fat around the bowel is noted during laparotomy.
   (E) All of the above.

5. A 19-year-old man presents to the emergency department with a 24-h history of right lower quadrant abdominal pain, fever to 100.5°F, anorexia, and two loose, non-bloody stools. He undergoes surgical exploration for a presumed diagnosis of appendicitis. In the operating room, the appendix and cecum appear completely normal, but the terminal ileum is inflamed. What is the most appropriate next step in his management?
   (A) Proceed with appendectomy.
   (B) Perform an ileocecectomy with ileostomy.
   (C) Perform full abdominal exploration to evaluate for further obvious lesions and obtain a colonoscopy prior to discharge.
   (D) Nothing. The patient's incision should be closed, and postoperatively there should be a GI consult for a presumed diagnosis of Crohn's disease.
   (E) Perform a subtotal colectomy.

417

6. Indications for surgical intervention in Crohn's disease include which of the following?
   (A) Postoperative enterocutaneous fistulas (ECFs)
   (B) Duodenal obstruction refractory to medical management
   (C) Small bowel obstruction that has not improved with nonoperative management
   (D) Child with secondary growth retardation related to CD
   (E) All of the above

7. A 48-year-old woman with human immunodeficiency virus (HIV) complains of severe right lower quadrant abdominal pain. Her initial lab work was significant for a white blood cell (WBC) count of 1.3. The remainder of her complete blood cell count (CBC) and chemistry panel was unremarkable. A computed tomographic (CT) scan revealed nonspecific enteritis and a normal appendix. Stool cultures were positive for cytomegalovirus (CMV), and she was diagnosed with CMV enteritis. What is the appropriate treatment for CMV enteritis?
   (A) Ganciclovir
   (B) Prednisone
   (C) Oseltamivir
   (D) Alfa interferon
   (E) Infliximab

8. Which of the following treatments for Crohn's disease is useful in maintaining remission?
   (A) Prednisone
   (B) Infliximab
   (C) Azathioprine
   (D) Interleukin (IL) 10 analogue
   (E) All of the above

9. Which clinical scenario should be managed operatively as soon as appropriate resuscitative measures have been initiated?
   (A) A 68-year-old man with metastatic pancreatic cancer presents with 18 h of nausea, vomiting, and crampy abdominal pain. His abdominal x-rays demonstrate multiple air-fluid levels and stairstepping pattern.
   (B) A 68-year-old woman postoperative day 5 status after colostomy takedown and reanastomosis presents with nausea, vomiting, and abdominal distension. Her abdominal x-rays demonstrate multiple air-fluid levels and stairstepping pattern.
   (C) A 68-year-old man status postprostatectomy and radiation therapy 6 years ago for prostate cancer now has a 24-h history of nausea, vomiting, and dull abdominal pain. His abdominal x-rays demonstrate multiple air-fluid levels and stairstepping pattern.

   (D) A 68-year-old woman status after colostomy takedown 1 year ago presents with 24-h history of nausea, feculent vomiting, fever to 100.2°F, tachycardia, persistent abdominal pain, and a mild leukocytosis. Her abdominal x-rays demonstrate multiple air-fluid levels and stairstepping pattern.
   (E) All of the above.

10. A 62-year-old man with a history of chronic obstructive pulmonary disease (COPD) due to 35 years of heavy smoking presents to the emergency department with nausea, occasional nonbilious emesis, loose stools, and nonspecific abdominal pain. On examination, his abdomen is distended, but soft, and mildly tender to deep palpation. A CT scan of the abdomen and pelvis reveals pneumatosis intestinalis and air within the falciform ligament, but no free intraperitoneal air or portal venous gas. What is the most appropriate next step in management of this patient?
    (A) If the patient is able to tolerate a diet, discharge him from the emergency department and have him follow up with his primary care physician if his symptoms do not improve.
    (B) Perform an emergent exploratory laparotomy.
    (C) Admit the patient for observation and a brief period of bowel rest.
    (D) Give the patient broad-spectrum intravenous antibiotics.

11. Which of the following factors is likely to prevent spontaneous fistula closure?
    (A) High-output fistula (>500 mL per day)
    (B) Radiation enteritis
    (C) Active inflammatory bowel disease (IBD) of fistulized segment
    (D) Fistula tract less than 2.5 cm in length
    (E) All of the above

12. The most common presentation of a Meckel's diverticulum in an adult is which of the following?
    (A) GI bleed
    (B) Intussusception
    (C) Littre's hernia
    (D) Diverticulitis

13. Superior mesenteric artery (SMA) syndrome is associated with which of the following?
    (A) Radiation enteritis
    (B) Coronary artery disease
    (C) Hypothyroidism
    (D) Rapid weight loss
    (E) All of the above

14. The preferred treatment of acute SMA syndrome is which of the following?
    (A) Billroth II reconstruction
    (B) Nutritional support
    (C) Duodenojejunostomy
    (D) SMA bypass
    (E) Strong's procedure

15. A 25-year-old man with schizophrenia presents to the emergency department 2.5 h after he was seen ingesting a razor blade. His abdominal exam is benign, and his WBC count is 8000. An abdominal x-ray demonstrates a razor blade in the patient's midabdomen (Fig. 19-1). The most appropriate next step in his management is which of the following?

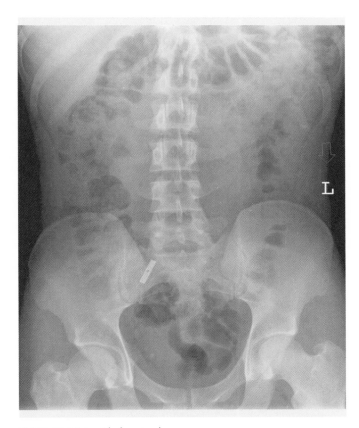

FIGURE 19-1. Abdominal x-ray.

    (A) Give milk of magnesia to speed excretion of the razor blade
    (B) Urgent exploratory laparotomy
    (C) Admit the patient for serial x-rays and serial abdominal examinations
    (D) GI consult to retrieve the razor blade by enteroscopy

16. The percentage of cardiac output delivered to the small bowel at rest is which of the following?
    (A) 10–15%
    (B) 20–25%
    (C) 30–35%
    (D) 45–50%

17. While in the operating room performing a laparotomy for mesenteric ischemia, a long segment of "dusky" small bowel is identified. There is some improvement after the application of warm laparotomy pads to the dusky-appearing bowel for 10–15 min. Which of the following is the best method for assessing/managing the viability of the segment of bowel in question in this patient?
    (A) Doppler ultrasound
    (B) Oximetry
    (C) Fluorescein administration followed by Wood's lamp examination
    (D) Plan for a second-look surgery within the next 36 h

18. Which of the following is true regarding the management of the bowel obstruction secondary to gallstone ileus that is depicted in Fig. 19-2?

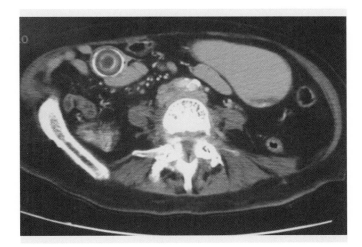

FIGURE 19-2. Gallstone ileus.

    (A) The gallbladder and fistula tract do not need to be dealt with at the time of laparotomy if the gallstone is impacted in the terminal ileum.
    (B) Recurrent gallstone ileus is rare, even when cholecystectomy is not performed.
    (C) If the gallstone is impacted in the colon, the stone should be excised via a colotomy.
    (D) All of the above.

19. Which of the following regarding the etiology of intussusception in adults is correct?
    (A) Intussusception is infrequently caused by benign small bowel tumors.
    (B) Reduction of intussusception in adults should not be attempted by air or contrast enema.
    (C) Intussusception does not occur episodically in Peutz-Jeghers–associated hamartomas.
    (D) Intussusception is frequently caused by primary malignant small bowel tumors.
    (E) All of the above.

20. Which of the following is true of malignant small bowel neoplasms?
    (A) Small bowel adenocarcinoma comprises greater than 30% of small bowel malignancies and rarely presents with metastatic disease.
    (B) Small bowel GI stromal tumors (GISTs) comprise 20% of small bowel malignancies and spread hematogenously to the liver and lungs and by local invasion.
    (C) Primary small bowel lymphomas rarely present with indolent symptoms.
    (D) Patients with primary small bowel lymphomas frequently have constitutional symptoms at the time of presentation.
    (E) All of the above.

21. Which of the following is true of carcinoid tumors?
    (A) Carcinoid syndrome is frequently seen in patients with carcinoid tumors.
    (B) The small bowel is the second-most-common site for carcinoid tumors of the GI tract.
    (C) Carcinoid syndrome is commonly seen in patients with carcinoid tumors localized to the small bowel.
    (D) In comparison with other small bowel malignancies, carcinoid tumors carry a considerably worse prognosis.
    (E) All of the above.

22. Which of the following adenomas can be managed endoscopically?
    (A) A 3-cm pedunculated adenoma in the second segment of the duodenum
    (B) A 3-cm tubulovillous adenoma in the second segment of the duodenum
    (C) A 3-cm villous adenoma in the second segment of the duodenum
    (D) All of the above can be managed endoscopically

23. A 52-year-old man is hospitalized with recurrent pancreatitis. He has no history of alcohol use, cholelithiasis, or hypertriglyceridemia. On endoscopic retrograde cholangiopancreatography (ERCP), he was found to have a moderate-size duodenal diverticulum located approximately 1 cm from the ampulla of Vater. What is the most appropriate next step in management?
    (A) Pancreaticoduodenectomy
    (B) Sphincterotomy and stent placement
    (C) Choledochoduodenostomy
    (D) Duodenectomy with duodenojejunal anastomosis

24. A 57-year-old man with no past surgical history presents to the emergency room with a small bowel obstruction. On CT, the transition point appears to be associated with a soft tissue mass. At laparotomy, a partially obstructing mass that is approximately 5 cm in diameter involving the wall of the distal jejunum is identified. A small bowel resection is performed, and the tumor is completely excised. Final pathology reveals that the mass is a GIST. What is the most likely mechanism of distal recurrence for this patient?
    (A) Lymphatic spread
    (B) Direct invasion
    (C) Hematogenous spread
    (D) Resection is curative as GISTs do not spread
    (E) All of the above

25. The patient from question 24 returns 3 years later with local recurrence and multiple liver metastases. His disease is not surgically resectable, and he is started on imatinib mesylate. What is imatinib mesylate's mechanism of action?
    (A) Cross-links DNA through alkylation
    (B) Inhibits a tyrosine kinase receptor
    (C) Inhibits ribonucleotide reductase
    (D) Inhibits mitosis by binding microtubules
    (E) Inhibits topoisomerase II

26. An otherwise-healthy 28-year-old woman undergoes an open appendectomy for perforated appendicitis. On postoperative day 3, she complains of nausea and abdominal distension. She has not passed flatus or had a bowel movement since surgery. An acute abdominal series is significant for gas throughout the small bowel and colon, consistent with ileus. Her current medications include oxycodone and ibuprofen. Lab values include WBC 11,000 mm^3, hemoglobin (Hb) 13 g/dL, Na 134 mmol/L, K 4.0 mmol/L, Cl 109 mmol/L, HCO$_3$ 26 mmol/L, and Cr 0.9 mg/dL. Which of the following is likely contributing to her ileus?
    (A) Intra-abdominal inflammation
    (B) Narcotic pain medication
    (C) Hyponatremia
    (D) Postoperative status
    (E) All of the above

27. Which of the following treatments have been proven to reduce the duration of postoperative ileus in the clinical setting?
    (A) Epidural local anesthetics
    (B) Postoperative nasogastric (NG) decompression of the GI tract
    (C) Aggressive pain control with intravenous narcotics
    (D) Erythromycin administration
    (E) Starting total parenteral nutrition immediately after surgery

28. Intra-abdominal adhesions following abdominal surgery have been associated with which of the following?
    (A) Small bowel obstruction
    (B) Infertility
    (C) Chronic pelvic pain
    (D) Increased risk for enterotomy on subsequent laparotomy
    (E) All of the above

29. A 76-year-old woman with a history of hypertension, tobacco use, and peripheral vascular disease presents to her primary care physician complaining of intermittent epigastric abdominal pain and nausea. Her symptoms started 4 months ago and have been increasing in severity. The abdominal pain is dull and "gnawing." It starts approximately 30 minutes after meals and lasts for 2–4 h at a time. The pain is sometimes accompanied by nausea. She denies vomiting, diarrhea, hematochezia, and melena. She fears eating and has lost 18 lb since her symptoms began. Her surgical history is significant for a right carotid endarterectomy. Her abdominal exam is unremarkable, and her routine laboratory values are normal except for hypoalbuminemia. A right upper quadrant ultrasound, esophagogastroduodenoscopy (EGD), and colonoscopy are all normal. Which of the following is true regarding the most likely diagnosis?
    (A) Mesenteric duplex ultrasound is not a helpful screening tool in symptomatic patients.
    (B) Postprandial abdominal pain is rarely present.
    (C) The most common cause is atherosclerosis.
    (D) Endovascular interventions for this condition are more durable than open techniques.
    (E) All of the above.

30. A 57-year-old man presents to the emergency department with sudden-onset, severe, epigastric pain that began approximately 8 h ago. The pain is constant, does not radiate, and is worse with movement. He denies any other symptoms but does report a history of episodic vague upper abdominal pain. He takes no medications but has used over-the-counter antacid tablets in the past. On physical exam his abdomen is distended, tympanic to percussion, and diffusely tender with peritoneal signs. An acute abdominal series is significant for free air under the diaphragm. During exploratory laparotomy, he is found to have a 3-mm perforated duodenal ulcer involving the anterior aspect of the first portion of the duodenum with minimal intraperitoneal soilage. Which of the following is true regarding the further surgical and medical management of this patient's disease?
    (A) *Helicobacter pylori* infection and Zollinger-Ellison syndrome are the two most common causes of duodenal ulcer disease.
    (B) Based on this ulcer's location, the patient will not require *H. pylori* testing.
    (C) A laparoscopic approach to this problem is contraindicated.
    (D) Appropriate surgical management is primary closure and abdominal washout.
    (E) The procedure of choice is antrectomy with truncal vagotomy.

31. Which of the following is true regarding bowel resections and short bowel syndrome?
    (A) Common nutrient deficiencies include iron, magnesium, zinc, copper, and vitamins.
    (B) The small bowel is unable to increase its absorptive capacity following significant small bowel resections.
    (C) Distal small bowel resections are better tolerated than proximal small bowel resections.
    (D) If the terminal ileum and ileocecal valve are preserved, resection of up to 35% of the small bowel can typically be tolerated.
    (E) All of the above.

ANSWERS AND EXPLANATIONS

1. **(E)** Cholecystokinin is a peptide hormone predominantly produced by I cells in the duodenum and jejunum in response to the ingestion of fats, peptides, and amino acids. Trypsin and bile acids inhibit its release. The overall function of CCK is to improve digestion and absorption of key nutrients.

   Cholecystokinin stimulates contraction of the gallbladder and relaxation of the sphincter of Oddi, making it useful in assessing for biliary dyskinesia with CCK hepatic iminodiacetic acid (HIDA) scans. It also stimulates secretion of enzymes by pancreatic acinar cells and slows gastric emptying by affecting muscular contraction of the pylorus. CCK has a trophic effect on small bowel mucosa and on pancreas cells, and it may also play a role in intestinal motility and insulin release. Finally, CCK acts to produce a sense of satiety.

BIBLIOGRAPHY

McKenzie S, Evers BM. Small intestine. In: Townsend CM, Beauchamp RD, Evers BM, et al., eds. *Sabiston Textbook of Surgery.* 19th ed. Philadelphia, PA: Elsevier Saunders; 2012:1234–1236.

Miller LJ. Gastrointestinal hormones and receptors. In: Yamada T, Alpers DH, Kaplowitz N, et al., eds. *Textbook of Gastroenterology.* 4th ed. Philadelphia, PA: Lippincott Williams & Wilkins; 2003:62–64.

Simeone DM. Anatomy and physiology of the small intestine. In: Greenfield L, Mulholland M, Oldham K, et al., eds. *Surgery: Scientific Principles and Practice.* 3rd ed. Philadelphia, PA: Lippincott Williams & Wilkins; 2001:797–798.

2. **(B)** The nonimmunologic defenses of the gut include epithelial tight junctions, endogenous bacteria, mucin production, gastric acid, proteolytic enzymes, and peristalsis.

   The gut has a complex array of defense mechanisms to protect it against constant pathogens. Its first line of defense is nonimmunologic barriers; these include gastric acid and proteolytic enzymes that directly degrade pathogens, the inhibition of bacterial growth by a mucinous coat on the epithelial cells, the spatial inhibition of exogenous bacteria by the presence of native bacteria, epithelial tight junctions' prevention of invasion of the epithelium by pathogens, and peristalsis to prevent stagnation of pathogens or carcinogens on the gut mucosa.

The immunologic barriers are vast. Gut-associated lymphoid tissue comprises a major division of the body's immune system, with approximately 70% of all IgA synthesis occurring in the intestinal tract (Fig. 19-3). Intraepithelial lymphocytes (IELs) live between gut epithelial cells in the crypts of the villi and primarily serve as cytolytic T cells during illness with a high CD8 expression; however, during health, they serve to secrete cytokines, such as interferon-gamma (IFN-γ.) Another function of IELs during health is that of immunosurveillance, ensuring against abnormal epithelial cells and inducing apoptosis in them. The lamina propria houses a number of unaggregated lymphoid cells, including B and T cells, presumably migrants from Peyer's patches, macrophages, neutrophils, eosinophils, and mast cells. The lamina propria B cells and plasma cells are the primary producers of IgA.

The lamina propria also is home to Peyer's patches, lymphoid nodules without capsules comprised primarily of B and T cells. These are found on the antimesenteric border of the ileum. Peyer's patches are covered by microfold cells (M cells). These cells allow the lymphoid cells selective exposure to intraluminal antigens by transporting endocytosed antigens transcellularly to the Peyer's patches. Once these cells are "educated," they travel to other areas of the lymph system.

Gut plasma cells produce a significant amount of IgA, which confers great protection for the intestinal tract.

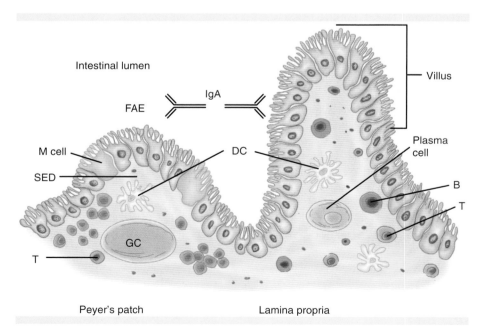

FIGURE 19-3. Gut-associated lymphoid tissue (from Brunicardi FC, Andersen DK, Billiar TR, et al., eds. *Schwartz's Principles of Surgery.* 10th ed. New York, NY: McGraw-Hill; 2014: Fig. 28-10. Copyright © The McGraw-Hill Companies, Inc. All rights reserved).

IgA occurs in monomeric and polymeric forms; 50% of gut IgA is polymeric, with its monomers connected by a J chain. The IgA and J chain are produced in the plasma cell and transported to the cell border to interact and complex with the epithelial polymeric immunoglobulin receptor (pIgR). This complex is endocytosed and transported to the epithelial surface to be secreted as secretory IgA (sIgA). Secretory IgA protects the mucosa against bacterial adherence and colonization. It neutralizes bacterial toxins and viral activity and prohibits absorption of intraluminal antigens. Unlike other immunoglobulins, however, it does *not* activate complement or cell-mediated opsonization.

BIBLIOGRAPHY

Blumberg RS, Stenson WF. The immune system and gastrointestinal inflammation. In: Yamada T, Alpers DH, Kaplowitz N, et al., eds. *Textbook of Gastroenterology.* 4th ed. Philadelphia, PA: Lippincott Williams & Wilkins; 2003:127–130.

McKenzie S, Evers BM. Small intestine. In: Townsend CM, Beauchamp RD, Evers BM, et al., eds. *Sabiston Textbook of Surgery.* 19th ed. Philadelphia, PA: Elsevier Saunders; 2012:1236.

Simeone DM. Anatomy and physiology of the small intestine. In: Greenfield L, Mulholland M, Oldham K, et al., eds. *Surgery: Scientific Principles and Practice.* 3rd ed. Philadelphia, PA: Lippincott Williams & Wilkins; 2001:795–797.

3. **(A)** The overall incidence of CD is three to seven new cases per year per 100,000 people. The prevalence is 80–120 per 100,000. It is more common in Europe and North America than in other parts of the world and occurs in individuals moving to these endemic areas at the same rate that is seen in those areas, suggesting an environmental component to CD. CD has a bimodal pattern of onset, with the first peak incidence seen in individuals in the second and third decade of life and a second, smaller peak occurring in the sixth decade. CD is more common in urban areas than rural areas.

The incidence of CD is the same in men and women. Jews of European decent are at significantly higher risk than similar age- and gender-matched Americans and Europeans. Smokers have twice the risk of developing CD as nonsmokers. First-degree relatives of Crohn's patients are at 13-fold greater risk, while siblings carry a risk increased by 30-fold.

BIBLIOGRAPHY

McKenzie S, Evers BM. Small intestine. In: Townsend CM, Beauchamp RD, Evers BM, et al., eds. *Sabiston Textbook of Surgery.* 19th ed. Philadelphia, PA: Elsevier Saunders; 2012:1244–1254.

Michelassi F, Hurst RD. Crohn's disease. In: Greenfield L, Mulholland M, Oldham K, et al., eds. *Surgery: Scientific Principles and Practice.* 3rd ed. Philadelphia, PA: Lippincott Williams & Wilkins; 2001:813.

4. **(A)** This patient's presentation is typical for that of IBD, both CD and UC. Periods of colicky, sharp abdominal pain, diarrhea, weight loss, and malaise alternate with periods of normalcy, but over time the symptomatic times become more frequent and prolonged. Diagnosis of IBD is made using endoscopy along with careful history and physical examination with possible computed tomographic (CT) scan and barium studies.

In early diagnosis of IBD, distinguishing between CD and UC can be difficult, but time will permit a nearly indisputable diagnosis (Fig. 19-4). CD typically presents with aphthous ulcers, lesions a few millimeters in diameter surrounded by thickened edematous mucosa, which can involve any part of the GI tract. The rectum, however, is usually spared. The ulcers traverse perpendicular to the mucosal plain. There are typically multiple foci of ulcers with intervening normal mucosa, known as skip lesions. The ulcers can form crossing linear tracts, creating the cobblestoning that can be seen on barium examination. Anal involvement includes deep perianal fissures, fistulas, and abscesses that result in severe limitations in defecation. Pathologic examinations of endoscopically obtained biopsies demonstrate transmural involvement containing all types of acute and chronic inflammatory cells.

Ulcerative colitis typically affects the rectum and distal colon first in a continuous fashion, with diffuse erythema and edema accompanied by frequent crypt abscesses and loss of mucin production. On pathologic exam, the crypt base demonstrates a loss of goblet cells and basal plasmacytosis, and the lamina propria is infiltrated by inflammatory cells. It usually is limited to the colon. The anus is usually spared. However, early UC may defy these generalizations and initially spare the rectum; backwash ileitis and spared areas may also be present, and the anus can have superficial ulcers that act like perianal fistulas.

BIBLIOGRAPHY

Finkelstein SD, Sasatomi E, Regueiro M. Pathologic features of early inflammatory bowel disease. *Gastroenterol Clin North Am* 2002;31:133–145.

McKenzie S, Evers BM. Small intestine. In: Townsend CM, Beauchamp RD, Evers BM, et al., eds. *Sabiston Textbook of Surgery.* 19th ed. Philadelphia, PA: Elsevier Saunders; 2012: 1244–1254.

Rubesin SE, Scotiniotis I, Birnbaum BA, et al. Radiologic and endoscopic diagnosis of Crohn's disease. *Surg Clin North Am* 2001;81:39–70.

Stenson WF, Korzenik J. Inflammatory bowel disease. In: Yamada T, Alpers D, Kaplowitz N, et al., eds. *Textbook of Gastroenterology.* 4th ed. Philadelphia, PA: Lippincott Williams & Wilkins; 2003:1713–1714.

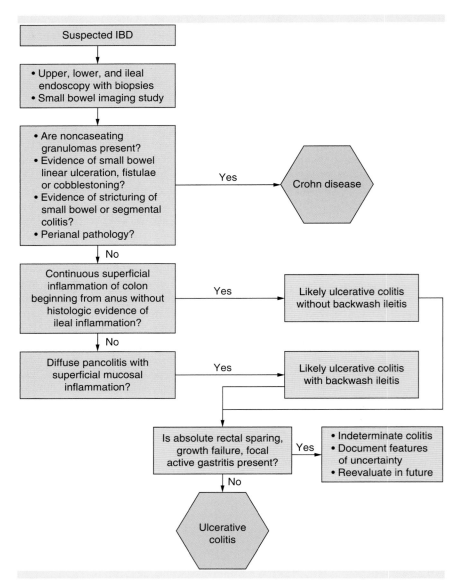

FIGURE 19-4. Diagnostic algorithm to differentiate Crohn's disease from ulcerative colitis (from Ziegler MM, Azizkhan RG, von Allmen D, Weber TR, eds. *Operative Pediatric Surgery*. 2nd ed. New York, NY: McGraw-Hill Education; 2014: Fig. 49-1. Copyright © The McGraw-Hill Companies, Inc. All rights reserved).

5. **(A)** This patient has acute ileitis. This may or may not be related to Crohn's (and most often is not related to CD). The correct procedure in this case is appendectomy only. Although the appendix appears normal on direct examination, the right lower quadrant wound or the laparoscopic wounds that the patient already has would be confusing in the future. Therefore, removing the appendix is appropriate to eliminate it as a source of abdominal pain in the future as long as there is no significant inflammatory involvement of the appendix or the base of the cecum. There is no indication for an ileocecectomy as

this is an infectious process and will heal with antibiotics. If this is in fact an initial presentation of CD, additional therapy will be required, but it will heal without surgery.

Acute ileitis presents with right lower quadrant pain, fever, and anorexia much the same as acute appendicitis. It is often caused by *Campylobacter* or *Yersinia* species. These can be cultured from the appendix and from the patient's stool. Although acute terminal ileitis can present as appendicitis and appear to be early Crohn's, the majority of instances have infectious etiologies.

BIBLIOGRAPHY

McKenzie S, Evers BM. Mark. Small intestine. In: Townsend CM, Beauchamp RD, Evers BM, et al., eds. *Sabiston Textbook of Surgery*. 19th ed. Philadelphia, PA: Elsevier Saunders; 2012:1244–1254.

6. **(E)** Unfortunately, surgery cannot cure CD. It does, however, address Crohn's complications and provide palliation of symptoms. Approximately 80% of patients with CD will require surgery at some point during the course of their disease. The most common operations performed are intestinal resections, stricturoplasties, and intestinal bypasses. The most common indications for surgery are failure of medical therapy, intestinal obstruction, enteric fistulas, growth retardation, abscess formation, and cancer. The primary strategy in operating for CD must be to operate only on the complicating segment of bowel. Resection must not extend to all areas that are grossly diseased but must be limited to the area of abscess, fistula, or obstruction.

Enterocutaneous fistulas most frequently occur postoperatively, either immediately or even after significant delay. They rarely occur spontaneously and rarely affect a clean, unscarred abdominal wall. A trial of total parenteral nutrition (TPN) and bowel rest is legitimate and will be effective if the drainage is limited and the CD well controlled medically; but, most others require surgery, especially in the face of CD unresponsive to medical therapy. Excision of the fistula tract and the diseased segment of bowel with reanastomosis is the preferred procedure.

Duodenal CD causing obstruction or severe symptoms frequently requires intestinal bypass for management. Fewer than 2% of patients with CD have duodenal disease, but 30% of these require surgery at some point. Intestinal bypass was once a mainstay of surgical therapy in CD, but complications (e.g., bacterial overgrowth and cancer) in the excluded segment caused limitation of this technique to the one area where it was effective and relatively complication free: the duodenum.

Patients with intestinal obstruction related to CD flare should be managed initially with intensive medical therapy, bowel rest, nutritional support, and NG decompression. This will often be adequate for initial management of the obstruction and allow the intestinal tract to undergo further radiographic evaluation. When high- or midgrade obstructions are present, surgery is indicated, with the preference for operating after the acute exacerbation of CD has subsided. The presence of multiple or single strictures, the presence of abscesses or fistulas, and the patient's prior operative history determine the necessary operation. Intestinal resection should be minimized

given the severe morbidity resulting from short bowel syndrome. Stricturoplasty has been an excellent choice for conservation of intestinal length.

Growth retardation has been a consistent finding in children diagnosed with CD and has even been noticed prior to the onset of intestinal symptoms. As many as 85% of children with CD will suffer from weight loss or lack of weight gain. Most children resume appropriate growth rates after surgical resection of diseased segments and occasionally experience a growth spurt following surgery; however, over time these children remain slightly smaller than the average American as adults. Using this as a sole indication for surgery has not been studied, but most children with CD do require surgery and experience this benefit. When the growth retardation is severe, some authors advocate surgery but do not recommend an exact length or criteria for intestinal resection. The cause of the slowed growth is attributed to increased metabolic rate, loss of protein and nutrients, growth hormone deficiency, and lack of appropriate response to growth hormone.

BIBLIOGRAPHY

Day AS, Ledder O, Leach ST, Lemberg DA. Crohn's and colitis in children and adolescents. *World J Gastroenterol* 2012;18(41):5862–5869.

Dokucu AI, Samacki S, Michel JL, et al. Indications and results of surgery in patients with Crohn's disease with onset under 10 years of age: a series of 18 patients. *Eur J Pediatr Surg* 2002;12:180–185.

McKenzie S, Evers BM. Small intestine. In: Townsend CM, Beauchamp RD, Evers BM, et al., eds. *Sabiston Textbook of Surgery*. 19th ed. Philadelphia, PA: Elsevier Saunders; 2012: 1244–1254.

Michelassi F, Hurst RD. Crohn's disease. In: Greenfield L, Mulholland M, Oldham K, et al., eds. *Surgery: Scientific Principles and Practice*. 3rd ed. Philadelphia, PA: Lippincott Williams & Wilkins; 2001:820–822.

Roses R, Rombeau J. Recent trends in the surgical management of inflammatory bowel disease. *World J Gastroenterol* 2008;14(3):408–412.

7. **(A)** Patients who are severely immunosuppressed as a result of HIV/AIDS, chemotherapy, or a solid organ transplant are subject to a host of GI diseases that are extremely rare in the immunecompetent (Fig. 19-5). CMV enteritis, GI tuberculosis, *Shigella*, and *Salmonella* are a few of the opportunistic pathogens that occasionally masquerade as an acute abdomen in immunocompromised patients demonstrating fever, severe abdominal pain, anorexia, and occasionally diarrhea.

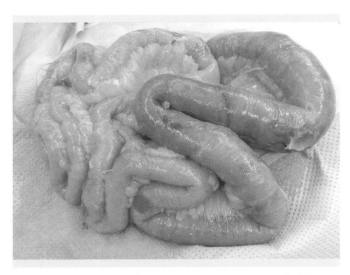

FIGURE 19-5. *Aspergillus* enteritis in a patient with AIDs and an example of neutropenic enteritis.

Cytomegalovirus enteritis most frequently attacks the distal ileum and right colon, but it can occur anywhere along the GI tract. Hemorrhagic ulcerated lesions are often seen during endoscopy. The diagnosis is made by culture or by seeing the characteristic nuclear inclusions (the "owl's eye") on cytology. Treatment consists of either ganciclovir or foscarnet. Both of these drugs are viridostatic, so complete elimination of the virus can be difficult.

Prednisone and infliximab (an anti–tumor necrosis factor alpha [TNF-α] antibody) are used in the management of IBD and do not play a role in the management of CMV enteritis. Oseltamivir is a neuraminidase inhibitor that is used in treatment of seasonal influenza and similarly has no role in treating CMV enteritis. Alfa interferon is an immunomodulatory cytokine that is used in the treatment of chronic hepatitis C virus infection.

BIBLIOGRAPHY

McKenzie S, Evers BM. Small intestine. In: Townsend CM, Beauchamp RD, Evers BM, et al., eds. *Sabiston Textbook of Surgery*. 19th ed. Philadelphia, PA: Elsevier Saunders; 2012: 1254–1255.

Smith PD, Janoff EN. Gastrointestinal complications of the acquired immunodeficiency syndrome. In: Yamada T, Alpers D, Kaplowitz N, et al., eds. *Textbook of Gastroenterology*. 4th ed. Philadelphia, PA: Lippincott Williams & Wilkins; 2003: 2567–2579.

8. **(C)** The medical therapy of CD is one fraught with frustration on many fronts because of the side effects of many of the effective drugs and the limited choices of drugs that are effective. Of the choices discussed, all are regularly used in the treatment of CD except IL-10, which is currently under study.

The most useful agent for maintaining remission for CD at this time is azathioprine. Azathioprine and its metabolite 6-mercaptopurine (6-MP) block lymphocyte proliferation, activation, and efficacy. Their efficacy is not realized until 3–4 months after treatment has begun; therefore, it is started concurrently with steroids and then continued well beyond the steroid taper. Azathioprine then is continued indefinitely; relapse rate in patients on this regimen remains about 30%, while 75% of those not taking the drug relapse. Leukopenia and pancreatitis are its primary toxicities, both of which resolve once the drug is stopped. Other maintenance drugs include various 5-aminosalicylic acid (5-ASA) preparations (most effective in ileal and colonic CD), methotrexate, and cyclosporine.

Steroids play a key role in the treatment of CD in bringing about a remission. Steroids are effective enterally and parenterally. They are effective in preventing or suppressing the inflammatory response in both early stages of inflammation (vascular permeability, vasodilatation, and neutrophil invasion) and the late stages of inflammation (vascular proliferation, collagen deposition, and activation of fibroblasts). However, in addition to their multiple side effects, corticosteroids do not bring about mucosal healing, and they are not effective in maintaining remission. Unfortunately, there are no good studies elucidating the best dosing strategies or timing of the steroid taper. Most determine the taper based on symptomatic improvements; this frequently does not correlate with endoscopic improvements. The majority of patients can be weaned from steroids after remission has been achieved, but about 25% will require lifetime steroids as they have symptomatic flares each time the steroids are discontinued, in spite of combination therapy with 5-ASA, 6-MP, methotrexate, or cyclosporine.

Infliximab, a mouse-human chimeric IgG antibody against TNF-α, has been effective in inducing remission and in treating fistulas. Clinical benefits of remission and decreased fistula drainage can be maintained with the infusion of infliximab every 8 weeks. The fistulas, once closed, remain closed for approximately 12 weeks and then usually require definitive treatment. Unfortunately, toxicity increases with increased number of infliximab infusions. Some develop human antichimeric antibodies and sustain acute and delayed hypersensitivity reactions. Infliximab has also been associated with varicella zoster, *Candida* esophagitis, and tuberculosis. Also, patients can develop intestinal strictures as a result of rapid healing of ulcers. Once again, the optimal timing of infliximab treatment has not been studied, so much remains to be learned about this treatment.

BIBLIOGRAPHY

Harrison J, Hanauer SB. Medical treatment of Crohn's disease. *Gastroenterol Clin North Am* 2002;31:167–184.

Stenson WF, Korzenik J. Inflammatory bowel disease. In: Yamada T, Alpers D, Kaplowitz N, et al., eds. *Textbook of Gastroenterology*. 4th ed. Philadelphia, PA: Lippincott Williams & Wilkins; 2003:1726–1740.

9. **(D)** A 68-year-old woman status after colostomy takedown 1 year ago presents with 24-h history of nausea, feculent vomiting, fever to 100.2°F, tachycardia, persistent abdominal pain, and a mild leukocytosis. Her abdominal x-rays demonstrate multiple air-fluid levels and stairstepping pattern.

   Small bowel obstructions are caused by intestinal adhesive disease in 60–80% of cases. Other causes include neoplasms (~20%), hernias (~10%), CD (~5%), volvulus, intussusception, and radiation enteritis. Although all abdominal surgeries cause adhesions, those resulting in obstruction most frequently occur after pelvic procedures such as appendectomies, abdominal hysterectomies, and abdominopelvic resections. Adhesive obstructions occur in 5% of patients with previous laparotomies; however, most of these resolve with nonoperative management.

   Patients present with varying degrees of nausea, vomiting, abdominal distension, and abdominal pain. These symptoms are often more acute and severe in closed-loop obstructions and strangulating obstructions. Patients with strangulation frequently demonstrate peritonitis and systemic signs of illness (i.e., fever, tachycardia, leukocytosis, and decreased urine output). These patients require emergent operation *after adequate resuscitation* and correction of electrolyte abnormalities for relief of the obstruction as mortality significantly increases with delay of surgery.

   Obstructions in the early postoperative period should be managed nonoperatively with bowel rest, NG decompression, and fluid resuscitation. These are often partial obstructions, and more than 90% will resolve spontaneously over time with nonoperative management. Enteroclysis, small bowel follow-through, or CT scan may be helpful in demonstrating the cause and degree of obstruction when these are persistent. Abdominal radiographs are rarely helpful as most have a similar appearance to postoperative ileus. If the early postoperative obstruction is complete or if systemic symptoms ensue, it must be managed surgically similar to other complete obstructions.

   Obstruction resulting from recurrent cancer and peritoneal studding is a special situation. One-third of these patients actually have adhesive disease and can be palliated or even cured with surgery. However, an extended opportunity for resolution of the obstruction with conservative management is warranted in the case of recurrent malignancy to spare the patient an additional laparotomy. Systemic symptoms, as before, warrant immediate surgery if the patient agrees. Malignant obstruction can be treated with intestinal bypass. If carcinomatosis is encountered, tube gastrostomy may prove palliative to avoid frequent NG intubation.

   Radiation enteritis also presents a difficult situation. These obstructions also will frequently resolve with nonoperative management. If surgery is necessary, it carries a significant morbidity as suturing bowel scarred by chronic inflammation can result in fistulas, abscesses, and anastomotic leaks.

BIBLIOGRAPHY

McKenzie S, Evers BM. Small intestine. In: Townsend CM, Beauchamp RD, Evers BM, et al., eds. *Sabiston Textbook of Surgery*. 19th ed. Philadelphia, PA: Elsevier Saunders; 2012: 1236–1244.

Maglinte D, Kelvin F, Rowe M. Small bowel obstruction: optimizing radiologic investigation and nonsurgical management. *Radiology* 2001;218:39–46.

Pickelman J. Small bowel obstruction. In: Cameron J, ed. *Current Surgical Therapy*. 7th ed. St. Louis, MO: Mosby; 2001:122–128.

Soybel D. Ileus and bowel obstruction. In: Greenfield L, Mulholland M, Oldham K, et al., eds. *Surgery: Scientific Principles and Practice*. 3rd ed. Philadelphia, PA: Lippincott Williams & Wilkins; 2001:798–812.

10. **(C)** This patient has pneumatosis intestinalis (PI) or air within the wall of the bowel (Fig. 19-6). PI is not a diagnosis in itself, so its significance and prognosis depend on the underlying cause. This finding has a wide range of possible causes and potential outcomes. PI can be primary, usually occurring in the distal large bowel, or secondary, which occurs more commonly in the small bowel. Secondary PI can be associated with iatrogenic injury from endoscopy or invasive radiologic examination, autoimmune or infectious diseases, ischemia, scleroderma, chemotherapy, trauma, or COPD, among others. Presenting complaints include diarrhea, abdominal pain and distension, vomiting, weight loss, and hematochezia. Physical examination may demonstrate abdominal distension or mass. If pneumoperitoneum results from PI, it is usually sterile, the examination remains benign, and no surgical treatment is required unless signs of peritonitis are present.

    Pneumatosis intestinalis frequently appears as air-filled cysts on radiologic examination. These can occur from the esophagus to the anus and can also occur in the mesentery, the omentum, and the falciform ligament. The cysts usually occur in the subserosa near the mesenteric border and in the submucosa. They can range in

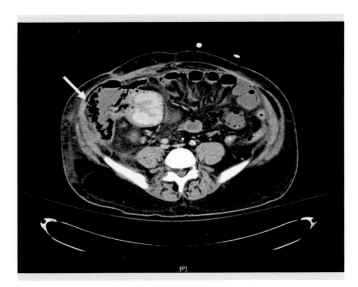

FIGURE 19-6. Pneumatosis intestinalis on CT with abdominal windows (from Brunicardi FC, Andersen DK, Billiar TR, et al., eds. *Schwartz's Principles of Surgery*. 10th ed. New York, NY: McGraw-Hill; 2014: Fig. 28-15. Copyright © The McGraw-Hill Companies, Inc. All rights reserved).

size from a few millimeters to several centimeters and can involve very short or very lengthy segments of bowel. Pneumoperitoneum frequently is seen. The presence of portal venous gas is most frequently associated with ischemia and is often indicative of more urgent need for surgical intervention.

The cysts contain pressurized gas from three possible sources: intraluminal GI gas, pulmonary gas, or gas produced by bacteria. Many theories exist regarding the exact etiology/pathogenesis of intramural gas. Many contend that the gas became intramural as a result of severe COPD with alveolar rupture and dissection from the mediastinum to the retroperitoneum by way of the great vessels through the mesentery and into the serosa. The mechanical theory purports that mucosal defects allow pressurized gas, as in endoscopy, trauma, or obstruction, to dissect into the bowel wall. The bacterial theory postulates that gas-forming organisms invade the wall of the mucosa, especially during times of immunosuppression or neutropenia, allowing cysts to form. However, each of these theories is significantly flawed. In the pulmonary theory, many patients do not have any evidence of pneumomediastinum, pneumothorax, or pneumoretroperitoneum. The mechanical theory does not explain the high hydrogen content of the cyst gas compared with air or usual intestinal gas. And, the bacterial theory does not explain the sterile pneumoperitoneum that exists when the cysts rupture. Thus, the true pathophysiology of PI remains a mystery.

Treatment is based on the underlying problem. Ischemia, acidosis, fever, peritonitis, leukocytosis, and clinical decline clearly necessitate intervention. However, PI can frequently be treated with minimal intervention. Overall, PI can often be managed expectantly except in the case of ischemia.

BIBLIOGRAPHY

Balledux J, McCurry T, Zeiger M, Coleman JJ, Sood R. Pneumatosis intestinalis in a burn patient: case report and literature review. *J Burn Care Res* 2006;27(3):399–403.

McKenzie S, Evers BM. Small intestine. In: Townsend CM, Beauchamp RD, Evers BM, et al., eds. *Sabiston Textbook of Surgery*. 19th ed. Philadelphia, PA: Elsevier Saunders; 2012:1272–1273.

St. Peter S, Abbas M, Kelly K. The spectrum of pneumatosis intestinalis. *Arch Surg* 2003;138:68–75.

11. **(E)** Enterocutaneous fistulas are often disheartening postoperative complications. As many as 75–80% of ECFs are the result of intraoperative iatrogenic injuries. They can be caused by technical errors such as missed enterotomies, anastomotic tension, or compromised blood supply at an anastomosis, resulting in its breakdown. Erosion into the bowel by foreign bodies such as suction catheters or nearby abscesses can also cause ECFs. Spontaneous ECFs result from CD, neoplasms, or radiation injury.

Fistula output (volume) and the length of the fistula tract are fundamentally important factors in determining the likelihood that an ECF will close spontaneously. Other factors that prevent the spontaneous closure of ECFs include **f**oreign body within the fistula tract, **r**adiation enteritis, active **i**nflammatory bowel disease or infection, **e**pithelialization of the fistula tract, **n**eoplasm, and **d**istal obstruction (FRIEND). Fistulas with an output of less than 500 mL per day are three times more likely to close than fistulas producing more than 500 mL per day. Fistulas that are less than 2.5 cm in length decrease the likelihood of closure over longer tracts because these are more likely to epithelialize to the skin and result in less resistance to flow. Patients with obstructions distal to the fistula tract, active IBD, active infection, presence of a foreign body within the fistula tract, large abdominal wall defects, or involved neoplasms are unlikely to experience spontaneous fistula closure. Finally, patients who are malnourished (albumin < 2.5, transferrin < 200) or septic are unlikely to resolve fistulas with nonoperative management.

An ECF should be considered in postoperative patients with fever and an erythematous wound. Once the wound is opened, the drainage of bilious or feculent contents confirms the diagnosis. Occasionally, ECFs may present with overt peritonitis and sepsis, although this is uncommon. In either case, treatment begins with fluid resuscitation and electrolyte replacement. In the event of ongoing sepsis and clinical decline, emergent operation is indicated with resection of the fistulized segment of small bowel. If the abdomen has marked contamination/inflammation such that the diseased segment cannot be clearly delineated, a proximal stoma or intestinal bypass is indicated. This avoids resecting a lengthy segment of bowel and causing short bowel syndrome.

If the patient is clinically stable, nonoperative management can begin with TPN, electrolyte replacement, and wound care. CT scan to delineate the location of the original fistula is often helpful. CT-guided placement of percutaneous drains may be needed to control an undrained enteric leak. A fistulogram may be needed to assess the length of the ECF tract and its exact location in the GI tract. An enterostomal therapist should become involved to assist devising a method to keep enteric contents from causing skin breakdown. Pharmacologic agents can also be employed to decrease fistula drainage, such as H_2 blockers to decrease gastric acid output and octreotide to decrease bilious and pancreatic output. Although octreotide has been shown to decrease the volume of output from ECFs, it has not been definitively shown to improve the rate of spontaneous closure. Maintaining adequate nutrition is imperative in fistula management to improve the likelihood for spontaneous closure or to improve outcome should surgery be needed. Some carefully selected ECF patients may receive enteral nutrition, but bowel rest and TPN should be the mainstay in early fistula management.

If an ECF is to close spontaneously, more than 90% are likely to do so within the first month of treatment. Fewer than 10% of ECFs present for greater than 2 months close spontaneously. By 3 months, ECFs are extremely unlikely to close spontaneously if they have not already done so. If surgical management is ultimately required, one must carefully plan this difficult operation using contrast studies of the fistula and GI tract. Also, nutritional status must be optimized. Delayed repair is often advocated, waiting 3–6 months or longer to pursue surgical management to allow for intra-abdominal inflammation to resolve and for adhesions to stabilize. However, no level 1 data exist exist that support any specific time period proceeding with repair. Fistulectomy with primary end-to-end anastomosis is the preferred surgical treatment, and one must carefully avoid additional enterotomies that would predispose to future ECFs.

BIBLIOGRAPHY

Davis K, Johnson E. Controversies in the care of enterocutaneous fistula. *Surg Clin North Am* 2013;93(1):231–250.

Denham D, Fabri P. Enterocutaneous fistula. In: Cameron J, ed. *Current Surgical Therapy*. 7th ed. St. Louis, MO: Mosby; 2001:156–161.

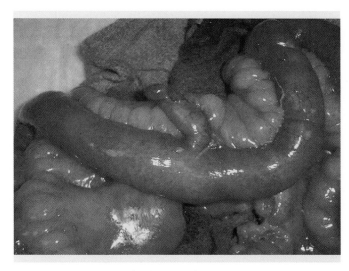

FIGURE 19-7. Meckel's diverticulum.

McKenzie S, Evers BM. Small intestine. In: Townsend CM, Beauchamp RD, Evers BM, et al., eds. *Sabiston Textbook of Surgery*. 19th ed. Philadelphia, PA: Elsevier Saunders; 2012: 1273–1274.

12. **(A)** Meckel's diverticulum (Fig. 19-7) is the most common congenital abnormality of the GI tract. The rule of 2s is helpful in remembering some important facts about this pathology, including that it is present in 2% of the population, symptomatic in 2%, twice as common in males than females, located within 2 feet of the ileocecal valve (on the antimesenteric border), approximately 2 inches in length, and generally presents with one of two complications (bleeding or obstruction). A Meckel's diverticulum is a remnant of the vitelline duct, a structure initially connecting the primitive gut to the fetal yolk sac. It usually obliterates by the seventh to eighth week of gestation. The remnant may endure as a fibrous band connecting the ileum to the umbilicus, as a fistulous tract to the umbilicus, or as a true diverticulum containing all layers of the small bowel wall. The vitelline duct contains pluripotent cells; it is therefore not uncommon to find heterotopic tissue within a Meckel diverticulum. Gastric mucosa is present in about 50% of Meckel's diverticula, and pancreatic mucosa is present in approximately 5%. Rarely, colonic mucosa may be present as well.

Complicated Meckel's diverticula most frequently contain gastric mucosa. These cells produce gastric acid and result in ileal ulcers that eventually bleed. Adults present with painless melena in this case, while children generally present with bright red blood per rectum. Hemorrhage is the most common complication, occurring in 30–50% of Meckel's complications. Obstruction can be the result of a number of mechanisms: intussusception, volvulus, strangulation related to the fibrous band attached to the umbilicus, or rarely a Littre's hernia, which is the incarceration of the Meckel's diverticulum in an inguinal hernia. Meckel's diverticulitis accounts for 10–20% of presentations. This should be considered in patients with right lower quadrant pain and a normal appendix at exploration.

Diagnosis of Meckel's is difficult, so high clinical suspicion is necessary. Technetium-99 can be used to identify normal and ectopic gastric mucosa; this is occasionally helpful, especially in children. Arteriography is useful if brisk bleeding is occurring.

Treatment of symptomatic Meckel's diverticula involves surgical resection. If bleeding is the presenting symptom, a segmental bowel resection should be performed. This is because the source of bleeding is typically an ulceration of the small bowel opposite the opening of the diverticulum due to chronic acid exposure from the gastric mucosa within the diverticulum. For nonbleeding Meckel's, diverticulectomy can also be performed. The management of incidentally found Meckel's diverticula remains controversial, although it is reasonable to manage them nonoperatively. This is especially true in adults, for whom the rate of the Meckel's becoming symptomatic is not markedly different from the rate of complications from a resection.

BIBLIOGRAPHY

McKenzie S, Evers BM. Small intestine. In: Townsend CM, Beauchamp RD, Evers BM, et al., eds. *Sabiston Textbook of Surgery*. 19th ed. Philadelphia, PA: Elsevier Saunders; 2012:1268–1270.

Rubin D. Small intestine: anatomy and structural abnormalities. In: Yamada T, Alpers DH, Kaplowitz N, et al., eds. *Textbook of Gastroenterology*. 4th ed. Philadelphia, PA: Lippincott Williams & Wilkins; 2003:1473–1474.

13. **(D)**

14. **(B)**

Explanation for questions 13 and 14

Superior mesenteric artery syndrome, also known as cast syndrome, chronic duodenal ileus, or Wilkie's syndrome, is a rare cause of duodenal obstruction. The third portion of the duodenum is compressed by the SMA as it branches from the aorta and passes over the duodenum at a sharp angle. The SMA typically has a 45-degree angle to the aorta, but in SMA syndrome the angle is decreased to 6–25 degrees. The aortomesenteric distance has also been found to be shorter. The increased acuity of this angle is associated with a period of rapid weight loss in adults, including eating disorders, burns, or neoplasms, or a period of rapid growth in children; these result in

decreased retroperitoneal or mesenteric fat. Other associated conditions include severe scoliosis, body casts that increase spinal lordosis, and large abdominal aortic aneurysms. Symptoms of SMA syndrome are somewhat vague. Postprandial epigastric pain, abdominal distension, nausea, and vomiting partially digested food are common presenting complaints. Patients may have some symptomatic relief in a knee-to-chest position. CT scan will demonstrate the acute angle of the SMA. Barium upper GI series show the abrupt obstruction of the third portion of the duodenum, with some relief of the obstruction in the left lateral decubitus position (Fig. 19-8). Arteriography adds little to the CT scan, but the acute angle can also be seen in the lateral view. Endoscopy demonstrates retained food in the stomach and a dilated duodenum with extrinsic compression easily noted at its third segment.

Treatment of SMA syndrome includes a trial of nonoperative management with fluid resuscitation, electrolyte replacement, and nutritional support. Nutritional support can consist of initiating multiple small feedings, a liquid diet, nasojejunal feeding, or TPN. This is most often effective in patients with more of an acute onset of symptomatology. If this results in weight gain, the symptoms gradually subside. If an adult has had symptoms chronically or if nonoperative management fails, surgical therapy is often necessary. Surgical options include duodenojejunostomy, gastrojejunostomy, and Strong's procedure. Duodenojejunostomy is thought to have the best results for surgical management of SMA syndrome, although it does carry a risk of blind-loop syndrome if the fourth portion of the duodenum is not divided. Gastrojejunostomy allows gastric decompression, but it does not address the duodenal obstruction and may result in recurrent symptoms. It also may lead to blind-loop

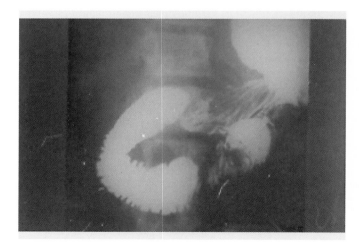

FIGURE 19-8. Duodenal C sweep with significant proximal dilatation due to obstruction by the SMA.

syndrome. Strong's procedure involves division of the ligament of Treitz, which allows the duodenum to fall away from the aorta. This procedure has the benefit of not requiring a new anastomosis; however, it has a failure rate as high as 25%. If SMA syndrome is the result of an abdominal aortic aneurysm, repair of the aneurysm will likely be necessary.

BIBLIOGRAPHY

Baltazar U, Dunn J, Floresguerra C, et al. Superior mesenteric artery syndrome: an uncommon cause of intestinal obstruction. *South Med J* 2000;93:606–608.

McKenzie S, Evers BM. Small intestine. In: Townsend CM, Beauchamp RD, Evers BM, et al., eds. *Sabiston Textbook of Surgery*. 19th ed. Philadelphia, PA: Elsevier Saunders; 2012:1276.

Merrett ND, Wilson RB, Cosman P, Biankin AV. Superior mesenteric artery syndrome: diagnosis and treatment strategies. *J Gastrointest Surg* 2008;13(2):287–292.

Raufman J. Stomach: anatomy and structural abnormalities. In: Yamada T, Alpers DH, Kaplowitz N, et al., eds. *Textbook of Gastroenterology*. 4th ed. Philadelphia, PA: Lippincott Williams & Wilkins; 2003:1290.

Richardson W, Surowiec W. Laparoscopic repair of superior mesenteric artery syndrome. *Am J Surg* 2001;181:377–378.

15. **(C)** Both children and adults ingest foreign objects accidentally and adults as a result of mental illness, for secondary gain, or in an effort to smuggle illicit drugs. Frequently ingested objects include paper clips, razor blades, safety pins, chicken bones, coins, toys, and batteries. Seventy-five percent of impactions occur in the esophagus. If this is the case, endoscopy is indicated for removal. Surgery would be necessary only if endoscopy were unsuccessful, as in the case of a large object that could not be snared. Endoscopy is indicated emergently for sharp objects or batteries in the esophagus or if the patient has airway compromise. If the foreign objects progress to the stomach, endoscopic removal is indicated if the foreign body is larger than 5 cm by 2 cm or if it is sharp; otherwise, serial films can be obtained with observation for up to 3 weeks or the patient experiences symptoms.

Most foreign bodies will pass without difficulty. Serial examinations and serial abdominal films can be used to follow the passage of even sharp objects. However, the patient must be monitored carefully for any signs of peritonitis, fever, or leukocytosis, at which time, emergent laparotomy would be required. Laparotomy is also indicated for small bowel obstruction because of the presence of the foreign objects. Cathartic agents are absolutely contraindicated with ingestion of sharp objects because of the increased risk of perforation.

Two special cases must be discussed regarding foreign bodies: battery ingestion and "body packers." In the case of disk batteries, leakage of their alkaline compounds can result in corrosion of esophageal, gastric, or intestinal mucosa. They can also lead to pressure necrosis or low-voltage burns. Batteries must be removed immediately if lodged in the esophagus; they can be monitored for up to 48 h in the stomach in the asymptomatic patient but should be endoscopically removed after this time. Serial films should ensure the ongoing progression of the battery through the GI tract if the battery is in the small intestine on presentation. Surgery should commence with any abdominal symptoms or leukocytosis or if the battery has remained stagnant for 48 h as the battery may have eroded into the bowel, eventually leading to perforation.

Body packers are those who ingest small plastic bags of illicit drugs for smuggling. These can frequently result in severe small bowel obstruction or drug overdose should the packing material break down. Physical examination is typical for small bowel obstruction, but x-ray demonstrates small dense packets surrounded by crescents of air (called the "double condom sign"). The bowel obstruction is managed nonoperatively with NG decompression, fluid resuscitation, and bowel rest. Surgery is indicated if the bowel appears to be compromised or if the patient shows signs of drug overdose. This is especially necessary in the case of cocaine smuggling because of its life-threatening consequences. Laparotomy may be complicated by the need for multiple enterotomies to extract each bag individually as they become adherent to the bowel mucosa.

BIBLIOGRAPHY

Faigel D. Miscellaneous diseases of the esophagus: systemic, dermatologic disease, foreign bodies and physical injury. In: Yamada T, Alpers D, Kaplowitz N, et al., eds. *Textbook of Gastroenterology*. 4th ed. Philadelphia, PA: Lippincott Williams & Wilkins; 2003:1262.

Greenberg R, Greenberg Y, Kaplan O. "Body packer" syndrome: characteristics and treatment—case report and review. *Eur J Surg* 2000;166:89–91.

McKenzie S, Evers BM. Small intestine. In: Townsend CM, Beauchamp RD, Evers BM, et al., eds. *Sabiston Textbook of Surgery*. 19th ed. Philadelphia, PA: Elsevier Saunders; 2012:1270.

Rabine J, Nostrant T. Miscellaneous diseases of the stomach. In: Yamada T, Alpers D, Kaplowitz N, et al., eds. *Textbook of Gastroenterology*. 4th ed. Philadelphia, PA: Lippincott Williams & Wilkins; 2003:1460.

16. **(A)** At rest, the small bowel receives 10–15% of a patient's cardiac output. This increases to up to 50% during digestion. Of the cardiac output received, 70–90% goes to mucosa and submucosa; the remainder goes to the muscularis. Ischemic injury can therefore be caused by a number of conditions that result in decreased cardiac output seen by the small bowel. These include, but are not limited to, bleeding, myocardial infarction,

pericardial tamponade, and hypovolemia. This is often referred to as nonocclusive mesenteric ischemia (NOMI). Initial treatment should be focused on restoring cardiac output by addressing the underlying cause; enteral feeding should also be discontinued to minimize the metabolic demand and subsequent proportion of cardiac output required by the small bowel. Some degree of reperfusion injury is likely to occur depending on the period of insult. This will result in edema, subsequent mucosal sloughing with possible hemorrhage, and possible loss of intestinal epithelial integrity.

Another cause of mesenteric ischemia includes mesenteric arterial embolus or thrombus causing acute disruption in splanchnic flow. This is especially true in patients with known arrhythmias or severe atherosclerotic disease. Acute disruption can also result from drugs such as cyclosporine that prohibit release of local vasodilators. Finally, reflex splanchnic arterial vasospasm occurs with venous thrombosis (as in patients with portal hypertension or a hypercoagulable state) and with digitalis toxicity that may result in mesenteric ischemia. Approximately 20% of cases of mesenteric ischemia are due to NOMI, 50% from arterial embolization, 25% from arterial thrombosis, and 5% from venous thrombosis (Fig. 19-9).

BIBLIOGRAPHY

Gatt M, JacFie J, Anderson AD, et al. Changes in superior mesenteric artery blood flow after oral, enteral, and parental feedings in humans. *Crit Care Med* 2009;37(1):171–176.

Gelabert H. Mesenteric vascular disease of the small bowel. In: Cameron J, ed. *Current Surgical Therapy*. 7th ed. St. Louis, MO: Mosby; 2001:149–156.

Melis M, Fichera A, Ferguson MK. Bowel necrosis associated with early jejunal tube feeding. *JAMA Surg* 2006;141(7):701–704.

17. **(D)** Once mesenteric ischemia has been diagnosed, mesenteric blood flow must be optimized. Adequate hydration, cardiac output optimization, and revascularization accomplish this goal. The next step is determination of viable bowel to determine margins for resection. Many options exist to accomplish this goal, including clinical judgment, Doppler ultrasound, oximetry, fluorescein, and second-look surgery. The best method to ensure remaining bowel is viable while minimizing the extent of resection is to plan a return trip to the operating room for second-look surgery.

Second-look surgery is the best option to prevent resection of potentially viable bowel if extensive areas of small bowel are compromised by embolus, venous

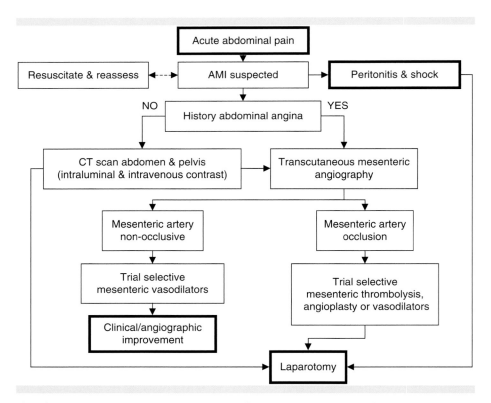

FIGURE 19-9. Algorithm for the diagnosis and investigation of mesenteric ischemia (from Hall JB, Schmidt GA, Wood LDH, eds. *Principles of Critical Care*. 3rd ed. New York, NY: McGraw-Hill Professional; 2005: Fig. 86-2).

thrombosis, or NOMI. This should be planned at the time of initial operation to take place within 12–36 h of the initial operation, although the return to the operating room may be necessary sooner in the event of clinical deterioration suggestive of ongoing or worsening ischemia.

Using clinical judgment alone is 90% accurate in assessing bowel viability. Bowel that peristalses, bleeds at its cut edge, and is pink in color is indeed viable. Unfortunately, we are not as accurate in assessing potentially salvageable bowel. Using clinical judgment alone can lead to significantly greater resection than necessary.

Doppler ultrasound is an easily accessible tool to assess viability. Early studies reported that bowel was viable within 1 cm of the last Doppler signal obtained at the bowel wall, making it accurate in assessing viable bowel. Once again, the problem arises in judging bowel that can be salvaged. It cannot determine microvascular circulation or accurately detect flow on the antimesenteric side of the bowel.

Fluorescein can be given intraoperatively (15 mg/kg or 1 g IV) and used to assess bowel under a Wood's lamp. Viable bowel becomes fluorescent yellow quickly, while nonviable bowel has no or patchy or delayed fluorescence. This method has been shown to be more accurate than clinical judgment or Doppler. Unfortunately, fluorescein dye can only be used once in a 24- to 48-h period, and some people have allergic reactions to the dye. Fluorescein dye test is the second-best option to second-look surgery.

Oximetry, similar to the usual pulse oximetry, requires a probe to assess venous saturations of oxygen in the intestinal wall. Although the concept is familiar, it requires special equipment in the operating room to be accurate.

BIBLIOGRAPHY

Belkin M, Whittemore AD, Donaldson MC, et al. Peripheral arterial occlusive disease. In: Townsend CM, Beauchamp RD, Evers BM, et al., eds. *Sabiston Textbook of Surgery*. 16th ed. Philadelphia, PA: Saunders; 2001:1398–1401.

Sise, MJ. Acute mesenteric ischemia. *Surg Clin North Am* 2014;94:165–181.

Zelenek GB. Visceral occlusive disease. In: Greenfield L, Mulholland M, Oldham K, et al., eds. *Surgery: Scientific Principles and Practice*. 3rd ed. Philadelphia, PA: Lippincott Williams & Wilkins; 2001:1700–1702.

18. **(D)** Gallstone ileus is the cause of less than 3% of small bowel obstructions. However, it is the source of nearly 25% of nonstrangulated small bowel obstructions in the elderly and has a 3:1–5:1 predominance in females. Gallstone ileus occurs as a result of biliary enteric fistulas. These develop when the inflammation associated with cholecystitis causes erosion of the gallbladder into an adjacent hollow viscus, most commonly duodenum, hepatic flexure of the colon, stomach, or jejunum. The stones then empty into the viscus and travel downstream. The "ileus" that results is actually a mechanical obstruction that develops as stones greater than 2.5 cm in diameter become impacted at the terminal ileum, in the sigmoid colon, or at the gastric outlet. Gallstone impaction at the gastric outlet is referred to as Bouveret's syndrome. These fistula tracts generally heal once the gallbladder has decompressed.

Patients present with usual signs of a small bowel obstruction, including abdominal pain, nausea, vomiting, and abdominal distension. However, symptoms may vary based on the site of impaction. Patients occasionally have a history of episodic, right upper quadrant postprandial abdominal pain, which may predate their presentation with a small bowel obstruction by weeks, months, or even years. On presentation, the usual workup, including detailed history and physical examination, chemistries, CBC, and acute abdominal series, should be done. The abdominal plain films can be diagnostic of gallstone ileus when Rigler's triad of dilated small bowel loops, air in the biliary tree, and an ectopic gallstone is seen. Also, this diagnosis should be strongly considered in elderly females with no prior surgical history and no apparent hernia who present with a small bowel obstruction. If the diagnosis remains in question, a CT scan or contrasted upper GI study can be diagnostic.

Initial treatment should be initiated as in any small bowel obstruction, with fluid resuscitation, correction of electrolyte abnormalities, and NG decompression of the GI tract. At laparotomy, the abdomen should be thoroughly explored. If a stone is lodged in the terminal ileum, it should be milked proximally to an area of bowel that is not edematous and removed through an enterotomy, which can then be closed primarily. Stone removal may require excision via an enterotomy at the point of impaction. In some cases, a segmental bowel resection with primary anastomosis may be necessary. If the stone is impacted in the colon, the stone should be milked proximally to normal colon and removed through a colotomy, which can then be closed primarily. As in the small bowel, a colotomy at the site of impaction or a segmental resection may be necessary. Proximal diversion via ileostomy or colostomy is at the discretion of the operating surgeon.

Management of the fistula and the gallbladder does not need to be done at the time of the initial operation, if at all. As many as 80% of these fistulas may close spontaneously, especially in the absence of residual cholelithiasis. In addition, repeat episodes of gallstone ileus occur in less than 5% of postoperative patients with their gallbladder left in place, with 80% of these recurrent obstructions resolving spontaneously. The decision to proceed with cholecystectomy at the time of initial operation should be carefully considered, as most cases of gallstone ileus do not necessitate cholecystectomy, and studies have shown a significantly higher mortality rate for patients undergoing definitive biliary management at the time of initial operation.

BIBLIOGRAPHY

Bailey E, Sharp K. Gallstone ileus. In: Cameron J, ed. *Current Surgical Therapy.* 11th ed. Philadelphia, PA: Elsevier Saunders; 2014:424–426.

Lee S, Ko C. Gallstones. In: Yamada T, Alpers DH, Kaplowitz N, et al., eds. *Textbook of Gastroenterology.* 4th ed. Philadelphia, PA: Lippincott Williams & Wilkins; 2003:2188–2189.

19. **(B)** Intussusception in adults cause approximately 1% of all small bowel obstructions. Unlike pediatric intussusceptions, they all should be managed operatively, as more than 95% have related pathology, most frequently a mass, but adhesions have also been implicated. Air or barium contrast reduction is not an appropriate option for management of intussusception in adults. Diagnosis of intussusception is frequently made intraoperatively as patients present with signs and symptoms consistent with small bowel obstruction and may only have plain x-rays preoperatively. However, CT scans are also frequently obtained and are the most sensitive study for preoperative diagnosis. A "target lesion" noted on CT demonstrates thickened edematous bowel surrounding decompressed bowel. Occasionally, a mass is also identified on CT.

Intussusceptions require a lead point to occur. This is a mass lesion in more than half of cases. Benign lesions such as adenomas, lipomas, hamartomas, and neurofibromas most commonly serve as the lead point because they are asymmetric on the bowel and frequently pedunculated. Primary malignancies such as adenocarcinoma rarely cause intussusceptions because they are circumferential. Small bowel metastases, however, such as malignant melanoma metastases, can lead to intussusceptions.

Patients with Peutz-Jeghers syndrome frequently experience intermittent abdominal pain resulting from intermittent intussusceptions. Peutz-Jeghers syndrome is an autosomal dominant genetic disease associated with GI hamartomas, primarily involving the jejunum and ileum (but may involve the stomach and the rectum); melanotic pigmentations of the face, buccal mucosa, palms of hands and soles of feet; and an increased risk of cancer of the ovaries, breast, and pancreas. When these patients present with intussusception or hemorrhage, resection should be limited to the implicated short segment of bowel, as extensive resections do not result in cure and can carry significant morbidity.

BIBLIOGRAPHY

Bresalier RS, Ben-Menachem T. Tumors of the small intestine. In: Yamada T, Alpers DH, Kaplowitz N, et al., eds. *Textbook of Gastroenterology.* 4th ed. Philadelphia, PA: Lippincott Williams & Wilkins; 2003:1645.

McKenzie S, Evers BM. Small intestine. In: Townsend CM, Beauchamp RD, Evers BM, et al., eds. *Sabiston Textbook of Surgery.* 19th ed. Philadelphia, PA: Elsevier Saunders; 2012:1236–1245.

Pickelman J. Small bowel obstruction. In: Cameron J, ed. *Current Surgical Therapy.* 7th ed. St. Louis, MO: Mosby; 2001:127.

Potts J, Samaraee Al, El-Hakeem A. Small bowel intussusception in adults. *Ann R Coll Surg Engl* 2014;96:11–14.

20. **(B)** Primary small bowel malignancies typically present with nonspecific complaints, such as long-standing nonspecific abdominal pain, weight loss, and diarrhea from partial obstructions. They also generally present with advanced disease, with more than 50% of patients presenting with nodal or distant metastases. Surgery is the mainstay for treatment, but overall survival is poor.

Adenocarcinomas comprise approximately 37% of primary small bowel cancers. They are most common in the duodenum and proximal jejunum. In addition to the symptoms previously discussed, duodenal adenocarcinoma may also present with obstructive jaundice or pancreatitis. Treatment relies on wide surgical resection of the tumor and regional lymph nodes; however, only 50% of patients present with resectable lesions, making surgery only palliative in many cases.

Primary small bowel lymphoma (PSBL) makes up only 5% of lymphomas but comprises 7–30% of small bowel malignancies. Once again, presentation is indolent long-standing abdominal pain, weight loss, and diarrhea. Constitutional symptoms that are commonly seen with other lymphomas are not present in patients with small bowel lymphoma. Perforation, although rare, is a more common presentation than with adenocarcinoma. Treatment is often nonsurgical in patients with PSBL, particularly when patients are asymptomatic, as small bowel lymphomas may respond to chemotherapy without the need for surgery.

Small bowel GISTs occasionally present with massive hemorrhage in addition to the usual presentation. In the small bowel, they most frequently occur in the jejunum and the ileum of patients in their fifth and sixth decades of life and are slightly more common in males. They are also treated with resection. Imantinib, a tyrosine kinase inhibitor, is often used as adjuvant therapy for malignant GISTS, especially ones that are large or have high mitotic rates.

BIBLIOGRAPHY

Bresalier RS, Ben-Menachem T. Tumors of the small intestine. In: Yamada T, Alpers D, Kaplowitz N, et al., eds. *Textbook of Gastroenterology*. 4th ed. Philadelphia, PA: Lippincott Williams & Wilkins; 2003:1643–1657.
Kunitake H, Hodin R. The management of small bowel tumors. In: Cameron J, ed. *Current Surgical Therapy*. 11th ed. Philadelphia, PA: Elsevier Saunders; 2014:122–128.
McKenzie S, Evers BM. Small intestine. In: Townsend CM, Beauchamp RD, Evers BM, et al., eds. *Sabiston Textbook of Surgery*. 19th ed. Philadelphia, PA: Elsevier Saunders; 2012:1264.
Schrieber ML, Bass BL. Small intestinal neoplasms. In: Greenfield L, Mulholland M, Oldham K, et al., eds. *Surgery: Scientific Principles and Practice*. 3rd ed. Philadelphia, PA: Lippincott Williams & Wilkins; 2001:836–843.

21. **(B)** Carcinoid tumors of the small bowel are slow-growing tumors that arise from enterochromaffin cells. These tumors are characterized by their secretion of various humorally active peptides, including serotonin. GI carcinoids most frequently occur in the appendix (45%), followed by the ileum (30%) and rectum (15%). Most are asymptomatic and are discovered incidentally in the operating room. However, symptomatic carcinoids present in much the same way as other small bowel tumors, with vague abdominal pain, weight loss, and eventually obstructive symptoms. These can be discovered on imaging evaluating for the source of these symptoms. Five-year survival for patients with localized disease is 65%, and it is 36% in patients with metastases.

Malignant carcinoid syndrome occurs in less than 10% of patients with carcinoid tumors and is characterized by cutaneous flushing (80%), diarrhea (76%), hepatomegaly (71%), cardiac lesions such as valvular disease (41–70%), and asthma (25%). The syndrome is typically described in carcinoid tumors of the GI tract, but also occurs in cases involving the bronchi, pancreas, ovaries, or testes. The responsible vasoactive peptides are metabolized in the liver, making the presence of carcinoid syndrome indicative of extra-abdominal disease, metastatic disease, disease that bypasses the liver, or massive hepatic replacement by metastatic disease.

The appropriate surgical management depends on the size and location of the tumor. For tumors smaller than 1 cm in diameter with no evidence of regional lymph node metastases, segmental small bowel resection is appropriate. For tumors larger than 1 cm, multiple tumors, or

regional lymph node involvement, wide excision of the small bowel and mesentery is required. Lesions of the terminal ileum are often best handled via right hemicolectomy. Given the slow-growing nature of carcinoid tumors, there is a legitimate role for palliative debulking operations if possible.

Carcinoid tumors have the best prognosis of all small bowel malignancies, with nearly a 100% survival rate in patients undergoing resection with disease localized to the primary site. Patients with regional disease have an approximately 65% five-year survival rate, and patients with distantly metastatic disease have a 25–35% five-year survival.

BIBLIOGRAPHY

McKenzie S, Evers BM. Small intestine. In: Townsend CM, Beauchamp RD, Evers BM, et al., eds. *Sabiston Textbook of Surgery*. 19th ed. Philadelphia, PA: Elsevier Saunders; 2012:1259–1262.
Schrieber ML, Bass BL. Small intestinal neoplasms. In: Greenfield L, Mulholland M, Oldham K, et al., eds. *Surgery: Scientific Principles and Practice*. 3rd ed. Philadelphia, PA: Lippincott Williams & Wilkins; 2001:839–841.

22. **(A)** Simple tubular pedunculated adenomas (those with narrow, well-defined stalks) can be managed endoscopically as they also have minimal malignant potential. The exception to this rule is in the case of a true surgical emergency, such as intussusception or massive hemorrhage.

Duodenal tubulovillous and villous adenomas frequently occur at the papilla. This is especially true for patients with inherited colonic polyposis syndromes. These have a high malignant potential, with 30% of those greater than 3 cm having foci of invasive disease. These may be excised endoscopically when smaller than 3 cm, but the recurrence rate is approximately 25%. Of these recurrences, 40% are malignant. Patients are therefore better served with a surgical resection in these cases. Pancreaticoduodenectomy is indicated in patients with large villous adenomas near the papilla (Fig. 19-10). Brunner's gland adenomas result from glandular hyperplasia of Brunner's glands, normally found throughout the duodenal submucosa. These glands secrete alkaline substances and bicarbonate, which serves to neutralize gastric acid. These adenomas have negligible malignant potential and can be managed at any size with local resection surgically or endoscopically to prevent obstruction or intussusception.

BIBLIOGRAPHY

Bresalier RS, Ben-Menachem T. Tumors of the small intestine. In: Yamada T, Alpers D, Kaplowitz N, et al., eds. *Textbook of Gastroenterology*. 4th ed. Philadelphia, PA: Lippincott Williams & Wilkins; 2003:1647–1649.

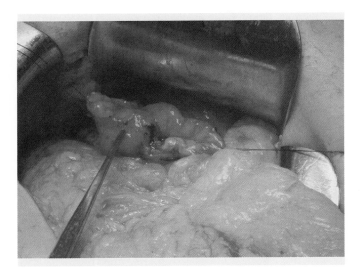

FIGURE 19-10. Benign duodenal neoplasm *in situ*.

Campbell KA. Small bowel tumors. In: Cameron J, ed. *Current Surgical Therapy*. 7th ed. St. Louis, MO: Mosby; 2001:139–141.
Schrieber ML, Bass BL. Small intestinal neoplasms. In: Greenfield L, Mulholland M, Oldham K, et al., eds. *Surgery: Scientific Principles and Practice*. 3rd ed. Philadelphia, PA: Lippincott Williams & Wilkins; 2001:833–835.

23. **(B)** Duodenal diverticular disease is relatively common, although few diverticula are clinically significant. Duodenal diverticula can be congenital or acquired, with congenital diverticula true diverticula and acquired diverticula false. Acquired duodenal diverticula rarely occur before the age of 40 (Fig. 19-11). The overall prevalence of duodenal diverticula is approximately 25% in both autopsy studies and ERCP studies. Approximately 75% occur within 2–3 cm of the ampulla of Vater (juxtapapillary diverticula) or contain the ampulla (intradiverticular papilla). These diverticula result from the relative decrease in number of muscle fibers in the periampullary region, more frequent migrating motor complexes, and increased contraction pressure in the duodenum.

    Complications of duodenal diverticula include pancreatitis, cholangitis, hemorrhage, and perforation. Presenting symptoms include early satiety, nausea, epigastric pain radiating to the back, vomiting, and melena. Hemorrhage results from inflammation and eventual erosion into a branch of the SMA. Perforation is rare. Pancreaticobiliary complications are most common. Pancreatitis may result from sphincter dysfunction because of the proximity of the ampulla to the diverticulum or from compression on the pancreatic duct by a diverticulum distended with food.

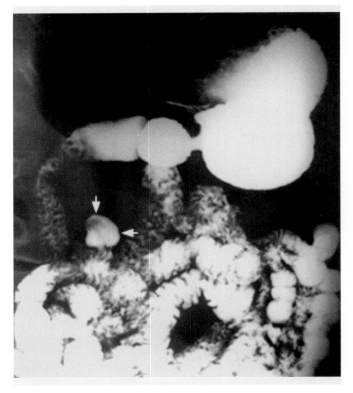

FIGURE 19-11. Duodenal diverticulum on contrast radiology (from Brunicardi FC, Andersen DK, Billiar TR, Dunn DL, Hunter JG, Matthews JB, et al., eds. *Schwartz's Principles of Surgery*. 9th ed. New York, NY: McGraw-Hill; 2010: Fig. 28-6).

Diagnosis is frequently made by EGD or ERCP. Barium studies can also be used but are much less sensitive and specific. Symptomatic duodenal diverticula are best treated nonoperatively with ERCP, sphincterotomy, and stent placement. Care must be taken to prevent iatrogenic perforation or hemorrhage in these cases. Surgery should be avoided because of its high rate of pancreaticobiliary complications and associated morbidity. Asymptomatic, incidental duodenal diverticula are an absolute contraindication to surgery.

If surgery must be undertaken due to unsatisfactory symptom control, several options exist and must be tailored to the patient. Diverticulectomy with or without transduodenal sphincterotomy is an option for anterior and posterior diverticula when a wide Kocher maneuver is performed. The diverticulum is excised, and the duodenum is closed in two layers in a direction that will not stricture the duodenum. This is an especially good option for hemorrhaging or perforated diverticula. Roux-en-Y duodenojejunostomy is used to exclude the diverticulum from the food stream, thereby preventing stasis and subsequent pancreatitis. Bile may also be diverted with a choledochojejunostomy at the same time.

BIBLIOGRAPHY

Lobo D, Balfour T, Iftikar S, et al. Periampullary diverticula and pancreaticobiliary disease. *Br J Surg* 1999;86:588–597.
McKenzie S, Evers BM. Small intestine. In: Townsend CM, Beauchamp RD, Evers BM, et al., eds. *Sabiston Textbook of Surgery*. 19th ed. Philadelphia, PA: Elsevier Saunders; 2012:1265–1266.

24. **(C)** Up to 30% of GISTs will demonstrate malignant behavior. Typically, GISTs invade locally and spread via direct extension into adjacent tissues or via hematogenous spread to the liver, lungs, and bones. Lymphatic spread is rare.

    The GISTs represent 2–3% of all GI neoplasms and approximately 20% of small bowel malignancies. They typically present in adulthood, with a peak incidence in the fifth and sixth decades. They are slightly more common in males. Clinical signs and symptoms tend to be nonspecific and vary by tumor location. The most common symptoms include nausea/vomiting, abdominal pain, and GI bleeding. Very rarely, GISTs may be associated with a tumor syndrome. Grossly, GISTs vary greatly in size and in morphologic appearance. They are usually well circumscribed and can be found in a submucosal, intramural, or subserosal location. Depending on the degree of hemorrhage or necrosis, the tumor may vary from completely solid to partially cystic.

BIBLIOGRAPHY

McKenzie S, Evers BM. Small intestine. In: Townsend CM, Beauchamp RD, Evers BM, et al., eds. *Sabiston Textbook of Surgery*. 19th ed. Philadelphia, PA: Elsevier Saunders; 2012:1264.
Miettinen M, Majidi M, Lasota J. Pathology and diagnostic criteria of gastrointestinal stromal tumors (GISTs): a review. *Eur J Cancer* 2002;38(Suppl 5):S39–S51.

25. **(B)** Imatinib mesylate is an orally administered tyrosine kinase inhibitor. This functions by blocking unregulated mutant c-kit tyrosine kinases and inhibits the BCR-ABL and platelet-derived growth factor tyrosine kinases. Adjuvant therapy with imantinib mesylate is now the standard of care for malignant GISTs, especially those larger than 5 cm and with high mitotic rates.

    Alkylating agents such as cyclophosphamide add alkyl groups to DNA, which causes cross-linkage. Hydroxyurea inhibits ribonucleotide reductase, which normally converts ribonucleotides into deoxyribonucleotides. Vinca alkaloids (vincristine and vinblastine) bind tubulin and inhibit microtubule assembly. Paclitaxel and docetaxel stabilize formed microtubules and prevent their disassembly. Both actions prevent completion of mitosis. Anthracyclines such as doxorubicin inhibit topoisomerase II, which normally repairs breaks in DNA.

BIBLIOGRAPHY

McKenzie S, Evers BM. Small intestine. In: Townsend CM, Beauchamp RD, Evers BM, et al., eds. *Sabiston Textbook of Surgery*. 19th ed. Philadelphia, PA: Elsevier Saunders; 2012:1264.
Sausville EA, Longo DL. Principles of Cancer Treatment. In: Kasper D, Fauci A, Hauser S, Longo D, Jameson J, Loscalzo J. eds. *Harrison's Principles of Internal Medicine, 19e*. New York, NY: McGraw-Hill; 2015.

26. **(E)** Ileus after abdominal surgery is the dysmotility of the bowel in the absence of a mechanical obstruction. Ileus can be defined as normal postoperative ileus or as paralytic ileus. If a normal postoperative ileus lasts longer than 5 days, it is considered a prolonged ileus. Risk factors for ileus include narcotic use, peritoneal or retroperitoneal inflammation, sepsis, severe pelvic fractures, and spinal cord injury. Metabolic derangements may also play a role, with hypomagnesemia, hypermagnesemia, hypercalcemia, hyponatremia, and hypokalemia playing a role. Numerous nonnarcotic medications may also contribute to the pathogenesis of an ileus.

BIBLIOGRAPHY

Clark J. Motility disorders of the stomach and small bowel. In: Cameron J, ed. *Current Surgical Therapy*. 11th ed. Philadelphia, PA: Elsevier Saunders; 2014:136–137.

27. **(A)** Postoperative ileus is a normal occurrence after abdominal surgery and is the subject of ongoing investigation. The use of epidural analgesia has been shown to be beneficial in reducing the duration of postoperative ileus, likely secondary to a decreased systemic narcotic requirement to adequately control postoperative pain. Other treatments that have shown promise for decreasing ileus include early feeding postoperatively, gum chewing, and peripherally acting μ-opioid receptor antagonists.

    Nasogastric decompression has not been shown to reduce the duration of postoperative ileus and is supported by multiple randomized clinical trials. It may, however, provide symptomatic relief for selected patients, particularly in the setting of postoperative ileus with nausea and abdominal distention. Erythromycin is a macrolide antibiotic known to bind to the motilin receptor on GI smooth muscle. Despite this action, a randomized controlled trial showed no effect of erythromycin on duration of ileus. Similarly, TPN has not been shown to decrease the length of postoperative ileus and thus is not indicated.

BIBLIOGRAPHY

Asao T, Kuwano H, Nakamura J, et al. Gum chewing enhances recovery from postoperative ileus after laparoscopic colectomy. *J Am Coll Surg* 2002;195(1):30–32.

Clark J. Motility disorders of the stomach and small bowel. In: Cameron J, ed. *Current Surgical Therapy*. 11th ed. Philadelphia, PA: Elsevier Saunders; 2014:136–137.

Luckey A, Livingston E, Tache Y, et al. Mechanisms and treatment of postoperative ileus. *Arch Surg* 2003;138(2):206–214.

Miedema B, Johnson J. Methods for decreasing postoperative gut dysmotility. *Lancet* 2003;4:365–372.

Van Bree S, Nemethova A, Cailotto C, Gomez-Pinilla PJ, Matteoli G, Boeckxstaens GE. New therapeutic strategies for postoperative ileus. *Nat Rev Gastroenterol Hepatol* 2012;9:675–683.

28. **(E)** As many as 95% of patients may develop intra-abdominal adhesions following laparotomy. Although the majority of patients will not develop any clinical sequelae from these adhesions, there are significant morbidities that are associated with their development. Other etiologies of intra-abdominal adhesions include infections/abscesses, anastomotic leaks, carcinomatosis, and other inflammatory processes.

Intra-abdominal adhesions are responsible for 75% of all cases of small bowel obstructions. After some open abdominal operations, the lifetime risk of developing an adhesion-related small bowel obstruction has been reported to be between 4 and 30%. Among individuals who have been admitted to the hospital with an adhesive small bowel obstruction, recurrence rates are nearly 30%, regardless of whether their initial small bowel obstruction was managed operatively or nonoperatively. In addition, as the number of previous admissions for small bowel obstructions increases, the likelihood of recurrence does as well, with studies demonstrating a greater than 50% recurrence rate for individuals who have been admitted with three small bowel obstructions in the past. Infertility and chronic pain can also occur secondary to adhesions. The presence of intra-abdominal adhesions can also significantly complicate future operations and places these patients at risk for unintended enterotomies during future abdominal surgeries.

BIBLIOGRAPHY

Diamond M, Wexner S, diZereg GS, et al. Adhesion prevention and reduction: current status and future recommendations of a multinational interdisciplinary consensus conference. *Surg Innov* 2010;17(3):183–188.

Kodadek L, Makary M. Small bowel obstruction. In: Cameron J, ed. *Current Surgical Therapy*. 11th ed. Philadelphia, PA: Elsevier Saunders; 2014:109–113.

Miller G, Boman J, Shrier I, Gordon PH. Natural history of patients with adhesive small bowel obstruction. *Br J Surg* 2000;87:1240–1247.

Reijnen M, Bleichrodt R, van Goor H. Pathophysiology of intra-abdominal adhesion and abscess formation, and the effect of hyaluronan. *Br J Surg* 2003;90:533–541.

Sulaiman H, Gabella G, Davis C, et al. Presence and distribution of sensory nerve fibers in human peritoneal adhesions. *Ann Surg* 2001;234(2):256–261.

29. **(C)** The most common cause of chronic mesenteric ischemia is atherosclerosis. This disease typically takes on one of three varieties: occlusions of the visceral arteries at their aortic orifices, occlusions involving long segments of the main trunks of the visceral arteries, and occlusions involving branches of the visceral arteries. The hallmark of chronic mesenteric ischemia is postprandial abdominal pain. This results in "food fear," which contributes to the progressive and often severe weight loss that is seen in patients with this disease. Given the significant collateral blood flow to the viscera, occlusion of two of the three main visceral artery trunks is typically necessary for symptoms to develop, typically the celiac artery and SMA. Inferior mesenteric artery (IMA) involvement produces symptoms in a less-predictable manner.

Symptoms of chronic mesenteric ischemia commonly include postprandial abdominal pain, fear of eating, and weight loss. Diarrhea, nausea and vomiting, and constipation are less-common symptoms. Abdominal pain is the most consistent symptom and typically occurs 15–60 min after a meal and lasts several hours. It is generally described as midabdominal, aching or cramping in quality, and worsening in severity as the disease progresses. Some patients will naturally reduce the size of their meals, which may at least initially decrease their symptoms.

Diagnosis of chronic mesenteric ischemia can be made based on history, exam, and imaging. CT scans, magnetic resonance imaging, and mesenteric duplex ultrasounds are all imaging modalities that can be useful in making the diagnosis of chronic mesenteric ischemia. Mesenteric duplex ultrasound is a good screening test for symptomatic patients before progressing to angiography. It is inexpensive and noninvasive and has a sensitivity of 87% for celiac stenosis and 92% for SMA stenosis. Disadvantages are that it requires expertise to both perform and interpret, and the IMA can be difficult to visualize.

Once the diagnosis of chronic mesenteric ischemia is made, treatment focuses on restoring mesenteric blood flow. This can be done endovascularly, via endarterectomy, or via bypass. The decision regarding which modality to use often is based on the location and extent of disease and which option is most likely to have success. Endovascular techniques carry lower morbidity and mortality rates; however, they also have been shown to be less durable over time than open techniques.

BIBLIOGRAPHY

Chandra A, Quinones-Baldrich W. Chronic mesenteric ischemia: how to select patients for invasive treatment. *Semin Vasc Surg* 2010;23(1):21–28.

Reilly L. The management of chronic mesenteric ischemia. In: Cameron J, ed. *Current Surgical Therapy*. 11th ed. Philadelphia, PA: Elsevier Saunders; 2014:947–953.

30. **(D)** Duodenal ulcer disease is responsible for approximately 60,000 patients annually and is associated with an in-hospital mortality rate of 3.7%. Of individuals hospitalized with duodenal ulcers, only 10% will ultimately require surgery. The most frequent causes of duodenal ulcers are *H. pylori* infection and recent non-steroidal anti-inflammatory drug use. Together, these are responsible for 90% of duodenal ulcers. Other important etiologies include gastrinoma (Zollinger-Ellison syndrome), smoking, and steroid or cocaine use. All patients with duodenal ulcers should be tested for *H. pylori* and treated as needed.

Surgical management of duodenal ulcers is most frequently indicated for bleeding, perforation, and obstruction. Perforated duodenal ulcers typically present with sudden-onset severe abdominal pain and abdominal sepsis. Most perforations occur on the anterior service of the first portion of the duodenum and are less than 5 mm in diameter, as is the case in this patient. For individuals presenting with less than 24 h of symptoms and ulcers less than 5 mm in diameter, primary repair with abdominal washout is appropriate. For larger ulcers or for individuals who have had symptoms for greater than 24 h, an omental patch is recommended. In the hands of an experienced laparoscopic surgeon, this can be performed safely laproscopically.

The most common reasons for operative intervention are bleeding, perforation, and obstruction.

BIBLIOGRAPHY

Beaulieu R, Eckhauser F. The management of duodenal ulcers. In: Cameron J, ed. *Current Surgical Therapy*. 11th ed. Philadelphia, PA: Elsevier Saunders; 2014:76–80.

31. **(A)** Short bowel syndrome occurs when the total length of small bowel is inadequate to support an individual's nutritional needs. Approximately 75% of cases of short bowel syndrome result from massive intestinal resections, which in adults are often due to mesenteric ischemia, midgut volvulus, and trauma to the superior mesenteric vessels. Multiple sequential resections, such as those occurring in individuals with CD, are responsible for most of the remaining 25% of cases.

The consequences of short bowel syndrome can be severe and most often include diarrhea, fluid and electrolyte deficiencies, and significant malnutrition. Gallstones and nephrolithiasis also occur due to the disruption of enterohepatic circulation and hyperoxaluria, respectively. Nutrient deficiencies that are common in short bowel syndrome include those for iron, magnesium, zinc, copper, and certain vitamins. Therefore, in patients with short bowel syndrome, these must be monitored.

The absolute length of small bowel that can be resected before a patient develops short bowel syndrome is unclear, as there is significant variation from person to person. The location of the resection within the GI tract plays a significant role in the clinical consequences for the patient. The small bowel has the ability to increase its absorptive capacity following significant small bowel resections. Interestingly, the distal small bowel, specifically the ileum, can increase its absorption capability better than the jejunum. This is in part why proximal small bowel resections are often better tolerated than distal small bowel resections. In addition, the distal two-thirds of the ileum and the ileocecal valve are key in absorbing bile salts and vitamin B_{12}. If these are resected, patients often suffer from diarrhea and anemia. If the terminal ileum and ileocecal valve are preserved, resection of up to 70% of the small bowel can typically be tolerated.

BIBLIOGRAPHY

American Gastroenterological Association. AGA technical review on short bowel syndrome and intestinal transplantation. *Gastroenterology* 2003;124:1111–1134.

Evers B, Townsend C, Thompson J. Small intestine. In: Schwartz S, Shires G, Spencer F, et al., eds. *Principles of Surgery*. 7th ed. New York, NY: McGraw-Hill; 1999:1217–1263.

McKenzie S, Evers BM. Small intestine. In: Townsend CM, Beauchamp RD, Evers BM, et al., eds. *Sabiston Textbook of Surgery*. 19th ed. Philadelphia, PA: Elsevier Saunders; 2012: 1274–1276.

MINIMALLY INVASIVE SURGERY AND BARIATRICS

THOMAS WADE AND J. CHRISTOPHER EAGON

QUESTIONS

1. Which of the following statements correctly identifies a component of the National Institutes of Health (NIH) Consensus Statement on qualification for bariatric surgery?
   - (A) Body mass index (BMI) greater than 35 kg/m² with a medical comorbidity related to morbid obesity or BMI greater than 40 kg/m²
   - (B) BMI greater than 35 kg/m²
   - (C) Age less than 60
   - (D) Significant weight loss with nonsurgical methods such as dieting, exercise, and behavioral modifications

2. Which patient qualifies for bariatric surgery based on NIH guidelines?
   - (A) 40-year-old female with no medical comorbidities and a BMI of 38 kg/m²
   - (B) 55-year-old male with insulin-dependent diabetes mellitus, a BMI of 38 kg/m², and failed nonsurgical weight loss techniques for 12 months
   - (C) 48-year-old male with BMI of 35 kg/m² who suffers from arthritis, sleep apnea, and gastroesophageal reflux and has no history of structured weight loss techniques
   - (D) 16-year-old female with BMI of 40 kg/m² with depression and hyperparathyroidism

3. Several surgical weight loss procedures have been performed during the development of bariatric surgery. Roux-en-Y gastric bypass procedure (GBP) is the most commonly performed bariatric procedure in the United States. Outcomes following weight loss procedures are frequently reported in excess body weight (EBW) loss. EBW is equal to the difference of a patient's presurgical weight and his or her ideal body weight. How much EBW can a patient expect to lose at 2 years following a Roux-en-Y GBP?

   - (A) 15%
   - (B) 31%
   - (C) 65%
   - (D) 86%
   - (E) 100%

4. Adjustable gastric banding (AGB) is performed around the world for treatment of clinically severe obesity. Benefits of the AGB include
   - (A) Greater weight loss than gastric bypass
   - (B) Decreased need for surgical revision
   - (C) Limited risk of malnutrition and vitamin deficiencies
   - (D) No risk of gastrointestinal leak
   - (E) Equal success in all patient populations

5. Which of the following patients is most appropriate for a laparoscopic inguinal hernia repair?
   - (A) 45-year-old woman with unilateral right side hernia
   - (B) 68-year-old man with unilateral left side hernia and history of open prostatectomy
   - (C) 85-year-old man with bilateral partially reducible inguinal hernia, history of congestive heart failure (CHF) with an ejection fraction (EF) of 35%
   - (D) 40-year-old man without significant comorbidities with a recurrent right inguinal hernia after open repair
   - (E) 85-year-old woman with a small asymptomatic and reducible left inguinal hernia

6. Which of the following statements regarding laparoscopic sleeve gastrectomy (LSG) is true?
   - (A) LSG is associated with greater weight loss than laparoscopic gastric bypass (LGB).
   - (B) LSG results in a greater long-term risk of internal hernia than LGB.
   - (C) LSG may worsen gastroesophageal reflux disease (GERD) symptoms.
   - (D) Weight loss with LSG is similar to that for gastric band.
   - (E) LSG has a lower staple line leak rate than gastric bypass.

7. A 35-year-old female with a BMI of 45 kg/m^2 and no significant medical comorbidities underwent Roux-en-Y GBP. On the morning of postoperative day 1, she has a heart rate of 110 bpm and a temperature of 38.5°C. Oxygen saturation on 2 L per nasal cannula is 98%, and her blood pressure is 140/80 mmHg. What is the most appropriate first step in management of this patient?
   (A) Administer an acetaminophen suppository per rectum, monitor the patient's vital signs, and encourage incentive spirometry
   (B) Start a clear liquid diet without concentrated sweets
   (C) Perform an exploratory laparotomy to identify and treat a gastrointestinal leak
   (D) Obtain a computerized tomographic (CT) scan to evaluate for intra-abdominal abscess or fluid collection
   (E) Schedule an immediate water-soluble contrast study to evaluate postoperative anatomy

8. According to institutional protocol, the patient in question 7 undergoes a Gastrografin swallow approximately as shown in Fig. 20-1. The patient's heart rate remains

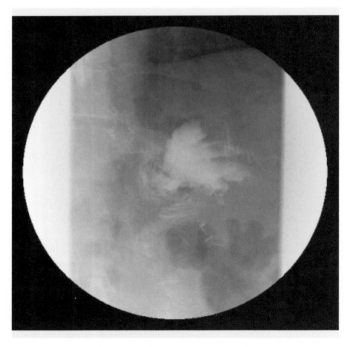

FIGURE 20-1. Gastrografin swallow study from patient 1 day after Roux-en-Y gastric bypass.

elevated at 125 bpm, and her temperature is 38.2°C. Her oxygen saturation is 96% on 4 L per nasal cannula, and her blood pressure is 100/60 mmHg. What is the next step in management of this patient?

   (A) An upper endoscopy is necessary to identify and treat the source of these findings.
   (B) Surgical exploration is needed to evaluate, drain, and possibly repair the swallow study findings.
   (C) CT-guided placement of percutaneous drainage catheters is needed.
   (D) Administer broad-spectrum intravenous antibiotics and begin total parenteral nutrition (TPN).
   (E) Insert a nasogastric tube to decompress the gastric pouch and proximal small intestine.

9. Four weeks after undergoing a laparoscopic Roux-en-Y GBP, a 38-year-old man develops intolerance to solids and most liquids. Preoperatively, he weighed 127 kg (280 lb), and he had a BMI of 42.5 kg/m^2. His current weight is 114 kg (251 lb), and his BMI is 38 kg/m^2. Consumption of a 2-oz meal leads to dysphagia and subsequent emesis. Upper endoscopy is performed. The endoscopic image is shown in Fig. 20-2. Which of the following is the most appropriate therapy?

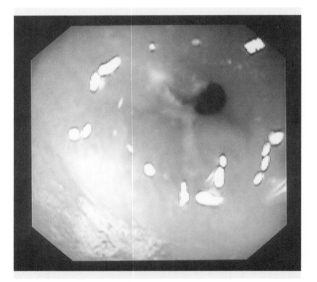

FIGURE 20-2. Upper endoscopic image following gastric bypass.

   (A) Nasogastric decompression of the gastric pouch and proximal small intestine
   (B) Take down of the GBP with reestablishment of normal anatomical intestinal continuity
   (C) Insertion of central venous access with administration of TPN
   (D) Dilation of the gastrojejunostomy anastomosis followed by observation and supportive care
   (E) Administration of a proton pump inhibitor and antibiotic therapy for *Helicobacter pylori*

10. A 28-year-old man underwent laparoscopic Roux-en-Y GBP and cholecystectomy 18 months prior to his presentation to an emergency room for sudden onset of abdominal pain. His preoperative weight was 185 kg, and his BMI was 58.5 kg/m^2. He now weighs 101 kg with a BMI of 32 kg/m^2. He is compliant and has kept appropriate postoperative follow-up appointments, takes his supplements, and maintains an active lifestyle. He has no other health problems. The pain extends "like a band" across his midabdomen and causes him to double over. Abdominal examination demonstrates minimal tenderness in the left upper quadrant of the abdomen and no signs of peritonitis. A kidney, ureter, and bladder (KUB) x-ray is shown in Fig. 20-3. Lab tests, including complete blood cell count and comprehensive chemistry panel are normal. What is the most likely cause for his pain?

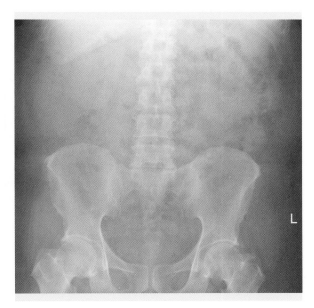

FIGURE 20-3. Abdominal flat plate film for patient after Roux-en-Y gastric bypass.

    (A) Anastomotic stricture
    (B) Internal herniation
    (C) Marginal ulcer
    (D) Dumping syndrome
    (E) Gastrointestinal leak

11. A 26-year-old woman presents 2 years after Roux-en-Y gastric bypass complaining of fatigue and muscle weakness. Laboratory studies reveal a macrocytic anemia. A deficiency in which of the following vitamins or minerals is most likely responsible for her symptoms?
    (A) Calcium
    (B) Iron

    (C) Vitamin K
    (D) Folic acid
    (E) Vitamin B$_{12}$

12. Which of the following medications is used postoperatively to prevent gallstone formation after bariatric surgery?
    (A) Cholestyramine
    (B) Ursodiol
    (C) Octreotide
    (D) Simvastatin
    (E) Misoprostol

13. A 43-year-old woman undergoes an uneventful laparoscopic insertion of an AGB. Her band reservoir is left empty on insertion. She undergoes a postoperative swallow study as demonstrated in Fig. 20-4. Her preoperative weight was 286 lb with a BMI of 46.3 kg/m^2. She now weighs 253 lb with a BMI of 41 kg/m^2 1 year after surgery. Her weight loss has reached a plateau. She presents for a band adjustment. Fluoroscopic evaluation is performed, including a barium swallow. Figure 20-4 is an image from the study. The patient has no complaints, excluding her inability to continue to lose weight. Which

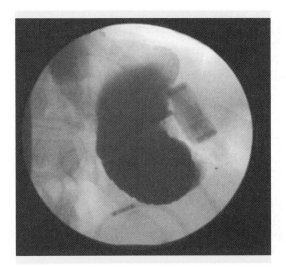

FIGURE 20-4. Swallow study following adjustable gastric band placement.

of the following has most likely led to this patient's weight plateau?
    (A) Maladaptive eating behavior
    (B) Band slippage
    (C) Gastrogastric fistula
    (D) Inadequate band reservoir inflation
    (E) Esophageal dilatation

14. A 65-year-old man presents to clinic with complaints of progressive dysphagia. Upper gastrointestinal, EGD, and esophageal manometry are consistent with achalasia. Which of the following options has the highest chance of success at 5 years:
    (A) Botox injection
    (B) Endoscopic dilation
    (C) Laparoscopic Heller myotomy
    (D) Nissen fundoplication
    (E) Diet modification

15. Although multiple variations of bariatric procedures are performed around the world, four basic procedures are performed commonly: Roux-en-Y GBP, sleeve gastrectomy, AGB, and biliopancreatic diversion (BPD). What is the appropriate order of average percentage excess weight loss 1 year after laparoscopic surgery for a patient with a BMI greater than 50?
    (A) SG > GBP > AGB > BPD
    (B) GBP > SG > BPD > AGB
    (C) AGB > GBP > SG > BPD
    (D) BPD > GBP > SG > AGB
    (E) None of the above

16. During insufflation of the abdomen, your anesthesiologist notices that the patient has become more cyanotic and is having ventricular arrhythmias, and the end-tidal CO_2 value on the monitor has decreased. What is the most likely cause?
    (A) CO_2 embolism
    (B) Vagal response to insufflation
    (C) Pulmonary embolism
    (D) Myocardial infarction
    (E) Trocar injury

17. What is the most appropriate initial step in management of the patient in question 16?
    (A) Cessation of insufflation
    (B) Hyperventilation
    (C) Aspiration of gas through central venous catheter
    (D) Positioning the patient head down and right lateral decubitus
    (E) Initiation of cardiopulmonary resuscitation

18. A pneumoperitoneum of less than 20 mmHg is associated with which of the following observed changes in the following cardiac parameters: mean arterial pressure (MAP), systemic vascular resistance (SVR), and central venous pressure (CVP)?
    (A) Increased MAP, increased SVR, increased CVP
    (B) Decreased MAP, decreased SVR, increased CVP
    (C) Increased MAP, decreased SVR, decreased CVP
    (D) Decreased MAP, decreased SVR, decreased CVP
    (E) Increased MAP, increased SVR, decreased CVP

19. You are insufflating the abdomen of an otherwise-healthy 35-year-old female for laparoscopic cholecystectomy when the patient becomes severely bradycardic. What should be your next course of action?
    (A) Continue with laparoscopic cholecystectomy
    (B) Administer 1 mg epinephrine
    (C) Deflate the abdomen
    (D) Place the patient in Trendelenburg position
    (E) Administer 10 mg rocuronium

20. Insufflation of the peritoneum with increasing pressures of CO_2 has several effects on CO_2 excretion and arterial CO_2. Which of the following effects is correct?
    (A) Linearly increasing CO_2 excretion; linearly increasing $PaCO_2$
    (B) Increase, then plateau of CO_2 excretion; linearly increasing $PaCO_2$
    (C) Increase, then plateau of CO_2 excretion; increase, then plateau of $PaCO_2$
    (D) Unchanged CO_2 excretion; unchanged $PaCO_2$
    (E) Decreased CO_2 excretion; increasing $PaCO_2$

21. Correct Veress needle placement may be confirmed by
    (A) Crepitus of neck, face, perineum, or extremities
    (B) Opening pressure between 10 and 15 mmHg
    (C) Positive saline drop test
    (D) Identification of four distinct abdominal wall layers during entry

22. While performing a laparoscopic Nissen fundoplication, the patient becomes markedly hypotensive, hypoxic, and difficult to ventilate. The anesthesiologist notes that the patient's breath sounds are now diminished on the left. What is the first step in management?
    (A) Placement of the patient in left lateral decubitus position
    (B) Placement of a left tube thoracostomy
    (C) Desufflation of the abdomen and placement of an angiocatheter in the left chest
    (D) Dissection through the diaphragmatic crura into the parietal pleura
    (E) Obtaining a chest x-ray

23. While performing a laparoscopic cholecystectomy for acalculous cholecystitis, you see an adhesion between the gallbladder and the duodenum. You take down the adhesion with electrocautery. The remainder of the cholecystectomy is uneventful. Five days after discharge, the patient presents to the emergency room with severe epigastric pain, rigid abdomen, and fever. Which of the following is the most likely cause of this patient's illness?
    (A) Duodenal necrosis
    (B) Gallstone pancreatitis
    (C) Localized ileus
    (D) Mallory-Weiss tear
    (E) Barrett's esophagus

24. A 48-year-old woman presents with long-term history of GERD despite maximal medical therapy. Esophageal manometry is within normal limits, and her upper gastrointestinal image is shown in Fig. 20-5. What is the most appropriate management strategy?
   (A) Nissen fundoplication
   (B) Laparoscopic hiatal hernia repair with fundoplication

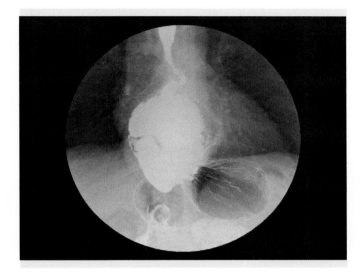

FIGURE 20-5. Upper GI imaging for patient with gastroesophageal reflux disease. Used with permission from Saurabh Khandelwal, MD, University of Washington.

   (C) Endoscopic fundoplication
   (D) Open hiatal hernia repair with fundoplication
   (E) Esophageal disconnect with Roux-en-Y reconstruction

25. You are performing a laparoscopic cholecystectomy for a patient with suspected choledocholithiasis, and, on performing an intraoperative cholangiogram, you notice a filling defect proximal to the duodenum. Which of the following options should be considered for relief of biliary obstruction intraoperatively?
   (A) Lithotripsy
   (B) Glucagon administration
   (C) Holmium laser stone obliteration
   (D) Endoscopic retrograde cholangiopancreatography (ERCP)
   (E) None of the above

26. A 24-year-old woman presents with right lower quadrant tenderness and guarding, fever, anorexia, and leukocytosis of 17,000. She is also in the second trimester of her pregnancy. Ultrasound is highly suspicious for appendicitis. You consider laparoscopic appendectomy. Which of the following statements is true regarding laparoscopic appendectomy during pregnancy?
   (A) Laparoscopic appendectomy is contraindicated in pregnancy.
   (B) The patient should be positioned with her left side down.
   (C) Pneumoperitoneum pressure should reach 15 mmHg.
   (D) Laparoscopic appendectomy cannot be performed in the second trimester.
   (E) Fetal loss is 10% in nonperforated appendicitis.

27. A 47-year-old man presents to your office 3 months after laparoscopic Nissen fundoplication with symptoms of dysphagia. An esophagogastroduodenoscopy (EDG) is performed and is shown in Fig. 20-6. What is the most likely etiology of his dysphagia?

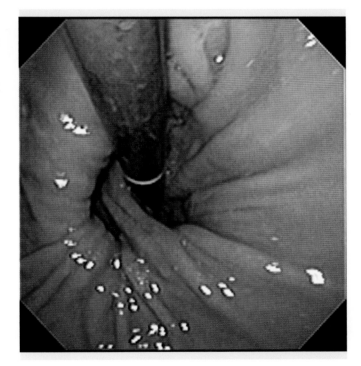

FIGURE 20-6. Esophagogastroduodenoscopy image for the patient in question 27 (from Sugarbaker DJ, Bueno R, Krasna MJ, Mentzer SJ, Zellos L, eds. *Adult Chest Surgery.* 2nd ed. New York, NY: McGraw Hill; 2013: Fig. 24-4. Copyright © The McGraw-Hill Companies, Inc. All rights reserved).

   (A) Hiatal hernia
   (B) Shortened esophagus
   (C) Slipped Nissen
   (D) Too tight Nissen fundoplication
   (E) Esophageal stricture

28. A 53-year-old woman with a BMI of 41 presents to clinic with continued reflux symptoms despite a Nissen fundoplication and two revisions. During the course of workup, it is evident that the fundoplication has failed again. What is the best option for this patient?
    (A) Laparoscopic Nissen revision
    (B) Laparoscopic revision of Nissen to gastric bypass
    (C) Conversion of the Nissen to a Toupet fundoplication
    (D) Esophageal dilation
    (E) Truncal vagotomy with gastric resection

29. Which of the following structures forms the medial border of the "triangle of doom" to be avoided in laparoscopic inguinal herniorrhaphy?
    (A) Inferior epigastric vessels
    (B) Vas deferens
    (C) Spermatic vessels
    (D) Iliac vessels
    (E) Lateral femoral cutaneous nerve

ANSWERS AND EXPLANATIONS

1. **(A)**

2. **(B)**

Explanation for questions 1 and 2

The NIH Consensus Development Conference Statement summarizes the conclusions obtained following a 2-day conference in March 1991. Several basic patient selection criteria were recommended, including the following: BMI $\geq$ 40 kg/m^2 or BMI $\geq$ 35 kg/m^2 with a minimum of one medical comorbidity related to obesity (e.g., sleep apnea, Pickwickian's syndrome, diabetes mellitus, joint disease, GERD, and so on), a demonstrated low probability to be successful with nonsurgical weight loss measures, and demonstrated ability to participate and maintain follow-up on a long-term basis.

The consensus panel did not provide guidelines regarding surgical weight loss treatment of children or adolescents, even subjects with BMI > 40 kg/m^2. Several centers perform weight loss surgery on adolescents, and guidelines have been proposed that are similar to the NIH guidelines. These guidelines, however, have not been incorporated into the NIH guidelines. Continued study to include randomized trials is necessary.

BIBLIOGRAPHY

Brolin RE., *NIH consensus conference. Gastrointestinal surgery for severe obesity.* Nutrition. 1996 Jun;12(6):403-4
Nguyen NT, DeMaria EJ, Hutter MM, eds. *The SAGES Manual: A Practical Guide to Bariatric Surgery.* New York, NY: Springer; 2008.

Pratt JS, Lenders CM, Dionne EA, et al. Best practice updates for pediatric/adolescent weight loss surgery. *Obesity (Silver Spring)* 2009;17(5):901–910.

3. **(C)** The common goal for all bariatric surgical procedures is achieving weight loss and obtaining its beneficial effects on the treatment or prevention of obesity-related medical comorbidities, including hypertension, coronary artery disease, and diabetes mellitus. Roux-en-Y GBP, initially described by Mason and Ito, is currently the most commonly performed bariatric procedure. It uses a restrictive gastric pouch with a small outlet. This pouch is drained by a Roux intestinal limb that causes malabsorption as food bypasses the distal stomach, entire duodenum, and proximal jejunum. Although both a traditional open and a laparoscopic approach are available, weight loss results appear to be similar.

On average, patients experience an initial loss of approximately 60–70% EBW at 2 years after the procedure. The most precipitous weight loss occurs during the first 6–12 months. This is followed by a slower period of weight loss or even a plateau. Long-term results suggest a slight weight gain several years following the procedure. Patients may experience a gain of 10–15% weight at 5 years following the procedure.

BIBLIOGRAPHY

Brolin RE. Gastric bypass. *Surg Clin North Am* 2001;81(5):1077–1095.
Cottam DR, Mattar SG, Schauer PR. Laparoscopic era of operations for morbid obesity. *Arch Surg* 2003;138:367–375.
Mason EE, Ito C. Gastric bypass. *Ann Surg* 1969;170(3):329–336.
Nguyen NT, Scott-Conner C, eds. *The SAGES Manual Vol. 2 Advanced Laparoscopy and Endoscopy.* New York, NY: Springer; 2012: Chapter 1.

4. **(C)** Adjustable gastric banding (AGB) was first described by Kuzmak in the early 1980s, but it was not commonly performed until it was adapted to a laparoscopic approach in the early 1990s. An AGB is a synthetic plastic ring with an inflatable balloon that allows the internal diameter to be altered for differing degrees of gastric restriction. More inflation leads to more restriction and more weight loss.

Many controversies surround the use of AGB for clinically severe obesity. The excellent results of weight loss following insertion of AGB in patients at large European and Australian centers are not reproducible at centers in the United States. Failure of weight loss in specific patient groups, including sweet eaters, and frequent revision operations needed to reposition or remove the band have caused many surgeons to limit the use of AGB.

However, AGB has benefits over other bariatric procedures. AGB does not involve division of the gastrointestinal tract. Therefore, gastrointestinal leak occurs infrequently. Removal of the band can be performed laparoscopically and essentially leads to reversibility of the restrictive procedure. Increased inflation of the band balloon leads to a small internal band diameter and greater restriction. This can effectively allow adjustability to modulate weight loss. Micronutrient malnutrition and dumping syndrome are not a significant concern after AGB because no segment of intestine is bypassed.

BIBLIOGRAPHY

Nguyen NT, DeMaria EJ, Hutter MM, eds. *The SAGES Manual: A Practical Guide to Bariatric Surgery.* New York, NY: Springer; 2008: Chapters 13, 18.

O'Brien PE, Dixon JB, Brown W, et al. The laparoscopic adjustable gastric band (Lap-Band®): a prospective study of medium-term effects on weight, health and quality of life. *Obes Surg* 2002;12:652–660.

Zinzindohoue F, Chevallier JM, Douard R, et al. Laparoscopic gastric banding: a minimally invasive surgical treatment for morbid obesity. *Ann Surg* 2003;237(1):1–9.

5. **(D)** Laparoscopic inguinal hernia repair is most appropriate for the patient with a history of prior open inguinal hernia repair. In this setting, the laparoscopic approach avoids the risks of reoperative surgery and risk of nerve injury. Laparoscopic repair may also be preferred in patients requiring bilateral inguinal hernia repair. It is not favored in patients with a history of open prostatectomy due to violation of the preperitoneal space or major medical comorbidity. Unilateral inguinal hernia repair may be approached via an open or laparoscopic approach.

BIBLIOGRAPHY

Pisanu A, Podda M, Saba A, Porceddu G, Uccheddu A. Meta-analysis and review of prospective randomized trials comparing laparoscopic and Lichtenstein techniques in recurrent inguinal hernia repair. *Hernia* 2015;19(#):355–366.

Takata MC, Duh QY. Laparoscopic inguinal hernia repair. *Surg Clin North Am* 2008 Feb;88(1):157–178.

6. **(C)** Laparoscopic sleeve gastrectomy is an increasingly common bariatric surgery procedure. Data from the American College of Surgeons Bariatric Surgery Center Network have indicated that sleeve gastrectomy results in more weight loss than the adjustable gastric band but with increased risk. The sleeve gastrectomy results in lower weight loss than gastric bypass but with lower overall complication rate. The risk of postoperative GERD may be higher after sleeve gastrectomy than Roux-en-Y gastric bypass and should be discussed during preoperative counseling.

BIBLIOGRAPHY

Hutter MM, Schirmer BD, Jones DB, et al. First report from the American College of Surgeons Bariatric Surgery Center Network: laparoscopic sleeve gastrectomy has morbidity and effectiveness positioned between the band and the bypass. *Ann Surg* 2011 Sep;254(3):410–420.

Nguyen NT, DeMaria EJ, Hutter MM, eds. *The SAGES Manual: A Practical Guide to Bariatric Surgery.* New York, NY: Springer; 2008: Chapter 2.

7. **(E)**

8. **(B)**

Explanation for questions 7 and 8

This patient has undergone a Roux-en-Y GBP. An infrequent, but life-threatening, complication is a gastrointestinal leak. Obese patients make physical examination a difficult and inaccurate method of determining intra-abdominal processes. Therefore, postoperative recovery with abnormal findings requires a high index of suspicion for complications, especially a gastrointestinal leak.

Initially, this patient demonstrated tachycardia, fever, and diminished respiratory capacity. These physical findings are common in obese patients with gastrointestinal leak following GBP; however, they are also associated with multiple benign postoperative sources, including atelectasis and postoperative pain. It is imperative that an immediate fluoroscopic water-soluble contrast swallow study is performed to assist with the diagnosis of a leak. It is important to recognize that this study is not helpful in evaluating the enteroenterostomy or distal anastomosis in a Roux limb.

This patient's study demonstrated a leak of contrast from the region of the proximal stomach or gastrojejunostomy. Treatment in this patient, who is beginning to demonstrate signs of sepsis, includes resuscitation and reoperation. During the reoperation, attempts to define the leak are performed, but they are frequently unsuccessful. If a leak is identified, primary repair may be performed. Extensive internal drainage is necessary. During the same surgical reexploration, many surgeons will introduce an enteral feeding tube in the distal stomach or jejunum. With restricted oral intake, proper internal drainage, and supplemental enteral tube feeding or parenteral alimentation, patients with a leak from the proximal stomach or gastrojejunostomy will frequently experience spontaneous resolution of the leak without further surgical intervention.

BIBLIOGRAPHY

Byrne TK. Complications of surgery for obesity. *Surg Clin North Am* 2001;81(5):1181–1193.

Hamilton EC, Sims TL, Hamilton TT, et al. Clinical predictors of leak after laparoscopic Roux-en-Y gastric bypass for morbid obesity. *Surg Endosc* 2003;17(5):679–684.

Marshall JS, Srivastava A, Gupta SK, et al. Roux-en-Y gastric bypass leak complications. *Arch Surg* 2003;138:520–524.

Nguyen NT, DeMaria EJ, Hutter MM, eds. *The SAGES Manual: A Practical Guide to Bariatric Surgery.* New York, NY: Springer; 2008: Chapters 22–26.

9. **(D)** One of the most common complications following Roux-en-Y GBP is stricture of the gastrojejunostomy. It occurs in from 3–12% of patients following open and laparoscopic GBP. Patients frequently present with an increasing or even sudden inability to tolerate solids or even liquids. Patients experience earlier-than-normal satiety and vomiting. Mechanisms to obtain a diagnosis include upper gastrointestinal swallow study; however, upper endoscopy is helpful in making a diagnosis, ruling out marginal ulcer, and treating the stricture with balloon dilation.

The image in Fig. 20-7 of the strictured gastrojejunostomy is stereotypic. As shown, balloon dilation of a stenotic anastomosis is efficient and effective. Rigid dilators passed transorally may also be used to dilate the anastomosis, but these dilators are difficult to pass and must be inserted blindly. Balloon dilation is effective and can be performed quickly with limited sequela and immediate symptomatic relief.

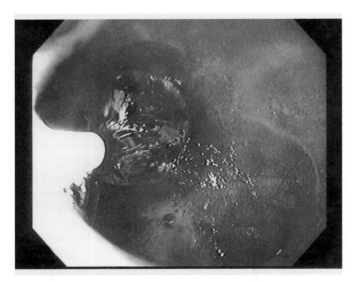

FIGURE 20-7. Balloon dilation of gastrojejunostomy stricture following Roux-en-Y gastric bypass.

BIBLIOGRAPHY

Byrne TK. Complications of surgery for obesity. *Surg Clin North Am* 2001;81(5):1181–1193.

Cottam DR, Mattar SG, Schauer PR. Laparoscopic era of operations for morbid obesity. *Arch Surg* 2003;138:367–375.

Nguyen NT, DeMaria EJ, Hutter MM, eds. *The SAGES Manual: A Practical Guide to Bariatric Surgery.* New York, NY: Springer; 2008: Chapters 22–26.

10. **(B)** All of the complications listed occur following Roux-en-Y GBP and are associated with abdominal pain; however, gastrointestinal leak typically occurs within a 1- to 2-week period following surgery. Dumping syndrome is associated with flushing, abdominal cramping, nausea, headache, and diarrhea. This patient does not carry the stereotypical presentation for dumping syndrome.

Anastomotic stricture frequently occurs during the healing phase of the gastrojejunostomy. During the initial 4–8 weeks after GBP, the gastrojejunostomy stoma may diminish in diameter from larger than 1 cm to only millimeters; however, after the initial 8 weeks following surgery, anastomotic stricture is an uncommon occurrence. In addition, a stricture is typically not associated with abdominal pain. It causes vomiting and inability to tolerate oral intake.

Marginal ulcer may be associated with abdominal pain that is often insidious in onset, although ulcer perforations can cause sudden severe abdominal pain in association with abdominal free air. Ulcers may be associated with gastrointestinal bleeding, melena, or gastric pouch outlet obstruction. Again, this patient's symptoms and x-ray are not consistent with an ulcer.

Internal herniation occurs in varying degrees following GBP and may occur in different locations based on the technique used. Patients may present with radiographic findings consistent with a small bowel obstruction, as in this case, although often radiographic findings are absent or more subtle and seen only on CT scan. It occurs in approximately 2.5–5% of patients following GBP. The most common locations of internal hernia occur in the mesocolic window following a retrocolic Roux limb creation or through Petersen's defect following an antecolic Roux limb creation. Petersen's defect is defined by the Roux limb mesentery sweeping over the transverse colon and its mesentery (Fig. 20-8). Figures 20-6 and 20-9 demonstrate the mesenteric window created by the antecolic Roux limb. Weight loss during the 18 months after surgery allows the potential defect to enlarge and permit passage of intestine as shown in Fig. 20-6. Treatment requires surgical intervention to reduce the hernia and close the defect.

BIBLIOGRAPHY

Al Harakeh AB. Complications of laparoscopic Roux-en-Y gastric bypass. *Surg Clin North Am* 2011 Dec;91(6):1225–1237.

Cottam DR, Mattar SG, Schauer PR. Laparoscopic era of operations for morbid obesity. *Arch Surg* 2003;138:367–375.

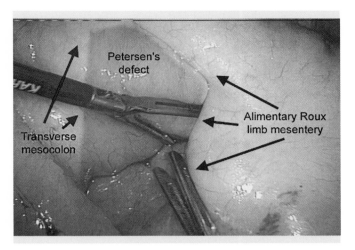

FIGURE 20-8. Demonstration of Petersen's defect after Roux-en-Y gastric bypass.

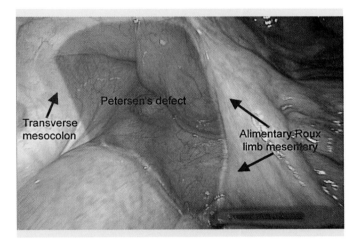

FIGURE 20-9. Demonstration of massive Petersen's defect created from weight loss following Roux-en-Y gastric bypass.

Higa KD, Boone KB, Ho TC. Complications of the laparoscopic Roux-en-Y gastric bypass: 1,040 patients—what have we learned? *Obes Surg* 2000;10:509–513.

Nguyen NT, DeMaria EJ, Hutter MM, eds. *The SAGES Manual: A Practical Guide to Bariatric Surgery.* New York, NY: Springer; 2008: Chapters 22–26.

11. **(E)** Roux-en-Y GBP leads to weight loss with both a restrictive component and a malabsorptive component. The removal of the distal stomach, duodenum, and proximal duodenum has important effects on vitamin and mineral absorption. Vitamin B_{12} is absorbed after binding with intrinsic factor produced by the parietal cells of the stomach. A deficiency in B_{12} results in fatigue, weakness, and macrocytic anemia.

A deficiency in iron results in microcytic anemia. Deficiency in calcium will result in osteopenia. Folate deficiency is also possible after gastric bypass, but is less common than vitamin B_{12} deficiency. Vitamin K is not at major risk of deficiency after gastric bypass surgery.

BIBLIOGRAPHY

Elliot K. Nutritional considerations after bariatric surgery. *Crit Care Nurs Q* 2003;26(2):133–138.

MacLean LD, Rhode BM, Shizgal HM. Nutrition following gastric operations for morbid obesity. *Ann Surg* 1983;198(3):347–354.

Nguyen NT, DeMaria EJ, Hutter MM, eds. *The SAGES Manual: A Practical Guide to Bariatric Surgery.* New York, NY: Springer; 2008: Chapter 5.

12. **(B)** Bypass of the gastric body and duodenum leads to biliary stasis. Biliary stasis, in conjunction with the rapid weight loss observed following Roux-en-Y GBP, leads to a high rate of gallstone formation in postoperative patients. Controversy remains over the most appropriate management of preoperative cholelithiasis; however, study results recommend the use of medical therapy postoperatively to prevent the development of gallstones.

A randomized controlled trial demonstrated that ursodeoxycholic acid, or ursodiol, at a dose of 300 mg administered orally twice daily, was effective at limiting the development of gallstones during the rapid weight loss seen following GBP. Although currently produced in the laboratory, ursodeoxycholic acid was originally obtained from the gallbladder of the Chinese black bear. It has been used for centuries to treat liver disease. The structure of ursodiol is demonstrated in Fig. 20-10. Its mechanism of action is twofold. It inhibits synthesis of cholesterol in the liver and limits the intestinal absorption of cholesterol. These two actions lead to decreased release of cholesterol by the liver and prevent cholesterol

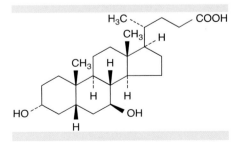

FIGURE 20-10. Molecular diagram of ursodiol, commonly used to prevent development of gallstones following weight loss surgery.

stone formation in the gallbladder. Ursodiol is also used to treat primary biliary cirrhosis, congenital cholestasis, viral hepatitis, and many other hepatic pathologies.

BIBLIOGRAPHY

Sugerman HJ, Brewer WH, Brolin RE, et al. A multicenter, placebo-controlled, randomized, double-blind, prospective trial of prophylactic ursodiol for the prevention of gallstone formation following gastric-bypass-induced rapid weight loss. *Am J Surg* 1995;169(1):91–97.

Uy MC, Talingdan-Te MC, Espinosa WZ, Daez ML, Ong JP. Ursodeoxycholic acid in the prevention of gallstone formation after bariatric surgery: a meta-analysis. *Obes Surg* 2008 Dec;18(12):1532–1538.

13. **(B)** Laparoscopic insertion of an AGB has been a commonly performed procedure abroad and in the United States since 2001. One of the concerns about AGB is that studies have shown a higher need for surgical intervention in managing complications of the AGB.

One of the main reasons for reoperation is gastric band slippage. Band slippage occurs when the gastric wall herniates through the band and allows the proximal gastric pouch to enlarge, as demonstrated in the swallow study. The enlarged pouch not only can lead to vomiting but also paradoxically can lead to less restriction of oral intake and diminished weight loss. An enlarged gastric pouch and AGB slippage are demonstrated in Fig. 20-4. Normal alignment of an AGB provides a small gastric pouch, as demonstrated by the barium swallow seen in Fig. 20-11.

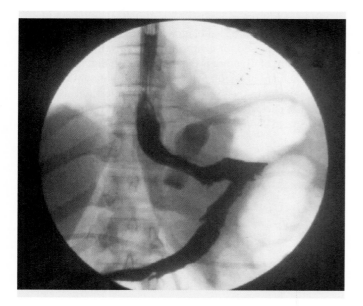

FIGURE 20-11. Barium swallow demonstrating normal alignment of adjustable gastric band and size of small gastric pouch.

During the early and mid-1990s, AGBs were inserted following creation of a transmesenteric window adjacent to the lesser gastric curve. In addition, the lesser peritoneal sac was routinely entered and the band was secured only in an anterior location with a limited number of sutures. During the late 1990s, a significant shift in surgical technique led to creation of the transmesenteric window through the pars flaccida, and dissection was limited to the retroperitoneal space above the lesser sac. In addition, several sutures were used to secure the band anteriorly. All of these changes have significantly reduced the rate of reoperation for slippage and improved results, although reoperation for other indications remains higher than in other bariatric procedures.

BIBLIOGRAPHY

Angrisani L, Furbeta F, Doldi SB, et al. Lap Band® adjustable gastric banding system: the experience with 1863 patients operated on 6 years. *Surg Endosc* 2003;17:409–412.

Nguyen NT, DeMaria EJ, Hutter MM, eds. *The SAGES Manual: A Practical Guide to Bariatric Surgery.* New York, NY: Springer; 2008: Chapter 13.

Weiner R, Blanco-Engert R, Weiner S, et al. Outcome after laparoscopic adjustable gastric banding—8 years experience. *Obes Surg* 2003;13:427–434.

14. **(C)** The intervention for a patient with achalasia and acceptable medical comorbidities with the highest odds of long-term success is laparoscopic Heller myotomy. The success rate with Heller myotomy is approximately 90% at 2-year follow-up. This is in comparison with dilation, which is around 75% successful with initial intervention but is less commonly used today due to concerns about perforation and poor longevity. Botox requires repeat intervention as its effect is temporary. Nissen fundoplication is contraindicated due to the nature of the disease process of achalasia: hypertensive lower esophageal sphincter. Diet modification is not an adequate treatment option for advanced achalasia.

BIBLIOGRAPHY

Boeckxstaens GE, Annese V, des Varannes SB, et al. and the European Achalasia Trial Investigators. Pneumatic dilation versus laparoscopic Heller's myotomy for idiopathic achalasia. *N Engl J Med* 2011 May 12;364(19):1807–1816.

Schoenberg MB, Marx S, Kersten JF, et al. Laparoscopic Heller myotomy versus endoscopic balloon dilatation for the treatment of achalasia: a network meta-analysis. *Ann Surg* 2013 Dec;258(6):943–952.

Weber CE, Davis CS, Kramer HJ, Gibbs JT, Robles L, Fisichella PM. Medium and long-term outcomes after pneumatic dilation or laparoscopic Heller myotomy for achalasia: a meta-analysis. *Surg Laparosc Endosc Percutan Tech* 2012 Aug;22(4):289–296.

15. **(D)** By convention, obesity is measured by BMI, and weight loss is reported as change in BMI and percentage of EBW loss. EBW is the difference of ideal body weight from the patient's preoperative weight.

Each of the listed procedures leads to weight loss in different ways. AGB is a gastric restrictive procedure. A synthetic band with an inflatable balloon allows adjustment of the internal diameter with injection of saline through a subcutaneous reservoir. The band is placed high on the stomach and creates a proximal gastric pouch approximately 10–30 mL in size. Injection of saline leads to a reduced internal diameter of the ring, more restriction on oral intake, and slower gastric pouch emptying. More restriction limits oral caloric intake, and weight loss occurs. Sleeve gastrectomy is a restrictive procedure as well. The creation of a small-diameter gastric tube, 32–40F catheter, results in restriction.

The GBP uses both a restrictive and a malabsorptive method of weight loss. A small gastric pouch approximately 20–30 mL in size is drained by a Roux-en-Y limb. The pouch restricts oral intake, and the stoma between the gastric pouch and the small intestine slows pouch emptying. Malabsorption is accomplished by bypassing the duodenum and proximal jejunum. The two methods of restriction and malabsorption cause weight loss.

Finally, the BPD leads to weight loss with both restriction and a larger contribution from malabsorption. Two forms of the BPD are currently performed. The classic form of BPD includes a hemigastrectomy drained by a Roux limb that causes bypass of the entire duodenum, jejunum, and proximal ileum. Pancreatic juices and bile mix with food in a short segment of terminal ileum that measures 50–100 cm long. A duodenal switch is another popular form of the BPD that includes formation of a gastric sleeve and division of the duodenum 1–2 cm from the pylorus. The proximal duodenal stump is drained by the distal Roux limb that bypasses the remaining duodenum, jejunum, and proximal ileum. Both forms of BPD limit digestion of oral intake, cause malabsorption, and lead to weight loss.

Patients lose weight precipitously following GBP, sleeve gastrectomy, and BPD. At 1 year, patients with AGB experience approximately 40% EBW loss. Patients with LSG experience approximately 55% EBW loss, those with GBP experience a 60–70% EBW loss, while patients with BPD experience 70–80% EBW loss.

BIBLIOGRAPHY

Anthone GJ, Lord RVN, DeMeester TR, et al. The duodenal switch operation for the treatment of morbid obesity. *Ann Surg* 2003;238(4):618–628.

Hutter MM, Schirmer BD, Jones DB, et al. First report from the American College of Surgeons Bariatric Surgery Center Network: laparoscopic sleeve gastrectomy has morbidity and effectiveness positioned between the band and the bypass. *Ann Surg* 2011 Sep;254(3):410–420.

Kim WW, Gagner M, Kini S, et al. Laparoscopic vs. open biliopancreatic diversion with duodenal switch: a comparative study. *J Gastrointest Surg* 2003;7:552–557.

Nguyen NT, Scott-Conner C, eds. *The SAGES Manual Vol. 2. Advanced Laparoscopy and Endoscopy.* New York, NY: Springer; 2012: Chapters 1–4.

Schauer PR, Ikramuddin S, Gourash W, et al. Outcomes after laparoscopic Roux-en-Y gastric bypass for morbid obesity. *Ann Surg* 2000;232(4):515–529.

Weiner R, Blanco-Engert R, Weiner S, et al. Outcome after laparoscopic adjustable gastric banding—8 year experience. *Obes Surg* 2003;13:427–434.

Zinzindohoue F, Chevallier JM, Douard R, et al. Laparoscopic gastric banding: a minimally invasive surgical treatment for morbid obesity. *Ann Surg* 2003;237(1):1–9.

16. **(A)**

17. **(A)**

Explanation for questions 16 and 17

The scenario illustrated is of CO_2 embolism caused by direct injection of CO_2 into the venous circulation. The hallmarks are cardiovascular collapse, including cyanosis, increased venous pressures, pulmonary edema, ventricular arrhythmias, and decreased end-tidal CO_2. The initial step in management is stopping gas insufflation. The patient should be hyperventilated, placed in Trendelenburg position, and the gas aspirated via central catheter to remove it from the circulation. A high clinical suspicion should lead to immediate measures for diagnostic confirmation, including transesophageal echocardiography, which may be performed during the surgical procedure with limited morbidity and good sensitivity.

BIBLIOGRAPHY

Schmandra TC, Mierdl S, Bauer H, et al. Trans-esophageal echocardiography shows high risk of gas embolism during laparoscopic hepatic resection under carbon dioxide pneumoperitoneum. *Br J Surg* 2002;89:870–876.

Zucker K. *Surgical Laparoscopy.* 2nd ed. Philadelphia, PA: Lippincott Williams & Wilkins; 2001: Chapters 2, 18.

18. **(A)** Creation of pneumoperitoneum to an intra-abdominal pressure of less than 20 cm H_2O is associated in the supine position with increased MAP, SVR, and cardiac filling pressures. These effects stem from direct mechanical effects of the pneumoperitoneum, myocardial and vasodilatory effects of carbon dioxide, and sympathetic stimulation.

The increased cardiac filling pressures are reflective of increased preload. CVP, pulmonary artery wedge pressure, and pulmonary vascular resistance; all increase secondary to increased intrathoracic pressure transmitted via the elevated diaphragm from the increased intra-abdominal pressure created during pneumoperitoneum. Although the filling pressures appear to have increased, in fact, they are decreased. True filling pressures are determined by calculating the difference of the intrathoracic pressure from the observed CVP. The increase in intrathoracic pressure is greater than the increase in CVP leads to decreased filling pressures.

The SVR increases secondary to increased venous resistance, compression of the intra-abdominal arterial tree by the pneumoperitoneum, and sympathetic or other chemical actions leading to increased afterload. Increased SVR helps create an increased MAP.

In addition to these changes, cardiac output is decreased. Stroke volume is limited secondary to chemical mediators, specifically hypercarbia, that restrict cardiac contractility. For all these reasons, laparoscopic surgery with pneumoperitoneum is still used cautiously in frail and elderly patients with limited cardiac or respiratory reserve.

BIBLIOGRAPHY

Chandrakanth A, Talamini MA. Current knowledge regarding the biology of pneumoperitoneum-based surgery. *Probl Gen Surg* 2001;18(1):52–63.
Zucker K. *Surgical Laparoscopy.* 2nd ed. Philadelphia, PA: Lippincott Williams & Wilkins; 2001: Chapters 2, 16.

19. **(C)** The scenario presented depicts a vagal response to the stimulation created during peritoneal insufflation. This may result in bradycardia and even asystole or atrioventricular block. The first course of action is to stop the procedure and desufflate the abdomen to remove the source of vagal stimulation. An anticholinergic agent, such as glycopyrrolate, may be administered for vagolytic activity.

One study, performed on gynecologic patients, described regular use of preemptive glycopyrrolate prior to insufflation of the abdomen. This is not regularly performed because bradycardia is an uncommon occurrence. In addition, it frequently resolves after the initial attempt to insufflate the abdomen. Simply desufflating the abdomen, allowing the patient to recover, and performing another attempt to insufflate, perhaps with a lower pressure limit, is generally sufficient to prevent another vagal response.

BIBLIOGRAPHY

Ambrose C, Buggy D, Farragher R, et al. Pre-emptive glycopyrrolate 0.2 mg and bradycardia during gynaecological laparoscopy with mivacurium. *Eur J Anaesthesiol* 1998;15(6):710–713.
Zucker K. *Surgical Laparoscopy.* 2nd ed. Philadelphia, PA: Lippincott Williams & Wilkins; 2001: Chapters 2, 16.

20. **(B)** Excretion of CO_2 increases as insufflation pressure increases from 0 to 10 mmHg, but then plateaus with insufflation pressure greater than 10 mmHg. CO_2 excretion is proportionally related to absorption, and the increase and plateau in CO_2 excretion may be caused by the initial increase in peritoneal surface area exposed to the CO_2, which then stabilizes as the peritoneum becomes distended and has no more surface area to absorb additional CO_2. $PaCO_2$, however, increases continuously as insufflation increases from 0–25 mmHg as dead space increases.

BIBLIOGRAPHY

Zucker K. *Surgical Laparoscopy.* 2nd ed. Philadelphia, PA: Lippincott Williams & Wilkins; 2001: Chapters 2, 21, 22.

21. **(C)** Placement of the Veress needle may be confirmed with a saline drop test: Saline in the needle should flow freely into the peritoneal cavity but will not if the needle is in soft tissue. In addition, an opening pressure of less than 8 is consistent with correct placement; however this number may be higher in obese patients. The presence of crepitus is consistent with incorrect placement into the subcutaneous tissue. In general, the three layers felt on Veress needle placement are anterior fascia, posterior fascia, and peritoneum.

BIBLIOGRAPHY

Soper N, Scott-Conner C, eds. *The SAGES Manual Vol. 1. Basic Laparoscopy and Endoscopy.* 3rd ed. New York, NY: Springer; 2012: Chapter 5.

22. **(C)** The scenario described is that of a tension pneumothorax, which may be secondary to intra-abdominal gas passing through diaphragmatic defects into the pleural or mediastinal space. Deflation of the abdomen is indicated, as well as standard treatment of a pneumothorax, including placing a needle into the chest or placing a chest tube thoracostomy. Nitrous oxide should be discontinued and the patient placed on 100% oxygen. Entering the parietal pleura may not relieve the pneumothorax and may actually lead to parenchymal injury of the lung, worsening the situation.

Pneumothorax is a common complication following advanced laparoscopic foregut procedures. Hemodynamic compromise is a rare occurrence. Intraoperative care routinely includes increased percentage of inspired oxygen, as mentioned, with completion of the procedure at a lower-pressure pneumoperitoneum. Patients are monitored postoperatively with continuous oxygen saturation, and the pneumothorax resolves without further intervention.

BIBLIOGRAPHY

Jager RM, Wexner SD, eds. *Laparoscopic Colorectal Surgery. Anesthetic and Positional Complications.* New York, NY: Churchill Livingstone; 1996:47.

Leong LM, Ali A. Carbon dioxide pneumothorax during laparoscopic fundoplication. *Anaesthesia* 2003;58(1):97.

Pohl D, Eubanks TR, Omelanczuk PE, Pellegrini CA. Management and outcome of complications after laparoscopic antireflux operations. *Arch Surg* 2001;136(4):399–404.

23. **(A)** Inadvertent injury from errant grounding of electrocautery may present as a delayed complication following laparoscopic procedures. Damaged insulation or movement outside the videoscopic field with electrified instruments may lead to intestinal or other injuries. Full-thickness wounds may demonstrate immediate leak of intestinal contents; however, partial-thickness burns of the intestinal wall may progress to full thickness over the course of several days and provide a delayed presentation.

Along these lines, duodenal necrosis can occur from electrocautery injury, especially if the adhesion is narrowly based at the duodenum and widely based at the gallbladder. In this case, current travels to both the gallbladder and duodenum but is concentrated at the duodenum. The resulting burn injury takes a few days to cause necrosis of the duodenum, which may then perforate.

BIBLIOGRAPHY

Wu MP, Ou CS, Chen SL, et al. Complications and recommended practices for electrosurgery in laparoscopy. *Am J Surg* 2000;179(1):67–73.

Zucker K. *Surgical Laparoscopy.* 2nd ed. Philadelphia, PA: Lippincott Williams & Wilkins; 2001: Chapters 5, 56, 57.

24. **(B).** The patient in this scenario has a type III paraesophageal hernia with GERD symptoms (Fig. 20-12). This hernia cannot be repaired with endoscopic fundoplication because the stomach must be reduced back into the abdominal cavity. Similarly, a Nissen fundoplication alone is not the correct operation for this patient. The patient requires paraesophageal hernia repair, and fundoplication is appropriate due to her normal manometry. The laparoscopic approach is favored to open due to its lower-morbidity profile.

BIBLIOGRAPHY

Nguyen NT, Scott-Conner C, eds. *The SAGES Manual Vol. 2. Advanced Laparoscopy and Endoscopy.* 3rd ed. New York, NY: Springer; 2012: Chapter 12.

Swantsrom LL, Soper NJ, eds. *Mastery of Endoscopic and Laparoscopic Surgery.* 4th ed. Philadelphia, PA: Lippincott Williams and Wilkins; 2014: Chapter 13.

25. **(B)** Glucagon administration is the easiest intraoperative measure to relieve biliary obstruction by relaxing the sphincter of Oddi. Following administration of 1 mg of glucagon, normal saline administered through the cholangiogram catheter may be used to flush the common bile duct. A repeat cholangiogram is then performed to reassess the duct. Simple flushing with saline is frequently unsuccessful in clearing the duct of stones. A common bile duct exploration is then necessary to clear the stones. This is a technically demanding procedure when performed both open and laparoscopically. Laparoscopic techniques include a transcystic duct approach. This frequently involves insertion of wire stone retrieval baskets through the cystic duct. The baskets are followed with fluoroscopic guidance. The stones are either withdrawn through the cystic duct or pushed into the duodenum. Other methods include creation of a choledochotomy with insertion of a flexible choledochoscope, allowing direct visualization of the stone for removal. In skilled hands, series have demonstrated a 75% or greater success rate at clearance of the common duct. Lithotripsy and holmium laser therapy are not typically used for gallstones but are useful for nephrolithiasis. ERCP may be performed postoperatively but is not typically performed during laparoscopic cholecystectomy.

BIBLIOGRAPHY

Ferguson CM. Laparoscopic common bile duct exploration: practical application. *Arch Surg* 1998;133(4):448–451.

Lauter DM, Froines EJ. Laparoscopic common duct exploration in the management of choledocholithiasis. *Am J Surg* 2000;179(5):372–374.

Zucker K. *Surgical Laparoscopy.* 2nd ed. Philadelphia, PA: Lippincott Williams & Wilkins; 2001: Chapters 10, 127, 128.

26. **(B)** The patient should be placed with left side down to avoid vena cava compression. Laparoscopic appendectomy is reasonable in the first two trimesters, and there is no increase in fetal or maternal morbidity; however, fetal loss is reported to be 1.5% in nonperforated appendicitis but as much as 35% in perforated appendicitis. When performing laparoscopic appendectomy, placement of the umbilical trocar should be performed using open technique, and the pneumoperitoneum pressure should be 10 mmHg to avoid injury to the gravid uterus and prevent impediment to placental blood flow.

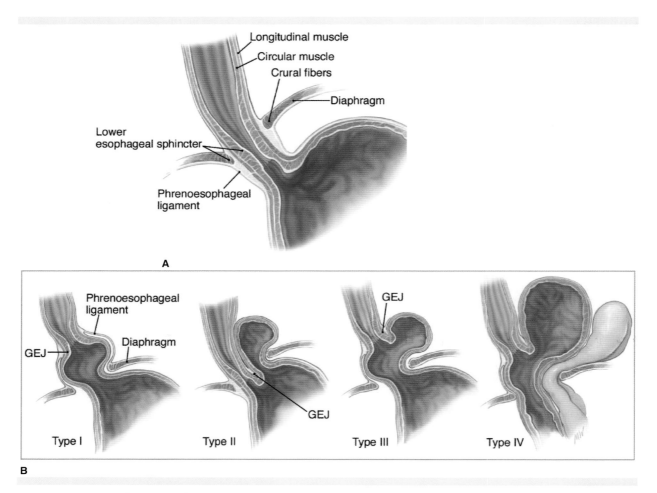

FIGURE 20-12. A. Normal paraesophageal anatomy. **B.** Classification of paraesophageal hernias; GEJ = gastroesophageal junction (from Sugarbaker DJ, Bueno R, Krasna MJ, Mentzer SJ, Zellos L, eds. *Adult Chest Surgery*. 2nd ed. New York, NY: McGraw Hill; 2013: Fig. 46-1. Copyright © The McGraw-Hill Companies, Inc. All rights reserved).

BIBLIOGRAPHY

Curet MJ. Special problems in laparoscopic surgery: previous abdominal surgery, obesity, and pregnancy. *Surg Clin North Am* 2000;80(4):1093–1110.

Soper NJ, Scott-Conner CEH, eds. *The SAGES Manual Vol. 1. Basic Laparoscopy and Endoscopy*. New York, NY: Springer; 2012: Chapter 14.

Zucker K. *Surgical Laparoscopy*. 2nd ed. Philadelphia, PA: Lippincott Williams & Wilkins; 2001:235.

27. **(C)** A slipped wrap occurs when proximal stomach slips proximal to the wrap, resulting in an hourglass-shaped stomach. It is commonly associated with short-ened esophagus or failure or breakdown of sutures tying down the fundoplication to the distal esophagus. The most common complaints include heartburn or dysphagia, while bloating, nausea and vomiting, diarrhea, chest pain, abdominal pain, or shoulder pain is also possible, although less common. Symptoms of a slipped wrap progress rather than diminish over time, so early surgical intervention is warranted to prevent worsening of the disorder. The swallow study demon-strates a Nissen wrap that has slipped into the chest (Fig. 20-13).

BIBLIOGRAPHY

Hunter JG, Smith D, Branum GD, et al. Laparoscopic fundoplication failures: patterns of failure and response to fundoplication revi-sion. *Ann Surg* 1999;230(4):595–606.

Soper NJ, Dunnegan D. Anatomic fundoplication failure after laparoscopic antireflux surgery. *Ann Surg* 1999;229(5):669–677.

Zucker K. *Surgical Laparoscopy*. 2nd ed. Philadelphia, PA: Lippincott Williams & Wilkins; 2001:458–459.

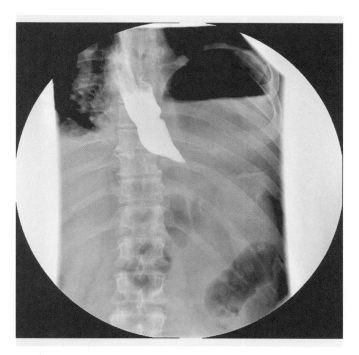

FIGURE 20-13. Gastrografin swallow following laparoscopic Nissen fundoplication with dehiscence of cruroplasty and slippage of the stomach into the chest.

28. **(B)** The patient in this question would benefit the most from a Roux-en-Y gastric bypass. This procedure will decrease GERD symptoms due to the disconnection of the gastric pouch from the remainder of the acid-producing stomach. In addition, weight loss will be beneficial in this patient with a BMI of 41. Repeat Nissen fundoplication or Toupet fundoplication is less likely to offer long-term success in reflux control. Esophageal dilation is not indicated for this patient.

BIBLIOGRAPHY

El-Hadi M, Birch DW, Gill RS, Karmali S. The effect of bariatric surgery on gastroesophageal reflux disease. *Can J Surg* 2014 Apr;57(2):139–144.

Tai CM, Lee YC, Wu MS, et al. The effect of Roux-en-Y gastric bypass on gastroesophageal reflux disease in morbidly obese Chinese patients. *Obes Surg* 2009 May;19(5):565–570.

29. **(B)** When looking toward the pelvis during extraperitoneal inguinal herniorrhaphy, the triangle of doom is bordered medially by the vas deferens, laterally by the spermatic vessels, and inferiorly by the iliac vessels. The inferior epigastric vessels lie superior to the triangle of doom, while the lateral femoral cutaneous nerve is lateral to the epigastric vessels. While not part of the triangle of doom, they should be avoided as well. In addition, the space lateral to the triangle of doom along the anterior surface of the psoas muscle contains the genitofemoral and iliophypogastric nerves. Dissection in this region may lead to paresthesias or numbness.

BIBLIOGRAPHY

Townsend CM, ed. *Sabiston Textbook of Surgery*. 19th ed. Philadelphia, PA: Saunders; 2012: Chapter 46.

CHAPTER 21

BILIARY TRACT

AMY LIGHTNER HILL AND WALDO CONCEPCION

1. Regarding the extrahepatic biliary and vascular anatomy, which of the following is true?
   (A) The cystic artery usually arises from the left hepatic artery.
   (B) The common duct courses downward posterior to the portal vein in the free edge of the lesser omentum.
   (C) The right branch of the hepatic artery crosses the main bile duct posteriorly.
   (D) The cystic artery usually crosses the common hepatic duct posteriorly.

2. The borders of the triangle of Calot consist of
   (A) Cystic duct, cystic artery, and inferior edge of the liver
   (B) Cystic artery, port vein, and cystic duct
   (C) Cystic duct, common hepatic duct, and inferior edge of the liver
   (D) Common bile duct (CBD), cystic duct, and inferior edge of the liver

3. Which of the following is a function of the gallbladder?
   (A) Absorption
   (B) Acidification of bile
   (C) Secretion
   (D) Storage of bile
   (E) All of the above

4. Which hormone is released by the duodenal mucosa in response to a meal and leads to release of bile from the gallbladder?
   (A) Cholecystokinin
   (B) Motilin
   (C) Somatostatin
   (D) Secretin

5. Which of the following is a function of bile?
   (A) Absorption of bile salt
   (B) Absorption of cholesterol
   (C) Absorption of lipid
   (D) Absorption of proteins
   (E) Absorption of vitamin B_{12}

6. What is the normal amount of bile produced by the liver daily?
   (A) 500–1000 mL
   (B) 1000–2000 mL
   (C) 1000–1500 mL
   (D) 200–400 mL

7. Which of the following is correct regarding the enterohepatic circulation?
   (A) Terminal ileum resection will result in an increase in the bile salt pool.
   (B) A patient with an external biliary fistula will have increased synthesis of bile by the liver.
   (C) During long fasting periods, the gallbladder becomes void of bile acid.
   (D) Bacterial action in the colon over the primary bile salts (cholate and lithocholate) results in the formation of secondary bile salt (chenodeoxycholate and deoxycholate).

8. Which of the following is correct regarding the function of the sphincter of Oddi?
   (A) Antral distention in response to food causes both gallbladder contraction and sphincter relaxation.
   (B) The phase III of the migrating motor complex (MMC) causes an increase in the sphincter pressure during fasting.
   (C) Cholecystokinin action increases the activity of the sphincter of Oddi.
   (D) Sphincter pressure elevates in response to a meal, preventing regurgitation of duodenal contents.

9. What is the most common type of gallstone in the United States?
   (A) Pigmented stones
   (B) Mixed cholesterol/Ca$^+$
   (C) Cholesterol stones
   (D) Ca$^+$ stones

10. Which of the following is correct regarding cholesterol gallstone pathogenesis?
   (A) Changes in the equilibrium between the amount of cholesterol and bile saturation capacity play a major role in stone formation.
   (B) Increased gallbladder motility results in less bile available for cholesterol solubilization, predisposing to crystal formation.
   (C) The formation of cholesterol stones is the result of specific alterations, congenital or acquired, in the hepatic metabolism.
   (D) Mucin production in the gallbladder is known to be a pronucleating factor that protects against stone formation.

11. A 30-year-old white male with a known hemolytic disorder comes to the surgery clinic with an ultrasound (US) that shows gallstones. What type of gallstones would you expect to find in this patient?
   (A) Cholesterol stones
   (B) Mixed cholesterol/Ca$^+$ stones
   (C) Brown pigmented stones
   (D) Black pigmented stones
   (E) Ca$^+$ stones

12. A 42-year-old white female presents to the emergency room (ER) with a 24-h history of right upper quadrant (RUQ) pain, fever, and a white blood cell (WBC) count of 16,000. What is the initial imaging study of choice?
   (A) ^{99m}-Tc hepatobiliary scintigraphy (hepatic iminodiacetic acid, HIDA) scan
   (B) Computed tomographic (CT) scan of abdomen
   (C) Kidney, ureter, and bladder (KUB) radiograph
   (D) Abdominal ultrasonography
   (E) Magnetic resonance cholangiopancreatography (MRCP)

13. Regarding the management of acute calculus cholecystitis, which of the following is correct?
   (A) Open cholecystectomy is the standard of care.
   (B) Postoperative endoscopic retrograde cholangiopancreatography (ERCP) is inappropriate management in the setting of a CBD stone.
   (C) Laparoscopic cholecystectomy should be attempted as soon as possible after the diagnosis is made unless critically ill with significant hemodynamic instability.

(D) Cholecystectomy should be delayed until the patient is afebrile and has a normal WBC.

14. What is the "critical view of safety"?
   (A) Gallbladder neck and portal triad
   (B) Liver edge, gallbladder, and cystic duct
   (C) Liver edge, duodenum, hepatic artery
   (D) Gallbladder neck, cystic duct, cystic artery

15. A patient is postoperative day 2 from a laparoscopic cholecystectomy and presents with RUQ pain, fever, and vomiting. Ultrasound is performed and shows a biloma. What is the best method of treatment?
   (A) Intravenous fluids, intravenous antibiotics, and bowel rest
   (B) ERCP with stenting of the CBD
   (C) Interventional radiology (IR) drainage of biloma
   (D) Intravenous antibiotics and drainage of biloma

Questions 16 and 17

A 43-year-old white female comes to the ER complaining of abdominal pain, fever up to 102°F, yellow coloration of the skin, and dark urine for 36 h.

16. The patient undergoes an ERCP study (Fig. 21-1). What is the most likely diagnosis?

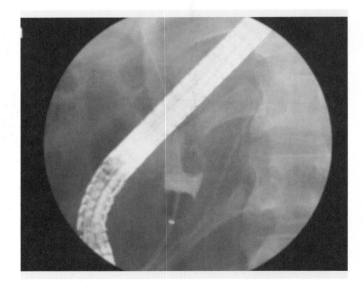

FIGURE 21-1. Endoscopic retrograde cholangiopancreatography.

   (A) Acute cholangitis secondary to periampullary tumor
   (B) Acute cholangitis secondary to a biliary duct tumor
   (C) Acute cholangitis secondary to a biliary-enteric fistula
   (D) Acute cholangitis and cholecystitis secondary to hepatic duct obstruction

17. What is the most appropriate treatment?
    (A) Endoscopic sphincterotomy
    (B) Percutaneous transhepatic placement of biliary drainage
    (C) Open cholecystectomy and CBD exploration
    (D) Laparoscopic cholecystectomy and CBD exploration

18. A 42-year-old white female comes to the ER complaining of RUQ abdominal pain for the last 36 h, associated with fever up to 39°C, bilious emesis, and jaundice. The following are the returning lab values: direct bilirubin 2.2, alkaline phosphatase 450, WBC 19,000, AST 24, ALT 19. What is the most probable diagnosis?
    (A) Acute cholecystitis
    (B) Acute cholangitis
    (C) Pancreatic cancer
    (D) Choledochal cyst
    (E) Acute hepatitis

19. What would be the most common etiology for the diagnosis made in question 18?
    (A) Primary pigment stones
    (B) Secondary CBD stones
    (C) Congenital abnormal development of the CBD
    (D) Hepatitis virus
    (E) Adenocarcinoma

20. How many patients with acute cholangitis present with Charcot's triad?
    (A) 1–2%
    (B) 5%
    (C) 20%
    (D) 50%
    (E) Nearly 100%

21. What is the most common organism isolated from bile and blood cultures in patients with acute cholangitis?
    (A) *Enterobacter* spp.
    (B) *Bacteroides* spp.
    (C) *Escherichia coli*
    (D) *Enterococcus* spp.
    (E) *Candida albicans*

22. What would be the most appropriate antibiotic therapy for the patient in question 18?
    (A) Gram-negative coverage alone
    (B) Gram-positive coverage
    (C) Double coverage for *Pseudomonas*
    (D) Gram-positive and gram-negative coverage, especially for *Enterococcus* spp.
    (E) Gram-positive, gram-negative, and antifungal coverage

23. The patient is not responding to resuscitation and intravenous antibiotics. Unfortunately, you are at a center without access to endoscopic ERCP. What is the next best step in treatment?
    (A) Abdominal ultrasound
    (B) CT scan of the abdomen with intravenous contrast
    (C) MRCP to better delineate the ductal anatomy
    (D) Percutaneous transhepatic cholangiography (PTC)

24. Which of the following is considered a complication of cholangitis?
    (A) Liver abscess
    (B) Secondary sclerosing cholangitis
    (C) Portal vein thrombosis
    (D) Pancreatitis
    (E) Sepsis
    (F) All of the above

25. What is the most sensitive test for the diagnosis of biliary dyskinesia?
    (A) Abdominal CT scan
    (B) ERCP
    (C) Cholecystokinin-Tc-HIDA scan
    (D) Abdominal US
    (E) MRCP

26. Which of the following patients most likely has biliary dyskinesia?
    (A) 43-year-old black female with 24 h of abdominal pain, fever, and gallstones by US
    (B) 60-year-old white male with RUQ pain, WBC 16, and diarrhea
    (C) 45-year-old white female with recurrent abdominal pain, gallbladder ejection fraction of 50% at 20 min
    (D) 30-year-old white female with chronic RUQ pain, normal US, and 30% ejection fraction at 20 min

27. What is the appropriate treatment for biliary dyskinesia?
    (A) Fat-free diet and decrease weight
    (B) ERCP with sphincteroplasty
    (C) Cholecystectomy
    (D) Prokinetic agents
    (E) Nothing by mouth, antibiotics, and cholecystectomy

28. Regarding choledochal cysts, which of the following is correct?
    (A) The most common presentation in children is RUQ abdominal pain and fevers.
    (B) The most common type of choledochal cyst is confined to the intrahepatic biliary tree.
    (C) Caroli's disease is defined as dilatation of the intra- and extrahepatic biliary tree.
    (D) There are two histologic types of choledochal cyst: glandular and fibrotic.
    (E) They are benign and do not progress to cholangiocarcinoma.

29. What is the most common type of choledochal cyst?
    (A) Type I
    (B) Type II
    (C) Type III
    (D) Type IV
    (E) Type V

30. Which of the following is the most useful for mapping the anatomy of the distal bile duct in the setting of a choledochal cyst?
    (A) Radionuclide hepatobiliary scan
    (B) CT scan
    (C) Percutaneous transhepatic cholangiogram
    (D) Plain abdominal x-ray
    (E) ERCP

31. What type of choledochal cyst is seen in the ERCP study shown in Fig. 21-2?

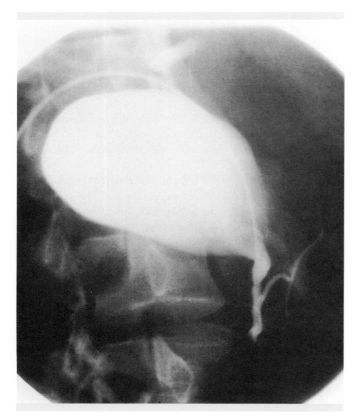

FIGURE 21-2. Choledochal cyst (from Zinner MJ, Ashley SW, eds. *Maingot's Abdominal Operations*. 12th ed. New York, NY: McGraw-Hill; 2013: Fig. 50-4. Copyright © The McGraw-Hill Companies, Inc. All rights reserved).

    (A) Type I
    (B) Type II

    (C) Type III
    (D) Type IV
    (E) Type V

32. What would be the surgical management of the cyst seen in Fig. 21-2?
    (A) Duodenopancreatectomy
    (B) Hemihepatectomy
    (C) Liver transplant
    (D) Cystectomy and biliary-enteric Roux-en-Y anastomosis
    (E) Transduodenal sphincteroplasty

33. Concerning Caroli's disease, which of the following is correct?
    (A) It is characterized by intrahepatic bile duct atresia.
    (B) Abdominal mass and weight loss are the most common initial symptoms.
    (C) It is a developmental anomaly of the ductal plate characterized by saccular dilatations of the large bile ducts.
    (D) It is more commonly seen in adult females.
    (E) It is a risk factor for the development of cystadenocarcinoma of the bile duct.

34. Which of the following is a complication of Caroli's disease?
    (A) Renal disorders
    (B) Recurrent cholecystitis
    (C) Nephrospongiosis
    (D) Cholangiocarcinoma
    (E) Enteric fistula

35. A 30-year-old white male was recently diagnosed with Caroli's disease limited to the right lobe of the liver. The most appropriate management of this disease is
    (A) Hepatic lobectomy
    (B) Resection of the CBD and Roux-en-Y hepaticojejunostomy
    (C) Internal drainage of the cyst into a Roux-en-Y jejunal limb
    (D) Resection of the extrahepatic biliary duct and hepaticoduodenostomy
    (E) Choledochal cyst resection

36. What is the etiology of cholangiocarcinoma?
    (A) Primary sclerosing cholangitis
    (B) Caroli's disease
    (C) Choledochal cyst
    (D) Biliary atresia
    (E) Unknown

37. What is the most common location of a cholangiocarcinoma?
    (A) Right hepatic duct
    (B) Left hepatic duct
    (C) Hepatic ducts' confluence
    (D) CBD

38. What is the appropriate treatment for a cholangiocarcinoma of the hepatic bifurcation?
    (A) Right hepatic lobectomy
    (B) Left hepatic lobectomy
    (C) Pancreaticoduodenectomy (Whipple)
    (D) Bile duct resection and hepaticojejunostomy plus partial hepatectomy
    (E) Radiation therapy plus bile duct stenting

39. How many patients undergoing cholecystectomy are found to have a gallbladder carcinoma?
    (A) 0.1%
    (B) 1%
    (C) 10%
    (D) 25%
    (E) 35%

40. What is the most common gallbladder tumor?
    (A) Adenocarcinoma
    (B) Papillary carcinoma
    (C) Mucinous carcinoma
    (D) Squamous cell carcinoma
    (E) Oat cell carcinoma

41. After an uneventful laparoscopic cholecystectomy in a 55-year-old white male, the pathology review demonstrates a gallbladder carcinoma invading, but not penetrating, the muscularis layer. What is the most appropriate next step in the management of this patient?
    (A) No more treatment needed
    (B) *En bloc* resection of gallbladder bed, including segments four to five of the liver and regional lymph nodes
    (C) Postoperative chemotherapy
    (D) Biliary stent placement to prevent future biliary obstruction
    (E) Biliary-enteric bypass

42. A 50-year-old white male underwent a laparoscopic cholecystectomy for symptomatic gallstones. On postoperative day 4, he complains of abdominal pain and nausea. Laboratory studies show WBC 10,000, direct bilirubin 2.5. What is the most appropriate first study?
    (A) Magnetic resonance cholangiography
    (B) Abdominal US
    (C) ERCP

    (D) HIDA scan
    (E) Percutaneous transhepatic cholangiogram

43. The patient described in Question 42 undergoes a PTC study (Fig. 21-3). What is the most appropriate initial management?

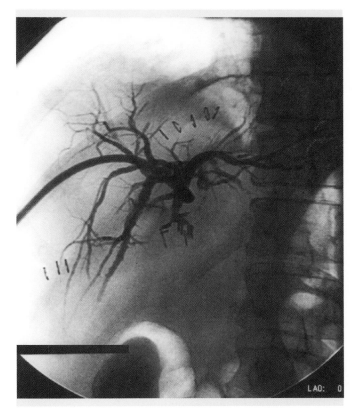

FIGURE 21-3. Postcholecystectomy PTC (from Zinner MJ, Ashley SW, eds. *Maingot's Abdominal Operations.* 12th ed. New York, NY: McGraw-Hill; 2013: Fig. 50-14. Copyright © The McGraw-Hill Companies, Inc. All rights reserved).

    (A) Total parenteral nutrition and antibiotics
    (B) Urgent laparotomy and bile duct reanastomosis
    (C) Percutaneous transhepatic cholangiogram and percutaneous biliary stents
    (D) Sphincterotomy

44. What is the most appropriate treatment for the biliary injury seen in Fig. 21-3?
    (A) End-to-end anastomosis of the bile duct
    (B) Roux-en-Y hepaticojejunostomy
    (C) Choledochoduodenostomy
    (D) Choledochojejunostomy
    (E) ERCP and stent placement

45. A 60-year-old white female presents to the ER complaining of abdominal distention and intermittent abdominal pain for 4 days. A CT scan of the abdomen was obtained (Fig. 21-4).

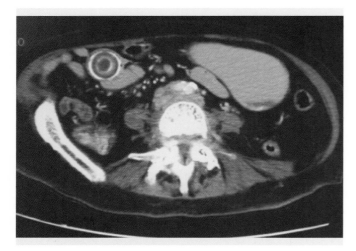

FIGURE 21-4. Abdominal CT.

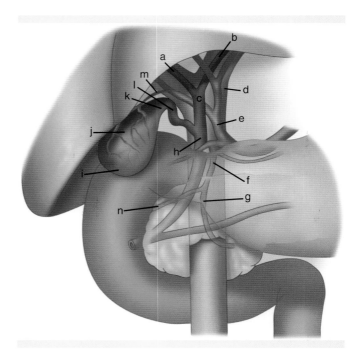

FIGURE 21-5. Biliary anatomy. Reprinted from Gunn A, Keddie N. Some clinical observations on patients with gallstones. *Lancet.* 1972;300(7771):239-241, Copyright 1972, with permission from Elsevier.

What should be avoided during the initial operation?
(A) Milking of the stone until passing the ileocecal valve
(B) Pushing the stone proximally to a less-edematous portion of intestine, then enterotomy and extraction
(C) Extraction of the stone through an enterotomy and primary repair
(D) Biliary-enteric fistula repair
(E) Nasogastric tube decompression

ANSWERS AND EXPLANATIONS

1. **(C)**

2. **(C)**

Explanations 1 and 2

The extrahepatic bile ducts are represented by the extrahepatic segments of the right and left hepatic ducts joining to form the biliary confluence and the main biliary channel training to the duodenum (Fig. 21-5). The accessory biliary apparatus comprises the gallbladder and the cystic duct. The confluence of the right and left hepatic ducts takes place at the right of the hilar fissure of the liver anterior to the portal venous bifurcation and overlying the origin of the right branch of the portal vein.

The main bile duct, the mean diameter of which is about 6 mm, is divided in two segments: the proximal segment (common hepatic duct) above the cystic duct and the CBD distal to the cystic duct. The latter courses downward anterior to the portal vein in the free edge of the lesser omentum and is closely applied to the hepatic artery, which runs upward on its left, giving rise to the right branch of the hepatic artery, which crosses the main bile duct posteriorly, although in about 20% of the cases anteriorly.

The cystic artery arises from the right hepatic artery in 95% of the population and may cross the common hepatic duct posteriorly or anteriorly (Fig. 21-6). The triangle of Calot is made up of the edge of liver, common hepatic duct, and cystic duct. Dissection of Calot's triangle is of key significance during cholecystectomy because in this triangle runs the cystic artery, often the right branch of the hepatic artery, and occasionally a bile duct. There are a large number of ductal and arterial anatomical variances. The most common ductal variant is that 20% of people have a right anterior duct directly. The most common vascular variant is that 20% will have a replaced left hepatic artery coming off the left

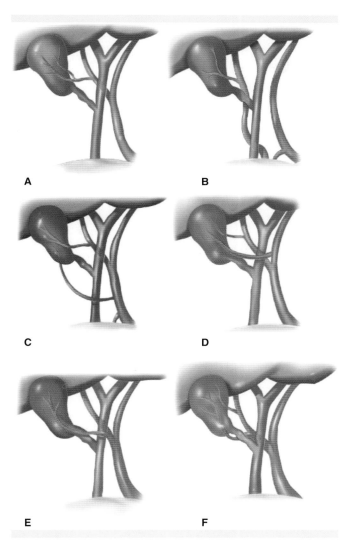

A   **B**

C   **D**

E   **F**

FIGURE 21-6. Variations in biliary anatomy (from Brunicardi FC, Andersen DK, Billiar TR, et al., eds. *Schwartz's Principles of Surgery*. 10th ed. New York, NY: McGraw-Hill; 2014: Fig. 32-4. Copyright © The McGraw-Hill Companies, Inc. All rights reserved).

gastric artery and transverses through the hepatogastric ligament.

BIBLIOGRAPHY

Blumgart LH. Surgical and biologic anatomy of the liver and biliary tracts. In: Blumgart LH, Fong Y, eds. *Surgery of the Liver and Biliary Tract*. 5th ed. London, England: Saunders; 2012:3–33.

Jackson PG, Evans SR. Biliary system. In: Townsend CM, Beauchamp RD, Evers BM, Mattox KL, eds. *Sabiston's Textbook of Surgery: The Biological Basis of Modern Surgical Practice*. 19th ed. Philadelphia, PA: Elsevier; 2012:1476–1514.

Klein AS, Lillemoe KD. Liver, biliary tract, and pancreas. In: O'Leary JP, ed. *The Physiologic Basis of Surgery*. 4th ed. Baltimore, MD: Williams & Wilkins; 2008:441–478.

Porrett PM, Frederick JR, Roses RE, Kaiser LR. The hepatobiliary system. In: Porrett PM, ed. *The Surgical Review*. 3rd ed. Philadelphia, PA: Lippincott Williams & Wilkins; 2010:159–175.

3. **(E)**

4. **(A)**

Explanation for questions 3 and 4

The main function of the gallbladder is to concentrate and store hepatic bile during the fasting state, allowing for its coordinated release in response to a meal. It also has absorptive, secretory, and motor capabilities. The usual gallbladder capacity is only 40–50 mL. Its absorptive capacity allows the gallbladder to manage the 600 mL of bile produced by the liver daily. The gallbladder mucosa has the greatest absorptive capacity per unit area of any structure in the body. Bile can be concentrated up to 10-fold by the absorption of water and electrolytes. The gallbladder epithelial cells secrete two important products: glycoproteins and hydrogen ions. They protect the mucosa against the effect of the highly concentrated bile. The acidification of the bile caused by the H$^+$ ions promotes Ca solubility, thereby preventing its precipitation as calcium salts. The release (motor activity) of stored bile from the gallbladder requires a coordinated motor response of gallbladder contraction and sphincter of Oddi relaxation. This is mediated by humoral and neural factors. The main stimulus for emptying is cholecystokinin, which is released by the duodenal mucosa in response to a meal. Vagal stimulation results in gallbladder contraction, while splanchnic sympathetic activity results in relaxation. Between meals, the gallbladder empties as a result of phase III MMC secondary to the action of motilin. Defects in gallbladder motility and increasing residence time of bile in the gallbladder play central roles in the pathogenesis of gallstones.

5. **(C)**

6. **(A)**

7. **(B)**

8. **(A)**

Explanation for questions 5 through 8

The formation of bile by the hepatocyte serves two main purposes. First, bile transport allows for the excretion of toxins and normal cellular metabolites because the liver is a major site of detoxification. Second, bile salts have a critical role in lipid absorption.

The major organic solutes in bile are bilirubin, bile salt, phospholipids, and cholesterol. The primary bile salts in humans, cholic and chenodeoxycholic acid, undergo bacterial conjugation in the intestine to form the secondary bile salts deoxycholate and lithocholate. The function of the bile salts is to solubilize lipids and facilitate their absorption.

The normal volume of bile secreted daily by the liver is 500–1000 mL. Bile flow depends on neurogenic, humoral, and chemical control. Vagal stimulation promotes bile secretion, while splanchnic stimulation causes vasoconstriction, decreases blood flow to the liver, and thus diminishes bile secretion. Secretin, cholecystokinin, gastrin, and glucagon all increase bile flow, primarily by increasing water and electrolyte secretion.

The most important factor that regulates bile volume is the rate of bile synthesis by the liver, which is regulated by the return of bile salt to the liver by the enterohepatic circulation. The enterohepatic circulation provides an important negative-feedback system on bile synthesis. If the recirculation is interrupted by resection of the terminal ileum or by primary ileal disease, large losses of bile salts can occur. The same happens if a large external biliary fistula is present. The hepatocyte regulates itself to maintain a constant bile salt pool size so synthesis matches losses. During fasting periods, 90% of the bile acid pool is sequestered in the gallbladder.

The sphincter of Oddi is a complex structure that is separated from the duodenal musculature (Fig. 21.7). It creates a high-pressure zone between the bile duct and the duodenum. It regulates the flow of bile and pancreatic juice and prevents the regurgitation of duodenal contents. Neural and humoral factors influence its function. Under the effect of cholecystokinin after a meal, the sphincter relaxes, allowing the passage of bile and pancreatic secretions to the duodenum. During fasting (phase III MMC), the sphincter relaxes as the gallbladder contracts to allow the passive flow of bile into the duodenum. Antral distention stimulates the secretion of cholecystokinin, causing contraction of the gallbladder and relaxation of the sphincter.

BIBLIOGRAPHY

Jackson PG, Evans SR. Biliary system. In: Townsend CM, Beauchamp RD, Evers BM, Mattox KL, eds. *Sabiston's Textbook of Surgery: The Biological Basis of Modern Surgical Practice*. 19th ed. Philadelphia, PA: Elsevier; 2012:1476–1514.

Klein AS, Lillemoe KD. Liver, biliary tract, and pancreas. In: O'Leary JP, ed. *The Physiologic Basis of Surgery*. 4th ed. Baltimore, MD: Williams & Wilkins; 2008:441–478.

9. **(B)**

10. **(A)**

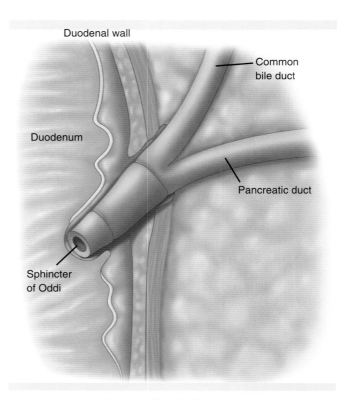

FIGURE 21-7. Sphincter of Oddi (from Brunicardi FC, Andersen DK, Billiar TR, et al., eds. *Schwartz's Principles of Surgery*. 10th ed. New York, NY: McGraw-Hill; 2014: Fig. 32-3. Copyright © The McGraw-Hill Companies, Inc. All rights reserved).

11. **(D)**

Explanation for questions 9 through 11

Gallstones represent a failure to maintain certain biliary solutes, primarily cholesterol and Ca^+, in a solubilized state. They are classified by their cholesterol content as either cholesterol or pigment stones (black or brown). Pure cholesterol stones are uncommon (<10%), and there are mixed cholesterol/Ca^+ (70–80%) and pigment (20–30%) stones. The pathogenesis of cholesterol gallstones is multifactorial, involving three stages: cholesterol saturation, nucleation, and stone growth. The hepatic metabolism is not involved in the pathogenesis of gallstones.

The process begins with excess cholesterol secretion, which surpasses the ability of the mixed micelles and cholesterol–phospholipid vesicles (carriers) to maintain cholesterol in solution, resulting in cholesterol supersaturation and subsequent precipitation. Additional factors must be present to allow for gallstone formation. First is nucleation, the process in which cholesterol crystals form and conglomerate. This process occurs more frequently in the gallbladder, where the bile is more concentrated. Second is the actual stone growth. Growth of stones may occur in two ways: progressive enlargement of stones by deposition of additional insoluble precipitate or fusion of individual crystals or stones to form a larger conglomerate.

Pigment stones are classified as brown and black. The brown stones are more common in Asia and are similar in composition to primary CBD stones; they occur as a result of infection. Bacteria are found in the brown stone matrix but are consistently absent from either black pigment or cholesterol stones. Black stones are typically found in patients with hemolytic disorders or cirrhosis. This results from an excessive load of bilirubin presented to the liver for excretion.

BIBLIOGRAPHY

Jackson PG, Evans SR. Biliary system. In: Townsend CM, Beauchamp RD, Evers BM, Mattox KL, eds. *Sabiston's Textbook of Surgery: The Biological Basis of Modern Surgical Practice*. 19th ed. Philadelphia, PA: Elsevier; 2012:1476–1514.

Klein AS, Lillemoe KD. Liver, biliary tract, and pancreas. In: O'Leary JP, ed. *The Physiologic Basis of Surgery*. 4th ed. Baltimore, MD: Williams & Wilkins; 2008:441–478.

12. **(D)** Ultrasonography is a useful examination during the initial evaluation of a patient with suspected cholecystitis. The ultrasound will show gallstones, gallbladder wall thickening (considered 4 mm or greater), and pericholecystic fluid, the combination of which is highly suggestive of acute cholecystitis. The ultrasound can also be used to detect CBD stones or dilation. This test, however, is operator dependent.

A HIDA scan is physiologic and demonstrates when the gallbladder does not fill (>2 h after injection of iminodiacetic acid), suggesting cystic duct obstruction consistent with acute cholecystitis. It may also be useful postoperatively in identifying leaks or obstruction of the biliary tree. Injection during the scan can demonstrate physiologic ejection of the gallbladder.

A CT scan is not a first-line test for the diagnosis of cholelithiasis or cholecystitis. It is useful when the concern is extrahepatic obstruction owing to causes other than choledocholithiasis. Limiting factors include patient exposure to ionizing radiation and cost.

MRCP is useful in delineating the anatomy of the intra- and extrahepatic biliary tree and pancreas. Most patients do not need such fine detail to alter management.

KUB radiography is not particularly useful since gallstones are rarely seen on plain films and, if seen, do not typically change management.

BIBLIOGRAPHY

Jackson PG, Evans SR. Biliary system. In: Townsend CM, Beauchamp RD, Evers BM, Mattox KL, eds. *Sabiston's Textbook of Surgery: The Biological Basis of Modern Surgical Practice*. 19th ed. Philadelphia, PA: Elsevier; 2012:1476–1514.

Van Arendonk KJ, Duncan MD. Acute cholecystitis. In: Cameron JL, Cameron AM, eds. *Current Surgical Therapy*. 10th ed. Philadelphia, PA: Elsevier; 2011:338–342.

13. **(C)**

14. **(B)**

Explanation for questions 13 and 14

The number of absolute and relative contraindications to performing laparoscopic cholecystectomy have decreased over the past 10 years as minimally invasive surgical equipment and skills have improved. Absolute contraindications include inability to tolerate general anesthesia or laparotomy, refractory coagulopathy, diffuse peritonitis with hemodynamic compromise, and potentially curable gallbladder cancer. Laparoscopic cholecystectomy has become the standard of care, with lower conversion rates as surgeons have become more experienced.

A cholecystectomy should be performed as soon as the patient is diagnosed as long as the patient is not critically ill with hemodynamic instability. Historically, it was thought patients should "cool off" for a period of up to 36 h, but there has been clear documentation that early cholecystectomy does not have higher rates of conversion or morbidity/mortality than waiting weeks prior to an operation.

When performing a laparoscopic cholecystectomy, it is important to achieve the "critical view of safety" prior to transection of the cystic duct (Fig. 21-8). This view is the liver edge, gallbladder, and cystic duct. This is done to prevent injury to the CBD, which can happen in multiple settings, including a short cystic duct. If an injury is made to the CBD, it should be repaired with a Roux-en-Y hepaticojejunostomy. If a biliary surgeon is not available who can perform this operation, the patient should be immediately transferred to a tertiary center with surgical and radiological experience in biliary tract injuries.

BIBLIOGRAPHY

Van Arendonk KJ, Duncan MD. Acute cholecystitis. In: Cameron JL, Cameron AM, eds. *Current Surgical Therapy*. 10th ed. Philadelphia, PA: Elsevier; 2011:338–342.

15. **(B)** Although laparoscopic cholecystectomies are often association with excellent outcomes, complications include a cystic duct stump leak with resulting biloma in 0.3% of cases. Leaks may occur when the surgical clip on the cyst duct stump slips off. Patients typically present with fever, RUQ pain, and vomiting. A CT scan or US may show RUQ fluid collection. HIDA or ERCP can confirm the cystic duct leak. ERCP and stenting of the CBD with or without percutaneous drainage of the biloma is the preferred method of treatment (Fig. 21-9).

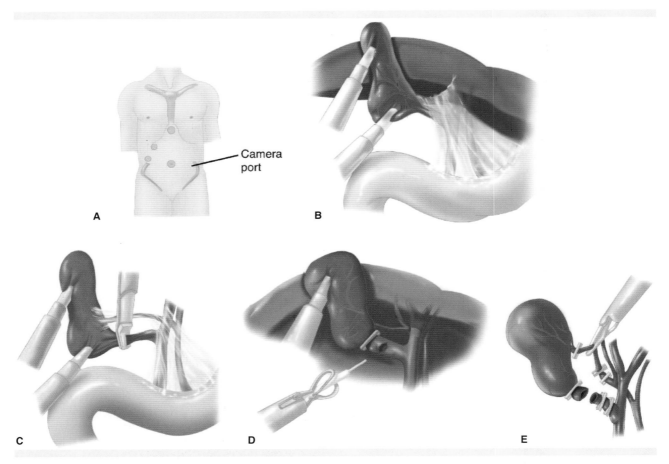

Camera port

A

B

C

D

E

FIGURE 21-8. Laparoscopic cholecystectomy (from Brunicardi FC, Andersen DK, Billiar TR, et al., eds. *Schwartz's Principles of Surgery.* 10th ed. New York, NY: McGraw-Hill; 2014: Fig. 32-18. Copyright © The McGraw-Hill Companies, Inc. All rights reserved).

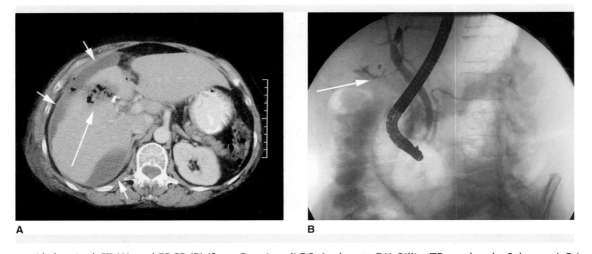

A

B

FIGURE 21-9. Abdominal CT (A) and ERCP (B) (from Brunicardi FC, Andersen DK, Billiar TR, et al., eds. *Schwartz's Principles of Surgery.* 10th ed. New York, NY: McGraw-Hill; 2014: Fig. 32-4. Copyright © The McGraw-Hill Companies, Inc. All rights reserved).

BIBLIOGRAPHY

Porrett PM, Frederick JR, Roses RE, Kaiser LR. The hepatobiliary system. In: Porrett PM, ed. *The Surgical Review*. 3rd ed.
Philadelphia, PA: Lippincott Williams & Wilkins; 2010:159–175.

16. **(D)**

17. **(C)**

Explanation for questions 16 and 17

Mirizzi's syndrome can be caused by a single large stone
or multiple small stones impacted in Hartmann's pouch
of the gallbladder or in the cystic duct. A long cystic duct
parallel to the bile duct predisposes to the development
of this syndrome. Recurrent attacks of cholecystitis may
cause inflammation and adhesions in the CBD and may
contribute to develop cholangitis. Either way, the CBD
becomes obstructed from the impingement of the stone
pushing on the duct or the resultant inflammatory process. Effectively, the CBD is obstructed, and there is a
resultant rise in total bilirubin and potential development
of acute cholangitis. ERCP can establish the diagnosis and
determine if there is a cholecystocholedochal fistula.

The differential diagnosis includes cholangiocarcinoma, gallbladder carcinoma, pancreatic cancer, and
sclerosing cholangitis. Surgery remains the treatment
of choice for Mirizzi's syndrome. The kind of surgery is
determined by whether a fistula is present. The common
approach is laparotomy, cholecystectomy if possible, and
CBD exploration. If the CBD viability is questionable, a
T tube, choledochoduodenostomy, and choledochojejunostomy are the recommended procedures. In any case,
excellent drainage should be achieved.

BIBLIOGRAPHY

Jackson PG, Evans SR. Biliary system. In: Townsend CM, Beau-
champ RD, Evers BM, Mattox KL, eds. *Sabiston's Textbook of
Surgery: The Biological Basis of Modern Surgical Practice*. 19th ed.
Philadelphia, PA: Elsevier; 2012:1476–1514.

18. **(B)**

19. **(B)**

20. **(D)**

21. **(C)**

22. **(D)**

23. **(D)**

24. **(F)**

Explanation for questions 18 through 24

Acute cholangitis is an inflammatory/infectious process
that develops as a result of bacterial colonization and
overgrowth within an obstructed biliary system. The
obstruction and cholangitis result from impacted stones
in 80% of the cases in the Western world. Such stones
most commonly originate from the gallbladder (secondary to CBD stones). Primary stones, most commonly
pigmented, are seen in the East Asian countries. Other
causes are benign strictures, neoplasms, papillary stenosis, sclerosing cholangitis, and foreign bodies. Biliary
instrumentation and malignant biliary strictures are risk
factors for the development of ascending cholangitis,
especially in the setting of an indwelling biliary drain or
stent, which serves as a potential nidus for infection.

Of the patients, 50–70% will present with the Charcot's
triad (abdominal pain, fever, and jaundice). The combination of change in mental status, hypotension, and the
Charcot's triad constitutes Reynold's pentad, which predicts a higher rate of fatality. Only 5% of patients present
with Reynold's pentad.

Chronic biliary obstruction may lead to liver abscesses
and secondary biliary cirrhosis. Organ failure and sepsis, sclerosing cholangitis, and strictures may develop.
Spread of the infection into the portal vein can cause
pyelophlebitis and portal vein thrombosis.

Analysis of the bile and blood in prospective studies
found that most patients have a polymicrobial infection,
with *E. coli* the most commonly identified gram-negative
bacteria (25–50%), and then *Klebsiella* spp. (15–20%),
Enterobacter spp. (5–10%), and *Enteroccocus* spp. (10–20%).

Antimicrobial agents should be administered to
patients as soon as acute cholangitis is suspected and
tailored appropriately on return of culture results. The
antibiotics initially used should target gram-positive and
gram-negative bacteria, especially *Enterococcus* sp.

A combination of abdominal US, CT scan, and cholangiography complements and confirms the clinical
diagnosis of cholangitis. Direct cholangiography (ERCP)
is the gold standard for diagnosing acute cholangitis and
is the most useful intervention when the patient is failing
medical management for biliary decompression. ERCP
is less invasive and has the advantage that offers therapeutic measures, including stone extraction and biliary
drainage (Fig. 21-10). PTC is used when ERCP fails or in
patients with previous biloenteric anastomosis or in centers unable to perform ERCP.

Chronic biliary obstruction may lead to liver abscesses
and secondary biliary cirrhosis. Organ failure and sepsis, sclerosing cholangitis, and strictures may develop.
Spread of the infection into the portal vein can cause
pyelophlebitis and portal vein thrombosis.

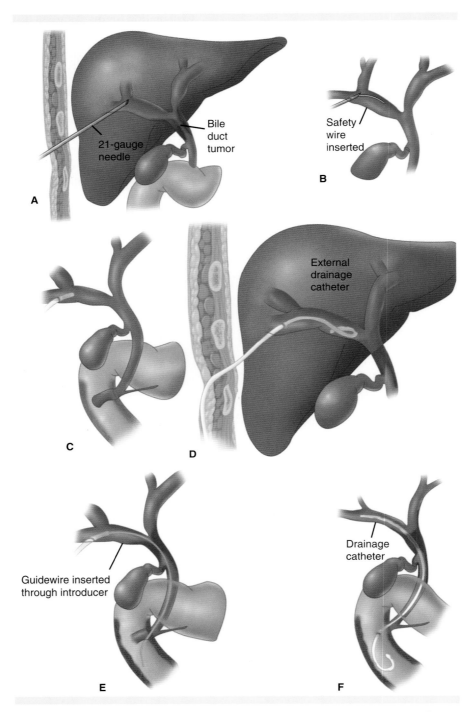

FIGURE 21-10. Schematic diagram of percutaneous transhepatic cholangiogram and drainage (from Brunicardi FC, Andersen DK, Billiar TR, et al., eds. *Schwartz's Principles of Surgery*. 10th ed. New York, NY: McGraw-Hill; 2014: Fig. 32-8. Copyright © The McGraw-Hill Companies, Inc. All rights reserved).

BIBLIOGRAPHY

Jackson PG, Evans SR. Biliary system. In: Townsend CM, Beauchamp RD, Evers BM, Mattox KL, eds. *Sabiston's Textbook of Surgery: The Biological Basis of Modern Surgical Practice.* 19th ed. Philadelphia, PA: Elsevier; 2012:1476–1514.

Jonnalagadda S, Strasberg SM. Acute cholangitis. In: Cameron JL, Cameron AM, eds. *Current Surgical Therapy.* 10th ed. Philadelphia, PA: Elsevier; 2011:345–348.

Yu AS, Leung JW. Acute cholangitis. In: Clavien PA, Baillie J, eds. *On Diseases of the Gallbladder and Bile Ducts.* Oxford, England: Blackwell Science; 2001:205–225.

25. **(C)**

26. **(D)**

27. **(C)**

Explanation for questions 25 through 27

Biliary dyskinesia is characterized by the presence of the typical symptoms of biliary colic, including postprandial RUQ pain, fatty food intolerance, and nausea without the identification of gallstones. These patients do not have gallstone disease on US examination. The cholecystokinin-Tc-HIDA scan has been useful in identifying patients with this disorder. Cholecystokinin is administered intravenously after the gallbladder is filled with the radionuclide. Twenty minutes after the injection, a gallbladder ejection fraction is calculated. An ejection fraction of less than 35% at 20 min is considered abnormal.

Patients with a symptomatic and abnormal gallbladder ejection fraction should be managed with laparoscopic cholecystectomy. Of patients with diagnosed biliary dyskinesia, 85% will improve or show resolution after the cholecystectomy.

BIBLIOGRAPHY

Jackson PG, Evans SR. Biliary system. In: Townsend CM, Beauchamp RD, Evers BM, Mattox KL, eds. *Sabiston's Textbook of Surgery: The Biological Basis of Modern Surgical Practice.* 19th ed. Philadelphia, PA: Elsevier; 2012:1476–1514.

28. **(D)**

29. **(A)**

30. **(E)**

31. **(D)**

32. **(D)**

Explanation for questions 28 through 32

A choledochal cyst is defined as an isolated or combined congenital dilatation of the extrahepatic or intrahepatic biliary tree (Fig. 21-11). In children, the classic findings include a RUQ abdominal mass, jaundice, and abdominal pain. In adults, it is usually confused with benign biliary and pancreatic diseases.

The most common type is confined to the extrahepatic biliary tree, starting just below the hepatic ducts bifurcation and extending into or near the pancreas (type I). Other types include the following:

Type II: saccular diverticulum of the extrahepatic bile duct

Type III: dilatation of the extrahepatic bile duct within the duodenum (choledochocele)

Type IVa: combined intra- and extrahepatic bile duct dilatation

Type IVb: multiple extrahepatic cysts

Type V: isolated intrahepatic biliary tree dilatation (Caroli's disease)

Histologically, two types of cysts are described: glandular, characterized by a chronic inflammatory cell infiltrate; and fibrotic, for which the bile duct is thickened with well-developed collagen fibers and less inflammation.

Because CT scanning is liberally used currently, most are suspected/noted initially on CT scan. The diagnosis is further classified by MRCP. MRCP helps create a complete cholangiogram. Because the distal duct is hard to see on MRCP, ERCP is the most useful test to evaluate the anatomy of the distal bile duct.

Choledochal cyst excision, with reconstruction via a Roux-en-Y hepaticojejunostomy, is the procedure of choice for most types of choledochal cysts. One exception is the type III (choledochocele) cyst, which can be treated with transduodenal sphincteroplasty or sphincterotomy. Also, an exception is type V (Caroli's disease). If it is localized to one lobe, hepatectomy is the preferred treatment, and if it is bilateral, liver transplantation is the procedure of choice.

The incidence of malignancy in patients with biliary cysts ranges from 10 to 30%. The entire biliary tree is at risk, even the nondilated portions of the biliary tree. Thus, complete excision does not completely eliminate the risk of subsequent development of cholangiocarcinoma.

BIBLIOGRAPHY

Jackson PG, Evans SR. Biliary system. In: Townsend CM, Beauchamp RD, Evers BM, Mattox KL, eds. *Sabiston's Textbook of Surgery: The Biological Basis of Modern Surgical Practice.* 19th ed. Philadelphia, PA: Elsevier; 2012:1476–1514.

33. **(C)**

34. **(D)**

35. **(A)**

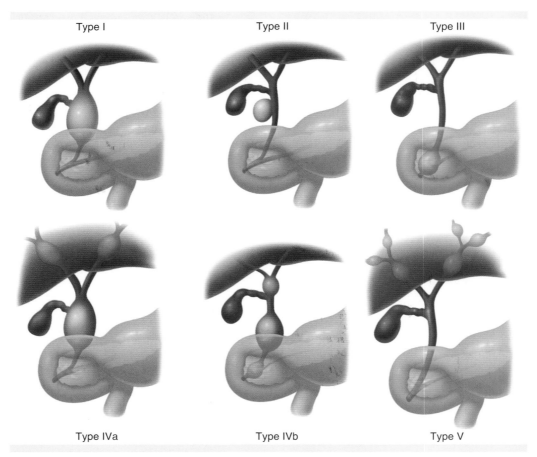

FIGURE 21-11. Choledochal cyst classification (from Brunicardi FC, Andersen DK, Billiar TR, et al., eds. *Schwartz's Principles of Surgery.* 10th ed. New York, NY: McGraw-Hill; 2014: Fig. 32-22. Copyright © The McGraw-Hill Companies, Inc. All rights reserved).

Explanation for questions 33 through 35

Caroli's disease (Fig. 21-12) is an abnormal development of the intrahepatic bile ducts without an obstructive cause, characterized by saccular dilatations, resembling a picture of multiple cyst-like structures of varying size. Two types have been described: a type with bile duct abnormalities alone and a type with bile duct abnormality combined with periportal fibrosis, similar to congenital hepatic fibrosis. This combined type is also known as Caroli's syndrome and has been reported more frequently than the pure type, or Caroli's disease.

Caroli's disease is anatomically characterized for saccular dilatations of the bile ducts more frequently seen in the left side of the liver. In 30–40% of the cases, these are confined to one segment of one side of the liver. Bilateral abnormalities are more common in Caroli's syndrome.

The most common complications are cholangitis, septicemia, amyloidosis, and cholangiocarcinoma (7–10% of patients). Caroli's syndrome is associated with renal disorders such as renal cysts and nephrospongiosis, seen in

30–40% of patients. These disorders have not been seen in Caroli's disease.

The diagnosis is made by radiologic studies, such as US, CT scan, ERCP, MRI, where saccular or cystically dilated intrahepatic ducts are seen. Surgical treatment is indicated to reduce the risk of recurrent cholangitis, biliary cirrhosis, or cholangiocarcinoma. Hepatic lobectomy is indicated for localized bile duct abnormalities (Caroli's disease), while liver transplantation should be considered in selected patients with generalized disease or concomitant liver fibrosis and portal hypertension (Caroli's syndrome).

BIBLIOGRAPHY

Porte R, Clavien PA. Cystic diseases of the biliary system. In: *On Diseases of the Gallbladder and Bile Ducts.* Oxford, England: Blackwell Science; 2001:216–225.

36. **(E)**

37. **(C)**

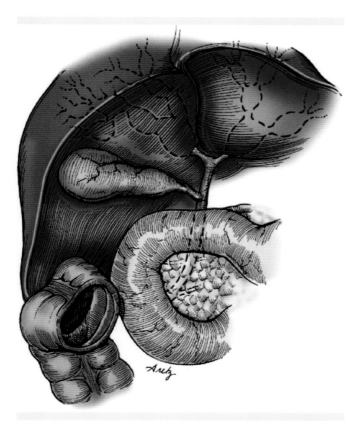

FIGURE 21-12. Caroli's disease (from Zinner MJ, Ashley SW, eds. *Maingot's Abdominal Operations*. 12th ed. New York, NY: McGraw-Hill; 2013: Fig. 50-1E. Copyright © The McGraw-Hill Companies, Inc. All rights reserved).

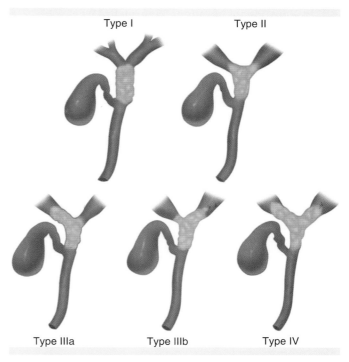

FIGURE 21-13. Bismuth classification (from Brunicardi FC, Andersen DK, Billiar TR, et al., eds. *Schwartz's Principles of Surgery*. 10th ed. New York, NY: McGraw-Hill; 2014: Fig. 32-26. Copyright © The McGraw-Hill Companies, Inc. All rights reserved).

38. **(D)**

Explanation for questions 36 through 38

Cholangiocarcinoma is an uncommon cancer with a dismal prognosis (Fig. 21-13). The etiology is unknown, but the risk seems to correlate with chronic inflammation in the biliary tree. Therefore, choledochal cysts, infection with the liver flukes *Clonorchis sinensis* and *Opisthorchis viverrini*, recurrent pyogenic cholangitis, and primary sclerosing cholangitis are some of the risk factors for the development of cholangiocarcinoma.

Historically, the bile duct was divided into thirds, but the middle third is so infrequently affected that treatment now focuses on tumors of the perihilar bifurcations (Klatskin tumors) or the periampullary region.

There are three distinct pathologic subtypes: sclerosing, nodular, and papillary cholangiocarcinoma. Sclerosing occurs in the proximal ducts, whereas nodular and papillary occur in the distal ducts.

Patients typically present with hyperbilirubinemia and an elevated alkaline phosphatase level. Ultrasound may show ductal dilation. CT allows assessment for metastatic disease as well as resectability. But, CT is typically not sufficient for assessment for determining resectability. MRCP, PTC, and ERCP also help delineate the anatomy. ERCP, however, can introduce infection. Brushings, biopsy, and cytology are not reliable or useful in the diagnosis.

Distal cholangiocarcinoma is best managed by pancreaticoduodenectomy. Proximal cholangiocarcinoma is best managed by resection of the CBD with hepatic parenchyma until the margins are negative. Chemotherapy and radiation have not been shown to improve survival.

BIBLIOGRAPHY

Jackson PG, Evans SR. Biliary system. In: Townsend CM, Beauchamp RD, Evers BM, Mattox KL, eds. *Sabiston's Textbook of Surgery: The Biological Basis of Modern Surgical Practice*. 19th ed. Philadelphia, PA: Elsevier; 2012:1476–1514.

39. **(B)**

40. **(A)**

41. **(A)**

Explanation for questions 39 through 41

Carcinoma of the gallbladder is a rare and fatal disease, with only 5% of patients surviving beyond 5 years. The association between cancer of the gallbladder and gallstones is well known. Ninety-five percent of the patients with cancer have gallstones. A gallbladder tumor will be found in 1% of all cholecystectomy specimens. Porcelain gallbladder and gallbladder polyps larger than 1 cm are risk factors for the development of carcinoma (Fig. 21-14).

The majority of gallbladder cancers are adenocarcinoma. A small subset of patients will have papillary cancer, which has markedly improved survival compared to all other histologic types.

A cure for gallbladder cancer can only be achieved by complete surgical resection. The extent of surgery for many stages of gallbladder cancer remains controversial.

The American Joint Committee on Cancer (AJCC) TMN and staging criteria are shown in Table 21-1. The most accepted recommendations are as follows:

Stage 1 tumors (T1, N0, M0): confined to muscularis propria: simple cholecystectomy

Stage 2, 3, and 4a (T4, N0, M0): en bloc resection of the gallbladder, segments 4 and 5 of the liver, and regional lymph node dissection

Stage 4b (distant metastases): palliation

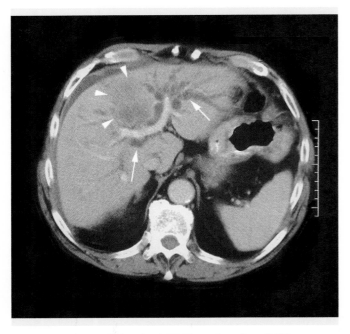

FIGURE 21-14. Abdominal CT (from Brunicardi FC, Andersen DK, Billiar TR, et al., eds. *Schwartz's Principles of Surgery*. 10th ed. New York, NY: McGraw-Hill; 2014: Fig. 32-25. Copyright © The McGraw-Hill Companies, Inc. All rights reserved).

Patients with T1 tumor and cholecystectomy have a 5-year survival rate close to 100%. Cholecystectomy alone in T2 tumors offers a 40% survival rate and no survival for T3 lesions. Performance of a radical second operation improves the T2 5-year survival rate to 90%. Because of the small number of patients, there is no definitive conclusion regarding improvement survival after radical surgery for T3 and T4 patients.

There are no prospective, randomized studies examining the utility of adjuvant therapy. The tumor has been resistant to most forms of chemotherapy, and the mode of spread does not lend itself to radiation.

BIBLIOGRAPHY

Jackson PG, Evans SR. Biliary system. In: Townsend CM, Beauchamp RD, Evers BM, Mattox KL, eds. *Sabiston's Textbook of Surgery: The Biological Basis of Modern Surgical Practice*. 19th ed. Philadelphia, PA: Elsevier; 2012:1476–1514.

Sicklick JK, Fong Y. Management of gallbladder cancer. In: Cameron JL, Cameron AM, eds. *Current Surgical Therapy*. 10th ed. Philadelphia, PA: Elsevier; 2011: Chapter 87.

42. **(B)** Several modalities of radiologic and endoscopic investigation are available to evaluate symptoms suggestive of postcholecystectomy biliary injury. Ninety percent of cholecystectomies are done laparoscopically, and most patients are discharged to home within 24 h of surgery. Immediate postoperative complications include hemorrhage, infection, bile leak, or bile duct injury. Initial investigation includes complete blood cell count (CBC), liver function tests, and serum amylase evaluation.

Abdominal US is the most useful imaging study in the early postoperative period; it will reveal fluid collections, abscess, bile leakage, and biliary dilatation. Patients with large fluid collections and dilated bile ducts should undergo biliary imaging by PTC or ERCP. ERCP has become the preferred technique for biliary duct visualization once the diagnosis of bile leak is made, allowing not only knowing what kind of injury is present but also performing therapeutic interventions, such as stone extraction, stent placement, and sphincterotomy.

Magnetic resonance cholangiography is a noninvasive technique, with no need of intravenous contrast. It allows detection of biliary and pancreatic pathology with a high degree of sensitivity (88%) and specificity (93%). Although its use during the evaluation of biliary injuries has not been fully investigated yet, it will probably become a strong tool for screening, avoiding the complications of ERCP.

TABLE 21-1 Gallbladder Cancer Staging: TNM Definitions

Primary tumor (T)	
TX	Primary tumor cannot be assessed
TO	No evidence of primary tumor
Tis	Carcinoma in situ
T1	Tumor invades lamina propria or muscular layer
T1a	Tumor invades lamina propria
T1b	Tumor invades muscular layer
T2	Tumor invades perimuscular connective tissue; no extension beyond serosa or into liver
T3	Tumor perforates the serosa (visceral peritoneum) and/or directly invades the liver and/or one other adjacent organ or structure, such as the stomach, duodenum, colon, pancreas, omentum, or extrahepatic bile ducts
T4	Tumor invades main portal vein or hepatic artery or invades two or more extrahepatic organs or structures

Regional lymph nodes (N)	
NX	Regional lymph nodes cannot be assessed
NO	No regional lymph node metastasis
N1	Metastases to nodes along the cystic duct, common bile duct, hepatic artery, and/or portal vein
N2	Metastases to periaortic, pericaval, superior mesentery artery, and/or celiac artery lymph nodes

Distant metastasis (M)	
MO	No distant metastasis
M1	Distant metastasis

Stage grouping			
Stage 0	Tis	NO	MO
Stage I	T1	NO	MO
Stage II	T2	NO	MO
Stage IIIA	T3	NO	MO
Stage IIIB	T1-3	N1	MO
Stage IVA	T4	NO-1	MO
Stage IVB	Any T	N2	MO
	AnyT	Any N	M1

From Edge SB, Byrd DR, Compton CC, et al., eds. *AJCC Cancer Staging Manual.* 7th ed. New York: Springer; 2010.

BIBLIOGRAPHY

Beckingham IJ, Rowlands BJ. Postcholecystectomy problems. In: Blumgart LH, Fong Y, eds. *On Surgery of the Liver and Biliary Tract.* 3rd ed. Philadelphia, PA: 2000:799–809.

43. **(C)**

44. **(B)**

Explanation for questions 43 and 44

Once a biliary injury is diagnosed and identified, every attempt should be made to define the biliary anatomy by PTC and to control the bile leak with percutaneous biliary drainage. Immediate reexploration should be avoided. The inflammation associated with bile spillage and the retracted proximal bile duct make recognition and repair difficult and unsafe. Delaying reconstruction by weeks, helped by percutaneous biliary decompression, allows for optimal surgical results. The goal of operative management is the establishment of bile flow into the bowel in a way in which stone formation, cholangitis, stricture development, and biliary cirrhosis are prevented (Fig. 21-15).

To obtain optimal results, healthy, nonischemic proximal bile duct and intestinal anatomy suitable for a Roux-en-Y anastomosis should be available to create a mucosal-mucosal biliary-enteric anastomosis (ERCP in Fig. 21-6).

Simple end-to-end anastomosis of the bile duct is difficult to accomplish secondary to fibrosis associated with the injury.

A hepaticojejunostomy constructed to a Roux-en-Y intestinal limb is the procedure of choice with a success rate greater than 90%.

Preoperative placement of percutaneous biliary catheters is essential not only in the early management of this patient but also in the intraoperative identification and manipulation of the proximal, injured bile duct. It is also important in the early postoperative period to allow decompression of the biliary tree, protection for possible bile leak, and ability to provide access for cholangiography.

BIBLIOGRAPHY

Lillemoe KD. Benign biliary stricture. In: Cameron JL, ed. *Current Surgical Therapy*. 7th ed. Baltimore, MD: Mosby; 2001:454–461.

45. **(D)** Gallstone ileus is a mechanical intestinal obstruction secondary to an impacted gallstone (Fig. 21-16). The gallstone enters the bowel lumen through a biliary-enteric fistula. It accounts for 3% of all intestinal obstructions. A biliary-enteric fistula is a prerequisite for gallstone ileus. It results from a chronic inflammation of the gallbladder, causing necrosis of the gallbladder wall with perforation into the duodenum, colon, or small bowel. Only large stones (>2.5 cm) can become impacted in the relatively narrow terminal ileum.

Abdominal pain, distention, cramping, nausea, and vomiting that appear intermittently over several days may correlate with the "tumbling" of the stone as it moves distally. Bouveret's syndrome occurs when the stone impacts into the duodenum; nausea, nonbilious vomiting, and no abdominal distention are the classical symptoms.

Multiple diagnostic tools are available, starting with an abdominal plain film that shows a classic obstructive pattern, pneumobilia (40%), and radiopaque stones (20%).

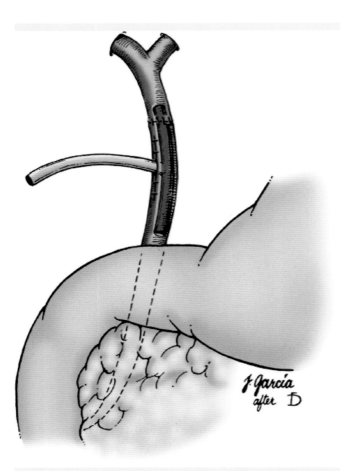

FIGURE 21-15. Schematics of biliary repair over T tube (from Zinner MJ, Ashley SW, eds. *Maingot's Abdominal Operations*. 12th ed. New York, NY: McGraw-Hill; 2013: Fig. 50-15. Copyright © The McGraw-Hill Companies, Inc. All rights reserved).

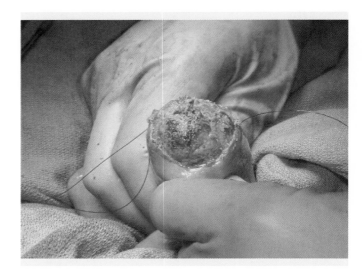

FIGURE 21-16. Gallstone ileus.

A CT scan can be helpful when the KUB radiography is not diagnostic; it is able to show air in the bile ducts and visualize the stone.

Exploratory laparotomy is the best approach. An RUQ dissection should be avoided unless the obstruction is at the level of the duodenum (Bouveret's syndrome); in that case, pushing the stone into the stomach, gastrotomy, and extraction are recommended.

If the stone is impacted distally, it should be extracted through an enterotomy, bowel resection (if not viable), or by "milking" it until passing the ileocecal valve.

Failure to remove all the stones increases recurrence rates. Management of the biliary-enteric fistula at the time of the initial surgery is not recommended. Most fistulas close spontaneously. Repairing of the fistula increases operative time and morbidity.

BIBLIOGRAPHY

Vagefi PA, Berger DL. Gallstone ileus. In: Cameron JL, Cameron AM, eds. *Current Surgical Therapy*. 10th ed. Philadelphia, PA: Elsevier; 2011: Chapter 88.

CHAPTER 22

LIVER

STEPHEN J. KAPLAN AND RAVI MOONKA

1. The obliterated ductus venosus
   - (A) Divides the left lateral and left medial sections of the liver
   - (B) Joins the left portal and left hepatic veins
   - (C) Anchors the liver to the retroperitoneum
   - (D) Travels within the falciform ligament
   - (E) Can recannulate with portal hypertension

2. In the most common variant of hepatic arterial anatomy,
   - (A) The affected artery passes posterior and lateral to the portal vein
   - (B) All hepatic arterial supply is received via branches from the superior mesenteric artery
   - (C) All hepatic arterial supply is received via branches from the celiac trunk
   - (D) 50% of hepatic blood flow is arterial
   - (E) The left liver receives hepatic arterial blood via branches from the left gastric artery

3. The middle hepatic vein
   - (A) Travels within the same anatomic space defining Cantlie's line
   - (B) Drains the right posterior and left medial sections
   - (C) Often drains into the right hepatic vein rather than directly into the inferior vena cava (IVC)
   - (D) Is contained within the falciform ligament
   - (E) Obliterates early in infancy

4. During a left hepatectomy,
   - (A) The liver is divided just lateral to the falciform ligament
   - (B) The liver is divided just medial to the falciform ligament
   - (C) Middle hepatic vein ligation is required
   - (D) Segment I resection is required
   - (E) Division is carried between the gallbladder fossa and the IVC

5. Which of the following is a contraindication to hepatectomy?
   - (A) Planned future liver remnant less than 40% of total liver volume
   - (B) Evidence of liver cirrhosis
   - (C) Portal hypertension
   - (D) Comorbid diabetes mellitus
   - (E) Presence of liver metastases

6. A 52-year-old man with hepatocellular carcinoma (HCC) and Child's A cirrhosis is undergoing preoperative planning for right hepatectomy. His predicted future liver remnant volume (FLRV) is estimated to be 35%. The next appropriate step for this patient would be to
   - (A) Undergo the planned right hepatectomy
   - (B) Cancel the operation and pursue nonsurgical management
   - (C) Place a transjugular intrahepatic portosystemic shunt (TIPS)
   - (D) Embolize his right portal vein
   - (E) Repeat imaging in 3 months for reconsideration of resection

7. Which of the following observations regarding ascites in the context of cirrhosis is true?
   - (A) Periodic large-volume paracentesis is a recognized treatment modality for ascites but is associated with an increased risk of spontaneous bacterial peritonitis.
   - (B) Isolated portal vein thrombosis (PVT) not associated with cirrhosis and is as likely to cause ascites as Budd-Chiari syndrome (BCS).
   - (C) Transjugular intrahepatic portosystemic shunting can successfully treat ascites and is not associated with the encephalopathy often seen with surgical shunts.
   - (D) Levine shunts presently have no role in the treatment of patients with ascites due to the high risk of shunt failure within 1 year of placement.
   - (E) Hepatic hydrothorax can complicate ascites due to the movement of fluid through full-thickness defects in the diaphragm.

8. Unexpected parenchymal bleeding during hepatic resection can be controlled by
   (A) Rapidly decreasing central venous pressure (CVP) with additional anesthesia
   (B) Ligation of common hepatic artery
   (C) Portal triad clamping
   (D) Induction of hypothermia
   (E) Venovenous bypass

9. The portal vein anatomy is uniquely important during right hepatectomy because
   (A) Left portal vein ligation is often necessary
   (B) Right portal and right hepatic veins appear similar on ultrasound
   (C) The right posterior branch of the portal vein commonly originates from the left portal vein
   (D) The caudate branch of the portal vein often branches posteriorly from the right portal vein
   (E) The right portal vein usually bifurcates into anterior and posterior branches deep within the parenchyma

10. Portal hypertension–related morbidity and mortality is primarily related to
    (A) Reversed blood flow from coronary and short gastric veins
    (B) Poor coagulation factor synthesis
    (C) Platelet sequestration
    (D) Limited toxin clearance
    (E) Recannulation of the umbilical vein

11. With regard to hepatic vein anatomy,
    (A) Intrahepatically, the hepatic veins parallel the hepatic arteries
    (B) The middle and right hepatic veins commonly join prior to terminating at the IVC
    (C) Segment 1 primarily drains directly into the IVC
    (D) 25% of venous drainage is through right, left, and middle hepatic veins
    (E) The three main hepatic veins travel superficially, paralleling the liver capsule

12. Hypoxic injury first affects hepatocytes located in
    (A) Acinar zone 1
    (B) Acinar zone 2
    (C) Acinar zone 3
    (D) The area closest to portal venules
    (E) The center of individual segments

13. After resection, the remaining healthy liver
    (A) Regenerates through hepatocyte hypertrophy
    (B) Takes at least 5 years to regenerate 75% of the preoperative volume
    (C) Begins regenerating within days
    (D) Completes cell division within 1 month
    (E) Begins regeneration in centrilobular areas

14. During fasting, the liver first provides energy and substrates for metabolism through
    (A) Glycogenolysis
    (B) Gluconeogenesis
    (C) Lipolysis
    (D) Glycolysis
    (E) The urea cycle

15. Liver function histology and cellular physiology are characterized by
    (A) Different hepatocyte functions depending on histological location
    (B) Bile acid secretion into the space of Disse
    (C) A rich microcirculation with direct hepatocyte-blood contact
    (D) An intrinsic dependence on glucose metabolism
    (E) Cell-cell interaction at the level of the sinusoidal membrane

16. Kupffer cells are a type of
    (A) Dendritic cell
    (B) Macrophage
    (C) Stellate cell
    (D) Endothelial cell
    (E) Hepatocyte

17. Drug and toxin metabolism in the liver occurs primarily via
    (A) Phagocytosis by Kupffer cells
    (B) Hepatocyte-mediated biotransformation
    (C) Hydrolysis in the space of Disse
    (D) Conjugation with chenodeoxycholic acid
    (E) Oxidation by sinusoidal endothelial cells

18. During an inflammatory state, synthesis of which protein will be diminished?
    (A) Fibrinogen
    (B) Ceruloplasmin
    (C) Factor VII
    (D) Transferrin
    (E) C-reactive protein

19. A 65-year-old man presents to the emergency room with a 3-day history of fever, chills, and right upper quadrant pain. He is otherwise healthy and gives a history of prior cholecystectomy in the distant past. On physical examination, he is not jaundiced. He is febrile, tachycardic, and has significant tenderness over the right upper quadrant. He denies any history of alcohol use or recent travel. An ultrasound is obtained and shows a hypoechoic intrahepatic lesion. The most likely diagnosis is
    (A) Hepatocellular carcinoma
    (B) Liver hemangioma
    (C) Acute hepatitis
    (D) Pyogenic liver abscess
    (E) Cholangitis

20. With the presumptive diagnosis of a pyogenic liver abscess, the initial management should include
    (A) Open incision and drainage
    (B) Laparoscopic exploration
    (C) Endoscopic retrograde cholangiopancreatography decompression
    (D) Liver resection
    (E) Radiographically guided percutaneous drainage

21. A 16-year-old male is referred for a 1-week history of progressively worsening right upper quadrant pain, fever, and leukocytosis. He has recently returned from school trip to Central America. Serum antibody test is positive for *Entamoeba histolytica*. Initial management of this patient should include
    (A) Laparoscopic drainage
    (B) Open incision and drainage
    (C) Endoscopic retrograde cholangiopancreatography decompression
    (D) Radiographically guided percutaneous drainage
    (E) Antibiotics alone

22. A 45-year-old man is found to have a 6-cm calcified cystic liver lesion containing daughter cysts in the right lobe of the liver. The initial preferred treatment includes
    (A) Open incision and drainage
    (B) Pericystectomy
    (C) A 2-week course of metronidazole
    (D) Percutaneous catheter drainage
    (E) Laparoscopic drainage

23. A 20-year-old is referred for progressively worsening abdominal pain over the past several years. He has marked hepatosplenomegaly on examination, along with prominent abdominal wall veins. He has never used alcohol or drugs. Hepatitis serologies are negative, and liver enzymes are normal. Ultrasound reveals periportal fibrosis. His condition is
    (A) Limited to immunocompromised hosts
    (B) Caused by to trophozoite venule obstruction
    (C) The most common cause of portal hypertension worldwide
    (D) Treated with mebendazole
    (E) Treated with liver resection

24. A 26-year-old female is brought to the emergency department with altered mental status. Her family reports she has been having a notable amount of pain, which she has been treating with acetaminophen, related to her third-trimester pregnancy. A rapid progression of mental status changes prompted their visit today. She is confused, with a Glasgow Coma Scale (GCS) score of 11. Workup reveals a lactate level of 2.8 mg/dL, arterial pH of 7.32, normal complete blood cell count (CBC),

elevated liver transaminases in the 3000s, and an international normalized ratio (INR) of 4.0. In this patient, what most portends a poor prognosis?
    (A) Elevated lactate
    (B) Elevated ALT (alanine aminotransferase) and AST (aspartate aminotransferase)
    (C) Coagulopathy
    (D) Mental status
    (E) Current pregnancy

25. A 28-year-old woman presents with abdominal pain and anorexia, both progressively worsening over the past week. She is 3 weeks postpartum from her first childbirth. Her examination is notable for abdominal distention, ascites, hepatomegaly, and severe right upper quadrant tenderness. Laboratory values are as follows: hematocrit 32%, platelets 150×10^9/L, ALT 600 units/L, AST 400 units/L, and total bilirubin 2.5 mg/dL. The liver portion of an abdominal ultrasound study will likely reveal
    (A) A thrombus within the sublobular hepatic veins
    (B) Surface nodularity with segmental hypertrophy and atrophy
    (C) A thrombus within the portal vein
    (D) A thrombus within the main hepatic veins
    (E) Intrahepatic bile duct dilation

26. An otherwise-healthy 40-year-old woman with polycystic liver disease presents with acute gastroesophageal variceal bleeding. Endoscopic management is unsuccessful. The next step in definitive management includes
    (A) TIPS placement
    (B) Liver transplantation
    (C) Luminal tamponade
    (D) Surgical portacaval shunting
    (E) Gastric devascularization and splenectomy

27. A 32-year-old surgery resident is evaluated for malaise, fatigue, myalgia, and low-grade fever. He was previously well and denies illicit drug use, transfusions, or recent travel. He does, however, admit to a needlestick injury several weeks ago. Physical examination reveals icteric sclera. AST is elevated at 500 U/L. Serological assays reveal immunoglobulin (Ig) G anti-HAV (hepatitis A virus) positive, IgM anti-HAV negative, hepatitis B surface antigen (HBsAg) negative, anti-HBs (hepatitis A surface) negative, anti-HBc (hepatitis B core) positive, anti-HCV (hepatitis C virus) negative. Which condition most likely explains these findings?
    (A) Acute hepatitis A
    (B) Acute hepatitis B
    (C) Chronic hepatitis B
    (D) Expected hepatitis B immunity
    (E) Acute hepatitis C

28. A 55-year-old man presents with tea-colored urine, jaundice, fatigue, and anorexia 6 weeks following a motor vehicle collision causing splenic rupture, for which he required massive blood transfusion and splenectomy. Examination shows icteric sclera and mild hepatomegaly. Laboratory investigation reveals the following: bilirubin 3 mg/dL, AST 550 U/L, and ALT 650 U/L. Serum assay tests for HBsAg, anti-HBc, anti-HAV, and anti-HCV are all negative. The most likely diagnosis is
    (A) Acute viral hepatitis A
    (B) Acute viral hepatitis B
    (C) Acute viral hepatitis C
    (D) Acute viral hepatitis D
    (E) Acute viral hepatitis E

29. Which of the following is true regarding risk factors for HCC?
    (A) Hepatitis B must produce cirrhosis to predispose patients to HCC.
    (B) The ability of HCV to integrate into the cellular genome partially explains its oncogenic properties.
    (C) Cirrhosis from NASH (nonalcoholic steatohepatitis) does not predispose to HCC.
    (D) Cirrhosis underlies the development of HCC in 90% of cases.
    (E) Ingestion of aflatoxin is now no longer considered a risk factor for HCC.

30. Which of the following statements concerning the presentation of HCC is true?
    (A) In patients with cirrhosis, HCC usually causes deterioration of liver function that is generally readily discernible early in the disease course.
    (B) Screening patients at high risk for HCC has not been shown to provide an improvement in survival.
    (C) Screening for HCC is most strongly indicated for patients with Child's C cirrhosis due to the increased risk of HCC in more severe liver disease.
    (D) Screening for HCC consists of a liver ultrasound and transaminase determinations every 6 months.
    (E) Any liver lesion over 1 cm in diameter seen on screening ultrasound requires four-phase liver computed tomography (CT) for follow-up.

31. Which of the following statements concerning HCC diagnosis and management is true?
    (A) Enlarged portal lymph nodes are a contraindication to extirpative surgery unless proven benign by tissue biopsy.
    (B) An image-guided biopsy is performed prior to treatment for primary HCC to avoid treating benign regenerative nodules.
    (C) A CT scan can anatomically define an abnormal nodule but provides no information on hepatic function.
    (D) HCC will demonstrate greater enhancement than surrounding liver on the arterial phase of a four-phase liver CT.
    (E) An MRI can sometimes provide information not provided with a CT scan and does not require intravenous contrast.

32. A 66-year-old male patient is evaluated for jaundice and is found to have a hepatic mass. He has a history of long-term exposure to vinyl chloride. The most likely diagnosis is
    (A) Angiosarcoma
    (B) Angiomyolipoma
    (C) Epithelioid hemangioendothelioma
    (D) Undifferentiated sarcoma
    (E) Rhabdomyosarcoma

33. Most primary and metastatic tumors to the liver derive nearly all their vascular inflow from branches of the
    (A) Portal vein
    (B) Collateral circulation
    (C) Hepatic arteries
    (D) Hepatic veins
    (E) De novo vasogenesis

34. Regarding hepatic hemangioma:
    (A) Resection is indicated in asymptomatic hemangiomas over 5 cm in diameter to prevent spontaneous or traumatic rupture.
    (B) Resection should be carried out with a 1-cm margin to prevent local recurrence.
    (C) Most patients with a hemangioma are asymptomatic.
    (D) Kasabach-Merritt is an unusual clinical syndrome associated with large hemangiomas that can result in thrombocytosis.
    (E) These tumors generally require biopsy to rule out hepatic malignancies or precancerous lesions.

35. Which of the following is true regarding focal nodular hyperplasia (FNH)?
    (A) It usually causes symptoms.
    (B) It can be distinguished from a hepatic adenoma on magnetic resonance imaging (MRI) with a proper protocol.
    (C) It is associated with a risk of spontaneous rupture and bleeding.
    (D) It undergoes malignant transformation in 10% of cases.
    (E) It is associated with the use of oral contraceptives.

36. A 44-year-old man is found to have an incidental 5-cm cystic liver lesion without internal septations on abdominal ultrasound. The patient is otherwise healthy and has no prior medical history. The next step should be
    (A) Elective open wedge resection
    (B) Laparoscopic biopsy of the cyst wall
    (C) Laparoscopic marsupialization
    (D) Observation
    (E) Percutaneous aspiration

37. Which of the following regarding treatment options for HCC is true?
    (A) CT-guided radio-frequency ablation is not effective for tumors in close proximity to major branches of the portal or hepatic veins.
    (B) Resection for HCC has a better oncologic outcome compared to radio-frequency ablation for lesions 2 cm or less in diameter.
    (C) Portal hypertension is not a contraindication to resection for HCC.
    (D) According to the Barcelona Clinic Liver Cancer algorithm, resection can be undertaken in patients with Child's A and B cirrhosis only.
    (E) A patient with one hepatoma 2 cm in diameter and another hepatoma 3.5 cm in diameter is within Milan criteria for liver transplantation.

38. In an otherwise-healthy man with colorectal cancer and a 2-cm lesion metastatic to the liver, the treatment of choice is
    (A) Arterial chemoembolization
    (B) Cryoablation
    (C) Resection
    (D) Ethanol injection
    (E) Radio-frequency ablation

39. A hepatic adenoma
    (A) Cannot be distinguished from FNH on core biopsy
    (B) Should be removed if it is greater than 5 cm in diameter
    (C) Is not associated with the use of oral contraceptives
    (D) Has a benign natural history
    (E) Can be associated with various patterns of genetic mutation, but these patterns do not have an impact on the treatment

40. Alpha fetoprotein (AFP) is most likely to be elevated in the presence of
    (A) Hepatocellular carcinoma
    (B) Focal nodular hyperplasia
    (C) Hepatic adenoma
    (D) Hepatic angiosarcoma
    (E) Cholangiocarcinoma

41. A 66-year-old man is found to have an elevated carcinoembryonic antigen (CEA) value 2 years after uneventful resection of a colon carcinoma. Resectable metastatic liver lesions are identified. Which statement regarding the workup, prognosis, and treatment options is true?
    (A) Neoadjuvant chemotherapy is contraindicated due to the hepatotoxic effects.
    (B) Preoperative imaging evaluation that includes a positron emission tomographic (PET) scan obviates the need for intraoperative ultrasound.
    (C) A longer disease-free interval between the treatment of the primary lesion and the diagnosis of metastatic disease is associated with decreased survival following liver resection.
    (D) An isolated lung metastasis is a contraindication to liver resection.
    (E) Laparoscopic staging has been shown to identify disease that leads to the abandonment of the planned resection.

42. Fibrolamellar and typical HCC
    (A) Share similar prognoses when matched by stage
    (B) Have comparable elevated levels of AFP
    (C) Are both disproportionately more prevalent in males
    (D) Are both associated with cirrhosis
    (E) Have peak incidences in the same age group

ANSWERS AND EXPLANATIONS

1. **(B)** The ligamentum venosum, or Arantius's ligament, is formed early in infancy by the obliteration of the ductus venosus, which shunts blood from the left umbilical vein via the left portal vein to the IVC via the left hepatic vein. It travels within a deep visceral surface plane, attaching to lesser omentum and dividing the caudate lobe (segment 1) from the left lateral section (segments 2 and 3). The ligamentum teres hepatis, or round ligament, forms from obliteration of the umbilical vein. It travels within the falciform ligament and divides left lateral (segments 2 and 3) and left medial (segments 4A and 4B) sections. Under pressure, such as that observed in portal hypertension, the ligamentum teres hepatis can recannulate. The inferior portion of the coronary ligament, as it extends beyond the right triangular ligament to the right kidney, anchors the peritoneum in the posterior, inferior aspect to the retroperitoneum.

BIBLIOGRAPHY

Blumgart LH, Hann LE. Surgical and radiologic anatomy of the liver, biliary tract, and pancreas. In: Jarnagin WR, Belghiti J, Büchler MW, et al., eds. *Blumgart's Surgery of the Liver, Biliary Tract and Pancreas.* 5th ed., Vol. 1. Philadelphia, PA: Saunders; 2012: Chapter 1B.

Cheng EY, Zarrinpar A, Geller DA, Goss JA, Busuttil RW. Liver. In: Brunicardi FC, Andersen DK, Billiar TR, et al., eds. *Schwartz's Principles of Surgery*. 10th ed. New York, NY: McGraw-Hill; 2015: Chapter 31.

Skandalakis JE, Branum GD, Colborn GL, et al. Liver. In: Skandalakis JE, Colburn GL, Weidman TA, et al., eds. *Skandalakis' Surgical Anatomy: The Embryologic and Anatomic Basis of Modern Surgery*. Athens, Greece: Paschalidis Medical Publications; 2004.

2. **(A)** The hepatic arterial supply is usually derived from the celiac axis by way of the common hepatic artery, which becomes the proper hepatic artery after giving off the gastroduodenal branch posterior and superior to the duodenum. It accounts for 25% of hepatic blood flow, the remainder being supplied by the portal vein. It subsequently bifurcates into the right and left hepatic branches within the hepatoduodenal ligament (Fig. 22-1).

The extrahepatic arterial system does not parallel the portal channels, although the intrahepatic system does. Over 50% of the population has the same anatomic pattern. There are, however, significant variations in hepatic arterial anatomy. In 15–20% of individuals, the right hepatic artery arises from the superior mesenteric artery and is found in the posterolateral aspect of the hepatoduodenal ligament rather than its usual antero-medial course. In 3–10% of individuals, the left hepatic artery originates from the left gastric artery and is located in the gastrohepatic ligament. Both replacements occur in 1–2% of individuals. Complete replacement of the common hepatic artery, originating from the superior mesenteric artery, occurs in 1–2% of individuals.

The most common situations in which variations of hepatic arterial anatomy may be problematic are during cholecystectomy when an aberrant right hepatic artery is mistaken for the cystic artery; during liver transplantation when aberrant branches are not recognized when coming off the aorta, superior mesenteric, or gastric arteries; and during hepatobiliary resections or repairs when a replaced hepatic artery is erroneously ligated.

BIBLIOGRAPHY

Cheng EY, Zarrinpar A, Geller DA, Goss JA, Busuttil RW. Liver. In: Brunicardi FC, Andersen DK, Billiar TR, et al., eds. *Schwartz's Principles of Surgery*. 10th ed. New York, NY: McGraw-Hill; 2015: Chapter 31.

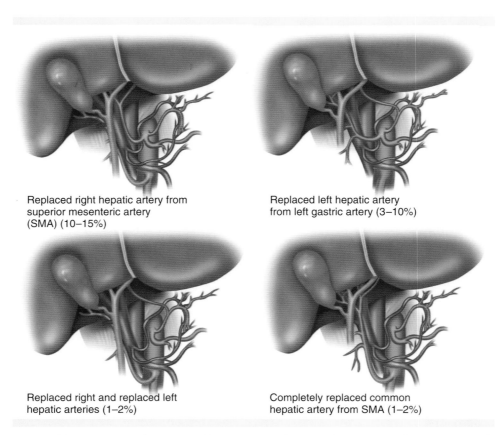

Replaced right hepatic artery from superior mesenteric artery (SMA) (10–15%)

Replaced left hepatic artery from left gastric artery (3–10%)

Replaced right and replaced left hepatic arteries (1–2%)

Completely replaced common hepatic artery from SMA (1–2%)

FIGURE 22-1. Variations of hepatic arterial anatomy (from Brunicardi FC, Andersen DK, Billiar TR, et al., eds. *Schwartz's Principles of Surgery*. 10th ed. New York, NY: McGraw-Hill; 2014: Fig. 31-5. Copyright © The McGraw-Hill Companies, Inc. All rights reserved).

Skandalakis JE, Branum GD, Colborn GL, et al. Liver. In: Skandalakis JE, Colburn GL, Weidman TA, et al., eds. *Skandalakis' Surgical Anatomy: The Embryologic and Anatomic Basis of Modern Surgery.* Athens, Greece: Paschalidis Medical Publications; 2004.

3. **(A)** Although described with some variability through history, the current surgical anatomy of the liver, as defined by the Brisbane 2000 terminology, is based on the branching of hepatic and portal veins into eight segments, as described by the French surgical anatomist, Claude Couinaud (Fig. 22-2). The main (portal) fissure passes from the left side of the gallbladder fossa to the left side of the IVC, dividing the liver into right and left; this is also referred to as *Cantlie's line* or the *midplane of the liver*. The left liver is further divided into two sections, medial (segment 4) and lateral (segments 2 and 3), by the left fissure, which notably contains the falciform ligament, pars umbilicus portion of the portal vein, and proximal left hepatic vein. The right liver is divided into anterior (segments 5 and 8) and posterior (segments 6 and 7) sections by the right fissure, which contains the right hepatic vein. Segment 1 corresponds to the caudate lobe and is considered anatomically independent of the right and left lobes, as it receives separate portal and arterial branches from both sides and drains directly into the IVC.

Of note, an alternative grouping of Couinaud segments into *sectors* (rather than sections) is based on portal vein divisions. The right liver is divided into a right anterior/paramedian sector (segments 5 and 8) and a right posterior/lateral sector (segments 6 and 7); these are anatomically identical to right anterior

and posterior sections, respectively. The left liver is divided into a left posterior/lateral sector (segment 2) and left medial/paramedian sector (segments 3 and 4, which are separated by the left fissure); these are distinctly different from the left liver sections. Care should be taken when referring to segments, sections, and sectors of the liver.

The middle, left, and right hepatic veins provide venous drainage for the liver to the IVC and travel within intersegmental planes. These veins are important anatomical landmarks for liver resections. Usually, the middle hepatic vein drains into the left hepatic vein rather than directly into the IVC.

BIBLIOGRAPHY

Blumgart LH, Hann LE. Surgical and radiologic anatomy of the liver, biliary tract, and pancreas. In: Jarnagin WR, Belghiti J, Büchler MW, et al., eds. *Blumgart's Surgery of the Liver, Biliary Tract and Pancreas.* 5th ed., Vol. 1. Philadelphia, PA: Saunders; 2012: Chapter 1B.

Cheng EY, Zarrinpar A, Geller DA, Goss JA, Busuttil RW. Liver. In: Brunicardi FC, Andersen DK, Billiar TR, et al., eds. *Schwartz's Principles of Surgery.* 10th ed. New York, NY: McGraw-Hill; 2015: Chapter 31.

Skandalakis JE, Branum GD, Colborn GL, et al. Liver. In: Skandalakis JE, Colburn GL, Weidman TA, et al., eds. *Skandalakis' Surgical Anatomy: The Embryologic and Anatomic Basis of Modern Surgery.* Athens, Greece: Paschalidis Medical Publications; 2004.

Terminology Committee of the International Hepato-Pancreato-Biliary Association. The Brisbane 2000 terminology of liver anatomy and resections. *HPB* 2000;2(3):333–339.

4. **(E)** The Brisbane 2000 terminology for hepatic resections reconciles nomenclature differences between the anatomic descriptions of Couinaud, Bismuth, Goldsmith, and Woodburne. There are three categories of resection: first, second, and third order. First-order resections refer to left and right hepatectomies (also called hemihepatectomies), with the dividing line through the midplane of the liver, with or without resection of segment 1. As the middle hepatic vein provides drainage for both left and right livers, preservation is generally performed during these procedures (Fig. 22-3).

Second-order resections involve the four sections and are referred to as *sectionectomies*. These divisions are performed through the intersectional planes. Alternatively, *sectorectomies* refer to resection of anatomical sectors as delineated by hepatic veins rather than portal watershed areas.

Third-order resections are *segmentectomies*. While resection of two contiguous segments within the same section or sector could be referred to as either a sectionectomy or sectorectomy, they also fall into the category of *bisegmentectomies*. In addition, resection of contiguous segments not within the same section or sector

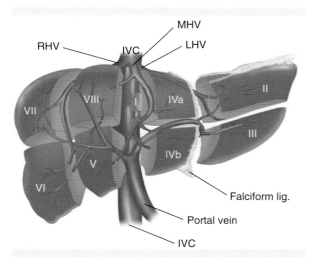

FIGURE 22-2. Couinaud segments of the liver and venous supply; LHV = left hepatic vein; MHV = middle hepatic vein; RHV = right hepatic vein (from Brunicardi FC, Andersen DK, Billiar TR, et al., eds. *Schwartz's Principles of Surgery.* 10th ed. New York, NY: McGraw-Hill; 2014: Fig. 31-21. Copyright © The McGraw-Hill Companies, Inc. All rights reserved).

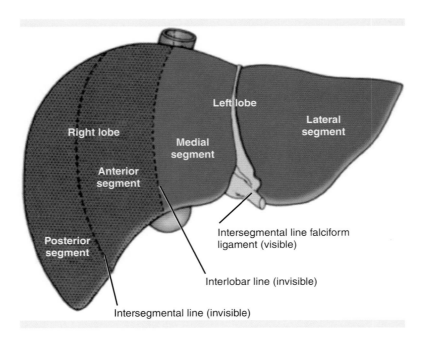

FIGURE 22-3. Liver sections and sectors. Note, the left liver is divided into lateral and medial sections, while the right is divided into anterior and posterior sections. Couniard segments are labelled 1 though 8. Cross-sectional anatomy of segments are labeled 7a though 7d. LHV = left hepatic vein; MHV = middle hepatic vein; RHV = right hepatic vein (from Ziegler MM, Azizkhan RG, von Allmen D, Weber TR, eds. *Operative Pediatric Surgery*. 2nd ed. New York, NY: McGraw-Hill; 2014: Fig. 93-7. Copyright © The McGraw-Hill Companies, Inc. All rights reserved).

(such as segments 5 and 6) would also be referred to as a *bisegmentectomy*.

Resection of three contiguous sections is preferentially termed *trisectionectomy*, with right trisectionectomy referring to resection of segments 4–8 and left trisectionectomy to segments 2–5 and 8. While the term *extended hepatectomy* is adequate, it is not preferred.

BIBLIOGRAPHY

Blumgart LH, Hann LE. Surgical and radiologic anatomy of the liver, biliary tract, and pancreas. In: Jarnagin WR, Belghiti J, Büchler MW, et al., eds. *Blumgart's Surgery of the Liver, Biliary Tract and Pancreas*. 5th ed., Vol. 1. Philadelphia, PA: Saunders; 2012: Chapter 1B.

Cheng EY, Zarrinpar A, Geller DA, Goss JA, Busuttil RW. Liver. In: Brunicardi FC, Andersen DK, Billiar TR, et al., eds. *Schwartz's Principles of Surgery*. 10th ed. New York, NY: McGraw-Hill; 2015: Chapter 31.

Skandalakis JE, Branum GD, Colborn GL, et al. Liver. In: Skandalakis JE, Colburn GL, Weidman TA, et al., eds. *Skandalakis' Surgical Anatomy: The Embryologic and Anatomic Basis of Modern Surgery*. Athens, Greece: Paschalidis Medical Publications; 2004.

Terminology Committee of the International Hepato-Pancreato-Biliary Association. The Brisbane 2000 terminology of liver anatomy and resections. *HPB*. 2000;2(3):333–339.

5. **(C)** A noncirrhotic, healthy liver may tolerate a resection of up to 75–85% of its volume, which is expected to regenerate within weeks after major resection. In addition to the general condition of the patient and tumor resectability, preoperative hepatic function and future liver remnant are primary prognostic factors. Postoperative liver volume is predicted through cross-sectional imaging, most commonly CT. Future liver remnant for patients with cirrhosis should be greater than 40%. However, this assessment method does not offer measurement of hepatic function. Some centers assess function with indocyanine green (ICG-R15) clearance, with normal retention at 15 min being less 10%. Resection is contraindicated when retention exceeds 20%. Clinically, hepatic function is usually assessed by the Child-Turcotte-Pugh scoring system (Table 22-1). Mortality and morbidity are more significant in patients with Child's B or C than those with Child's A liver function. Moreover, serum bilirubin above 2 mg/mL, clinically detectable ascites, and portal hypertension are general contraindications to liver resection. Cirrhosis is not an absolute contraindication, but it entails much less-effective liver regeneration and greater impairment of future liver function. Diabetes mellitus is not a contraindication provided that glycemic control is adequate. However, severe comorbidities, such as congestive heart failure

TABLE 22-1 Child-Turcotte-Pugh Scoring System

Points	1	2	3
Ascites	None	Small or diuretic controlled	Tense
Encephalopathy	Absent	Mild	Significant
Albumin (g/L)	>3.5	2.8–3.5	<2.8
Bilirubin (mg/dL)	<2	2–3	>3
PT (seconds > control) *or*	<4	4–6	>6
INR	<1.7	1.7–2.3	>2.3

INR, international normalized ratio; PT, prothrombin time; class A, 5 to 6 points; class B, 7 to 9 points; class C, 10 to 15 points.

and chronic kidney disease, are generally considered contraindications. Liver metastases, especially colorectal in origin, are an indication for resection provided other criteria for resection are met.

BIBLIOGRAPHY

Belghiti J, Dokmak S. Liver resection in cirrhosis. In: Jarnagin WR, Belghiti J, Büchler MW, et al., eds. *Blumgart's Surgery of the Liver, Biliary Tract and Pancreas*. 5th ed., Vol. 2. Philadelphia, PA: Saunders; 2012: Chapter 90F.

Cha C. Assessment of hepatic function: implications for the surgical patient. In: Jarnagin WR, Belghiti J, Büchler MW, et al., eds. *Blumgart's Surgery of the Liver, Biliary Tract and Pancreas*. 5th ed., Vol. 1. Philadelphia, PA: Saunders; 2012: Chapter 2.

Cheng EY, Zarrinpar A, Geller DA, Goss JA, Busuttil RW. Liver. In: Brunicardi FC, Andersen DK, Billiar TR, et al., eds. *Schwartz's Principles of Surgery*. 10th ed. New York, NY: McGraw-Hill; 2015: Chapter 31.

Maithel SK, Jarnagin WR, Belghiti J. Hepatic resection for benign disease and for liver and biliary tumors. In: Jarnagin WR, Belghiti J, Büchler MW, et al., eds. *Blumgart's Surgery of the Liver, Biliary Tract and Pancreas*. 5th ed., Vol. 2. Philadelphia, PA: Saunders; 2012: Chapter 90B.

Welling TH. Hepatectomy. In: Minter RM, Doherty GM, eds. *Current Procedures: Surgery*. New York, NY: McGraw-Hill; 2010: Chapter 14.

6. **(D)** Preoperative portal vein embolization (PVE) is a strategy for increasing FLRV prior to resection. The intervention is predicated the portal vein-dominant hepatic circulation with resultant physiologic hypertrophy in the nonembolized portion of the liver. For planned resections that would leave suboptimal FLRVs (less than 25% for healthy livers, less than 40% for diseased livers), PVE can increase the FLRV by 10 to 15%. Access to the portal vein is achieved most commonly through a percutaneous transhepatic approach. Atrophy of the embolized liver and hypertrophy of the preserved liver should occur within 4 weeks.

BIBLIOGRAPHY

Aoki T, Imamura H, Kokudo N, Makuuchi M. Preoperative portal vein embolization: rationale, indications, and results. In: Jarnagin WR, Belghiti J, Büchler MW, et al., eds. *Blumgart's Surgery of the Liver, Biliary Tract and Pancreas*. 5th ed., Vol. 2. Philadelphia, PA: Saunders; 2012: Chapter 93A.

Belghiti J, Dokmak S. Liver resection in cirrhosis. In: Jarnagin WR, Belghiti J, Büchler MW, et al., eds. *Blumgart's Surgery of the Liver, Biliary Tract and Pancreas*. 5th ed., Vol. 2. Philadelphia, PA: Saunders; 2012: Chapter 90F.

Cheng EY, Zarrinpar A, Geller DA, Goss JA, Busuttil RW. Liver. In: Brunicardi FC, Andersen DK, Billiar TR, et al., eds. *Schwartz's Principles of Surgery*. 10th ed. New York, NY: McGraw-Hill; 2015: Chapter 31.

Madoff DC. Preoperative portal vein embolization: technique. In: Jarnagin WR, Belghiti J, Büchler MW, et al., eds. *Blumgart's Surgery of the Liver, Biliary Tract and Pancreas*. 5th ed., Vol. 2. Philadelphia, PA: Saunders; 2012: Chapter 93B.

7. **(E)** As the Child's Pugh classification suggests, the presence or absence of ascites and its responsiveness to management are significant prognostic indicators for patients with cirrhosis. If the first-line treatment of diuresis fails, large-volume paracentesis is second-line therapy and is not associated with an increased risk of peritonitis. Ascites is a manifestation of increased pressure in the hepatic sinusoids, so PVT is less often associated with ascites. TIPS provides excellent control of ascites in many cases refractory to less-invasive management but is associated with the neurological deterioration seen in all portosystemic shunts. The role of Levine shunts in the modern management of ascites is limited to patients who are not candidates for TIPS or transplantation. Finally, egress of fluid through defects in the diaphragm can cause a transudative pleural effusion, which will generally respond to the same interventions as ascites (Fig. 22-4).

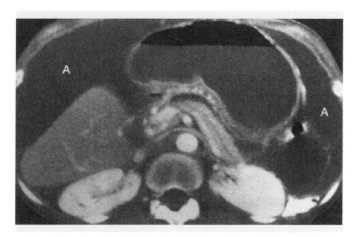

FIGURE 22-4. Abdominal ascites (A) (from Chen MYM, Pope TL, Ott DJ, eds. *Basic Radiology*. 2nd ed. New York, NY: McGraw-Hill; 2007: Fig. 11-43. Copyright © The McGraw-Hill Companies, Inc. All rights reserved).

BIBLIOGRAPHY

Caserta MP, Chaudhry F, Bechtold RE. Liver, biliary tract, and pancreas. In: Chen MYM, Pope TL, Ott DJ, eds. *Basic Radiology*. 2nd ed. New York, NY: McGraw-Hill; 2007: Chapter 11.

Cheng EY, Zarrinpar A, Geller DA, Goss JA, Busuttil RW. Liver. In: Brunicardi FC, Andersen DK, Billiar TR, et al., eds. *Schwartz's Principles of Surgery*. 10th ed. New York, NY: McGraw-Hill; 2015: Chapter 31.

Korenblat K. Management of ascites in cirrhosis and portal hypertension. In: Jarnagin WR, Belghiti J, Büchler MW, et al., eds. *Blumgart's Surgery of the Liver, Biliary Tract and Pancreas*. 5th ed., Vol. 2. Philadelphia, PA: Saunders; 2012: Chapter 74.

8. **(C)** Bleeding from the hepatic veins and the vena cava during hepatic resection is a major concern. This is more likely to occur during parenchymal transection for high and posteriorly located tumors that are closely adherent or adjacent to the vena cava. A variety of intraoperative techniques have been developed in an attempt to avoid such complications. Clamping of the portal triad or the hepatic pedicle, the so-called Pringle maneuver (Fig. 22-5), interrupts the arterial and venous inflow to the liver but has no effect on back bleeding from branches of the hepatic veins. It is indicated for both minor and major hepatic resections. This technique can be applied in either a continuous fashion until the hepatic parenchymal transection is finished or in an intermittent fashion with 15–20 min of clamping followed by 5 min of unclamping. Although the liver tolerates better the intermittent strategy, blood loss is usually more significant because of parenchymal bleeding when the clamp is released. Yet, the more important issue is tolerance of the liver to clamping, especially in patients with abnormal liver parenchyma (e.g., fatty liver and cirrhosis). Intermittent clamping is better tolerated and is

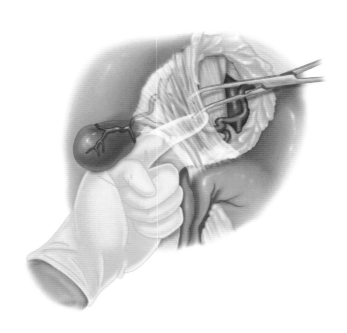

FIGURE 22-5. Pringle maneuver. In this fig., control is obtained by accessing the foramen of Winslow (epiploic foramen) under the hepatoduodenal ligament manually to provide compression prior to occlusion with a vascular clamp (from Brunicardi FC, Andersen DK, Billiar TR, et al., eds. *Schwartz's Principles of Surgery*. 10th ed. New York, NY: McGraw-Hill; 2014: Fig. 32-1. Copyright © The McGraw-Hill Companies, Inc. All rights reserved).

usually recommended to avoid deterioration of postoperative liver function.

Persistent bleeding during a Pringle maneuver is usually secondary to incomplete inflow occlusion or back bleeding from the hepatic veins. Backflow bleeding can be minimized in the majority of cases by maintaining the CVP below 5 mmHg, which can be achieved through less-aggressive fluid administration rather than more anesthesia.

Occlusion of the portal triad can be safely performed for up to 60 min under normothermic conditions and results in minimal hemodynamic changes and does not require any specific anesthetic management. However, in patients with right heart failure, pulmonary hypertension, or significant tricuspid insufficiency who are preload dependent, a low CVP strategy may not be tolerated, and total vascular exclusion should be considered.

Outflow control could be achieved by precise extrahepatic dissection of the major hepatic veins or by total vascular isolation techniques that obviate the risk of hemorrhage associated with hepatic venous control. Total hepatic vascular isolation requires occlusion of the IVC above and below the liver in addition to the Pringle maneuver and may not be hemodynamically tolerated by some patients. Venovenous bypass has been commonly used during hepatic transplantation and used in rare circumstances for hepatic resections.

BIBLIOGRAPHY

Burlew CC, Moore EE. Trauma. In: Brunicardi FC, Andersen DK, Billiar TR, et al., eds. *Schwartz's Principles of Surgery*. 10th ed. New York, NY: McGraw-Hill; 2015: Chapter 7.

Cheng EY, Zarrinpar A, Geller DA, Goss JA, Busuttil RW. Liver. In: Brunicardi FC, Andersen DK, Billiar TR, et al., eds. *Schwartz's Principles of Surgery*. 10th ed. New York, NY: McGraw-Hill; 2015: Chapter 31.

Maithel SK, Jarnagin WR, Belghiti J. Hepatic resection for benign disease and for liver and biliary tumors. In: Jarnagin WR, Belghiti J, Büchler MW, et al., eds. *Blumgart's Surgery of the Liver, Biliary Tract and Pancreas*. 5th ed., Vol. 2. Philadelphia, PA: Saunders; 2012: Chapter 90B.

9. **(D)** The portal vein provides about 75% of the liver's blood supply. It is formed by the junction of the superior mesenteric and splenic veins, dorsal to the neck of the pancreas. It ascends dorsal to the common bile duct and hepatic artery in the hepatoduodenal ligament. It has no valves, which has several important clinical implications: Portal vein pressure is similar to the pressure in portal vein tributaries, and the intrahepatic portal vein's low resistance sustains a large amount of flow.

The portal trunk divides into left and right hepatic branches in the main or portal fissure. The right portal vein divides into anterior and posterior branches approximately at the point of entry into the liver parenchyma, with both further dividing into superior and inferior branches. Of note, the caudate branch usually originates from the posterior aspect of the right portal vein. Care must be taken not to avulse this branch during exposure of the right portal vein for right hepatectomy.

The left portal vein is longer and has two portions: a longer transverse portion (pars transversus) that traverses the base of segment 4B and the pars umbilicus, which angulates anteriorly into the umbilical fissure, where it first branches laterally to segment 2, then bifurcates laterally to segment 3 and medially to segments 4A and 4B.

The right portal system is more variable than the left. More than 86% of livers have classic anatomy. About 6% have a trifurcation of the main portal vein into left, right anterior, and right posterior branches; in 7% of individuals, the right anterior branch originates from the left portal vein.

The portal vein and its branches (Fig. 22-6) have prominent hyperechoic walls on ultrasound. This has been attributed to the accompanying intrahepatic branches of the hepatic artery and bile duct, which are not usually individually seen on external ultrasound. In contrast, the hepatic veins are hypoechoic walls that increase in caliber as they course toward the IVC. Portal venous flow is normally toward the liver, is a continuous forward flow during diastole, and is of low velocity. On the other hand, flow in the hepatic veins is away from the liver and varies with the cardiorespiratory cycle.

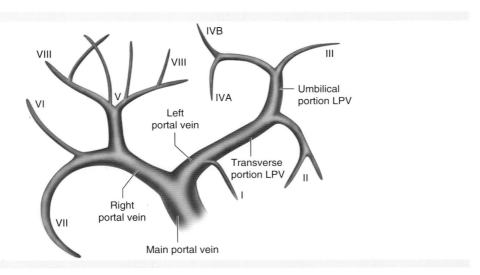

FIGURE 22-6. Further delineation of branches with associated liver segments; LPV= left portal vein (from Brunicardi FC, Andersen DK, Billiar TR, et al., eds. *Schwartz's Principles of Surgery*. 10th ed. New York, NY: McGraw-Hill; 2014: Fig. 31-7. Copyright © The McGraw-Hill Companies, Inc. All rights reserved).

BIBLIOGRAPHY

Cheng EY, Zarrinpar A, Geller DA, Goss JA, Busuttil RW. Liver. In: Brunicardi FC, Andersen DK, Billiar TR, et al., eds. *Schwartz's Principles of Surgery*. 10th ed. New York, NY: McGraw-Hill; 2015: Chapter 31.

Maithel SK, Jarnagin WR, Belghiti J. Hepatic resection for benign disease and for liver and biliary tumors. In: Jarnagin WR, Belghiti J, Büchler MW, et al., eds. *Blumgart's Surgery of the Liver, Biliary Tract and Pancreas*. 5th ed., Vol. 2. Philadelphia, PA: Saunders; 2012: Chapter 90B.

Skandalakis JE, Branum GD, Colborn GL, et al. Liver. In: Skandalakis JE, Colburn GL, Weidman TA, et al., eds. *Skandalakis' Surgical Anatomy: The Embryologic and Anatomic Basis of Modern Surgery*. Athens, Greece: Paschalidis Medical Publications; 2004.

10. **(A)** Gastroesophageal varices are the most common cause of morbidity and mortality related to portal hypertension and are present in 30–60% of patients with cirrhosis. One-third of varices will have clinically significant bleeding, which is associated with a 20–30% mortality risk and 70% risk of recurrent bleeding within 2 years among survivors. While poor coagulation factor synthesis and thrombocytopenia may also be present in and worsen variceal bleeding in patients with liver cirrhosis, the cause of these problems is not portal hypertension.

Numerous tributaries of the portal vein connect outside the liver with the systemic venous system. They have no physiologic importance under normal circumstances but will develop into large channels with increased collateral flow in the setting of portal hypertension. Portosystemic anastomoses of the most clinical importance include the following:

1. Submucosal veins of the esophagus and proximal stomach, which can receive blood from the coronary and short gastric veins to drain into the azygos veins. This pathway forms the basis of gastric and esophageal varices in portal hypertension (Fig. 22-7).

2. The superior hemorrhoidal vein, which communicates with the middle and inferior hemorrhoidal veins of the systemic circulation and may result in large hemorrhoids and significant hemorrhage.

3. Umbilical and periumbilical veins, which are recanalized from the obliterated umbilical vein in the ligamentum teres hepaticus. These account for the physical finding of caput medusae or the Cruveilhier-Baumgarten bruit in portal hypertension.

4. Collateral veins between splenic vein and left renal vein.

BIBLIOGRAPHY

Cheng EY, Zarrinpar A, Geller DA, Goss JA, Busuttil RW. Liver. In: Brunicardi FC, Andersen DK, Billiar TR, et al., eds. *Schwartz's*

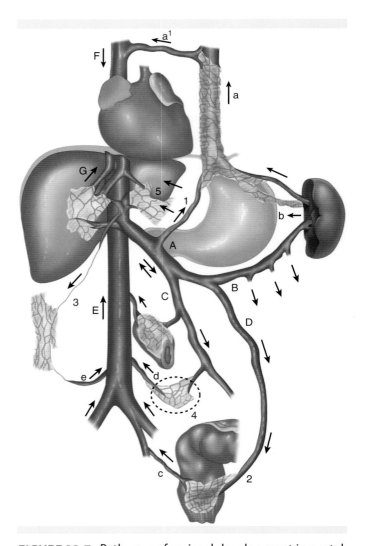

FIGURE 22-7. Pathways of variceal development in portal hypertension: 1, coronary vein; 2, superior hemorrhoidal veins; 3, paraumbilical veins; A, portal vein; B, splenic vein; C, superior mesenteric vein; D, inferior mesenteric vein; E, inferior vena cava; F, superior vena cava; G, hepatic veins; a, esophageal veins; a[1], azygos system; b, vasa brevia; c, middle and inferior hemorrhoidal veins; d, intestinal; e, epigastric veins (4, Retzius's veins; and 5, veins of Sappey, are of debatable significance) (from Brunicardi FC, Andersen DK, Billiar TR, et al., eds. *Schwartz's Principles of Surgery*. 10th ed. New York, NY: McGraw-Hill; 2014: Fig. 31-14. Copyright © The McGraw-Hill Companies, Inc. All rights reserved).

Principles of Surgery. 10th ed. New York, NY: McGraw-Hill; 2015: Chapter 31.

Pai RK, Brunt EM. Cirrhosis and portal hypertension: pathologic aspects. In: Jarnagin WR, Belghiti J, Büchler MW, et al., eds. *Blumgart's Surgery of the Liver, Biliary Tract and Pancreas*. 5th ed., Vol. 2. Philadelphia, PA: Saunders; 2012: Chapter 70A.

11. **(C)** The hepatic venous drainage is through the three major hepatic veins: right, middle, and left (Figs. 22-8 and 22-9). These begin in the liver lobules as the central veins and coalesce to form the major venous outflow.

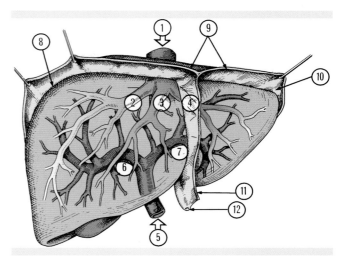

FIGURE 22-9. Venous drainage of the liver and associated relevant anatomy: (1) inferior vena cava; (2) right hepatic vein; (3) middle hepatic vein; (4) left hepatic vein; (5) portal vein; (6) right branch portal vein; (7) left branch portal vein; (8) right triangular ligament; (9) coronary ligament; (10) left triangular ligament; (11) falciform ligament; (12) ligamentum teres (from Mattox KL, Moore EE, Feliciano DV, eds. *Trauma.* 7th ed. New York, NY: McGraw-Hill Education/ Medical; 2012: Fig. 29-1. Copyright © The McGraw-Hill Companies, Inc. All rights reserved).

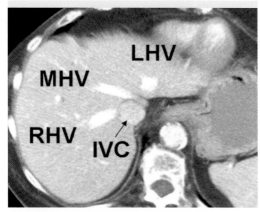

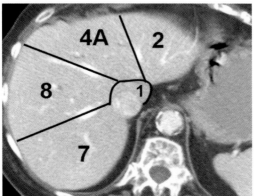

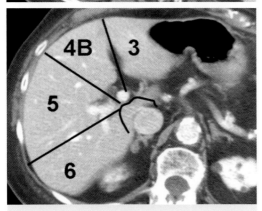

FIGURE 22-8. Venous-phase CT images demonstrating relationship of hepatic veins within liver segments. The left, middle, and right hepatic veins are converging on the inferior vena cava in the top panel, with liver segments annotated in the middle and lower panels (from Brunicardi FC, Andersen DK, Billiar TR, et al., eds. *Schwartz's Principles of Surgery.* 10th ed. New York, NY: McGraw-Hill; 2014: Fig. 31-11. Copyright © The McGraw-Hill Companies, Inc. All rights reserved).

Unlike portal veins and bile ducts, they do not parallel hepatic arteries intrahepatically. Under normal physiologic circumstances, all hepatic venous drainage flows through the hepatic veins to the IVC.

Each vein has a short extrahepatic course before draining in the IVC. They are of surgical importance because they define the three vertical fissures (or scissura) of the liver and because the short extrahepatic segment makes surgical accessibility difficult, particularly for control of traumatic hemorrhage. The right vein is the largest and drains most of the right hemiliver: segments 6, 7, and some of segments 5 and 8. The left vein drains the lateral section of the left hemiliver (segments 2 and 3) and a portion of the medial section (segments 4A and 4B) as well. The left hepatic vein is joined by the middle hepatic vein 80% of the time. The middle hepatic vein lies in the portal fissure and drains portions of segments 4, 5, and 8.

Additional posterior inferior draining hepatic veins with a short course into the anterior surface of the IVC are sometimes encountered and may be large. These accessory veins should be recognized prior to liver resection and can be visualized on cross-sectional imaging. Exact knowledge of the hepatic venous anatomy is critical for successful liver resection. A precise partial hepatectomy depends on control of the inflow vasculature, draining bile ducts, and outflow hepatic veins. Liver regeneration will be prompt if the remaining liver segment has an excellent hepatic arterial and portal venous supply, as well as biliary drainage and unobstructed hepatic venous outflow.

The caudate lobe's venous drainage is through short vessels draining posteriorly from the caudate directly into the IVC.

BIBLIOGRAPHY

Blumgart LH, Hann LE. Surgical and radiologic anatomy of the liver, biliary tract, and pancreas. In: Jarnagin WR, Belghiti J, Büchler MW, et al., eds. *Blumgart's Surgery of the Liver, Biliary Tract and Pancreas*. 5th ed., Vol. 1. Philadelphia, PA: Saunders; 2012: Chapter 1B.

Cheng EY, Zarrinpar A, Geller DA, Goss JA, Busuttil RW. Liver. In: Brunicardi FC, Andersen DK, Billiar TR, et al., eds. *Schwartz's Principles of Surgery*. 10th ed. New York, NY: McGraw-Hill; 2015: Chapter 31.

Skandalakis JE, Branum GD, Colborn GL, et al. Liver. In: Skandalakis JE, Colburn GL, Weidman TA, et al., eds. *Skandalakis' Surgical Anatomy: The Embryologic and Anatomic Basis of Modern Surgery*. Athens, Greece: Paschalidis Medical Publications; 2004.

12. **(C)** The liver consists of histological divisions of cells situated around terminal portal venules (acini) or central hepatic venules (lobules). Lobules are hexagon shaped, anatomic regions defined by venous inflow; acini are diamond-shaped regions defined by blood flow and metabolism (Fig. 22-10). In the acinus, a hepatic arteriole, a bile ductule, a lymphatic, and nerves accompany a portal venule. Blood flows from the terminal portal venule into the hepatic sinusoids, where it comes in contact with hepatocytes within the unit. It then drains into the terminal hepatic venule at the periphery of the acinar

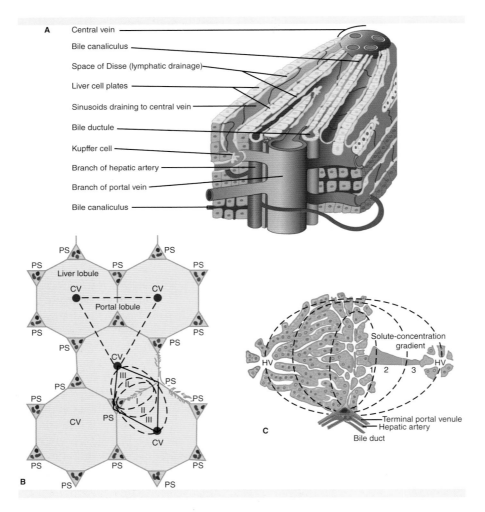

FIGURE 22-10. (A) Detailed structure of the liver lobule. (B) Relationship of lobule to acinus; CV = central vein; PS = portal space (or triad). (C) Hepatic acinus, with acinar zones 1, 2, and 3 annotated by the dashed lines; HV = hepatic venule. Reproduced with permission from Gumucio JJ. Hepatic transport. In: Kelley WN, ed. *Textbook of Medicine*. Lippincott; 1989.

unit. The hepatic venules are at the center of the histologic lobule.

Solute concentration diminishes gradually toward the central veins as they are removed by hepatocytes along the way. The hepatocytes of the acinus are divided into three zones, with zone 1 the area closest to the afferent portal venule where the sinusoids are smaller in diameter and have many collaterals. Zones 2 and 3 are farther away from the portal venule, with zone 3 closest to the central hepatic venule.

Within the acinus, there is a gradient of solute concentration and oxygen tension that is greatest near the portal venules at the center of the acinus. Hepatocytes in zone 1 receive blood with the highest concentration of oxygen, followed by zone 2 and then zone 3. Therefore, hepatocytes in zone 3 are the first to be compromised in low-flow or low-oxygenation states. This concept explains the centrilobular necrosis seen with hypotension. Zone 3 hepatocytes may also be less resistant to hepatotoxins because they receive nutritionally depleted blood. This heterogeneity in liver cells around the portal venule axis is reflected by the intracellular arrangement as well, with hepatocytes in zone 1 richer in Golgi apparatus, a requirement for bile salt transport.

BIBLIOGRAPHY

Cheng EY, Zarrinpar A, Geller DA, Goss JA, Busuttil RW. Liver. In: Brunicardi FC, Andersen DK, Billiar TR, et al., eds. *Schwartz's Principles of Surgery*. 10th ed. New York: McGraw-Hill; 2015.

Glasgow RE, Mulvihill SJ. Liver, Biliary Tract, and Pancreas. In: O'Leary JP, Tabuenca A, Capote LR, eds. *The Physiologic Basis of Surgery*. 4th ed. Philadelphia: Lippincott, Williams, and Wilkins; 2008.

Khalili M, Burman B. Liver Disease. In: Hammer GD, McPhee SJ, eds. *Pathophysiology of Disease: An Introduction to Clinical Medicine*. 7th ed. New York: McGraw-Hill; 2014.

Rocha FG. Liver Blood Flow: Physiology, Measurement, and Clinical Relevance. In: Jarnagin WR, Belghiti J, Büchler MW, et al., eds. *Blumgart's Surgery of the Liver, Biliary Tract and Pancreas*. 5th ed. Philadelphia: Saunders; 2012.

13. **(C)** Following hepatectomy, the liver can regain its normal size through regeneration even if 75–85% has been resected, provided that the liver remnant is normal. Hepatocytes constitute the main cellular elements of the liver and up to 95% of liver mass. They are highly differentiated cells, but not terminally differentiated, and have the capacity to proliferate. Nonparenchymal liver cells (such as biliary, endothelial, and Kupffer cells) also possess the ability to proliferate. During the midlife of humans, the liver regenerates to a volume of 25 ± 1.2 mL/kg; however, the exact time course for this is not known, and regeneration to roughly 75% of the preoperative liver volume within 1 year is expected. It is also known that small livers will grow to the expected liver/body ratio after liver transplantation into a larger recipient based on proliferation termination pathways.

Actual cell division occurs within days of resection, and is nearly complete within 3 months of hepatectomy in most circumstances. At the histological level, centrilobular regions (acinar zone 3) are the slowest to regenerate due to the lower oxygen delivery.

BIBLIOGRAPHY

De Jonge J, Olthoff KM. Liver regeneration: mechanisms and clinical relevance. In: Jarnagin WR, Belghiti J, Büchler MW, et al., eds. *Blumgart's Surgery of the Liver, Biliary Tract and Pancreas*. 5th ed., Vol. 1. Philadelphia, PA: Saunders; 2012: Chapter 5.

Glasgow RE, Mulvihill SJ. Liver, biliary tract, and pancreas. In: O'Leary JP, Tabuenca A, Capote LR, eds. *The Physiologic Basis of Surgery*. 4th ed. Philadelphia, PA: Lippincott, Williams, and Wilkins; 2008.

Khalili M, Burman B. Liver disease. In: Hammer GD, McPhee SJ, eds. *Pathophysiology of Disease: An Introduction to Clinical Medicine*. 7th ed. New York, NY: McGraw-Hill; 2014: Chapter 14.

14. **(A)** The liver plays a pivotal role in energy metabolism. It helps maintain homeostasis by detecting and altering components of both splanchnic and systemic blood. Indeed, most of the body's metabolic needs are regulated by the liver to some extent. The liver expends nearly 20% of the body's energy to accomplish this task, although it only constitutes 4–5% of the body weight.

In the fasting state, the liver maintains homeostasis first by glycogenolysis. The breakdown of stored glycogen will provide glucose, a critical energy source for red blood cells and the central nervous system. However, after glycogen stores are depleted, usually within 1 day of fasting commencement, the liver relies on other sources to generate glucose. Gluconeogenesis begins shortly after with the use of lactate, glycerol, and amino acids to serve as carbon sources. Lactate produced by anaerobic metabolism is metabolized only in the liver. It will be converted to pyruvate and subsequently back to glucose. This shuttling of glucose and lactate between the liver and the peripheral tissues is part of Cori's cycle.

Lipolysis occurs during prolonged fasting. The liver will oxidize fatty acids released from adipose stores into ketone bodies. These are important alternative sources of fuel for the brain and muscle. The urea cycle prepares nitrogen for excretion as urea.

BIBLIOGRAPHY

Cheng EY, Zarrinpar A, Geller DA, Goss JA, Busuttil RW. Liver. In: Brunicardi FC, Andersen DK, Billiar TR, et al., eds. *Schwartz's Principles of Surgery*. 10th ed. New York, NY: McGraw-Hill; 2015: Chapter 31.

Glasgow RE, Mulvihill SJ. Liver, biliary tract, and pancreas. In: O'Leary JP, Tabuenca A, Capote LR, eds. *Physiologic Basis of Surgery.* 4th ed. Philadelphia, PA: Lippincott, Williams, and Wilkins; 2008.

Khalili M, Burman B. Liver disease. In: Hammer GD, McPhee SJ, eds. *Pathophysiology of Disease: An Introduction to Clinical Medicine.* 7th ed. New York, NY: McGraw-Hill; 2014: Chapter 14.

15. **(A)** The liver collects and transforms plasma substrates and proteins to meet the fuel requirement of other tissues in response to various metabolic signals. It is the only organ that produces acetoacetate, for use by brain, kidney, and muscle. The liver also uses little glucose for its own metabolism.

The functional histologic unit of the liver is the acinus, at the center of which is a terminal branch of the hepatic arteriole, bile ductule, and portal vein. The acinar unit allows each cell to be in contact with sinusoidal blood and, at the same time, has an excretory pathway via a separate biliary component. The sinusoids are the major site for regulation of hepatic blood flow and solute exchange between the hepatocyte and blood. They are a low-resistance system and are lined by Kupffer cells along the luminal surface of the endothelium. Hepatocytes and membrane microvilli project through fenestrations in the endothelial cells, allowing significant access to blood and plasma. The fenestrae allow for free passage of plasma into the perisinusoidal space of Disse, where it contacts the hepatocyte membrane. Zone 1 hepatocytes, exposed to high oxygen concentrations, participate in gluconeogenesis, oxidative metabolism, and urea synthesis. Zone 3 hepatocytes are more involved in lipolysis and glycolysis.

The sinusoidal membrane that borders the perisinusoidal space of Disse is covered with microvilli that project into the perisinusoidal space. Proteins, solutes, and other substances are actively transported across. On the other hand, the flat basolateral membrane connects the hepatocyte to adjacent cells and is essential for cell-to-cell interaction. Another specialized section of the hepatocyte membrane is the canalicular membrane, which is involved in bile formation and excretion of various substances into bile. It comprises around 15% of the hepatocyte membrane and has a microvillous structure where enzymes such as alkaline phosphatase and 5′-nucleotidase are found. About 90% of bile is recirculated from enteric reabsorption, leaving just 10% that is synthesized de novo.

Perisinusoidal cells consist of the Kupffer cells, important in phagocytosis and antigen presentation; Ito cells or fat-storing cells important in collagen metabolism and vitamin A storage; and the rare pit cells, which have neuroendocrine and natural killer activity (Fig. 22-11).

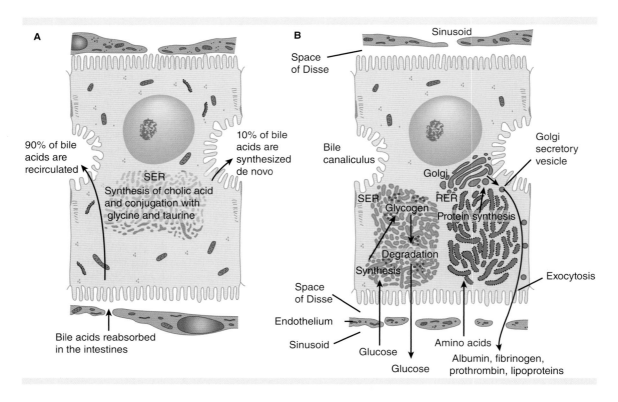

FIGURE 22-11. Perisinusoidal cells (from Hammer GD, McPhee SJ, eds. *Pathophysiology of Disease: An Introduction to Clinical Medicine.* 7th ed. New York, NY: McGraw-Hill; 2014.

BIBLIOGRAPHY

Cheng EY, Zarrinpar A, Geller DA, Goss JA, Busuttil RW. Liver. In: Brunicardi FC, Andersen DK, Billiar TR, et al., eds. *Schwartz's Principles of Surgery*. 10th ed. New York, NY: McGraw-Hill; 2015: Chapter 31.

Glasgow RE, Mulvihill SJ. Liver, biliary tract, and pancreas. In: O'Leary JP, Tabuenca A, Capote LR, eds. *The Physiologic Basis of Surgery*. 4th ed. Philadelphia, PA: Lippincott, Williams, and Wilkins; 2008.

Khalili M, Burman B. Liver disease. In: Hammer GD, McPhee SJ, eds. *Pathophysiology of Disease: An Introduction to Clinical Medicine*. 7th ed. New York, NY: McGraw-Hill; 2014: Chapter 14.

16. **(B)** The reticuloendothelial system of the liver clears the circulation of particulate matter and bacteria. Splanchnic blood returns to the liver, where initial host defenses become activated. The resultant defense mechanisms occur via Kupffer cells, neutrophils, Ito cells, endothelial cells, or the hepatocytes themselves.

Kupffer cells are liver macrophages primarily responsible for the reticuloendothelial function of the liver, and in addition to producing and controlling various cytokine and inflammatory regulators such as tumor necrosis factor and interleukin, they orchestrate the immunologic response by other cells. They also have a phagocytic function and engulf endotoxins or other microbials. They are primarily located along hepatic sinusoids.

Hepatic stellate cells, also called Ito cells, lipocytes, or fat-storing cells, line the space of Disse and play an early role in cytokine and prostaglandin production, in addition to vitamin A storage. They also contribute to the pathogenesis of cirrhosis through collagen deposition and fibrosis. Liver sinusoidal endothelial cells promote migration and sequestration of other immune cells while selectively allowing passage of antigens. Dendritic cells in the liver augment immune function via multiple pathways, including proliferation of suppressive regulatory T cells. Hepatocytes produce and degrade key cytokines and growth factors. These cells, acting in concert, constitute the hepatic defense against toxins and other pathogens.

BIBLIOGRAPHY

Bamboat ZM, Pillarisetty VG, DeMatteo RP. Liver immunology. In: Jarnagin WR, Belghiti J, Büchler MW, et al., eds. *Blumgart's Surgery of the Liver, Biliary Tract and Pancreas*. 5th ed., Vol. 1. Philadelphia, PA: Saunders; 2012: Chapter 9.

Cheng EY, Zarrinpar A, Geller DA, Goss JA, Busuttil RW. Liver. In: Brunicardi FC, Andersen DK, Billiar TR, et al., eds. *Schwartz's Principles of Surgery*. 10th ed. New York, NY: McGraw-Hill; 2015: Chapter 31.

Glasgow RE, Mulvihill SJ. Liver, biliary tract, and pancreas. In: O'Leary JP, Tabuenca A, Capote LR, eds. *The Physiologic Basis of Surgery*. 4th ed. Philadelphia, PA: Lippincott, Williams, and Wilkins; 2008.

Khalili M, Burman B. Liver disease. In: Hammer GD, McPhee SJ, eds. *Pathophysiology of Disease: An Introduction to Clinical Medicine*. 7th ed. New York, NY: McGraw-Hill; 2014: Chapter 14.

Rocha FG. Liver blood flow: physiology, measurement, and clinical relevance. In: Jarnagin WR, Belghiti J, Büchler MW, et al., eds. *Blumgart's Surgery of the Liver, Biliary Tract and Pancreas*. 5th ed., Vol. 1. Philadelphia, PA: Saunders; 2012: Chapter 4.

17. **(B)** Drug and toxin metabolism is primarily a hepatic function. Indeed, the liver is responsible for the biotransformation of endogenous and exogenous substances. For the most part, this is a protective function that detoxifies substances or biotransforms them to facilitate their elimination; however, in some instances, the by-products of hepatic metabolism are more toxic metabolites (e.g., acetaminophen toxicity).

Biotransformation performed by the liver primarily occurs in hepatocyte smooth endoplasmic reticulum and is categorized broadly into two groups:

1. Phase I reactions include oxidation, reduction, and hydrolysis. These are catalyzed by an enzyme system known as the cytochrome P-450 system. This pathway produces more hydrophilic molecules.
2. Phase II reactions are conjugation reactions, during which a compound is combined with an endogenous molecule to convert compounds from hydrophobic into hydrophilic. This conjugate is more easily excreted in bile or urine. These reactions involve an array of different enzymes.

The cytochrome P-450 system of enzymes can be upregulated or downregulated by different drugs, significantly affecting the metabolism of other concomitantly administered medications. This is termed *enzyme induction and inhibition*.

Kupffer cells are primarily involved in liver immunity. Chenodeoxycholic and cholic acids are primary bile salts that are conjugated with glycine or taurine to form conjugated bile salts.

BIBLIOGRAPHY

Cheng EY, Zarrinpar A, Geller DA, Goss JA, Busuttil RW. Liver. In: Brunicardi FC, Andersen DK, Billiar TR, et al., eds. *Schwartz's Principles of Surgery*. 10th ed. New York, NY: McGraw-Hill; 2015: Chapter 31.

Glasgow RE, Mulvihill SJ. Liver, biliary tract, and pancreas. In: O'Leary JP, Tabuenca A, Capote LR, eds. *The Physiologic Basis of Surgery*. 4th ed. Philadelphia, PA: Lippincott, Williams, and Wilkins; 2008.

Khalili M, Burman B. Liver disease. In: Hammer GD, McPhee SJ, eds. *Pathophysiology of Disease: An Introduction to Clinical Medicine*. 7th ed. New York, NY: McGraw-Hill; 2014: Chapter 14.

Rocha FG. Liver blood flow: physiology, measurement, and clinical relevance. In: Jarnagin WR, Belghiti J, Büchler MW, et al., eds. *Blumgart's Surgery of the Liver, Biliary Tract and Pancreas*. 5th ed., Vol. 1. Philadelphia, PA: Saunders; 2012: Chapter 4.

18. **(D)** The liver is the only organ that produces albumin and alpha globulins and is responsible for most of the urea synthesis in the body. It is the principal site for conversion of ammonia to urea via the urea cycle.

Often used as an index of liver synthetic capacity, albumin is the most abundant serum protein, and its level in the blood is determined by liver function, nutritional state, thyroid hormone, insulin, glucagon, and cortisol. The half-life of albumin is about 20 days, which is relatively long compared to other serum proteins. Albumin loss is augmented in certain disease states, such as sepsis, burn, nephrotic syndrome, and protein-losing enteropathies.

Transferrin and transthyretin (also called prealbumin) are also synthesized in the liver and have shorter half-lives than albumin (8–10 days and 2–3 days, respectively). Changes in transferrin and transthyretin levels therefore more accurately reflect acute changes in liver function than do changes in albumin level. However, in inflammatory states, synthesis of acute-phase proteins, such as C-reactive protein, fibrinogen, haptoglobin, and ceruloplasmin, are favored over synthesis of transferrin, transthyretin, and albumin. Of note, transferrin, transthyretin, and albumin are also used to assess nutritional status.

Several proteins involved in the coagulation cascade are also synthesized in the liver, including fibrinogen (factor I), the vitamin K–dependent factors (II, VII, IX, X), and nearly all of the procoagulation factors. Factor VII has the shortest half-life (5–7 hours), and in patients with liver dysfunction, the synthetic ability of the liver can be assessed by monitoring the prothrombin time. Like albumin, prothrombin time can be influenced by several extrahepatic factors that must be taken into account when evaluating liver synthesis.

BIBLIOGRAPHY

Cheng EY, Zarrinpar A, Geller DA, Goss JA, Busuttil RW. Liver. In: Brunicardi FC, Andersen DK, Billiar TR, et al., eds. *Schwartz's Principles of Surgery*. 10th ed. New York, NY: McGraw-Hill; 2015: Chapter 31.

Glasgow RE, Mulvihill SJ. Liver, biliary tract, and pancreas. In: O'Leary JP, Tabuenca A, Capote LR, eds. *The Physiologic Basis of Surgery*. 4th ed. Philadelphia, PA: Lippincott, Williams, and Wilkins; 2008.

Khalili M, Burman B. Liver disease. In: Hammer GD, McPhee SJ, eds. *Pathophysiology of Disease: An Introduction to Clinical Medicine*. 7th ed. New York, NY: McGraw-Hill; 2014: Chapter 14.

Martindale RG, Zhou M. Nutrition and metabolism. In: O'Leary JP, Tabuenca A, Capote LR, eds. *The Physiologic Basis of Surgery*. 4th ed. Philadelphia, PA: Lippincott, Williams, and Wilkins; 2008.

Rocha FG. Liver blood flow: physiology, measurement, and clinical relevance. In: Jarnagin WR, Belghiti J, Büchler MW, et al., eds. *Blumgart's Surgery of the Liver, Biliary Tract and Pancreas*. 5th ed., Vol. 1. Philadelphia, PA: Saunders; 2012: Chapter 4.

19. **(D)** Pyogenic liver abscesses are relatively rare, accounting for about 20 hospital admissions per 100,000. They are almost always secondary to monobacterial infection, although occasionally fungal or polymicrobial infections may be the culprit, with the underlying organism usually being specific to etiology. Positive cultures are documented in the majority of cases and mostly reveal intestinal organisms, including *Escherichia coli*, *Klebsiella*, and *Proteus*. *Staphylococcus* and *Streptococcus* occur in the setting of a skin-source infection, such as an indwelling catheter or injection drug use.

Pyogenic liver abscesses result from the following:

1. Diseases of the biliary tract, such as cholangitis and periampullary tumors.

2. Infectious gastrointestinal disorders spreading via the portal vein. These are mostly accounted for by diverticulitis, perforated ulcers, and appendicitis.

3. Hematogenous spread via the hepatic artery. This occurs in the setting of systemic bacteremia, as in subacute bacterial endocarditis.

4. Traumatic insult, either mechanical (collision, fall) or iatrogenic (chemoembolization, radio-frequency ablation)

5. Direct extension from adjacent intra-abdominal pathology, such as acute cholecystitis or colonic perforation.

6. An unknown source. These are termed *cryptogenic* pyogenic liver abscesses.

Diseases of the biliary tract are the most common cause of pyogenic liver abscesses. They account for about 20–40% of cases. Biliary obstruction from stones, strictures, or tumors leads to ascending cholangitis, resulting in multiple liver abscesses. Some cases remain of unknown etiology and are referred to as cryptogenic abscesses. These still account for up to 20 to 67% of cases. The right lobe is affected in 58–72% of cases. Diabetes mellitus is implicated in up to 40% of cases, with an associated 10-fold risk of abscess formation compared to individuals with diabetes.

A liver abscess forms once the offending organism overwhelms the hepatic defense systems. Bacteria entering the portal system are usually engulfed by Kupffer cells in the liver. Once the organisms exceed the capacity of Kupffer cells, or if the host is immunocompromised, a liver abscess may form.

Patients most commonly present with fever and chills. Other common manifestations include right upper quadrant pain, abdominal pain, jaundice, weight loss, nausea, and vomiting. Occasionally, patients present with peritonitis after intra-abdominal rupture.

Up to one-quarter of patients will be septic. Leukocytosis and elevated transaminases are common laboratory findings.

Plain abdominal films may show gas in the abscess cavity in 10–20% of cases and elevation of the right hemidiaphragm; however, ultrasonography should be the preferred initial diagnostic study when this entity is clinically suspected (Fig. 22-12A). Sonographic findings include a hypoechoic lesion with a smooth wall. The presence of gas within the abscess cavity can also frequently been seen. Ultrasound also offers evaluation of the gallbladder, biliary tract, and portal vein.

Computed tomography has the advantage of detecting intrahepatic collections as small as 0.5 cm (Fig. 22-12B). This is essential in patients with multiple small pyogenic abscesses. The lesions on CT scan are seen as well-defined round or oval cavities or poorly marginated lobulated lesions. Abscesses usually have a low internal density with circumferential contrast enhancement. MRI is another well-established sensitive modality for the diagnosis of liver abscesses. However, it does not offer clear advantages over CT or ultrasound and is usually more expensive and not as readily available.

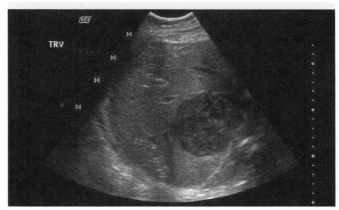

A

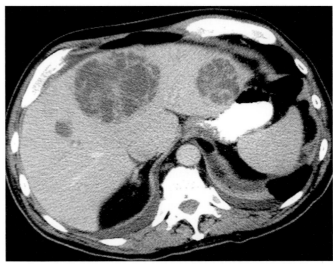

B

FIGURE 22-12. (A) Ultrasound demonstrating heterogeneous, well-circumscribed hypoechoic fluid collection consistent with liver abscess (from Zinner MJ, Ashley SW, eds. *Maingot's Abdominal Operations*. 12th ed. New York, NY: McGraw-Hill; 2013: Fig. 43-3A. Copyright © The McGraw-Hill Companies, Inc. All rights reserved). (B) CT scan with multiple loculated liver abscesses (from Brunicardi FC, Andersen DK, Billiar TR, et al., eds. *Schwartz's Principles of Surgery*. 10th ed. New York, NY: McGraw-Hill; 2014: Fig. 31-6. Copyright © The McGraw-Hill Companies, Inc. All rights reserved).

BIBLIOGRAPHY

Cheng EY, Zarrinpar A, Geller DA, Goss JA, Busuttil RW. Liver. In: Brunicardi FC, Andersen DK, Billiar TR, et al., eds. *Schwartz's Principles of Surgery*. 10th ed. New York, NY: McGraw-Hill; 2015: Chapter 31.

Christians KK, Pitt HA. Hepatic abscess and cystic disease of the liver. In: Zinner MJ, Ashley SW, eds. *Maingot's Abdominal Operations*. 12th ed. New York, NY: McGraw-Hill; 2013: Chapter 43.

Mazza OM, Santibañes ED. Pyogenic liver abscess. In: Jarnagin WR, Belghiti J, Büchler MW, et al., eds. *Blumgart's Surgery of the Liver, Biliary Tract and Pancreas*. 5th ed., Vol. 2. Philadelphia, PA: Saunders; 2012: Chapter 66.

20. **(E)** The mainstay of treatment of liver abscesses is drainage and systemic antibiotic therapy.

Drainage has been accomplished either surgically via an open or laparoscopic technique or percutaneously. Anesthetic risk of the patient, the presence or absence of coexisting intra-abdominal pathology, and the local expertise in the different available modalities are factors that determine the selection of drainage modality.

Ultrasonography or CT-directed percutaneous drainage is considered the treatment of choice for patients without surgically correctable disease, with failure rates around 10%.

Surgical drainage is indicated in cases of multiple abscesses, loculated abscesses, underlying surgically amenable disease, limited percutaneous access, and inadequate response to percutaneous drainage. Intraoperative ultrasound may be helpful in localization during the procedure. Laparoscopic drainage has also been advocated, with a reported success rate of 85% in selected patient populations. Intraoperative ultrasound should be utilized for abscess localization and complete liver examination.

Endoscopic biliary decompression is indicated in patients with abscesses that communicate with the biliary tree in the setting of biliary obstruction, but this is generally not considered as an initial management strategy as it is primarily employed to ensure antegrade biliary flow in concert with another drainage modality.

No prospective randomized trials have compared the different modalities. The choice of drainage modality should therefore be individualized depending on the source and the patient's underlying clinical condition.

Broad-spectrum coverage should be initiated on suspicion of pyogenic liver abscess, with targeted therapy following aspiration Gram stain and culture results. Empiric coverage should be directed at likely sources, taking into consideration local microbial resistance. Antibiotic therapy could be used as the only treatment modality in cases with solitary or microabscesses smaller than 2 cm in diameter, in patients in good clinical condition. The length of therapy should be individualized according to the clinical response and the number of abscesses.

Optimal management of pyogenic abscesses, however, involves not only treatment of the abscess but also correction of the underlying source.

BIBLIOGRAPHY

Cheng EY, Zarrinpar A, Geller DA, Goss JA, Busuttil RW. Liver. In: Brunicardi FC, Andersen DK, Billiar TR, et al., eds. *Schwartz's Principles of Surgery*. 10th ed. New York, NY: McGraw-Hill; 2015: Chapter 31.

Christians KK, Pitt HA. Hepatic abscess and cystic disease of the liver. In: Zinner MJ, Ashley SW, eds. *Maingot's Abdominal Operations*. 12th ed. New York, NY: McGraw-Hill; 2013: Chapter 43.

Mazza OM, Santibañes ED. Pyogenic liver abscess. In: Jarnagin WR, Belghiti J, Büchler MW, et al., eds. *Blumgart's Surgery of the Liver, Biliary Tract and Pancreas*. 5th ed., Vol. 2. Philadelphia, PA: Saunders; 2012: Chapter 66.

21. **(E)** Liver abscess complicates intestinal amebiasis in 3–10% of cases. Amebiasis is a disease with the highest incidence in subtropical and tropical climates and in areas with poor sanitation. It is more common in males and affects a younger population than pyogenic abscesses. It occurs as a result of infestation with *Entamoeba histolytica* via fecal-oral transmission. The cystic form of *E. histolytica* gains access to the host by oral ingestion of contaminated food or water. The trophozoites are then released into the gastrointestinal tract and can reach the liver via the portal system by entering the mesenteric venules. An amebic liver abscess results as the trophozoites cause cellular necrosis. It is usually solitary and surrounded by a thin-walled granulation tissue. The right lobe is most commonly involved. These abscesses are usually sterile unless secondary bacterial contamination occurs.

Signs and symptoms are similar to those seen with pyogenic liver abscesses. The patients are usually younger, however, and have a history of travel to endemic areas. The most common symptoms are fever and abdominal pain. Diarrhea is present in 20–30% of cases. The most common signs include hepatomegaly and right upper quadrant tenderness.

Serology is the diagnostic test of choice. Indirect hemagglutination and gel diffusion precipitation are the most commonly used tests, with a reported 85–95% sensitivity and specificity. Stool testing will show the cyst of the protozoon in only one-fourth of cases.

Imaging studies are essential to make the diagnosis. Ultrasonography reveals a round or oval hypoechoic lesion with well-defined margins in the setting of amebic liver abscess. CT findings include a low-density lesion with smooth margins.

The most common complication of amebic liver abscesses is secondary infection. It occurs in 10–20% of cases. Amebic abscesses can rupture into the pleura, lung, pericardium, or peritoneum. Those located in the dome of the liver may rupture through the diaphragm and result in empyema, pleural effusions, or bronchopleural fistula in up to 7% of cases. Conversely, those located on the inferior surface tend to rupture into the peritoneal cavity in 7–11% of cases.

The first line of treatment of an amebic liver abscess is pharmacologic therapy. Metronidazole is the drug of choice and is effective against both the intestinal and hepatic phases. The dose is 750 mg three times a day and should be given for 7–10 days. The response to treatment is determined by the size of the abscess. Abscesses smaller than 5 cm in diameter respond better to metronidazole therapy. Pharmacologic therapy is still the treatment of choice in the setting of uncomplicated perforation, when the abscess perforates into the pleural or pericardial cavity, or even into the peritoneal cavity if there is no peritonitis.

Routine abscess aspiration is not recommended. It may be required for the treatment of larger abscesses and may be done under ultrasound or CT guidance (Fig. 22-13).

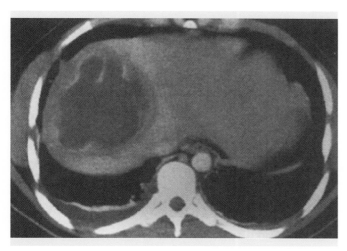

FIGURE 22-13. Amoebic abscess on CT with irregular, peripherally enhancing fluid collection within the liver; it is difficult to distinguish from a pyogenic abscess (from Chen MYM, Pope TL, Ott DJ, eds. *Basic Radiology*. 2nd ed. New York, NY: McGraw-Hill; 2007: Fig. 11-29. Copyright © The McGraw-Hill Companies, Inc. All rights reserved).

Surgical open drainage is reserved for patients with complicated amebic liver abscesses with secondary infection or perforation with peritoneal irritation or in patients who fail to respond to conservative methods.

Mortality for uncomplicated amebic abscesses should be less than 5%, in contrast to the 15–20% reported mortality rates for pyogenic abscesses.

BIBLIOGRAPHY

Caserta MP, Chaudhry F, Bechtold RE. Liver, biliary tract, and pancreas. In: Chen MYM, Pope TL, Ott DJ, eds. *Basic Radiology*. 2nd ed. New York, NY: McGraw-Hill; 2007: Chapter 11.

Cheng EY, Zarrinpar A, Geller DA, Goss JA, Busuttil RW. Liver. In: Brunicardi FC, Andersen DK, Billiar TR, et al., eds. *Schwartz's Principles of Surgery*. 10th ed. New York, NY: McGraw-Hill; 2015: Chapter 31.

Christians KK, Pitt HA. Hepatic abscess and cystic disease of the liver. In: Zinner MJ, Ashley SW, eds. *Maingot's Abdominal Operations*. 12th ed. New York, NY: McGraw-Hill; 2013: Chapter 43.

Dabbous H, Shokouh-Amiri H, Zibari G. Amebiasis and other parasitic infections. In: Jarnagin WR, Belghiti J, Büchler MW, et al., eds. *Blumgart's Surgery of the Liver, Biliary Tract and Pancreas*. 5th ed., Vol. 2. Philadelphia, PA: Saunders; 2012: Chapter 67.

22. **(B)** Hydatid disease is a zoonotic infection caused by the larval stage of the tapeworm *Echinococcus* (Fig. 22-14A). The disease has a worldwide distribution but is endemic in the Mediterranean and Baltic areas, Middle and Far East, South America, and South Africa. The only species of importance in human disease are *Echinococcus granulosus* and *Echinococcus multilocularis*. Infection occurs by fecal-oral transmission and is acquired by ingestion of the parasite eggs released in the feces of the definite host (carnivores and rodents) that harbors the adult worm in its gut. The eggs hatch after being ingested by the intermediate host (usually herbivores, accidentally humans). They migrate into different tissues and form multilayer cysts.

The liver is the most commonly involved organ in adults (50–70%). Lungs are the second-most-common site. In children, pulmonary involvement is the most common.

Clinical manifestations occur after an asymptomatic phase of variable duration. Symptoms are secondary to compression or complicated disease resulting in rupture or infection. Cyst rupture is a serious complication and can result in dissemination and hypersensitivity or anaphylactic reaction. Rupture most commonly occurs in the biliary tree and is the most common complication overall (25%). It can cause biliary obstruction by daughter cysts. There are no pathognomonic physical signs. Yet, the findings of fever, jaundice, right upper quadrant pain, and weight loss in endemic areas should raise the suspicion of hydatidosis.

Diagnosis is usually made by serologic testing. Indirect hemagglutination has good sensitivity and has largely replaced the use of the complement fixation test. The mainstay of radiologic diagnosis is by ultrasound because of its wide availability, low cost, and high diagnostic rate. CT scan of the chest and abdomen is not routinely done but is essential in planning for surgery as it gives a better definition of cyst size, number, and relation to surrounding structures (Fig. 22-14B).

Surgical therapy is the only curative approach, yet it is usually not necessary in very small cysts or calcified dead cysts. Cysts could be radically excised by a partial hepatectomy or by a pericystectomy, which involves a nonanatomic liver resection.

The laparoscopic approach has several drawbacks, primarily related to difficulty controlling spillage and the risk of recurrence. When attempted, the cyst is aspirated with subsequent injection of scolicidal agent to reduce spillage of live organisms. These agents include 70–90% ethanol, 15–20% hypertonic saline, or 0.5% silver nitrate and hydrogen peroxide. Scolicidal use in the presence of a cystobiliary fistula, which occurs 20% of the time, could result in chemical cholangitis and subsequent sclerosing cholangitis.

Albendazole is the drug of choice and is used in preparation for surgery, presumably to reduce the incidence of spillage and recurrence.

BIBLIOGRAPHY

Cheng EY, Zarrinpar A, Geller DA, Goss JA, Busuttil RW. Liver. In: Brunicardi FC, Andersen DK, Billiar TR, et al., eds. *Schwartz's Principles of Surgery*. 10th ed. New York, NY: McGraw-Hill; 2015: Chapter 31.

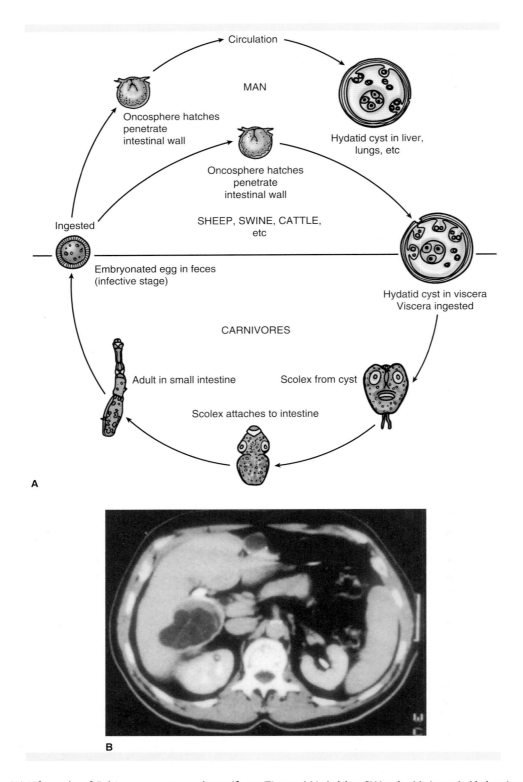

FIGURE 22-14. (A) Life cycle of *Echinococcus granulosus* (from Zinner MJ, Ashley SW, eds. *Maingot's Abdominal Operations.* 12th ed. New York, NY: McGraw-Hill; 2013: Fig. 43-8. Copyright © The McGraw-Hill Companies, Inc. All rights reserved). (B) CT scan demonstrating a heavily calcified hydatid cyst on the right and a second lightly calcified cyst on the left (from Zinner MJ, Ashley SW, eds. *Maingot's Abdominal Operations.* 12th ed. New York, NY: McGraw-Hill; 2013: Fig. 43-9B. Copyright © The McGraw-Hill Companies, Inc. All rights reserved).

Christians KK, Pitt HA. Hepatic abscess and cystic disease of the liver. In: Zinner MJ, Ashley SW, eds. *Maingot's Abdominal Operations.* 12th ed. New York, NY: McGraw-Hill; 2013: Chapter 43.

Krige J, Bornman PC, Belghiti J. Hydatid disease of the liver. In: Jarnagin WR, Belghiti J, Büchler MW, et al., eds. *Blumgart's Surgery of the Liver, Biliary Tract and Pancreas.* 5th ed., Vol. 2. Philadelphia, PA: Saunders; 2012: Chapter 68.

23. **(C)** Schistosomiasis is a disease caused by trematodes belonging to the family Schistosomatidae. Three principal species are implicated in human disease: *Schistosoma mansoni*, prevalent in Africa, the Arabian Peninsula, Brazil, and Puerto Rico; *Schistosoma japonicum*, found mainly in the Far East (Japan, China, Taiwan, and the Philippines); and *Schistosoma haematobium*, centered in the Nile valley and Africa. It is estimated that more than 200 million of the world's population are affected with this disease.

Humans acquire the disease by exposure to water contaminated by the cercaria form of the organism, which emerges in large numbers from the snail host. Conditions that contribute to the prevalence of the disease include poor sanitation, contaminated water, and a snail host required to complete the life cycle. They penetrate the human skin and enter the peripheral venules. They are carried as metacercariae to the right side of the heart and lungs and subsequently enter the systemic circulation. They mature into the adult form after they reach the hepatic bed.

In endemic areas, the schistosome is the most frequent cause of hepatic fibrosis associated with portal hypertension and is the most common cause of portal hypertension worldwide. It is mainly associated with *S. mansoni* and *S. japonicum*. Eggs that lodge in the portal areas form granuloma-like lesions, which, with the accompanying fibrosis, produce presinusoidal obstruction. Therefore, the wedged hepatic vein pressure will be normal. The disease course is slow and progressive, and many patients are actually asymptomatic. Characteristic findings are hepatosplenomegaly and, in advanced stages, variceal bleeding associated with portal hypertension.

During the acute stage, the diagnosis may be made by finding the ova in freshly passed stools. A skin test and several serologic tests are available for diagnosis. The best is the complement fixation test; however, the reliance on serologic testing alone for diagnosis is hazardous because of the significant false-positive and false-negative reactions. In patients with liver involvement, needle biopsy will reveal portal and septal fibrosis and granulomatous lesions in association with the ova. The characteristic lesion is referred to as "pipe-stem" fibrosis because of the extensive portal tract fibrosis.

Liver function, despite widespread involvement, appears to be much better than in other forms of cirrhosis. Treatment with praziquantel may reverse this fibrosis.

Surgical portal decompression may be considered for advanced stages with portal hypertension and recurrent bleeding varices.

BIBLIOGRAPHY

Cheng EY, Zarrinpar A, Geller DA, Goss JA, Busuttil RW. Liver. In: Brunicardi FC, Andersen DK, Billiar TR, et al., eds. *Schwartz's Principles of Surgery.* 10th ed. New York, NY: McGraw-Hill; 2015: Chapter 31.

Dabbous H, Shokouh-Amiri H, Zibari G. Amebiasis and other parasitic infections. In: Jarnagin WR, Belghiti J, Büchler MW, et al., eds. *Blumgart's Surgery of the Liver, Biliary Tract and Pancreas.* 5th ed., Vol. 2. Philadelphia, PA: Saunders; 2012: Chapter 67.

24. **(D)** Acute liver failure (ALF), also termed fulminant hepatic failure, is an uncommon manifestation of liver disease that constitutes a medical emergency. ALF is defined by three criteria: (1) rapid development of hepatocellular dysfunction; (2) encephalopathy within 26 weeks of injury; and (3) no prior history of liver disease. It is a clinical syndrome that encompasses a variety of disease entities, all of which cause liver injury. It is usually the end stage of hepatic cellular necrosis but could on occasion be the result of massive hepatocellular replacement, as seen with malignant infiltration.

The most common cause of ALF in the United States is drug related. It results from acetaminophen overdose, which is directly hepatotoxic and predictably produces hepatocellular necrosis with overdose (>12 g). ALF can even occur at recommended therapeutic doses (as low as 4 g) in patients with chronic alcohol abuse or those who chronically use drugs that induce cytochrome oxidases. Other drugs implicated include halothane, isoniazid, valproic acid, sulfonamides, phenytoin, and propylthiouracil.

Viral hepatitis is another major cause of ALF. Infection with HAV rarely leads to ALF, and when it does, the prognosis is usually good. HBV is the most common viral cause, yet this is an uncommon manifestation. Hepatitis D virus infection has also been implicated and requires coinfection with HBV. It can account for more than one-third of cases in patients seropositive for HBV. In specific endemic regions, infection with hepatitis C or hepatitis E has been implicated.

Other etiologies of ALF include pregnancy (usually in the third trimester, in the setting of hemolysis, elevated liver enzymes, and low platelets [HELLP] syndrome); Wilson disease; *Amanita* mushroom poisoning; autoimmune hepatitis; BCS; malignant infiltration (usually lymphoma); and ischemic hepatitis. Pediatric ALF etiologies overlap significantly with those mentioned, with the addition of metabolic diseases.

Prognosis in ALF correlates with the course of encephalopathy (Table 22-2). Liver transplantation should be considered if certain indicators of poor

TABLE 22-2 Hepatic Encephalopathy Grades

Grade	Description
0	Minimal changes in behavior and cognition
1	Notable changes in behavior, sleep pattern, and mood; normal level of consciousness
2	Disorientation, drowsiness, inappropriate behavior, slurred speech, asterixis
3	Confusion, incoherent speech, lethargy but arousable to verbal stimuli
4	Comatose, posturing, no response to verbal stimuli

prognosis are met (Table 22-3). Intensive medical management is usually required, with emphasis on identification of the etiology and prognosis evaluation. Common complications include infection, hemodynamic instability, renal failure, coagulopathy, and poor nutrition.

BIBLIOGRAPHY

Cheng EY, Zarrinpar A, Geller DA, Goss JA, Busuttil RW. Liver. In: Brunicardi FC, Andersen DK, Billiar TR, et al., eds. *Schwartz's Principles of Surgery*. 10th ed. New York, NY: McGraw-Hill; 2015: Chapter 31.

TABLE 22-3 Indicators of a Poor Prognosis in Acute Liver Failure

Acetaminophen-Induced ALF
Arterial pH < 7.3, *OR* Lactate > 3.5 or > 3.0 mg/dL after adequate fluid resuscitation, *OR* All of the following: • INR > 6.5 • Creatinine > 3.4 mg/dL • Grade 3 or 4 encephalopathy

Non–Acetaminophen-Induced ALF
INR > 6.5, *OR* Acute presentation of Wilson disease, *OR* Any three of the following: • Cryptogenic or drug (nonacetaminophen) etiology • Age < 10 years or > 40 years • Time from jaundice onset to encephalopathy > 7 days • Serum bilirubin > 17 mg/dL (300 μmol/L) • INR > 3.5

Source: Modified from the King's College Criteria.

O'Grady JG. Management of liver failure. In: Jarnagin WR, Belghiti J, Büchler MW, et al., eds. *Blumgart's Surgery of the Liver, Biliary Tract and Pancreas*. 5th ed., Vol. 2. Philadelphia, PA: Saunders; 2012: Chapter 72.

25. **(D)** Budd-Chiari syndrome encompasses a variety of problems that result in obstruction of hepatic outflow at the main hepatic veins (right, left, and/or middle), the IVC, or both. The three primary pathogenic pathways by which this occurs are trauma, thrombosis (e.g., thrombophilic disorders or underlying conditions such as infection or malignancy), or tumor (i.e., direct mechanical obstruction of the veins), although there are other causes. One rare, but notable, cause of BCS most prevalent in the Eastern Hemisphere is membranous obstruction of the vena cava (MOVC). Up to 15% of BCS cases occur during pregnancy or the postpartum period. Signs and symptoms nearly always include abdominal distention, hepatomegaly, pain, ascites, weakness, and anorexia. Patients may also present with jaundice, lower extremity edema, and similar findings as that of portal hypertension. Angiography of the IVC and hepatic veins with pressure measurements is the best diagnostic test in BCS. However, other tests, such as ultrasound and CT, may be adequate to make the diagnosis. Management of BCS is aimed at correcting thrombophilia, relieving hepatic venous pressure, preventing thrombus extension, and reversing ascites; however, prognosis for nonoperative approaches (e.g., thrombolytic therapy) remains poor. Thus, operative treatment is generally indicated and includes portacaval or cavoatrial shunting, except for MOVC, for which angioplasty or membranotomy is needed.

    Sinusoidal obstruction syndrome (SOS), formerly called hepatic veno-occlusive disease, is similar to BCS in that it involves obstruction of hepatic outflow. However, the level of obstruction is more proximal, involving the sublobular and central hepatic vein branches and sinusoids. SOS occurs most commonly after bone marrow transplantation, chemotherapy, or ingestion of pyrrolizidine alkaloids, such as certain types of traditional teas, all of which contribute to subendothelial sclerosis. In contrast to BCS, jaundice is almost always present in SOS, but laboratory abnormalities do not otherwise differ that greatly from BCS. Although thrombosis extending from the sinusoids to central veins to sublobular veins occurs, this would not likely be appreciated on ultrasound. Rather, many findings would mimic that of BCS: portal vein dilation with flow reversal and elevated hepatic artery resistive index. The key finding differentiating SOS from BCS is the absence of main hepatic vein or IVC thrombus. Management is aimed at preventing further liver damage, with consideration of anticoagulation, antithrombotics, and portacaval shunting.

Portal vein thrombosis (PVT) may exist concurrently in some patients with BCS, but this finding is not the most likely, and PVT alone would not produce hepatomegaly and severe right upper quadrant tenderness.

BIBLIOGRAPHY

Cheng EY, Zarrinpar A, Geller DA, Goss JA, Busuttil RW. Liver. In: Brunicardi FC, Andersen DK, Billiar TR, et al., eds. *Schwartz's Principles of Surgery*. 10th ed. New York, NY: McGraw-Hill; 2015: Chapter 31.

Orloff MJ, Orloff MS, Orloff SL. Budd-Chiari syndrome and venoocclusive disease. In: Jarnagin WR, Belghiti J, Büchler MW, et al., eds. *Blumgart's Surgery of the Liver, Biliary Tract and Pancreas*. 5th ed., Vol. 2. Philadelphia, PA: Saunders; 2012: Chapter 77.

26. **(D)** Emergency management of acute variceal bleeding includes standard support measures, transfusion of red blood cells to a goal hemoglobin of 8 mg/dL, antibiosis, and reduction of splanchnic blood flow with octreotide and vasopressin. Endoscopic therapy includes sclerosing and banding of bleeding varices.

Although luminal tamponade via Sengstaken-Blakemore or Minnesota tube is effective for 90% of patients with variceal bleeding, it is only a temporizer for definitive therapy.

Surgical shunting (Fig. 22-15) is performed for management of variceal bleeding when TIPS is not available or contraindicated, such as is the case with polycystic liver disease due to the profound anatomical distortions and high risk for intracystic hemorrhage (although the procedure has been reported in selected patients with cystic livers). A variety of surgical shunts have been described, all with the primary purpose of reducing portal venous pressure while balancing the known complication of hepatic encephalopathy. Distal splenorenal shunts are most commonly performed due to the preservation of portal anatomy for later transplantation, preservation of portal blood flow, and decreased risk of hepatic encephalopathy.

Liver transplantation is likely needed for this patient, but will not rectify her active bleeding in a timely manner. The nonshunting surgical interventions, such as the modified Sugiura procedure, involve splenectomy, gastric devascularization, and esophageal transection. They have the benefit of preserving portal flow, which obviates the increased risk of hepatic encephalopathy encountered in shunting procedures. However, these procedures are rarely performed in the United States as a primary choice in definitive management.

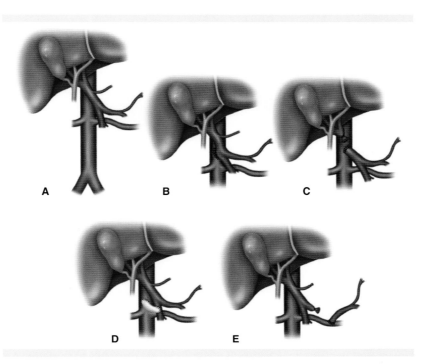

FIGURE 22-15. Surgical shunts for portal hypertension. Types of portacaval anastomoses: A, normal anatomy; B, side-to-side portacaval shunt; C, end-to-side portacaval shunt; D, mesocaval shunt; E, distal splenorenal (Warren) shunt (from Brunicardi FC, Andersen DK, Billiar TR, et al., eds. *Schwartz's Principles of Surgery*. 10th ed. New York, NY: McGraw-Hill; 2014: Fig. 31-15. Copyright © The McGraw-Hill Companies, Inc. All rights reserved).

BIBLIOGRAPHY

Awad J, Wattacheril J. Esophageal varices: acute management of portal hypertension. In: Jarnagin WR, Belghiti J, Büchler MW, et al., eds. *Blumgart's Surgery of the Liver, Biliary Tract and Pancreas.* 5th ed., Vol. 2. Philadelphia, PA: Saunders; 2012: Chapter 75B.

Cheng EY, Zarrinpar A, Geller DA, Goss JA, Busuttil RW. Liver. In: Brunicardi FC, Andersen DK, Billiar TR, et al., eds. *Schwartz's Principles of Surgery.* 10th ed. New York, NY: McGraw-Hill; 2015: Chapter 31.

Hsieh CB, Hsu KF. Esophageal varices: operative devascularization and splenectomy. In: Jarnagin WR, Belghiti J, Büchler MW, et al., eds. *Blumgart's Surgery of the Liver, Biliary Tract and Pancreas.* 5th ed., Vol. 2. Philadelphia, PA: Saunders; 2012: Chapter 75C.

Knechtle SJ, Galloway JR. Location of portosystemic shunting. In: Jarnagin WR, Belghiti J, Büchler MW, et al., eds. *Blumgart's Surgery of the Liver, Biliary Tract and Pancreas.* 5th ed., Vol. 2. Philadelphia, PA: Saunders; 2012: Chapter 76A.

27. **(B)** Hepatitis B virus is primarily transmitted by parenteral and mucous membrane exposure to infectious body fluids such as blood, serum, semen, and saliva. Risk factors include close personal or intimate exposure to an infected household contact or sexual partner, intravenous drug use, tattooing and body piercing, unapparent blood inoculations as with shared razor blades, blood transfusion or exposure to blood products, hemophilia and hemodialysis, and work in the health care profession.

Diagnosis of acute hepatitis depends on the results of specific antiviral serology (Fig. 22-16). Hospitalization is warranted for intractable symptoms of anorexia, vomiting, or severe impairment of liver function. Other symptoms include jaundice, weight loss, and malaise. Severe hepatic dysfunction manifests as renal failure, metabolic acidosis, encephalopathy, variceal bleeding, or ascites.

In adults, more than 90% of HBV infection results in self-limited acute hepatitis with subsequent resolution of the disease in 3–6 months. Approximately 10% of patients will develop chronic hepatitis, and fewer than 1% will progress to fulminant hepatitis.

Detection of the IgM antibody to hepatitis B core antigen is the most specific marker for diagnosis of acute hepatitis B. Development of antibodies to HBsAg signifies resolution of the acute infection and is the marker for cure and immunity to HBV infection. The pattern of negative HBsAg, positive anti-HBsAg, and positive anti-HBc assays is seen during the recovery phase following

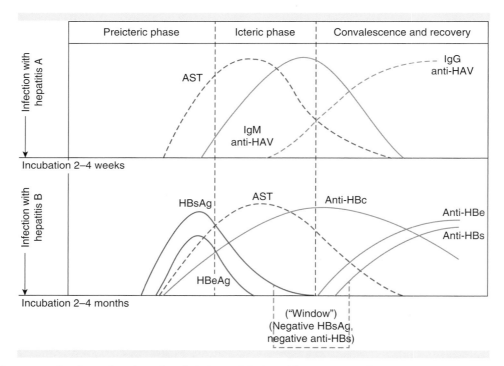

FIGURE 22-16. Serum antibody and antigen levels in hepatitis A and hepatitis B; AST = aspartate aminotransferase, a marker for hepatocellular injury and necrosis; IgM anti-HAV, early antibody response to hepatitis A infection; IgG anti-HAV, late antibody response to hepatitis A infection; HBsAg = hepatitis B surface antigen, a marker of active viral gene expression; HBeAg = hepatitis B early antigen, a marker of infectivity. Antibodies to the surface or early antigens (anti-HBs or anti-HBe) indicate immunity (Hammer GD, McPhee SJ, eds. *Pathophysiology of Disease: An Introduction to Clinical Medicine.* 7th ed. New York: McGraw-Hill; 2014).

acute hepatitis B. This antibody pattern may persist for years and is not associated with liver disease or infectivity. Coinfection with delta agent, an incomplete virus requiring HBsAg for replication, is associated with severe hepatitis and higher likelihood of fulminant hepatic failure. During acute infection, there may be a window period wherein surface antibodies remain negative and the surface antigen becomes undetectable, yet the core antibody is positive. This occurs when antibodies are bound to antigen, thus preventing detection of both.

Treatment is primarily supportive and consists of rest, fluids, and maintenance of adequate nutrition. Antiviral therapy is currently not recommended for acute hepatitis B in patients with preexisting HBsAg or anti-HBs. In patients with parenteral and sexual exposure, blood should therefore be tested for HBsAg and antibody to HBsAg prior to hepatitis B immune globulin (HBIG) administration.

Coadministration of hepatitis B vaccine with HBIG is recommended for susceptible individuals sustaining parenteral or sexual exposure and for all neonates born to HBV-positive mothers as this population is at higher risk for progressing to chronic hepatitis B.

Vaccination with the hepatitis B vaccine (genetically manufactured HBsAg particles with HBV DNA or core antigen) is universally indicated, with the initial dose given at birth and repeated at 1 and 6 months of age. It is associated with the development of anti-HBs antibody alone.

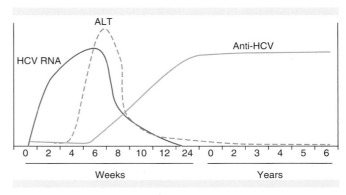

FIGURE 22-17. Acute HCV infection course; ALT = alanine aminotransferase; HCV RNA = hepatitis C viral load; anti-HCV = HCV antibody. Adapted from Hoofnagle JH. Course and outcome of hepatitis C. *Hepatology*. 2002 Nov;36(5 Suppl 1):S21–9.

BIBLIOGRAPHY

Ahmad N, Drew WL, Lagunoff M. Hepatitis viruses. In: Ryan KJ, Ray CG, eds. *Sherris Medical Microbiology.* 6th ed. New York, NY: McGraw-Hill; 2014: Chapter 13.

Cheng EY, Zarrinpar A, Geller DA, Goss JA, Busuttil RW. Liver. In: Brunicardi FC, Andersen DK, Billiar TR, et al., eds. *Schwartz's Principles of Surgery.* 10th ed. New York, NY: McGraw-Hill; 2015: Chapter 31.

Khalili M, Burman B. Liver disease. In: Hammer GD, McPhee SJ, eds. *Pathophysiology of Disease: An Introduction to Clinical Medicine.* 7th ed. New York, NY: McGraw-Hill; 2014: Chapter 14.

Shimoda M, Wands JR. Molecular biology of liver carcinogenesis and hepatitis. In: Jarnagin WR, Belghiti J, Büchler MW, et al., eds. *Blumgart's Surgery of the Liver, Biliary Tract and Pancreas.* 5th ed., Vol. 1. Philadelphia, PA: Saunders; 2012: Chapter 8C.

28. **(C)** Acute hepatitis C infection presents within a few months of exposure, if at all, because most cases of acute hepatitis C are asymptomatic (Fig. 22-17). Anti-HCV antibody is commonly not detectable until up to 6 months after the onset of symptoms. While anti-HCV is usually negative, HCV RNA is usually detectable within days to weeks following exposure. Subsequent seroconversion to positive anti-HCV confirms the diagnosis.

Transfusion of blood products was once a major risk factor for transmission of HCV. With the introduction of screening measures for potential donors and donated blood, this mode of transmission has virtually disappeared as a cause of hepatitis C. Currently, intravenous drug use accounts for the majority of new cases of acute HCV infections.

Prevention and universal precautions remain the most effective means of combating the disease. HCV exposure remains an important occupational hazard for practicing health care providers.

BIBLIOGRAPHY

Ahmad N, Drew WL, Lagunoff M. Hepatitis viruses. In: Ryan KJ, Ray CG, eds. *Sherris Medical Microbiology.* 6th ed. New York, NY: McGraw-Hill; 2014: Chapter 13.

Cheng EY, Zarrinpar A, Geller DA, Goss JA, Busuttil RW. Liver. In: Brunicardi FC, Andersen DK, Billiar TR, et al., eds. *Schwartz's Principles of Surgery.* 10th ed. New York, NY: McGraw-Hill; 2015: Chapter 31.

Khalili M, Burman B. Liver disease. In: Hammer GD, McPhee SJ, eds. *Pathophysiology of Disease: An Introduction to Clinical Medicine.* 7th ed. New York, NY: McGraw-Hill; 2014: Chapter 14.

Shimoda M, Wands JR. Molecular biology of liver carcinogenesis and hepatitis. In: Jarnagin WR, Belghiti J, Büchler MW, et al., eds. *Blumgart's Surgery of the Liver, Biliary Tract and Pancreas.* 5th ed., Vol. 1. Philadelphia, PA: Saunders; 2012: Chapter 8C.

29. **(D)** Viral hepatitis worldwide is the most common risk factor for the development of HCC. Unlike most causes of cirrhosis, hepatitis B infection does not require cirrhosis as an intermediary in the development of HCC, presumably due to the genetic derangements associated

with its integration into cellular DNA. Hepatitis C is an RNA virus that does not integrate into the genome and causes HCC by first causing inflammation and fibrosis of the liver. NASH is a risk factor for both cirrhosis and HCC and is in fact evolving into the leading risk factor for both in the United States. Almost all cases of HCC occur in the setting of cirrhosis. Aflatoxin ingestion, as well as cigarette smoking, remains important risk factors for HCC.

BIBLIOGRAPHY

Cheng EY, Zarrinpar A, Geller DA, Goss JA, Busuttil RW. Liver. In: Brunicardi FC, Andersen DK, Billiar TR, et al., eds. *Schwartz's Principles of Surgery*. 10th ed. New York, NY: McGraw-Hill; 2015: Chapter 31.

Shimoda M, Wands JR. Molecular biology of liver carcinogenesis and hepatitis. In: Jarnagin WR, Belghiti J, Büchler MW, et al., eds. *Blumgart's Surgery of the Liver, Biliary Tract and Pancreas*. 5th ed., Vol. 1. Philadelphia, PA: Saunders; 2012: Chapter 8C.

30. **(E)** Hepatocellular carcinoma can cause signs and symptoms, but they often overlap with cirrhosis and generally are seen late in the disease evolution. Screening improved survival in patients with hepatitis B in a randomized, controlled trial from China. Screening with a combination of ultrasound and serial serum AFP measurements is considered the standard strategy in patients with cirrhosis, although the usefulness of AFP has been recently called into question. Transaminases play no role in the screening process. Screening is not indicated in patients who are not candidates for treatment, such as patients with Child's class C cirrhosis or patients with poor performance status. A four-phase CT scan is the appropriate follow-up study for lesions seen on ultrasound over 1 cm in size.

BIBLIOGRAPHY

Cheng EY, Zarrinpar A, Geller DA, Goss JA, Busuttil RW. Liver. In: Brunicardi FC, Andersen DK, Billiar TR, et al., eds. *Schwartz's Principles of Surgery*. 10th ed. New York, NY: McGraw-Hill; 2015: Chapter 31.

Forner A, Reig ME, Lopes CRD, Bruix J. Hepatocellular carcinoma. In: Jarnagin WR, Belghiti J, Büchler MW, et al., eds. *Blumgart's Surgery of the Liver, Biliary Tract and Pancreas*. 5th ed., Vol. 2. Philadelphia, PA: Saunders; 2012: Chapter 80.

Shimoda M, Wands JR. Molecular biology of liver carcinogenesis and hepatitis. In: Jarnagin WR, Belghiti J, Büchler MW, et al., eds. *Blumgart's Surgery of the Liver, Biliary Tract and Pancreas*. 5th ed., Vol. 1. Philadelphia, PA: Saunders; 2012: Chapter 8C.

31. **(D)** The CT scan is the defining examination for a patient with a suspected hepatic malignancy (Fig. 22-18). Enlarged lymph nodes in the porta hepatis are common and are not a contraindication to curative treatment unless necrotic or in some other way worrisome. The diagnosis

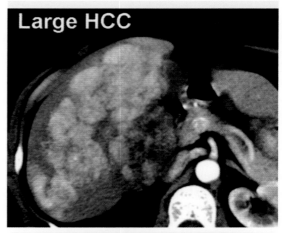
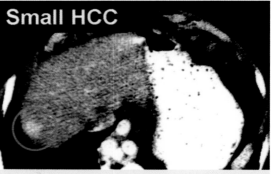

FIGURE 22-18. Abdominal CT with large and small hepatocellular carcinoma and characteristic hypervascular appearance (from Brunicardi FC, Andersen DK, Billiar TR, et al., eds. *Schwartz's Principles of Surgery*. 10th ed. New York, NY: McGraw-Hill; 2014: Fig. 31-19. Copyright © The McGraw-Hill Companies, Inc. All rights reserved).

of HCC can be made by imaging alone, and a biopsy is usually contraindicated to avoid needle tracking of the tumor. The tumor classically is more contrast enhanced than nonneoplastic liver on the arterial phase and is less enhanced on the venous or delayed phase. The CT scan can also characterize aspects of liver dysfunction relevant to surgical planning, such as ascites and portal hypertension. An MRI can serve as an adjunct to CT scanning, but intravenous contrast is required to optimize the study.

BIBLIOGRAPHY

Cheng EY, Zarrinpar A, Geller DA, Goss JA, Busuttil RW. Liver. In: Brunicardi FC, Andersen DK, Billiar TR, et al., eds. *Schwartz's Principles of Surgery*. 10th ed. New York, NY: McGraw-Hill; 2015: Chapter 31.

Shimoda M, Wands JR. Molecular biology of liver carcinogenesis and hepatitis. In: Jarnagin WR, Belghiti J, Büchler MW, et al., eds. *Blumgart's Surgery of the Liver, Biliary Tract and Pancreas*. 5th ed., Vol. 1. Philadelphia, PA: Saunders; 2012: Chapter 8C.

32. **(A)** Primary angiosarcoma of the liver accounts for up to 2% of all primary liver tumors and is the second-most-common primary malignant neoplasm of the liver. Approximately 25 new cases are diagnosed every year in the United States. Hepatic angiosarcoma is three to four times more prevalent in men than in women, most commonly occurring in adults, often in the sixth and seventh decades of life. Occurrence in children is rare. Thorotrast, arsenic, or vinyl chloride are identified as causative factors in the development of hepatic angiosarcoma in 25–40% of cases.

The overall prognosis is poor, with a median survival of only 6 months. While surgical resection provides long-term survival, the tumor is often unresectable at diagnosis, with more than half of patients presenting with distant metastases. The roles of radiotherapy and chemotherapy are limited. Transplantation offers minimal survival benefit with a high rate of recurrence.

Epithelioid hemangioendotheliomas are low-grade malignant tumors that present with a small female preference, usually between ages 30 and 50. They generally involve the entire liver with multiple nodules. The course is usually indolent, even when metastatic. Although vinyl chloride has been associated with epithelioid hemangioendotheliomas, the association is not nearly as robust as for angiosarcoma.

The other mesenchymal tumors of the hepatobiliary system are not associated with the same carcinogen exposure as that of angiosarcoma. Angiomyolipomas are benign tumors occurring primarily in middle-aged women and can be associated with tuberous sclerosis. There are three components of the tumor, as suggested by the name: (1) tortuous vessels; (2) myoid cells; and (3) fat. Undifferentiated, or embryonal, sarcoma is the third-most-common hepatic malignancy in children (following hepatoblastoma and HCC). It is aggressive, often with direct extension, and carries a poor prognosis. Rhabdomyosarcomas usually occur in children and arise from the common bile duct.

BIBLIOGRAPHY

Bedossa P, Paradis V. Tumors of the liver: pathologic aspects. In: Jarnagin WR, Belghiti J, Büchler MW, et al., eds. *Blumgart's Surgery of the Liver, Biliary Tract and Pancreas*. 5th ed., Vol. 2. Philadelphia, PA: Saunders; 2012: Chapter 78.

Cho CS, Fong Y. Benign and malignant primary liver neoplasms. In: Zinner MJ, Ashley SW, eds. *Maingot's Abdominal Operations*. 12th ed. New York, NY: McGraw-Hill; 2013: Chapter 44.

33. **(C)** The portal vein provides three-fourths of the liver's blood supply; the rest is supplied by the hepatic artery. Metastatic tumors make up the largest group of malignant tumors in the liver and reach the liver mostly as the result of shedding into the vascular system. This is most commonly caused by bronchogenic carcinoma, followed by carcinoma of the prostate, colon, breast, pancreas, stomach, kidney, and cervix. This is explained by the fact that primary tumors that drain into the portal system contribute more hepatic metastases than tumors arising outside the portal drainage system. However, in contrast to liver parenchyma, liver metastases derive nearly all their vascular inflow from branches of the hepatic artery. The same concept applies to primary liver malignancies. This difference in blood supply between normal liver and malignant liver lesion is the basis for the use of dynamic CT scans for the detection of hepatic tumors.

BIBLIOGRAPHY

Cheng EY, Zarrinpar A, Geller DA, Goss JA, Busuttil RW. Liver. In: Brunicardi FC, Andersen DK, Billiar TR, et al., eds. *Schwartz's Principles of Surgery*. 10th ed. New York, NY: McGraw-Hill; 2015: Chapter 31.

Rocha FG. Liver blood flow: physiology, measurement, and clinical relevance. In: Jarnagin WR, Belghiti J, Büchler MW, et al., eds. *Blumgart's Surgery of the Liver, Biliary Tract and Pancreas*. 5th ed., Vol. 1. Philadelphia, PA: Saunders; 2012: Chapter 4.

34. **(C)** Cavernous hemangiomas are more clinically relevant because of the associated symptoms and potential complications. They occur in all age groups but are mostly seen in the third to fifth decades of life and have a predilection for women. They are found in 2–7% of livers at autopsy, making this the most common liver tumor encountered coincidentally at laparotomy. The origin is unclear, however, and it is thought to represent progressive growth of congenital lesions.

This lesion can range in size from less than 1 mm to 30–40 cm, forming a so-called giant hemangioma. It is usually well demarcated from the surrounding liver tissue and may be partly necrotic or fibrotic. The lesions have a sponge-like appearance and do not usually present a diagnostic dilemma. They are typically expansive rather than infiltrating, leading to compression of surrounding structures along the edge of the tumor, and forming a fibrous tissue plane for dissection. No resection margin is needed.

Most patients with liver hemangiomas are asymptomatic and are diagnosed only at autopsy. Pain is usually the most common symptom, although other presentations have been reported, such as nausea, vomiting, early satiety, increased abdominal girth, and fever. Some of these symptoms can be secondary to distension of Glisson's capsule or infarction within the tumor. Biliary-related symptoms seldom occur secondary to extrinsic compression by the tumor and include obstructive jaundice and biliary colic. The great concern about spontaneous rupture with life-threatening hemorrhage is unfounded because few such cases have been reported in the literature. Moreover, acute symptoms from a hepatic hemangioma are rare and are usually because of rapid expansion with stretching of the liver capsule or thrombosis within the tumor.

Hemangiomas are occasionally present as nontender palpable masses when they reach a large size, but the physical examination is usually unremarkable. A bruit can sometimes be heard over the liver on auscultation.

Diagnosis is usually made by noninvasive radiographic imaging and has largely replaced the need for biopsy. Ultrasonography is usually the first study performed and shows a hyperechoic lesion clearly demarcated from the surrounding liver. CT scan is typically the next study obtained and shows a characteristic pattern of peripheral enhancement after contrast injection (Fig. 22-19). Delayed imaging after several minutes shows central filling of the lesion. The most sensitive test is MRI and has largely replaced hepatic angiography and ^{99}Tc red blood cell scans. A hemangioma will yield a hyperintense pattern on T2-weighted images. The classic appearance of rim enhancement with centripetal filling on delayed images during the arterial phase is also demonstrated.

Resection is indicated for clearly symptomatic lesions. Kasabach-Merritt syndrome is a rare clinical entity consisting of intravascular coagulation within the hemangioma, which can result in thrombocytopenia. This is cured by resection.

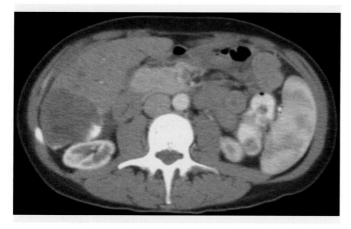

FIGURE 22-19. Arterial-phase abdominal CT with hemangioma, characterized by peripheral enhancement (from Zinner MJ, Ashley SW, eds. *Maingot's Abdominal Operations.* 12th ed. New York, NY: McGraw-Hill; 2013: Fig. 44-2. Copyright © The McGraw-Hill Companies, Inc. All rights reserved).

BIBLIOGRAPHY

Bedossa P, Paradis V. Tumors of the liver: pathologic aspects. In: Jarnagin WR, Belghiti J, Büchler MW, et al., eds. *Blumgart's Surgery of the Liver, Biliary Tract and Pancreas.* 5th ed., Vol. 2. Philadelphia, PA: Saunders; 2012: Chapter 78.

Belghiti J, Dokmak S, Vilgrain V, Paradis V. Benign liver lesions. In: Jarnagin WR, Belghiti J, Büchler MW, et al., eds. *Blumgart's Surgery of the Liver, Biliary Tract and Pancreas.* 5th ed., Vol. 2. Philadelphia, PA: Saunders; 2012: Chapter 79A.

Cheng EY, Zarrinpar A, Geller DA, Goss JA, Busuttil RW. Liver. In: Brunicardi FC, Andersen DK, Billiar TR, et al., eds. *Schwartz's Principles of Surgery.* 10th ed. New York, NY: McGraw-Hill; 2015: Chapter 31.

Cho CS, Fong Y. Benign and malignant primary liver neoplasms. In: Zinner MJ, Ashley SW, eds. *Maingot's Abdominal Operations.* 12th ed. New York, NY: McGraw-Hill; 2013: Chapter 44.

35. **(B)** Focal nodular hyperplasia is a benign, tumor-like condition that is predominantly (80–95%) diagnosed in women during their third to fifth decade of life, although it has been described in women in other age groups and in men as well.

Focal nodular hyperplasia is the second-most-common benign tumor of the liver and, like hepatic adenoma, is most often found in women of reproductive age. It is usually asymptomatic and usually discovered incidentally. The association with oral contraceptives is not well established, and other than anecdotal reports, no firm data link pregnancy and changes in the size or symptoms of FNH.

Focal nodular hyperplasia and hepatic adenoma are not always easily differentiated. An MRI with hepatocyte avid contrast can distinguish the two because the abnormal cells of an adenoma will not take up the contrast agent, but FNH hepatocytes will (Fig. 22-20). FNH can sometimes, but not always, demonstrate characteristic findings on a four-phase CT, including a central stellate scar. Similarly, the Kupffer cells generally present in an FNH will produce a warm or hot spot on a liver-spleen scan, and the absence of those cells in an adenoma will produce a cold or photopenic defect. The two lesions can generally, but not always, be distinguished on a core biopsy. It is important that the two lesions be distinguished from one another as FNH carries little, if any, risk of spontaneous rupture and no risk of malignant transformation compared to hepatic adenoma, which can rupture and can undergo malignant transformation.

Symptoms and inability to exclude malignancy are the most common indications for resection. If the diagnosis is known, enucleation is sufficient. Otherwise, a formal resection is required.

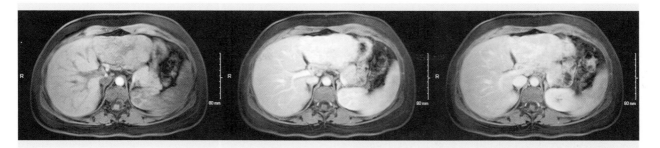

FIGURE 22-20. Magnetic resonance imaging demonstrating focal nodular hyperplasia with gradual contrast washout from the lesion and enhancement of the central scar on delayed sequences (from Zinner MJ, Ashley SW, eds. *Maingot's Abdominal Operations*. 12th ed. New York, NY: McGraw-Hill; 2013: Fig. 44-3. Copyright © The McGraw-Hill Companies, Inc. All rights reserved).

BIBLIOGRAPHY

Belghiti J, Dokmak S, Vilgrain V, Paradis V. Benign liver lesions. In: Jarnagin WR, Belghiti J, Büchler MW, et al., eds. *Blumgart's Surgery of the Liver, Biliary Tract and Pancreas*. 5th ed., Vol. 2. Philadelphia, PA: Saunders; 2012: Chapter 79A.

Cheng EY, Zarrinpar A, Geller DA, Goss JA, Busuttil RW. Liver. In: Brunicardi FC, Andersen DK, Billiar TR, et al., eds. *Schwartz's Principles of Surgery*. 10th ed. New York, NY: McGraw-Hill; 2015: Chapter 31.

Cho CS, Fong Y. Benign and malignant primary liver neoplasms. In: Zinner MJ, Ashley SW, eds. *Maingot's Abdominal Operations*. 12th ed. New York, NY: McGraw-Hill; 2013: Chapter 44.

36. **(D)** The vast majority of benign liver masses are discovered incidentally during the course of a patient's evaluation for unrelated symptoms. The majority of benign hepatic lesions will be one of the following: a cyst, a hemangioma, FNH, or a liver cell adenoma. Based on characteristic radiologic appearance, it is almost always possible to make an accurate diagnosis without the need for a liver biopsy. A biopsy, whether percutaneous or radiographically guided, is often dangerous and contraindicated in these patients.

Liver lesions more likely to cause symptoms are usually large, extend to the liver surface, occupy a large volume of the left lateral segment, or press on other viscera. In the absence of such features, the patient's symptoms are unlikely to be attributed to the liver mass, and the search for other pathology should continue.

In general, benign liver tumors should undergo operative resection when they are symptomatic, actively bleeding or present a substantial risk for bleeding, at risk for malignant transformation, or when a malignancy cannot be confidently excluded either radiologically or by biopsy when indicated.

Liver cysts are generally benign (Fig. 22-21). They may be solitary or multiple and may or may not communicate with the hepatic ductal system. They are most commonly found in the right lobe of the liver and are more frequent in males. They are usually small and asymptomatic, yet some can be quite large and can cause symptoms such as increased abdominal girth, vague pain, and rarely obstructive jaundice.

Incidentally discovered small cysts require no treatment. Simple large cysts that cause symptoms usually never require resection because most can be adequately treated by laparoscopic marsupialization or sclerotherapy (e.g., ethanol injection). If pathology of a simple cyst wall reveals evidence of ovarian stroma, it is diagnostic

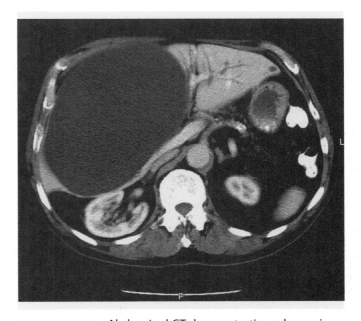

FIGURE 22-21. Abdominal CT demonstrating a large simple liver cyst with compression of the IVC, hepatic veins, and portal veins (from Zinner MJ, Ashley SW, eds. *Maingot's Abdominal Operations*. 12th ed. New York, NY: McGraw-Hill; 2013: Fig. 43-11. Copyright © The McGraw-Hill Companies, Inc. All rights reserved).

of cystadenoma, and resection is indicated because of the risk of malignant degeneration. Complex cysts with internal septae or fronds are indicative of cystadenoma or cystadenocarcinoma, and resection is advised.

BIBLIOGRAPHY

Belghiti J, Dokmak S, Vilgrain V, Paradis V. Benign liver lesions. In: Jarnagin WR, Belghiti J, Büchler MW, et al., eds. *Blumgart's Surgery of the Liver, Biliary Tract and Pancreas*. 5th ed., Vol. 2. Philadelphia, PA: Saunders; 2012: Chapter 79A.

Cheng EY, Zarrinpar A, Geller DA, Goss JA, Busuttil RW. Liver. In: Brunicardi FC, Andersen DK, Billiar TR, et al., eds. *Schwartz's Principles of Surgery*. 10th ed. New York, NY: McGraw-Hill; 2015: Chapter 31.

Christians KK, Pitt HA. Hepatic abscess and cystic disease of the liver. In: Zinner MJ, Ashley SW, eds. *Maingot's Abdominal Operations*. 12th ed. New York, NY: McGraw-Hill; 62013: Chapter 43.

Farges O, Vilgrain V. Simple cysts and polycystic liver disease: clinical and radiographic features. In: Jarnagin WR, Belghiti J, Büchler MW, et al., eds. *Blumgart's Surgery of the Liver, Biliary Tract and Pancreas*. 5th ed., Vol. 2. Philadelphia, PA: Saunders; 2012: Chapter 69A.

37. **(A)** The treatment for HCC must be informed by the anatomic specifics of the tumor, the degree of hepatic functional impairment, and the limitations of each treatment modality (Fig. 22-22). Radio-frequency ablation has equivalent oncologic outcomes compared to resection for tumors less than or equal to 2 cm; however, it will not adequately heat a tumor that is close to a major intrahepatic vessel. Resection cannot be offered to many patients with HCC because candidates must have an isolated lesion, no portal hypertension, and cirrhosis limited to Child's class A. Patients with a single tumor under 5 cm in diameter or up to three tumors each under 3 cm in diameter meet Milan criteria, which are typically used to determine eligibility for transplantation.

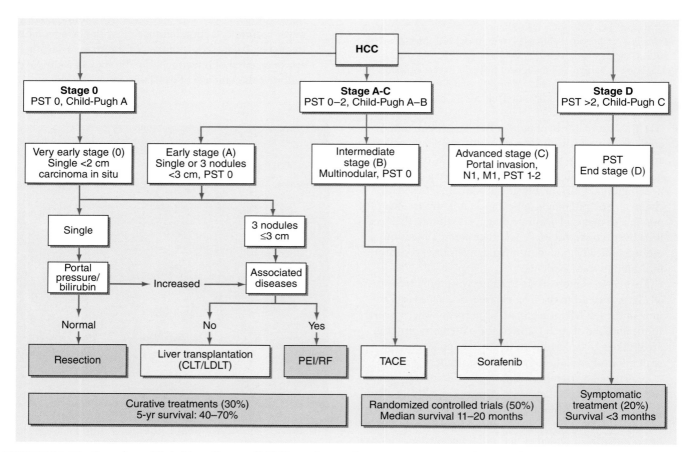

FIGURE 22-22. Barcelona Clinic Liver Cancer (BCLC) staging and treatment strategy; CLT = cadaveric liver transplantation; HCC = hepatocellular carcinoma; LDLT = living donor liver transplantation; LT = liver transplantation; PEI = percutaneous ethanol injection; PST = Performance Status Test; RF = radio-frequency ablation; TACE = transcatheter arterial chemoembolization; Used with permission from Llovet JM, et al. Design and endpoints of clinical trials in hepatocellular carcinoma. *JNCI J Natl Cancer Inst.* 2008; 100(10):698–711.

BIBLIOGRAPHY

Belghiti J, Dokmak S. Liver resection in cirrhosis. In: Jarnagin WR, Belghiti J, Büchler MW, et al., eds. *Blumgart's Surgery of the Liver, Biliary Tract and Pancreas*. 5th ed., Vol. 2. Philadelphia, PA: Saunders; 2012: Chapter 90F.

Carr BI. Tumors of the liver and biliary tree. In: Kasper D, Fauci A, Hauser S, Longo D, Jameson JL, Loscalzo J, eds. *Harrison's Principles of Internal Medicine*. 19th ed. New York, NY: McGraw-Hill; 2015: Chapter 92.

Cheng EY, Zarrinpar A, Geller DA, Goss JA, Busuttil RW. Liver. In: Brunicardi FC, Andersen DK, Billiar TR, et al., eds. *Schwartz's Principles of Surgery*. 10th ed. New York, NY: McGraw-Hill; 2015: Chapter 31.

Forner A, Reig ME, Lopes CRD, Bruix J. Hepatocellular carcinoma. In: Jarnagin WR, Belghiti J, Büchler MW, et al., eds. *Blumgart's Surgery of the Liver, Biliary Tract and Pancreas*. 5th ed., Vol. 2. Philadelphia, PA: Saunders; 2012: Chapter 80.

Llovet JM, Di Bisceglie AM, Bruix J, et al. Design and endpoints of clinical trials in hepatocellular carcinoma. *J Natl Cancer Inst.* 2008;100(10):698–711.

Maithel SK, Jarnagin WR, Belghiti J. Hepatic resection for benign disease and for liver and biliary tumors. In: Jarnagin WR, Belghiti J, Büchler MW, et al., eds. *Blumgart's Surgery of the Liver, Biliary Tract and Pancreas*. 5th ed., Vol. 2. Philadelphia, PA: Saunders; 2012: Chapter 90B.

38. **(C)** Resection, if possible, remains the treatment of choice for metastatic colorectal cancer to the liver and is associated with low operative morbidity and mortality and a concomitant long-term survival benefit. Indeed, without resection, median survival is less than 1 year, with 3-year survival approaching zero. However, 5-year survival after resection of metastatic lesions from a colorectal primary tumor is well documented in the 20% to 40% range, with selected patients approaching 70%.

When a synchronous hepatic metastasis is found during operation with a primary colorectal malignancy, the hepatic lesion may be removed simultaneously or during a separate procedure. This decision depends on the magnitude of the planned procedure as well as the extent of hepatic metastases, the general health status of the patient, and the experience of the surgeon with liver resections. In general, contraindications to major hepatic resection for metastatic disease include total hepatic replacement, advanced cirrhosis, invasion of the portal vein or vena cava, and extrahepatic metastasis.

Complete resection of hepatic metastases can be achieved in only 10–20% of patients, and palliative resection has shown no survival benefit. Nonresective destructive techniques such as cryoablation, ethanol injection, and radio-frequency ablation are currently being used to focally ablate hepatic metastases via a percutaneous or laparoscopic approach. The benefits include improved operative morbidity and mortality and less destruction of normal hepatic parenchyma. They may also allow curative resections to be performed in patients with multiple tumors or tumors involving both hepatic lobes. In addition, up to 50% of patients presenting with liver metastases will have a significant radiologic response following preoperative chemotherapy, thus converting many patients' disease from unresectable to resectable (Fig. 22-23).

BIBLIOGRAPHY

Cheng EY, Zarrinpar A, Geller DA, Goss JA, Busuttil RW. Liver. In: Brunicardi FC, Andersen DK, Billiar TR, et al., eds. *Schwartz's Principles of Surgery*. 10th ed. New York, NY: McGraw-Hill; 2015: Chapter 31.

Choti MA. Hepatic colorectal metastases: resection, pumps, and ablation. In: Zinner MJ, Ashley SW, eds. Maingot's Abdominal Operations. 12th ed. New York, NY: McGraw-Hill; 2013: Chapter 45.

Winter J, Auer RAC. Metastatic malignant liver tumors: colorectal cancer. In: Jarnagin WR, Belghiti J, Büchler MW, et al., eds. *Blumgart's Surgery of the Liver, Biliary Tract and Pancreas*. 5th ed., Vol. 2. Philadelphia, PA: Saunders; 2012: Chapter 81A.

39. **(B)** Hepatic adenomas (Fig. 22-24) are often found incidentally, but they can rupture and bleed and can degenerate into HCC; therefore, they must be thoughtfully evaluated. The diagnosis can sometimes be made through imaging alone, although there is overlap of imaging characteristics with both FNH and HCC. A biopsy is sometimes required, which will reveal an absence of portal triads, distinguishing the lesion from FNH. An absence of severe atypia and the presence of trabeculation distinguish the lesion from HCC. The association between the use of oral contraceptive pills (OCPs) and the development of hepatic adenomas is now well established, and the risk correlates with the duration of use and age above 30. Other risks factors are the use of anabolic steroids and certain glycogen storage diseases. In patients who have used OCPs for more than 2 years, the incidence is 3–4 per 100,000. About 90% of patients diagnosed with a hepatic adenoma have used OCPs in the past. The risk may indeed vary among different OCPs and depends on the amount of estrogen in the preparation. Hepatic adenomas usually persist, even after stopping OCP use. Although regression of the liver lesion has been documented, this is not universal.

Resection is generally indicated for tumors greater than 5 cm in diameter to prevent rupture. Similarly, certain genotypes and histologic phenotypes are associated with an increased risk of complications. Beta-catenin mutations that result in nuclear translocation of the protein product increase the risk of malignant degeneration and are a relative indication for resection. Plans for future pregnancy can also have an impact on the decision to resect.

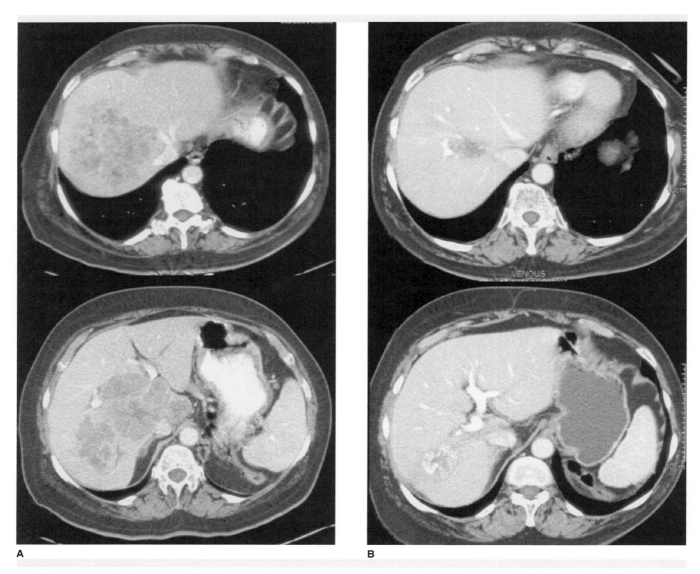

FIGURE 22-23. Abdominal CT demonstrating liver metastases from a primary colorectal cancer. (A) Before chemotherapy, unresectable tumor burden. (B) Same patient after chemotherapy, now with resectable disease (from Zinner MJ, Ashley SW, eds. *Maingot's Abdominal Operations.* 12th ed. New York, NY: McGraw-Hill; 2013: Figs. 45-3A, B. Copyright © The McGraw-Hill Companies, Inc. All rights reserved).

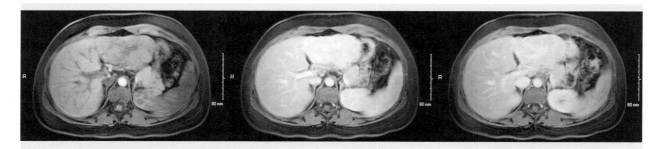

FIGURE 22-24. Computed tomography with hepatic adenoma. Hyperenhancement on arterial phase (left panel) with contrast washout seen on delayed images (middle and right panels) (from Zinner MJ, Ashley SW, eds. *Maingot's Abdominal Operations.* 12th ed. New York, NY: McGraw-Hill; 2013: Fig. 44-4. Copyright © The McGraw-Hill Companies, Inc. All rights reserved).

BIBLIOGRAPHY

Belghiti J, Dokmak S, Vilgrain V, Paradis V. Benign liver lesions. In: Jarnagin WR, Belghiti J, Büchler MW, et al., eds. *Blumgart's Surgery of the Liver, Biliary Tract and Pancreas.* 5th ed., Vol. 2. Philadelphia, PA: Saunders; 2012: Chapter 79A.

Cheng EY, Zarrinpar A, Geller DA, Goss JA, Busuttil RW. Liver. In: Brunicardi FC, Andersen DK, Billiar TR, et al., eds. *Schwartz's Principles of Surgery.* 10th ed. New York, NY: McGraw-Hill; 2015: Chapter 31.

Cho CS, Fong Y. Benign and malignant primary liver neoplasms. In: Zinner MJ, Ashley SW, eds. *Maingot's Abdominal Operations.* 12th ed. New York, NY: McGraw-Hill; 2013: Chapter 44.

40. **(A)** Alpha fetoprotein is a tumor marker in HCC and nonseminomatous testicular cancer. Although abnormal serum levels usually occur in malignant neoplasms, benign disease of endodermally derived organs, including hepatitis, inflammatory bowel disease, and cirrhosis, can cause increased levels. It was once used as a screening test for HCC, but due to poor sensitivity and specificity, the practice is controversial. However, levels above 200 µg/L have a high positive predictive value, and levels above 400 µg/L are diagnostic for HCC.

    Pronounced elevation of AFP can also be seen with teratocarcinoma, yolk sac tumors, fulminant hepatitis B infection, and occasionally metastatic pancreatic or gastric carcinoma. Mild elevation may be found in patients with chronic liver disease, acute viral hepatitis, and metastatic cancer. Elevation in the presence of hepatic adenoma is abnormal and can herald malignant transformation.

    Routine use of AFP as a screening test is controversial, although some centers still continue to do so, augmenting the recommended 6- to 12-month ultrasound screening for patients at high risk for developing HCC. Serum levels of AFP may return to normal after liver resection and is a useful marker to follow.

BIBLIOGRAPHY

Belghiti J, Dokmak S, Vilgrain V, Paradis V. Benign liver lesions. In: Jarnagin WR, Belghiti J, Büchler MW, et al., eds. *Blumgart's Surgery of the Liver, Biliary Tract and Pancreas.* 5th ed., Vol. 2. Philadelphia, PA: Saunders; 2012: Chapter 79A.

Carr BI. Tumors of the liver and biliary tree. In: Kasper D, Fauci A, Hauser S, Longo D, Jameson JL, Loscalzo J, eds. *Harrison's Principles of Internal Medicine.* 19th ed. New York, NY: McGraw-Hill; 2015: Chapter 92.

Cho CS, Fong Y. Benign and malignant primary liver neoplasms. In: Zinner MJ, Ashley SW, eds. *Maingot's Abdominal Operations.* 12th ed. New York, NY: McGraw-Hill; 2013: Chapter 44.

Forner A, Reig ME, Lopes CRD, Bruix J. Hepatocellular carcinoma. In: Jarnagin WR, Belghiti J, Büchler MW, et al., eds. *Blumgart's Surgery of the Liver, Biliary Tract and Pancreas.* 5th ed., Vol. 2. Philadelphia, PA: Saunders; 2012: Chapter 80.

41. **(E)** Irinotecan and oxaliplatin are commonly used medications in the treatment of colon cancer and have deleterious impacts on the liver histologically. However, the impact on clinical hepatic function is not great enough to preclude their use in downstaging metastases of questionable resectability.

    Intraoperative ultrasound is somewhat redundant with the other imaging modalities but can find previously occult lesions missed by CT and MRI (Fig. 22-25). It can also prove useful in the technical conduct of the operation by identifying major vascular structures.

    Many factors have an impact on long-term survival after resection of hepatic metastases from colon cancer, including the size and the number of lesions, the node status of the original tumor, and the serum CEA. The longer the disease-free interval between the primary and the development of metastases, the better the prognosis. However, even patients with a very poor projected prognosis can be long-term survivors after resection.

    Lung and other solid-organ metastases are not a contraindication to liver resection, assuming the extrahepatic disease is resectable. Long-term survivorship of 20 to 30% in this cohort is described.

    Laparoscopic evaluation is used to assess the liver surface and intra-abdominal tumor spread and can detect lesions as small as 1 mm. Because approximately 90% of

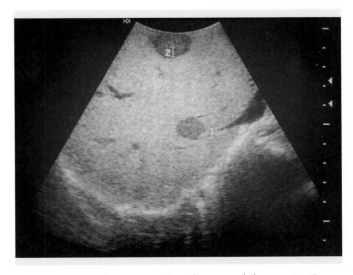

FIGURE 22-25. Intraoperative ultrasound demonstrating metastases. Used with permission from van Vledder MG, Pawlik TM, Munireddy S, Hamper U, de Jong MC, Choti MA. Factors determining the sensitivity of intraoperative ultrasonography in detecting colorectal liver metastases in the modern era. *Ann Surg Oncol.* 2010 Oct;17[10]:2756–2763.

liver metastases are present on the surface, diagnostic laparoscopy is an essential tool for evaluation prior to hepatic resection. The addition of laparoscopic ultrasound will contribute further to the prevention of unnecessary laparotomies for unresectable lesions.

BIBLIOGRAPHY

Cheng EY, Zarrinpar A, Geller DA, Goss JA, Busuttil RW. Liver. In: Brunicardi FC, Andersen DK, Billiar TR, et al., eds. *Schwartz's Principles of Surgery*. 10th ed. New York, NY: McGraw-Hill; 2015: Chapter 31.

Choti MA. Hepatic colorectal metastases: resection, pumps, and ablation. In: Zinner MJ, Ashley SW, eds. Maingot's Abdominal Operations. 12th ed. New York, NY: McGraw-Hill; 2013: Chapter 45.

Winter J, Auer RAC. Metastatic malignant liver tumors: colorectal cancer. In: Jarnagin WR, Belghiti J, Büchler MW, et al., eds. *Blumgart's Surgery of the Liver, Biliary Tract and Pancreas*. 5th ed., Vol. 2. Philadelphia, PA: Saunders; 2012: Chapter 81A.

42. **(A)** The fibrolamellar variant of HCC is relatively uncommon and accounts for less than 5% of noncirrhotic HCCs. It primarily occurs in middle-aged adults with noncirrhotic livers as a bulky lesion. Whereas standard HCC has a strong male predominance, the fibrolamellar variant affects females and males equally.

Unlike conventional HCC, the serum AFP level is rarely elevated in patients with fibrolamellar HCC. No specific risk factors for fibrolamellar HCC have been identified.

Histologically, it consists of sheets of well-differentiated hepatocytes separated by fibrous tissue. Gross features include a solitary mass sharply demarcated with scalloped borders. The lesion occurs in the left lobe in two-thirds of cases and has a central scar reminiscent of that seen in the benign process of FNH.

Fibrolamellar HCC is a slow-growing and often well-circumscribed tumor that develops in a noncirrhotic liver, allowing a successful hepatic resection in many cases. Fibrolamellar HCC carries the same prognosis as typical HCC stage per stage. The presumed better prognosis likely associated with fibrolamellar HCC is because the slow-growing tumor is often detected at an earlier stage.

BIBLIOGRAPHY

Bedossa P, Paradis V. Tumors of the liver: pathologic aspects. In: Jarnagin WR, Belghiti J, Büchler MW, et al., eds. *Blumgart's Surgery of the Liver, Biliary Tract and Pancreas*. 5th ed., Vol. 2. Philadelphia, PA: Saunders; 2012: Chapter 78.

Cho CS, Fong Y. Benign and malignant primary liver neoplasms. In: Zinner MJ, Ashley SW, eds. *Maingot's Abdominal Operations*. 12th ed. New York, NY: McGraw-Hill; 2013: Chapter 44.

CHAPTER 23

PANCREAS

KATHRYN SCHMIDT AND FABIAN JOHNSTON

QUESTIONS

1. Which of the following statements regarding pancreatic anatomy is true?
   (A) The majority of the pancreas is drained through the major papilla by the duct of Santorini.
   (B) The minor papilla communicates with the small duct of Wirsung, draining the inferior head and uncinate process.
   (C) Nervous innervation of the pancreas arises in the superior mesenteric ganglion.
   (D) Venous drainage of the pancreas is into the inferior vena cava.
   (E) Arterial supply is from branches of the celiac axis and superior mesenteric artery (SMA).

2. Which of the following is correct regarding pancreatic exocrine secretion?
   (A) The total daily volume of pancreatic secretion can be as much as 6 L.
   (B) Changes in chloride and bicarbonate concentrations in pancreatic fluid depend on the rate and volume of pancreatic secretion.
   (C) Cholecystokinin (CCK) stimulates gallbladder contraction and inhibits pancreatic enzyme secretion.
   (D) Secretin, released in response to duodenal acidification, stimulates activation of trypsinogen.
   (E) Somatostatin stimulates pancreatic enzyme secretion.

3. Which of the following is true regarding the exocrine function of the pancreas?
   (A) Starches are broken down by lipase.
   (B) Fatty acids are hydrolyzed by amylase.
   (C) Proteins are broken down by enterokinase.
   (D) Enterokinase activates trypsin (from trypsinogen), which in turn activates other digestive proenzymes.
   (E) Enzymes, in an inactive form, are made by the alpha, beta, and delta cells and are released into the pancreatic duct as zymogen granules.

4. Which of the following is true regarding the islets of Langerhans?
   (A) Alpha cells produce glucagon and comprise the innermost portion of the islet.
   (B) Beta cells produce insulin and are the smallest component of the islet volume.
   (C) Delta cells produce somatostatin and contain a subtype that is responsible for producing vasoactive intestinal peptide (VIP).
   (D) Islets account for 25% of the total pancreatic mass.
   (E) Islets in the head and uncinate process are replete with alpha cells but poor in pancreatic polypeptide (PP) cells. The converse is true of islets in the body and tail.

5. Which is of the following statements about pancreatic adenocarcinoma is true?
   (A) The 5-year survival for pancreatic cancer is 15%.
   (B) The US incidence of pancreatic cancer is approximately 100,000 cases per year.
   (C) Chronic pancreatitis is a risk factor for developing pancreatic cancer.
   (D) There is no association between cigarette smoking and pancreatic cancer.
   (E) Pain, jaundice, and weight loss are rarely presenting signs of pancreatic cancer.

6. Which of the following computed tomographic (CT) scan findings does not rule out resectability of a pancreatic head mass?
   (A) Encasement of the SMA or celiac axis
   (B) Dilated intra- and extrahepatic biliary ducts, with an engorged gallbladder
   (C) Encasement of the confluence of the superior mesenteric vein (SMV) and portal vein
   (D) Evidence of extrapancreatic disease
   (E) Absence of a fat plane between the tumor and the SMA

7. Which of the following statements regarding the pathology of pancreatic cancer is true?
   (A) The minority of pancreatic exocrine tumors arise from ductal cells.
   (B) Ductal cells constitute approximately 80% of the total mass of the pancreas.
   (C) More than three-fourths of pancreatic cancers are adenocarcinoma.
   (D) Approximately 30% of pancreatic adenocarcinomas arise in the head of the gland.
   (E) Mutations of the tumor suppressor genes p53, p16, and DPC4 are early events.

8. Which of the following is true regarding the diagnosis of acute pancreatitis?
   (A) Lipase levels normalize within 5 days of the onset of pain.
   (B) Amylase levels normalize within 48 h of the onset of pain.
   (C) Amylase levels are more sensitive than lipase levels for the diagnosis of pancreatitis.
   (D) Lipase levels are more specific than amylase levels for the diagnosis of pancreatitis.
   (E) CT findings of pancreatic inflammation are required for diagnosis.

9. Which of the following statements is *false* concerning modalities for staging pancreatic cancer?
   (A) A CT scan is extremely sensitive and specific for demonstrating nonresectable disease.
   (B) Laparoscopic staging is useful to differentiate between equivocal and resectable pancreatic cancer.
   (C) In defining respectability, laparoscopic staging combined with laparoscopic US is superior to laparoscopy alone.
   (D) A CT-guided fine-needle biopsy should be performed prior to laparoscopic staging to confirm the diagnosis.
   (E) When selecting resectable pancreatic tumors, a CT scan is sensitive in the identification of vascular invasion.

10. A 64-year-old woman has an incidentally noted 3.0-cm pancreatic cyst in the uncinate process of the pancreas. The cyst is homogeneous, with no evidence of internal septations or adjacent organ invasion. Which of the following statements is true regarding this patient's disease?
   (A) Multiple, small, well-defined cystic loculations with a central stellate scar on CT are highly suggestive of a mucinous cyst.
   (B) Mucinous cystic lesions of the pancreas are uncommon in women.

   (C) The patient should undergo a pancreaticoduodenectomy given that this type of cyst has significant malignant potential.
   (D) The CT should be repeated in 3 months and evaluated for change before surgically intervening.
   (E) Cholelithiasis is a risk factor; the patient should undergo cholecystectomy.

11. Which is true about pancreatic serous cystic neoplasms?
   (A) Serous neoplasms are distributed evenly throughout the pancreas.
   (B) CT findings are nonspecific.
   (C) Communication with the main pancreatic duct occurs in 30% of patients.
   (D) They are more common in men than women.
   (E) They stain negative with a periodic acid–Schiff (PAS) test.

12. Which of the following is true of intraductal papillary mucinous neoplasms (IPMNs)?
   (A) Pancreatitis is more common in patients with branch duct-type lesions.
   (B) Main duct-type lesions are most frequently discovered incidentally.
   (C) Branch duct-type IPMNs are more likely to demonstrate the development of malignancy.
   (D) Endoscopic retrograde cholangiopancreatography (ERCP) is the diagnostic modality of choice.
   (E) Resection is indicated for all main duct IPMN with pancreatic duct dilatation greater than or equal to 1 cm.

13. In comparing the classic, non–pylorus-preserving, pancreaticoduodenectomy to pylorus-preserving pancreaticdodenectomy (PPPD), which of the following statements is true?
   (A) The gastric emptying time is faster in the early postoperative period for PPPD.
   (B) PPPD is associated with higher surgical morbidity.
   (C) PPPD is more commonly associated with dumping syndrome at 6 months.
   (D) When performed for pancreatic adenocarcinoma, there is no difference in survival between the classic pancreaticoduodenectomy and PPPD.
   (E) In the 6-month perioperative period, the patients classically treated demonstrate improved nutritional parameters.

14. Which of the following statements is most accurate regarding chemoradiotherapy patients with pancreatic cancer?
   (A) Neoadjuvant therapy is associated with a lower rate of lymph node positivity.
   (B) Preoperative chemoradiation increases the perioperative morbidity of pancreaticoduodenectomy.

(C) Of patients who undergo neoadjuvant chemora-diation, 50% develop metastatic disease prior to surgery.
(D) Adjuvant 5-fluorouracil (5-FU) alone is the stand-ard adjuvant therapy.
(E) Adjuvant chemoradiotherapy provides a survival advantage.

15. Which of the following is true with regard to palliative strategies for unresectable pancreatic cancer?
(A) Pancreatic adenocarcinoma is an asymptomatic disease.
(B) Celiac axis neurolysis is effective in 90% of patients over the short term.
(C) Gastric outlet obstruction (GOO) in the pres-ence of unresectable disease is best treated with gastrostomy.
(D) The presence of biliary obstruction is best treated with biliary-enteric anastomosis.
(E) Prophylactic gastrojejunal anastomosis is highly recommended.

16. A 54-year-old male with a history of multiple prior admissions for exacerbations of chronic alcoholic pancreatitis comes to clinic requesting your opin-ion regarding surgical treatment for his pancreatitis. Which of the following sequelae of chronic pancreatitis would prevent him from being a candidate for longi-tudinal pancreaticojejunostomy (modified Puestow procedure)?
(A) Disabling pain requiring the use of high doses of narcotics
(B) Obstruction of the intrapancreatic common bile duct
(C) Dilated (6 mm) pancreatic duct with no strictures
(D) Diabetes
(E) Multiple strictures along the entire length of a 9-mm duct

17. A 45-year-old female with a history of gallstone pan-creatitis presents to the emergency department with abdominal pain, early satiety, nausea, and vomiting. A CT scan of the abdomen is performed, revealing a large collection of fluid within the lesser sac. Which statement is true regarding this patient's condition?
(A) The cyst wall has an epithelial lining.
(B) Pseudocyst Intraductal pappilary mucnous neo-plasm (IPMN) Mucinous cystic neoplasm (MCN) Serous cystadenoma are the most common cystic lesions of the pancreas.
(C) This fluid collection would only be called a pseu-docyst if it persists 4 weeks after an attack of acute pancreatitis.

(D) Percutaneous drainage is the preferred therapy.
(E) It is recommended that a 12-week period pass between the onset of pancreatitis and attempted surgical or endoscopic drainage.

18. Which of the following is true?
(A) The insulin gene is located on chromosome 9.
(B) Endogenous enzymatic cleavage of proinsu-lin yields equimolar amounts of insulin and C-peptide.
(C) Commercially available pharmaceutical insulin con-tains 25–50% C-peptide.
(D) The half-life of endogenous insulin is 30–60 min.
(E) There is a greater rise in plasma insulin follow-ing intravenous glucose administration than there is following an equivalent oral glucose administration.

19. A psychiatrist refers a 47-year-old female to you. She has experienced early morning confusion and weakness, followed by paroxysms of extreme anxiety and palpita-tions. She has been treated for anxiety for approximately 2 years with no improvement. She notes that frequent meals obviate these symptoms. Her serum glucose is 40 mg/dL, and contrast CT of the abdomen shows a 3-cm hyperattenuating mass. Which of the following is true regarding this condition?
(A) Elevated C-peptide levels confirm diagnosis.
(B) Hypoglycemia after a 24-h fast occurs in 95% of patients.
(C) Insulin/glucose ratio is greater than 0.3.
(D) The majority of tumors are located in the pancreatic tail.
(E) Fifty percent of tumors are benign.

20. You believe that the patient from question 19 is mani-festing Whipple's triad. The patient undergoes a super-vised 72-h fast, during which time serum glucose and insulin levels are measured every 6 h. The fast is termi-nated at 14 h because the patient develops symptoms of visual disturbances, confusion, and weakness. Blood and urine samples are obtained, and intravenous glu-cose is administered. Which of the following findings in this patient is *not* consistent with the diagnosis of insulinoma?
(A) Blood glucose of 38 mg/dL
(B) Elevated plasma insulin levels (≥6 μU/mL) during hypoglycemia
(C) Elevated C-peptide levels (≥1.2 ng/mL)
(D) Detectable urinary sulfonylurea
(E) Symptoms of confusion, amnesia, and diplopia

21. Laboratory values from the patient's 72-h fast reveal an elevated insulin-to-glucose ratio, as well as elevated pro-insulin and C-peptide levels. No urinary sulfonylurea is detected. With the patient's history and these findings, you diagnose the patient with insulinoma and schedule her for surgery. Which of the following is *false* regarding the localization of insulinomas?
    (A) Approximately two-thirds are located to the left of the SMA in the body or tail of the pancreas.
    (B) Intraoperative ultrasound can localize small tumors and their relationship to vascular and ductal structures.
    (C) Transhepatic portal venous sampling can be used to differentiate between localized and diffuse hyperinsulinism.
    (D) Because insulinomas have a poor blood supply, selective arteriography has never been useful.
    (E) Selective arterial calcium injection with hepatic venous sampling can help locate the region of the insulinoma.

22. A 35-year-old man, with a history of primary hyperparathyroidism and treated with a subtotal (three and one-half glands) parathyroidectomy, presents with a recent onset of severe gastroesophageal reflux disease (GERD) and diarrhea. A secretin stimulation test is performed, yielding an elevated serum gastrin level, approximating 500 pg/mL over baseline. Somatostatin receptor scintigraphy suggests that the patient has a pancreatic tumor. Which of the following statements regarding this disease is true?
    (A) A double-spiral CT scan is the imaging modality of choice for localizing these abdominal tumors, especially when they are smaller than 1 cm.
    (B) These tumors arise in the head of the pancreas and commonly metastasize to the duodenum.
    (C) Ninety percent of these tumors are benign.
    (D) Diarrhea associated with this syndrome can be ameliorated by nasogastric suction.
    (E) Seventy-five percent of these tumors are found in association with multiple endocrine neoplasia (MEN) 1.

23. A 55-year-old woman presented to her family doctor with an extremely pruritic rash of the groin and lower extremities. Topical treatments were ineffective. Several weeks later, she developed deep venous thrombosis and was admitted to a university hospital. During this admission, she was also diagnosed with diabetes. A plasma glucagon level is obtained and found to be markedly elevated. Which of the following is true of this patient's condition?
    (A) These are twice as common in women.
    (B) The majority are located in the pancreatic head
    (C) Malignancy is rare.

(D) Diabetes develops in 30% of patients,
(E) Diagnosis is established with plasma glucose levels.

24. A 66-year-old male undergoes a pancreaticoduodenectomy (Whipple procedure) for obstructive jaundice from a periampullary tumor. Immunohistochemical staining of the tumor is strongly positive for somatostatin. Which of the following is true of somatostatinomas?
    (A) Tumors are most commonly found in the tail of the pancreas.
    (B) They are associated with MEN 2A.
    (C) Most commonly, there are multiple tumors.
    (D) An elevated fasting somatostatin level of greater than 14 mol/L is diagnostic.
    (E) These are rarely malignant.

25. A patient is admitted to the emergency room with severe, watery diarrhea and acute renal failure. The diarrhea exceeds 3 L per day and is found to be secretory in nature. The diarrhea is also recalcitrant to standard medical therapy. As part of the workup, a plasma VIP level is obtained and found to be greater than 10 times the normal level. Which of the following is true of this diarrhea-related syndrome?
    (A) CT scan is the most sensitive imaging method.
    (B) Surgical resection is first-line treatment.
    (C) Hypokalemia and achlorhydria are common abnormalities.
    (D) Tumors are most commonly located in the pancreatic head.
    (E) Thirty percent of tumors are malignant.

26. Which of the following is true about the condition shown in Fig. 23-1?
    (A) Pancreas divisum is an anatomic variant that occurs from fusion of the ventral and dorsal pancreatic ducts.
    (B) Endoscopic stenting through the lesser papilla is curative.
    (C) Pancreas divisum is the most common congenital anomaly involving the pancreas.
    (D) The majority of patients develop pancreatitis.
    (E) The entire pancreas is drained by the duct of Wirsung.

27. Which of the following statements is most accurate regarding pancreatic fistula following pancreatic surgery?
    (A) Randomized prospective studies using octreotide have conclusively shown it prevents pancreatic fistula.
    (B) Postoperative pancreatic fistulas have been reported to occur in as many as 30% of patients.
    (C) Surgical sealants or glues to occlude pancreatic fistulas remain experimental.

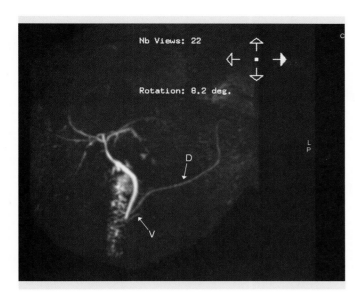

FIGURE 23-1. Magnetic resonance imaging (MRI) of classic pancreas divisum. V indicates the ventral duct draining through the major papilla and a larger dorsal duct (D) draining through the minor papilla (from Butler KL, Harisinghani M, eds. *Acute Care Surgery: Imaging Essentials for Rapid Diagnosis*. New York, NY: McGraw-Hill Education; 2014: Fig. 14-13. Copyright © McGraw-Hill Education. All rights reserved).

    (D) Reoperation is almost always contraindicated.
    (E) CT scanning of the abdomen is not essential if a fistula develops.

28. Which statement is true concerning the surgical anatomy of the pancreas?
    (A) The head lies over the first lumbar vertebra.
    (B) The lesser duct enters the third part of the duodenum.
    (C) The superior mesenteric vessels pass behind the uncinate process.
    (D) The SMA lies to the right of the SMV.
    (E) The SMV joins the portal vein behind the head of the pancreas.

29. During an exploratory laparotomy to determine the mechanism of injury by a low-velocity gunshot wound to the abdomen, the surgeon finds duodenal disruption with necrosis of the middle segment and distal bile duct disruption within the head of the pancreas. The patient is hemodynamically stable. Which of the following procedures is most appropriate?
    (A) Whipple
    (B) Duodenojejunostomy with placement of drains around the pancreas and bile duct

    (C) Pyloric exclusion, gastrojejunostomy, and wide pancreatic biliary drainage
    (D) Cholecystojejunostomy, ligation of the distal bile duct, and wide pancreatic biliary drainage
    (E) Near-total pancreatectomy and biliary-enteric reconstruction

30. A 10-year-old child develops severe abdominal pain while in the hospital for a viral syndrome. She experiences less pain when she sits up and leans forward. Laboratory studies reveal an amylase level of 180 and white blood cell (WBC) count of 15,000. A CT scan of the abdomen further reveals an edematous pancreatic gland and retroperitoneal stranding. What is the most likely cause of her pancreatitis?
    (A) Gallstone pancreatitis
    (B) Coxsackie virus infection
    (C) Heterotopic pancreas
    (D) Drug-induced pancreatitis
    (E) Spherocytosis

ANSWERS AND EXPLANATIONS

1. **(E)** The majority of the pancreas is drained through the minor papilla, rather than the major papilla, by the duct of Santorini. The major papilla communicates with the small duct of Wirsung, draining the inferior head and uncinate process. Nervous innervation of the pancreas is both sympathetic from the splanchnic nerves and parasympathetic from the vagus. The main pathways for pain sensation are the sympathetic nerves from the celiac ganglion (Fig. 23-2); therefore, splanchnicectomy targets the sympathetic nerves to alleviate pain from chronic pancreatitis.

    Arterial supply to the pancreas is from branches of the celiac artery and SMA, which converge via the superior and inferior pancreaticoduodenal arteries. The celiac axis arises from the abdominal aorta and most commonly gives rise to the splenic artery, the left gastric artery, and the common hepatic artery. The splenic artery courses along the posterior surface of the pancreatic body and tail and gives rise to branches that supply the pancreatic body and tail. The gastroduodenal artery (GDA) is the first branch off the common hepatic artery. Distal to the first portion of the duodenum, the GDA becomes the superior pancreaticoduodenal artery, which divides into anterior and posterior branches.

    The SMA gives rise to the inferior pancreaticoduodenal artery, which also divides into anterior and posterior branches. The inferior and superior pancreaticoduodenal arcades form an extensive collateral network with the superior pancreaticoduodenal arcades, supplying both the duodenum and head of the pancreas.

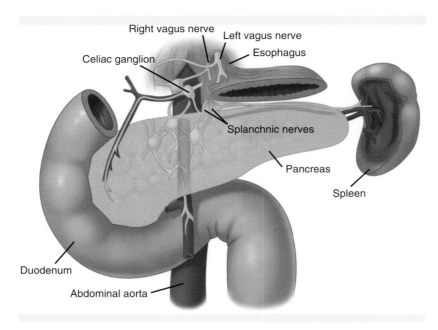

FIGURE 23-2. Pancreatic innervation. Reproduced with permission from Bell RH Jr. Atlas of pancreatic surgery. In: Bell RH Jr, Rikkers LF, Mulholland MW, eds. *Digestive Tract Surgery: A Text and Atlas*. Philadelphia: Lippincott-Raven; 1996:p 969.

Venous drainage of the pancreas is into the portal vein (Fig. 23-3). The superior venous arcades drain the pancreatic head either directly into the suprapancreatic portal vein or laterally into the retropancreatic portal vein. The anterior and inferior pancreaticoduodenal arcades drain the pancreatic head directly into the infrapancreatic SMV. The body and tail of the pancreas are drained into the splenic vein, which joins the SMV posterior to the pancreatic neck, forming the portal vein. The three named tributaries of the splenic are the inferior

pancreatic vein, the caudal pancreatic vein, and the great pancreatic vein. The inferior mesenteric vein does not drain the pancreas but joins the splenic vein posterior to the pancreatic body.

BIBLIOGRAPHY

Jensen E, Borja-Cacho D, Al-Refaie W, Vickers S. Exocrine pancreas. In: Townsend C Jr, Beauchamp R, Evers B, Mattox K, eds.

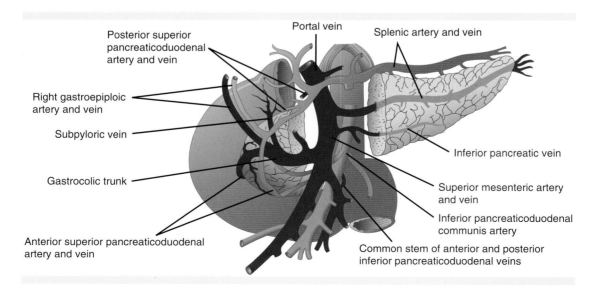

FIGURE 23-3. Pancreas blood supply (from Doherty GM, ed. *Current Diagnosis and Treatment: Surgery*. 14th ed. New York, NY: McGraw-Hill Education; 2015: Fig. 26-2. Copyright © McGraw-Hill Education. All rights reserved).

Sabiston Textbook of Surgery. The Biological Basis of Modern Surgical Practice. Philadelphia, PA: Saunders; 2012:1515–1547.
Mulvihill S. Pancreas. In: Norton J, Bollinger R, Chang A, et al., eds. Essential Practice of Surgery. New York, NY: Springer-Verlag; 2003:199–218.

2. **(B)** The total volume of pancreatic secretion is variable and ranges from 1.5 to 3 L per day. Tonic inhibition by somatostatin minimizes pancreatic enzyme secretion between meals. Fat or amino acids in the duodenum after a meal lead to the release of CCK, which then stimulates gallbladder contraction and pancreatic enzyme secretion. Activated trypsin in the duodenum, conversely, inhibits CCK release.

Secretin, found in the duodenal epithelium, is released in response to acid and is the most potent stimulant of bicarbonate secretion. Although the concentration of the cations (sodium and potassium) is not related to the rate of pancreatic fluid secretion, the concentration of the anions (chloride and bicarbonate) does change with the secretory rate. Chloride concentration is inversely related to the bicarbonate concentration and volume of pancreatic secretion (Fig. 23-4).

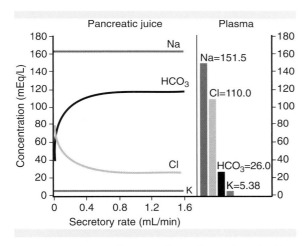

FIGURE 23-4. Pancreatic secretions. Reproduced with permission from Bro-Rasmussen F, et al. The composition of pancreatic juice as compared to sweat, parotid saliva, and tears. *Acta Phys Scandinav.* 1956;37:97–113.

BIBLIOGRAPHY

Jensen E, Borja-Cacho D, Al-Refaie W, Vickers S. Exocrine pancreas. In: Townsend C Jr, Beauchamp R, Evers B, Mattox K, eds. Sabiston Textbook of Surgery. The Biological Basis of Modern Surgical Practice. Philadelphia, PA: Saunders; 2012:1515–1547.
Mulvihill S. Pancreas. In: Norton J, Bollinger R, Chang A, et al., eds. Essential Practice of Surgery. New York, NY: Springer-Verlag; 2003:199–218.

3. **(D)** The digestive enzymes (amylase, lipase, trypsin, and chymotrypsin) function to digest, respectively, the starches, fatty acids, and proteins. These proteases are made and stored in the pancreas as inactive proenzymes. They are then packaged into zymogen granules and released into the central ductule of the acinus. Trypsin, for example, is the activated form of trypsinogen, which is cleaved by the enterokinase enzyme embedded in the duodenal brush border. Trypsin, in turn, activates chymotrypsinogen, which becomes chymotrypsin, as well as activates the other proenzymes. The inactive form of enzymes are not made by alpha, beta, and delta cells. Rather, these cells make up the islets of Langerhans and play a role in endocrine secretion, related to glucose homeostasis.

BIBLIOGRAPHY

Jensen E, Borja-Cacho D, Al-Refaie W, Vickers S. Exocrine pancreas. In: Townsend C Jr, Beauchamp R, Evers B, Mattox K, eds. Sabiston Textbook of Surgery. The Biological Basis of Modern Surgical Practice. Philadelphia, PA: Saunders; 2012:1515–1547.
Mulvihill S. Pancreas. In: Norton J, Bollinger R, Chang A, et al., eds. Essential Practice of Surgery. New York, NY: Springer-Verlag; 2003:199–218.
Riall T, Townsend C Jr. Endocrine pancreas. In: Townsend C Jr, Beauchamp R, Evers B, Mattox K, eds. Sabiston Textbook of Surgery. The Biological Basis of Modern Surgical Practice. Philadelphia, PA: Saunders; 2012:944–962.

4. **(C)** Alpha cells comprise 5–20% of the islet, produce glucagon, and are found in the outermost aspect of the islet. Beta cells make up 50–80% of the islet volume, produce insulin, and are found in the core of the islet. Delta cells make up less than 5% of the islet volume, produce somatostatin, and are found at the interface of the alpha and beta cells. A subtype of the delta cells, D₂ cells, make VIP. PP cells comprise 10–35% of the islet, make the inactive PP, and are found at the periphery of the islet. Islets occupy only approximately 2% of the pancreatic mass. Fortunately, for patients who undergo a Whipple pancreaticoduodenectomy, islets in the head and uncinate process are rich in PP cells but poor in alpha cells. Islets in the body and tail are rich in valuable glucagon-producing alpha cells but poor in PP cells.

BIBLIOGRAPHY

Hidalgo M. Pancreatic cancer. *N Engl J Med.* 2010;362:1605–1617.
Riall T, Townsend C Jr. Endocrine pancreas. In: Townsend C Jr, Beauchamp R, Evers B, Mattox K, eds. Sabiston Textbook of Surgery. The Biological Basis of Modern Surgical Practice. Philadelphia, PA: Saunders; 2012:944–962.

5. **(C)** The 5-year survival for patients diagnosed with pancreatic adenocarcinoma is approximately 6%.

Approximately 44,000 Americans develop pancreatic cancer each year. Worldwide, over 265,000 people contract this disease annually; of these individuals, 74% die within the first year after diagnosis. In the United States, it represents only 2% of all cancer cases but accounts for 5% of all cancer deaths. It is the fourth leading cause of cancer death, ranking only behind lung cancer, colorectal cancer, and breast cancer. Approximately 30% of pancreatic cancer cases are related to cigarette smoking. Chronic pancreatitis and diabetes have also been shown to be associated with the development of pancreatic cancer. Between 5 and 8% of pancreatic cancers are familial.

About two-thirds of pancreatic adenocarcinomas arise within the head or uncinate process of the pancreas. Tumors in the pancreatic body (15–20%) and tail (5–10%) are generally larger at the time of diagnosis. Tumors in the head of the pancreas typically cause obstructive jaundice, but ampullary carcinomas, carcinomas of the distal bile duct, and periampullary duodenal adenocarcinomas generally cause earlier obstruction of the bile duct and accordingly have a slightly better prognosis. Pain and jaundice are the most common presenting signs of pancreatic cancer.

BIBLIOGRAPHY

Fisher WE, Andersen DK, Windsor JA, Saluja AK, Brunicardi F. Pancreas. In: Brunicardi F, Andersen DK, Billiar TR, et al., eds. *Schwartz's Principles of Surgery*. 10th ed. New York, NY: McGraw-Hill; 2014: Chapter 33.

6. **(B)** A multidetector, dynamic, contrast-enhanced CT scan is the current diagnostic test of choice for pancreatic cancer (Fig. 23-5).

    Findings on the CT that indicate that the tumor is not resectable include the presence of extrapancreatic disease; involvement of 180 degrees or more of the celiac axis, hepatic or SMA; enlarged lymph nodes outside the boundaries of resection; ascites; or occlusion of the SMV–portal vein junction.

    Borderline resectable findings include tumors with abutment of 180 degrees or less of the circumference of the SMA, celiac axis, or hepatic artery; those with a short segment of vein occlusion; or those with lesions too small for biopsy but suspicious for metastatic disease. Tumors adjacent to the portal vein, splenic vein, or SMV can sometimes be resected along with a portion of the portal vein.

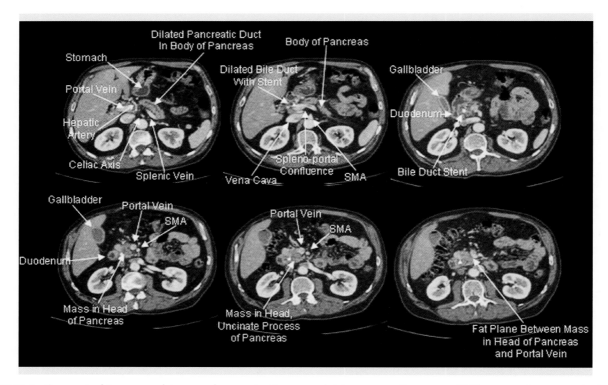

FIGURE 23-5. Computed tomographic scan demonstrating resectable pancreatic cancer; SMA = superior mesenteric artery from Brunicardi FC, Andersen DK, Billiar TR, et al., eds. *Schwartz's Principles of Surgery*. 10th ed. New York, NY: McGraw-Hill; 2015: Fig. 33-66. Copyright © The McGraw-Hill Companies, Inc. All rights reserved.

Endoscopic ultrasound is also valuable in the diagnosis and staging of pancreatic cancer and in assessing the relationship between the neoplasm and SMA, SMV, and portal vein.

BIBLIOGRAPHY

Hidalgo M. Pancreatic cancer. *N Engl J Med.* 2010;362:1605–1617.

Jensen E, Borja-Cacho D, Al-Refaie W, Vickers S. Exocrine pancreas. In: Townsend C Jr, Beauchamp R, Evers B, Mattox K, eds. *Sabiston Textbook of Surgery. The Biological Basis of Modern Surgical Practice.* Philadelphia, PA: Saunders; 2012:1515–1547.

7. **(C)** Only 5% of the pancreatic mass is composed of ductal cells, even though the majority (80–90%) of pancreatic neoplasms arise from these cells and have characteristics consistent with adenocarcinoma. In contrast, approximately 80% of the gland is composed of acinar cells, and acinar cell carcinoma is rare. Pancreatic cancer development arises via progressive dysplasia of duct epithelium. Dysplasia is associated with accumulation of kRAS mutations, and progressive genetic damage leads to the development of premalignant intraepithelial pancreatic neoplasms.

   The phenotypic changes are associated with mutation of the *K-ras* oncogene as an early event and mutations of the tumor suppressor genes p53, p16, and DPC4 as later events. The diagnosis of ductal adenocarcinoma rests on the identification of mitoses, nuclear and cellular pleomorphism, discontinuity of ductal epithelium, and evidence of perineural, vascular, or lymphatic invasion. Approximately 75% of pancreatic adenocarcinomas arise in the head of the gland, 15–20% arise in the body, and 5–10% arise in the tail.

BIBLIOGRAPHY

Hidalgo M. Pancreatic cancer. *N Engl J Med.* 2010;362:1605–1617.

Jensen E, Borja-Cacho D, Al-Refaie W, Vickers S. Exocrine pancreas. In: Townsend C Jr, Beauchamp R, Evers B, Mattox K, eds. *Sabiston Textbook of Surgery. The Biological Basis of Modern Surgical Practice.* Philadelphia, PA: Saunders; 2012:1515–1547.

Shroff RT, Wolff RA, Javle MM. Pancreatic cancer. In: Kantarjian HM, Wolff RA, Koller CA, eds. *The MD Anderson Manual of Medical Oncology.* 2nd ed. New York, NY: McGraw-Hill; 2011: Chapter 18.

8. **(D)** With pancreatic injury, a variety of digestive enzymes escape from acinar cells and enter the systemic circulation. Serum lipase is more sensitive and specific than amylase for diagnosis of acute pancreatitis. Serum amylase and lipase are both elevated early in the course of acute pancreatitis (within 4–12 h). Amylase levels rise within several hours after onset of symptoms. However, because of the short serum half-life of amylase (10 h), levels usually normalize 3 to 5 days after disease onset. Lipase has a longer serum half-life than amylase, returning to baseline within 8 to 14 days, and may be useful for diagnosing acute pancreatitis late in the course of an episode (at which time serum amylase concentrations may have already normalized). The magnitude of the increases in amylase or lipase concentrations has no correlation with the severity of pancreatitis.

   The diagnosis of acute pancreatitis requires two of the following three criteria:

   - sudden onset of characteristic abdominal pain
   - elevation of serum amylase or lipase above three times normal
   - findings of pancreatic inflammation noted on imaging (CT, MRI, or ultrasound)

   Imaging is not required for diagnosis of acute pancreatitis in patients who present with characteristic abdominal pain and elevated serum amylase or lipase. Early CT scans often fail to identify developing necrosis until 2–3 days after the initial clinical onset of symptoms.

BIBLIOGRAPHY

Clancy TE, Ashley SW. Management of acute pancreatitis. In: Zinner MJ, Ashley SW, eds. *Maingot's Abdominal Operations.* 12th ed. New York, NY: McGraw-Hill; 2013: Chapter 54.

Singh A, Gelrud A. Acute pancreatitis. In: Hall JB, Schmidt GA, Kress JP, eds. *Principles of Critical Care.* 4th ed. New York, NY: McGraw-Hill; 2015: Chapter 108.

9. **(D)** Computed tomography is an adept modality for identifying patients with advanced or metastatic pancreatic adenocarcinoma that precludes staging laparotomy. CT demonstration of vascular invasion, or peritoneal or hepatic metastases, excludes patients from undergoing surgical exploration for staging. Laparoscopic staging techniques have been developed to mimic "open" staging laparotomy while obviating the need for a laparotomy. Advantages of laparoscopic staging that have been well described include direct vision biopsies, identification of subcentimeter disease, reduced length of hospital stay, and decreased interval until the commencement of chemotherapy. Although the routine use of laparoscopy and laparoscopic ultrasound in pancreatic cancer surgery is not universally supported, it is sometimes used for detection of liver metastases. While CT-guided biopsy may be a useful technique to establish a diagnosis, this should be reserved for patients for whom resectability has been excluded (Fig. 23-6).

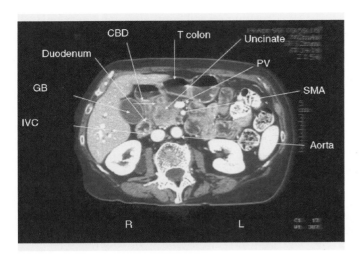

FIGURE 23-6. Computed tomographic demonstration of anatomy at the level of the pancreas in the evaluation of potential resectability. IVC = inferior vena cava, GB = gallbladder, CBD = common bile duct, T colon = transverse colon, PV = portal vein, SMA = superior mesenteric artery.

BIBLIOGRAPHY

Piccolboni P. Laparoscopic ultrasound: a surgical "must" for second line intra-operative evaluation of pancreatic cancer resectability. *G Chir*. 2015 Jan–Feb;36(1):5–8.

10. **(D)**

11. **(A)**

Explanations 10 and 11

Pancreatic cystic neoplasms are divided into three categories: malignant tumors (*in situ* or invasive), borderline (uncertain malignant potential), and benign (adenomas). Microcystic, glycogen-rich, serous tumors are almost universally benign, and macrocystic, mucinous tumors are accepted as either malignant or premalignant.

Benign variants of pancreatic cysts include serous oligocystic or macrocystic and microcystic adenoma. Serous neoplasms account for 1–2% of all pancreatic tumors. They are most commonly diagnosed incidentally on imaging. They occur more frequently in women than men and are distributed evenly throughout the pancreas. CT scan will reveal a thin-walled, multilocular mass with a sunburst pattern of calcification and honeycomb-like cysts less than 2 cm in diameter. There is no communication with the main pancreatic duct. Serous neoplasms have glycogen-rich clear cytoplasm that stains positive with a PAS test.

Mucinous cysts are typically spherical, thick-walled, septated or unilocular cysts with a tall, columnar, mucin-producing epithelium. They exhibit characteristics of an adenoma-carcinoma sequence and are classified as mucinous cystadenomas, borderline lesions, *in situ* lesions, or invasive cystadenocarcinoma. The vast majority occur in perimenopausal women. CT or MRI will demonstrate large septated cysts with thick irregular walls. Abdominal pain is the presenting symptom in over 70% of patients.

Differentiating between serous cystic lesions and mucinous neoplasms (cystadenoma or carcinoma and IPMN) is crucial due to the radically different biological characteristics exhibited by these two neoplasms. Endoscopic ultrasound may be useful at defining the contents of the cyst, and if indicated, it may be used to aspirate cyst contents for cytologic examination. Fluid aspirated from mucinous cystic neoplasms (MCNs) will often exhibit low amylase and lipase levels, but high carcinoembryonic antigen (CEA), CA19-9, and cancer antigen (CA) 125 levels. On the other hand, IPMNs show not only variable levels of amylase and lipase but also higher levels of CEA and CA19-9. However, because these values are often not consistent, the true benefit of fine-needle aspiration is controversial.

Surgical treatment is indicated for symptomatic serous neoplasms, as well as with growth of serous neoplasms greater than 0.6 cm per year or tumors more than 4 cm in size.

BIBLIOGRAPHY

Kimura W, Moriya T, Hirai I, et al. Multicenter study of serous cystic neoplasm of the Japan pancreas society. *Pancreas*. 2012;41(3):380–387.

Talukdar R, Nageshwar Reddy D. Treatment of pancreatic cystic neoplasm: surgery or conservative? *Clin Gastroenterol Hepatol*. 2014;12(1):145–151.

Verbesey JE, Munson JL. Pancreatic cystic neoplasms. *Surg Clin North Am*. 2010;90(2):411–425.

12. **(E)** The IPMNs are defined as papillary mucin-producing neoplasms that arise in the main pancreatic duct or major branches. They include a range of neoplastic lesions that can be benign or malignant and may be cystic or solid.

The first report of an IPMN was in the 1980s, and it was formally recognized by the World Health Organization (WHO) as a distinct entity in 1996. IPMNs represent 1% of all pancreatic neoplasms and 25% of cystic neoplasms. Females and males have an equal risk. The proliferation of mucinous cells may involve the main pancreatic duct (main duct type) or be confined to the branch ducts (branch duct type) or show a pattern spanning both areas in a combined type (40% of all IPMNs). Clinical recognition of the disease is often delayed because it is confused with chronic pancreatitis or cystic neoplasms of the pancreas.

Main duct type and combined main duct and branch duct type lesions are more likely to present with symptoms, while branch duct type IPMNs are more frequently

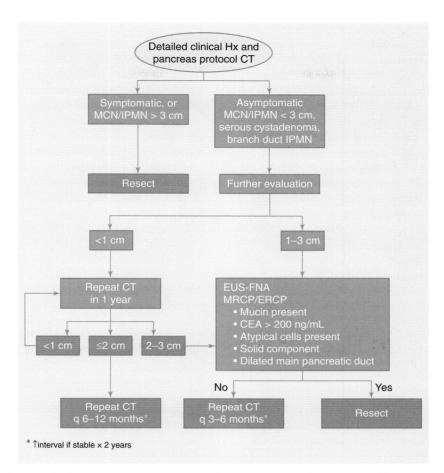

FIGURE 23-7. Approach to cystic lesions of the pancreas; EUS = endoscopic ultrasound; FNA = fine-needle aspiration; Hx = history (from Brunicardi FC, Andersen DK, Billiar TR, et al., eds. *Schwartz's Principles of Surgery*. 10th ed. New York, NY: McGraw-Hill; 2015: Fig. 33-75. Copyright © The McGraw-Hill Companies, Inc. All rights reserved).

detected incidentally in younger asymptomatic patients on cross-sectional imaging.

Multiple radiologic modalities can be used to make the diagnosis of a pancreatic cystic neoplasm, including ultrasound, CT, MRI/magnetic resonance cholangiopancreatography (MRCP), ERCP, arteriography, and endoscopic ultrasound (Fig. 23-7). IPMNs characteristically appear as cystic masses resulting from dilatation of the main pancreatic duct or side branch ducts.

Histologic features include a tall, columnar epithelium with marked mucin production and cystic transformation of either the main pancreatic duct or one of its side branches. IPMNs demonstrate a progressive precursor model of carcinogenesis similar to that seen in colon cancer. IPMN adenomas are well differentiated with no or low-grade dysplasia, whereas IPMNs with carcinoma *in situ* have severe dysplastic changes.

The International Association of Pancreatology guidelines for the management of IPMN (Sendai guidelines) recommend the resection for all IPMN of a main

duct type and mixed variants. For patients with IPMN of branch duct type, indications for resection are more conservative. High-risk stigmata include enhanced solid component and Main pancreatic duct (MPD) size of 10 mm or more. Worrisome features include cysts 3 cm or larger, thickened enhanced cyst walls, nonenhanced mural nodules, MPD size of 5–9 mm, abrupt change in the MPD caliber with distal pancreatic atrophy, and lymphadenopathy.

BIBLIOGRAPHY

Maley WR, Yeo CJ. Cystic neoplasms of the pancreas. In: Zinner MJ, Ashley SW, eds. *Maingot's Abdominal Operations*. 12th ed. New York, NY: McGraw-Hill; 2013: Chapter 58.

Tanaka M, Fernandez-del Castillo C, Adsay V, et al. International consensus guidelines 2012 for the management of IPMN and MCN of the pancreas. *Pancreatology*. 2012 May–Jun;12(3):183–197.

Verbesey JE, Munson JL. Pancreatic cystic neoplasms. *Surg Clin North Am*. 2010;90(2):411–425.

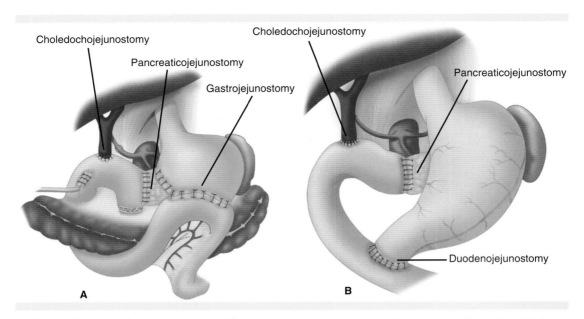

FIGURE 23-8. Classic (A) and pylorus-preserving (B) pancreaticoduodenectomy. Reproduced from Gaw JU, Andersen DK. Pancreatic surgery. In: Wu GY, Aziz K, Whalen GF, eds. *An Internist's Illustrated Guide to Gastrointestinal Surgery.* Totowa: Humana Press; 2003:229, with permission of Springer.

13. **(D)** The PPPD was first described by Watson in 1944 and was reintroduced by Traverso and Longmire in 1978 to improve the nutritional deficiencies associated with the classic Whipple (Fig. 23-8).

Delayed gastric emptying is found to be twice as common after PPPD (20–30%) compared to the classic Whipple. PPPD is associated with several theoretical nutritional advantages, including reduced likelihood of marginal ulceration, dumping, and bile reflux gastritis; however, the nutritional advantages are most evident in the early postsurgical period and become equivalent between operations over time. Operating time and intra-operative blood loss are significantly reduced with PPPD. Unfortunately, there is no difference in mortality, morbidity, or survival between the procedures performed for pancreatic adenocarcinoma.

BIBLIOGRAPHY

Diener MK, Fitzmaurice C, Schwarzer G, et al. Pylorus-preserving pancreaticoduodenectomy (pp Whipple) versus pancreaticoduo-denectomy (classic Whipple) for surgical treatment of periampul-lary and pancreatic carcinoma. *Cochrane Database Syst. Rev* 2014 Nov 11;11:CD006053. doi:10.1002/14651858.CD006053.pub5.

Matsumoto I, Shinzeki M, Asari S, et al. A prospective random-ized comparison between pylorus- and subtotal stomach-preserving pancreatoduodenectomy on postoperative delayed gastric emptying occurrence and long-term nutritional status.

J Surg Oncol. 2014 Jun;109(7):690–696. doi:10.1002/jso.23566. Epub 2014 Mar 12.

14. **(A)** Neoadjuvant therapy is given before an attempt at surgical resection. In patients with pancreatic cancer, advantages include reduced tumor burden, increased rate of resectability, and lower rate of lymph node positivity. As many as 20% of patients treated with neoadjuvant chemoradiation develop meta-static disease, detected by restaging CT, and do not go on to surgery. For those patients who do go on to resection, preoperative chemoradiation does not increase the perioperative morbidity or mortality of pancreaticoduodenectomy.

Adjuvant therapy is given following surgical resec-tion. In patients with pancreatic cancer, gemcitabine has replaced 5-FU as standard therapy. Several studies have demonstrated a beneficial role for neoadjuvant or adjuvant therapy to reduce the rate of local recur-rence; however, the rate of distant metastases has been unaltered. Extended lymphadenectomy is suggested to provide a more complete and accurate staging of the disease for stratification of prognosis, but no survival advantage has been demonstrated. The most recent European Study Group for Pancreatic Cancer trial showed no survival benefit for adjuvant chemoradio-therapy but revealed a potential benefit for adjuvant chemotherapy, justifying the need for further con-trolled trials.

BIBLIOGRAPHY

Fisher WE, Andersen DK, Windsor JA, Saluja AK, Brunicardi F. Pancreas. In: Brunicardi F, Andersen DK, Billiar TR, et al., eds. *Schwartz's Principles of Surgery*. 10th ed. New York, NY: McGraw-Hill; 2014: Chapter 33.

Iott M, Neben-Wittich M, Quevedo JF, et al. Adjuvant chemoradiotherapy for resected pancreas cancer. *World J Gastrointest Surg*. 2010;2(11):373–380.

15. **(B)** At first presentation, approximately 80% of patients with pancreatic cancer have advanced unresectable disease; 40% will exhibit local spread, and 50% demonstrate distant disease. Pain is reported by 75% of patients. Transmission of painful sensation is via T5 to T11 through the sympathetic chain celiac ganglion. Neurolytic celiac plexus block is used to treat refractory cancer-associated pain of the upper abdomen because narcotic analgesics achieve satisfactory pain control for only 50% of patients. Pain relief is effective in the short term (3–6 months) for 90% of patients and in the long term for 23% of patients. In regard to obstructive jaundice, the data suggest an improved benefit from stent-biliary decompression rather than surgical bypass. This has been a paradigm shift as plastic stents have been replaced with metallic expandable wall stents. Metallic biliary stents have several advantages over plastic stents. They have a lower occlusion rate and a lower intervention rate. Wall stents allow for balloon tumorectomy or can be bypassed by placement of a second stent; however, metallic stents cannot be removed as easily as plastic stents.

In contrast, gastric bypass remains controversial. The rate of GOO ranges from 3 to 19%. It is important to be aware that prophylactic gastric bypass for GOO remains recommended for laparotomy-based staging but not for laparoscopy-based staging. However, in the presence of unresectable pancreatic cancer, with a demonstrated mechanical GOO, gastrojejunostomy is the procedure of choice.

BIBLIOGRAPHY

Schnelldorfer T, Gagnon AI, Birkett RT, et al. Staging laparoscopy in pancreatic cancer: a potential role for advanced laparoscopic techniques. *J Am Coll Surg*. 2014;218(6):1201–1206.

16. **(B)** Patients with chronic pancreatitis commonly seek medical attention for pain. Surgical treatment for pancreatitis is indicated in cases of severe disabling pain and obstruction of adjacent hollow viscera.

The two main categories of operations for chronic pancreatitis are designed to decompress the obstructed ductal system or resect diseased tissue. "Hybrid" procedures include both decompressive and resectional components. Surgical options include the longitudinal pancreaticojejunostomy (modified Puestow procedure), caudal pancreaticojejunostomy (Duval procedure), pancreatic head resection (Beger and Frey procedures), pancreaticoduodenectomy (Whipple procedure), and various partial pancreatic resections.

The longitudinal pancreatectomy is indicated in patients with disabling pain who have a dilated (>6 mm) pancreatic duct with or without strictures. In the longitudinal pancreaticojejunostomy, the surface of the pancreas is exposed, and the pancreatic duct is identified and opened along its length. An anastomosis is created between the opened duct and a Roux-en-Y limb. Relief of pain is anticipated in 80–90% of patients, especially if patients refrain from alcohol. Diabetes does not typically occur until 80% of the pancreas is destroyed; however, endocrine insufficiency is not a contraindication to surgery. Further loss of exocrine or endocrine function may, in fact, be delayed by performing a drainage procedure. Patients with obstruction of adjacent hollow viscera, such as the common bile duct or duodenum, are candidates for resectional surgery.

BIBLIOGRAPHY

Andersen DK, Frey CF. The evolution of the surgical treatment of chronic pancreatitis. *Ann Surg*. 2010;251(1):18–32.

17. **(B)** Pseudocysts are defined as persistent, contained collections of pancreatic fluid that remain for 4 weeks following an attack of acute pancreatitis. Pseudocysts are the result of a pancreatic duct disruption and can occur in as many as 10% of patients following an episode of acute alcoholic pancreatitis. Pseudocysts may occur within the pancreatic parenchyma or outside the pancreas in an adjacent space. The cyst is formed by inflammation within the surrounding structures walling off the fluid. Pancreatic pseudocysts lack the epithelial lining that defines true cysts and account for three-quarters of all encountered cystic lesions of the pancreas (Fig. 23-9).

Asymptomatic, uncomplicated, acute pseudocysts should be expected to resolve with nonoperative treatment. Chronic pseudocysts, with a mature cyst wall, at presentation are less likely to resolve spontaneously.

For symptomatic pancreatic pseudocysts adjacent to the stomach, open cystgastrostomy has been the traditional treatment approach. However, recent data have confirmed the efficacy and safety of laparoscopic cystgastrostomy and endoscopic transmural cystgastrostomy, with reported advantages including shorter operative times, lower complication rates, and more rapid return to full function compared with the

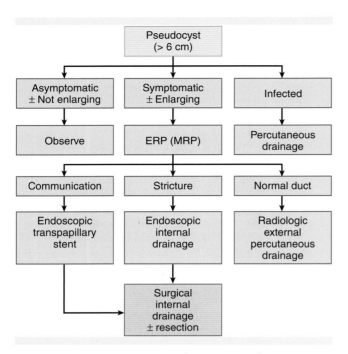

FIGURE 23-9. Investigation and treatment of pancreatic pseudocysts ; ERP = endoscopic retrograde cholangiopancreatography, MRP = magnetic resonance cholangiopancreatography (from Zinner MJ, Ashley SW, eds. *Maingot's Abdominal Operations.* 12th ed. New York, NY: McGraw-Hill; 2013: Fig. 55-6. Copyright © The McGraw-Hill Companies, Inc. All rights reserved).

open approach. In the setting of suspected infection, aspiration can be performed under CT or ultrasound guidance.

Endoscopic retrograde cholangiopancreatography is used to define the ductal anatomy prior to the chosen intervention. Transpapillary drainage may be successful where communication of the pseudocyst with the duct system is demonstrated and can be left across the area of suspected duct leakage to facilitate decompression and cyst drainage.

For pseudocysts that fail to resolve with conservative therapy, the preferred management is internal drainage to avoid the complication of pancreaticocutaneous fistula. Internal drainage may be performed endoscopically or surgically via cystogastrostomy, Roux-en-Y cystojejunostomy, or cystoduodenostomy.

BIBLIOGRAPHY

Fisher WE, Andersen DK, Windsor JA, Saluja AK, Brunicardi F. Pancreas. In: Brunicardi F, Andersen DK, Billiar TR, et al., eds. *Schwartz's Principles of Surgery.* 10th ed. New York, NY: McGraw-Hill; 2014: Chapter 33.

Jensen E, Borja-Cacho D, Al-Refaie W, Vickers S. Exocrine pancreas. In: Townsend C Jr, Beauchamp R, Evers B, Mattox K, eds. *Sabiston Textbook of Surgery. The Biological Basis of Modern Surgical Practice.* Philadelphia, PA: Saunders; 2012:1515–1547.

18. **(B)** The gene that encodes insulin is located on chromosome 11 at 11p15. Preproinsulin is cleaved into proinsulin while still in the endoplasmic reticulum. In the rough endoplasmic reticulum and Golgi, proinsulin is cleaved into insulin and C-peptide. Equimolar amounts of insulin and C-peptide, along with a small amount of proinsulin, are released by exocytosis (Fig. 23-10). Mature insulin is then stored in secretory granules as inactive zinc-insulin crystals. Consumption of carbohydrates triggers a rapid insulin secretory response that is greater than an equivalent intravenous glucose administration. Hyperglycemia stimulates insulin secretion through a complex signaling pathway. GLUT2 transports glucose into the cell where it is phosphorylated by glucokinase. Adenosine triphosphate (ATP) is generated by the glycolytic pathway. As its intracellular concentration increases, the ATP-sensitive potassium channel is inhibited, leading to depolarization of the cell membrane, an increase in cytoplasmic calcium, and exocytosis of the insulin secretory crystals. Insulin is cleared from circulation by the liver and kidney, with a half-life of about 3–6 min. C-peptide has a longer half-life than insulin, resulting in a ratio of about 5:1 of plasma C-peptide to insulin. Commercially available insulin contains no C-peptide.

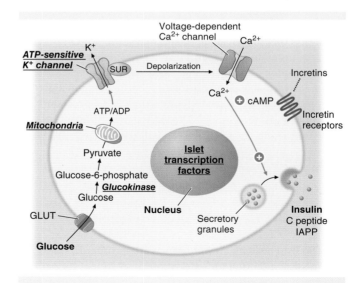

FIGURE 23-10. Pathways of insulin regulation; ADP = adenosine diphosphate; cAMP, cyclic adenosine monophosphate (from Kasper D, Fauci A, Hauser S, Longo D, Jameson JL, Loscalzo J, eds. *Harrison's Principles of Internal Medicine.* 18th ed. New York, NY: McGraw-Hill; 2012: Fig. 344-4. Copyright © The McGraw-Hill Companies, Inc. All rights reserved).

BIBLIOGRAPHY

Kacsoh B. The endocrine pancreas. In: Dolan J, ed. *Endocrine Physiology*. St. Louis, MO: McGraw-Hill; 2000:189–250.

19. **(C)**

20. **(D)**

21. **(D)**

Explanations 19 to 21

Whipple proposed his triad prior to the development of laboratory testing more sophisticated than the measurement of serum glucose. The eponymous triad consists of symptoms of hypoglycemia, low blood glucose (<50 mg/dL in men, <45 mg/dL in women), and relief of symptoms by administration of glucose. Insulinoma cells do not respond to the normal regulatory pathways, leading to tumor overproduction of proinsulin and high circulating levels of insulin. Although elevated plasma insulin is a component of the diagnosis for insulinoma, it is not a component of Whipple's triad.

Approximately 90% of insulinomas are benign. The diagnosis of insulinoma is made with a monitored 72-h fast. Hypoglycemia occurs in 95% of patients after a 72-h fast, and 75% of patients after 24 h. Serum insulin levels greater than 7 μU/mL in the presence of hypoglycemia are highly suggestive of an insulinoma; the insulin/glucose ratio is greater than 0.3 in this setting. C-peptide levels should be measured if there is any suspicion of hypoglycemia from surreptitious insulin injections. C-peptide levels of greater than 1.2 μg/mL with a glucose level less than 40 mg/dL confirm an endogenous source of insulin.

Contrast-enhanced CT, ultrasonographic imaging, and somatostatin receptor scintigraphy have permitted successful localization in about 80% of patients. Intraoperative palpation with adjunctive intraoperative ultrasonography has been used when preoperative localization fails; pancreatic endocrine tumors are hyperattenuating when compared to surrounding pancreatic tissue. Despite the predominance of beta cells in the body and tail of the pancreas, 97% of insulinomas are located in the pancreas with equal distribution in the head, body, and tail. The remaining 3% of insulinomas are located in the duodenum, splenic hilum, or gastrocolic ligament. Localization of insulinomas should not be attempted prior to establishing a biochemical diagnosis (Fig. 23-11).

Intraoperative ultrasound, when combined with palpation of the pancreas, is the most effective and cost-effective method to localize insulinomas; however, because there is an equal probability that these tumors will be found in any of the three regions of the pancreas, many surgeons desire preoperative regional localization. Multiple preoperative strategies have been employed in an attempt to localize these tumors, but most results have been unsatisfying. Unlike gastrinomas, insulinomas have few somatostatin receptors. CT, MRI, transabdominal ultrasound, and octreotide scans are rarely useful. CT and MRI, however, provide good studies for evaluation of hepatic metastases. Endoscopic ultrasound has been shown to have a sensitivity of up to 85% and a specificity of up to 95% in the identification of pancreatic insulinomas in highly specialized centers. Insulinomas have a rich blood supply, and because of their rich vascularity, they can demonstrate a blush on selective arteriography. Because insulinomas (and other APUD tumors) are stimulated to release hormone by calcium injection, selective arterial calcium injection with hepatic venous sampling has been employed to localize these tumors. Success in localizing insulinomas using this modality has been nearly 90% in some series.

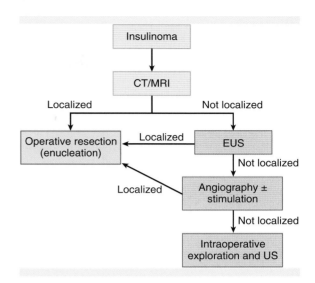

FIGURE 23-11. Localization of insulinomas (from Zinner MJ, Ashley SW, eds. *Maingot's Abdominal Operations.* 12th ed. New York, NY: McGraw-Hill; 2013: Fig. 60-13A. Copyright © The McGraw-Hill Companies, Inc. All rights reserved).

BIBLIOGRAPHY

Riall T, Townsend C Jr. Endocrine pancreas. In: Townsend C Jr, Beauchamp R, Evers B, Mattox K, eds. *Sabiston Textbook of Surgery. The Biological Basis of Modern Surgical Practice.* Philadelphia, PA: Saunders; 2012:944–962.

Riall TS, Evers B. Endocrine tumors of the pancreas. In: Zinner MJ, Ashley SW, eds. *Maingot's Abdominal Operations.* 12th ed. New York, NY: McGraw-Hill; 2013: Chapter 60.

22. **(D)** Zollinger and Ellison first reported the association of peptic ulcer disease with gastric acid hypersecretion and tumors of the islets of Langerhans in 1955. The gastrinoma, which causes Zollinger-Ellison's syndrome (ZES), produces excessive amounts of gastrin, thereby stimulating gastric acid secretion and causing the ulcer diathesis. ZES is rare, but it should be suspected in patients with peptic ulcer disease or GERD in association with diarrhea. Most patients in current series present with abdominal pain, diarrhea, heartburn, nausea, and weight loss. The diarrhea associated with gastrinomas (40% of patients) is secretory and stops with nasogastric suctioning.

Of gastrinomas, 75 to 80% are sporadic. About 20% of gastrinomas are associated with MEN 1 syndrome, and at least two-thirds of patients with MEN 1 have pancreatic neuroendocrine tumors (the majority of which are gastrinomas). The diagnosis is confirmed by documenting a marked increase (more than 10 times normal) of serum gastrin levels in patients with a gastric pH less than 2.1. CT scan can be useful to document the presence of the tumor. However, greater than 90% of gastrinomas express receptors for somatostatin; thus somatostatin receptor scintigraphy is the test of choice for localizing gastrinomas. Endoscopic ultrasonography is a useful adjunct. Approximately 80% of gastrinomas are found in the gastrinoma triangle. The duodenum is the primary site in 45–60% of patients. Approximately 70% of duodenal gastrinomas are located in the first portion and 20% in the second portion.

Resection involves open laparotomy, mobilization of the pancreas and duodenum, and careful palpation of the pancreas. Duodenotomy with palpation of the duodenal wall and examination with ultrasound should be performed in all cases, with enucleation of all discovered pancreatic and duodenal tumors. In patients for whom the tumor is not found, excision of the lymph nodes in the region of the pancreas and duodenum or performance of a highly selective vagotomy are supported. Long-term survival is good, with many series reporting 10-year survivals of more than 90%. Although they are slow growing, approximately 60% are malignant. Lymph node, liver, and distant metastases are not uncommon.

BIBLIOGRAPHY

Riall T, Townsend C Jr. Endocrine pancreas. In: Townsend C Jr, Beauchamp R, Evers B, Mattox K, eds. *Sabiston Textbook of Surgery. The Biological Basis of Modern Surgical Practice.* Philadelphia, PA: Saunders; 2012:944–962.

23. **(A)** Glucagonomas are rare tumors of the alpha cells of the pancreatic islets that produce a distinct syndrome, characterized by diabetes, migrating skin rash (necrolytic migratory erythema), deep vein thrombosis, and depression. Skin manifestations resolve with institution of total parenteral nutrition and are thought to arise from amino acid deficiency and trace element deficiency. These patients are at high risk for the development of deep venous thrombosis and should undergo prophylactic anticoagulation. Diagnosis of glucagonoma is established by measuring plasma glucagon levels; levels greater than 1000 pg/mL or a fasting glucagon level greater than 50 pmol/L are diagnostic. Diabetes develops in 76–94% of patients with glucagonoma at some point during their illness, and 38% of patients will demonstrate an elevated glucose level at initial presentation.

Imaging by CT scanning or somatostatin receptor scintigraphy is frequently successful in localizing primary and metastatic disease. Preoperative management includes the use of somatostatin analogues and nutritional supplementation. More than 50% of glucagonomas are malignant, and they tend to be larger than other pancreatic endocrine tumors, averaging 5–10 cm at presentation. They are two to three times more common in women, and 65–75% are found in the body or tail of the pancreas, corresponding to distribution of alpha cells.

BIBLIOGRAPHY

Abood GJ, Go A, Malhotra D, et al. The surgical and systemic management of neuroendocrine tumors of the pancreas. *Surg Clin North Am.* 2009;89(1):249–266, x.

Riall TS, Evers B. Endocrine tumors of the pancreas. In: Zinner MJ, Ashley SW, eds. *Maingot's Abdominal Operations.* 12th ed. New York, NY: McGraw-Hill; 2013: Chapter 60.

24. **(D)** Somatostatinomas are rare tumors that produce somatostatin. Over 60% of tumors are located in the head of the pancreas and the remainder in the duodenum or small intestine. Diabetes, cholelithiasis, and steatorrhea comprise the classic triad of somatostatinoma syndrome. The diagnosis can be confirmed preoperatively by measuring elevated plasma levels of somatostatin. An elevated fasting somatostatin level of greater than 14 mol/L is diagnostic. These tumors frequently (>50%) have nodal and liver metastases at the time of diagnosis. Patients with localized disease should undergo pancreaticoduodenectomy. Somatostatinomas are rarely associated with MEN 1 but are associated with von Recklinghausen's disease and pheochromocytomas.

BIBLIOGRAPHY

Abood GJ, Go A, Malhotra D, et al. The surgical and systemic management of neuroendocrine tumors of the pancreas. *Surg Clin North Am.* 2009;89(1):249–266, x.

Riall TS, Evers B. Endocrine tumors of the pancreas. In: Zinner MJ, Ashley SW, eds. *Maingot's Abdominal Operations*. 12th ed. New York, NY: McGraw-Hill; 2013: Chapter 60.

25. **(C)** Tumors that elaborate VIP are rare. The syndrome caused by excessive VIP secretion is known as Verner-Morrison's syndrome or WDHA syndrome (acronym for watery diarrhea, hypokalemia, and achlorhydria). The diagnosis is made by demonstrating an elevated fasting level of VIP concomitant with secretory diarrhea (>700 mL per day) and a pancreatic tumor. Flushing is sometimes seen because of the direct vasodilation effect of the hormone. Unlike other neuroendocrine tumors, diabetes is not a feature of this syndrome. Achlorhydria results from the direct inhibitory effect that VIP has on gastric acid secretion.

Imaging by CT scanning or somatostatin receptor scintigraphy is frequently successful in localizing primary and metastatic disease. However, endoscopic ultrasound is the most sensitive imaging modality. Although VIP is a neuropeptide that is normally distributed in the central and peripheral nervous systems, the majority of VIPomas are found in the body or tail of the pancreas or, rarely, the duodenum. About 60 to 80% of VIPomas are malignant, and 75% have metastasized by the time of resection. Treatment should be initiated with volume resuscitation and electrolyte (hypokalemia) normalization. Octreotide is commonly used preoperatively to reduce diarrhea volume and facilitate fluid and electrolyte replacement. Complete resection is curative, but electrolyte abnormalities need to be corrected prior to definitive surgical management.

BIBLIOGRAPHY

Abood GJ, Go A, Malhotra D, et al. The surgical and systemic management of neuroendocrine tumors of the pancreas. *Surg Clin North Am.* 2009;89(1):249–266, x.

Fisher WE, Andersen DK, Windsor JA, Saluja AK, Brunicardi F. Pancreas. In: Brunicardi F, Andersen DK, Billiar TR, et al., eds. *Schwartz's Principles of Surgery*. 10th ed. New York, NY: McGraw-Hill; 2014: Chapter 33.

Riall TS, Evers B. Endocrine tumors of the pancreas. In: Zinner MJ, Ashley SW, eds. *Maingot's Abdominal Operations*. 12th ed. New York, NY: McGraw-Hill; 2013: Chapter 60.

26. **(C)** Pancreas divisum is the most common congenital variant of pancreatic anatomy (Fig. 23-12). The lesser duct (duct of Santorini) usually drains the head, communicates with the duct of Wirsung, and drains separately via a minor papilla located 2 cm proximal to the ampulla of Vater. Pancreas divisum occurs when the ventral and dorsal pancreatic ducts fail to fuse, resulting in drainage of the major portion of the pancreatic exocrine secretions by the lesser duct and minor papilla.

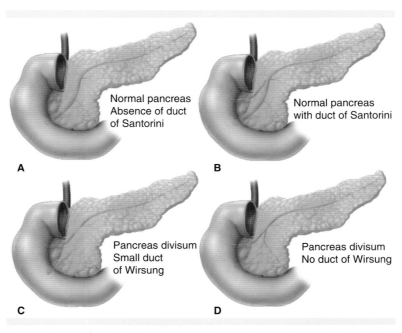

FIGURE 23-12. Pancreas divisum. Reproduced with permission of Wiley-Blackwell. From Warshaw.118/Warshaw AL: Pancreas divisum and pancreatitis. In: Beger HG, eds., et al. *The Pancreas*. London: Blackwell-Science; 1998:364.

Pancreas divisum is estimated to be present in 10% of all patients, and affected patients demonstrate a higher incidence of pancreaticobiliary anomalies. Most patients are asymptomatic and completely unaffected by the condition; however, 5% present with recurrent attacks of acute pancreatitis. The initial treatment of choice in patients is ERCP. Endoscopic stenting through the lesser papilla may result in temporary relief of symptoms; minor papillotomy and temporary stent insertion have greater than 80% long-term success. If sphincterotomy and stent placement fail, operative pancreatic resection or ductular drainage by longitudinal pancreaticojejunostomy may be required.

BIBLIOGRAPHY

Bondoc A, Tiao GM. Chronic pancreatitis in the pediatric population. In: Ziegler MM, Azizkhan RG, Allmen D, Weber TR, eds. *Operative Pediatric Surgery.* 2nd ed. New York, NY: McGraw-Hill; 2014: Chapter 58.

Jensen E, Borja-Cacho D, Al-Refaie W, Vickers S. Exocrine pancreas. In: Townsend C Jr, Beauchamp R, Evers B, Mattox K, eds. *Sabiston Textbook of Surgery. The Biological Basis of Modern Surgical Practice.* Philadelphia, PA: Saunders; 2012:1515–1547.

Lal G, Clark OH. Endocrine surgery. In: Gardner DG, Shoback D, eds. *Greenspan's Basic and Clinical Endocrinology.* 9th ed. New York, NY: McGraw-Hill; 2011: Chapter 26.

27. **(B)** Presence of pancreatic fistulas as a complication following pancreatic operation have been reported to be as high as 30%. Pancreatic fistulas may be internal (pancreatic ascites and pleural effusion) or external (pancreaticocutaneous fistula). External fistulas occur as a result of percutaneous drainage of pseudocysts or peripancreatic fluid collections. Those that drain less than 200 cc/L over 24 h are defined as low output, while those that drain more than 200 cc/L are high output. Complications include sepsis, fluid and electrolyte abnormalities, and skin excoriation.

    Computed tomography and MRCP document the anatomy of the pancreatic fluid collection, confirm the location and anatomic features of a pseudocyst, and define the pancreatic ductal anatomy. ERCP is most sensitive at demonstrating pancreatic duct connection or disruption. Sphincterotomy and ductal stenting can relieve ductal obstruction and reestablish normal enteric drainage for pancreatic secretions.

    Initial treatment for pancreatic fistula is consistent with other manifestations of duct leak: bowel rest, parenteral nutrition, and octreotide, which may reduce the volume of pancreatic secretions and assist in maintenance of electrolyte balance, increasing the chance of spontaneous closure. Percutaneous image-guided techniques are useful for draining peripancreatic fluid collections. Fibrin sealant and glues have not been demonstrated to be beneficial. Surgical closure of the fistula is indicated primarily in the setting of an infected fluid collection. Secondary indications include enlarging fluid collections despite conservative management, external fistulas, and recurrent pain or pancreatitis during recurrent attempts at refeeding.

BIBLIOGRAPHY

Larsen M, Kozarek R. Management of pancreatic ductal leaks and fistulae. *J Gastroenterol Hepatol.* 2014;29(7):1360–1370.

28. **(D)** The pancreas is a retroperitoneal organ at the level of L2, posterior to the stomach and anterior to the vertebrae. The head of the pancreas is the portion between the duodenum and the superior mesenteric vessels. The superior mesenteric vessels lie anterior to the uncinate process, and the neck overlies the SMV (Fig. 23-13).

    The exocrine drainage system comprises the main duct and the lesser duct. The main pancreatic duct drains the tail, body, and most of the head of the pancreas. The lesser duct drains the superior pancreatic head into the second portion of the duodenum via the lesser papilla, which is approximately 2 cm superior to the ampulla of Vater (Fig. 23-14).

BIBLIOGRAPHY

Jensen E, Borja-Cacho D, Al-Refaie W, Vickers S. Exocrine pancreas. In: Townsend C Jr, Beauchamp R, Evers B, Mattox K, eds. *Sabiston Textbook of Surgery. The Biological Basis of Modern Surgical Practice.* Philadelphia, PA: Saunders; 2012:1515–1547.

29. **(A)** Most pancreatic and duodenal injuries can be handled by simple repair and drainage. Injuries involving both organs that cannot be repaired require pancreaticoduodenectomy. Mortality is related to hemorrhage and associated injuries; therefore, hemostasis is of paramount importance. The surgeon should perform only the essential resections needed to obtain hemostasis and close the gastrointestinal tract. Postoperatively, hypovolemia, hypothermia, acidosis, and coagulopathy can be corrected. Definitive reconstruction, when the patient has stabilized, can be done in a delayed fashion. In other words, one should resect as necessary and stabilize, then reconstruct. In this patient, a Whipple procedure is the most appropriate option when nonsalvageable duodenal injuries and pancreatic duct injury occur, especially in a hemodynamically stable patient.

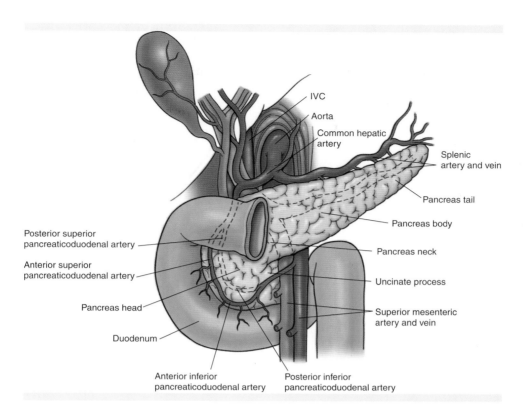

FIGURE 23-13. Pancreas *in situ* (from Mattox KL, Moore EE, Feliciano DV, eds. *Trauma*. New York, NY: McGraw-Hill; 2013. Copyright © The McGraw-Hill Companies, Inc. All rights reserved).

BIBLIOGRAPHY

Degiannis E1, Glapa M, Loukogeorgakis SP, Smith MD. Management of pancreatic trauma. *Injury*. 2008 Jan;39(1):21-9. Epub 2007 Nov 9.

30. **(B)** Although biliary disease is a common cause of pancreatitis, cholelithiasis is an uncommon cause of pancreatitis in young children (Table 23-1). Specific hematologic disorders, such as hereditary spherocytosis or sickle cell anemia, may predispose patients to early gallstone formation; however, pancreatitis is an uncommon presentation. Heterotopic pancreatic tissue or drug-induced pancreatitis are also reported but uncommon causes of pancreatitis in children. The most likely

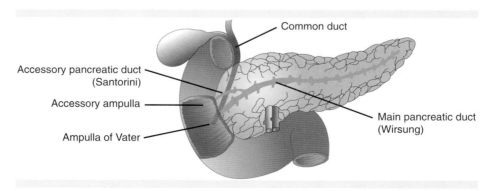

FIGURE 23-14. Pancreas ductal anatomy (from Doherty GM, ed. *Current Diagnosis and Treatment: Surgery*. 13th ed. New York, NY: McGraw-Hill Education; 2010: Fig. 26-1. Copyright © McGraw-Hill Education. All rights reserved).

TABLE 23-1 Etiology of Acute Pancreatitis in Children

Acute Pancreatitis	
Drugs	Salicylates Paracetamol Cytotoxic drugs (i.e., L-asparaginase) Corticosteroids Immunosuppressives (particularly azathioprine and 6-MP) Thiazides Sodium valproate Tetracycline (particularly if aged) Erythromycin
Periam-pullary obstruction	Gallstones Choledochal cyst Pancreatic duct obstruction Congenital anomalies of pancreas (especially pancreas divisum) Enteric duplication cysts
Infections	Epstein-Barr virus Mumps Measles Cytomegalovirus Influenza A Mycoplasma Leptospirosis Malaria Rubella Ascariasis Cryptosporidium
Trauma	Blunt injury (handlebar, child abuse, etc.) ERCP
Metabolic	α-1 Antitrypsin deficiency Hyperlipidemias Hypercalcemia
Toxin	Scorpion, Gila monster, tropical marine snakes
Miscellaneous	Refeeding pancreatitis
Inflamma-tory/systemic disease	Hemolytic-uremic syndrome Reye's syndrome Kawasaki disease Inflammatory bowel disease Henoch-Schonlein purpura SLE

ERCP, endoscopic retrograde cholangiopancreatography; G-MP, 6-mercaptopurine; SLE, systemic lupus erythematosus. Reprinted with permission from Nydegger et al. Childhood pancreatitis. *J Gastroenterol Hepatol*. 2006.

etiology in this young patient is coxsackie viral pancreatitis. There are two dozen viruses that may be associated with clinical pancreatitis, and this uncommon syndrome may be associated with viral syndromes or vaccinations against specific viruses (i.e., mumps). Treatment is supportive and conservative.

BIBLIOGRAPHY

Bondoc A, Tiao GM. Chronic pancreatitis in the pediatric population. In: Ziegler MM, Azizkhan RG, Allmen D, Weber TR, eds. *Operative Pediatric Surgery*. 2nd ed. New York, NY: McGraw-Hill; 2014: Chapter 58.

CHAPTER 24

SPLEEN

LISA M. MCELROY AND TRAVIS P. WEBB

QUESTIONS

1. Morphologic alterations in erythrocytes seen in individuals after splenectomy include all of the following *except*
   - (A) Howell-Jolly's bodies
   - (B) Heinz's bodies
   - (C) Pappenheimer's bodies
   - (D) Stippling
   - (E) Dohle's bodies

2. In agnogenic myeloid metaplasia, splenectomy
   - (A) Results in long-term improvement in thrombocytopenia and anemia in most cases
   - (B) Alleviates portal hypertension and lowers risk of variceal bleeding
   - (C) Has little proven benefit
   - (D) Results in resolution of the primary disease
   - (E) Is most commonly performed for life-threatening thrombocytopenia

3. In type I Gaucher's disease,
   - (A) Most patients eventually require splenectomy
   - (B) Recent advances in medical therapies have largely obviated the need for surgical intervention
   - (C) Although partial splenectomy reduces the risk of overwhelming postsplenectomy sepsis (OPSI), it does not significantly affect glycolipid deposition in bone marrow
   - (D) Most common clinical symptoms are related to hepatic cirrhosis and portal hypertension
   - (E) Genetic transmission is X-linked recessive

4. An 18-year-old male underwent splenectomy for hereditary spherocytosis. He returned a month later with complaints of diffuse abdominal pain, diarrhea, vomiting, and fever. Examination revealed a lack of peritonitis or significant distention, and amylase and lipase values were within normal limits. Blood cultures were negative. A computed tomographic (CT) scan of the abdomen and pelvis is shown in Fig. 24-1.

The following therapy should be initiated:
   - (A) Bowel rest
   - (B) Exploratory laparotomy
   - (C) Observation
   - (D) Acid suppression therapy
   - (E) Systemic heparinization

5. Isolated splenic vein thrombosis
   - (A) Commonly presents with isolated esophageal varices
   - (B) Is usually accompanied by cirrhosis and portal venous hypertension
   - (C) Is usually a consequence of pancreatic pathology
   - (D) Should be managed initially with a course of thrombolytic therapy followed by systemic anticoagulation
   - (E) Is usually accompanied by hypersplenism and thrombocytopenia

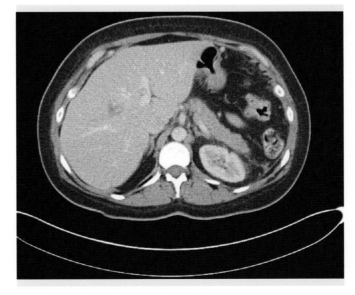

FIGURE 24-1. Abdominal CT scan (from Zinner MJ, Ashley SW, eds. *Maingot's Abdominal Operations.* 12th ed. New York, NY: McGraw-Hill; 2013. Copyright © The McGraw-Hill Companies, Inc. All rights reserved).

6. The most common indication for splenectomy for a red cell enzymatic defect is
   (A) Hereditary spherocytosis
   (B) Glucose-6-phosphate dehydrogenase deficiency
   (C) Pyruvate kinase deficiency
   (D) Hereditary high red blood cell phosphatidylcholine anemia
   (E) Cold-agglutinin syndrome

7. Which of the following is an indication for splenectomy in patients with Felty syndrome?
   (A) Splenomegaly
   (B) Chronic pain
   (C) Asymptomatic neutropenia
   (D) Recurrent infections
   (E) Thrombocytosis

8. A 25-year-old man presents with splenomegaly. He is asymptomatic except for mild fatigue. He denies any personal history of alcohol abuse, hematologic dysfunction, or travel. He was adopted as an infant, and family history is unknown. All laboratory studies, including peripheral smear, angiotensin-converting enzyme levels, autoimmune antibody panel, hepatic panel, sickle cell and thalassemia assays, and human immunodeficiency virus tests are normal. Platelet count is mildly depressed. A CT scan of the abdomen was performed and was completely unremarkable except for a large spleen. The next step in this patient's workup is
   (A) Splenectomy
   (B) Fine-needle aspiration
   (C) Abdominal ultrasound
   (D) Intravenous antibiotics
   (E) Corticosteroid therapy

9. Each of the following is true regarding splenic circulation *except*:
   (A) The splenic vein and superior mesenteric vein join to form the portal vein.
   (B) The splenic vein typically runs superior to the artery.
   (C) The splenic artery gives rise to the left gastroepiploic artery.
   (D) The splenorenal ligament is the double-layered sheath containing the splenic vessels.
   (E) The inferior mesenteric vein usually empties into the splenic vein.

10. A 24-year-old woman presents with complaints of intermittent chronic abdominal pain for 3 months but no other significant problems. On abdominal examination, you notice that she has a nontender mobile mass in the

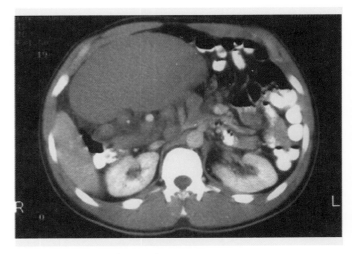

FIGURE 24-2. Abdominal CT scan.

left lower quadrant. Her CT abdomen scan is shown in Fig. 24-2.

Which of the following statements regarding this disease are correct:
(A) The underlying defect involves absence or hyperlaxity of the ligamentous attachments of the spleen to the retroperitoneum, colon, and diaphragm.
(B) A shortened vascular mesentery confines the organ to the upper abdomen.
(C) It occurs most commonly among men.
(D) Treatment of choice is splenectomy.
(E) Complications are rare.

11. You are evaluating a 3-month-old patient with polysplenia for surgery. Which of the following anomalies is classically associated with this syndrome?
    (A) Choanal atresia
    (B) Necrotizing enterocolitis
    (C) Common atrioventricular canal
    (D) Bilateral trilobed lungs
    (E) Normal liver

Scenario for Questions 12 and 13
A 19-year-old woman presents with intermittent episodes of acute knife-like midepigastric and left upper quadrant abdominal pain, nausea, and vomiting that have persisted over the last year. She also reports early satiety and progressive weight loss as well as the sensation of a heavy abdominal mass that is especially noticeable when she is supine. She denies any history of abdominal trauma, travel, medication use, or any other significant medical history. Except for a palpable spleen,

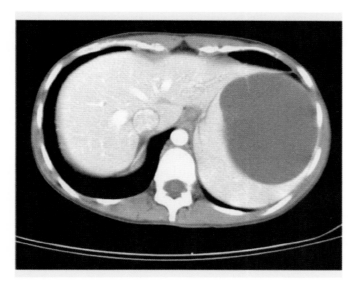

FIGURE 24-3. Splenic mass.

her physical examination is unremarkable. CT of the abdomen is obtained (Fig. 24-3).

12. Which of the following is true?
    (A) The incidence of secondary pseudocysts has increased in recent years.
    (B) Laboratory analysis is unlikely to change management.
    (C) An inherited defect in p53 function is likely.
    (D) Epstein-Barr virus Ig M titer is likely elevated.
    (E) Open splenectomy is the treatment of choice.

13. The following must be performed prior to operation:
    (A) *Echinococcus* serology
    (B) EBV IgM titer
    (C) Evaluation for a primary source of infection
    (D) Trial of medical therapy with bowel rest and total parenteral nutrition
    (E) Bone marrow biopsy

14. A 65-year-old intoxicated male driver is brought to the trauma bay after a motor vehicle collision. He is confused and combative with obvious head trauma to the right occipital region. He has obvious instability of his left lower rib cage, but he is oxygenating well, with breath sounds bilaterally. His blood pressure is 80/30 mmHg, and the heart rate is 140 bpm. On infusion of 2 L of crystalloid, blood pressure improves to 110/60 mmHg, and the heart rate drops to 100 bpm. The patient remains hemodynamically stable for the next 20 min, and you decide to send the patient to the CT scanner to evaluate his head, chest, and abdomen. The most reliable

predictor for the success of nonoperative treatment of splenic trauma in this patient is
    (A) Hemodynamic status
    (B) Grade of injury
    (C) Degree of hemoperitoneum on the abdominal CT
    (D) Coexistent head trauma
    (E) Contrast blush on vascular phase of CT scan

15. Which of the following is true regarding partial splenectomy?
    (A) A minimally invasive approach is contraindicated.
    (B) Retained phagocytic function of splenic tissue is an indicator of intact immunologic function.
    (C) Partial splenic resection is preferred to total splenectomy for hereditary spherocytosis.
    (D) It is primarily indicated for prevention of postsplenectomy sepsis.
    (E) Immunization against encapsulated bacteria in a patient who undergoes partial splenectomy of 80% of original splenic mass is not warranted.

16. Splenectomy may increase long-term risk of all of the following *except*
    (A) Hypercoagulability
    (B) Secondary atherosclerotic events
    (C) Pancreatic cancer
    (D) Pulmonary hypertension
    (E) Pancreatitis

17. A 23-year-old woman in the first trimester of her pregnancy presents to the emergency department with complaints of acutely worsening left upper quadrant abdominal pain, nausea, and dizziness. She denies any fever, emesis, or any changes in bowel movements. She admits to a 5-month history of similar pain in her midepigastrium and left upper abdomen, which was treated with antacids. She appears uncomfortable but is normotensive and only mildly tachycardic. Her abdomen is moderately tender in the left upper quadrant and epigastrium. Laboratory studies are unremarkable. You obtain an abdominal series. The upright film is shown in Fig. 24-4. Which of the following is true?
    (A) She should have a splenectomy performed electively following delivery of her baby.
    (B) Among patients with this problem, she is at relatively low risk for complications.
    (C) The lesion poses a significant threat to the survival of the fetus.
    (D) The most common time for complications to occur is at the time of labor and delivery.
    (E) This lesion develops most commonly in patients with an alcohol abuse history or gallstones.

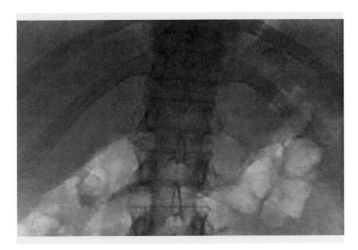

FIGURE 24-4. Abdominal plain film.

18. Which of the following statements regarding immune (or idiopathic) thrombocytopenic purpura (ITP) is true?
    (A) Most adult patients respond to medical therapy.
    (B) Most patients undergoing splenectomy for ITP require additional medical treatment.
    (C) Short-term thrombocytotic response to splenectomy is not a reliable predictor of long-term success or therapy.
    (D) Laparoscopic splenectomy has a higher incidence of missed accessory spleen than open splenectomy.
    (E) Persistent postoperative thrombocytopenia mandates reinstituting aggressive medical therapy.

19. A 6-year-old male is found to have bilirubinate stones at the time of laparoscopic cholecystectomy. Abdominal CT obtained during a previous admission for abdominal pain shows a small, shrunken spleen. This patient most likely has
    (A) Thalassemia
    (B) Sickle cell disease
    (C) Thrombotic thrombocytopenic purpura with hemolytic-uremic syndrome
    (D) Autoimmune hemolytic anemia
    (E) Hereditary spherocytosis

20. Splenosis
    (A) Usually results from failure of embryonic splenic lobules to fuse
    (B) Results in splenetic tissue that in most cases derives its blood supply from a tributary of the splenic artery
    (C) Results in tissue that differs histologically from the parent organ
    (D) Often results in sufficient splenic tissue to clear intraerythrocytic inclusion bodies from the bloodstream
    (E) Offers significant protection against OPSI

21. Which of the following factors does not correlate with increased morbidity in laparoscopic splenectomy?
    (A) Splenic mass
    (B) Blood transfusion
    (C) HIV status
    (D) Hematologic malignancy
    (E) Age

22. Which of the following splenectomized patients is at lowest risk for overwhelming postsplenectomy infection?
    (A) 25-year-old man who had a splenectomy for traumatic rupture in a motor vehicle collision
    (B) 20-year-old man who had a splenectomy for sequelae of thalassemia major
    (C) 5-year-old boy who had a splenectomy for ITP
    (D) 56-year-old man who had a splenectomy for staging of lymphoma
    (E) 25-year-old man who had a splenectomy 8 years ago for hereditary spherocytosis

23. Immunizations for patients undergoing elective splenectomy
    (A) Do not require boosters
    (B) Are equally effective regardless of their timing in relation to the operation
    (C) Are equally effective regardless of the age of the patient
    (D) Provide complete protection against the major pathogens responsible for OPSI
    (E) Can be improved by conjugation of polysaccharides to peptide adjuvants

24. Splenectomy is performed primarily for palliation in all of the following *except*
    (A) Non-Hodgkin's lymphoma
    (B) Hodgkin's lymphoma
    (C) Chronic lymphocytic leukemia
    (D) Chronic myeloid leukemia
    (E) Hairy cell leukemia

25. You are asked to evaluate a 50-year-old kidney transplant patient hospitalized with recurrent sigmoid diverticulitis. After initial improvement, the patient's condition deteriorated, requiring transfer to the intensive care unit, intubation, and pressors. White blood cell (WBC) count was 30,000. CT scan of the abdomen was obtained, demonstrating a unilocular heterogeneous fluid collection in the splenic parenchyma. The following considerations are true regarding the appropriate management of this patient *except* which of the following?
    (A) This patient will likely require surgical intervention.
    (B) This patient will likely require colectomy in conjunction with management of splenic disease.

(C) Broad-spectrum antibiotics including an antifungal agent are mandatory.

(D) This process is likely a complication of diverticulitis.

(E) Immunosuppression was a key predisposing factor in development of this problem.

ANSWERS AND EXPLANATIONS

1. **(E)** The spleen is responsible for removal of senescent and defective RBCs. In contrast to other organs in which the diameter of the smallest capillaries is slightly larger than that of RBCs, the splenic capillary bed terminates in the red pulp, a sieve-like network of sinuses and cords filled with macrophages through which only the most plastic of cells may pass. Here, the circulation stagnates and permits prolonged contact of the bloodstream with cordal macrophages. Senescent cells are destroyed (culling), and weathered red cells that are salvageable are remodeled and repaired (pitting) as intracellular inclusion bodies are removed.

After splenectomy, leukocytosis and thrombocytosis may develop in some patients, but blood counts usually normalize within the first 3 weeks. Although other macrophage-filled organs continue to remove damaged erythrocytes so that the overall survival of RBCs does not increase, less-damaged cells are not remodeled in the absence of the splenic filter. The result is characteristic differences on peripheral blood smears of splenectomized individuals:

Howell-Jolly bodies are small, spherically shaped nuclear remnants of RBCs. They arise from nuclear fragmentation or incomplete expulsion of the nucleus during normal RBC maturation. They are also seen in patients with megaloblastic anemia and hyposplenic states.

Heinz bodies are composed of denatured proteins—principally hemoglobin—that form in RBCs as a result of chemical injury, hereditary defects of the hexose monophosphate shunt, thalassemia, and inherited syndromes of unstable hemoglobin.

Pappenheimer bodies are a type of siderosome (iron body) commonly found in reticulocytes.

Target cells, also known as codocytes, are characterized by relative membrane excess because of either increased red cell surface area or decreased intracellular hemoglobin. They are seen in obstructive liver disease, hemoglobinopathies (S and C), thalassemia, iron deficiency, the postsplenectomy period, and lecithin cholesterol acetyltransferase deficiency. They are bell-shaped cells that assume a target-like appearance on a laboratory slide.

Spur cells, also known as acanthocytes, result from accumulation of cholesterol in the RBC membrane due to elevated plasma cholesterol/lipoprotein ratios. Acanthocytosis, or spur cell anemia, is most commonly seen in patients with end-stage liver disease.

Basophilic stippling refers to deep blue granules composed of clumped ribosomes, degenerating mitochondria, and siderosomes. They are also seen in lead intoxication and thalassemia.

Dohle's bodies are cytoplasmic inclusion bodies found in neutrophils in the setting of inflammatory diseases, infections, myelocytic leukemia, burns, cyclophosphamide therapy, and myeloproliferative syndromes.

BIBLIOGRAPHY

Beauchamp RD, Holzman MD, Fabian TC. Spleen. In: Townsend CM, Beauchamp RD, Evers BM, et al., eds. *Textbook of Surgery: The Biological Basis of Modern Surgical Practice*. 16th ed. Philadelphia, PA: Saunders; 2001:1144–1164.

Bull BS, Herrmann PC. Morphology of the erythron. In: Lichtman MA, Kipps TJ, Seligsohn U, Kaushansky K, Prchal JT, eds. *Williams Hematology*. 8th ed. New York, NY: McGraw-Hill; 2010: Chapter 29.

Gallagher PG. The red blood cell membrane and its disorders: hereditary spherocytosis, elliptocytosis, and related diseases. In: Lichtman MA, Kipps TJ, Seligsohn U, Kaushansky K, Prchal JT, eds. *Williams Hematology*. 8th ed. New York, NY: McGraw-Hill; 2010: Chapter 45.

Henry PH, Longo DL. Enlargement of lymph nodes and spleen. In: Longo DL, Fauci AS, Kasper DL, Hauser SL, Jameson J, Loscalzo J, eds. *Harrison's Principles of Internal Medicine*. 18th ed. New York, NY: McGraw-Hill; 2012: Chapter 59.

2. **(B)** Agnogenic myeloid metaplasia, or primary myelofibrosis, is a chronic, malignant hematologic disease associated with splenomegaly, the presence of RBC and white blood cell progenitors in the bloodstream, marrow fibrosis, and extramedullary hematopoiesis. The exact mechanisms are unclear, but the disease process appears to involve dysregulated secretion of growth factors with clonal proliferation of hematopoietic stem cells.

Patients are usually in the fifth decade of life, with complaints of fatigue, weight loss, and vague abdominal fullness or discomfort. Splenomegaly is virtually universal; 50–75% of patients also develop hepatic fibrosis with consequent portal hypertension, hepatomegaly, varices, and ascites. Patients are anemic and may have either elevated or depressed leukocyte and platelet counts, and peripheral blood smear is diagnostic.

The most common indications for splenectomy in patients with myelofibrosis are (1) painful enlarged spleen (~50% of patients), (2) excessive transfusion requirements or refractory hemolytic anemia (~25% of patients), (3) portal hypertension (~15% of patients), and (4) severe thrombocytopenia (~10% of patients). Extensive preoperative workup is required, with particular attention paid to correction of any coagulopathies. Approximately 75% of patients respond to splenectomy. The leading causes of perioperative morbidity are bleeding, infection, and thrombosis, and preoperative thrombocytopenia is an independent predictor of mortality.

BIBLIOGRAPHY

Akpek G, McAneny D, Weintraub L. Risks and benefits of splenectomy in myelofibrosis with myeloid metaplasia: a retrospective analysis of 26 cases. *J Surg Oncol.* 2001;77:42–48.

Lichtman MA, Tefferi A. Primary myelofibrosis. In: Lichtman MA, Kipps TJ, Seligsohn U, Kaushansky K, Prchal JT, eds. *Williams Hematology.* 8th ed. New York, NY: McGraw-Hill; 2010: Chapter 91.

Mesa RA, Nagorney DS, Schwager S, et al. Palliative goals, patient selection, and perioperative platelet management: outcomes and lessons from three decades of splenectomy for myelofibrosis with myeloid metaplasia at the Mayo Clinic. *Cancer.* 2006;107:361–370.

Park AE, Targarona EM, Belyansky I. Spleen. In: Brunicardi F, Andersen DK, Billiar TR, et al., eds. *Schwartz's Principles of Surgery.* 10th ed. New York, NY: McGraw-Hill; 2014: Chapter 34.

3. **(B)** Gaucher disease is an autosomal recessive lysosomal storage disorder resulting from an inherited deficiency in β-glucosidase, the enzyme responsible for degrading glococerebroside. The result is an accumulation of undegraded glycolipids in the white pulp of the spleen, liver, and bone marrow. Patients characteristically present with bleeding from hypersplenism-related thrombocytopenia, fatigue, anemia, and early satiety and weight loss because of mechanical compression of the stomach by the enlarged spleen. Gaucher's disease type I most commonly presents in patients under age 20, with a more pronounced hepatosplenomegaly and variable anemia and thrombocytopenia. The primary treatment is enzyme replacement therapy. Splenectomy is effective for treatment of hematologic abnormalities and mechanical symptoms of splenomegaly but does not correct the underlying disease. Partial splenectomy is sufficient to correct the symptoms of splenomegaly, while the remnant spleen provides a site for further deposition of lipid that is protective of the liver and bone. The disadvantage of partial splenectomy is the risk of enlargement accompanied by recurrent symptoms.

BIBLIOGRAPHY

Doherty GM. Spleen. In: Doherty GM, ed. *Current Diagnosis and Treatment: Surgery.* 14th ed. New York, NY: McGraw-Hill; 2014: Chapter 27.

Hopkin R, Grabowski GA. Lysosomal storage diseases. In: Longo DL, Fauci AS, Kasper DL, Hauser SL, Jameson J, Loscalzo J, eds. *Harrison's Principles of Internal Medicine.* 18th ed. New York, NY: McGraw-Hill; 2012: Chapter 361.

Park AE, Targarona EM, Belyansky I. Spleen. In: Brunicardi F, Andersen DK, Billiar TR, et al., eds. *Schwartz's Principles of Surgery.* 10th ed. New York, NY: McGraw-Hill; 2014: Chapter 34.

Vellodi A. Lysosomal storage disorders. *Br J Haematol.* 2005; 128(4):413–431.

4. **(E)** Portal vein thrombosis following splenectomy has become more common with the increasing popularity of laparoscopic splenectomy. The risk of thrombosis is higher with splenectomy than with other upper abdominal operations. It is most commonly associated with splenectomy for myeloproliferative and hematologic indications but occurs also in the setting of splenectomy performed for trauma. In addition to the underlying indication for splenectomy, risk factors include hypercoagulable state and splenomegaly. Other causes of stasis include increased viscosity associated with leukocytosis and thrombocytosis and decreased plasticity of erythrocytes from the high number of nuclear remnants in the absence of the filtering spleen. Although many patients remain asymptomatic and never come to clinical attention, others present with abdominal pain, diarrhea, nausea, vomiting, or fever or several years later with variceal bleeding because of portal hypertension. Occasionally, the syndrome presents with extensive intestinal gangrene, leading to death.

Patency of veins may be assessed by abdominal ultrasound with color flow Doppler imaging with a specificity of 99% and sensitivity of 93%. CT is more sensitive but also exposes the patient to additional radiation. Surveillance imaging is not standard practice, however.

Treatment involves systemic heparinization followed by long-term oral anticoagulation. Some studies report use of thrombolytic therapy with success. Overall, successful recanalization appears to depend on prompt recognition and initiation of treatment. Approximately 80% of patients experience partial or complete thrombus dissolution following anticoagulation therapy.

BIBLIOGRAPHY

Lai W, Lu S-C, Li G-Y, et al. Anticoagulation therapy prevents portal-splenic vein thrombosis after splenectomy with gastroesophageal devascularization. *World J Gastroenterol.* 2012;18(26):3443.

Tavakkoli A. The spleen. In: Zinner MJ, Ashley SW, eds. *Maingot's Abdominal Operations*. 12th ed. New York, NY: McGraw-Hill; 2013: Chapter 62.

5. **(C)** Isolated thrombosis of the splenic vein occurs most commonly as a consequence of an underlying pancreatic inflammatory process or from infiltration by a neighboring pancreatic malignancy. Other causes include idiopathic retroperitoneal fibrosis and iatrogenic causes, such as splenectomy, gastrectomy or splenorenal shunt. In pancreatitis, the close proximity of the splenic vein to the pancreatic tail leads to local prothrombotic inflammatory change in the vascular endothelium. External compression of the vein occurs by glandular enlargement, adjacent pseudocyst, or fibrosis and encasement by surrounding tissues. In addition to a primary tumor, enlarged lymph nodes may cause external compression.

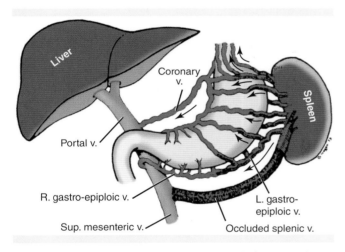

FIGURE 24-5. Splenic vein occlusion; L. = left; R. = right; Sup. = superior; v. = vein (from Skandalakis JE, Colburn GL, Weidman TA, et al., eds. *Skandalakis' Surgical Anatomy: The Embryologic and Anatomic Basis of Modern Surgery*. Athens, Greece: Paschalidis Medical Publications; 2004: Copyright © The McGraw-Hill Companies, Inc. All rights reserved).

Following obstruction with thrombus, flow is most commonly diverted to the short gastric veins with dilation of the cardiac and fundal submucosal venous plexus (Fig. 24-5). While many patients remain asymptomatic, a significant proportion develop sinistral (left-sided) portal hypertension with isolated gastric varices. Esophageal varices can also develop if the coronary vein joins the splenic vein proximal to the point of obstruction.

Most patients are asymptomatic with normal liver function at the time of diagnosis. When symptoms develop, the most common clinical presentation is with acute upper gastrointestinal bleeding from gastric varices, often with the patient in extremis.

In the case of acute bleeding, the diagnostic test of choice is upper endoscopy, especially in patients with known chronic pancreatitis because of alcohol abuse who need evaluation for more common etiologies as the cause of hemorrhage. Isolated gastric varices on endoscopy are pathognomonic. Ultrasound is a good preliminary test for patients not in extremis, as visualization of the splenic vein makes the diagnosis unlikely. Splenic vein thrombosis is often an incidental finding on abdominal CT performed for other reasons. Magnetic resonance imaging (MRI) may also be used to establish the diagnosis and has the advantage of allowing detailed imaging of the stomach and pancreas. Endoscopic ultrasound is a good adjunct when the etiology is unclear. Evaluation for coexistent pancreatic pathology should also be strongly considered if an underlying etiology is not evident because of the potential for a malignant cause of the occlusion.

Splenectomy is indicated in all patients with splenic vein thrombosis and a history of bleeding gastric varices. Splenectomy is curative and results in reversal of the sequelae of sinistral hypertension, including varices, by elimination of blood flow into the spleen. Asymptomatic patients with incidentally discovered splenic vein thrombosis do not require elective splenectomy, as the risk of gastric variceal hemorrhage is less than 5%. Splenic artery embolization is an alternative for the poor operative candidate or unstable patient but frequently results in extensive splenic infarction with subsequent splenic abscess development.

BIBLIOGRAPHY

Butler JR, Eckert GJ, Zyromski NJ, Leonardi MJ, Lillemoe KD, Howard TJ. Natural history of pancreatitis-induced splenic vein thrombosis: a systematic review and meta-analysis of its incidence and rate of gastrointestinal bleeding. *HPB (Oxford)* 2011 Dec;13(12):839–845.

Shirley LA, Bloomston M. Splenic vein thrombosis. In: Dean SM, Satiani B, Abraham WT, eds. *Color Atlas and Synopsis of Vascular Diseases*. New York, NY: McGraw-Hill; 2014: Chapter 49.

Skandalakis PN, Skandalakis LJ, Kingsnorth AN, et al. Spleen. In: Skandalakis JE, Colburn GL, Weidman TA, et al., eds. *Skandalakis' Surgical Anatomy*. New York, NY: McGraw-Hill; 2004: Chapter 22.

6. **(C)** The major categories of anemia that benefit from splenectomy are membrane abnormalities (hereditary elliptocytosis and spherocytosis); enzyme defects; hemoglobinopathies (thalassemias, sickle cell); and autoimmune hemolytic anemias. Although they are common indications for splenectomy, neither hereditary spherocytosis nor β-thalassemia is an enzymatic disorder. Cold-agglutinin syndrome (IgM autoimmune hemolytic anemia) is an immunologic disorder, and splenectomy is of no benefit.

Mature erythrocytes rely solely on the anaerobic metabolism of glucose through glycolysis (Embden-Meyerhof's pathway; Fig. 24-6) as their source of energy. Defects in the enzymes that catalyze these reactions may have profound effects on the energetics and behavior of erythrocytes. The most common hereditary enzymatic red cell defect is G6PD deficiency. G6PD catalyzes the oxidation of glucose-6-phosphate to 6-phosphogluconolactone as the first step in the hexose monophosphate pathway. NADP+ (nicotinamide adenine dinucleotide

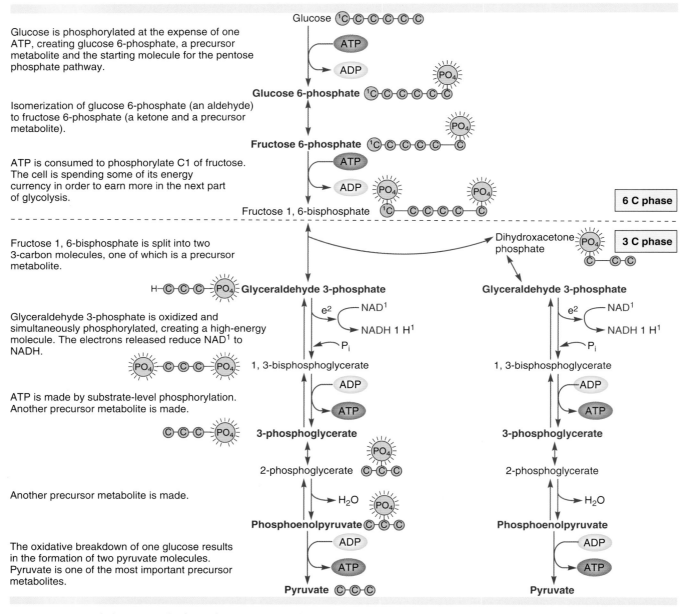

FIGURE 24-6. Embden-Meyerhof's pathway; ADP = adenosine diphosphate; ATP = adenosine triphosphate (from Brooks GF, Carroll KC, Butel JS, Morse SA, Mietzner TA, eds. *Jawetz, Melnick & Adelberg's Medical Microbiology.* 26th ed. New York, NY: McGraw-Hill; 2013: Fig. 6-22. Copyright © The McGraw-Hill Companies, Inc. All rights reserved).

phosphate) is reduced to reduced (hydrogenated) NADP (NADPH) in the reaction, generating 1 mol of NADPH. The primary manifestation is nonspherocytic hemolytic anemia; splenomegaly is rare, and splenectomy is not beneficial.

The second-most-common hereditary enzymatic red cell defect is pyruvate kinase deficiency. Pyruvate kinase catalyzes the conversion of phosphoenolpyruvate to pyruvate in glycolysis, which generates ATP. Four isoenzymes exist: PK-M1 (skeletal muscle); PK-M2 (leukocytes, kidney, adipose tissue, and lungs); PK-L (liver); and PK-R (erythrocytes). Inheritance is autosomal recessive. Patients often have mild-to-moderate splenomegaly because of sequestration of the less-deformable cells. Splenectomy has been shown to decrease transfusion requirements, presumably by preventing the trapping of reticulocytes and young red cells. The procedure should be delayed until after age 3 owing to the immunosuppressive effect of the surgery.

HPCHA is a rare hematologic disorder characterized by chronic hemolytic anemia of autosomal dominant inheritance. Levels of erythrocyte phosphatidylcholine are elevated, while plasma levels are normal. In this situation, splenectomy is not indicated because, while the hemolysis remains unaffected, the anemia worsens.

BIBLIOGRAPHY

Tavakkoli A. The spleen. In: Zinner MJ, Ashley SW, eds. *Maingot's Abdominal Operations*. 12th ed. New York, NY: McGraw-Hill; 2013: Chapter 62.

van Solinge WW, van Wijk R. Disorders of red cells resulting from enzyme abnormalities. In: Lichtman MA, Kipps TJ, Seligsohn U, Kaushansky K, Prchal JT, eds. *Williams Hematology*. 8th ed. New York, NY: McGraw-Hill; 2010: Chapter 46.

7. **(D)** Felty syndrome refers to the clinical triad of chronic severe rheumatoid arthritis with associated neutropenia and splenomegaly. The specific membrane protein in Felty syndrome is not known, but accumulation of anti-CCP IgG on the surface of granulocytes has been observed, indicating the presence of a specific membrane antigen. Splenic changes in these patients include a relatively hypertrophic white pulp on gross examination with elevated concentrations of neutrophils in the white pulp, T-cell zone, and red pulp on microscopy.

Clinical findings include leukopenia, neutropenia, and splenomegaly. Approximately one-third of patients develop lymphocytic leukemia. Although a majority of patients are symptomatic, neutropenia (<2000 neutrophils/mm^3) increases the risk for recurrent infection.

Treatment of Felty syndrome is directed at the underlying arthritis, usually with corticosteroids and methotrexate. Splenectomy is reserved for patients with symptomatic neutropenia who fail to respond to medical treatment. Following splenectomy, neutropenia resolves in most patients within 2–3 days, with greater than 80% of patients experiencing a sustained increase in white blood count and concomitant decrease in infections. The arthritis is unaffected by splenectomy.

BIBLIOGRAPHY

O'Dell JR, Imboden JB, Miller LD. Rheumatoid arthritis. In: Imboden JB, Hellmann DB, Stone JH, eds. *Current Rheumatology Diagnosis and Treatment*. 3rd ed. New York, NY: McGraw-Hill; 2013: Chapter 15.

Park AE, Targarona EM, Belyansky I. Spleen. In: Brunicardi F, Andersen DK, Billiar TR, et al., eds. *Schwartz's Principles of Surgery*. 10th ed. New York, NY: McGraw-Hill; 2014: Chapter 34.

Tavakkoli A. The spleen. In: Zinner MJ, Ashley SW, eds. *Maingot's Abdominal Operations*. 12th ed. New York, NY: McGraw-Hill; 2013: Chapter 62.

8. **(A)** The normal spleen weighs less than 250 g and decreases in size with age. It normally lies entirely within the rib cage, and a palpable spleen may be the only physical sign in patients with splenomegaly. Splenomegaly by itself does not indicate disease, with estimates of disease-free asymptomatic splenomegaly at approximately 30% of the US population and higher in tropical countries.

Three basic mechanisms lead to splenomegaly:

Hyperplasia or hypertrophy is usually related to splenic function, such as reticuloendothelial hyperplasia (work hypertrophy), and is seen in diseases such as hereditary spherocytosis or thalassemia syndromes that require removal of large numbers of defective RBCs.

Passive congestion is due to decreased blood flow from the spleen in conditions that produce portal hypertension, such as congestive heart failure.

Infiltrative diseases, such as lymphomas or myeloproliferative disorders, enlarge the spleen via mass effect.

Workup for splenomegaly should include a thorough history, including family history, past medical history, and history of substance abuse, travel or residence in a foreign country, medications, as well as a history of any constitutional symptoms or history of bleeding. Early satiety or other mechanical symptoms may be reported if significant splenomegaly is present, the most common of which are pain and early satiety.

Laboratory evaluation is of limited value initially, although complete blood cell count may reveal cytopenias suggestive of hypersplenism. The need for additional laboratory studies is dictated by the differential diagnosis of the underlying disease (Table 24-1).

Fine-needle aspiration is not routinely used for evaluation without a focal mass because of the potential for

TABLE 24-1 Diseases Associated With Splenomegaly Grouped by Pathogenic Mechanism

Enlargement Due to Increased Demand for Splenic Function	Enlargement Due to Abnormal Splenic or Portal Blood Flow	Infiltration of the Spleen
Reticuloendothelial system hyperplasia (for removal of defective erythrocytes)	Cirrhosis	Intracellular or extracellular depositions
Spherocytosis	Hepatic vein obstruction	Amyloidosis
Early sickle cell anemia	Portal vein obstruction, intrahepatic or extrahepatic	Gaucher's disease
Ovalocytosis	Cavernous transformation of the portal vein	Niemann-Pick disease
Thalassemia major	Splenic vein obstruction, splenic artery aneurysm	Tangier disease
Hemoglobinopathies	Hepatic schistosomiasis	Hurler's syndrome and other mucopolysaccharidoses
Paroxysmal nocturnal hemoglobinuria	Congestive heart failure	Hyperlipidemias
Pernicious anemia	Hepatic echinococcosis	Benign and malignant cellular infiltrations
Immune hyperplasia	Portal hypertension (any cause, including the above): "Banti's disease"	Leukemias (acute, chronic, lymphoid, myeloid, monocytic)
Response to infection (viral, bacterial, fungal, parasitic)		Lymphomas
Infectious mononucleosis		Hodgkin's disease
AIDS	Unknown etiology	Myeloproliferative syndromes (e.g., polycythemia vera, essential thrombocytosis)
Viral hepatitis	Idiopathic splenomegaly	Angiosarcomas
Cytomegalovirus	Berylliosis	Metastatic tumors (melanoma is most common)
Subacute bacterial endocarditis	Iron-deficiency anemia	Eosinophilic granuloma
Bacterial septicemia		Histiocytosis X
Congenital syphilis		Hamartomas
Splenic abscess		Hemangiomas, fibromas, lymphangiomas
Tuberculosis		Splenic cysts
Histoplasmosis		
Malaria		
Leishmaniasis		
Trypanosomiasis		
Ehrlichiosis		
Disordered immunoregulation		
Rheumatoid arthritis (Felty's syndrome)		
Systemic lupus erythematosus		

(Continued)

TABLE 24-1 Differential Diagnosis: Splenomegaly Diseases Associated With Splenomegaly Grouped by Pathogenic Mechanism (*Continued*)

Enlargement Due to Increased Demand for Splenic Function	Enlargement Due to Abnormal Splenic or Portal Blood Flow	Infiltration of the Spleen
Collagen vascular diseases		
Serum sickness		
Immune hemolytic anemias		
Immune thrombocytopenias		
Immune neutropenias		
Drug reactions		
Angioimmunoblastic lymphadenopathy		
Sarcoidosis		
Thyrotoxicosis (benign lymphoid hypertrophy)		
Interleukin 2 therapy		
Extramedullary hematopoiesis		
Myelofibrosis		
Marrow damage by toxins, radiation, strontium		
Marrow infiltration by tumors, leukemias, Gaucher's disease		

Source: Longo DL, Fauci AS, Kasper DL, Hauser SL, Jameson J, Loscalzo J, eds. *Harrison's Principles of Internal Medicine*. 18th ed. New York, NY: McGraw-Hill; 2012: Table 59-2. Copyright © The McGraw-Hill Companies, Inc. All rights reserved.

misdiagnosis among the diseases associated with isolated splenomegaly. Laparoscopic evaluation with biopsy and positron emission tomographic (PET) scanning are options to consider, but further study is needed to determine their effectiveness. Imaging may be nondiagnostic or may show a nonhomogeneous texture on radionuclide studies, ultrasonography, or CT scan.

Splenectomy is infrequently performed for diagnostic purposes.

BIBLIOGRAPHY

Henry PH, Longo DL. Enlargement of lymph nodes and spleen. In: Longo DL, Fauci AS, Kasper DL, Hauser SL, Jameson J, Loscalzo J, eds. *Harrison's Principles of Internal Medicine*. 18th ed. New York, NY: McGraw-Hill; 2012: Chapter 59.

Motyckova G, Steensma DP. Why does my patient have lymphadenopathy or splenomegaly? *Hematol Oncol Clin North Am*. 2012 Apr;26(2):395–408.

Tavakkoli A. The spleen. In: Zinner MJ, Ashley SW, eds. *Maingot's Abdominal Operations*. 12th ed. New York, NY: McGraw-Hill; 2013: Chapter 62.

9. **(B)** The splenic artery arises as one of the three branches from the celiac axis and courses laterally along the posterior wall of the omental bursa mostly external to the parenchyma of the pancreas, through the splenorenal (lienorenal) ligament and into the splenic hilum, where it divides into six or more branches. The left gastroepiploic (gastro-omental) artery originates from the splenic artery near the hilum. A massively enlarged spleen may parasitize vessels from the mesocolon of the splenic flexure or the diaphragm or from the omentum.

The splenic vein emerges from the confluence of six or more veins from the splenic hilum. It then passes behind the pancreas inferior to the artery and joins the superior mesenteric vein behind the pancreas to form the portal vein. The portal and systemic circulations intermingle through collateral vessels in this area, and this becomes clinically significant in portal hypertension. In the case of splenic vein occlusion or thrombosis with associated sinistral (left-sided) portal hypertension, drainage of the splenic outflow is diverted to the short gastric veins with subsequent dilation of the cardiac and fundal submucosal venous plexus resulting in isolated gastric

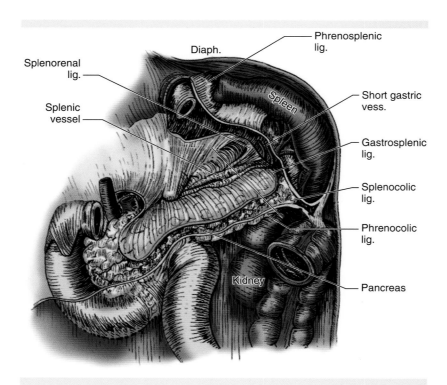

FIGURE 24-7. Ligaments (lig.) of the spleen; Diaph. = diaphragm; vess. = vessel (from Zinner MJ, Ashley SW, eds. *Maingot's Abdominal Operations*. 12th ed. New York, NY: McGraw-Hill; 2013: Fig. 62-3. Copyright © The McGraw-Hill Companies, Inc. All rights reserved).

varices. Esophageal varices are not typical because, in the presence of normal portal pressures and patent coronary vein, the esophageal bed is unaffected, but they can occur if drainage of the coronary vein is distal to the point of obstruction in the splenic vein.

The spleen is affixed to the left upper quadrant by the splenorenal (lienorenal), gastrosplenic (gastrolienal), and splenocolic suspensory ligaments and more variably by the spleno-omental and splenophrenic (phrenicolienal) attachments (Fig. 24-7). The splenogastric ligament forms the mesentery between the spleen and stomach and contains the short gastric and left gastroepiploic vessels. The splenorenal ligament attaches the spleen to Gerota's fascia of the upper left kidney and contains the main splenic artery and vein. The splenophrenic, spleno-omental, and splenocolic are considered relatively avascular but must be divided carefully because of small vessels that are often present, especially in disease states.

BIBLIOGRAPHY

Mirjalili SA, McFadden SL, Buckenham T, Stringer MD. A reappraisal of adult abdominal surface anatomy. *Clin Anat.* 2012 Oct;25(7):844–850.

Skandalakis PN, Skandalakis LJ, Kingsnorth AN, et al. Spleen. In: Skandalakis JE, Colburn GL, Weidman TA, et al., eds. *Skandalakis' Surgical Anatomy.* New York, NY: McGraw-Hill; 2004: Chapter 22.

Tavakkoli A. The spleen. In: Zinner MJ, Ashley SW, eds. *Maingot's Abdominal Operations.* 12th ed. New York, NY: McGraw-Hill; 2013: Chapter 62.

10. **(A)** Wandering spleen, also called ectopic spleen, is a rare anomaly that results from absence or hyperlaxity of the normal ligamentous attachments to the retroperitoneum and neighboring structures that affix the organ in the left upper quadrant. The splenorenal and gastrosplenic ligaments are particularly critical in immobilizing the spleen.

Clinical presentation varies considerably. Patients frequently present with an asymptomatic abdominal mass or abdominal pain that ranges from chronic intermittent and mild-to-acutely toxic with frank peritonitis because of torsion, infarction, and splenic necrosis. GI symptoms such as vomiting are also common. Characteristically, the vascular mesentery is elongated and serves as the sole attachment to the spleen, predisposing the organ to axial torsion and infarction. Acute pancreatitis from involvement of the tail of the pancreas in torsion has also been reported.

Symptoms of pain may also develop chronically when capsular stretching leads to venous engorgement during intermittent episodes of mild torsion.

Computed tomographic scan or ultrasonography can be used to establish a diagnosis. Decreased or absent flow may be present on Doppler examination and signifies torsion. That 70–80% of patients are women of childbearing age supports the theory that hormonal changes lead to an acquired increased laxity of ligaments and excess mobility; however, a developmental etiology in which failure of dorsal mesogastrium fusion to the posterior abdominal wall during embryogenesis results in a wandering spleen is equally plausible because its incidence is well documented among children. In addition, its association with gastric volvulus in children has been well documented in the literature, suggesting a common etiology. The mechanical stress placed on attachments by enlarged spleens may also play a role; however, not all cases exhibit splenomegaly.

Treatment is with splenectomy or splenopexy. Prior to discovery of the associated immunologic consequences, splenectomy was routinely performed; however, splenopexy is currently the procedure of choice in the absence of infarction or necrosis and can be performed by formation of a retroperitoneal pouch, by suturing the spleen to the abdominal wall or diaphragm directly, or by using synthetic or bioabsorbable mesh. Laparoscopic splenopexy has also been performed with success. Splenectomy is reserved for cases in which the spleen is nonviable. Conservative management carries a complication rate of 65%.

BIBLIOGRAPHY

Magowska A. Wandering spleen: a medical enigma, its natural history and rationalization. *World J Surg.* 2013 Mar;37(3):545–550.

Park AE, Targarona EM, Belyansky I. Spleen. In: Brunicardi F, Andersen DK, Billiar TR, et al., eds. *Schwartz's Principles of Surgery.* 10th ed. New York, NY: McGraw-Hill; 2014: Chapter 34.

Skandalakis PN, Skandalakis LJ, Kingsnorth AN, et al. Spleen. In: Skandalakis JE, Colburn GL, Weidman TA, et al., eds. *Skandalakis' Surgical Anatomy.* New York, NY: McGraw-Hill; 2004: Chapter 22.

11. **(C)** Visceral heterotaxia, also known as heterotaxy syndrome, is a congenital defect characterized by loss of normal orientation of the viscera in the chest and abdomen with respect to the left-right axis. The heart is the most commonly affected organ. In contrast to *situs solitus*, or normal orientation of viscera and vasculature, and *situs inversus*, the complete mirror image of normal, any other arrangement is considered "situs ambiguous" or heterotaxy. Visceral organization in heterotaxy is disorderly and variable among individuals along a wide spectrum.

The syndrome likely results from a disrupted lateralization leading to abnormal chiral development; inheritance appears to be multifactorial. Embryologically, the event occurs at 20–30 days' gestation when the primitive heart and venous connections are forming, accounting for the high incidence of anomalies of the heart and great vessels. Other associated abnormalities include bronchial isomerism, biliary atresia, intestinal malrotation, a bridging (midline) liver, asplenia, and polysplenia.

Asplenia has a stronger association with complex cyanotic cardiac malformations, while anomalies in polysplenic patients are generally less severe, most commonly atrioventricular canal defects. In asplenia (right isomerism, bilateral right-sidedness, double right-sidedness, Ivemark's syndrome), classically both lungs are trilobar with bilateral minor fissures and eparterial bronchi. Absence or hypofunction of the spleen (despite polysplenia) in patients with heterotaxia render them susceptible to infection, especially with encapsulated organisms.

Polysplenia (left isomerism, bilateral left-sidedness) is associated with bilateral bilobar lungs, intestinal malrotation, and interrupted inferior vena cava with azygous or hemiazygous continuation. Polysplenia is also associated with abnormal splenic function in certain children.

Evaluation should include chest x-ray, echocardiography, abdominal ultrasound, and upper GI series. Certain structures must be evaluated to define situs: the atria; the aorta and great veins below the diaphragm with regard to their relationship to midline; the stomach and small bowel for the presence of malrotation; liver and gallbladder; location of the cardiac apex; the spleen or spleens; and lungs. Congenital asplenia should be suspected in any infant with abnormal abdominal viscera or complex congenital heart disease. Diagnosis may be established in a newborn by documentation of Howell-Jolly's bodies on peripheral smear in combination with scintigraphy. Prophylactic antibiotics and vaccination are recommended to treat asplenic patients. Ladd's procedure should be performed in all stable patients with associated malrotation to prevent future midgut volvulus.

BIBLIOGRAPHY

Christison-Lagay E, Langer JC. Intestinal rotation abnormalities. In: Ziegler MM, Azizkhan RG, Allmen D, Weber TR, eds. *Operative Pediatric Surgery.* 2nd ed. New York, NY: McGraw-Hill; 2014: Chapter 41.

Crary SE. The spleen and lymph nodes. In: Rudolph CD, Rudolph AM, Lister GE, First LR, Gershon AA, eds. *Rudolph's Pediatrics.* 22nd ed. New York, NY: McGraw-Hill; 2011: Chapter 440.

Kothari SS. Non-cardiac issues in patients with heterotaxy syndrome. *Ann Pediatr Cardiol.* 2014 Sep;7(3):187–192.

Ruppel KM. Genetics of heart disease. In: Rudolph CD, Rudolph AM, Lister GE, First LR, Gershon AA, eds. *Rudolph's Pediatrics.* 22nd ed. New York, NY: McGraw-Hill; 2011: Chapter 481.

12. **(A)**

13. **(A)**

Explanation for questions 12 and 13

Cysts of the spleen may be classified into primary or secondary (pseudocysts). Secondary pseudocysts do not have an epithelial lining and usually result from trauma. Primary cysts are further classified into parasitic or nonparasitic. Nonparasitic cysts include simple cysts, epidermoid cysts, and dermoid cysts. Paracytic cysts include hydatid disease, most commonly from *Echinococcus granulosis.* CT scan is the best modality for diagnosis of a splenic cyst, and the incidence has risen in recent years because of the increased use of CT scanning and more widespread use of a nonoperative approach to blunt splenic injury. Generally, symptoms are caused by the mass effect of the cyst, so that cysts less than 8 cm are usually asymptomatic. Patients may present with abdominal fullness, left shoulder or back pain, early satiety, shortness of breath, pleuritic chest pain, or renal symptoms from mass effect. Complications include acute hemorrhage, rupture, or infection.

Nonparasitic true cysts and pseudocysts should be treated if greater than 10 cm or symptomatic. Symptomatic pseudocysts should be managed operatively or through percutaneous drainage. *Echinococcus* serology (enzyme-linked immunosorbent assay [ELISA] or Western blot) must be performed prior to any invasive intervention to rule out a parasitic etiology because of the risk of anaphylactic shock with intra-abdominal spillage of infective scolices. Patients should undergo splenectomy with intraoperative injection of hypertonic saline, alcohol, or silver nitrate prior to removal.

Traditionally, splenectomy has been the standard of care for splenic cysts; however, spurred by the increased awareness of the immunologic consequences surrounding splenectomy and the rising popularity of minimally invasive surgery, techniques of splenic preservation are being used more frequently, with encouraging results. Partial splenectomy, percutaneous aspiration, decapsulation, and partial cystectomy have all been used successfully to treat nonparasitic true cysts and pseudocysts; however, recurrence of epidermoid cysts following incomplete removal of the epithelial lining with partial cystectomy and marsupialization has been reported. Resected tissue should be evaluated by pathology because both benign and malignant primary cystic tumors of the spleen, although extremely rare, can mimic epidermoid cysts.

Splenic abscess is a rare but potentially lethal condition. Immunocompromised patients and patients who abuse intravenous drugs are particularly susceptible. They develop by four basic mechanisms: metastatic hematogenous spread from a distant source such as osteomyelitis or infective endocarditis; following trauma or iatrogenic injury, especially with increasing use of nonoperative management; secondary infection following splenic infarction such as in sickle cell and splenic embolization; and by extension from a contiguous infective source, such as a perinephric, pancreatic, or diverticular abscess. They are primarily unilocular in adults but multilocular in children. *Staphyloccoccus* and *Streptococcus* species account for 30% of cases; other common organisms include *Enterococcus, Salmonella,* and *Escherichia coli.* They tend to have a heterogeneous appearance on CT, while cysts tend to be homogeneous. Patients should be treated promptly with broad-spectrum antibiotics. Unilocular abscesses may be percutaneously aspirated, but multilocular abscesses usually require splenectomy. Partial splenectomy, splenotomy with drainage, and laparoscopic splenectomy have all been used with success. They may be complicated by intraperitoneal rupture or rupture into adjacent organs and with possible subsequent formation of a fistula. Given the patient's history and homogeneous appearance of the cyst on CT scan, a splenic abscess is highly unlikely.

The p53 and EBV IgM titer are not involved in the pathogenesis and are not routinely evaluated in such a patient. Infectious mononucleosis may manifest with splenomegaly, fever, and adenopathy but rarely produces a cystic mass except possibly in the case of a traumatic pseudocyst resulting from subcapsular rupture. Again, the CT scan does not support this diagnosis or suggest a hematologic malignancy.

BIBLIOGRAPHY

Skandalakis PN, Skandalakis LJ, Kingsnorth AN, et al. Spleen. In: Skandalakis JE, Colburn GL, Weidman TA, et al., eds. *Skandalakis' Surgical Anatomy.* New York, NY: McGraw-Hill; 2004: Chapter 22.

Tavakkoli A. The spleen. In: Zinner MJ, Ashley SW, eds. *Maingot's Abdominal Operations.* 12th ed. New York, NY: McGraw-Hill; 2013: Chapter 62.

14. **(A)** Nonoperative management has become more common over the past decade and is considered a reasonable treatment option for hemodynamically stable patients (Fig. 24-8). The current Eastern Association for the Study of Trauma guidelines for management of blunt injury to the spleen state the following recommendations:

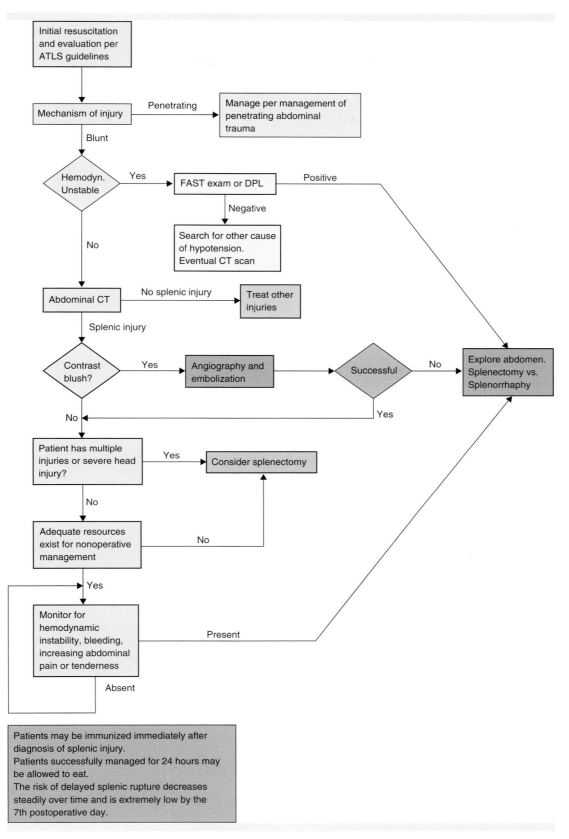

FIGURE 24-8. Approach to splenic injury; hemodyn. = hemodynamics (from Mattox K, Moore E, Feliciano D, eds. *Trauma*. 7th ed. New York, NY: McGraw-Hill; 2013: Fig. 30-6. Copyright © The McGraw-Hill Companies, Inc. All rights reserved).

Level 1: Patients who have diffuse peritonitis or who are hemodynamically unstable after blunt abdominal trauma should be taken urgently for laparotomy.

Level 2:

1. A routine laparotomy is not indicated in the hemodynamically stable patient without peritonitis presenting with an isolated splenic injury.

2. The severity of splenic injury (as suggested by CT grade or degree of hemoperitoneum), neurologic status, age greater than 55, and/or the presence of associated injuries are not contraindications to a trial of nonoperative management in a hemodynamically stable patient.

3. In the hemodynamically normal blunt abdominal trauma patient without peritonitis, an abdominal CT scan with intravenous contrast should be performed to identify and assess the severity of injury to the spleen.

4. Angiography should be considered for patients with American Association for the Surgery of Trauma (AAST) grade of greater than III injuries, presence of a contrast blush, moderate hemoperitoneum, or evidence of ongoing splenic bleeding.

5. Nonoperative management of splenic injuries should only be considered in an environment that provides capabilities for monitoring, serial clinical evaluations, and an operating room available for urgent laparotomy. Absolute contraindications to nonoperative management of splenic injuries include hemodynamic instability and concomitant serious intra-abdominal injuries that require surgery. Major disruption of hilar vessels is another contraindication for splenic salvage. In addition, institutional resources such as operating personnel and facilities and the ability for critical care monitoring should be available in case of acute bleeding requiring splenectomy.

Hemodynamic status of a patient is the single most reliable criteria predicting the success of nonoperative therapy and in initial stages should be monitored continuously. Other indices, such as age of the patient and the presence of a contrast blush on CT abdomen, are also associated with an increased risk of failure but are less predictive and should not exclude a patient from a trial of conservative therapy. Grade of injury, hemoperitoneum on abdominal CT, as well as concomitant head injury or extra-abdominal injury are not accurate predictors of the outcome of nonoperative management.

While diagnostic peritoneal lavage, laparoscopy, and ultrasound have all been used successfully in the assessment of splenic injury, the most specific, sensitive, and accurate modality for determination of the severity and extent of injury is CT scan, which also provides the additional benefit of assessment of retroperitoneal injuries.

BIBLIOGRAPHY

Stassen NA, Bhullar I, Cheng JD, et al. Selective nonoperative management of blunt splenic injury: an Eastern Association for the Surgery of Trauma practice management guideline. *J Trauma Acute Care Surg.* 2012 Nov;73(5 Suppl 4):S294–S300.

Wisner DH. Injury to the spleen. In: Mattox KL, Moore EE, Feliciano DV, eds. *Trauma.* 7th ed. New York, NY: McGraw-Hill; 2013: Chapter 30.

15. **(D)** Phagocytosis accounts for the spleen's ability to remove intraerythrocytic inclusion bodies from red cells as they pass through its filter; splenectomy results in characteristic changes in the peripheral smear in the absence of this function. The primary immunologic defect in the asplenic state is in antibody-mediated destruction of encapsulated bacteria. Antibody function and production and phagocytosis are independent functions of the spleen.

Partial splenectomy is primarily indicated to minimize the risk of OPSI and preserve splenic function. Following partial splenectomy, hypertrophy of the remaining segment is the norm and occurs primarily during the first year after surgery. Even with regrowth to 75–100% of the original size of the spleen, hemolysis does not necessarily recur. Partial splenectomy can also reduce transfusion requirements in children with thalassemia, but the results are temporary, and symptoms recur with splenic remnant hypertrophy.

Partial splenectomy involves selective ligation of some of the splenic arteries to induce a large splenic infarct; however, this technique does not consistently result in a predictable amount of residual splenic mass because of the absence of discrete splenic lobules and the prevalence of aberrant arterial supply to the various segments. Because of the technically challenging nature of the operation, all patients should also provide consent for total splenectomy and preoperatively receive immunizations against *Pneumococcus*, *Neisseria meningitides*, and *Haemophilus influenzae*, optimally at least 2 weeks prior to surgery.

BIBLIOGRAPHY

Caro J, Outschoorn U. Hypersplenism and hyposplenism. In: Lichtman MA, Kipps TJ, Seligsohn U, Kaushansky K, Prchal JT, eds. *Williams Hematology.* 8th ed. New York, NY: McGraw-Hill; 2010: Chapter 55.

Park AE, Targarona EM, Belyansky I. Spleen. In: Brunicardi F, Andersen DK, Billiar TR, et al., eds. *Schwartz's Principles of Surgery*. 10th ed. New York, NY: McGraw-Hill; 2014: Chapter 34.

16. **(E)** The most common short-term complications related to splenectomy are atelectasis, pancreatitis, and hemorrhage. In addition to the risk of overwhelming septicemia from encapsulated bacteria, splenectomy may increase the long-term risk for a variety of other conditions.

Hypercoagulable states and thromboembolic disease appear to occur more frequently in a variety of inherited human hemolytic diseases and in a murine model of hereditary spherocytosis.

The increased risk of death from ischemic heart disease after splenectomy has been recognized since the 1970s. The exact pathophysiology is not known, but a number of factors are reasonable: the increased hematocrit, mild-to-moderate thrombocytosis, and elevated cholesterol levels in those with hereditary spherocytosis following splenectomy. In one review of 144 men with hereditary spherocytosis, a long-term increased incidence of arteriosclerotic events, such as stroke, myocardial infarction, and coronary or carotid artery surgery, was shown.

The incidence of pulmonary hypertension may be increased as a result of splenectomy. The underlying mechanism of disease remains unclear.

Although pancreatitis occurs in the immediate postoperative period in as many as 7% of cases, no association between splenectomy and the long-term risk of pancreatitis has been shown to exist. However, there is a significantly increased risk of malignancy, including liver, colon and pancreas cancer.

BIBLIOGRAPHY

Doherty GM. Spleen. In: Doherty GM, ed. *Current Diagnosis and Treatment: Surgery*. 14th ed. New York, NY: McGraw-Hill; 2014: Chapter 27.

Kristinsson SY, Gridley G, Hoover RN, Check D, Landgren O. Long-term risks after splenectomy among 8,149 cancer-free American veterans: a cohort study with up to 27 years follow-up. *Haematologica*. 2014 Feb;99(2):392–398.

Simonneau G, Gatzoulis MA, Adatia I, et al. Updated clinical classification of pulmonary hypertension. *J Am Coll Cardiol*. 2013;62(25):D34–D41.

17. **(C)** Aneurysms of the splenic artery are the most prevalent splanchnic artery aneurysm, accounting for 60% of cases. Although rare, improvements in radiologic imaging have resulted in an increased awareness of their significance. They are four times more common among women and occur in almost 10% of patients with portal hypertension, with equal distribution among genders. Rarely, they may occur as a result of congenital anomalies of the foregut circulation. They occur most often external to the pancreatic parenchyma except when induced by periarterial chronic pancreatitis.

Three factors have been identified as fundamental to the development of these lesions: arterial fibrodysplasia, pregnancy with its hemodynamic changes and estrogen-related effects on elastic vascular tissue, and cirrhosis with portal hypertension. Pregnancy, especially with multiparity, is a major risk factor for both the development and rupture of aneurysms, with a rate of rupture approaching 95% in lesions identified during pregnancy. Aneurysms less commonly result from penetrating trauma, periarterial inflammation as in the case of chronic pancreatitis, or a systemic vasculitic process. They are predominantly saccular, occur at vessel bifurcations, and occur multiply in 20% of cases. Pancreatic lesions tend to be solitary and occur proximally. Aneurysms are usually found incidentally during studies performed for other reasons and can be diagnosed with arteriography, MRI, color flow Doppler ultrasound, and CT scan. When seen on plain abdominal films, they classically appear as signet ring calcifications in the left upper quadrant.

Patients may be asymptomatic, or they may present with midepigastric or left upper quadrant pain. On rupture, patients may remain hemodynamically stable if the bleeding remains confined to the lesser sac, or they may present in extremis with free intraperitoneal rupture. Less commonly, GI bleeding may be the presentation, resulting either from rupture of a pancreatitis-induced aneurysm into adjacent hollow viscera or from esophageal varices that form after rupture of the aneurysm into the neighboring splenic vein produces an arteriovenous fistula. Pregnancy-related lesions have a much higher rate of rupture compared to the 2% risk in other populations. Rupture typically occurs during the third trimester, with a very high mortality rate for both the mother and fetus, thus mandating operative intervention.

Treatment of choice is simple aneurysm ligation or exclusion with vascular reconstruction. Distal pancreatectomy may be needed for the aneurysm embedded within the pancreas. Distal lesions in close proximity to the splenic hilum should be treated with concomitant splenectomy. An excellent prognosis follows elective treatment. Splenic artery embolization has been used to treat splenic artery aneurysm, but painful splenic infarction and abscess may follow. Endovascular treatment appears to have better short-term results compared with open repair, including significantly lower perioperative mortality. However, open repair is associated with fewer late complications and fewer reinterventions.

BIBLIOGRAPHY

Hogendoorn W, Lavida A, Hunink MG, et al. Open repair, endovascular repair, and conservative management of true splenic artery aneurysms. *J Vasc Surg.* 2014 Dec;60(6):1667–76.e1.

Park AE, Targarona EM, Belyansky I. Spleen. In: Brunicardi F, Andersen DK, Billiar TR, et al., eds. *Schwartz's Principles of Surgery.* 10th ed. New York, NY: McGraw-Hill; 2014: Chapter 34.

18. **(D)** Immune thrombocytopenic purpura is an autoimmune disorder in which the antibody targets platelet membrane glycoprotein IIb/IIIa. Women are affected twice as frequently as men. Approximately 50% of patients are children, characteristically presenting abruptly after a viral illness. Among adults, patients are typically in their 20s or 30s and clinically unremarkable except for nosebleeds, petechiae, or other mucocutaneous bleeding with minor trauma. Splenomegaly is uncommon except in children. The diagnosis is difficult to establish and remains one of exclusion. In adults, an underlying cause should be sought, including evaluation for other autoimmune diseases, lymphoproliferative disease, and viral infection. Certain medications, such as quinidine and heparin, are other etiologies of secondary ITP.

Medical therapy consists of high-dose corticosteroids and intravenous immune globulin. In selected patients, anti-D immune globulin may be helpful. ITP is typically self-limited in children and in most cases resolves within 12 months with medical management and activity restriction; 10–30% of cases become chronic but respond well to splenectomy. Only 15% of adult patients respond to medical interventions and thus most require splenectomy.

Splenectomy is currently indicated in patients who fail to respond to steroid treatment within 6 weeks, who recur after steroid taper, who respond to medical therapy but cannot tolerate the side effects, or who develop intracranial bleeding or profound GI bleeding and do not respond to intensive medical treatment. A favorable response to splenectomy is obtained in 85% of patients undergoing surgery. Predictors of success include initial response to medical therapy, younger age, short duration of disease, and prompt thrombocytosis after surgery.

Laparoscopic management has proven to be safe and cost-effective, with less postoperative pain, earlier return to regular diet, and shorter hospitalization compared to the open procedure; results in ITP also compare favorably with laparoscopic splenectomy performed for other hematologic indications. The procedure has been reported to have a higher incidence of missed accessory spleens; thus, a careful exploration should be performed at the start of the procedure. Any postoperative persistent thrombocytopenia should prompt careful workup with red cell scintigraphy to evaluate for residual splenic tissue before aggressive medical therapy is resumed. Reexploration for a missed accessory spleen appears to be effective with minimal associated morbidity. Preoperative scintigraphy and CT scanning for detection of accessory spleens has not proven sufficiently sensitive to be a cost-effective modality and is not recommended.

BIBLIOGRAPHY

Allshouse MJ. The spleen. In: Ziegler MM, Azizkhan RG, Allmen D, Weber TR, eds. *Operative Pediatric Surgery.* 2nd ed. New York, NY: McGraw-Hill; 2014: Chapter 59.

Cines DB, Blanchette VS. Immune thrombocytopenic purpura. *N Engl J Med.* 2002;346(13):995–1008.

Konkle B. Disorders of platelets and vessel wall. In: Longo DL, Fauci AS, Kasper DL, Hauser SL, Jameson J, Loscalzo J, eds. *Harrison's Principles of Internal Medicine.* 18th ed. New York, NY: McGraw-Hill; 2012: Chapter 115.

Tavakkoli A. The spleen. In: Zinner MJ, Ashley SW, eds. *Maingot's Abdominal Operations.* 12th ed. New York, NY: McGraw-Hill; 2013: Chapter 62.

19. **(B)** Hemolytic anemia is an important cause of cholelithiasis, and discovery of bilirubinate stones in a previously undiagnosed patient should prompt a search for an underlying etiology. Hemolysis can be diagnosed by the presence of reticulocytosis in the absence of bleeding. Other tests, such as serum haptoglobin, are less specific and are supplementary. Screening for sickle hemoglobinopathies is now routinely included in most neonatal screening programs.

The spleen often plays an important role in hemolytic disease, frequently sequestering abnormal or misshapen cells, leading to their early destruction. In sickle cell anemia, cells occlude the sinusoids and lead to splenomegaly, abscess formation, and infarction. After multiple episodes, the spleen may fibrose and cease to function. This is known as *autosplenectomy* and frequently occurs in children affected with sickle cell anemia by 1 year of age. Patients with sickle cell anemia are at extremely high risk for septicemia and must be treated as asplenic patients with careful attention to prophylactic oral penicillin and immunization against encapsulated bacteria. Prophylactic penicillin may reduce the risk of sepsis by as much as 84%.

β-Thalassemia is a heritable disorder that in its homozygous form is the most common cause of transfusion-dependent anemia in children worldwide. The primary defect is a quantitative deficiency in globin chain production that leads to accumulation of intracellular particles that contribute to accelerated RBC destruction in the spleen. The thalassemia minor heterozygote is asymptomatic. Thalassemia major is characterized by chronic anemia and jaundice. Anemia develops after 3–4 months of life with the decline in production of fetal hemoglobin. Associated splenic manifestations include compressive splenomegaly, transfusion-dependent anemia, and splenic infarction. Gallstones occur in about one-fourth of these patients. Diagnosis is by peripheral blood smear and hemoglobin electrophoresis. Treatment is primarily supportive with iron chelation and transfusion to maintain a hemoglobin of 9–10 g/dL. High transfusion requirements (greater than 200–250 mL/kg per year) often result in hypersplenism; requirements may be reduced significantly with splenectomy. Even with appropriate immunization and penicillin prophylaxis, among asplenic patients, these individuals have one of the highest rates of postsplenectomy sepsis.

In autoimmune hemolytic anemia, the body produces IgG or IgM directed against the Rh antigen or against one of the minor Rh determinants (c or e), which shortens the life of RBCs. The majority of cases involve autoantibodies optimally reactive in warm temperatures (>37°C), termed *warm-agglutinin* disease. Splenectomy is indicated in patients who require chronic steroid therapy in doses greater than 15 mg/day or experience persistent or worsening anemia with medical therapy; a favorable response is achieved in 50–80% of patients. Surgery plays no role in the management of cold-agglutinin hemolytic anemia.

Thrombotic thrombocytopenic purpura (TTP) is a form of thrombotic microangiopathy that results in microvascular occlusion by subendothelial and luminal deposition of hyaline material. It is postulated to arise from unregulated von Willebrand factor–dependent platelet thrombosis. Hemolytic uremic syndrome is frequently associated with TTP and refers to thrombotic microangiopathy that mainly affects the kidney and usually causes oliguric or anuric renal failure. The classic clinical pentad consists of fever, hemolytic anemia, purpura, neurologic symptoms, and renal failure. Management relies on plasma exchange to remove antibody inhibitors and replenish deficient enzymes, although splenectomy may reduce the frequency of relapses for some patients with TTP who are refractory to plasma exchange or immunosuppressive therapy.

Hereditary spherocytosis is an autosomal dominant disorder caused by a defect in spectrin, a membrane protein in RBCs. It is the most common hemolytic anemia for which splenectomy is performed. Cells are less plastic and pass through the spleen with difficulty; trapping and sequestration result in mild-to-moderate hemolytic anemia, jaundice, and splenomegaly. Incidence of pigmented

gallstones is estimated at 30–60%, and in many patients cholecystectomy is performed at the time of splenectomy. Although splenectomy does not correct the membrane defect, anemia resolves because the hemolysis is stopped. Because of concerns of postsplenectomy sepsis, splenectomy should be postponed until children are 6 years old or above.

Of the listed hemolytic disorders, sickle cell anemia alone characteristically results in a shrunken spleen. The others typically have a normal spleen or mild splenomegaly.

BIBLIOGRAPHY

Allshouse MJ. The spleen. In: Ziegler MM, Azizkhan RG, Allmen D, Weber TR, eds. *Operative Pediatric Surgery.* 2nd ed. New York, NY: McGraw-Hill; 2014: Chapter 59.

Benz EJ Jr. Disorders of hemoglobin. In: Longo DL, Fauci AS, Kasper DL, Hauser SL, Jameson J, Loscalzo J, eds. *Harrison's Principles of Internal Medicine.* 18th ed. New York, NY: McGraw-Hill; 2012: Chapter 104.

Packman CH. Hemolytic anemia resulting from immune injury. In: Lichtman MA, Kipps TJ, Seligsohn U, Kaushansky K, Prchal JT, eds. *Williams Hematology.* 8th ed. New York, NY: McGraw-Hill; 2010: Chapter 53.

Sadler J, Poncz M. Antibody-mediated thrombotic disorders: thrombotic thrombocytopenic purpura and heparin-induced thrombocytopenia. In: Lichtman MA, Kipps TJ, Seligsohn U, Kaushansky K, Prchal JT, eds. *Williams Hematology.* 8th ed. New York, NY: McGraw-Hill; 2010: Chapter 133.

20. **(D)** Splenosis is the traumatic displacement, autotransplantation, and proliferation of fragmented splenic tissue on peritoneal surfaces. It may occur in as many as 75% of cases of traumatic rupture of the spleen. In elective splenectomy, splenosis correlates with splenic disruption and peritoneal contamination because of poor technique, especially during morcellation and extraction, and can be avoided by careful dissection and handling of tissues. This condition is distinguished from accessory spleen and from polysplenia by its acquired nature. Histologically, the splenetic tissue resembles the parent organ in that all components are present: white pulp, red pulp, and marginal zones. In addition, the fragments retain the ability to clear intraerythrocytic inclusion bodies. Although splenosis appears to correlate with elevated tuftsin levels, it does not appear to protect meaningfully against OPSI. Most patients are asymptomatic, but the implants stimulate adhesion formation and may lead to bowel obstruction.

Polysplenia is a congenital abnormality found in some cases of heterotaxy, or situs ambiguus, the malposition and dysmorphism of viscera in the chest and abdomen. In contrast to situs solitus, or normal orientation of viscera and vasculature, and situs inversus, the complete mirror image of normal, visceral organization in hetero-taxia is disorderly and variable among individuals along a wide spectrum. Patients with polysplenia have bilateral left-sidedness (left isomerism) and usually have other abnormalities, such as bilateral bilobar lungs, congenital heart disease, and intestinal malrotation. Splenic elements each tend to be more substantial than in splenosis or accessory spleens; however, polysplenia may result in abnormal splenic function in certain children.

Accessory spleens result from incomplete embryologic fusion of splenic elements and have been reported to occur in as many as 15–40% of patients. Failure of splenectomy to treat hematologic disorders such as ITP is frequently because of a missed accessory spleen; thus, a careful exploration should be performed at the start of the procedure. Any postoperative persistent thrombo-cytopenia should prompt careful workup with red cell scintigraphy to evaluate for residual splenic tissue before aggressive medical therapy is resumed. Preoperative scintigraphy and CT scanning for detection of accessory spleens has not proven sufficiently sensitive to be a cost-effective modality and is not recommended.

BIBLIOGRAPHY

Doherty GM. Spleen. In: Doherty GM, ed. *Current Diagnosis and Treatment: Surgery*. 14th ed. New York, NY: McGraw-Hill; 2014: Chapter 27.

Skandalakis PN, Skandalakis LJ, Kingsnorth AN, et al. Spleen. In: Skandalakis JE, Colburn GL, Weidman TA, et al., eds. *Skandalakis' Surgical Anatomy*. New York, NY: McGraw-Hill; 2004: Chapter 22.

21. **(C)** Laparoscopic splenectomy has rapidly become the standard of care for benign splenic disease in the last decade in both children and adults. Advantages include reduced postoperative pain, earlier mobilization, shorter hospitalization, reduced severity of wound-related complications, and improved postoperative pulmonary toilet. It has proved to be therapeutically equivalent to the open procedure and cost-effective. Lateral positioning, development of bipolar electrocautery and the harmonic scalpel, and standardization of techniques have all contributed to its success.

The application in treatment of malignant disease has been received less enthusiastically, particularly in cases of massive splenomegaly (spleen weight > 1000 g). Increased splenic mass even in the absence of a malignant diagnosis substantially increases the technical difficulty of both the open and laparoscopic approaches. In addition, there is concern for tumor spillage in cases of primary or metastatic tumors of the spleen. Hand assistance is generally recommended in these cases.

Blood transfusion also appears to correlate directly as an independent risk factor with the incidence of infectious complications in a linear, dose-dependent fashion. Other factors, such as active perisplenitis, splenic infection, severe obesity, and abdominal adhesions, also increase the difficulty of the procedure.

Splenectomy is often performed in HIV-positive patients for HIV-related ITP. HIV-positive status does not appear to adversely affect outcomes, and splenectomy has proven effective therapy, with a 93% remission rate in autoimmune thrombocytopenia. Of note, HIV-positive patients appear to improve following splenectomy, likely because of elimination of the large viral load carried by splenic lymphocytes, and have been observed to experience delay in onset of AIDS and elevation of $CD4^+$ counts.

BIBLIOGRAPHY

Gamme G, Birch DW, Karmali S. Minimally invasive splenectomy: an update and review. *Can J Surg*. 2013 Aug;56(4):280–285.

Katz SC, Pachter HL. Indications for splenectomy. *Am Surg*. 2006;72:565–580.

Tavakkoli A. The spleen. In: Zinner MJ, Ashley SW, eds. *Maingot's Abdominal Operations*. 12th ed. New York, NY: McGraw-Hill; 2013: Chapter 62.

22. **(A)** Overwhelming postsplenectomy infection, otherwise known as postsplenectomy sepsis, occurs in asplenic and hyposplenic patients. Encapsulated bacteria are most often responsible, with *Streptococcus pneumoniae* estimated to account for 50–90% of cases, but a wide range of other microorganisms, such as *E. coli*, *Enterococcus*, *Salmonella*, *Staphylococcus*, and *Clostridium* species, as well as nonbacterial organisms have been implicated. The lifetime risk ranges from 1 to 5%, but does not appear to diminish with time; cases several decades after splenectomy have been reported.

The spleen plays an important role in sequestration of microorganisms in the primary exposure to an antigen, and prolonged contact with immune cells in the splenic sinusoids facilitates the prompt manufacture of specific antibodies early in the course of infection and subsequent phagocytosis. Patients without a spleen have delayed amplification of the immune response in both primary and subsequent exposures and are thus highly susceptible to infections by potent, rapidly disseminating organisms such as *S. pneumoniae*. In addition, while complement effectively opsonizes unencapsulated bacteria for uptake in the liver, complement bound to the cell wall in encapsulated bacteria is buried under the capsule and is thus inaccessible to hepatic phagocytes.

The principal determinant of risk for OPSI is reason for splenectomy, with patients who undergo splenectomy for hematologic disease at greatest risk. The lowest incidence is observed in patients who undergo splenectomy for trauma or incidentally as part of other procedures, such as gastrectomy. Clinically, the disposition of patients with congenital absence of the spleen and sickle cell disease to developing OPSI is indistinguishable from that of postsurgical patients, and these patients should be protected in a similar manner.

Children under 5 years of age and adults over 50 are also at risk. The increased susceptibility in children stems partly from the relative naiveté of their immune systems from lack of exposure to a sufficient range of antigens prior to the time of the hyposplenic or asplenic state. In addition, children do not appear to respond as efficiently to vaccination, indicating the involvement of factors innate to the developing immune system. For these reasons, splenectomy is delayed or avoided as much as possible, and current recommendations advocate oral penicillin prophylaxis.

BIBLIOGRAPHY

Di Sabatino A, Carsetti R, Corazza GR. Post-splenectomy and hyposplenic states. *Lancet.* 2011;378:86–97.

Park AE, Targarona EM, Belyansky I. Spleen. In: Brunicardi F, Andersen DK, Billiar TR, et al., eds. *Schwartz's Principles of Surgery.* 10th ed. New York, NY: McGraw-Hill; 2014: Chapter 34.

23. **(E)** Immunity is serotype specific because specific antibodies are required to confer protection against each serotype. In addition, vaccines protect poorly against less-immunogenic serotypes, so that individuals remain susceptible despite careful adherence to protocols. Children under 2 years of age have suboptimal antibody responses to vaccination regardless of timing of vaccination because of the immaturity of their immune systems.

Conjugate vaccines are particularly effective in children and other patients with suboptimal immune competence. They are engineered using additional peptide adjuvants to a polysaccharide antigen to enhance immunogenicity. The current *Pneumococcus* vaccine incorporates 23 capsular polysaccharides responsible for 85% of infections and is estimated to have a 57% overall protective efficacy in patients over 5 years of age. A conjugated form is not currently available. Asplenic patients who received the earlier 14-valent vaccine should be revaccinated. In addition, data show a decline over time in antibody titers, particularly in young children, and individuals should receive booster revaccination for *Pneumococcus* every 3–5 years, depending on the individual's degree of risk.

The conjugate *H. influenzae* type B vaccine has enhanced T cell–dependent characteristics over the original unconjugated vaccine, with excellent immunologic response even in infants. Integration of this vaccine in pediatric vaccination protocols has virtually eradicated invasive disease in young children, and all previously unvaccinated adults should be immunized prior to splenectomy.

The vaccine against *Meningococcus* is a conjugate vaccine against four of the major capsular antigens: A, C, Y, and W135. Response to immunization against *Meningococcus* is more uniformly effective among all populations, even among children under 2 years of age. Serotype B is poorly immunogenic, and although the incidence is approximately 60% of isolates, no vaccine exists at present. Data currently do not support booster revaccination with *Meningococcus* or *H. influenzae* vaccines.

Although most patients have some degree of response to vaccines, data indicate that the response in asplenic individuals is subnormal, and thus current guidelines for vaccination recommend immunization of patients at the earliest possible time, at a minimum of 2 weeks prior to elective splenectomy. In patients immunized postoperatively following emergent splenectomy for trauma, delay of pneumococcal vaccination to 14 days postsplenectomy appeared to correlate with better functional antibody response against a number of serotypes. This benefit should be carefully weighed against the potential for loss to follow-up.

In addition to these measures, patients should receive annual influenza vaccination. Children should receive daily oral penicillin or erythromycin chemoprophylaxis. A high level of suspicion must be maintained for OPSI, and with any evidence of febrile illness, patients should be hospitalized and managed empirically with broad-spectrum systemic antibiotics while cultures are pending.

None of these measures protects completely against OPSI, and numerous cases of sepsis have been reported even with strict compliance with prescribed regimens. These interventions have, however, markedly reduced the incidence of OPSI.

BIBLIOGRAPHY

Davies JM, Lewis MPN, Wimperis J, Rafi I, Ladhani S, Bolton-Maggs HB. Review of guidelines for the prevention and treatment of infection in patients with an absent or dysfunctional spleen: prepared on behalf of the British Committee for Standards in Haematology by a Working Party of the Haemato-Oncology Task Force. *Br J Haematol.* 2011;155(3):308–317.

Schuchat A, Jackson LA. Immunization principles and vaccine use. In: Longo DL, Fauci AS, Kasper DL, Hauser SL, Jameson J, Loscalzo J, eds. *Harrison's Principles of Internal Medicine.* 18th ed. New York, NY: McGraw-Hill; 2012: Chapter 122.

24. **(B)** The primary indications for splenectomy in the management of myeloproliferative and lymphoproliferative malignancies are symptomatic splenomegaly, cytopenias associated with hypersplenism, relief of pain from splenic infarction, and staging to determine the need for chemotherapy. With the exception of diagnostic applications in Hodgkin's lymphoma, surgical intervention is therefore primarily palliative. Splenomegaly is common and frequently results in hypersplenism, cellular trapping, and sequestration that lead to splenic enlargement, thrombocytopenia, and anemia. Patients tend to be older with greater morbidity and debilitation and are at higher risk for bleeding and complications than individuals undergoing splenectomy for benign causes. The increased risk of bleeding is related both to preexistent cytopenias and to organomegaly. Some degree of immunosuppression is in most cases inherent in the primary disease process, and these patients are at particularly high risk for postsplenectomy sepsis. Nevertheless, splenectomy often provides significant relief as well as improvement in cytopenias and should be considered in symptomatic patients and those with refractory cytopenia.

Non-Hodgkin's lymphoma is distinguished from Hodgkin's lymphoma in that progression does not occur in a predictable stepwise fashion, and frequently patients present with disseminated disease. Approximately 75% have hypersplenism, and many experience correction of hematologic depression following splenectomy. Only in rare cases lymphoma may be limited to the splenic parenchyma and may require no further intervention beyond splenectomy. More commonly, patients have splenic-predominant features and low-grade disease; in these patients, splenectomy may improve short-term survival.

Although splenectomy is primarily of palliative value for relief of pain and cytopenia in all of the indications mentioned, only in Hodgkin's lymphoma does it play a substantial role in diagnosis. The disease spreads in a predictable anatomic stepwise progression among nodal beds from cranial to caudal in 90% of patients. Staging laparotomy with splenectomy may be of benefit in selected early-stage patients to help determine the need for systemic treatment for chemotherapy.

BIBLIOGRAPHY

Beauchamp RD, Holzman MD, Fabian TC. Spleen. In: Townsend CM, Beauchamp RD, Evers BM, et al., eds. *Textbook of Surgery: The Biological Basis of Modern Surgical Practice.* 16th ed. Philadelphia, PA: Saunders; 2001:1144–1164.

Fraker DL. Spleen. In: Greenfield LJ, Mulholland MW, Oldham KT, et al., eds. *Scientific Principles and Practice of Surgery.* 3rd ed. Philadelphia, PA: Lippincott Williams & Wilkins; 2001:1236–1259.

Harris JA, Gadacz TR. Tumors, cysts, and abscesses of the spleen. In: Cameron JL, ed. *Current Surgical Therapy.* 7th ed. St. Louis, MO: Mosby; 2001:591–595.

25. **(E)** Splenic abscess is a rare but potentially lethal condition. Immunocompromised patients and patients who abuse intravenous drugs are particularly susceptible. The abscesses develop by four basic mechanisms: metastatic hematogenous spread from a distant source, such as osteomyelitis or infective endocarditis; following trauma or iatrogenic injury, especially with increasing use of nonoperative management; secondary infection following splenic infarction, such as in sickle cell and splenic embolization; and by extension from a contiguous infective source, such as a perinephric, pancreatic, or diverticular abscess. They may also develop in patients undergoing chemotherapy for diseases such as leukemia. They are primarily unilocular in adults but multilocular in children. *Staphyloccoccus* and *Streptococcus* species account for 30% of cases; other common organisms include *Enterococcus, Salmonella,* and *E. coli.* The growing population of immunosuppressed patients has increased the frequency of atypical pathogens, such as *Mycobacterium* and *Actinomycoses* species, as well as fungal infections with *Candida, Cryptococcus,* and *Aspergillus.*

The most common presenting symptoms are fever and abdominal pain in the left upper quadrant. Patients also frequently have splenomegaly, leukocytosis, and bacteremia. In the face of such a nonspecific presentation, imaging should be performed early for diagnosis, especially in the intensive care unit (ICU) setting and in immunosuppressed patients.

The imaging modality of choice is CT scan, on which lesions tend to have a heterogeneous appearance while cysts tend to be homogeneous. Ultrasound may be helpful where CT is unavailable. Patients should be hospitalized and treated promptly with broad-spectrum systemic antibiotics, including coverage for fungal agents if immunosuppressed. Unilocular abscesses may be percutaneously aspirated; however, contents may be thick and tenacious, and with failure of percutaneous drainage, operative intervention should be performed early to avoid significant increases in morbidity and mortality. Percutaneous drainage has the advantage of splenic conservation with all of the associated immunologic implications, especially in young patients. Multilocular abscesses and those originating from a contiguous source usually require splenectomy. Relative contraindications to percutaneous management also include refractory coagulopathy, ascites, rupture with hemorrhage, and need for surgical intervention for another associated problem. Partial splenectomy, splenotomy with drainage, and laparoscopic splenectomy have all been used with success. Splenic abscesses may be complicated by intraperitoneal rupture, by rupture into adjacent organs, and with possible subsequent formation of a fistula.

Although immunosuppressed patients are at higher risk for development of splenic abscesses, this patient is clearly able to mount an immune response judging from the marked leukocytosis and the recent history of clinical improvement of the diverticulitis. Depressed immune function would first manifest increased bacterial translocation across the gut mucosa into the portal system, and the presence of an isolated splenic abscess with no hepatic disease or other foci suggesting hematogenous dissemination further discounts this mechanism. More plausibly, this process is a result of direct local extension of the sigmoid disease into the spleen or from rupture of a previously contained abscess.

BIBLIOGRAPHY

Beauchamp RD, Holzman MD, Fabian TC. Spleen. In: Townsend CM, Beauchamp RD, Evers BM, et al., eds. *Textbook of Surgery: The Biological Basis of Modern Surgical Practice*. 16th ed. Philadelphia, PA: Saunders; 2001:1144–1164.

Harris JA, Gadacz TR. Tumors, cysts, and abscesses of the spleen. In: Cameron JL, ed. *Current Surgical Therapy*. 7th ed. St. Louis, MO: Mosby; 2001:591–595.

Ooi LLPJ, Leong SS. Splenic abscesses from 1987 to 1995. *Am J Surg*. 1997;174:87–93.

Phillips GS, Radosevich MD, Lipsett PA. Splenic abscesses: another look at an old disease. *Arch Surg*. 1997;132:1331–1336.

CHAPTER 25

ADRENAL GLAND

ELLIOT A. ASARE, JOHN T. MIURA, AND AZADEH A. CARR

QUESTIONS

1. A computed tomography (CT) scan is obtained on a 60-year-old patient with suspected acute diverticulitis. In addition to findings consistent with diverticulitis of the sigmoid colon, he is found to have a 2-cm homogeneous left adrenal mass, as seen in Fig. 25-1. Which of the following is true concerning the further workup of the adrenal mass?

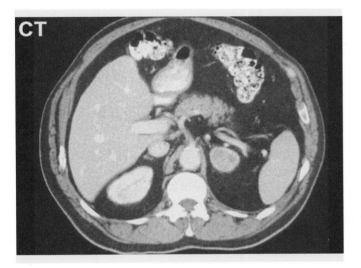

FIGURE 25-1. CT scan of a left-sided, benign adrenal adenoma.

(A) Biopsy should be performed, followed by biochemical workup.
(B) Given the patient's age, this is likely a metastatic lesion from a nonadrenal primary.
(C) Normal serum aldosterone, in the face of normokalemia and normal blood pressure, essentially rules out functional aldosteronoma.
(D) Normal plasma cortisol level essentially rules out cortisol-producing adrenocortical adenoma.

2. In the patient from question 1, you have demonstrated that this is a nonfunctional adrenal mass, and you have no suspicion of it being metastatic. Which of the following is the most appropriate management?
(A) Biopsy via fine-needle aspiration
(B) Laparoscopic adrenalectomy
(C) Repeat imaging with CT scan in 3–6 months
(D) Transabdominal adrenalectomy with exploration of the contralateral adrenal gland for occult tumor

3. A 22-year-old woman with hypertension refractory to medical management is referred to you after a CT scan was obtained that demonstrated a 3-cm mass in the right adrenal gland (Fig. 25-2). The initial diagnostic test of choice is
(A) Measurement of plasma free metanephrines and normetanephrines
(B) Magnetic resonance imaging (MRI)
(C) Measurement of catecholamines and metanephrines in a morning serum sample
(D) High-dose dexamethasone suppression test

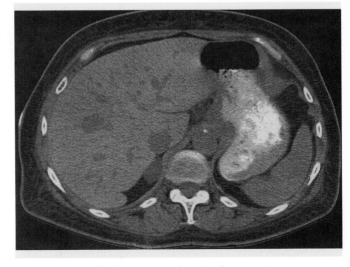

FIGURE 25-2. Right benign adrenal adenoma. Image courtesy of Fergus Coakley, MD, UCSF Radiology Department.

4. Which of the following is false about the perioperative management of pheochromocytoma?
   (A) Use of a long-acting alpha-adrenergic antagonist preoperatively
   (B) Initiation of β-adrenergic blockers before starting long-acting α-adrenergic antagonists
   (C) Ligation of the adrenal vein(s) before the adrenal artery(ies)
   (D) Surgical debulking even if the pheochromocytoma is deemed unresectable on exploration

5. You have been asked to see a full-term infant born yesterday with ambiguous genitalia. There is a small urethral phallus, apparent hypertrophy of a clitoris, and near fusion of the labioscrotal folds. The neonatologist tells you that this child has elevated 17-hydroxyprogesterone. Which of the following is true?
   (A) The most likely cause is 17-hydroxylase deficiency.
   (B) The sex of this patient is usually male (XY chromosomes).
   (C) Serum levels of cortisol will be higher than normal.
   (D) If the sex is female, then ovaries and uterus will likely develop normally.

6. Among adrenal tumors that hypersecrete sex steroids,
   (A) Most are feminizing tumors as opposed to virilizing tumors that develop normally.
   (B) Almost all virilizing tumors are malignant.
   (C) Open adrenalectomy is the preferred procedure of choice for tumors that secrete sex steroids.
   (D) Virilizing tumors may be detected with 24-h urine dehydroepiandrosterone (DHEA), dehydroepiandrosterone sulfate (DHEA-S), or testosterone.

7. Which of the following is true regarding the anatomy of the adrenal glands?
   (A) Venous drainage of the right adrenal gland is predominantly into the right renal vein.
   (B) Both adrenal glands receive significant blood supply from branches of the superior mesenteric artery.
   (C) Venous drainage of both adrenal glands is directly into the inferior vena cava.
   (D) Both adrenal glands receive significant blood supply from their corresponding renal arteries.

8. In which one of the following patients is laparoscopic adrenalectomy contraindicated?
   (A) A 40-year-old male with a 7-cm homogeneous, well-defined, nonfunctional left adrenal mass with previous surgical history of open cholecystectomy
   (B) A 20-year-old female with a 3-cm well-defined mass in the right adrenal gland with episodes of hypertension, whose father died of thyroid carcinoma and apparently had also undergone adrenalectomy at a young age

   (C) A 60-year-old female with back pain and a 7-cm left adrenal mass with irregular borders and possible tumor extension into renal vein
   (D) A 30-year-old male with a 5-cm smooth-bordered right adrenal mass with a 3-month history of diastolic hypertension and elevated serum aldosterone

9. Which of the following is *false* concerning laparoscopic adrenalectomy?
   (A) It is associated with a lower hospital cost compared to open adrenalectomy.
   (B) It is an acceptable technique to remove small hereditary pheochromocytoma.
   (C) It is associated with longer operating room times.
   (D) It is associated with a reduced rate of perioperative blood transfusions.

10. A 55-year-old male undergoes workup for recent onset of diastolic hypertension, polyuria, and fatigue. The diagnosis of hyperaldosteronism is considered. The diagnostic test(s) of choice is (are) which of the following?
    (A) CT scan with special attention to the adrenal glands and kidneys
    (B) Low-dose dexamethasone suppression test
    (C) MRI of the abdomen
    (D) Serum potassium, aldosterone, and renin levels

11. You have diagnosed hyperaldosteronism in the patient in question 10. You obtain a CT scan, which shows bilateral adrenal nodules or bilateral adrenal hyperplasia. Your next step in the management of this patient should be
    (A) Magnetic resonance imaging
    (B) Bilateral adrenalectomy
    (C) Selective adrenal venous sampling
    (D) Medical therapy with spironolactone, triamterene, or amiloride

12. Which of the following is true concerning primary hyperaldosteronism?
    (A) Bilateral hyperplasia of the zona glomerulosa is about twice as likely as either adrenal adenoma or adrenal carcinoma to be responsible for primary hyperaldosteronism.
    (B) Unilateral adrenalectomy is usually curative for bilateral hyperplasia.
    (C) All patients are hypokalemic.
    (D) These patients may present with metabolic alkalosis.

13. Which of the following sites of steroid hormone synthesis is *incorrectly* matched with its product?
    (A) Aldosterone : zona fasciculata
    (B) Cortisol : zona fasciculata
    (C) Cortisol : zona reticularis
    (D) DHEA : zona reticularis

14. Which of the following is *false* concerning adrenal physiology?
    (A) The enzyme 17-alphahydroxylase is necessary to produce both cortisol and the adrenal androgen DHEA.
    (B) Steroid hormones exert their local effects so quickly because they bind directly to cell membrane receptors.
    (C) Cholesterol is either synthesized by the adrenal cortex or extracted from the plasma.
    (D) Cholesterol is the ultimate precursor of cortisol, aldosterone, and DHEA.

15. Which of the following is *not* an effect of the steroid hormone cortisol?
    (A) It curtails the inflammatory response by inhibiting the migration of monocytes and neutrophils.
    (B) It promotes hyperglycemia by both antagonizing glucose uptake peripherally and stimulating hepatic gluconeogenesis.
    (C) It sustains positive nitrogen balance by increasing amino acid delivery to the liver and by increasing peripheral protein synthesis.
    (D) It retards wound healing by impairing collagen formation and fibroblast activity.

16. Which of the following stimuli to adrenal aldosterone secretion is the weakest?
    (A) Long-standing unilateral renal artery stenosis that restricts blood supply by 80%
    (B) Acute hemorrhage from a gunshot wound to the chest in which 30% of total blood volume is lost
    (C) A rise in serum potassium from 4.0 to 4.3 mEq/L
    (D) A pituitary adenoma that secretes ACTH (corticotropin), with serum ACTH levels twice normal

17. Which of the following is true regarding adrenal production of androgens?
    (A) Production of adrenal DHEA is primarily under control of luteinizing hormone (LH) and follicle-stimulating hormone (FSH).
    (B) DHEA is converted to estrogen peripherally.
    (C) The presence of adrenal androgens in the developing fetus influences development of male genitalia.
    (D) In adults, excessive adrenal production of androgens is most likely secondary to an enzyme deficiency.

18. A 35-year-old male patient presents with signs and symptoms consistent with Cushing's syndrome. A low-dose dexamethasone suppression test shows no significant suppression of serum cortisol. Measurement of serum ACTH level demonstrates profoundly low levels of ACTH. A CT scan shows a 4-cm, well-circumscribed mass in the right adrenal gland. The best choice for further therapy is which one of the following?
    (A) Laparoscopic right adrenalectomy
    (B) Suppression of cortisol production with aminoglutethimide
    (C) CT scan of the head to delineate pituitary anatomy
    (D) CT-guided biopsy of the right adrenal mass

19. Which statement best describes the role of exogenous steroids in the perioperative period in the patient in question 18?
    (A) There is no role for exogenous steroids in this patient.
    (B) Exogenous steroids are indicated only if there is suspicion of an additional contralateral adrenal tumor.
    (C) Almost all patients undergoing surgery for this disease will require perioperative exogenous steroids.
    (D) The high-dose dexamethasone suppression test will determine whether this patient needs perioperative exogenous steroids.

20. A 35-year-old male patient presents with signs and symptoms consistent with Cushing's syndrome. A low-dose dexamethasone suppression test shows no significant suppression of serum cortisol. Measurement of serum ACTH demonstrates a level that is higher than normal. A high-dose dexamethasone suppression test reveals only partial suppression of serum cortisol levels. The next step should be which of the following?
    (A) MRI of the head
    (B) CT scan of the chest and abdomen
    (C) Bilateral adrenalectomy and lifelong exogenous steroid administration
    (D) Transsphenoidal resection of the pituitary gland

21. A 35-year-old male patient presents with signs and symptoms consistent with Cushing's syndrome. A low-dose dexamethasone suppression test shows no significant suppression of serum cortisol. Measurement of serum ACTH demonstrates a level that is higher than normal. The high-dose dexamethasone suppression test reveals no suppression of serum ACTH. Which of the following is *not* likely to be indicated?
    (A) CT scan of the abdomen and chest
    (B) Medical therapy with drugs such as aminoglutethimide or metyrapone if deemed inoperable
    (C) Administration of exogenous steroids to suppress ACTH production
    (D) Surgical debulking if deemed unresectable

22. Among the following, the first test of choice to diagnose Cushing's syndrome (hypercortisolism) is
    (A) Overnight low-dose dexamethasone suppression test
    (B) Plasma ACTH level
    (C) Corticotropin-releasing hormone (CRH) test
    (D) High-dose dexamethasone suppression test

23. Among the following, the first test in the process to diagnose adrenal insufficiency is
    (A) ACTH stimulation test
    (B) Low-dose dexamethasone suppression test
    (C) Measurement of plasma ACTH level
    (D) Measurement of morning levels of serum or salivary cortisol levels

24. Which of the following tests is *not* useful in differentiating between a pituitary and ectopic source of ACTH excess?
    (A) High-dose dexamethasone suppression test
    (B) Inferior petrosal venous sampling
    (C) ACTH stimulation test
    (D) MRI of the head

ANSWERS AND EXPLANATIONS

1. **(C)**

2. **(C)**

Explanation for questions 1 and 2

Adrenal incidentalomas are masses discovered on the adrenal gland during radiologic imaging for other reasons. The reported incidence is 5%. Among patients with adrenal incidentalomas, approximately 80% have non-functional adenomas, 5% have subclinical Cushing's syndrome, 5% have pheochromocytoma, fewer than 5% have adrenal cortical carcinoma, 2.5% have metastatic lesions, and the rest may be ganglioneuromas, myelolipomas, or benign cysts. Cortical adenomas are usually small and homogeneous, with a smooth, encapsulated margin on CT scan. They usually do not enhance with intravenous contrast and are usually low-attenuation lesions (less than 10 Hounsfield units) when intravenous contrast is not used. Important questions to address when evaluating an adrenal incidentaloma are as follows: (1) Functional status: Is the lesion hormonally active? (2) Radiologic characteristics: Does the lesion have radiographic features suggestive of a malignancy? (3) Medical history: Does the patient have a previous history of cancer?

Serum biochemical tests can rule out functional cortical adenomas. Functional aldosteronomas cause hypertension, hypokalemia, weakness, and polyuria. Laboratory abnormalities include elevated serum aldosterone, hypokalemia, and suppressed renin activity. Functional aldosteronoma is unlikely in a patient

without hypertension and with normal serum potassium. Functional cortisol-producing adenomas usually cause Cushing's syndrome, characterized by weight gain, hypertension, easy bruisability, diabetes mellitus, and centripetal obesity ("buffalo hump" and "moon face") (Fig. 25-3).

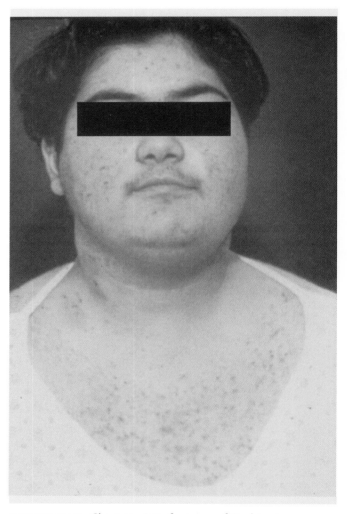

FIGURE 25-3. Characteristic features of Cushing's syndrome (from Brunicardi FC, Andersen DK, Billiar TR, et al., (eds.), *Schwartz's Principles of Surgery*. 9th ed. New York, NY: McGraw-Hill; 2010: Fig. 38-42. Copyright © The McGraw-Hill Companies, Inc., All rights reserved).

Because the total amount of daily cortisol secreted in these patients can be normal, 24-h urine collection for cortisol may be normal, and this test is not sensitive. Random serum tests for cortisol are not helpful, as these patients lose the normal diurnal variation in cortisol secretion. The simplest test to screen for functional cortisol-producing adenoma is the 1-mg overnight dexamethasone suppression test. Patients with functional cortisol-producing adenoma will fail to suppress the plasma cortisol level after a low dose of dexamethasone.

A late-night salivary cortisol level may be obtained. Further testing in the form of plasma ACTH level is then necessary to exclude a pituitary source. A hormonally active adenoma is an indication for adrenalectomy.

The most important tumor to exclude in the case of adrenal incidentaloma is pheochromocytoma. These are tumors of the chromaffin cells of the adrenal medulla. Pheochromocytomas are also relatively rare tumors unless there is a patient or family history of its predisposing syndromes: von Recklinghausen's neurofibromatosis, von Hippel–Lindau's (VHL) disease, and multiple endocrine neoplasia (MEN) syndromes 2A and 2B. All patients with an adrenal mass need to be biochemically tested for pheochromocytoma, which consists of checking plasma free metanephrines and normetanephrines.

Adrenocortical carcinomas (ACCs) are rare tumors. Approximately two-thirds of ACCs are functional and secrete cortisol, androgens, estrogens, aldosterone, or multiple hormones. One-third of patients manifest classic Cushing's syndrome. No biochemical or cytologic test can definitively predict ACC before surgical resection. The prevalence of ACC among incidentalomas larger than 6 cm is 25%. The concern for ACC is high when an adrenal mass has more than 10 Hounsfield units on noncontrast CT. They are inhomogeneous masses with irregular borders that enhance with intravenous contrast. For example, see Fig. 25-4 of a left-sided adrenal carcinoma. Surgery is

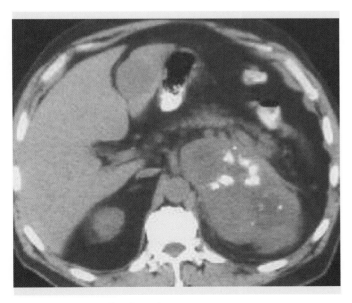

FIGURE 25-4. Left adrenal carcinoma.

the only possible cure for this rare entity. Biopsy should never be performed of a suspected ACC.

Primary tumors that metastasize to the adrenals include breast, lung, renal cell, melanoma, stomach, and lymphomatous cancers. In a patient with known

extra-adrenal malignancy and adrenal mass, this mass can be assumed to be metastatic. In a patient with a history of extra-adrenal malignancy but who is deemed disease free, the finding of an adrenal mass is the only case in which fine-needle aspiration biopsy may be warranted. This should never be done until the possibility of pheochromocytoma is excluded.

Once the entities of functional adenoma, metastatic lesion, pheochromocytoma, and carcinoma are ruled out, it is assumed that this is a nonfunctional adenoma. Because of the increased risk of malignancy with increased size, it is recommended that adrenalectomy be performed for lesions 4 or 5 cm in diameter or larger or if there is a suggestion of atypical features on CT or MRI. If the mass is less than 4–5 cm in diameter and its appearance is benign on imaging, repeat imaging should be performed at 3–6 months and annually for 1–2 years. Annual hormone evaluation should be performed for up to 5 years. Surgical excision is recommended if the lesion grows more than 1 cm or becomes hormonally active.

BIBLIOGRAPHY

Duh Q, Liu C, Tyrrell J. Adrenals. In: Doherty GM, (ed.), *Current Diagnosis & Treatment: Surgery*. 13e. New York, NY: McGraw-Hill; 2010: Chapter 33.

Kebebew E, Reiff E, Duh QY, Clark OH, McMillan A. Extent of disease at presentation and outcome for adrenocortical carcinoma: have we made progress? *World J Surg* 2006 May;30(5):872–878.

Lal G, Clark OH. Thyroid, parathyroid, and adrenal. In: Brunicardi F, Andersen DK, Billiar TR, et al., (eds.), *Schwartz's Principles of Surgery*. 9th ed. New York, NY: McGraw-Hill; 2010: Chapter 38.

Yeh M, Duh QY. The adrenal glands. In: Townsend CM, Beauchamp RD, Evers BM, Mattox KL, (eds.), *Sabiston Textbook of Surgery*. 19th ed. Philadelphia, PA: Saunders; 2012:963–992.

Zeiger MA, Thompson GB, Duh QY, et al. American Association of Clinical Endocrinologists and American Association of Endocrine Surgeons medical guidelines for the management of adrenal incidentalomas: executive summary of recommendations. *Endocr Pract* 2009 Jul–Aug;15(5):450–453.

3. **(A)**

4. **(B)**

Explanation for questions 3 and 4

There are multiple adrenal causes of surgically correctable hypertension, including functional aldosteronoma, cortisol-producing adenoma, and pheochromocytoma. It is imperative to rule out pheochromocytoma early. The most sensitive and specific test for pheochromocytoma is plasma free metanephrines and normetanephrines. Measurement of urinary fractionated metanephrines may be used as a confirmatory test or in borderline cases. Measurements of urinary vanillylmandelic acid and catecholamines (epinephrine, norepinephrine, and dopamine) are less sensitive and less specific.

Pheochromocytoma is a catecholamine-secreting tumor of the adrenal medulla chromaffin cells. Pheochromocytomas can also be extra-adrenal, occurring in sympathetic ganglia, most often the organ of Zuckerkandl, at which point they are called paragangliomas. These are rare tumors unless there exists a predisposing hereditary setting: MEN type 2A or 2B, von Recklinghausen's neurofibromatosis type 1, VHL disease, or succinate dehydrogenase (SDH) disease.

The often-cited "rule of tens"—pheochromocytomas are bilateral in 10%, extra-adrenal in 10%, familial in 10%, and malignant in 10% and occur in children in 10%—may no longer be valid due to advances in knowledge of the causes and incidence from genetic studies. Symptoms include palpitations, anxiety, headaches, and flushing. Hypertension is often present, paroxysmal in some and sustained in others.

The approach to evaluating a patient with suspected pheochromocytoma is shown in Fig. 25-5. Imaging studies to confirm the adrenal or extra-adrenal mass include CT and MRI, including down to the aortic bifurcation to examine the organ of Zuckerkandl. [131]Iodine-metaiodobenzylguanidine (MIBG) scanning is also available, and although less sensitive than MRI or CT, it is useful in detecting small or extra-adrenal pheochromocytomas. MIBG scanning is often indicated in patients at higher risk for multiple or extra-adrenal tumors, such as those with MEN syndrome. Positron emission tomography (PET) and PET-CT may also be used.

Surgical resection is indicated for pheochromocytoma. Preoperative medical management includes control of hypertension, alpha-adrenergic blockade to prevent hypertensive crisis intraoperatively, and maintenance of adequate fluid resuscitation. Phenoxybenzamine is the alpha-adrenergic antagonist of choice and is usually begun 10–14 days before surgery. Dose is titrated until normotension, well-controlled hypertension, or development of intolerable side effects: tachycardia, nasal congestion, or orthostatic hypotension. If tachycardia occurs, beta-adrenergic blockade is indicated, but only after sufficient alpha-adrenergic antagonism is confirmed. A beta-adrenergic antagonist administered to a patient with pheochromocytoma can result in unopposed alpha-adrenergic effects of the tumor products, precipitating hypertensive crisis. Selective alpha1-adrenergic antagonists such as prazosin, doxazosin, and terazosin may also be used.

There are several surgical approaches to pheochromocytoma. Laparoscopic adrenalectomy is the preferred method but is contraindicated if local invasion is suspected on radiographic imaging, in larger pheochromocytomas, or for paragangliomas in locations that are inaccessible laparoscopically. Modern imaging techniques are sensitive enough to preclude routine exploration of the contralateral adrenal gland. Transabdominal open adrenalectomy is excellent for exploration of bilateral or extra-adrenal tumors if necessary. Large, malignant tumors may best be approached via a thoracoabdominal approach. The posterior retroperitoneoscopic approach is less morbid than the transabdominal approach especially for bilateral disease, but exposure is limited, reserving this procedure for smaller tumors.

Management of pheochromocytoma in patients with hereditary endocrine syndromes, especially MEN syndrome and VHL, is complex. Of patients with MEN, regardless of type (2A or 2B), 30–40% develop pheochromocytomas. For unilateral disease, on presentation most centers perform unilateral adrenalectomy with close follow-up. In patients with bilateral pheochromocytomas who undergo bilateral total adrenalectomy, the risk of Addisonian crisis is 10–30%. Experienced centers may offer cortical-sparing adrenalectomy for initial unilateral procedure, initial bilateral procedure, or subsequent operation in contralateral adrenal. Cortical-sparing adrenalectomy may prevent the need for chronic corticosteroids, although there is an accepted risk of recurrence.

Malignant pheochromocytoma is diagnosed by demonstrating invasion of local structures or by proving metastasis. Therapy is surgical adrenalectomy and resection of metastases, with debulking. Radiation therapy may ameliorate pain from bone metastases. MIBG can

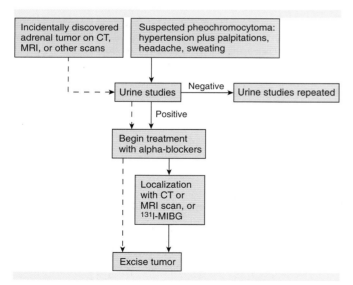

FIGURE 25-5. Approach to evaluation of a patient with suspected pheochromocytoma (from Doherty GM, (ed.), *Current Diagnosis and Treatment: Surgery.* 13th ed. New York, NY: McGraw-Hill; 2010: Fig. 33-2. Copyright © The McGraw-Hill Companies, Inc., All rights reserved).

be attempted as ablative therapy, and there exist chemo-therapy protocols. Five-year survival has been reported to be from 20 to 45%.

BIBLIOGRAPHY

Duh Q, Liu C, Tyrrell J. Adrenals. In: Doherty GM, (ed.), *Current Diagnosis & Treatment: Surgery.* 13e. New York, NY: McGraw-Hill; 2010: Chapter 33.

Grubbs EG, Rich TA, Ng C, et al. Long-term outcomes of surgical treatment for hereditary pheochromocytoma. *J Am Coll Surg* 2013 Feb;216(2):280–289.

Lal G, Clark OH. Thyroid, parathyroid, and adrenal. In: Brunicardi F, Andersen DK, Billiar TR, et al., (eds.), *Schwartz's Principles of Surgery.* 9th ed. New York, NY: McGraw-Hill; 2010: Chapter 38.

Olson JA, Scheri RP. Adrenal gland. In: Mulholland MW, Lillemoe KD, Doherty GM, Maier RV, Simeone DM, Upchurch GR, (eds.), *Surgery: Scientific Principles and Practice.* 5th ed. Philadelphia, PA: Lippincott, Williams & Wilkins; 2011:1325–1345.

Yeh M, Duh QY. The adrenal glands. In: Townsend CM, Beauchamp RD, Evers BM, Mattox KL, (eds.), *Sabiston Textbook of Surgery.* 19th ed. Philadelphia, PA: Saunders; 2012:963–992.

Zeiger MA, Thompson GB, Duh QY, et al. American Association of Clinical Endocrinologists and American Association of Endocrine Surgeons medical guidelines for the management of adrenal incidentalomas: executive summary of recommendations. *Endocr Pract* 2009 Jul–Aug;15(5):450–453.

5. **(D)** This infant most likely has congenital adrenal hyperplasia, which often presents as ambiguous genitalia in the newborn infant. The enzymatic defect in the steroidogenesis pathway causes a decrease in cortisol secretion, with consequent increased ACTH production, which acts in a vicious cycle to further drive the production of steroids in the pathway other than cortisol. These excess adrenal androgens are converted peripherally to testosterone.

The most common enzymatic deficiency is 21-hydroxylase deficiency, responsible for more than 90% of the congenital adrenal hyperplasias. In this deficiency, progesterone and 17-hydroxyprogesterone cannot be converted into 11-deoxycortisol and 11-deoxycorticosterone, respectively. There is therefore decreased production of both aldosterone and cortisol. In complete absence of 21-hydroxylase, there is androgen excess, salt wasting in the urine, diarrhea, hypovolemia, hyponatremia, hyperkalemia, and hyperpigmentation. Partial absence of the enzyme presents only as virilization and may not present itself until later in childhood. The high levels of ACTH are able to force production of cortisol and aldosterone into near-normal range. Virilization of the female fetus produces female pseudohermaphroditism: clitoral hypertrophy, labioscrotal fold fusion, and a urogenital sinus that appears as a phallic urethra. The ovaries, fallopian tubes, and uterus are not affected by androgens and thus develop normally. In fact, medical

control of the endocrine defect and surgical correction of the external genital abnormalities may allow these females to bear children. Virilization of the male fetus may not be detected unless the enzyme deficiency is complete, and thus salt-wasting is present. Partial deficiency in male infants may go undiagnosed until precocious puberty occurs. Diagnosis is easily confirmed by measuring the elevated plasma 17-hydroxyprogesterone. Treatment of this disorder consists of glucocorticoid and mineralocorticoid replacement. In the case of the female pseudohermaphrodite, the external genitalia are surgically modified to be female.

The second most common is 11-beta-hydroxylase deficiency. Without this enzyme, 11-deoxycorticosterone and 11-deoxycortisol cannot be converted to corticosterone or cortisol. In contrast to 21-hydroxylase deficiency, the mineralocorticoid 11-deoxycorticosterone is produced and in fact is overproduced as the decreased level of cortisol causes excess ACTH production. This overproduction of a mineralocorticoid causes hypokalemia and hypertension. 11-Beta-hydroxylase deficiency also causes androgen excess and thus virilization. Diagnosis is performed by measuring elevated 17-hydroxyprogesterone (as in 21-hydroxylase deficiency), and treatment is similar: replacement of glucocorticoids and surgical correction of ambiguous genitalia in female infants.

3-Beta-hydroxydehydrogenase deficiency reduces levels of glucocorticoids, mineralocorticoids, and androgens, shunting steroidogenesis to the production of 17-hydroxypregnenolone and DHEA, a weak androgen. Female infants show virilization, whereas male infants show incomplete virilization. These infants rarely survive because of profound salt wasting.

17-Hydroxylase deficiency results in decreased production of cortisol and androgens, with a concomitant overproduction of mineralocorticoids. Affected patients thus present with hypertension and hypokalemia. Treatment is with corticosteroid and androgen replacement.

BIBLIOGRAPHY

Olson JA, Scheri RP. Adrenal gland. In: Mulholland MW, Lillemoe KD, Doherty GM, Maier RV, Simeone DM, Upchurch GR, (eds.), *Surgery: Scientific Principles and Practice.* 5th ed. Philadelphia, PA: Lippincott, Williams & Wilkins; 2011:1325–1345.

Yeh M, Duh QY. The adrenal glands. In: Townsend CM, Beauchamp RD, Evers BM, Mattox KL, (eds.), *Sabiston Textbook of Surgery.* 19th ed. Philadelphia, PA: Saunders; 2012:963–992.

6. **(D)** Most adrenal tumors that hypersecrete sex steroids cause virilizing symptoms as opposed to feminizing symptoms. Adrenal neoplasms that cause feminizing symptoms are almost always carcinomas, while one-third of virilizing tumors are malignant. In children,

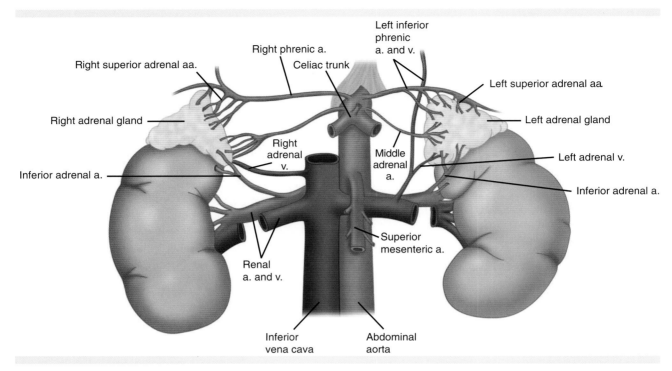

FIGURE 25-6. Adrenal gland anatomy; a. = artery; v. = vein (from Brunicardi FC, Andersen DK, Billiar TR, et al., (eds.), *Schwartz's Principles of Surgery*. 9th ed. New York, NY: McGraw-Hill; 2010: Fig. 38-38. Copyright © The McGraw-Hill Companies, Inc., All rights reserved).

adrenal neoplasms that cause virilization present as clitoral enlargement and pubic hair formation in girls and as hirsutism, enlarged penis, and small testes in boys. In adults, women present with hirsutism and other masculinizing features, and men often go unnoticed until the disease progresses to local tumor enlargement symptoms or metastasis. Biochemical tests to detect virilizing tumors include measurement of 24-h urine DHEA, DHEA-S and testosterone. Laparoscopic adrenalectomy is the procedure of choice unless there is high suspicion for malignancy. Malignancy is best determined by local invasion or distant metastases. Aminoglutethimide or mitotane may help ameliorate symptoms in patients with metastases or unresectable adrenal disease.

BIBLIOGRAPHY

Olson JA, Scheri RP. Adrenal gland. In: Mulholland MW, Lillemoe KD, Doherty GM, Maier RV, Simeone DM, Upchurch GR, (eds.), *Surgery: Scientific Principles and Practice*. 5th ed. Philadelphia, PA: Lippincott, Williams & Wilkins; 2011:1325–1345.
Yeh M, Duh QY. The adrenal glands. In: Townsend CM, Beauchamp RD, Evers BM, Mattox KL, (eds.), *Sabiston Textbook of Surgery*. 19th ed. Philadelphia, PA: Saunders; 2012:963–992.

7. **(D)** There are normally three main adrenal arteries to each gland. The superior adrenal artery is a branch from the inferior phrenic artery. The middle adrenal artery comes directly from the aorta on each side. The inferior adrenal artery arises from each gland's corresponding renal artery. The venous drainage is predominantly via one central vein. This vein drains into the vena cava on the right and into the left renal vein on the left (Fig. 25-6).

BIBLIOGRAPHY

Clemente C. *Anatomy. A Regional Atlas of the Human Body*. 6th ed. Philadelphia, PA: Lippincott Williams and Wilkins; 2011.
Yeh M, Duh QY. The adrenal glands. In: Townsend CM, Beauchamp RD, Evers BM, Mattox KL, (eds.), *Sabiston Textbook of Surgery*. 19th ed. Philadelphia, PA: Saunders; 2012:963–992.

8. **(C)**

9. **(C)**

Explanation for questions 8 and 9

With few exceptions, almost all adrenal tumors can be removed laparoscopically. Open adrenalectomy is recommended under the following circumstances:

Invasive adrenal cortical carcinoma

Tumor size greater than 8 cm (depends on surgeon's experience)

Evidence of clinical feminization

Hypersecretion of multiple sex hormones

Contraindication to laparoscopy

Suspicion for malignancy with possible local invasion

The only patient in the question 8 that portrays one of these contraindications is the 60-year-old woman with a likely invasive adrenal mass. It is currently recommended that likely invasive adrenal tumors be approached surgically with an open approach. Isolated well-defined adrenal metastases from other primary cancers may be removed laparoscopically. Pheochromocytomas can be removed laparoscopically if deemed benign on preoperative imaging. In fact, the laparoscopic approach may result in less hemodynamic instability than in open adrenalectomy. The surgeon's laparoscopic surgery experience should guide the decision regarding the choice of operative approach for tumors larger than 8 cm if none of the other criteria for open approach is met.

In comparison to any of the open approaches to adrenalectomy, laparoscopic adrenalectomy has been proven to result in shorter operative time, decreased postoperative analgesic use, shorter postoperative ileus time, faster rehabilitation times, less use of postoperative blood transfusions, and overall lower hospital costs.

BIBLIOGRAPHY

Duh Q, Liu C, Tyrrell J. Adrenals. In: Doherty GM, (ed.), *Current Diagnosis & Treatment: Surgery*. 13e. New York, NY: McGraw-Hill; 2010: Chapter 33.

Yeh M, Duh QY. The adrenal glands. In: Townsend CM, Beauchamp RD, Evers BM, Mattox KL, (eds.), *Sabiston Textbook of Surgery*. 19th ed. Philadelphia, PA: Saunders; 2012:963–992.

10. **(D)**

11. **(C)**

12. **(D)**

Explanation for questions 10 through 12

Aldosterone excess can be primary or secondary. Secondary hyperaldosteronism is caused by stimulation of the renin-angiotensin-aldosterone system, such as in renal artery stenosis, congestive heart failure, and normal pregnancy. Primary hyperaldosteronism occurs when aldosterone secretion by the adrenal gland becomes autonomous. In approximately two-thirds of cases, this is because of an aldosterone-producing adenoma, and in approximately one-third of cases, it is due to bilateral adrenal hyperplasia (often idiopathic in nature). In less than 1% of cases is aldosterone hypersecretion due to adrenal carcinoma. Most patients afflicted with primary aldosteronism have

some degree of diastolic hypertension because of sodium retention, and many (80%) have hypokalemia. Other signs and symptoms are secondary to potassium depletion and include muscle weakness, fatigue, polyuria, polydipsia, hyperglycemia, metabolic alkalosis, and impaired insulin secretion. Edema is characteristically absent. In a hypertensive patient with hypokalemia, primary hyperaldosteronism should be suspected.

The screening test of choice for hyperaldosteronism is measuring ambulatory plasma aldosterone concentration (PAC) and plasma renin activity (PRA). This test should be performed in the morning with the patient in the seated position. An aldosterone-to-renin ratio greater than 20, with PAC greater than 15 ng/dL is highly suggestive of primary hyperaldosteronism. Certain medications, such as spironolactone, must be discontinued for at least 4 weeks prior to measurement. Confirmation of the diagnosis can be performed by the saline infusion test, in which patients placed on a low-sodium diet for 3 days are then infused with 2 L of normal saline over 4 h, followed by measurement of plasma aldosterone levels. Alternatively, oral salt loading, which requires patients to consume 500 mg of salt daily for 3 days, can be performed. This is followed by measurement of 24-h urine aldosterone levels on day 3. Urine aldosterone greater than 14 µg/24 h after oral salt loading or plasma aldosterone greater than 10 ng/mL after saline infusion confirms the diagnosis of primary hyperaldosteronism.

Once primary hyperaldosteronism is diagnosed, the distinction between adrenal adenoma and bilateral adrenal hyperplasia must be made (Fig. 25-7). CT is an excellent test to determine this. When CT imaging shows bilateral adrenal nodules, bilateral adrenal hyperplasia should be in the differential. In this instance, bilateral adrenal venous sampling is used. In patients in whom adrenal vein sampling is unsuccessful, other tests are occasionally used. The posture stimulation test involves measuring plasma renin and aldosterone levels in both recumbent and upright positions and is based on the nonresponsiveness of aldosterone-producing adenomas to changes in angiotensin II that occur with standing. The NP-59 nuclear scintigraph scan may also be used to distinguish between aldosterone-producing adenomas and bilateral hyperplasia, although sensitivity is often dependent on size of the adenoma. The reason that the distinction between adenoma and bilateral hyperplasia must be made is that treatment is completely different for each. The treatment of choice for adenoma is surgical resection. Preoperative preparation of the patient may include spironolactone and potassium administration to replete potassium stores and correct any alkalosis. Because aldosterone-secreting adenomas are characteristically small and rarely malignant, these tumors are ideally suited to a laparoscopic approach in most cases. The treatment of choice for bilateral adrenal hyperplasia

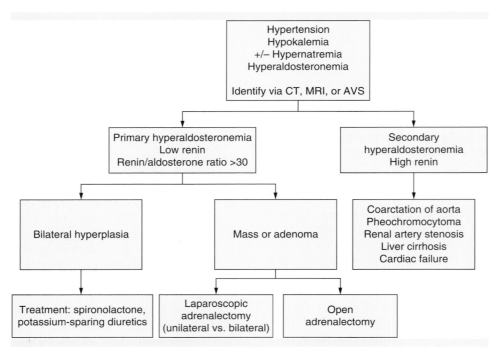

FIGURE 25-7. Approach to evaluation of primary hyperaldosteronism; AVS= adrenal venous sampling (from Morita SY, Dackiw APB, Zeiger MA, (eds.), *McGraw-Hill Manual: Endocrine Surgery*. New York, NY: McGraw-Hill; 2010: Fig. 13-2).

is medical and consists of spironolactone, triamterene, or amiloride. In the uncommon case of bilateral adrenal adenomas, medical therapy to control hypertension should be given, as this is usually much easier to do than treating adrenal insufficiency after bilateral adrenalectomy. Bilateral adrenalectomy is indicated if the hypertension associated with bilateral adrenal hyperplasia or bilateral adenomas is refractory to medical therapy.

BIBLIOGRAPHY

Funder JW, Carey RM, Fardella C, et al. Case detection, diagnosis, and treatment of patients with primary aldosteronism: an endocrine society clinical practice guideline. *J Clin Endocrinol Metab* 2008 Sep;93(9):3266–3281.

Olson JA, Scheri RP. Adrenal gland. In: Mulholland MW, Lillemoe KD, Doherty GM, Maier RV, Simeone DM, Upchurch GR, (eds.), *Surgery: Scientific Principles and Practice*. 5th ed. Philadelphia, PA: Lippincott, Williams & Wilkins; 2011:1325–1345.

Yeh M, Duh QY. The adrenal glands. In: Townsend CM, Beauchamp RD, Evers BM, Mattox KL, (eds.), *Sabiston Textbook of Surgery*. 19th ed. Philadelphia, PA: Saunders; 2012:963–992.

13. **(A)**

14. **(B)**

Explanation for questions 13 and 14

The adrenocortical hormones are all synthesized from cholesterol, which is either synthesized in the adrenal cortex or is extracted directly from the plasma. The cholesterol is transformed into delta-5-pregnenolone inside the mitochondria, and this molecule, which serves as the precursor for all of the adrenal steroid hormones, enters the smooth endoplasmic reticulum and is diverted into one of many possible pathways. The different zones of the adrenal cortex (zona glomerulosa, fasciculata, and reticularis) each have differing combinations and amounts of the enzymes necessary to form the adrenocortical steroids. All mineralocorticoids are synthesized within the zona glomerulosa. The glucocorticoids and the adrenal androgens are synthesized within both the zona fasciculata and the zona reticularis (Fig. 25-8).

The steroid hormones pass through the cell membrane and bind directly to cytosolic receptors. This steroid-receptor complex then translocates into the nucleus and binds to the DNA itself, affecting transcription of DNA. This chain of events is why the final physiologic effects of steroid hormones are delayed more than an hour after release into the bloodstream or after intravenous administration. This is in direct contrast to the products of the adrenal medulla—the catecholamines. The catecholamines dopamine, norepinephrine, and epinephrine

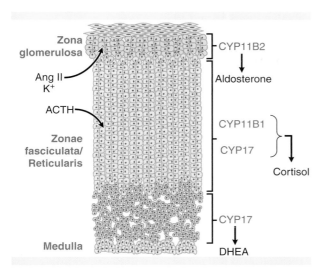

FIGURE 25-8. Major functional compartments of the adrenal cortex (from Brunton LL, Chabner BA, Knollmann BC, (eds.), *Goodman & Gilman's The Pharmacological Basis of Therapeutics.* 12th ed. New York, NY: McGraw-Hill; 2011. Copyright © The McGraw-Hill Companies, Inc., All rights reserved).

bind to specific cell membrane receptors that are coupled to their effector proteins via G proteins, which allows for fast actions once the catecholamine reaches its receptor.

The plasma half-life of cortisol is approximately 90 min, and it is the liver that transforms cortisol into its inactive metabolites, which are eventually secreted in the urine and can be detected as 17-hydroxycorticosteroids. The plasma half-life of aldosterone is approximately 15 min, and it is inactivated by the liver. DHEA is the major sex steroid secreted from the adrenal glands. DHEA is a weak androgen, and most of its virilizing effect is because of peripheral conversion to the more powerful androgen testosterone. It is important to remember that DHEA secretion is not regulated by the gonadotropins, as is testicular production of testosterone, but instead by ACTH.

BIBLIOGRAPHY

Olson JA, Scheri RP. Adrenal gland. In: Mulholland MW, Lillemoe KD, Doherty GM, Maier RV, Simeone DM, Upchurch GR, (eds.), *Surgery: Scientific Principles and Practice.* 5th ed. Philadelphia, PA: Lippincott, Williams & Wilkins; 2011:1325–1345.
Yeh M, Duh QY. The adrenal glands. In: Townsend CM, Beauchamp RD, Evers BM, Mattox KL, (eds.), *Sabiston Textbook of Surgery.* 19th ed. Philadelphia, PA: Saunders; 2012:963–992.

15. **(C)** The adrenal glucocorticoid cortisol has many effects on human physiology. It stimulates the release of glucagon, stimulates hepatic gluconeogenesis, and antagonizes insulin-stimulated glucose uptake in peripheral cells, all of which contribute to hyperglycemia. It decreases peripheral protein synthesis and amino acid uptake to increase the delivery of amino acids back to the liver for gluconeogenesis. Cortisol also stimulates peripheral lipolysis. The net effect of these metabolic regulatory functions is a catabolic state peripherally (skin, muscle, adipocytes, and the like) to provide glucose energy for the liver and brain. Cortisol stimulates angiotensinogen release, decreases capillary permeability, and inhibits the vasodilatory prostaglandin I_2, all in an effort to maintain adequate intravascular volume. Cortisol inhibits lymphocyte activation, suppresses interleukin 2 production, prevents neutrophil and monocyte migration, inhibits histamine release by mast cells, and prevents T-cell activation of B cells. These actions are responsible for cortisol's profound anti-inflammatory effect, which is increased greatly at higher doses, at which cortisol directly inhibits B-cell activation and proliferation. Cortisol negatively affects wound healing by impairing fibroblast activity, which reduces wound tensile strength and delays epithelialization, and by inhibiting osteoblast activity. Common side effects of hypercortisolism include proximal muscle weakness, insulin-resistant diabetes mellitus, truncal obesity ("buffalo hump" and "moon faces"), and psychological disturbances.

BIBLIOGRAPHY

Olson JA, Scheri RP. Adrenal gland. In: Mulholland MW, Lillemoe KD, Doherty GM, Maier RV, Simeone DM, Upchurch GR, (eds.), *Surgery: Scientific Principles and Practice.* 5th ed. Philadelphia, PA: Lippincott, Williams & Wilkins; 2011:1325–1345.
Yeh M, Duh QY. The adrenal glands. In: Townsend CM, Beauchamp RD, Evers BM, Mattox KL, (eds.), *Sabiston Textbook of Surgery.* 19th ed. Philadelphia, PA: Saunders; 2012:963–992.

16. **(D)** The major stimuli of aldosterone secretion are the renin-angiotensin system and the serum potassium concentration. Significant renal artery stenosis causes release of renin from the kidney's juxtaglomerular cells, thus invoking the renin-angiotensin system, resulting in a significantly higher release of adrenal aldosterone than normal. Acute hemorrhage with corresponding acute intravascular volume depletion also invokes the renin-angiotensin system by decreasing blood flow to the kidneys. Adrenal secretion of aldosterone is most strongly controlled by the plasma concentration of potassium. An increase in plasma potassium concentration by only 0.1 mEq/L will increase adrenal aldosterone secretion by more than 30%. Decreases in plasma potassium concentration have the converse effect: Lowering plasma

potassium concentration severely restricts the ability of the adrenal gland to secrete aldosterone. ACTH has a relatively mild effect as far as increasing adrenal aldosterone secretion.

BIBLIOGRAPHY

Olson JA, Scheri RP. Adrenal gland. In: Mulholland MW, Lillemoe KD, Doherty GM, Maier RV, Simeone DM, Upchurch GR, (eds.), *Surgery: Scientific Principles and Practice.* 5th ed. Philadelphia, PA: Lippincott, Williams & Wilkins; 2011:1325–1345.

Yeh M, Duh QY. The adrenal glands. In: Townsend CM, Beauchamp RD, Evers BM, Mattox KL, (eds.), *Sabiston Textbook of Surgery.* 19th ed. Philadelphia, PA: Saunders; 2012:963–992.

17. **(C)** The predominant sex steroid produced by the adrenal glands is DHEA, which is a relatively weak androgen compared to testosterone, produced mainly by the gonads. DHEA exerts its androgen effects after conversion to testosterone, occurring only peripherally. Unlike gonadal testosterone, the stimulation of DHEA release from the adrenal glands is by ACTH, not the gonadotropins LH and FSH. Adrenal androgens are important in fetal development, as they promote development of male external genitalia, male ductal structures (vas deferens, epididymis, seminal vesicles), and male prostate. If androgens are not circulating in the fetal bloodstream, female genitalia result. Excessive adrenal production of androgens in adults is likely because of carcinoma. Any enzyme deficiency responsible for excessive adrenal androgen production would almost certainly have been detected shortly after birth or at the time of puberty. (Androgen overproduction in male children may be overlooked until precocious puberty ensues.) Regardless of whether the patient with excessive adrenal androgen production is a child or adult, it is important to maintain a high suspicion for an ACC.

BIBLIOGRAPHY

Moley JF, Wells SA. Pituitary and adrenal glands. In: Townsend CM, Beauchamp RD, Evers BM, et al., (eds.), *Sabiston Textbook of Surgery.* 16th ed. Philadelphia, PA: Saunders; 2001:674.

Olson JA, Scheri RP. Adrenal gland. In: Mulholland MW, Lillemoe KD, Doherty GM, Maier RV, Simeone DM, Upchurch GR, (eds.), *Surgery: Scientific Principles and Practice.* 5th ed. Philadelphia, PA: Lippincott, Williams & Wilkins; 2011:1325–1345.

Yeh M, Duh QY. The adrenal glands. In: Townsend CM, Beauchamp RD, Evers BM, Mattox KL, (eds.), *Sabiston Textbook of Surgery.* 19th ed. Philadelphia, PA: Saunders; 2012:963–992.

18. **(A)**

19. **(C)**

Explanations 18 and 19

The clinical picture of Cushing's syndrome (hypercortisolism) (Fig. 25-9) should prompt the physician to test for elevated production of cortisol.

Testing random plasma cortisol levels is often not useful because of the episodic nature of cortisol secretion. The first diagnostic test is determination of 24-h urine free cortisol (at least two measurements) or a low-dose dexamethasone suppression test. In this test, the patient is administered 1–2 mg of oral dexamethasone at night, and then the cortisol level is measured the next morning by checking plasma cortisol. In normal individuals, this amount of synthetic glucocorticoid (dexamethasone) is able to suppress cortisol levels to less than half the normal value (less than 5 μg/dL), but in individuals with hypercortisolism, it will not be as significantly suppressed, as in the patient in questions 18 and 19. Depending on the clinical circumstances, a third diagnostic test that can be used is a late-night salivary cortisol level (two measurements). Once Cushing's syndrome is diagnosed, the cause must be sought. The best initial test is to determine the amount of plasma ACTH, which in the normal human is between 10 and 100 pg/mL. Suppression of ACTH to levels below 5 pg/mL is nearly diagnostic of an adrenocortical neoplasm (high levels of cortisol profoundly suppress ACTH production from the pituitary gland) (Fig. 25-10).

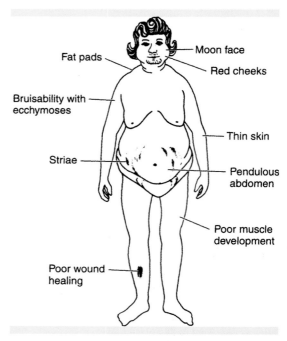

FIGURE 25-9. Principal clinical features of Cushing's syndrome. Reproduced with permission from Forsham PH: The adrenal cortex. In: Williams RH (ed.), *Textbook of Endocrinology.* 4th ed. Saunders, 1968.

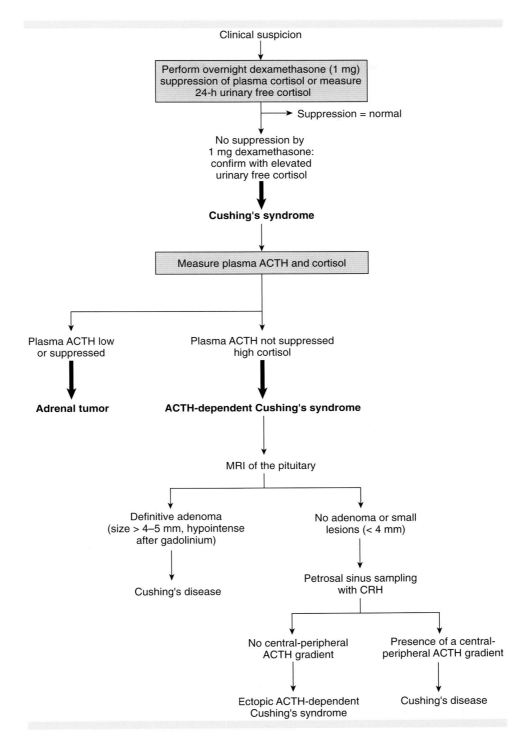

FIGURE 25-10. Diagnosis of Cushing's syndrome (from Doherty GM, (ed.), *Current Diagnosis and Treatment: Surgery*. 13th ed. New York, NY: McGraw-Hill; 2010: Fig. 33-3. Copyright © The McGraw-Hill Companies, Inc., All rights reserved).

Biochemical testing has thus essentially diagnosed the cause of hypercortisolism, and the CT scan has localized the adrenocortical neoplasm in this patient. The CT scan also suggests benign disease (well circumscribed, size less than 5 cm, no apparent extra-adrenal disease). Because this is a functional adrenocortical tumor, the therapy of choice is surgical adrenalectomy. Medical suppression of the adrenal gland with a drug such as aminoglutethimide or metyrapone is contraindicated unless this patient cannot withstand surgical intervention. Medical suppression may be indicated if surgery must be delayed for a substantial reason, but neither of these drugs will prevent growth of the neoplasm and carry multiple side effects. Biopsy of the adrenal mass is not indicated—this will not add any information that will change management of this patient. Imaging of the pituitary gland is not indicated because the finding of a low ACTH level has ruled out a pituitary source of hypercortisolism. For this patient, laparoscopic adrenalectomy would generally be recommended as there is no contraindication, although this is up to surgeon preference.

Prophylactic preoperative administration of glucocorticoids should be performed if adrenalectomy is contemplated or if there is suspicion of adrenal suppression. This patient presents with both—one assumes that the contralateral, "normal" adrenal gland is suppressed because of a profoundly low ACTH status. One regimen for steroid administration is 100 mg of hydrocortisone (or equivalent dose of another glucocorticoid) preoperatively and then every 6 h for the first 48 h postoperatively. This dose can be halved every 2–3 days if everything proceeds well, but depending on how long hypercortisolism has been present, the pituitary-adrenal axis can remain suppressed for up to 2 years. The duration of replacement steroid therapy can be guided by the ACTH stimulation test, in which ACTH is administered intravenously and plasma cortisol and aldosterone are measured. In patients with adequate adrenal function, both plasma cortisol and aldosterone will rise appropriately.

BIBLIOGRAPHY

Duh Q, Liu C, Tyrrell J. Adrenals. In: Doherty GM, (ed.), *Current Diagnosis & Treatment: Surgery*. 13e. New York, NY: McGraw-Hill; 2010: Chapter 33.

Nieman LK, Biller BMK, Findling JW, et al. The diagnosis of Cushing's syndrome: an Endocrine Society clinical practice guideline. *J Clin Endocrinol Metab* 2008 May;93(5):1526–1540.

Olson JA, Scheri RP. Adrenal gland. In: Mulholland MW, Lillemoe KD, Doherty GM, Maier RV, Simeone DM, Upchurch GR, (eds.), *Surgery: Scientific Principles and Practice*. 5th ed. Philadelphia, PA: Lippincott, Williams & Wilkins; 2011:1325–1345.

20. **(A)** In this patient with Cushing's syndrome, biochemical testing reveals elevated ACTH. Patients with pituitary neoplasms secreting ACTH (Cushing's disease) have serum values of ACTH over the upper limits of normal (100 pg/mL), often much higher than this. To further delineate the source of this exogenous ACTH, the high-dose dexamethasone suppression test is performed. In this test, 2 mg of dexamethasone are given orally every 6 h for 2–3 days. In the morning following the last day, the cortisol level is checked as serum cortisol, urine free cortisol, or urinary 17-hydroxycorticosteroids. In Cushing's disease (pituitary neoplasm), the cortisol level will be suppressed by at least 50% ("partial suppression"). Ectopic tumors that produce ACTH will not show any suppression with the high-dose dexamethasone suppression test, and neither will adrenal tumors.

At this point, the diagnosis rests on either pituitary neoplasm or ectopic tumor that produces ACTH. Because pituitary adenoma is much more likely in this young patient, the next-best test is MRI of the head to search for a pituitary adenoma. MRI for this purpose reaches 100% sensitivity, whereas CT scanning of the head approaches only half that sensitivity. Once diagnosed by imaging, the therapy of choice is transsphenoidal resection of the pituitary tumor. If inoperable or unsuccessful, irradiation and medical adrenalectomy are alternatives.

BIBLIOGRAPHY

Duh Q, Liu C, Tyrrell J. Adrenals. In: Doherty GM, (ed.), *Current Diagnosis & Treatment: Surgery*. 13e. New York, NY: McGraw-Hill; 2010: Chapter 33.

Olson JA, Scheri RP. Adrenal gland. In: Mulholland MW, Lillemoe KD, Doherty GM, Maier RV, Simeone DM, Upchurch GR, (eds.), *Surgery: Scientific Principles and Practice*. 5th ed. Philadelphia, PA: Lippincott, Williams & Wilkins; 2011:1325–1345.

21. **(C)** The absence of suppression after high-dose dexamethasone suppression testing coupled with an elevated serum ACTH in this patient with Cushing's syndrome points to an ectopic tumor that produces ACTH. The most likely sources are small cell carcinoma of the lung and bronchial carcinoid, although there are many other less-common sources from the abdomen. It is hoped that diagnosis is made by CT scanning. Surgical removal of the tumor is indicated, and debulking is indicated if deemed unresectable. Medical therapy is an option, with drugs such as aminoglutethimide or metyrapone. Bilateral adrenalectomy may be indicated if hypercortisolism cannot be controlled medically or if imaging techniques fail to discover the ectopic source. Giving the patient with an ectopic ACTH-producing tumor exogenous steroids would not help—the pituitary gland is already suppressed.

BIBLIOGRAPHY

Duh Q, Liu C, Tyrrell J. Adrenals. In: Doherty GM, (ed.), *Current Diagnosis & Treatment: Surgery*. 13e. New York, NY: McGraw-Hill; 2010: Chapter 33.

Olson JA, Scheri RP. Adrenal gland. In: Mulholland MW, Lillemoe KD, Doherty GM, Maier RV, Simeone DM, Upchurch GR, (eds.), *Surgery: Scientific Principles and Practice*. 5th ed. Philadelphia, PA: Lippincott, Williams & Wilkins; 2011:1325–1345.

22. **(A)**

23. **(D)**

24. **(C)**

Explanation for questions 22 through 24

No single test is specific for diagnosing Cushing's syndrome. A combination of tests must be used to arrive at a diagnosis. The first test of choice is the overnight low-dose dexamethasone suppression test, measurement of 24-h urine free cortisol, or late-night salivary cortisol. This avoids the episodic nature of cortisol secretion. The ACTH level can be elevated, suppressed, or normal in hypercortisolism. The CRH test is a test used to differentiate between a pituitary cause for hypercortisolism and other causes. The high-dose dexamethasone test separates a pituitary source of hypercortisolism from an ectopic source of ACTH.

The first step in diagnosing adrenal insufficiency is the measurement of morning serum or salivary cortisol levels. Serum cortisol levels of 15μg/dL or less or a salivary cortisol level of 5.8 ng/mL or less should raise concern for possible adrenal insufficiency, and the ACTH stimulation test should be performed. The low-dose dexamethasone suppression test is the first test of choice to diagnose hypercortisolism. Although plasma ACTH level will most likely be elevated in adrenal insufficiency, this test is not specific for this condition. Random serum cortisol levels are variable because of the episodic nature of cortisol secretion; however, early morning serum or salivary cortisol levels help determine if further testing with ACTH stimulation is needed.

Several tests are available to aid in differentiating between a pituitary neoplasm and an ectopic source of ACTH as the cause of hypercortisolism. These include MRI of the head and CT scanning of the chest and abdomen. Inferior petrosal sinus sampling for ACTH is an invasive but useful test to diagnose pituitary neoplasm as the source of elevated ACTH.

BIBLIOGRAPHY

Duh Q, Liu C, Tyrrell J. Adrenals. In: Doherty GM, (ed.), *Current Diagnosis & Treatment: Surgery*. 13e. New York, NY: McGraw-Hill; 2010: Chapter 33.

Olson JA, Scheri RP, Adrenal gland. In: Mulholland MW, Lillemoe KD, Doherty GM, Maier RV, Simeone DM, Upchurch GR (eds.), *Surgery: Scientific Principles and Practice*, 5th ed. Philadelphia, PA: Lippincott, Williams & Wilkins, 2011, 1325–1345.

Yeh M, Duh QY. The adrenal glands. In: Townsend CM, Beauchamp RD, Evers BM, Mattox KL, (eds.), *Sabiston Textbook of Surgery*. 19th ed. Philadelphia, PA: Saunders; 2012:963–992.

CHAPTER 26

ACUTE ABDOMEN AND THE APPENDIX

MARGARET RIESENBERG-KARGES AND DAVID C. BORGSTROM

QUESTIONS

1. A 23-year-old man presents to the emergency department (ED) with crampy, nonradiating abdominal pain in the right lower quadrant. He is taken to the operating room and found to have a normal-appearing appendix. On further evaluation, the distal ileum appears inflamed with fat wrapping. You notice the cecum is not involved. What is your management at this time?
   (A) Perform appendectomy
   (B) Close and consult gastroenterology
   (C) Perform appendectomy and resect the distal ileum
   (D) Perform appendectomy and stricturoplasty of the terminal ileum
   (E) Run the small bowel to rule out Meckel diverticulum

2. A 42-year-old man presents to the ED with complaints of abdominal pain, nausea, and vomiting. He states the pain is 8/10 in intensity and began early in the morning. The pain is located in the left upper quadrant (LUQ) without radiation and is described as being achy and dull. He also complains of a low-grade fever and having no bowel movements in the last 2 days. There is no other significant medical history. Lab work reveals white blood cell (WBC) count of 16,000 with left shift; urinalysis (UA) is negative. Physical examination reveals tenderness in the lower border of the LUQ, with some guarding but no rebound or rigidity. There are no palpable masses and no hepatosplenomegaly. A computed tomography (CT) of the abdomen revealed malrotation with appendicitis. What is the most appropriate surgical option?
   (A) Rocky-Davis incision with appendectomy
   (B) Lower midline incision with appendectomy
   (C) Laparoscopic appendectomy
   (D) Midline incision with appendectomy and lysis of Ladd's bands
   (E) Antibiotics and observation only

3. A 65-year-old woman comes to the ED with a 2-day history of mild right lower abdominal pain. She describes the pain as dull and persistent. She admits to a 4-day history of constipation, as well as nausea and vomiting. A mass is palpated in the right lower quadrant (RLQ), and CT of the abdomen and pelvis shows an enlarged appendix. The patient is taken to the operating room for an appendectomy. On gross examination, the tip of the appendix appears to be neoplastic, and a frozen section comes back as adenocarcinoma. What operative procedure is warranted?
   (A) Appendectomy with peritoneal fluid cytology
   (B) Appendectomy with frozen section of proximal margin
   (C) Convert to a midline incision and perform an abdominal exploration for metastasis followed by appendectomy
   (D) Extend the incision medially and perform right hemicolectomy and ileocolic anastomosis

4. A 15-year-old girl is referred to your surgery clinic by her family physician with a 5-day history of RLQ pain. She also complains of high-grade fevers of 39°C, which led her to see her primary care doctor earlier that morning. Lab reveals WBC of 18,000, urine pregnancy test is negative, and gynecology examination is negative. Her primary physician ordered a CT of the abdomen, which demonstrates a 6-cm abscess in the RLQ. What is the appropriate treatment for this patient?
   (A) Exploratory laparotomy with drainage of abscess and appendectomy
   (B) RLQ incision, drainage, and appendectomy
   (C) Percutaneous drainage, antibiotics, and elective appendectomy in 6–8 weeks
   (D) Conservative treatment with intravenous (IV) antibiotics
   (E) Laparoscopic drainage of abscess, appendectomy, and placement of drain

5. A 42-year-old woman presents to her primary physician with 5-hour history of nausea and vomiting accompanied by RLQ pain. She has just completed her menstrual cycle. She denies any changes of bowel habits or dysuria. She has a normal gynecologic examination. Lab studies come back normal. She is sent to the ED, where a CT of the abdomen and pelvis reveals enlargement of the distal appendix. After reviewing the studies, you take the patient to the operating room (OR). On opening the peritoneum via RLQ incision, no purulent fluid is observed, and there is a 2.5-cm mass visualized at the distal one-third of the appendix. You run the small bowel and find no areas to signify Meckel diverticulum, Crohn disease, or mesenteric lymphadenitis. There is no purulent material surrounding the ovary, and it is not cystic. What operation should you perform?

(A) Appendectomy
(B) Right hemicolectomy
(C) Extended right hemicolectomy
(D) Close RLQ incision, create a midline incision, and explore the abdomen for metastatic disease
(E) Close incision and consult oncology for chemoradiation

6. A 50-year-old man comes into the ED with upper gastrointestinal (GI) bleeding and hypotension. He has a 25-year history of alcohol abuse, which has led to cirrhosis and subsequent development of ascites. This is his first episode of GI bleeding. The patient is adequately resuscitated with lactated Ringer's and packed red blood cells (PRBCs). Endoscopic therapy fails to stop the esophageal variceal bleeding. What would be the next step for controlling the bleeding?

(A) Sengstaken–Blakemore tube
(B) Sugiura procedure
(C) Transjugular intrahepatic portosystemic shunt (TIPS)
(D) Warren shunt
(E) Octreotide

7. An 80-year-old diabetic woman presents to the ED with abdominal pain radiating to the right thigh, knee, and hip. She also has nausea and vomiting that is bilious in nature. Although this pain has been intermittent for the past year, she believes that this episode is more severe, which prompted her to seek assistance at the ED. She denies any history of prior surgery, but does have a history of a myocardial infarction in the past. On physical examination, the patient is tachycardic, normotensive, and afebrile. Abdominal examination reveals a distended abdomen, with guarding, rebound, diffuse tenderness, and high-pitched bowel sounds. No obvious umbilical or inguinal hernias were detected. A palpable mass was discovered high in the medial aspect of the right thigh. Two images from her CT scan are shown in Figs. 26-1 and 26-2. What is your diagnosis?

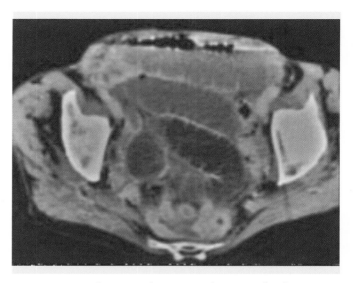

FIGURE 26-1. Computed tomography scan of pelvis.

(A) Femoral hernia
(B) Mesenteric ischemia
(C) Obturator hernia
(D) Ruptured appendicitis
(E) Lymphoma

8. A 65-year-old woman complains of recurrent bouts of gnawing, epigastric pain with occasional nausea and blood-streaked emesis despite taking a proton pump inhibitor (PPI) for several years. The pain has progressively worsened over the past 24 hours and is aggravated by food intake. An esophagogastroduodenoscopy shows an ulcer 1.5 cm distal to the gastroesophageal junction

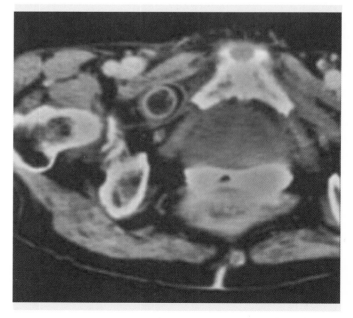

FIGURE 26-2. Computed tomography scan of pelvis.

with active bleeding that is poorly controlled with endoscopic measures. Choose the correct characteristic of the ulcer and operative management.

(A) Hyperacidity; truncal vagotomy and pyloroplasty
(B) Hyperacidity; vagotomy and antrectomy
(C) Normal acidity; vagotomy and antrectomy
(D) Normal acidity; Roux-en-Y gastrojejunostomy
(E) Hyperacidity; highly selective vagotomy

9. A 72-year-old woman with a history of gastroesophageal reflux disease (GERD) and atrial fibrillation presents to the ED with abdominal distention, retching, and complaints of chest pain. She also complains of an acute onset of epigastric pain, which she characterizes as sharp and 8 out of 10 in intensity. Attempts at passing a nasogastric tube (NGT) were unsuccessful. An upper GI is obtained, with the film shown in Fig. 26-3. She

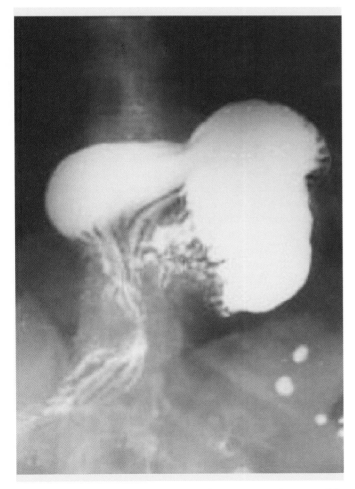

FIGURE 26-3. Upper gastrointestinal series. From Peterson RP, Pellegrini CA, Oelschlager BK. Hiatal hernia and gastroesophageal reflux disease. In: Townsend CM, Beauchamp RD, Evers M, Mattox KL (eds.), *Sabiston Textbook of Surgery*, 19th ed. Philadelphia, PA: WB Saunders Co.; 2012.

is febrile, tachycardic, and tachypneic. What is the next step in management?

(A) Esophageal stent placement
(B) Laparotomy
(C) Right thoracotomy and gastrectomy
(D) Median sternotomy
(E) Left thoracotomy

10. A 65-year-old man with a history of peptic ulcer disease presents with an acute onset of epigastric pain and hematemesis. He reports relief with antacids and PPIs for 1 year. His past medical history is significant for hypertension and coronary artery disease. On physical examination, the patient is hypotensive and tachycardic. His abdomen is soft and tender in the epigastric region, but otherwise benign. Endoscopy reveals a large amount of clot in the stomach with an active arterial bleed just distal to the duodenal bulb. Multiple attempts at endoscopic therapy failed, and he was taken to the operating room for laparotomy. A longitudinal incision through the pylorus, spanning 3 cm on each side of the great vein of Mayo, was created. Traction sutures were placed superiorly and inferiorly prior to the enterotomy. The ulcer was readily identified at the posterior duodenal bulb, and a clot was removed. What is the next step in the procedure?

(A) Sclerotherapy
(B) Perform a fig.-of-eight stitch
(C) Vasopressin infusion
(D) Three-stitch suture ligation
(E) Kocherize the duodenum and perform a Graham patch

11. A 50-year-old man presents to the ED with a history of melena and, most recently, three episodes of hematemesis. The patient denies reflux or a history of peptic ulcer disease. He has no other significant medical problems. He had a right inguinal hernia repair 10 years ago. The patient's vital signs are stable. Physical exam of the abdomen was unremarkable. Rectal examination reveals a positive fecal occult blood test. At this point in the exam, the patient retches and vomits approximately 250 mL of maroon emesis with specks of blood. Endoscopy reveals a large submucosal vessel along the lesser curvature that is actively bleeding (see Fig. 26-4). What is the management for this condition?

(A) Endoscopic cauterization
(B) Vagotomy and antrectomy
(C) Wedge resection of gastric wall
(D) Distal gastrectomy without vagotomy

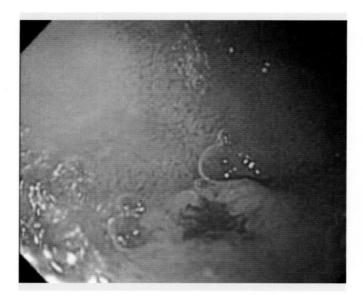

FIGURE 26-4. Esophagogastroduodenoscopy. From Tavakkolizadeh A, Ashley SW. Acute gastrointestinal hemorrhage. In: Townsend CM, Beauchamp RD, Evers M, Mattox KL (eds.), *Sabiston Textbook of Surgery*, 19th ed. Philadelphia, PA: WB Saunders Co.; 2012.

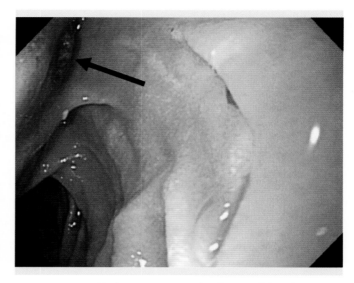

FIGURE 26-5. Endoscopic view; third part of duodenum. Used with permission from Neal Barshes, MD, MPH, Brigham and Women's Hospital, Boston, MA.

12. A 72-year old man presents with complaints of mild abdominal pain and two bowel movements with blood-streaked stool and clots. He characterizes the abdominal pain as diffuse and colicky, with some mild tenesmus. Past history is significant for peripheral vascular disease, coronary artery bypass graft, congestive heart failure, diabetes mellitus, chronic obstructive pulmonary disease (COPD), an abdominal aortic aneurysm repair, and left femoropopliteal bypass graft. On physical examination, he is normotensive and slightly tachycardic. Abdominal examination reveals no organomegaly, guarding, rebound, rigidity, or pulsatile mass. Rectal examination is heme positive without identification of any hemorrhoids. A nasogastric tube was passed, with only 50 mL of coffee-ground material aspirated. Endoscopy is performed (see Fig. 26-5). What is the next step in management?
    (A) Admit to floor, nothing by mouth (NPO), and fluid resuscitation
    (B) Laparotomy and repair of ulceration
    (C) Endoscopic cauterization of bleeding site
    (D) CT with oral (PO) and IV contrast
    (E) CT with IV contrast

13. A 30-year-old man complains of gnawing, epigastric abdominal pain, diarrhea, and a 20-lb weight loss in the last 6 months. Past medical history is significant for peptic ulcer disease, which has been previously treated with antacids and triple therapy for *Helicobacter pylori*. He has no history of prior surgery, alcohol intake, smoking, or recent travel. On physical examination, mild epigastric tenderness without rebound is noted. There is slight guarding in the hypogastric area. Esophagogastroduodenoscopy (EGD) showed esophagitis as well as ulcers in the second and third portions of the duodenum and gastric fundus. What is the imaging test of choice for localizing this condition?
    (A) Endoscopic ultrasound
    (B) Somatostatin receptor scintigraphy
    (C) CT scan
    (D) Magnetic resonance imaging (MRI)
    (E) Selective angiography

14. A 17-year-old male patient arrives at the ED with abdominal pain that began approximately 1 hour after leaving his wrestling practice at school. With the exception of a sore throat a few weeks ago (now resolved) and some fatigue over the last week, he has been in good health with no other medical or surgical history. On physical examination, his blood pressure is 90/67 mmHg with a heart rate (HR) of 120 bpm and a respiratory rate (RR) of 22 breaths/min. Abdominal examination reveals

a mildly distended abdomen, with guarding and rebound tenderness, no palpable masses, and hypoactive bowel sounds. Laboratory studies show a hemoglobin (Hgb) of 9 g/dL, with a normal WBC of 8000. The patient receives 2 L of normal saline, and his blood pressure normalizes. A CT scan of the abdomen and pelvis is performed (see Fig. 26-6). What is the treatment modality of choice?

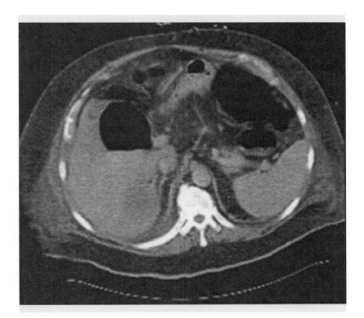

FIGURE 26-7. Computed tomography of abdomen. From Edil BH, Pitt HA. Hepatic abscess. In: Cameron JL, Cameron AM (eds.), *Current Surgical Therapy*, 10th ed. Philadelphia, PA: Elsevier Saunders; 2011.

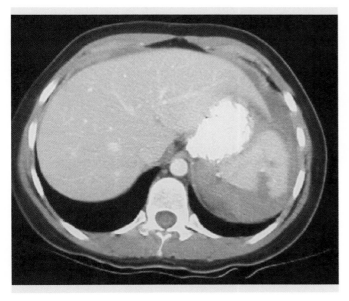

FIGURE 26-6. Computed tomography of the abdomen.

(A) Splenectomy
(B) IV fluids with continued observation
(C) Angiogram with embolization
(D) Laparoscopy
(E) Transfusion of two units of PRBCs

15. A 68-year-old woman with abdominal pain for about a week presents to the ED with fever and chills, increased abdominal pain, and lethargy. She had surgery for injury to her bile ducts after a complicated cholecystectomy 3 years earlier. Laboratory examination shows Hgb of 10 g/dL, WBC of 18,000 with a left shift, total bilirubin of 2 mg/dL, and an alkaline phosphatase of 320 U/100 mL. A CT of the abdomen and pelvis shows intrahepatic biliary dilatation and a fluid collection with an air-fluid level within the liver (see Fig. 26-7). Based on this clinical scenario, what is the most common organism causing this infection?
(A) *Staphylococcus*
(B) *Candida*
(C) *Pseudomonas*
(D) *Klebsiella*
(E) Cytomegalovirus (CMV)

16. A 65-year-old woman with hypertension and diabetes presents with abdominal pain of a few hours in duration, with accompanying hematemesis. On physical examination, her blood pressure is 160/90 mmHg, HR is 100 bpm, RR is 20 breaths/min, and she is afebrile. She has icteric sclera. Rectal examination is guaiac positive. She was admitted and made NPO. An elective EGD was performed the following day, which showed grade II esophagitis, normal stomach with some blood in the proximal duodenum, and no evidence of mucosal ulceration, but blood-tinged bile was noted from the sphincter of Oddi. Abdominal x-ray showed calcifications at the inferior edge of the liver. CT scan of the abdomen showed a 3-cm calcified common hepatic artery with no evidence of acute cholecystitis, no liver abscesses, and no other intra-abdominal pathology. What is the treatment of choice for this patient?
(A) Aneurysm resection
(B) Hepatic lobectomy
(C) Observation with follow-up
(D) Heparin
(E) Angiography and embolization

17. A 50-year-old man with a history of factor V Leiden deficiency presents with chronic abdominal pain with accompanying nausea. He denies any change in bowel habits, but admits to an increase in body weight in the last 3 months. His past medical history is significant for hypertension and coronary artery disease. He denies surgery in the past. On physical examination, his blood pressure is 160/90 mmHg, HR is 100 bpm, RR is 20 breaths/min, and he is afebrile. His abdomen is markedly distended with right upper quadrant (RUQ) tenderness without rebound, with spider angiomas, and with a palpable, nontender liver that spans 5 cm below the right subcostal margin. The patient also has a positive fluid wave. Initial laboratory examinations show elevated serum transaminases, Hgb of 17 g/dL, and prolonged coagulation studies. CT scan of the abdomen and pelvis shows massive ascites with hepatomegaly, especially in the caudate lobe, and pooling of IV contrast in the periphery of the liver. The hepatic vasculature was not well visualized. What would be the initial surgical management of this condition?
    (A) TIPS
    (B) Mesocaval shunt
    (C) Mesoatrial shunt
    (D) Hepatic resection
    (E) Denver shunt

18. A 65-year-old female nursing home resident presents with crampy abdominal pain, nausea, and vomiting. Her medical history is significant for a stroke 1 year ago with residual weakness of her left side, which has kept her bedridden, and previous cholecystectomy and total abdominal hysterectomy and bilateral salpingo-oophorectomy. On physical examination, blood pressure is 160/80 mmHg, HR is 110 bpm, RR is 20 breaths/min, and she is afebrile. Her abdomen is distended and diffusely tender with high-pitched bowel sounds. An abdominal x-ray reveals a "bent inner tube sign" directed to the RUQ. A rigid sigmoidoscopy was performed with successful decompression of the colon, and it showed no ischemic changes. What is the standard of care for this patient?
    (A) Observation and diet as tolerated
    (B) Repeated sigmoidoscopic decompression when it reoccurs
    (C) Placement of rectal tube with elective sigmoid colectomy during this admission
    (D) Hartmann's procedure on same day of hospitalization
    (E) Sigmoidectomy on same day of hospitalization

19. A 33-year-old man comes to the ED complaining of abdominal pain for the past 4 days; the pain was initially crampy, but now it is sharp and exacerbated with movement. He has a medical history that is significant for a factor V Leiden deficiency and a cerebrovascular accident a year ago secondary to occlusion of the vertebral artery. Abdominal examination reveals a distended abdomen that is diffusely tender with rebound tenderness. On laboratory examination, he has leukocytosis and acidosis. CT scan showed dilated loops of bowel with a thickened wall, and an enlarged portal and superior mesenteric vein with a central area of low attenuation. The patient was taken emergently for exploratory laparotomy. Intraoperatively, a 2-foot segment of small bowel was found to be necrotic and was resected. The patient was then transferred to the intensive care unit. What is the next step in the treatment for this patient?
    (A) Begin anticoagulation 2 days postoperatively
    (B) No anticoagulation required since the involved bowel segment has been already resected
    (C) Begin anticoagulation immediately postoperatively
    (D) Give aspirin per rectum until patient resumes oral intake

20. A 55-year-old woman presents with diffuse abdominal pain and nausea. Abdominal exam reveals RLQ tenderness, and a CT scan demonstrates an enlarged appendix. She is taken to the operating room for laparoscopic appendectomy. Upon entering the abdomen, she is found to have a cystic lesion of the appendix as well as diffuse intraperitoneal mucus. Which of the following is the appropriate management?
    (A) Laparoscopic appendectomy and peritoneal washings
    (B) Abort procedure and refer to surgical oncology
    (C) Laparoscopic appendectomy and abdominal exploration with removal of all mucus
    (D) Open appendectomy with abdominal exploration and removal of all mucus
    (E) Open right hemicolectomy with abdominal exploration and removal of all mucus

21. Which of the following is true regarding peritonitis?
    (A) The diagnosis of primary peritonitis is based on the presence of >1000 WBCs/mL on Gram stain of peritoneal fluid.
    (B) Primary peritonitis is often polymicrobial.
    (C) Secondary peritonitis is most commonly observed in immunocompromised patients.
    (D) Approximately one-third of patients with primary peritonitis have negative ascites fluid cultures.
    (E) Secondary peritonitis is rarely treated surgically.

ANSWERS AND EXPLANATIONS

1. **(A)** Historically, 20% of all explorations for appendicitis turn out to be negative; however, the negative appendectomy rate has decreased to less than 10% at some centers (possibly related to improvement in CT imaging). If appendicitis is not found at operation, other sources of pain must be sought. On exploration, the patient had classic findings of Crohn disease, including fat wrapping, which is pathognomonic for Crohn disease. Clinically, differentiating Crohn disease from appendicitis can be difficult, especially without preoperative imaging. If the history discloses previous episodes of colicky abdominal pain with bouts of diarrhea, it should lead to a suspected diagnosis of Crohn disease. Management of the disease intraoperatively is to perform an appendectomy if there is no cecal involvement in order to eliminate the diagnostic confusion of appendicitis versus Crohn flare in the future. If the cecum is involved, an appendectomy is not performed because of the risk of fistula formation. Stricturoplasty is not indicated secondary to the lack of obstructive symptoms.

BIBLIOGRAPHY

Maa J, Kirkwood KS. The appendix. In: Townsend CM, Beauchamp RD, Evers M, Mattox KL (eds.), *Sabiston Textbook of Surgery*, 19th ed. Philadelphia, PA: WB Saunders Co.; 2012.

2. **(D)** This is a rare presentation of appendicitis within this age group. Malrotation is most commonly found within the pediatric population and presents as obstruction. The duodenum and jejunum fail to rotate, whereas the ileum and cecum rotate only partially. Unfortunately, there is an attachment between the cecum and lateral abdominal wall that forms (Ladd's band). This band passes anterior to the duodenum and acts as a site of obstruction. This leads to the cecal fixation in the RUQ. Treatment consists of an appendectomy and Ladd's procedure. The Ladd's procedure consists of derotating the bowel in a counterclockwise rotation, if needed, and lysis of the Ladd's band (see Fig. 26-8). This is extremely difficult through a Rocky-Davis incision and thus best performed through a midline incision or laparoscopically.

BIBLIOGRAPHY

Chung DH. Pediatric surgery. In: Townsend CM, Beauchamp RD, Evers M, Mattox KL (eds.), *Sabiston Textbook of Surgery*, 19th ed. Philadelphia, PA: WB Saunders Co.; 2012.

3. **(D)** Primary appendiceal malignancies are rare and fall into one of the following categories: mucinous adenocarcinoma (38% of cases), adenocarcinoma (26%), carcinoid (17%), goblet cell carcinoma (15%), and signet ring cell carcinoma (4%). In regard to appendiceal adenocarcinomas, there are three histologic subtypes: mucinous adenocarcinoma, colonic adenocarcinoma, and adenocarcinoid. Typical presentation is that of appendicitis, which may also present with ascites or palpable mass. Recommended treatment is right hemicolectomy, which can be performed with medial extension of a Rocky-Davis incision through the anterior and posterior rectus sheaths. These tumors have a tendency for early perforation, although this does not necessarily worsen the prognosis. In regard to appendiceal adenocarcinomas, patients have a 55% 5-year survival. These patients are also at risk for synchronous and metachronous neoplasms within the GI tract. Ten percent of patients have metastases at diagnosis, which are not commonly diagnosed preoperatively. About half of patients present with acute appendicitis, and 15% have appendiceal abscesses. Five-year survival is 60% after a right hemicolectomy and 20% after appendectomy alone. The latter group includes patients with distant metastasis at the time of operative intervention.

BIBLIOGRAPHY

Liang MK, Andersson RE, Jaffe BM, Berger DH. The appendix. In: Brunicardi FC, Andersen DK, Billiar TR, et al. (eds.), *Principles of Surgery*, 10th ed. New York, NY: McGraw-Hill; 2014.

4. **(C)** Appendiceal abscesses <5 cm can be treated by conservative therapy consisting of antibiotics, IV fluids, and keeping the patient NPO. Larger abscesses should be managed via percutaneous drainage and antibiotic treatment, with interval appendectomy. Noncontained perforations should be treated by surgical therapy with or without appendectomy. Because of the risk of a perforated cecal carcinoma, people over 50 should undergo barium enema or colonoscopy prior to interval appendectomy. At colonoscopy, about 5% of individuals will have a malignancy found. About 15–25% of patients, particularly in the younger age group, develop recurrent appendicitis; hence, it is recommended that interval appendectomy be performed in children and at least discussed with adult patients.

BIBLIOGRAPHY

Liang MK, Andersson RE, Jaffe BM, Berger DH. The appendix. In: Brunicardi FC, Andersen DK, Billiar TR, et al. (eds.), *Principles of Surgery*, 10th ed. New York, NY: McGraw-Hill; 2014.
Maa J, Kirkwood KS: The appendix. In: Townsend CM, Beauchamp RD, Evers M, Mattox KL (eds.), *Sabiston Textbook of Surgery*, 19th ed. Philadelphia, PA: WB Saunders Co.; 2012.

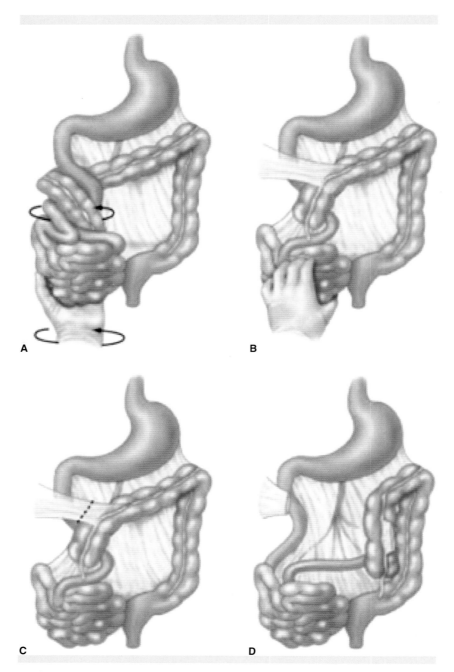

FIGURE 26-8. Ladd's procedure. **A.** Evisceration of bowel. **B.** Derotation of intestine in counterclockwise fashion. **C.** Division of Ladd's band (peritoneal attachment between cecum and retroperitoneum). **D.** Widening of mesenteric base and appendectomy. From Brunicardi F, Andersen DK, Billiar TR, et al. (eds.), *Schwartz's Principles of Surgery*, 10th ed. New York, NY: McGraw-Hill; 2014.

5. **(B)** This is an example of carcinoid tumor of the appendix, which is the second most common primary tumor of the appendix (behind mucinous tumors). Carcinoid tumors that arise at the base of the appendix should be treated with a right hemicolectomy; likewise, tumors that are greater than 2 cm or invade the mesentery should receive right hemicolectomy, regardless of location. Carcinoids that are located in the tip of the appendix and are less than 2 cm may be treated with appendectomy alone, which is curative in nearly 100% of patients. Widespread metastatic disease is found in 3% of patients with appendiceal carcinoid, which means carcinoid syndrome is rare in these patients. Over 15% have synchronous, noncarcinoid tumors at other sites. About one-quarter of patients found to have appendiceal carcinoid tumors receive the appropriate operation, according to the Surveillance, Epidemiology, and End Results database.

BIBLIOGRAPHY

Liang MK, Andersson RE, Jaffe BM, Berger DH. The appendix. In: Brunicardi FC, Andersen DK, Billiar TR, et al. (eds.), *Principles of Surgery*, 10th ed. New York, NY: McGraw-Hill; 2014.

Maa J, Kirkwood KS: The appendix. In: Townsend CM, Beauchamp RD, Evers M, Mattox KL (eds.), *Sabiston Textbook of Surgery*, 19th ed. Philadelphia, PA: WB Saunders Co.; 2012.

6. **(E)** Varices develop in about 30% of patients with cirrhosis and portal hypertension. About one-third of these patients will bleed, and the 6-week mortality of this subset is 20%. Once the patient is resuscitated and the diagnosis of esophageal varices is confirmed, the next therapeutic modality would be drug therapy. Vasopressin was the first medication used with successful results. It ceased active bleeding in about 50–70% of patients. Once the drug is halted, recurrent bleeding is common. Side effects of vasopressin are hypertension, bradycardia, arrhythmias, myocardial ischemia, acute pulmonary edema, and water retention. This was the reason why nitroglycerin was added to vasopressin infusion. The current drug of choice is somatostatin and its analogue octreotide. These have been shown to reduce blood flow and to decrease both portal venous pressure and glucagon levels in patients with cirrhosis. Side effects of these medications are minimal, which may be mild abdominal pain, hot flashes, and diarrhea. Both vasopressin and octreotide have equal efficacy.

BIBLIOGRAPHY

Tavakkolizadeh A, Ashley SW. Acute gastrointestinal hemorrhage. In: Townsend CM, Beauchamp RD, Evers M, Mattox KL (eds.), *Sabiston Textbook of Surgery*, 19th ed. Philadelphia, PA: WB Saunders Co.; 2012.

7. **(C)** Obturator hernias account for 0.1% of all hernias. The pubic and ischial rami form the obturator foramen, which is nearly closed by a membrane, with the exception of the cephalad portion, which is the obturator canal. The hernia passes through the obturator canal, along with obturator vessels and nerves that lie posterolateral to the hernia sac. There are four cardinal features of this hernia, with the most common being intestinal obstruction. Another is the Howship–Romberg sign (pain in the hip and medial thigh with external rotation and extension), which is found in 50% of patients. This is referred pain caused by compression of the obturator nerve by the hernia in the canal. The next feature is a palpable mass high in the medial aspect of the thigh at the origin of the adductor muscles. The mass is best felt with the thigh flexed, adducted, and rotated outward. The last feature is repeated attacks of intestinal obstruction that pass spontaneously. Treatment entails operative intervention as soon as possible, secondary to the high rate of strangulation. There are three general operative approaches for obturator hernia repair: the lower midline transperitoneal approach, which is used commonly in cases of incidental diagnosis at the time of laparotomy for small bowel obstruction; the lower midline extraperitoneal approach, which is preferred in cases where the diagnosis is made preoperatively; and the anterior thigh exposure with medial retraction of the adductor longus. The hernia can be repaired by suturing closed the membrane of the canal. The images show the radiologic findings of a small bowel obstruction (see Fig. 26-1) and an incarcerated obturator hernia (see Fig. 26-2).

BIBLIOGRAPHY

Ferguson CM, Meltzer AJ. Spigelian, lumbar and obturator hernias. In: Cameron JL, Cameron AM (eds.), *Current Surgical Therapy*, 10th ed. Philadelphia, PA: Elsevier Saunders; 2011.

Javid PJ, Greenberg JA, Brooks DC. Hernias. In: Zinner MJ, Ashley SW (eds.), *Maingot's Abdominal Operations*, 12th ed. New York, NY: McGraw-Hill; 2013:Chapter 7.

8. **(D)** Gastric ulcer disease is broken down into five types. Type 1 (60% of ulcers) is found in the lesser curvature at the incisura and is associated with normal acid production. Therapy is excision of the ulcer alone, but may require distal gastrectomy with Billroth I or II reconstruction. Type 2 ulcers (15%) are found in the body in combination with a duodenal ulcer and are associated with hyperacidity. Treatment is truncal vagotomy and antrectomy. Type 3 (20%) is found near the pylorus and is seen with hyperacidity. Treatment is also a truncal vagotomy and antrectomy. For both types 2 and 3, one may prefer to treat the patient with a PPI rather than performing a vagotomy. This is a decision that should be

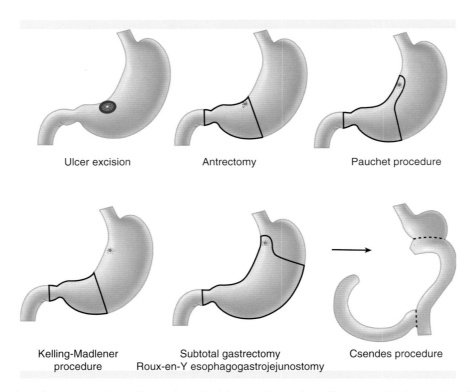

Ulcer excision   Antrectomy   Pauchet procedure

Kelling-Madlener   Subtotal gastrectomy   Csendes procedure
procedure   Roux-en-Y esophagogastrojejunostomy

FIGURE 26-9. Operations for gastric ulcers. Reproduced with permission from Seymour NE. Operations for peptic ulcer and their complications. In: Feldman M, Scharschmidt BF, Sleisenger MH, (eds.), *Gastrointestinal and Liver Disease,* 6th ed. Philadelphia: WB Saunders; 1998.

based on the patient's ability to comply with medical therapy and whether or not they have had a history of complicated gastric ulcers. Type 4 gastric ulcers make up less than 10% and are found high up the incisura by the gastroesophageal (GE) junction and are seen with normal acidity. Treatment depends on size, distance from the GE junction, and degree of inflammation (see Fig. 26-9). It is preferable to simply excise the ulcer, but it may require Roux-en-Y gastrojejunostomy (Csendes procedure). Type 5 ulcers can be found anywhere in the stomach and are associated with nonsteroidal anti-inflammatory drug (NSAID) use and normal acid levels. It is important to recognize that stricture, perforation, bleeding, or other serious complications will develop in 10–35% of patients diagnosed with gastric ulcers. Additionally, 10% of ulcers will harbor a malignancy, and thus one should consider performing a biopsy of the ulcer, especially if the patient does not have risk factors for gastric ulcers.

BIBLIOGRAPHY

Mahvi DM, Krantz SB. Stomach. In: Townsend CM, Beauchamp RD, Evers M, Mattox KL (eds.), *Sabiston Textbook of Surgery*, 19th ed. Philadelphia, PA: WB Saunders Co.; 2012.

Newman NA, Mufeed S, Makary MA. Benign gastric ulcer. In: Cameron JL, Cameron AM (eds.), *Current Surgical Therapy*, 10th ed. Philadelphia, PA: Elsevier Saunders; 2011.

Soriano IS, Dempsey DT. Benign gastric disorders. In: Zinner MJ, Ashley SW (eds.), *Maingot's Abdominal Operations*, 12th ed. New York, NY: McGraw-Hill; 2013:Chapter 21.

9. **(B)** This patient is suffering with gastric volvulus associated with paraesophageal hernia. Gastric volvulus can be recognized by Borchardt's triad (acute epigastric pain, violent retching, and inability to pass a nasogastric tube). The diagnosis is confirmed by the presence of a large, gas-filled viscus in the chest or abdomen on plain abdominal film. Confirmation is by barium swallow. Surgical treatment involves untwisting the stomach, checking for viability of the stomach, reducing the hernia, cruroplasty (primarily or with mesh), and fundoplication or tube gastrostomy. There are reports of endoscopic reduction followed by percutaneous endoscopic gastrostomy tube placement.

Type 2 paraesophageal hernia, or pure paraesophageal hernia, is found when the GE junction is kept within the abdomen by an intact phrenoesophageal ligament, while the fundus and body moves upward due to an anterior laxity. This type accounts for 3–5% of paraesophageal hernias. A volvulus of the stomach may occur along the organoaxial plane, which is a line drawn from the cardia to the pylorus over which the stomach flips. There are four types of hiatal hernias. Type 1 is a sliding hiatal hernia, which is an upward dislocation of the GE junction into the chest due to laxity of the phrenoesophageal ligament. This is the most common type, accounting for more than 90% of these hernias. It is associated with GERD. Type 3 paraesophageal hernia, or "mixed hernia," has the upward dislocation of both the cardia and fundus as well as the GE junction and is often associated with GERD. Type 4 paraesophageal hernia exists when any of the intra-abdominal organs, such as the colon, spleen, or small bowel, are present with the stomach in the hernia sac.

BIBLIOGRAPHY

Banki F, DeMeester TR. Paraesophageal hiatal hernia. In: Cameron JL, Cameron AM (eds.), *Current Surgical Therapy*, 10th ed. Philadelphia, PA: Elsevier Saunders; 2011.

Melvin WS, Perry KA. Paraesophageal hernia: open repair. In: Fischer JE, Jones DB, Pomposelli FB, et al. (eds.), *Mastery of Surgery*, 6th ed. Philadelphia, PA: Lippincott Williams & Wilkins; 2012.

Peterson RP, Pellegrini CA, Oelschlager BK. Hiatal hernia and gastroesophageal reflux disease. In: Townsend CM, Beauchamp RD, Evers M, Mattox KL (eds.), *Sabiston Textbook of Surgery*, 19th ed. Philadelphia, PA: WB Saunders Co.; 2012.

10. **(D)** This is an example of a bleeding duodenal ulcer in the posterior wall. There are some studies that state that the incidence of emergent or urgent operations for bleeding duodenal ulcers has remained unchanged over the past few years, despite the decrease in the numbers of elective cases performed. Hematemesis is the most common sign of a bleeding ulcer, and the diagnosis is supported by performing gastric lavage with a 32-F Ewald tube. Most patients are successfully treated with medical or endoscopic management. Endoscopy remains the initial standard of care for the diagnosis and treatment of bleeding duodenal ulcers. Indications for surgery for a bleeding ulcer include failure of endoscopic intervention, lack of availability of endoscopy, or hemodynamic instability. Antrectomy plus vagotomy is no longer considered the gold standard surgery because it is considered too risky to be performed in the setting of hemodynamic instability (due to complexity and anastomosis). If surgery is indicated, the three-suture technique should be performed because it has a significantly lower morbidity and mortality (see Fig. 26-10). This is performed by encompassing the proximal and distal branches of the gastroduodenal arteries and then using a U-type stitch to transfix the transverse branch of the pancreatic artery. If the patient's condition is stable, a pyloroplasty and truncal vagotomy could be considered after oversewing the ulcer. A highly selective vagotomy can be done for the young, hemodynamically stable patient with minimal comorbidities. Certainly, the last two procedures are primarily indicated for those who have failed medical management or who might be deemed unreliable with medical management.

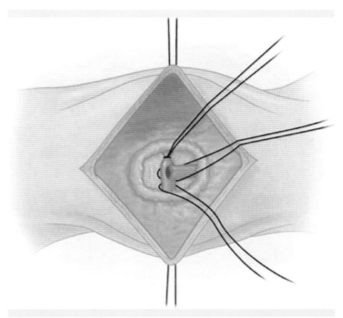

FIGURE 26-10. Three-stitch suture ligation of bleeding duodenal ulcer. From Schirmir BD. Bleeding duodenal ulcer. In: Fischer JE, Jones DB, Pomposelli FB, et al. (eds.), *Mastery of Surgery*, 6th ed. Philadelphia, PA: Lippincott Williams & Wilkins; 2012.

BIBLIOGRAPHY

Schirmir BD. Bleeding duodenal ulcer. In: Fischer JE, Jones DB, Pomposelli FB, et al. (eds.), *Mastery of Surgery*, 6th ed. Philadelphia, PA: Lippincott Williams & Wilkins; 2012.

11. **(A)** This is an example of a Dieulafoy lesion, which is a vascular malformation and a rare cause of upper GI hemorrhage, and is usually found within 6 cm of the GE junction. It is also called "caliber-persistent artery." The malformation is a submucosal or mucosal vessel 1–3 mm in size that may bleed when there is erosion into it. It is usually found along the lesser curvature and in middle-aged individuals and has no association with any vascular or peptic ulcer disease. The hemorrhage produced from the lesion can be massive and can cease spontaneously at times. It is difficult to diagnose endoscopically because there is no ulcer surrounding the lesion, and the mucosal erosion is only about 2–5 mm. Diagnosis is best achieved by performing endoscopy at the time of bleeding and visualizing a pinpoint mucosal defect with blood. Sclerosis or thermal therapy performed at endoscopy is able to successfully treat 80–100% of cases. The area should be marked with India ink in case endoscopic management fails. Usually the lesion may be oversewn, but if it is not identifiable, a partial gastrectomy may be necessary. Vagotomy is not required because it is not associated

with peptic ulcer disease. Surgery is required if there are recurrent bouts of hemorrhage. Angiography may also be considered as an option prior to taking a patient for surgery.

BIBLIOGRAPHY

Tavakkolizadeh A, Ashley SW. Acute gastrointestinal hemorrhage. In: Townsend CM, Beauchamp RD, Evers M, Mattox KL (eds.), *Sabiston Textbook of Surgery*, 19th ed. Philadelphia, PA: WB Saunders Co.; 2012.

12. **(E)** Aortoenteric fistula is a rare condition; it develops from an inflammatory tract between the aorta and GI tract most commonly caused by abdominal aortic aneurysm (AAA) repair with synthetic graft. It may also be caused by infectious aortitis or an inflammatory aortic aneurysm. Aortoenteric fistula complicates AAA repairs in up to 1% of patients and most commonly involves the proximal portion of the anastomosis with the third or fourth portion of the duodenum. Diagnosis must be considered in any patient with acute GI bleed and a history of AAA repair. The herald bleed or "sentinel bleed" is an episode of acute GI bleeding that ceases spontaneously. It occurs hours to days prior to the massive exsanguination that ensues if not diagnosed and treated urgently. Treatment requires proximal vascular control, with graft excision and extra-anatomic bypass (axillofemoral) with resection of the involved bowel. The aortic stump is debrided to viable tissue, closed in two layers with permanent monofilament suture, and buttressed with omentum. Aortic stump blowout is fatal; therefore, it may be necessary to sacrifice the kidneys in order to obtain viable aortic tissue for closure.

BIBLIOGRAPHY

Brady CM, Chaikof CL. Management of infected vascular grafts. In: Cameron JL, Cameron AM (eds.), *Current Surgical Therapy*, 10th ed. Philadelphia, PA: Elsevier Saunders; 2011.

13. **(B)** Zollinger–Ellison syndrome (ZES) "gastrinoma" was first reported in 1955 by Zollinger and Ellison. It is caused by a pancreatic or duodenal neuroendocrine tumor that elaborates excessive amounts of gastrin. It is usually diagnosed in the fourth decade and occurs in sporadic (75% of cases) and familial (25% of cases) forms. The latter is associated with multiple endocrine neoplasia type 1 (MEN1) syndrome. ZES accounts for 0.1–1% of cases with peptic ulcer disease (PUD). Seventy-five percent of patients have symptoms of PUD, and 25% have diarrhea. Eighty percent are found in the gastrinoma triangle (area to the right of superior mesenteric artery, below the head of the pancreas, and medial

to the duodenal wall), as well as stomach, spleen, ovary, and heart. The diagnosis is by EGD, gastrin levels (fasting serum gastrin levels >1000 pg/mL while off PPI), increased basal acid output (>15 mEq/h or >5 mEq/h with history of antiulcer surgery for PUD), and secretin stimulation test (increase in gastrin levels >200 pg/mL). One should be aware that serum gastrin levels may be normal. Localization procedures include ultrasound (specific but not sensitive), CT scan (can detect most lesions >2 cm), endoscopic ultrasound (sensitivity is 75–100% for pancreatic lesions, but much less for gastric), angiography, and somatostatin receptor scintigraphy (octreotide scan). Sensitivity and specificity of the octreotide scan are near 100% when the pretest probability of gastrinoma is high. Medical therapy includes a PPI, with intermittent measurements of basal acid output. Surgical management entails enucleation of the lesion or resection of the involved organ.

BIBLIOGRAPHY

Ellison EC. Zollinger–Ellison syndrome. In: Cameron JL, Cameron AM (eds.), *Current Surgical Therapy*, 10th ed. Philadelphia, PA: Elsevier Saunders; 2011.
Fisher WE, Anderson DK, Windsor JA, Saluja AK, Brunicardi FC. Pancreas. In: Brunicardi FC, Andersen DK, Billiar TR, et al. (eds.), *Principles of Surgery*, 10th ed. New York, NY: McGraw-Hill; 2014.
Kennedy EP, Brody JR, Yeo CJ. Neoplasms of the endocrine pancreas. In: Mulholland MW, Lillemoe KD, Doherty GM, Maier RV, Simeone DM, Upchurch DR (eds.), *Greenfield's Surgery: Scientific Principles and Practice*, 5th ed. Philadelphia, PA: Wolters Kluwer Health; 2011.

14. **(B)** This patient has a splenic laceration from his wrestling match. This was a consequence of the infectious mononucleosis he had 2 weeks prior (implied by sore throat and fatigue), with the subsequent development of splenomegaly. Patients who contract this disease are usually advised to avoid contact sports for at least 2–3 months. Criteria for consideration of nonoperative management in splenic injury include (1) absence of significant injury to another intra-abdominal organ, (2) absence of shock, (3) stabilization with 1–2 L of IV fluid resuscitation, and (4) no coagulopathy. Patients should be placed on bedrest with serial abdominal exams. The greatest bleeding risk is found within the first 48 hours; however, delayed bleeding is always a concern. Risk factors for failure of nonoperative management include injuries at the hilum, patients with other severe injuries, coagulopathy with grade 2 or higher splenic injuries, or splenic parenchyma that has been pulverized. With proper selection criteria, nonoperative management is successful in 90% of patients. Splenic artery embolization

has been an effective way to stop bleeding in selected patients, particularly those who have a vascular blush on CT scan.

BIBLIOGRAPHY

Burlew CC, Moore EE. Trauma. In: Brunicardi FC, Andersen DK, Billiar TR, et al. (eds.), *Principles of Surgery*, 10th ed. New York, NY: McGraw-Hill; 2014.

Wisner DH, Galante JM, Dolich MO, Hoyt DB. Abdominal trauma. In: Mulholland MW, Lillemoe KD, Doherty GM, Maier RV, Simeone DM, Upchurch DR (eds.), *Greenfield's Surgery: Scientific Principles and Practice*, 5th ed. Philadelphia, PA: Wolters Kluwer Health; 2011.

15. **(D)** This is an example of a hepatic pyogenic abscess. Common sources are the biliary tree, the portal vein (GI tract infections), hepatic artery, extension from nearby infections, trauma, or indeterminate causes. The biliary tree is the most common source, with trauma causing 5% of abscesses, and 20–40% of abscesses being cryptogenic. Patients at risk for developing pyogenic abscesses are male, are older than 50 years, have had a liver transplant, have diabetes, or have a malignancy. Patients undergoing biliary enteric bypass (choledocho-jejunostomy) are at increased risk of abscess formation even when there is no stricture at the anastomosis. This patient developed a stricture at the anastomotic site, which resulted in the intrahepatic biliary dilatation on CT scan as well as increased liver function tests (LFTs). Fevers and chills, malaise, weight loss, RUQ pain, jaundice, and anorexia are common symptoms. Fifty percent of patients with pyogenic abscesses have elevated LFTs and bilirubin. Chest and abdominal x-rays will show right-sided atelectasis and pleural effusion with an elevated hemidiaphragm in 50% or air in the abscess in 10–20% of patients. Ultrasonography can identify an abscess in about 90% of patients, but CT is most commonly used and can help with image-guided drainage procedures. Two-thirds of causative organisms are gram-negative aerobes (including *Escherichia coli, Klebsiella pneumoniae,* and *Proteus*), anaerobes are present in 30%, and 30% are streptococci. Biliary sources are often marked by the presence of *Enterococcus*, whereas the presence of anaerobes implies a colonic or pelvic source. Percutaneous drainage is preferred, but surgical drainage may be indicated with large or multiple abscesses, if the drainage route is transpleural, or if there is another intra-abdominal pathology that requires operation. Patients should undergo IV antibiotic therapy for 2 weeks and then receive oral agents for 1 month. Therapy should include ampicillin, an aminoglycoside, and metronidazole. A third-generation cephalosporin could replace the ampicillin and aminoglycoside. The mortality rate is 2.5–30%, and risk factors include multiple or large (>5 cm) abscesses, mixed bacterial and fungal abscesses, and the presence of organisms other than *K. pneumoniae.*

BIBLIOGRAPHY

Edil BH, Pitt HA. Hepatic abscess. In: Cameron JL, Cameron AM (eds.), *Current Surgical Therapy*, 10th ed. Philadelphia, PA: Elsevier Saunders; 2011.

Subramanian A, Gurakar A, Klein A, Cameron A. Hepatic infection and acute hepatic failure. In: Mulholland MW, Lillemoe KD, Doherty GM, Maier RV, Simeone DM, Upchurch DR (eds.), *Greenfield's Surgery: Scientific Principles and Practice*, 5th ed. Philadelphia, PA: Wolters Kluwer Health; 2011.

16. **(A)** Hepatic artery aneurysms make up 20% of all splanchnic artery aneurysms. The most common causes, in order of frequency, are medial degeneration (24%), trauma (22%), and infection (10%). Orthotopic liver transplantation has also been associated with 17% of hepatic artery aneurysms. Most patients are older than 50 years, if the etiology of the aneurysm is not due to trauma. Eighty percent are extrahepatic, and lesions larger than 2 cm are most commonly saccular. Those smaller than 2 cm are fusiform. Sixty-three percent arise in the common hepatic artery, 28% in the right hepatic artery, and 5% in the left hepatic artery. Patients may have RUQ or epigastric pain similar to biliary colic or chronic cholecystitis if the aneurysm is symptomatic but not ruptured. About 20% of these rupture, with a mortality rate of 35%. Rupture can occur into the peritoneal cavity or hepatobiliary tree. Rupture into the bile ducts can cause hemobilia, hematemesis, and jaundice. Treatment is surgery unless the patient is too ill to undergo operative management. Surgical management can include ligation of the aneurysm, aneurysmectomy with primary anastomosis, or aneurysmectomy with interposition graft.

BIBLIOGRAPHY

Upchurch GR Jr, Henke PK, Stanley JC. Treatment of splanchnic artery aneurysms. In: Fischer JE, Bland KI (eds.), *Mastery of Surgery*, 5th ed. Philadelphia, PA: Lippincott Williams & Wilkins; 2007.

17. **(A)** Budd-Chiari syndrome (BCS) is a rare condition, and its diagnosis is often missed. It results from hepatic vein occlusion secondary to thrombosis of the major hepatic veins. The most common causes are hypercoagulable states (chronic myeloproliferative disorders, paroxysmal nocturnal hemoglobinuria, factor V Leiden deficiency, protein C and S deficiency,

oral contraceptives, and pregnancy) and mechanical etiologies such as vena caval membranous webs (most commonly seen in the East) and extrinsic hepatic vein occlusion by liver tumors. Clinically, the patients present with an insidious course with ascites, hepatomegaly, and RUQ abdominal pain. Unexplained ascites should raise suspicion for BCS and lead to ultrasound of the hepatic veins and liver biopsy. Sudden occlusion presents with a more dramatic picture, with massive ascites, severe RUQ tenderness, and increased serum transaminases. Diagnostic evaluation is based on hepatic vein imaging and liver biopsy. Ultrasound of the hepatic veins would show a decreased flow in the hepatic veins and has a sensitivity of 85–95%. Liver biopsy must also be performed to determine the progression and severity of the disease. Surgical management is often indicated for BCS, because survival without it is 10%. If the patient has end-stage liver disease without a web, the treatment of choice is orthotopic liver transplant, with a 5-year survival of 34–88%. If the patient does not have cirrhosis, then a TIPS or shunt (side-to-side portosystemic) should be performed. With a surgical shunt, the 5-year survival rate is 60%, as long as liver function is preserved. A TIPS procedure can provide a 5-year survival of 74%, again if performed before cirrhosis develops. In fulminant hepatic failure, as seen in the patient described in this scenario, a TIPS is done as a bridge to orthotopic liver transplant (definitive therapy).

BIBLIOGRAPHY

Marvin MR, Emond JC. Cirrhosis and portal hypertension. In: Mulholland MW, Lillemoe KD, Doherty GM, Maier RV, Simeone DM, Upchurch DR (eds.), *Greenfield's Surgery: Scientific Principles and Practice*, 5th ed. Philadelphia, PA: Wolters Kluwer Health; 2011.

18. **(C)** Volvulus is derived from the Latin word *volvere*, which means "to twist upon." The colon must be mobile with sufficient length to rotate around the mesenteric base. The most common site involved is the sigmoid (65–80%), and sigmoid volvulus tends to occur in those in their 70s. Cecal volvulus is next most common (15–30%) and is found in younger, female patients (age 50). Volvulus accounts for 10–15% of colonic obstructions in the United States and 2–4% of obstructions overall. Risk factors include institutionalization (low-fiber diet, decreased mobility, and chronic constipation), megacolon (due to Parkinson disease, hypothyroidism, Hirschsprung disease), and pregnancy. Sigmoid volvulus is an acquired entity, whereas cecal volvulus is congenital (incomplete peritoneal fixation of the right colon). Clinically, it presents with crampy abdominal

pain, distention, and obstipation, whereas peritoneal signs and elevated WBC count suggest a gangrenous colon. The volvulus may act as a closed loop obstruction with increasing intraluminal pressure causing ischemia. Torsion may compromise the mesenteric vasculature. Abdominal x-rays may show the "bent inner tube sign" or "coffee bean sign." Barium enema shows "bird's beak" at the site of twisting. Treatment for sigmoid volvulus is decompression with endoscopy and placement of a rectal tube for maintenance of decompression if the patient does not have evidence of peritonitis and is hemodynamically stable. Elective sigmoid resection at the same hospitalization is preferable, as this will help reduce the risk of recurrence while waiting to undergo an elective resection. The recurrence rate with decompression alone ranges from 40 to 90%. If peritoneal signs and gangrenous colon are encountered, a Hartmann's procedure is performed, or the patient could be left in discontinuity and a primary anastomosis could be performed at the time of second look. Mortality rate in the setting of resection of gangrenous bowel ranges from 18 to 75%, versus 10% in the setting of viable bowel. Colopexy could be considered; however, it has a recurrence rate of up to 22% (vs 1% if resected). Cecal volvulus is usually treated by operation, because there is gangrenous colon in 23–100% of cases. The choices are detorsion alone (20–75% recurrence rate), detorsion with fixation (16% recurrence rate), or resection (no risk of recurrence). Resection is required for ischemic or perforated colon consisting of a right hemicolectomy.

BIBLIOGRAPHY

Cocanour CS. Colonic volvulus. In: Cameron JL, Cameron AM (eds.), *Current Surgical Therapy*, 10th ed. Philadelphia, PA: Elsevier Saunders; 2011.

19. **(C)** Mesenteric venous thrombosis (MVT) comprises 5–15% of cases of acute mesenteric ischemia. Symptoms include nausea, vomiting, diarrhea, and vague abdominal pain. CT has a sensitivity of more than 90%. Bowel wall thickening and ascites are also suggestive of MVT. Complete thrombosis of the superior mesenteric vein is seen in about 12% of patients who undergo laparotomy. Therapy includes immediate anticoagulation to minimize thrombus progression and bowel rest. If there is evidence of peritonitis on exam, emergent laparotomy should be performed, where the mesentery appears cyanotic in coloring and the distal mesenteric veins contain thrombus. In patients with a hypercoagulable state, long-term anticoagulation is suggested for this condition. Mortality is around 20–25%, and recurrent MVT presents in 50% of patients.

BIBLIOGRAPHY

Jundt JP, Liem TK, Moneta GL. Venous and lymphatic disease. In: Brunicardi FC, Andersen DK, Billiar TR, et al. (eds.), *Principles of Surgery*, 10th ed. New York, NY: McGraw-Hill; 2014.

20. **(D)** Mucinous neoplasms of the appendix include simple cysts, mucinous cystadenoma, mucinous cystadenocarcinoma, and pseudomyxoma peritonei. Mucoceles of the appendix typically remain asymptomatic due to slow-growing distension of the appendix and are frequently discovered incidentally as a mass on physical examination or abdominal imaging; wall calcification is characteristic on plain radiograph or CT. It is recommended that all mucinous appendiceal masses 2 cm or larger be surgically removed. For mucinous cystadenoma or simple cysts, appendectomy is sufficient if the lesion does not involve the appendiceal base. For ruptured benign mucoceles, appendectomy and removal of any residual mucin are curative; however, the procedure should be performed via traditional laparotomy because laparoscopic appendectomy increases the risk of spillage of mucin-secreting cells throughout the abdomen. In addition, a screening colonoscopy should be performed postoperatively due to the association with colon and rectal carcinoma. For patients with diffuse pseudomyxoma peritonei, the suspicion of malignancy is significantly higher; in one series, 95% of patients with pseudomyxoma had an associated mucinous cystadenocarcinoma. These patients should undergo right hemicolectomy with debulking of any gross spread of disease and removal of all mucin. For patients with malignant lesions diagnosed at the time of pathologic evaluation of the appendectomy specimen, reoperation with right hemicolectomy is recommended. Reported 5-year survival for mucinous cystadenocarcinoma is 75% after hemicolectomy and less than 50% after appendectomy alone.

BIBLIOGRAPHY

Peranteau WH, Smink DS. Appendix, Meckel's, and other small bowel diverticula. In: Zinner MJ, Ashley SW (eds.), *Maingot's Abdominal Operations*, 12th ed. New York, NY: McGraw-Hill; 2013:Chapter 31.

21. **(D)** Peritonitis is an inflammation of the peritoneum; it may be localized or diffuse in location, acute or chronic in natural history, and infectious or aseptic in pathogenesis.

Primary peritonitis occurs when microbes invade the peritoneal cavity via hematogenous dissemination from a distant source of infection or direct inoculation without an obvious source such as a gastrointestinal (GI) tract perforation. This most frequently occurs in patients who have ascites secondary to cirrhosis of the liver, congestive heart failure, or renal failure with peritoneal dialysis. Approximately one-third of patients with primary peritonitis have no signs or symptoms of abdominal sepsis. Diagnosis is based on clinical suspicion, the patient's presentation, and the Gram stain and culture results obtained from ascitic fluid aspiration. Culture of infected ascitic fluid usually yields aerobic enteric organisms; however, approximately 35% of patients with these diseases will have negative ascitic fluid cultures. Blood cultures are also frequently positive in these patients. Primary bacterial peritonitis may be assumed to be present when the ascitic fluid neutrophil count is >100–250/μL. Primary peritonitis rarely requires surgical intervention.

Secondary peritonitis is caused by contamination of the peritoneum from the gut lumen due to perforation or severe intra-abdominal organ infection, penetrating wound of the abdominal wall, or external introduction of a foreign object that is or becomes infected (e.g., a chronic peritoneal dialysis catheter). The conditions that most commonly result in the introduction of bacteria into the peritoneum are ruptured appendix, ruptured diverticulum, perforated peptic ulcer, incarcerated hernia, gangrenous gallbladder, volvulus, bowel infarction, cancer, inflammatory bowel disease, or intestinal obstruction. These infections are polymicrobial in accordance with the source. Patients with secondary bacterial peritonitis are unlikely to respond to antibiotic administration alone and usually require surgical treatment.

Tertiary peritonitis refers to recurrent intra-abdominal infection after therapy with antibiotics and drainage for secondary peritonitis. Abscess formation and resistance to first-line antibiotics are common. Most patients with tertiary peritonitis require one or more additional operative procedures to achieve control of their infection.

BIBLIOGRAPHY

Beilman GJ, Dunn DL. Surgical infections. In: Brunicardi F, Andersen DK, Billiar TR, et al. (eds.), *Schwartz's Principles of Surgery*, 10th ed. New York, NY: McGraw-Hill; 2014.

Bohnen JA, Mustard RA, Schouten BD. The acute abdomen and intra-abdominal sepsis. In: Hall JB, Schmidt GA, Wood LH (eds.), *Principles of Critical Care*, 3rd ed. New York, NY: McGraw-Hill; 2005:Chapter 89.

Doron S, Snydman DR. Peritonitis and intra-abdominal abscess. In: McKean SC, Ross JJ, Dressler DD, Brotman DJ, Ginsberg JS (eds.), *Principles and Practice of Hospital Medicine*. New York, NY: McGraw-Hill; 2012:Chapter 187.

Silen W. Acute appendicitis and peritonitis. In: Longo DL, Fauci AS, Kasper DL, Hauser SL, Jameson J, Loscalzo J (eds.), *Harrison's Principles of Internal Medicine*, 18th ed. New York, NY: McGraw-Hill; 2012:Chapter 300.

CHAPTER 27

ABDOMINAL WALL AND RETROPERITONEUM

DANIEL G. DAVILA AND TRAVIS P. WEBB

QUESTIONS

1. Which of the following is true regarding laparoscopic inguinal hernia repair?
    (A) There are three primary approaches.
    (B) The extraperitoneal approach has a higher rate of recurrence.
    (C) The abdominal approach makes use of a dissection balloon.
    (D) Pain levels on postoperative day 1 are increased compared to open hernia repair.
    (E) The extraperitoneal approach dissects between the peritoneum and transversalis fascia.

2. Which of the following is an absolute contraindication to laparoscopic inguinal hernia repair?
    (A) Urinary tract infection
    (B) Previous radical prostatectomy
    (C) Incarcerated hernia
    (D) Cirrhosis
    (E) Recurrence after open repair

3. Which of the following is characteristic of epigastric hernias?
    (A) They rarely contain preperitoneal fat.
    (B) The defect is usually large and solitary.
    (C) They occur as a defect in the aponeurotic fibers in between the rectus sheaths.
    (D) A true peritoneal sac is frequently found on exploration.
    (E) Ultrasound has no role in the diagnosis of epigastric hernias.

4. Umbilical hernias
    (A) Are present in one-third of all newborns
    (B) Will most likely spontaneously close by the age of 4 years if the defect is 3 cm or smaller
    (C) Are three times more likely to occur in males than females

    (D) Can be safely managed nonoperatively with abdominal binders if the patient is not a surgical candidate
    (E) If larger than 2 cm, warrant consideration for mesh repair

5. A 48-year-old alcoholic presents with massive ascites with a large umbilical hernia, with thin skin at the apex. There is a slow ooze of clear, odorless fluid from the hernia. Appropriate management is
    (A) Hernia repair with mesh after diuresis
    (B) Diuresis with observation
    (C) Paracentesis and abdominal binder
    (D) Peritovenous shunt
    (E) Diet modifications

6. Which of the following is the most common cause of lumbar hernias?
    (A) Partial nephrectomy via a flank incision
    (B) Congenital weakness of the lumbodorsal fascia
    (C) Drainage of a lumbar abscess
    (D) Stab injury to the flank
    (E) Iliac bone graft harvesting

7. The shelving portion of the inguinal ligament used for open inguinal hernia repair
    (A) Is formed from the external oblique aponeurosis
    (B) Arises from the transversalis fascia
    (C) Inserts directly onto the cremasteric fascia
    (D) Represents the superior border of the iliopubic tract
    (E) Is usually sutured to the transversus aponeurotic arch (falx inguinalis), which lies inferiorly to it, to complete a primary open repair

8. The median umbilical ligament is the remnant of which of the following fetal structures?
    (A) Vitelline duct
    (B) Urachus
    (C) Umbilical vein
    (D) Umbilical artery
    (E) Ductus venosus

9. Which of the following nerves is most commonly injured during laparoscopic inguinal hernia repair?
   (A) Ilioinguinal
   (B) Femoral
   (C) Obturator
   (D) Iliohypogastric
   (E) Genitofemoral

10. Which of the following is true concerning congenital abnormalities of the abdominal wall?
    (A) Diastasis recti is a weakness of the linea alba in the lower midline.
    (B) Gastroschisis occurs medial to the umbilicus and does not involve an amniotic sac.
    (C) A persistent omphalomesenteric duct has a low risk of intussusception or volvulus and should be managed conservatively.
    (D) Meckel diverticulum is a false diverticulum and represents persistent intestinal portion of the omphalomesenteric duct.
    (E) Chronic umbilical drainage may indicate the presence of a urachal sinus.

11. Retroperitoneal fibrosis
    (A) Is considered idiopathic in about one-third of all cases
    (B) Has been associated with hydralazine, ergotamine, methyldopa, and α-blocking agents
    (C) Is excluded if only one ureter appears to be involved
    (D) Can be treated surgically with ureteral transposition, renal autotransplantation, or omental encasement
    (E) Cannot be accurately diagnosed with intravenous pyelography

12. Which of the following is true regarding primary retroperitoneal tumors?
    (A) Malignant in 60–85% of all cases
    (B) Classified as either mesodermal or neurologic in origin, the latter of which comprises the majority of these tumors
    (C) Clearly defined with a combination of magnetic resonance imaging (MRI) and computed tomography (CT); angiography, but imaging is limited in determining resectability
    (D) Effectively treated with partial resection and chemotherapy, with a significant improvement in median survival at 5 years
    (E) Mostly found to have low histologic grade and be of small (<5 cm) size at the time of diagnosis

13. Which of the following correctly describes the management of retroperitoneal hematomas?
    (A) Zone 3 hematomas due to penetrating injury in a stable patient should be managed nonoperatively with pelvic angiography to determine potential sites for embolization.
    (B) Exploration of nonexpanding stable zone 2 hematomas due to blunt trauma increases the likelihood of renal injury and/or loss of the kidney.
    (C) Supramesocolic zone 1 hematomas should first be approached by gaining control of the abdominal aorta via the midline posterior peritoneum at the supraceliac aorta.
    (D) The most common site of blunt trauma to the abdominal aorta is at the origin of the superior mesenteric artery (SMA).
    (E) Infrarenal lacerations of the abdominal aorta are associated with the highest mortality rate.

14. Rectus sheath hematomas
    (A) Can be caused by coughing
    (B) Are rarely associated with anticoagulation therapy
    (C) Usually occur at the semicircular line of Douglas at the entry site of the superior epigastric artery into the rectus sheath
    (D) Are infrequently palpable on physical examination
    (E) Usually require operative drainage

15. The peritoneum
    (A) Can absorb isotonic fluids such as saline at a rate of approximately 90–100 mL/h
    (B) Contains a mesothelial lining that secretes fluid to lubricate the peritoneal surfaces, and normally 200–300 mL of free intraperitoneal fluid is present in an adult
    (C) Can reabsorb approximately 90% of the red blood cells in the peritoneal cavity intact via fenestrated lymphatic channels in the undersurface of the diaphragm
    (D) Normally contains air after laparotomy for 7–8 days
    (E) Can contain chylous ascites, which predisposes to intraperitoneal infection

16. Which of the following is true concerning primary peritonitis?
    (A) It occurs more frequently in adults than in children.
    (B) Pediatric patients with nephrotic syndrome and systemic lupus erythematosus (SLE) are at increased risk for this condition.
    (C) Risk in the pediatric population occurs at age 2–3 years.
    (D) It occurs when inflammation of the peritoneal cavity occurs with a documented source of contamination.
    (E) The bacteriostatic nature of ascites related to liver disease explains the decreased incidence of primary peritonitis in that patient population.

17. Which of the following is true concerning peritoneal fluid?
    (A) Chylous ascites increases the likelihood of infection due to its high fat content.
    (B) Vancomycin doses should be adjusted in patients with peritoneal dialysis.
    (C) Choleperitoneum can only occur as a result of injury to the biliary tract.
    (D) Intraperitoneal hemoglobin interferes with intraperitoneal bacterial clearance and thus interferes with the immune response.
    (E) Ruptured aortic aneurysm and traumatic vascular injuries are the most common causes of hemoperitoneum.

18. Mesenteric cysts
    (A) Are usually filled with bloody effluent
    (B) Are only embryonic or traumatic in origin
    (C) Are rarely palpable on physical examination
    (D) Usually present as nontender, asymptomatic abdominal masses
    (E) Have a characteristic lateral mobility on physical examination

19. A 76-year-old woman presents with abdominal pain, vomiting, and groin pain. Which of the following is true?
    (A) Femoral hernia is the most common abdominal wall hernia.
    (B) The anterior border of the femoral canal is Cooper's ligament.
    (C) Conservative management is indicated in patients over 70.
    (D) Postoperative bleeding is most commonly from the obturator artery.
    (E) Preperitoneal repair is contraindicated.

20. Testicular atrophy following inguinal hernioplasty is usually due to
    (A) Injury to the pampiniform plexus
    (B) Subacute orchitis
    (C) Damage to the external spermatic artery
    (D) Ligation of the vas deferens
    (E) Damage to the testicle from mobilization

Scenario for questions 21 through 24
    A 43-year-old man with a history of chronic pancreatitis, status post multiple pancreatic duct stent placements, presents to the emergency room with severe left lower quadrant abdominal pain. He notes increasingly frequent attacks of sharp pain in the past several days, with the pain on presentation being constant and having been present for 12 hours. He notes no emesis but has nausea, and notes no hematemesis or hematochezia. His last bowel movement was earlier in the day. Examination reveals severe left lower quadrant pain on palpation with evidence of guarding and equivocal signs of rebound. White blood cell (WBC) count is 13,000 with a left shift, and his temperature is 37.0°C. A CT scan is obtained, which shows the following (see Fig. 27-1):

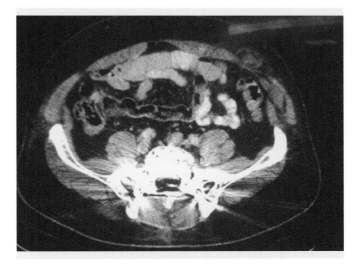

FIGURE 27-1. Computed tomography scan of abdomen.

21. Given the CT scan, what is the most likely diagnosis?
    (A) Recurrent pancreatitis
    (B) Biliary colic
    (C) Strangulated epigastric hernia
    (D) Incarcerated spigelian hernia
    (E) Incarcerated inguinal hernia

22. Which of the following is true concerning spigelian hernias?
    (A) Preoperative diagnosis of spigelian hernias is made in over 75% of cases.
    (B) Regardless of the technique of repair, the recurrence rate for spigelian hernias is less than 10%.
    (C) Similar symptoms of pain can be produced by entrapment of the anterior cutaneous nerves of T10–T12.
    (D) Although ultrasound has no role in diagnosis, CT scan can be helpful in detecting small spigelian hernias.
    (E) None of the above

23. Which of the following is true concerning the location of spigelian hernias?
    (A) They are more likely to occur below the semicircular line of Douglas because the aponeurotic fibers of the internal and external oblique muscles are parallel below the umbilicus.
    (B) They occur just medial to the semilunar line.
    (C) Spigelian hernias may occur inferior to the epigastric vessels.
    (D) A and B
    (E) B and C

24. Which of the following is true concerning repair of spigelian hernias?
    (A) Small spigelian hernias can most often be closed primarily.
    (B) Large hernias may require repair with prosthetic mesh.
    (C) Laparoscopic repair of nonincarcerated spigelian hernias is feasible, with a reduction in postoperative morbidity and length of hospital stay.
    (D) Some repairs may require reduction of herniated sigmoid colon.
    (E) All of the above

Scenario for questions 25 through 28

A 37-year-old white man is 24 hours post exploratory laparotomy for multiple gunshot wounds. Injuries required multiple bowel resections, repair of a liver laceration, and splenectomy; the patient has required over 10 L of fluid and blood product resuscitation. The patient is now oliguric with a tense, distended abdomen, and there is a high suspicion for abdominal compartment syndrome.

25. Which of the following would be the most likely set of findings for this patient?
    (A) Central venous pressure (CVP) 6, peak airway pressure of 24, systemic vascular resistance index (SVRI) 500
    (B) CVP 20, peak airway pressure of 24, SVRI 1400
    (C) CVP 20, peak airway pressure of 44, SVRI 1400
    (D) CVP 20, peak airway pressure of 44, SVRI 500
    (E) CVP 6, peak airway pressure of 44, SVRI 500

26. Which of the following is *not* true concerning the etiology of this condition?
    (A) Elevated intrathoracic pressure is the result of elevation of the diaphragms.
    (B) Decrease in venous return to the heart results from compression of the intra-abdominal inferior vena cava (IVC) and is magnified by elevated intrathoracic pressure.

    (C) Oliguria results from decreased renal blood flow as well as from compression of the ureters.
    (D) Elevated intracranial pressures are associated with this condition.
    (E) Patients with this condition have an increased likelihood of thrombophlebitis and pulmonary embolism.

27. In which situation should immediate decompression be most likely warranted?
    (A) Intravesicular pressure readings of 30 mmHg or 40 mmH$_2$O, urine output of 10 mL/h
    (B) Intravesicular pressure readings of 25 mmHg or 20 mmH$_2$O, urine output of 40 mL/h
    (C) Intravesicular pressure readings of 15 mmHg or 20 mmH$_2$O, urine output of 10 mL/h
    (D) A and B
    (E) A and C

28. Which of the following is *not* true about therapy for abdominal compartment syndrome?
    (A) Resolution of elevated peak airway pressures, decreased cardiac output, and oliguria always occurs immediately during operative intervention.
    (B) Frequently, fascial closure is not possible secondary to visceral and retroperitoneal edema.
    (C) If abdominal wall closure is not possible immediately, further attempts can reasonably be made within the following 3–4 days.
    (D) Abdominal closure techniques can include usage of sterile irrigation bags, polytetrafluoroethylene (PTFE) sheets, Vicryl mesh, and towel clip closure of the skin.
    (E) Abdominal wall component separation is a technique that can close a fascial defect of up to 15 cm.

Scenario for questions 29 through 32

A 54-year-old man is admitted to the hospital for suspected gallstone pancreatitis. CT scan on presentation reveals significant peripancreatic fluid, inflammation, and evidence of devitalized pancreatic tissue. He otherwise remains stable and afebrile and is maintained on total parenteral nutrition (TPN), intravenous (IV) broad-spectrum antibiotics, and bowel rest. After several weeks of stabilization, he is released to home with this continued therapy. Two weeks later, he presents with altered mental status, seizure activity, shortness of breath, substernal chest pain, and fever (39.0°C).

29. Which of the following is *not* part of the immediate workup?
    (A) CT scan of the head
    (B) CT scan of the chest and pulmonary embolus protocol
    (C) CT scan of the abdomen and pelvis
    (D) 12-lead electrocardiogram (ECG) and chest radiograph
    (E) Electroencephalogram (EEG)

30. With other workup being negative, clinical attention focuses on continued pancreatic *complications* with this patient. Which of the following is true concerning the treatment of severe pancreatitis?
    (A) Nasoduodenal feeding with nonelemental formulas is recommended, as gastric feedings can stimulate pancreatic secretion.
    (B) Total parenteral nutrition is not associated with increased likelihood of infectious complications.
    (C) Piperacillin–tazobactam has the best tissue penetration of the pancreatic parenchyma.
    (D) Fungal organisms are the most common organisms found on aspiration of pancreatic fluid collections.
    (E) None of the above

31. CT scan of the abdomen and pelvis reveals a large retroperitoneal fluid collection with evidence of air. Given the suspicion that this collection is infected, which of the following is true?
    (A) Pancreatic abscess, infected pseudocyst, and infected necrosis occur in up to 15% of patients with acute pancreatitis.
    (B) More than 50% of patients with six or more of Ranson's criteria will develop a pancreatic septic complication.
    (C) The double bubble sign signifies the presence of retroperitoneal, extraluminal air on plain abdominal radiograph.
    (D) CT scan is the gold standard for detecting pancreatic necrosis, with an accuracy of 95% when there is parenchymal necrosis of less than 10%.
    (E) None of the above

32. The patient undergoes laparotomy with debridement of the necrotic pancreas and infected retroperitoneal collection. Concerning this therapy, which of the following is true?
    (A) There should be a low threshold for formal anatomic resection of the pancreas if open debridement of the pancreas is necessary.
    (B) Following operative debridement with sump drainage, mortality occurs in 5–50% of patients, averaging 30%.

    (C) The majority of patients with this condition can be managed conservatively with percutaneous drainage and antibiotics.
    (D) Minimally invasive techniques for pancreatic drainage have been proven to provide effective debridement of infected peripancreatic infected necrosis.
    (E) A cholecystostomy tube should be placed if operative intervention is necessary for biliary associated pancreatitis.

33. The most common clinical presentation in patients with obturator hernia is
    (A) Groin pain
    (B) Intestinal obstruction
    (C) Pain along the medial surface of the thigh that may radiate to the knee and hip joints
    (D) History of repeated episodes of bowel obstruction that pass quickly and without intervention
    (E) Palpable mass in the proximal medial aspect of the thigh at the origin of the adductor muscles

34. Which of the following is true regarding the inguinal canal?
    (A) The anterior boundary is the external oblique muscle.
    (B) The posterior boundary is the internal oblique aponeurosis.
    (C) The superior boundary is the inguinal ligament.
    (D) The inferior boundary is the lacunar ligament.
    (E) The superficial border is the transversus abdominis muscle.

ANSWERS AND EXPLANATIONS

1. **(E)**

2. **(B)**

Explanation for questions 1 and 2

Laparoscopic inguinal hernia repair is a procedure that has been in common practice for over 10 years. The two most commonly performed types are the transabdominal preperitoneal (TAPP) and the totally extraperitoneal (TEP) approaches. The TAPP involves laparoscopic dissection of the peritoneum off of the pelvic floor and hernia sac, placement of mesh around the defect, and closure of the peritoneum over the mesh. The TEP involves dissection between the peritoneum and transversalis fascia with a dissecting balloon, with subsequent creation of a pneumoextraperitoneum to allow visualization, reduction of the hernia, and placement of mesh.

Regardless of the technique used, there are several contraindications to the laparoscopic technique. Of, course the patient must be able to hemodynamically tolerate both general anesthesia and the effects of pneumoperitoneum as with any laparoscopic surgery.

Previous preperitoneal surgery, history of radical prostatectomy, strangulation of the hernia, infection, and history of pelvic radiation secondary to the presence of scarred tissue in the preperitoneal space are contraindications to laparoscopic repair. Cirrhosis with portal hypertension and ascites is considered only a relative contraindication to laparoscopic repair.

Recurrence rate for both techniques range from 0 to 5%, and patients who undergo laparoscopic hernia repair experience less pain in the early postoperative period and have lower analgesic and narcotic requirements, better cosmesis, and earlier return to normal activities.

BIBLIOGRAPHY

Bathla L, Fitzgibbons RJ Jr. Perspective on hernias: laparoscopic inguinal hernia repair. In: Zinner MJ, Ashley SW (eds.), *Maingot's Abdominal Operations*, 12th ed. New York, NY: McGraw-Hill; 2013:Chapter 8B.
Sherman V, Macho JR, Brunicardi F. Inguinal hernias. In: Brunicardi F, Andersen DK, Billiar TR, et al. (eds.), *Schwartz's Principles of Surgery*, 9th ed. New York, NY: McGraw-Hill; 2010:Chapter 37.

3. **(C)** An epigastric hernia is a defect in the abdominal wall that occurs between the xiphoid process and the umbilicus. These hernias occur through defects of the linea alba, the aponeurotic fibers between the rectus sheaths, and most often contain preperitoneal fat. Epigastric hernias rarely have a peritoneal sac and are usually solitary and small in size compared with the herniated tissues. Incisional hernias may also occur above the umbilicus in the setting of previous trocar placement. These hernias usually will have a peritoneal sac and may involve other abdominal contents other than fat.

The most common presenting symptom is discomfort in the upper abdomen in the midline, and a bulge can often be palpated on physical examination. Ultrasound may be helpful in diagnosis, as well as upright positioning and Valsalva maneuvers.

BIBLIOGRAPHY

Javid PJ, Greenberg JA, Brooks DC. Hernias. In: Zinner MJ, Ashley SW (eds.), *Maingot's Abdominal Operations*, 12th ed. New York, NY: McGraw-Hill; 2013:Chapter 7.

4. **(E)**

5. **(A)**

Explanation for questions 4 and 5

Umbilical hernias are congenital in nature in children and most often acquired in the adult and occur in females at a ratio of 3:1. In children, failure of the umbilical ring to close produces the hernia, which may occur in as many as 20% of newborns. If the umbilical hernia

in the pediatric patient is less than 1.5 cm, it will more than likely close by the age of 4 years. Pediatric surgical candidates are patients with large, complicated, or incarcerated/strangulated hernias, as well as children over the age of 4 with a persistent umbilical hernia.

Adults usually acquire umbilical hernias from conditions that increase intra-abdominal pressure. Persistent coughing (smokers) or abdominal straining (chronic constipation) can provide enough force over time to produce the hernia. Patients with ascites also frequently develop umbilical hernias. Small hernias are usually more symptomatic than larger ones. Over time, the herniated contents, usually bowel or omentum, adhere to the peritoneal sac, leading to incarceration.

Management of umbilical hernias should favor surgical repair in patients who can tolerate it, so as to avoid the morbidity associated with strangulation. Usage of abdominal binders has not been shown to adequately manage these hernias nonoperatively and should be avoided. Surgical management classically involved the Mayo repair ("vest over pants"), but recent years have heralded tension-free repairs using mesh. This is especially true for large umbilical hernias over 2 cm in size. Abdominal binders may be used postoperatively and may aid in reducing seroma formation.

Umbilical hernia in a patient with ascites is a significant challenge, particularly in the setting of leaking abdominal ascites. These patients should be immediately admitted to the hospital and started on IV antibiotics to decrease the risk of bacterial peritonitis and/or hernia rupture. Umbilical hernia repair in cirrhotics with uncontrolled ascites is associated with a mortality rate of nearly 10%. For this reason, elective repair of umbilical hernias in decompensated cirrhotics with ascites is preferable to urgent repair. In the setting of urgent repair, an aggressive diuresis and sodium and fluid restriction are prudent, as is bedrest to remove undue strain on the weak and leaking site. If operation must be undertaken emergently (true rupture) or diuretic therapy fails to control the ascites, combined umbilical herniorrhaphy with a peritoneal-venous shunt is effective in achieving a stable repair with a relatively low morbidity.

BIBLIOGRAPHY

Javid PJ, Greenberg JA, Brooks DC. Hernias. In: Zinner MJ, Ashley SW (eds.), *Maingot's Abdominal Operations*, 12th ed. New York, NY: McGraw-Hill; 2013:Chapter 7.

6. **(A)** The lumbar hernia involves herniation of abdominal contents through either the superior lumbar (Grynfelt–Lesshaft) or inferior lumbar (Petit) triangles (see Fig. 27-2). The superior triangle is formed superiorly from the 12th rib, medially from the paraspinous muscles, and laterally

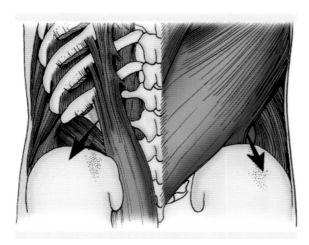

FIGURE 27-2. Anatomy of the lumbar triangle. Used with permission from Neal Barshes, MD, MPH, Brigham and Women's Hospital, Boston, MA.

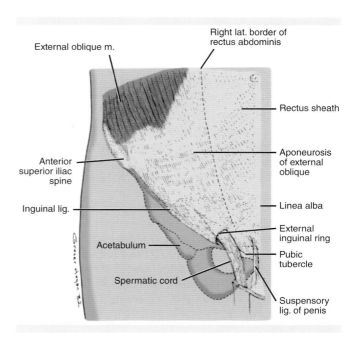

FIGURE 27-3. External oblique muscle and aponeurosis. From Skandalakis PN, Skandalakis JE, Colborn GL, Kingsnorth AN, Weidman TA, Skandalakis LJ. Abdominal wall and hernias. In: Skandalakis JE, Colburn GL, Weidman TA, et al. (eds.), *Skandalakis' Surgical Anatomy*. New York, NY: McGraw-Hill; 2004:Chapter 9, Fig. 9-3.

by the internal oblique muscle, with the floor of the space composed of the lumbodorsal fascia and covered by the latissimus dorsi muscle. The inferior lumbar triangle is formed by the latissimus dorsi medially, the external oblique muscle laterally, and the iliac crest inferiorly, with the floor again the lumbodorsal fascia, but covered only by subcutaneous tissue. Lumbar hernias are thought to occur more frequently through the superior lumbar triangle. Strangulation is rare in lumbar hernias since at least two of the three boundaries for the hernia defect are soft and muscular in origin.

Lumbar hernias are classified either as congenital or acquired, the latter being the result of trauma, surgery, or spontaneous development. Iatrogenic causes of these hernias are most commonly the result of retroperitoneal surgeries via a flank incision. Latissimus dorsi flaps, drainage of lumbar abscesses, iliac bone graft harvesting, and blunt/penetrating trauma are less common causes.

The most common symptom is pain, either a vague dullness in the flank or lower back or more focal pain associated with movement over the site of the defect. On physical examination, a soft swelling in the lower posterior abdomen will be found that is usually reducible without difficulty and increases with a Valsalva maneuver. Ultrasound or CT imaging can aid in diagnosis.

BIBLIOGRAPHY

Javid PJ, Greenberg JA, Brooks DC. Hernias. In: Zinner MJ, Ashley SW (eds.), *Maingot's Abdominal Operations*, 12th ed. New York, NY: McGraw-Hill; 2013:Chapter 7.

7. **(A)** The anatomy of the inguinal canal is best visualized by considering its borders: the aponeurotic arch of the

transversus abdominis (falx inguinalis) superiorly, the inguinal ligament inferiorly, the transversalis fascia posteriorly, and the external oblique aponeurosis anteriorly. The inguinal ligament runs from the anterior superior iliac spine laterally to the pubic tubercle medially. The shelving portion of the inguinal ligament is formed when the external oblique aponeurosis travels inferiorly and posteriorly, cradling the spermatic cord. It thus inserts into the inguinal ligament and runs along inferiorly to the iliopubic tract (see Fig. 27-3). The lacunar ligament is the medial extent of the inguinal ligament as it travels posteriorly to attach to the pectineal (Cooper's) ligament.

BIBLIOGRAPHY

Skandalakis PN, Skandalakis JE, Colborn GL, Kingsnorth AN, Weidman TA, Skandalakis LJ. Abdominal wall and hernias. In: Skandalakis JE, Colburn GL, Weidman TA, et al. (eds.), *Skandalakis' Surgical Anatomy*. New York, NY: McGraw-Hill; 2004:Chapter 9.

8. **(B)** The remnants of fetal structures and epigastric vessels are located in the extraperitoneal adipose layer of the abdominal wall between the endoabdominal fascia and the peritoneum (see Fig. 27-4).

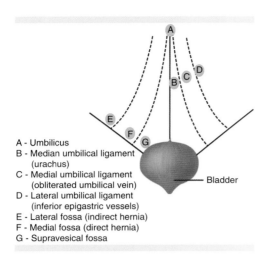

A - Umbilicus
B - Median umbilical ligament
    (urachus)
C - Medial umbilical ligament
    (obliterated umbilical vein)
D - Lateral umbilical ligament
    (inferior epigastric vessels)
E - Lateral fossa (indirect hernia)
F - Medial fossa (direct hernia)
G - Supravesical fossa

FIGURE 27-4. Posterior view of intraperitoneal folds and associated fossa. From Sherman V, Macho JR, Brunicardi F. Inguinal hernias. In: Brunicardi F, Andersen DK, Billiar TR, et al. (eds.), *Schwartz's Principles of Surgery*, 9th ed. New York, NY: McGraw-Hill; 2010:Chapter 37, Fig. 37-9.

The paired medial umbilical ligaments are remnants of the left and right umbilical arteries and lie between the epigastric vessels and the midline. The midline ligament, known as the median umbilical ligament, represents the obliteration of the urachus. The obliterated umbilical vein is located in the margin of the falciform ligament and is known as the ligamentum teres. The vitelline is a

fibrous band from the ileum to the umbilicus, although not usually present in adults. A patent vitelline sinus of the umbilicus with obliteration before connecting to the bowel, a persistent vitelline duct with connection to the bowel (and subsequent umbilical drainage), or most commonly as a Meckel's diverticulum.

These structures are important during transabdominal laparoscopic hernia repairs in identifying structures of the lower abdominal wall. Along the abdominal wall, the inferior epigastric vessels can be identified, traveling from the external iliac vessels to the rectus sheath (see Fig. 27-5).

The ductus venosus is a fetal vascular structure that connects the left umbilical vein to the upper inferior vena cava (IVC), allowing richly oxygenated placental blood to bypass the sinusoids of the liver. After birth, this structure, along with the umbilical vein, clots, and its obliteration eventually forms the ligamentum venosum within the falciform ligament.

BIBLIOGRAPHY

Colborn GL, Rogers RM Jr, Skandalakis JE, Badalament RA, Parrott TS, Weidman TA. Pelvis and perineum. In: Skandalakis JE, Colburn GL, Weidman TA, et al. (eds.), *Skandalakis' Surgical Anatomy*. New York, NY: McGraw-Hill; 2004:Chapter 28.

Sherman V, Macho JR, Brunicardi F. Inguinal hernias. In: Brunicardi F, Andersen DK, Billiar TR, et al. (eds.), *Schwartz's Principles of Surgery*, 9th ed. New York, NY: McGraw-Hill; 2010:Chapter 37.

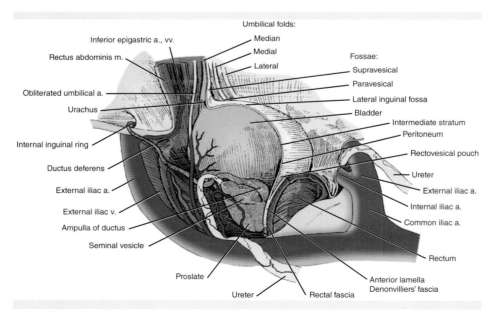

FIGURE 27-5. Peritoneal relationships in the male. From Colborn GL, Rogers RM Jr, Skandalakis JE, Badalament RA, Parrott TS, Weidman TA. Pelvis and perineum. In: Skandalakis JE, Colburn GL, Weidman TA, et al. (eds.), *Skandalakis' Surgical Anatomy*. New York, NY: McGraw-Hill; 2004:Chapter 28, Fig. 28-5.

9. **(E)** Nerve injuries during inguinal hernia repair can occur secondary to entrapment, electrocautery, and/or transection. The most commonly injured nerves are genitofemoral and lateral femoral cutaneous.

The most commonly injured nerves with open inguinal hernia repair are ilioinguinal, genital branch of the genitofemoral, and iliohypogastric. The triangle of pain is an imaginary triangle formed by the iliopubic tract inferolaterally and the gonadal vessels superomedially. Several nerves traverse the triangle that if injured can lead to postoperative pain. These include the lateral femoral cutaneous, anterior femoral cutaneous, femoral branch of genitofemoral, and femoral nerves.

The ilioinguinal nerve is at considerable risk to injury during closure of the external oblique aponeurosis. The ilioinguinal, along with the iliohypogastric nerve, may also become entrapped within the mesh in tension-free repairs. Laparoscopically, the lateral femoral cutaneous nerve and the genital and femoral branches of the genitofemoral nerve are at risk when placing lateral fixation tacks below the iliopubic tract, yet the lateral femoral cutaneous nerve may too be affected by mesh entrapment. Such injury to the lateral femoral cutaneous nerve will lead to meralgia paresthetica, a "pins and needles" sensation over the lateral aspect of the thigh. It also may be associated with a specific paresthesia known as formication, a sensation of insects crawling on or under the skin.

BIBLIOGRAPHY

Sherman V, Macho JR, Brunicardi F. Inguinal hernias. In: Brunicardi F, Andersen DK, Billiar TR, et al. (eds.), *Schwartz's Principles of Surgery*, 9th ed. New York, NY: McGraw-Hill; 2010:Chapter 37.

Skandalakis PN, Skandalakis JE, Colborn GL, Kingsnorth AN, Weidman TA, Skandalakis LJ. Abdominal wall and hernias. In: Skandalakis JE, Colburn GL, Weidman TA, et al. (eds.), *Skandalakis' Surgical Anatomy*. New York, NY: McGraw-Hill; 2004:Chapter 9.

10. **(E)** Diastasis recti is the protrusion of the abdominal wall in the midline above the umbilicus between the rectus abdominis muscles. Clinically, these patients present with a fusiform, linear bulge between the two rectus abdominis muscles without a discrete fascial defect. The cause is weakness of the linea alba and does not represent a true hernia. Repair should be avoided because there is no risk of incarceration, the fascial layer is weak, and the recurrence rate is high

Omphalocele is a congenital defect of the closure of the umbilical ring, classically represented by a midline herniation of abdominal contents within an amniotic sac. Gastroschisis is a congenital defect in the closure of the abdominal wall during development, leading to a lateral defect leading to herniation of abdominal contents without an amniotic sac.

The omphalomesenteric (vitelline) duct is an embryologic structure connecting the fetal midgut to the yolk sac, and it usually obliterates prior to birth. Remnants of the vitelline duct can present with a spectrum of conditions, from an umbilical polyp to a Meckel diverticulum.

Persistent vitelline ducts can be diagnosed by the passage of enteric contents via the umbilicus. Immediate laparotomy should be performed for excision to eliminate the high risk of intussusception or volvulus. Meckel diverticulum is a true diverticulum and is formed when the intestinal end of the vitelline duct persists. If discovered, treatment is excision.

The urachus is a fetal structure that connects the bladder to the umbilicus and also usually obliterates prior to birth. Urachal sinus presents with chronic umbilical drainage, as the umbilical end has not closed. Excision is warranted to avoid infection. Bladder diverticula may represent failure of closure of the bladder end of the urachus; these should also be excised once distal obstruction is ruled out. A persistent urachus is heralded by the leakage of urine from the umbilicus and should also warrant excision.

BIBLIOGRAPHY

Deveney KE. Hernias & other lesions of the abdominal wall. In: Doherty GM (eds.), *Current Diagnosis & Treatment: Surgery*, 13th ed. New York, NY: McGraw-Hill; 2010:Chapter 32.

Skandalakis PN, Skandalakis JE, Colborn GL, Kingsnorth N, Weidman TA, Skandalakis LJ. Abdominal wall and hernias. In: Skandalakis JE, Colburn GL, Weidman TA, et al. (eds.), *Skandalakis' Surgical Anatomy*. New York, NY: McGraw-Hill; 2004:Chapter 9.

11. **(D)** Retroperitoneal fibrosis is a class of disorders characterized by hyperproliferation of fibrous tissue in the retroperitoneum. When idiopathic in etiology, it is referred to as Ormond disease. It can also occur as a secondary reaction to inflammatory processes, malignancy, or various medications including methysergide, ergotamine, hydralazine, methyldopa, and β-blocking agents.

The key characteristic of retroperitoneal fibrosis is its effect on the ureters, which pass through it. Entrapment of the ureters by fibrotic tissue leads to constriction and eventual obstructive uropathy. Intravenous pyelogram (IVP) usually provides an accurate diagnosis, with characteristic signs of medial displacement, hydronephrosis/hydroureter proximal to the lesion, and a long segment of affected ureter. The strictures are bilateral and symmetrical in 67% of cases.

Mild cases with low-grade obstruction can be treated initially with steroids and cessation of any causative medications. High-grade or severe cases of obstruction will require surgical management and nephrostomy if indicated. Surgical management involves liberation of the ureters from the retroperitoneum. Concomitant intraperitoneal transposition of the ureters may be required, and encasement with omentum may also be necessary. Renal autotransplantation should also be considered.

BIBLIOGRAPHY

Seymour NE, Bell RL. Abdominal wall, omentum, mesentery, and retroperitoneum. In: Brunicardi F, Andersen DK, Billiar TR, et al. (eds.), *Schwartz's Principles of Surgery*, 9th ed. New York, NY: McGraw-Hill; 2010:Chapter 35.

12. **(A)** Retroperitoneal tumors are challenging both in diagnosis and in treatment. The majority of retroperitoneal tumors are malignant and discovered well after they have involved contiguous structures and organs. They are a rare phenomenon with an incidence of 0.3–3% and are classified as either mesodermal or neural in origin. Diagnosis and determination of resectability are based on a combination of CT, MRI, and angiography. Differential diagnosis includes primary germ cell tumor, lymphoma, and metastatic testicular cancer. Evaluation of retroperitoneal soft tissue sarcomas has shown that the approximately 50% are greater than 20 cm in size (60%) and have a high-grade histology (64%) at presentation. Most common presenting symptoms include a palpable abdominal mass, lower extremity neurologic symptoms, and pain.

Complete surgical resection of primary disease is the most effective treatment and provides a median survival time of 103 months, whereas incomplete or no resection provides a median survival of 18 months. Analysis of median survival times has shown that incomplete resection does not provide a significant increase in survival compared with chemotherapy (doxorubicin based) and/or radiation therapy for unresectable tumors. However, partial resection has been shown to provide some symptomatic relief and thus should be reserved for cases in which partial resection may provide palliation. Overall, high-grade histology, unresectability, and positive gross margin are the strongest factors negatively influencing survival for these tumors.

BIBLIOGRAPHY

Cormier JN, Pollock RE. Soft tissue sarcomas. In: Brunicardi F, Andersen DK, Billiar TR, et al. (eds.), *Schwartz's Principles of Surgery*, 9th ed. New York, NY: McGraw-Hill; 2010:Chapter 36.

13. **(B)** The retroperitoneum is roughly divided into three major anatomic zones (see Fig. 27-6). Zone 1 is the midline retroperitoneum and contains the suprarenal

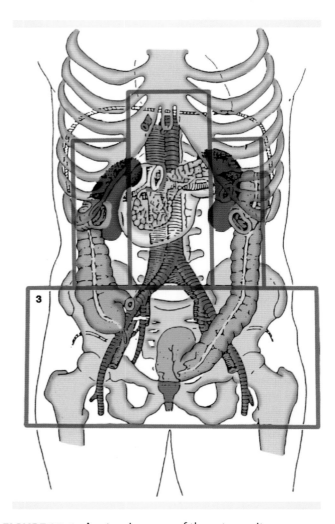

FIGURE 27-6. Anatomic zones of the retroperitoneum. From Skandalakis JE, Colborn GL, Weidman TA, et al. Retroperitoneum. In: Skandalakis JE, Colburn GL, Weidman TA, et al. (eds.), *Skandalakis' Surgical Anatomy*. New York, NY: McGraw-Hill; 2004:Chapter 11, Fig. 11-9.

abdominal aorta, IVC, superior mesenteric, and proximal renal arteries. A hematoma in this area should warrant exploration for both blunt and penetrating trauma, because the likelihood of major vessel injury is high.

Zone 2 of the retroperitoneum is comprised of the paired perinephric spaces containing the kidneys and renal vessels. Stable hematomas in zone 2 after blunt trauma can be observed, but expansion or instability warrants exploration.

Zone 3 is the pelvic retroperitoneum and contains the iliac vessels and the ureters. Blunt trauma resulting in nonexpanding stable hematomas is often secondary to pelvic fracture or bleeding, which is most likely best controlled by angiographic embolization, and thus should not be explored. Blunt expanding hematomas and all penetrating trauma-related hematomas in this area should be explored given the likelihood of iliac vessel injury.

BIBLIOGRAPHY

Dente CJ, Feliciano DV. Abdominal vascular injury. In: Mattox KL, Moore EE, Feliciano DV (eds.), *Trauma*, 7th ed. New York, NY: McGraw-Hill; 2013:Chapter 34.

Skandalakis JE, Colborn GL, Weidman TA, et al. Retroperitoneum. In: Skandalakis JE, Colburn GL, Weidman TA, et al. (eds.), *Skandalakis' Surgical Anatomy*. New York, NY: McGraw-Hill; 2004:Chapter 11.

14. **(A)** Rectus sheath hematomas are most commonly caused by bleeding from the inferior epigastric vessels rather than the rectus muscle. Trauma is the primary cause, and patients are frequently on anticoagulation therapy. Other causes include collagen vascular diseases and infectious diseases like typhoid fever.

Diagnosis can be made by palpation of a tender mass over the rectus abdominis muscle, with assistance from abdominal CT scanning or ultrasonography (see Fig. 27-7). Management is most often nonoperative, although continued expansion of the hematoma may warrant operative therapy. This should usually involve simple evacuation, control of hemorrhage, and closure without drainage. Operative therapy is also indicated if more serious intra-abdominal conditions cannot be excluded in the process of diagnosis.

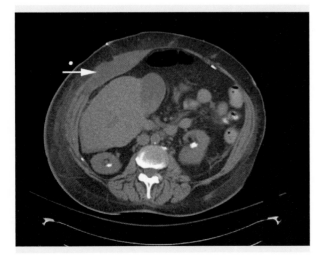

FIGURE 27-7. Rectus sheath hematoma. From Seymour NE, Bell RL. Abdominal wall, omentum, mesentery, and retroperitoneum. In: Brunicardi F, Andersen DK, Billiar TR, et al. (eds.), *Schwartz's Principles of Surgery*, 9th ed. New York, NY: McGraw-Hill; 2010:Chapter 35, Fig. 35-9.

BIBLIOGRAPHY

Seymour NE, Bell RL. Abdominal wall, omentum, mesentery, and retroperitoneum. In: Brunicardi F, Andersen DK, Billiar TR, et al. (eds.), *Schwartz's Principles of Surgery*, 9th ed. New York, NY: McGraw-Hill; 2010:Chapter 35.

15. **(A)**

16. **(B)**

17. **(D)**

Explanation for questions 15–17

The peritoneum is a semipermeable membrane that lines the peritoneal cavity and reflects onto the abdominal organs. Its relationship to intraperitoneal structures defines discrete compartments within which abscesses may form. The area is comparable to that of the cutaneous body surface and participates in fluid exchange with the extracellular fluid space at rates of 500 mL or more per hour. The peritoneal cavity is normally sterile with less than 50 mL of free peritoneal fluid, a transudate with the following characteristics: specific gravity below 1.016, protein concentration less than 3 g/dL, white blood cell count less than 3000/μL, complement-mediated antibacterial activity, and lack of fibrinogen-related clot formation.

The circulation of peritoneal fluid is directed toward lymphatics in the undersurface of the diaphragm. There, particulate matter—including bacteria up to 20 μm in size—is cleared via stomas in the diaphragmatic mesothelium and lymphatics and discharged mainly into the right thoracic duct.

The peritoneum is a mesodermally derived structure and serves many important functions. It provides a frictionless surface inside which intra-abdominal organs can be contained. It also can secrete lubricating fluid from its mesothelial lining to assist in free movement of viscera. Given its structure, it also has bidirectional transport capabilities for water and solutes. This is driven largely in part by osmolar gradients; however, experimentally isotonic saline has been shown to be absorbed at a rate of 25–30 mL/h. Overall, there is approximately 100 mL of fluid that is normally present in the peritoneal cavity. This transport property of the peritoneum is the basis for peritoneal dialysis.

Air and gases can also be absorbed by the peritoneum. Normally, intraperitoneal air left after laparotomy is almost completely absorbed by 4–5 days. Of note, intraperitoneal blood can also be reabsorbed. Fenestrated lymphatic channels underlying the diaphragms serve to reabsorb red blood cells, to an extent that 70% of intraperitoneal red blood cells are resorbed intact and with a normal circulatory survival time. The peritoneum has the capability of bidirectional transport, thus making it a medium via which dialysis can be performed. Water, electrolytes, and various drugs can thus be removed with peritoneal dialysis. Most antibiotics do not require adjustment of dosing with peritoneal dialysis; this includes vancomycin. Antibiotics such as aztreonam, amikacin, cefaclor, ceftazidime, fluconazole, gentamicin, isoniazid, and kanamycin do require dosage adjustments.

Peritonitis is an inflammatory or suppurative response of the peritoneal lining to direct irritation. Primary peritonitis is defined as the inflammation of the parietal peritoneum without an evident source of infection. It is a condition that occurs more frequently in children and females. Incidence in the pediatric population shows a bimodal distribution in the neonatal period and again at 4–5 years of age. Increased female incidence is thought to be the result of entry of organisms into the peritoneal cavity via the fallopian tubes. This condition is also associated with nephrotic syndrome and SLE in children; in adults, patients with liver disease have been shown to have an increased incidence of primary peritonitis. Also, previous upper respiratory tract infection or ear infection is not uncommonly found on taking the patient's history. Patients with this condition often present with fever, leukocytosis, and abdominal pain, which may be severe. Diagnosis can be made by paracentesis, culture, and exclusion of other sources of infection such as pneumonia or urinary tract infection. Organisms usually found with nephrotic syndrome or SLE are hemolytic streptococci or pneumococci. Liver disease is more often associated with gram-negative rather than gram-positive organisms. Distinction between primary and secondary peritonitis may be difficult to establish and sometimes may only be made after laparotomy or extensive investigation. Secondary peritonitis results from bacterial contamination originating from within viscera or from external sources.

Factors that influence the severity of peritonitis include the type of bacterial or fungal contamination, the nature and duration of the injury, and the host's nutritional and immune status. Clean (e.g., proximal gut perforations) or well-localized (e.g., ruptured appendix) contaminations progress to fulminant peritonitis relatively slowly (e.g., 12–24 hours), whereas bacteria associated with distal gut or infected biliary tract perforations quickly overwhelm host peritoneal defenses. This degree of toxicity is also characteristic of postoperative peritonitis due to anastomotic leakage or contamination. Conditions that ordinarily cause mild peritonitis may produce life-threatening sepsis in an immunocompromised host.

Choleperitoneum is often the result of trauma or iatrogenic biliary tract injury or postoperative leak; however, spontaneous rupture of the bile duct can be seen in both adults and infants and is the second most common cause of surgical jaundice in infancy. Bile produces an inflammatory response from the peritoneum due to its irritating properties. The increase of peritoneal fluid in response to bile is seen as biliary ascites. Infection of intraperitoneal bile requires urgent surgical intervention.

Chyloperitoneum, or chylous ascites, is the accumulation of free chyle, or lymph fluid, in the peritoneal cavity. The common causes of chylous ascites are from trauma, tumor involving lymphatic structures, spontaneous bacterial peritonitis, cirrhosis, abdominal surgery, tuberculosis, congenital defects, and peritoneal dialysis. Patients typically present with abdominal distention and pain along with vague constitutional symptoms. Milky ascitic fluid with high triglyceride count on paracentesis suggests the correct diagnosis.

Hemoperitoneum is most often caused by hepatic or splenic trauma, although ruptured aortic aneurysm and ectopic pregnancy are also common causes. Via the peritoneum, more than two-thirds of intraperitoneal red blood cells can be reabsorbed intact into the bloodstream. However, efforts to evacuate as much blood as possible from the abdomen should be made during surgery, because hemoglobin has been shown to interfere with clearance of intraperitoneal bacteria and thus impair the immune response to peritonitis.

BIBLIOGRAPHY

Doherty GM. Peritoneal cavity. In: Doherty GM (eds.), *Current Diagnosis & Treatment: Surgery*, 13th ed. New York, NY: McGraw-Hill; 2010:Chapter 22.

18. **(E)** The mesentery develops with the embryonic gut. After the fifth week of development, the gut extends into the umbilical cord. The SMA provides the axis around which the duodenum rotates 270 degrees counterclockwise on its reentry into the abdominal cavity. The right colon also does the same, giving the normal anatomic positioning of the intestines. After the 12th week, the mesentery of the rotated gut begins to adhere to the posterior abdominal wall, although this may not be completed until birth. The root of the mesentery is formed with this fixation, spanning the transverse mesocolon in the left upper abdomen to the ileocecal junction in the right lower quadrant, thereby eliminating the risk of volvulus.

Mesenteric cysts are congenital lymphatic spaces, are most often filled with lymphatic fluid, and enlarge in size over time. They have been classified by their etiologies, which include embryonic/congenital, traumatic/acquired, neoplastic, and infective/degenerative cysts. They are often present as symptomatic abdominal masses, with pain, nausea, and/or vomiting, and can often be palpated on physical examination. Lateral mobility is a characteristic finding on palpation. Treatment consists of surgical resection, although they may often require partial bowel resection due to their proximity to the vascular supply of the bowel.

BIBLIOGRAPHY

Seymour NE, Bell RL. Abdominal wall, omentum, mesentery, and retroperitoneum. In: Brunicardi F, Andersen DK, Billiar TR, et al. (eds.), *Schwartz's Principles of Surgery*, 9th ed. New York, NY: McGraw-Hill; 2010:Chapter 35.

19. **(D)** Femoral hernias make up only 5–10% of all hernias but are the second most common abdominal wall hernia. Femoral hernia is more common in females than in males, by a ratio of approximately 4:1, and have a high rate of incarceration and strangulation. The defect through which a femoral hernia occurs is in the medial femoral canal. The anterior boundary of this defect is the inguinal ligament, the lateral boundary the femoral vein, the posterior boundary the pubic ramus and Cooper's ligament, and the medial boundary the lacunar portion of the inguinal ligament (see Fig. 27-8). Treatment for femoral hernia is operative repair, and there is little to no role for conservative management.

    The repair is best approached via a transverse incision just below the inguinal ligament. The hernia sac can be found anterior to the inguinal ligament. Repair of the defect can be performed using a Cooper's ligament repair as described earlier, by affixing the transversalis fascia to the Cooper's ligament medially and the iliopubic tract laterally up to the internal ring. Alternatively, a simple suture repair can be performed by tacking the inguinal ligament

anteriorly to Cooper's ligament posteromedially to close the defect. A third option is a purse-string suture placed first anteriorly into the inguinal ligament, then through the lacunar ligament medially, the pectineal ligament posteriorly, and finally through the fascia medial to the femoral vein and back to the inguinal ligament. A unique complication from suture repair of the femoral hernia defect is bleeding from an aberrant obturator artery, which originates from the inferior epigastric artery and traverses a space medial to the femoral hernia defect adjacent to the pubic ramus. The medial suture placed in femoral hernia repair can injure an aberrant obturator artery if present.

BIBLIOGRAPHY

Javid PJ, Greenberg JA, Brooks DC. Hernias. In: Zinner MJ, Ashley SW (eds.), *Maingot's Abdominal Operations*, 12th ed. New York, NY: McGraw-Hill; 2013:Chapter 7.

20. **(A)** Testicular swelling and atrophy seen after inguinal hernia repair is referred to as ischemic orchitis. This is most commonly caused by injury to the pampiniform plexus, but also may be secondary to injury to the blood supply to the genitals during dissection and isolation of the cord. Ischemic orchitis usually presents within the first week following inguinal hernia repair. The patient may present with a low-grade fever, but more commonly presents with an enlarged, indurated, and painful testicle. This complication occurs in <1% of all herniorrhaphies but increases in the reoperations for recurrent inguinal hernias. A testicle that is tender on examination may require ultrasonographic imaging to rule out testicular torsion or a corresponding abscess.

BIBLIOGRAPHY

Javid PJ, Greenberg JA, Brooks DC. Hernias. In: Zinner MJ, Ashley SW (eds.), *Maingot's Abdominal Operations*, 12th ed. New York, NY: McGraw-Hill; 2013:Chapter 7.
Sherman V, Macho JR, Brunicardi F. Inguinal hernias. In: Brunicardi F, Andersen DK, Billiar TR, et al. (eds.), *Schwartz's Principles of Surgery*, 9th ed. New York, NY: McGraw-Hill; 2010:Chapter 37.

21. **(D)**

22. **(C)**

23. **(E)**

24. **(E)**

Explanation for questions 21–24

The abdominal CT scan reveals evidence of a spigelian hernia on the left. A variety of ventral hernias occur along the lateral edge of the rectus abdominis, medial to the semilunar line. Most often they occur inferior to the

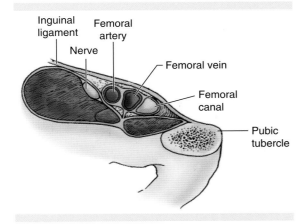

FIGURE 27-8. Anatomy of femoral hernia. From Javid PJ, Greenberg JA, Brooks DC. Hernias. In: Zinner MJ, Ashley SW (eds.), *Maingot's Abdominal Operations*, 12th ed. New York, NY: McGraw-Hill; 2013:Chapter 7, Fig. 7-6.

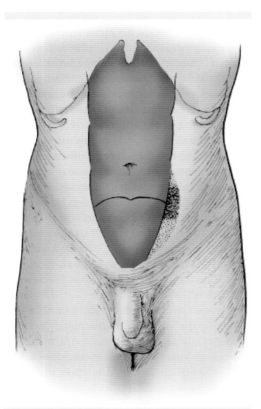

FIGURE 27-9. Anatomy of spigelian hernia. From Javid PJ, Greenberg JA, Brooks DC. Hernias. In: Zinner MJ, Ashley SW (eds.), *Maingot's Abdominal Operations*, 12th ed. New York, NY: McGraw-Hill; 2013:Chapter 7, Fig. 7-13.

junction of the semilunar line of the rectus abdominis and the semicircular line of Douglas (arcuate line) (see Fig. 27-9). This is consistent with the lack of posterior fascia below the arcuate line. They may occur at any level of the abdominal wall and may also dissect between the internal and external oblique muscle layers.

Presenting symptoms are similar to those of standard ventral hernias and most often include pain, palpable abdominal wall mass, and bowel obstruction. Entrapment of the anterior cutaneous nerves of T10–T12 can provide a similar distribution of pain. Preoperative diagnosis is usually possible in 50–75% of cases. Diagnosis is most often obtained by abdominopelvic CT scan; however, abdominal ultrasound can also provide the diagnosis. Sensitivity is increased with simultaneous Valsalva maneuver during diagnostic testing.

Open surgical repair has been the traditional method of treatment for spigelian hernias. Hernia contents have been found most often to be nothing, small bowel, omentum, cecum, and sigmoid colon, in order of decreasing frequency. The vast majority is amenable

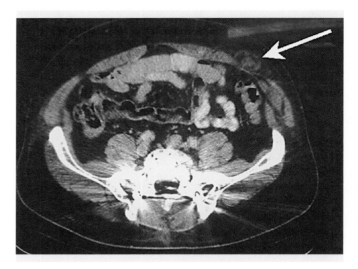

FIGURE 27-10. Abdominopelvic computed tomography scan showing a left-sided spigelian hernia. Note its position just lateral to the rectus abdominis. The hernia was found to contain fat and was closed primarily.

to primary repair, but large hernias may require mesh placement. An extraperitoneal laparoscopic repair has been shown to provide improved results for length of stay and morbidity and remains a viable option for elective repairs in the hands of the experienced surgeon. In a study of 76 patients, only 3 patients had recurrent hernias in an 8-year follow-up period (see Fig. 27-10).

BIBLIOGRAPHY

Javid PJ, Greenberg JA, Brooks DC. Hernias. In: Zinner MJ, Ashley SW (eds.), *Maingot's Abdominal Operations*, 12th ed. New York, NY: McGraw-Hill; 2013:Chapter 7.

25. **(C)**

26. **(C)**

27. **(E)**

28. **(A)**

Explanation for questions 25–28

Abdominal compartment syndrome (ACS) is used to describe the constellation of pulmonary, renal, and cardiac sequelae that results from increased abdominal pressure. Its etiology is multifactorial and has been shown to be associated with many clinical syndromes, including hemorrhage, dilatation of bowel, acute ascites, mesenteric venous thrombosis, pelvic/retroperitoneal hematoma, necrotizing pancreatitis, and massive fluid resuscitation. It is important to note that although ACS is related to mostly intra-abdominal processes, massive resuscitation alone from extremity or thoracic trauma, hypothermia, and sepsis may also be etiologic factors.

Conditions that increase abdominal wall compliance (e.g., prior pregnancy, obesity, and cirrhosis) appear to be protective, whereas inflexible surgical closures or scars increase risk. ACS most commonly occurs within 24–48 hours after injury, during the resuscitation period. The increased pressure is thought to produce several main effects: compression of both the kidneys and retroperitoneum and elevation of the diaphragms. Direct compression of the retroperitoneum causes decreased venous return via the IVC, which in turn will result in decreased preload, leading to decreased cardiac output and stroke volume, with a resultant increase in systemic vascular resistance. The increased intrathoracic pressure also contributes to this. Elevation of the diaphragms results in increased intrathoracic pressure, which in turn causes increased peak airway pressures and decreased lung compliance, leading eventually to hypoxemia. Compression of the kidneys results in increased renovascular resistance, leading to decreased renal blood flow. This, in combination with a mild relative venous outflow obstruction, leads to oliguria. There is no significant compressive effect on the ureters. Interestingly enough, there also appears to be an association between ACS and increased intracranial pressure. A number of surgical and nonsurgical conditions have been associated with intra-abdominal hypertension. Particularly at risk is the trauma patient requiring large-volume resuscitation and emergent abdominal surgery. Use of temporary closure techniques as an alternative to tight surgical closure increases abdominal wall compliance and minimizes intra-abdominal pressure in patients at risk.

Signs of ACS are abdominal distention, decreased cardiac output, oliguria, and elevated peak airway pressures. Diagnosis is made via measurement of intra-abdominal pressure via a Foley catheter. The bladder should be filled with approximately 50 mL of sterile saline with the drainage port clamped. Because the bladder acts as a passive reservoir due to its low muscular tone, intra-abdominal pressure can be measured with a manometer or by connecting a pressure transducer to the infusion port of the Foley catheter. The severity of ACS is based on a grading system: grade 1 (10–15 mmHg), grade 2 (16–25 mmHg), grade 3 (26–35 mmHg), and grade 4 (>35 mmHg) (see Fig. 27-11).

BIBLIOGRAPHY

Corbridge T, Wood LH. Restrictive disease of the respiratory system and the abdominal compartment syndrome. In: Hall JB, Schmidt GA, Wood LH (eds.), *Principles of Critical Care*, 3rd ed. New York, NY: McGraw-Hill; 2005:Chapter 42.

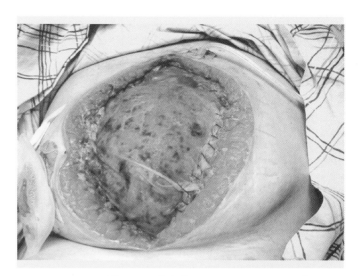

FIGURE 27-11. Closure of abdomen in a patient with abdominal compartment syndrome due to severe pancreatitis.

29. **(E)**

30. **(E)**

31. **(B)**

32. **(B)**

Explanation for questions 29 through 33

The standard treatment of acute pancreatitis is nonoperative; however, operative intervention may be warranted for several reasons: (1) uncertainty of diagnosis, (2) correction of associated biliary tract disease, (3) progressive clinical deterioration given maximum supportive care, and (4) treatment of secondary pancreatic infections.

The advent of abdominopelvic CT scanning has facilitated the nonoperative diagnosis of acute pancreatitis; however, given the situation, other surgical conditions cannot be excluded (perforated viscus or mesenteric ischemia, for instance), and laparotomy may be warranted to elucidate the patient's condition. In exploration of the lesser sac, the pancreas can be evaluated for evidence of pancreatitis or necrosis. Should noncomplicated acute pancreatitis exist, no further surgical intervention is warranted. If concomitant biliary disease is suspected, cholecystectomy and/or intraoperative cholangiography may be needed. Also, if noninfected necrotizing pancreatitis is found, then gentle debridement of the necrotic tissue with wide sump drainage should be performed. Note that formal pancreatic resection is rarely warranted. Regardless, thoughts to placement of gastrostomy and/or jejunostomy tubes should be considered at the time of laparotomy, because studies have proven that postpyloric (jejunal or nasoduodenal) enteral feeding is superior to total parenteral nutrition (TPN), given the higher incidence of pneumonia and infectious complications with TPN.

Secondary pancreatic infections are classified as pancreatic abscess, infected pancreatic pseudocyst, and infected pancreatic necrosis; overall, only 5% of patients with acute pancreatitis will develop an infectious pancreatic complication. Severity of pancreatitis is directly related to the incidence of infection. Patients with six or more Ranson's criteria have greater than 50% chance of developing pancreatic sepsis. The etiology is thought to derive from either hematogenous seeding or translocation of bacteria via adjacent bowel. Gram-negative organisms are most common, with fungal infections becoming more frequently identified. Imipenem has been shown to have the best parenchymal penetration of the pancreas and is commonly thought to be the first-line antibiotic of choice for prophylaxis.

Pancreatic sepsis should be considered in patients with known bacteremia, clinical deterioration after 7 days, or pancreatitis that does not resolve after 7–10 days. Patients frequently present with symptoms of fever, tachycardia, abdominal pain, and distention. Radiographic findings usually begin with peripancreatic and/or retroperitoneal fluid collections, which often on CT scan are shown to dissect behind the right and left colon. The finding of gas (the so-called "soap bubble sign") within these collections is pathognomonic. Overall, CT scan is considered the gold standard of radiographic analysis, because the sensitivity is greater than 90% when more than 30% of the pancreatic parenchyma is involved. Laboratory abnormalities almost always show leukocytosis with concomitant elevations of liver function tests and serum amylase. Guided percutaneous needle aspiration may be warranted. Although it can demonstrate the presence of bacteria from within a peripancreatic fluid collection, some clinicians are concerned with the likelihood of seeding a previously sterile peripancreatic fluid collection with a percutaneous procedure and often refrain from these invasive techniques to diagnose pancreatic infection.

Once the diagnosis is made, the treatment is primarily operative. Sometimes with well-defined pancreatic abscesses or infected pseudocysts, percutaneous drainage may be sufficient to adequately drain the lesion. There have also been efforts to endoscopically drain infected pancreatic necrosis. Often, however, there is a complex and loculated collection that is not amenable to these techniques alone. Open pancreatic debridement should be performed with several goals in mind: (1) debridement should be gentle, avoiding vigorous debridement of the retroperitoneum, which could cause injury of retroperitoneal vascular structures resulting in life-threatening hemorrhage; (2) formal resection of the pancreas should be avoided; (3) wide sump drainage of the retroperitoneum

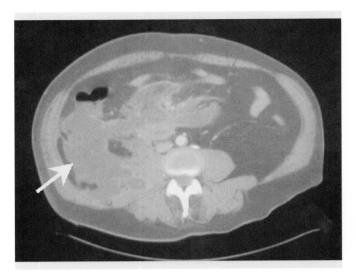

FIGURE 27-12. Abdominopelvic computed tomography scan showing a large peripancreatic fluid collection dissecting into the retroperitoneum behind the right colon. Note the absence of gas within this fluid collection.

via large-bore drains placed in dependent positions or open packing of the peripancreatic space should be performed; and (4) given the presence of associated biliary tract disease, cholecystectomy with or without intraoperative cholangiogram should be performed.

Overall, 16–40% of patients requiring operative intervention will require reoperation for continued sepsis, and the mortality rate has been reported to be between 5 and 50%, with an average of 30% (see Fig. 27-12).

BIBLIOGRAPHY

Blackbourne LH (ed.). *Surgical Recall*, 3rd ed. Philadelphia, PA: Lippincott, Williams & Wilkins; 2002.

Fink D, Alverdy JC. In: Cameron JL (ed.), *Current Surgical Therapy*, 7th ed. St. Louis, MO: Mosby; 2001.

Humar A, Dunn DL. Transplantation. In: Brunicardi F, Andersen DK, Billiar TR, et al. (eds.), *Schwartz's Principles of Surgery*, 9th ed. New York, NY: McGraw-Hill; 2010:Chapter 11.

Lewis JJ. Retroperitoneal soft-tissue sarcoma: analysis of 500 patients treated and followed at a single institution. *Ann Surg* 1998;228(3):355–365.

Moreno-Egea A, Flores B, Girela E, Martin JG, Aguayo JL, Canteras M. Spigelian hernia: bibliographical study and presentation of a series of 28 patients. *Hernia* 2002;6(4):167–170.

Steer ML. Exocrine pancreas. In: Sabiston DC Jr (ed.), *Sabiston Textbook of Surgery*, 16th ed. Philadelphia, PA: W.B. Saunders; 2001.

33. **(B)** The obturator foramen is formed by the ischial and pubic rami (see Fig. 27-13). The obturator membrane covers the majority of the foramen space, except for

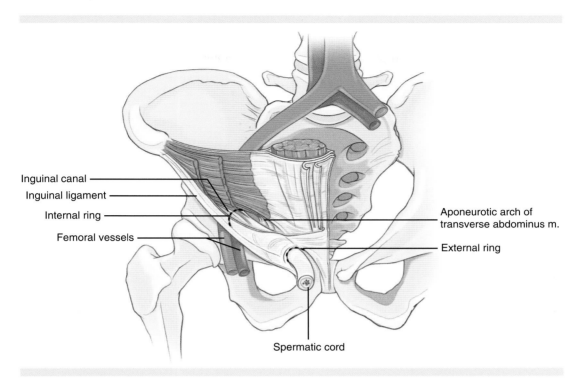

Inguinal canal
Inguinal ligament
Internal ring
Femoral vessels

Aponeurotic arch of
transverse abdominus m.

External ring

Spermatic cord

FIGURE 27-13. Diagrammatic representation of the inguinal canal. From Sherman V, Macho JR, Brunicardi F. Inguinal hernias. In: Brunicardi F, Andersen DK, Billiar TR, et al. (eds.), *Schwartz's Principles of Surgery*, 9th ed. New York, NY: McGraw-Hill; 2010:Chapter 37, Fig. 37-2.

a small portion through which the obturator vessels and nerve pass. The boundaries of the obturator canal are the obturator groove on the superior pubic ramus superiorly and the upper edge of the obturator membrane inferiorly. The hernia lies deep to the pectineus muscle and therefore is difficult to palpate on examination. Small bowel is the most likely intra-abdominal organ to be found in an obturator hernia, although rare cases have been reported of the appendix, Meckel diverticulum, omentum, bladder, and ovary incarcerated in the hernia.

Clinically, obturator hernia is associated with four cardinal findings:

1. Intestinal obstruction (80%)

2. Howship–Romberg sign: pain along the medial surface of the thigh that may radiate to the knee and hip joints (50%)

3. Intermittent bowel obstruction (30%)

4. A palpable mass in the proximal medial aspect of the thigh at the origin of the adductor muscles, best palpated with the thigh flexed, abducted, and rotated outward (20%)

In rare cases, ecchymoses may be noted in the upper medial thigh due to effusion from the strangulated hernia contents. The obturator hernia mass may also be palpated laterally on a vaginal examination.

BIBLIOGRAPHY

Javid PJ, Greenberg JA, Brooks DC. Hernias. In: Zinner MJ, Ashley SW (eds.), *Maingot's Abdominal Operations*, 12th ed. New York, NY: McGraw-Hill; 2013:Chapter 7.

34. **(D)**

- *Anterior:* The anterior boundary is the aponeurosis of the external oblique muscle and, more laterally, the internal oblique muscle. Remember, there are no external oblique muscle fibers in the inguinal area, only aponeurotic fibers.
- *Posterior:* In about three-fourths of patients, the posterior wall (floor) is formed laterally by the aponeurosis of the transversus abdominis muscle and the transversalis fascia; in the remainder, the posterior wall is transversalis fascia only. Medially, the posterior wall is reinforced by the internal oblique aponeurosis.

- *Superior:* The roof of the canal is formed by the arched fibers of the lower edge (roof) of the internal oblique muscle and by the transversus abdominis muscle and aponeurosis.
- *Inferior:* The wall of the canal is formed by the inguinal ligament (Poupart's) and the lacunar ligament (Gimbernat's) (see Fig. 27-13).

BIBLIOGRAPHY

Skandalakis PN, Skandalakis JE, Colborn GL, Kingsnorth AN, Weidman TA, Skandalakis LJ. Abdominal wall and hernias. In: Skandalakis JE, Colburn GL, Weidman TA, et al. (eds.), *Skandalakis' Surgical Anatomy*. New York, NY: McGraw-Hill; 2004:Chapter 9.

CHAPTER 28

COLON AND ANORECTAL DISEASE

CARLOS A. SAN MATEO AND JORGE MARCET

1. Which of the following statements regarding diverticular disease of the colon is true?
   (A) According to the Law of LaPlace, the intraluminal pressure is directly proportional to the radius of the lumen.
   (B) True diverticula involve all layers of the colon wall and are most commonly found in the cecum.
   (C) The lifetime recurrence rate of diverticulitis after the first attack managed conservatively is 80%.
   (D) Less than 1% of persons with diverticula develop diverticula-associated bleeding.
   (E) In a patient undergoing sigmoid colon resection for apparent isolated sigmoid diverticulitis, the recurrence rate for diverticulitis is 5%.

2. According to the Hinchey classification for diverticular disease of the colon, which of the following statements is correct?
   (A) Antibiotics are not indicated for stage I disease.
   (B) Antibiotics only are indicated for pericolic abscesses >4 cm.
   (C) All stages except stage I involve colonic wall perforation.
   (D) Hartmann's procedure is mandated for Hinchey stage II disease.
   (E) Sigmoid colectomy with primary anastomosis is the preferred elective procedure.

3. Which of the following statements regarding colonic physiology is true?
   (A) The colon is a major site for water absorption and electrolyte exchange due to extensive surface villi.
   (B) Following abdominal surgery, the colon is the first segment of the gastrointestinal tract to regain motility.
   (C) The primary fuel source for colonocytes is glutamine.
   (D) Colonic motility consists of intermittent contractions of either low or high amplitude.
   (E) The colon is the site of greatest water absorption in the gastrointestinal (GI) tract.

4. Which of the following regarding inflammatory bowel disease is true?
   (A) Distinguishing between Crohn disease and ulcerative colitis is impossible in approximately 15% of cases.
   (B) Bloody diarrhea is more common in Crohn disease than ulcerative colitis.
   (C) Crohn disease rarely spares the rectum.
   (D) Patients with ulcerative colitis are frequently anti–*Saccharomyces cerevisiae* antibody (ASCA) positive.
   (E) Perineal disease is more common in ulcerative colitis than Crohn disease.

5. Which of the following is *not* an indication for surgical intervention in ulcerative colitis?
   (A) Intractable bloody diarrhea
   (B) Perforation
   (C) Toxic colitis
   (D) Diagnosis of ulcerative colitis for more than 5 years
   (E) Poorly controlled extraintestinal manifestations

6. Regarding acute colonic pseudo-obstruction (Ogilvie syndrome), which of the following statements is *not* correct?
   (A) This condition is characterized by the radiographic appearance of a large bowel obstruction without mechanical etiology.
   (B) Cholinesterase inhibitors lead to symptom resolution in a majority of patients.
   (C) Ogilvie syndrome is associated with a number of neurologic disorders, including Alzheimer and Parkinson disease and elderly dementia.
   (D) Most cases of this disease are idiopathic in etiology.
   (E) The proximal and transverse portions of the colon tend to be more involved than the left or sigmoid colon.

7. Which of the following statements regarding *Clostridium difficile* is *not* true?
   (A) Ten percent of hospitalized patients have gut colonization with *C difficile*.
   (B) *C difficile* may colonize the upper and lower GI tract, but symptomatic infection appears to be isolated only to the colon.
   (C) Pseudomembranous colitis is caused by transmural translocation of *C difficile* bacteria with irritation of the muscularis propria.
   (D) The first treatment option for pseudomembranous colitis should be oral metronidazole.
   (E) Oral cholestyramine can be useful in controlling the effects of *C difficile* by intraluminal binding of clostridial toxin.

8. Which of the following is true regarding colonic volvulus?
   (A) It likely results from redundant sigmoid colon with a shortened mesocolon.
   (B) Fifty percent of colonic volvulus cases in the United States involve the sigmoid colon.
   (C) There appears to be a congenital predisposition to sigmoid volvulus.
   (D) Diagnostic x-ray for sigmoid volvulus shows a dilated loop of colon, which points toward the right upper quadrant.
   (E) Cecopexy is the preferred surgical intervention for cecal volvulus

9. Which of the following statements is *not* true regarding lower gastrointestinal hemorrhage (LGIH)?
   (A) The most common cause of a lower GI bleed in adults younger than age 60 is colonic diverticula.
   (B) The most common cause of a lower GI bleed in adults older than age 60 is colonic diverticula.
   (C) Lower GI bleeding because of arteriovenous malformations is much more common in older rather than younger persons.
   (D) The most common cause of LGIH in a child is inflammatory bowel disease.
   (E) Massive LGIH is generally defined as an acute requirement for more than 6 units of blood.

10. Which of the following statements regarding large bowel obstruction is *not* true?
    (A) The most common cause of colonic obstruction in adults is diverticulitis.
    (B) The ileocecal valve is incompetent in 10–20% of people.
    (C) Approximately 15% of intestinal obstructions occur in the large bowel.
    (D) The most common site of large bowel obstruction is the sigmoid colon.
    (E) Cecal perforation carries a 40% mortality rate.

11. According to the Haggitt classification for polyps, which of the following statements is *not* true?
    (A) A level 0 polyp refers to noninvasive carcinoma *in situ*.
    (B) All level IV polyps must be treated with segmental resection.
    (C) Endoscopic excision is adequate treatment for level I and level II polyps.
    (D) A wide-based sessile polyp with carcinoma at the tip of the polyp *only* is considered a level III polyp.
    (E) Carcinoma from a level I polyp invades the muscularis mucosa but remains contained within the head of the polyp.

12. Which of the following is a genetic mutation linked to colorectal cancer?
    (A) Activation of adenomatous polyposis coli (*APC*)
    (B) CAG triplicate repeat sequence
    (C) Inactivation of *K-ras*
    (D) Activation of *DCC/p53*
    (E) Inactivation of *hMLH1/hMSH2*

13. According to the tumor, node, metastasis (TNM) staging for colon cancer, which of the following is true?
    (A) All perforated colon cancers are considered T4.
    (B) N2 refers to involvement of greater than one regional lymph node.
    (C) T5 grade involves direct carcinoma invasion into adjacent solid organs.
    (D) MX indicates metastatic disease involvement of more than one additional organ system (e.g., liver, lung, brain).
    (E) Five-year survival for stage I colon cancer is approximately 75%.

14. Which of the following is associated with familial polyposis syndromes?
    (A) Gardner syndrome
    (B) Turcot syndrome
    (C) Hereditary nonpolyposis colorectal cancer (HNPCC)
    (D) Peutz-Jeghers syndrome
    (E) Juvenile polyposis syndrome

15. Which of the following statements is *not* true regarding familial adenomatous polyposis (FAP) syndrome?
    (A) All patients will eventually develop colon cancer.
    (B) Polyps >1 cm in these patients carry a 50% risk of carcinoma.
    (C) Ninety percent of these patients manifest polyps by age 10.
    (D) Medical treatment with sulindac/celecoxib decreases the number and size of polyps.
    (E) Sulindac and tamoxifen have been shown to be effective in the treatment of desmoid tumors.

16. Which of the following is true regarding the surgical management of colon cancer?
    (A) Colon carcinoma spreads primarily via lymphatics.
    (B) A 10-cm margin is required for adequate resection.
    (C) Perioperative mortality in patients with perforated colon cancer approaches 30%.
    (D) Patients presenting with an obstructing colon cancer have an in-hospital mortality rate of 50%.
    (E) Minimally invasive resections are contraindicated in patients with regional lymphadenopathy.

17. A previously healthy 22-year-old male college football player presents to your emergency department 24 hours after the homecoming football game with complaints of severe left lower quadrant abdominal pain, fever of 101°F, nausea, and vomiting. Laboratory findings include a white blood cell (WBC) count of 16,300 with 7% bands. On physical examination, his abdomen is soft, but he has marked tenderness in the left lower quadrant. Which of the following is the most appropriate next step in the management of this patient?
    (A) Computed tomography (CT) of abdomen and pelvis
    (B) Barium enema and intravenous (IV) antibiotics
    (C) Abdominal ultrasound and IV antibiotics
    (D) Immediate surgical intervention with intraoperative ultrasound
    (E) Diagnostic laparoscopy

18. A 72-year-old woman is hospitalized in the burn unit after sustaining 17% total body surface area (TBSA) flash burns in an explosion of methane fumes from a pile of manure. She undergoes uneventful excision and grafting of her burn wounds but postoperatively develops significant abdominal distension and obstipation. Plain films reveal markedly dilated small bowel and colon, with a cecal diameter of 9 cm. Appropriate management at this time involves
    (A) Urgent surgical intervention with resection and diverting ostomy
    (B) Nasogastric (NG) decompression, limitation of narcotic use, serial abdominal radiographs
    (C) Colonoscopic decompression
    (D) IV neostigmine
    (E) Placement of a rectal tube

19. A 92-year-old man presents to the local Veteran Affairs hospital from the nursing home where he resides and complains of new onset of abdominal distension, constipation, nausea, and vomiting. On physical examination, he has a distended abdomen but no evidence of peritonitis. Abdominal radiograph is obtained (see Fig. 28-1).

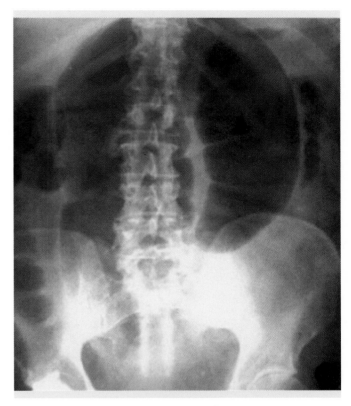

FIGURE 28-1. Abdominal radiograph.

   Regarding this patient's condition, which of the following statements is true?
    (A) A gastrografin enema is required to confirm the diagnosis.
    (B) Colonoscopic decompression is unlikely to be successful and may be dangerous.
    (C) The recurrence rate may be as high as 90%.
    (D) The patient should undergo emergent exploration and resection.

20. Which of the following statements is true regarding ischemic colitis?
    (A) Intestinal ischemia is more common in the small intestine than the large intestine.
    (B) Sigmoidoscopy is the preferred diagnostic tool.
    (C) The hepatic flexure is the most common site of ischemic colitis.
    (D) Plain abdominal radiographs may reveal thumb printing.
    (E) No follow-up care is required following definitive surgical treatment.

21. A 54-year-old man presents with complaints of a severe pain and tearing in his rectal area when he defecates. History elicits an occurrence of these same symptoms with partial resolution two times in the last year. His fiber intake is less than 10 g/d, and he drinks only coffee and cola beverages. Your examination reveals the following (see Fig. 28-2). *Initial* management should include

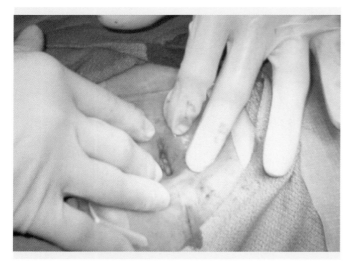

FIGURE 28-2. External anal examination.

   (A) Open or closed lateral internal sphincterotomy
   (B) Anoscopy with dilatation under general anesthesia
   (C) Dietary counseling to include 25–35 g of fiber per day, increasing intake of water, application of topical nitrates/calcium channel blockers, and sitz baths
   (D) Incision and drainage with seton placement
   (E) Fistulotomy and debridement

22. The same patient in Question 21 presents 2 months later with worsening pain and constipation. His physical examination has not significantly changed. The preferred treatment at this time is
   (A) Open or closed lateral internal sphincterotomy
   (B) Anoscopy with dilation under general anesthesia
   (C) Dietary counseling to include 25–35 g of fiber per day, increasing intake of water, application of topical nitrates/calcium channel blockers, and sitz baths
   (D) Incision and drainage with seton placement
   (E) Fistulotomy and debridement

23. A 22-year-old male construction worker is referred to your office complaining of an itching and burning rash around his anus that has worsened since he started putting an over-the-counter hemorrhoid cream on it. The patient is asked to lie on his left side, and examination

reveals a diffuse erythematous rash surrounding the anus. There are no masses, fistula, hemorrhoids, or fissures evident. The patient states that it is getting worse since he has been sweating a lot at work. Appropriate recommendations should include
   (A) Continue treating with over-the-counter hemorrhoidal cream for 6 weeks
   (B) Washing the affected area with warm water, patting dry, and applying a steroid-based cream daily until symptoms are resolved
   (C) Biopsy and preparation for wide local excision
   (D) Incision and drainage with wet to dry dressing changes
   (E) Colonic diversion

24. A 72-year-old woman was found on routine hemorrhoidectomy to have a 3-cm lesion in the anal canal (see Fig. 28-3). Biopsy of the lesion is positive for moderately differentiated squamous cell carcinoma. What is/are the appropriate step(s) in management?

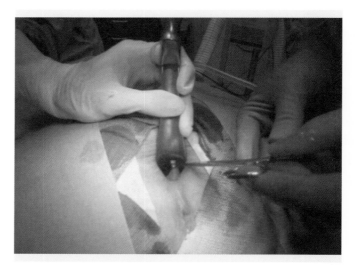

FIGURE 28-3. A 3-cm anal canal lesion.

   (A) Initial biopsy followed by chemoradiation therapy
   (B) Vigilant follow-up with repeat biopsy in 1 year after completion of therapy
   (C) Primary abdominal perineal resection for a 3-cm lesion at initial diagnosis
   (D) Resection for residual cancer after initial treatment
   (E) Quoting a 5-year survival rate of 45% with a complete response of patients with appropriate therapy

25. The use of endoscopic ultrasound (EUS) for staging of rectal cancer has increased in recent years. Which of the following is true regarding EUS?
    (A) EUS delineates five separate layers of the rectum including mucosal surface, mucosal/muscularis mucosa, submucosa, muscularis propria, and serosa and/or perirectal fat.
    (B) EUS cannot accurately predict lymph node involvement.
    (C) Most incorrect staging is secondary to understaging of lesions.
    (D) EUS is only useful in assessing rectal masses.
    (E) Pelvic CT is more accurate than EUS in assessing tumor depth in rectal cancer.

26. Choice of hemorrhoid treatment depends not only on the grade of the hemorrhoid but also the location. Which of the following statements about external versus internal hemorrhoids is correct?
    (A) External hemorrhoids are located in the anal canal and are of endodermal origin.
    (B) Banding of grade 2 internal hemorrhoids in an office setting is feasible because they are located below the dentate line.
    (C) Thrombosed hemorrhoids are typically located below the dentate line and can cause exquisite pain.
    (D) Grade 4 hemorrhoids can be easily controlled by simple ligation.
    (E) Initial treatment for grade 1 hemorrhoids should include primary operative intervention.

27. Which of the following statements is true regarding anal canal lesions?
    (A) Anal canal lesions are most successfully treated with abdominoperineal resection (APR).
    (B) Anal canal melanoma and mucinous adenocarcinoma are associated with a good prognosis.
    (C) Carcinoid tumors of anal canal less than 5 cm are best treated with wide local excision.
    (D) Anal canal squamous cell carcinoma should be initially treated with wide local excision.
    (E) Anal canal condylomas can be locally fulgurated.

28. Many anal margin lesions can be treated with wide local excision. For which of the following is wide local excision appropriate?
    (A) Melanoma of the anal margin
    (B) Bowen disease of the anal margin
    (C) Noninvasive Paget disease of the anal margin
    (D) Basal cell carcinoma of the anal margin
    (E) All of the above can be treated surgically with wide local excision

29. Concerning embryologic origin, innervation, and lymphatic and venous drainage of the anal canal versus the rectum, which of the following is correct?
    (A) The rectum is of ectoderm origin.
    (B) The anal canal below the dentate line is insensitive to pain.
    (C) The venous drainage for the rectum is the portal system.
    (D) The lymphatic drainage for the rectum is the inguinal lymphatic system.
    (E) The anal canal is lined with glandular mucosa.

30. A 33-year-old woman presents with a perirectal abscess. She is exquisitely tender, and you are unable to examine her adequately in the office. On evaluation under anesthesia, you find a fluctuant area surrounding an area of granulation tissue with associated purulence (see Fig. 28-4). Which of the following is correct?

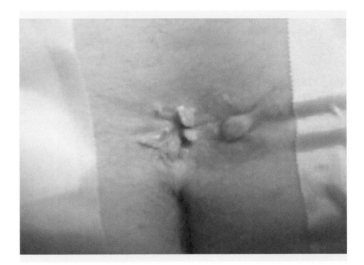

FIGURE 28-4. Perirectal abscess.

    (A) Perirectal abscess is the most common type of anorectal abscess accounting for approximately 40% of anorectal abscess.
    (B) All perirectal abscesses must be drained under general anesthesia.
    (C) Abscess and fistula do not occur with human immunodeficiency virus (HIV) because these patients are unable to mount a cellular response.
    (D) If perirectal erythema is present without an apparent fluctuant mass, no incision and drainage is needed.
    (E) Perirectal abscess is rare in hematologic abnormalities such as leukemia and lymphoma.

31. The same patient in Question 30 undergoes incision and drainage. After draining the abscess, anoscopy is performed and a fistula is identified (see Fig. 28-5). Which of the following is correct regarding anal fistula?

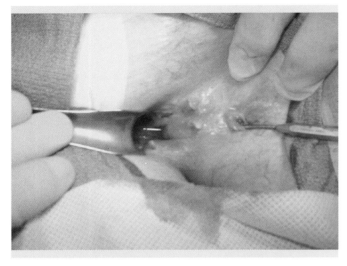

FIGURE 28-5. Chronic anal fistula with probe demonstrating the internal and external anal openings.

   (A) When the external opening lies anterior to the transverse plane, the internal opening usually is located in the anterior midline.
   (B) When the external opening lies posterior to the transverse plane, the internal opening tends to be located in the posterior midline.
   (C) Dye is the optimal method for identifying the internal opening of a fistula.
   (D) The internal opening should be easily identified by visualization alone.
   (E) Intersphincteric fistulas tend to be deep, and transphincteric fistulas characteristically tend to be superficial.

32. Which of the following is true regarding the principles of surgical treatment of anal fistula?
   (A) After identification of external and internal fistula openings, the tract should be incised unless excessive overlying muscle is present.
   (B) The granulation tissue exposed in the fistula tract should be left untreated.
   (C) Fistulotomy should be performed even if a portion of external sphincter is involved.
   (D) Treatment of horseshoe fistula-in-ano should include complete resection of the entire fistula tract regardless of the extent of soft tissue involvement.
   (E) Complex transphincteric fistulas require a cutting seton tightened over time.

33. A 52-year-old woman is referred to your office for evaluation of foul-smelling drainage from her vagina for 2 months. Pelvic examination revealed a small 2-mm opening in her vaginal vault with active drainage of stool consistency. Past surgical history was significant for an abdominal hysterectomy and bilateral oophorectomy for cervical cancer 3 years ago followed by radiation therapy. You are concerned about a rectovaginal fistula. Which of following is correct about rectovaginal fistulas?
   (A) A low rectovaginal fistula can be treated with a rectal advancement flap.
   (B) A high rectovaginal fistula should be treated with a rectal advancement flap.
   (C) Fistulotomy is sufficient to treat most rectovaginal fistulas.
   (D) Fibrin glue can be locally applied with good long-term results.
   (E) Etiology of rectovaginal fistulas is most often due to congenital causes.

34. Which of the following is correct regarding staging of anal canal cancer?
   (A) Stage I includes any tumor size less than 3 cm and no nodal involvement.
   (B) Stage II includes any T2 or T3 tumor with no nodal involvement.
   (C) Stage III includes any T stage with no nodal involvement.
   (D) Stage IV disease is most commonly associated with metastasis to the lungs.

35. Anorectal manometry can be used in the evaluation of fecal incontinence. Which of the following statements regarding anal manometry is true?
   (A) It is an objective method used to assess anal muscular tone, rectal compliance, and anorectal sensation.
   (B) There are strict universal guidelines for collection and analysis of anal manometry data for quality assurance.
   (C) Manometry can identify and document sphincter function before operative intervention that might require optimal continence.
   (D) All of the above are true.
   (E) Only A and C are true.

36. Regarding staging of rectal cancer, which of the following is true?
   (A) Stage I rectal cancer has a 70% 5-year survival rate.
   (B) In stage II rectal cancer, the primary tumor has extended either through the muscularis propria or into the pericolic fat with possible local extension into other organs.

(C) Metastatic nodal involvement in stage III rectal cancer is classified as either N1 or N2, describing the number of nodes positive for metastatic cancer in the inguinal region.

(D) Stage IV rectal cancer is limited to a T4 lesion with any local lymph node involvement and distant metastasis.

(E) The use of EUS is limited to measuring tumor depth.

37. Which of the following can be used to evaluate disorders of defecation?
(A) Anorectal manometry and EUS
(B) Radiologic studies such as plain films and fluoroscopy
(C) Defecography or evacuation proctography
(D) Bowel transit studies and biofeedback
(E) All of the above

38. Comparing the anorectal manifestation of Crohn disease and ulcerative colitis, which of the following is true?
(A) Perianal disease is less common in Crohn disease.
(B) Perirectal fistulas occur frequently in ulcerative colitis.
(C) Ulcerative colitis attacks rarely involve the rectum.
(D) Bloody stools are more common in Crohn disease than in ulcerative colitis.
(E) Granulomas are a common finding on rectal biopsy in Crohn disease.

39. A 60-year-old man with hypertension is referred to you for evaluation of rectal bleeding. He has had bloody diarrhea on and off for 6 weeks. He has lost 20 lb in the past 6 months but has been dieting. Antidiarrhea drugs have caused him to have crampy abdominal pain. Colonoscopy reveals a 4-cm lesion at 10 cm from the anal verge. Which of the following is appropriate for initial evaluation?
(A) Endoscopic biopsy for pathology from the edge of the mass
(B) Resection of the lesion with endoscopic snare
(C) Injection with hypertonic saline or alcohol for ablation
(D) Termination of colonoscopy as diagnosis has been made
(E) Application of methylene blue on the surface of the mass for easy intraoperative identification

40. Biopsy results of the lesion in the man in Question 39 reveal a poorly differentiated adenocarcinoma. Which of the following is useful in preoperative workup and staging of the cancer?

(A) Magnetic resonance imaging (MRI) of the abdomen and pelvis
(B) EUS examination
(C) Grade of the cancer
(D) CT of the abdomen and pelvis
(E) All of the above

41. The preoperative staging of the patient in Questions 39 and 40 is completed with perirectal lymphadenopathy but no distal metastatic lesions identified. What is important to consider in operative planning?
(A) Body habitus, gender, and age
(B) Comorbidities including cardiomyopathy, coronary artery disease, and obstructive pulmonary disease
(C) Distance of the tumor from the anal verge
(D) Metastatic disease
(E) All of the above

42. A 64-year-old woman presents at your office with complaints of bleeding hemorrhoids. She describes them as always falling out no matter how many times she replaces them manually. A full colonoscopy reveals no other source of bleeding. Physical examination reveals grade 3 hemorrhoids with redundant mucosal prolapse circumferentially. Which of the following options would be best for this patient?
(A) Dietary modification with increasing fiber and water intake
(B) Rubber band ligation to all the hemorrhoidal bundles
(C) Infrared coagulation (IRC) to all the hemorrhoidal bundles
(D) Circumferential hemorrhoidectomy with removal of all hemorrhoidal tissue
(E) A stapled procedure for both the prolapsed mucosa and hemorrhoidal bundles

43. Melanoma of the anal canal can be discovered incidentally in hemorrhoid specimens. Which of the following is true regarding melanoma?
(A) The anal canal is the most common site of the development of malignant melanoma of the alimentary tract.
(B) Ten percent of all melanomas occur in the anal canal.
(C) All melanomas-in-ano are characteristically pigmented.
(D) Abdominoperineal resection is the only surgical option for melanoma of the anal canal.
(E) Supplemental therapy with chemotherapy, radiotherapy, and immunotherapy significantly affects survival.

44. A 52-year-old man presents at your office with complaint of a lump in his anus. He has little physical mobility and is wheelchair bound from advanced arthritis. You attempt to examine him in the office, but he is unable to tolerate the examination without physical discomfort. He denies any other symptoms of rectal bleeding or constipation. He has no other medical problems. Colonoscopy under conscious sedation was undertaken in the last year, but the examination was incomplete. Completion barium enema was performed and read as normal. You schedule him for examination under anesthesia and excision of the lesion. Your initial physical examination is shown in Fig. 28-6. Anoscopy reveals a large skin tag with a grade 3 left lateral hemorrhoid (see Fig. 28-7). What is the next appropriate step?

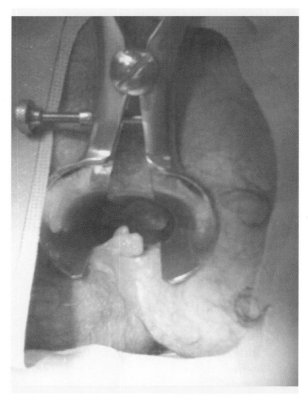

FIGURE 28-7. Anoscopy discovers a large left lateral grade 3 hemorrhoid with the preexisting skin tag.

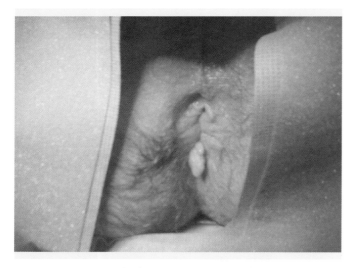

FIGURE 28-6. Initial physical inspection of the perineum.

(A) Biopsy the skin tag and perform IRC of the hemorrhoid.
(B) Band the hemorrhoid and leave the skin tag intact.
(C) Perform open or closed hemorrhoidectomy and resect the skin tag.
(D) Perform a stapled procedure for hemorrhoid and prolapse.
(E) Biopsy the skin tag and perform a lateral sphincterotomy.

45. Concerning local anesthesia and positioning for common anorectal procedures, which of the following is true?
(A) A perianal field block with bupivacaine and epinephrine is very effective at pain control and allows simple anorectal procedures to be done without general anesthesia.

(B) Prone jackknife position is advantageous for anterior rectal lesions as well as for many anorectal procedures such as hemorrhoidectomy; high lithotomy is advantageous for posterior rectal lesions.
(C) Open or closed hemorrhoidectomy can be performed under spinal anesthesia as well as general anesthesia.
(D) Lateral sphincterotomy can be easily preformed with a perianal field block and conscious sedation.
(E) All of the above are true.

ANSWERS AND EXPLANATIONS

1. **(B)** Only 1–2% of US adults age 30 and younger have diverticulosis, but this increases to >50% by age 50. Approximately 10–25% of US adults with diverticulosis will develop inflammation and infection associated with a diverticulum (diverticulitis). Symptoms range from mild left lower quadrant pain amenable to outpatient treatment to free perforation and peritonitis requiring emergency laparotomy.

   Colonic diverticula form primarily in the sigmoid colon and descending colon. The majority of these are false diverticula, involving herniation of the mucosa and

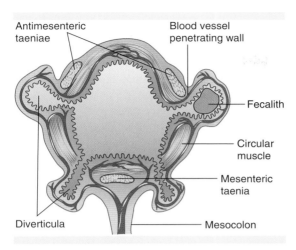

FIGURE 28-8. Cross-section of the colon depicting the sites where diverticula form. From Doherty GM (ed.). *Current Diagnosis & Treatment: Surgery*, 13th ed. New York, NY: McGraw-Hill; 2010:Fig. 30-12.

muscularis mucosa through the colonic wall between the teniae coli in areas of penetration of vasa rectum (see Fig. 28-8). True diverticula involve all layers of the colon wall, are most commonly found in the cecum, and are more common among Asians.

The pathophysiology of this diverticulosis is related to a lack of dietary fiber, which results in decreased colonic motility and a small stool volume, requiring high intraluminal pressure and high colonic wall tension for propulsion. According to the Law of LaPlace, the intraluminal pressure is inversely proportional to the radius of the lumen, whereas the wall tension is directly proportional to the pressure (pressure = tension/radius). The increased intraluminal pressure results in muscular hypertrophy and development of segmentation, where the colon acts like separate segments instead of functioning as a continuous tube. Segmentation results in the high intraluminal pressures being directed radially toward the colon wall.

Most patients with uncomplicated diverticulitis will recover without surgery, and 50–70% will have no further episode. However, the risk of complications increases with recurrent disease. Elective sigmoid colectomy should be considered after a second episode or complicated diverticulitis. Treatment of sigmoid diverticulitis with sigmoid colectomy is very effective, resulting in an overall lifetime recurrence rate of 20–25%.

BIBLIOGRAPHY

Bullard Dunn KM, Rothenberger DA. Colon, rectum, and anus. In: Brunicardi F, Andersen DK, Billiar TR, et al. (eds.), *Schwartz's Principles of Surgery*, 10th ed. New York, NY: McGraw-Hill; 2014.

Morris CR, Harvey IM, Stebbings WS, et al. Epidemiology of perforated colonic diverticular disease [Review]. *Postgrad Med J* 2002;78(925):654–658.

von Rahden BH, Germer CT. Pathogenesis of colonic diverticular disease. *Langenbecks Arch Surg* 2012;397(7):1025–1033.

2. **(E)** Diverticulitis can be classified as complicated or uncomplicated.

Uncomplicated diverticulitis is characterized by left lower quadrant pain and tenderness. Abdominal CT may reveal pericolic soft tissue stranding, colonic wall thickening, or phlegmon in association with colonic diverticula. Treatment consists of broad-spectrum oral antibiotics and a low-residue diet.

The Hinchey classification for *complicated* diverticular disease is as follows (see Fig. 28-9):

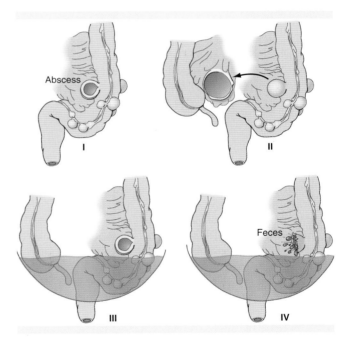

FIGURE 28-9. Hinchey classification of diverticulitis. From Gearhart SL. Diverticular disease and common anorectal disorders. In: Longo DL, Fauci AS, Kasper DL, Hauser SL, Jameson J, Loscalzo J (eds.), *Harrison's Principles of Internal Medicine*, 18th ed. New York, NY: McGraw-Hill; 2012: Chapter 297, Fig. 297-2.

Stage I: colonic inflammation with an associated pericolic abscess

Stage II: colonic inflammation with a retroperitoneal or pelvic abscess

Stage III: purulent peritonitis

Stage IV: feculent peritonitis

Surgical treatment is guided by the clinical status of the patient and the degree of peritoneal contamination. Stage I and II and small abscesses (<2 cm) may be treated with IV antibiotics and bowel rest. Larges abscesses warrant an attempt at CT-guided drainage in addition to antibiotics. Stages III and IV both involve diffuse peritonitis and require operative exploration and voluminous irrigation. It was previously thought that a Hartman's procedure was mandated in these cases, but recent studies have suggested that laparoscopic lavage and drainage without bowel resection may be safe in selected patients.

BIBLIOGRAPHY

Angenete E, Thornell A, Burcharth J, et al. Laparoscopic lavage is feasible and safe for the treatment of perforated diverticulitis with purulent peritonitis: the first results from the randomized controlled trial DILALA. *Ann Surg* Decemeber 8, 2014. [Epub ahead of print]

Bullard Dunn KM, Rothenberger DA. Colon, rectum, and anus. In: Brunicardi F, Andersen DK, Billiar TR, et al. (eds.), *Schwartz's Principles of Surgery*, 10th ed. New York, NY: McGraw-Hill; 2014.

Gearhart SL. Diverticular disease and common anorectal disorders. In: Longo DL, Fauci AS, Kasper DL, Hauser SL, Jameson J, Loscalzo J (eds.), *Harrison's Principles of Internal Medicine*, 18th ed. New York, NY: McGraw-Hill; 2012:Chapter 297.

3. **(D)** The colon has two primary functions: storage of stool and absorption of water and electrolytes. The surface of the colon consists of a columnar epithelium with no villi. However, the epithelial cells include absorptive cells and contain microvilli on their surface as well as mucus-secreting goblet cells. Sodium is actively transported across the cell membrane, and water accompanies the transported sodium and is absorbed passively along an osmotic gradient. Potassium is actively secreted into the colonic lumen and absorbed by passive diffusion. Chloride is absorbed actively via a chloride-bicarbonate exchange.

Because of the electrolyte exchange that occurs with water resorption in the colon, a high concentration of bicarbonate results. The colon secretes potassium and bicarbonate in exchange for chloride (and water) absorption. Therefore, with profuse diarrhea, a large volume of bicarbonate can be quickly lost from the colon and the patient can develop a relative acidosis (with hypokalemia). Although the primary function of the colon is water retention, the majority of water resorption occurs in the small bowel.

The primary fuel source for the colon is short-chain fatty acids, particularly butyric acid. Colonic motility is not cyclic as with the small intestine, because the migrating motor complex of the small bowel rarely continues into the colon. Instead, colonic contents are mixed by short duration or phasic contractions, and high-amplitude propagated contractions lead to mass movements through the colon. These phasic contractions normally occur approximately five times per day. Following abdominal surgery under general anesthesia, GI motility is first seen in the small bowel, followed by the stomach and then the colon.

BIBLIOGRAPHY

Bullard Dunn KM, Rothenberger DA. Colon, rectum, and anus. In: Brunicardi F, Andersen DK, Billiar TR, et al. (eds.), *Schwartz's Principles of Surgery*, 10th ed. New York, NY: McGraw-Hill; 2014.

Camilleri M, Murray JA. Diarrhea and constipation. In: Longo DL, Fauci AS, Kasper DL, Hauser SL, Jameson J, Loscalzo J (eds.), *Harrison's Principles of Internal Medicine*, 18th ed. New York, NY: McGraw-Hill; 2012:Chapter 40.

Priebe MG, Vonk RJ, Sun X, et al. The physiology of colonic metabolism. Possibilities for pre- and probiotics [Review]. *Eur J Nutr* 2002;41(S1):2–10.

Pryde SE, Duncan SH, Hold GL, et al. The microbiology of butyrate formation in the human colon [Review]. *FEMS Microbiol Lett* 2002;217(2):133–139.

4. **(A)** Distinguishing between ulcerative colitis and Crohn disease is impossible in up to 15% of cases upon initial diagnosis and in approximately 5% of gross colonic resection specimens (Table 28-1). These cases are termed indeterminate colitis. Distinguishing between ulcerative colitis and Crohn disease is less important during medical treatment, but of paramount importance in patients being considered for surgery because the ileoanal pouch procedure carries a high risk of recurrence and pouch failure in over one-third of patients with an ultimate diagnosis of Crohn disease.

BIBLIOGRAPHY

Friedman S, Blumberg RS. Inflammatory bowel disease. In: Longo DL, Fauci AS, Kasper DL, Hauser SL, Jameson J, Loscalzo J (eds.), *Harrison's Principles of Internal Medicine*, 18th ed. New York, NY: McGraw-Hill; 2012:Chapter 295.

Guy TS, Williams NN, Rosato EF. Crohn's disease of the colon [Review]. *Surg Clin North Am* 2001;81(1):159–168.

Roberts PL. Perspective on inflammatory bowel disease (ulcerative colitis and Crohn's disease). In: Zinner MJ, Ashley SW (eds.), *Maingot's Abdominal Operations*, 12th ed. New York, NY: McGraw-Hill; 2013:Chapter 35B.

5. **(D)** Ulcerative colitis typically manifests with periods of remission and exacerbations characterized by rectal bleeding and diarrhea. Because ulcerative colitis most commonly affects patients in their youth or early middle age, the disease can have serious long-term local and systemic consequences.

TABLE 28-1 Inflammatory Bowel Disease Characteristics

	Ulcerative Colitis	Crohn Disease
Clinical		
Gross blood in stool	Yes	Occasionally
Mucus	Yes	Occasionally
Systemic symptoms	Occasionally	Frequently
Pain	Occasionally	Frequently
Abdominal mass	Rarely	Yes
Significant perineal disease	No	Frequently
Fistulas	No	Yes
Small intestinal obstruction	No	Frequently
Colonic obstruction	Rarely	Frequently
Response to antibiotics	No	Yes
Recurrence after surgery	No	Yes
ANCA-positive	Frequently	Rarely
ASCA-positive	Rarely	Frequently
Endoscopic		
Rectal sparing	Rarely	Frequently
Continuous disease	Yes	Occasionally
"Cobblestoning"	No	Yes
Granuloma on biopsy	No	Occasionally
Radiographic		
Small bowel significantly abnormal	No	Yes
Abnormal terminal ileum	No	Yes
Segmental colitis	No	Yes
Asymmetric colitis	No	Yes
Stricture	Occasionally	Frequently

ANCA, antineutrophil cytoplasm antibody; ASCA, anti–*Saccharomyces cerevisiae* antibody.
Adapted from Friedman S, Blumberg RS. Inflammatory bowel disease. In: Longo DL, Fauci AS, Kasper DL, Hauser SL, Jameson J, Loscalzo J (eds.), *Harrison's Principles of Internal Medicine*, 18th ed. New York, NY: McGraw-Hill; 2012: Chapter 295, Table 295-5.

Indications for urgent surgical intervention in ulcerative colitis include acute colitis and toxic megacolon, particularly when accompanied by hemorrhage or perforation. Other indications for elective resection include intractable symptoms not controlled by medical management, dysplasia or cancer, stricture, or systemic symptoms. The reported risk of colorectal cancer is estimated to be 2% after 10 years, 8% after 20 years, and 18% after 30 years of the disease. Therefore, surgical intervention is commonly recommended beginning approximately 10 years after initial diagnosis.

BIBLIOGRAPHY

Azer SA. Overview of molecular pathways in inflammatory bowel disease associated with colorectal cancer development. *Eur J Gastroenterol Hepatol* 2013;25(3):271–281.

Campbell S, Ghosh S. Ulcerative colitis and colon cancer: strategies for cancer prevention [Review]. *Dig Dis* 2002;20(1):38–48.

Eaden JA, Mayberry JF. Colorectal cancer complicating ulcerative colitis: a review [Review]. *Am J Gastroenterol* 2000;95(10):2710–2719.

Forbes S, Messenger D, McLeod RS. Ulcerative colitis. In: Zinner MJ, Ashley SW (eds.), *Maingot's Abdominal Operations*, 12th ed. New York, NY: McGraw-Hill; 2013:Chapter 34.

6. **(D)** Acute colonic pseudo-obstruction is a functional disorder characterized by abdominal distention accompanied by colonic dilation, particularly involving the cecum and right colon. The syndrome develops as a result of decreased parasympathetic tone from the sacral nerves, resulting in severe adynamic ileus. It is associated with sepsis; respiratory failure; organic brain disorders; malignancy; trauma to the spine, retroperitoneum, and pelvis; burns; electrolyte disturbances; and a variety of medications including narcotics, calcium channel blockers, and cyclic antidepressants. Only a few cases of Ogilvie syndrome have been considered idiopathic in origin.

The diagnosis of the condition is through radiographic evidence of colonic obstruction without identifiable mechanical etiology. Evaluation of the markedly distended colon in the intensive care unit setting involves excluding mechanical obstruction and other causes of toxic megacolon such as *C difficile* infection, correcting electrolyte disturbances, and assessing for signs of ischemia and perforation.

The risk of colonic perforation in acute colonic pseudo-obstruction increases when cecal diameter exceeds 12 cm and when the distention has been present for greater than 6 days. Appropriate management includes supportive therapy and selective use of neostigmine (acetylcholinesterase inhibitor, which leads to resolution in approximately 90% of cases) and colonoscopy for decompression. Early recognition and management are critical in minimizing complications. Increasing age, cecal diameter, delay in decompression, and status of the bowel significantly influence mortality, which is approximately 40% when ischemia or perforation is present.

BIBLIOGRAPHY

Bullard Dunn KM, Rothenberger DA. Colon, rectum, and anus. In: Brunicardi F, Andersen DK, Billiar TR, et al. (eds.), *Schwartz's Principles of Surgery*, 10th ed. New York, NY: McGraw-Hill; 2014.

De Giorgio R, Knowles CH. Acute colonic pseudo-obstruction. *Br J Surg* 2009;96(3):229–239.

Ehrenpreis ED. Gut and hepatobiliary dysfunction. In: Hall JB, Schmidt GA, Wood LH (eds.), *Principles of Critical Care*, 3rd ed. New York, NY: McGraw-Hill; 2005:Chapter 81.

Valle RG, Godoy FL. Neostigmine for acute colonic pseudo-obstruction: a meta-analysis. *Ann Med Surg (Lond)* 2014;3(3):60–64.

7. **(C)** *C difficile* is present in 3% of the general population and 10% of hospitalized patients. It is the single most common cause of infectious diarrhea among all hospitalized patients and the major known etiology of nosocomial antibiotic-associated colitis.

C difficile is an obligate anaerobic gram-positive bacillus whose virulence is attributed to the production of extracellular toxins. Spores of toxigenic *C difficile* are ingested, survive gastric acidity, germinate in the small bowel, and colonize the lower intestinal tract. Toxin-negative strains of *C difficile* can be identified as part of the normal flora in patients without overt diarrheal disease; however, those strains that cause infectious symptoms elaborate two large toxins: toxin A (an enterotoxin) and toxin B (a cytotoxin). This is known as pseudomembranous colitis (PMC).

The pseudomembranes of PMC are confined to the colonic mucosa and initially appear as 1- to 2-mm whitish-yellow plaques. The intervening mucosa appears unremarkable, but as the disease progresses, the pseudomembranes coalesce to form larger plaques and become confluent over the entire colon wall (see Fig. 28-10). The whole colon is usually involved, but 10% of patients have rectal sparing.

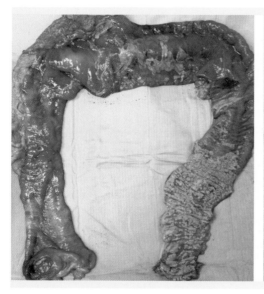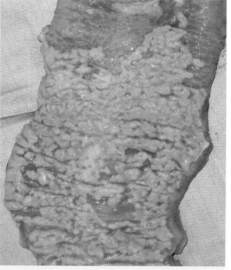

FIGURE 28-10. *Clostridium difficile.* Gross specimen. From Kaiser A. *McGraw-Hill Manual Colorectal Surgery.* New York, NY: McGraw-Hill; 2008.

The spectrum of disease ranges from watery diarrhea to fulminant, life-threatening colitis. Stools are almost never grossly bloody and range from soft and unformed to watery or mucoid in consistency, with a characteristic odor. Patients may have as many as 20 bowel movements per day, sometimes accompanied by fever (28% of cases), abdominal pain (22% of cases), and leukocytosis (50% of cases). Table 28-2 lists the sensitivity and specificity of diagnostic tests for *C difficile* infection.

In the mildest cases of *C difficile* infection, the discontinuation of antimicrobial agents alone may be sufficient to manage clinical illness without further therapy. The primary treatment for mild to moderate disease in a clinically stable patient is metronidazole, which may be administered orally or intravenously. Oral vancomycin and fidaxomicin are reserved for patients with one of the following: presence of important comorbidity, altered sensorium, unstable clinical course, confinement in an intensive care unit, renal failure (creatinine level ≥1.5 times the upper limit of normal), reduced serum albumin level (<2.5 g/dL), hypotension, or leukocytosis with a WBC count greater than 15,000/μL.

TABLE 28-2 Relative Sensitivity and Specificity of Diagnostic Tests for *Clostridium difficile* Infection (CDI)

Type of Test	Relative Sensitivity[a]	Relative Specificity[a]	Comment
Stool culture for *C difficile*	+ + + +	+ + +	Most sensitive test; specificity of + + + + if the *C difficile* isolate tests positive for toxin; with clinical data, is diagnostic of CDI; turnaround time too slow for practical use
Cell culture cytotoxin test on stool	+ + +	+ + + +	With clinical data, is diagnostic of CDI; highly specific but not as sensitive as stool culture; slow turnaround time
Enzyme immunoassay for toxin A or toxins A and B in stool	+ + to + + +	+ + +	With clinical data, is diagnostic of CDI; rapid results, but not as sensitive as stool culture or cell culture cytotoxin test
Enzyme immunoassay for *C difficile* common antigen in stool	+ + + to + + + +	+ + +	Detects glutamate dehydrogenase found in toxigenic and nontoxigenic strains of *C difficile* and other stool organisms; more sensitive and less specific than enzyme immunoassay for toxins; rapid results
Polymerase chain reaction for *C difficile* toxin B gene in stool	+ + + +	+ + + +	Detects toxigenic *C difficile* in stool; newly approved for clinical testing, but appears to be more sensitive than enzyme immunoassay toxin testing and at least as specific
Colonoscopy or sigmoidoscopy	+	+ + + +	Highly specific if pseudomembranes are seen; insensitive compared with other tests

Note: + + + +, >90%; + + +, 71–90%; + +, 51–70%; +, ~50%.
[a]According to both clinical and test-based criteria.
Adapted from Gerding DN, Johnson S. *Clostridium difficile* infection, including pseudomembranous colitis. In: Longo DL, Fauci AS, Kasper DL, Hauser SL, Jameson J, Loscalzo J (eds.), *Harrison's Principles of Internal Medicine*, 18th ed. New York, NY: McGraw-Hill; 2012:Chapter 129, Table 129–1.

BIBLIOGRAPHY

Dupont HL. Diagnosis and management of *Clostridium difficile* infection. *Clin Gastroenterol Hepatol* 2013;11(10):1216–1223.

Gerding DN, Johnson S. *Clostridium difficile* infection, including pseudomembranous colitis. In: Longo DL, Fauci AS, Kasper DL, Hauser SL, Jameson J, Loscalzo J (eds.), *Harrison's Principles of Internal Medicine*, 18th ed. New York, NY: McGraw-Hill; 2012:Chapter 129.

Weber SG. Gastrointestinal infections. In: Hall JB, Schmidt GA, Wood LH (eds.), *Principles of Critical Care*, 3rd ed. New York, NY: McGraw-Hill; 2005:Chapter 57.

8. **(D)** Volvulus represents an axial twist of the bowel and its mesentery. This entity is an infrequent cause of small or large bowel obstruction in the Western Hemisphere (see Figs. 28-11 and 28-12). Volvulus is encountered more frequently in the geriatric population, in individuals with a long history of constipation, and in institutionalized, neurologically impaired, or psychiatric patients.

Colonic volvulus comprises about 1–4% of all bowel obstructions and about 10–15% of all large bowel obstructions. The volvulized segment has to be relatively mobile to allow the degree of freedom necessary to permit an axial twist of the mesentery. Either the affected segment has an especially long, narrow mesentery (e.g., malrotation or cecal volvulus) and/or a lack of bowel wall fixation (floppy cecum syndrome) or one aspect of the affected segment is fixed, around which the contiguous segment can twist (e.g., a deep fibrous band fixing the other end of the segment).

Sigmoid and cecal volvulus are the most commonly encountered, although transverse colonic volvulus has also been reported. Sigmoid volvulus is felt to be "acquired" through accumulation of risk factors, whereas cecal volvulus is considered "congenital" because of individual anatomic variation. Both sigmoid and cecal volvulus demonstrate a large, dilated loop of colon on plain radiograph. The loop "points" to the left upper quadrant

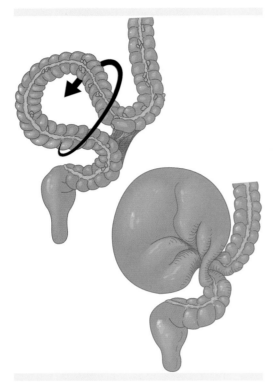

FIGURE 28-11. Schematic of sigmoid volvulus. From Doherty GM (ed.). *Current Diagnosis & Treatment: Surgery*, 13th ed. New York, NY: McGraw-Hill; 2010:Fig. 30-15.

of the abdomen with a cecal volvulus and to the right upper quadrant with a sigmoid volvulus. Radiologic imaging characteristic of sigmoid volvulus includes a dilated loop of colon pointing to the right upper quadrant on x-ray and a "bird's beak" deformity on contrast enema.

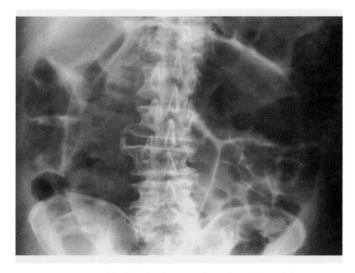

FIGURE 28-12. Abdominal x-ray showing sigmoid volvulus.

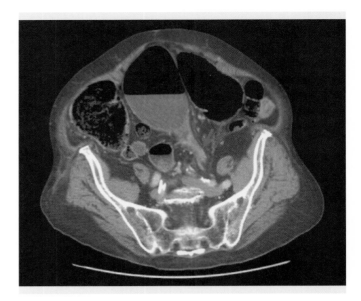

FIGURE 28-13. Abdominal computed tomography showing sigmoid volvulus. From Zinner MJ, Ashley SW (eds.). *Maingot's Abdominal Operations*, 12th ed. New York, NY: McGraw-Hill; 2013:Fig. 32-13.

CT findings also include a "bird beak whirl" or coffee bean sign (see Figs. 28-12 and 28-13).

The most common site of colonic volvulus is the sigmoid colon because of its inherent redundancy. Sigmoid volvulus accounts for 75% of all patients with volvulus. The development of sigmoid volvulus is associated with an elongated narrow mesocolon attached to a redundant sigmoid colon, which allows the elongated portion to rotate and twist on a narrow base (see Fig. 28-11). Sigmoid volvulus is more common in older, institutionalized patients with neurologic disorders or with chronic constipation. The initial management of sigmoid volvulus is resuscitation and endoscopic detorsion either with a rigid proctoscope, flexible sigmoidoscope, or colonoscope. A rectal tube may be inserted to maintain decompression, but the overall risk of recurrence is approximately 40%. For this reason, an elective sigmoid colectomy should be performed after the patient has been stabilized and undergone an adequate bowel preparation.

Cecal volvulus is the second most common site of colonic volvulus and the most common cause of large bowel obstruction in pregnancy. The "cecal bascule" is a somewhat unique, though less common, form of cecal volvulus that occurs when the true anatomic cecum (i.e., the part of the ascending colon that lies caudal to the entrance of the ileocecal valve) flops anteriorly over onto the ascending colon, obstructing the lumen. This form of cecal volvulus may be intermittent and recurrent and is often difficult to diagnose. Cecal volvulus can almost never be detorsed endoscopically. Moreover, because vascular compromise occurs early in the course of cecal volvulus, surgical exploration is necessary when the diagnosis is made. Right hemicolectomy with a primary ileocolic anastomosis can usually be performed safely and prevents recurrence. Although cecopexy has been well described and does have some success, the definitive treatment for cecal volvulus is right hemicolectomy with primary anastomosis in the appropriate setting with resection, ileostomy, and mucous fistula in the presence of perforation or peritonitis.

BIBLIOGRAPHY

Bullard Dunn KM, Rothenberger DA. Colon, rectum, and anus. In: Brunicardi F, Andersen DK, Billiar TR, et al. (eds.), *Schwartz's Principles of Surgery*, 10th ed. New York, NY: McGraw-Hill; 2014.

Halabi WJ, Jafari MD, Kang CY, et al. Colonic volvulus in the United States: trends, outcomes, and predictors of mortality. *Ann Surg* 2014;259(2):293–301.

Robinson RJ, Krishnamoorthy R. The role of endoscopy in the diagnosis and management of Crohn's disease. In: Rajesh A, Sinha R (eds.), *Crohn's Disease*. New York, NY: Springer International Publishing; 2015:23–32.

Sclabas GM, Sarosi GA, Khan S, Sarr MG, Behrns KE. Small bowel obstruction. In: Zinner MJ, Ashley SW (eds.), *Maingot's Abdominal Operations*, 12th ed. New York, NY: McGraw-Hill; 2013:Chapter 29.

9. **(D)** LGIH is defined as bleeding beyond the ligament of Treitz. Determination must be made between the small bowel and the colon as the etiology of the hemorrhage. The most common cause of LGIH in all adults is colonic diverticula. In adults younger than age 60, the next most common causes are cancer and inflammatory bowel disease. In adults older than age 60, the next most common causes are arteriovenous malformations and cancer. Among children, the most common cause of LGIH is a Meckel diverticulum, followed by inflammatory bowel disease and colonic polyps. Other common etiologies include hemorrhoidal bleeding and ischemic colitis. Blood loss requiring transfusion of more than 6 units of blood within a 24-hour period is considered "massive" bleeding and should prompt a mesenteric arteriogram or operative exploration.

BIBLIOGRAPHY

Feinman M, Haut ER. Lower gastrointestinal bleeding. *Surg Clin North Am* 2014;94(1):55–63.

Kodner IJ, Fry RD, Fleshman JW, et al. Colon, rectum, and anus. In: Schwartz SI, Spencer FC (eds.), *Schwartz: Principles of Surgery*, 7th ed. New York, NY: McGraw-Hill; 1999:1282–1284.

Tavakkolizadeh A, Ashley SW. Acute gastrointestinal hemorrhage. In: Townsend CM, Beauchamp RD, Evers BM, et al. (ed.), *Sabiston Textbook of Surgery*, 19th ed. Philadelphia, PA: Elsevier Saunders; 2012:1160–1181.

10. **(A)** Approximately 15% of all bowel obstructions occur in the large intestine. The most common site of obstruction is the sigmoid colon, with the right colon being much less likely to cause obstruction given its wider diameter. The most common cause of colonic obstruction in the adult is colon cancer, which accounts for approximately 60–70%. The next most common etiologies are diverticulitis (20%) and volvulus (5%). Adhesive bands, the most common etiology of obstruction in the small bowel, almost never cause colonic obstruction. The ileocecal valve is incompetent in 10–20% of persons, allowing colonic decompression in these individuals, which can be protective against perforation in cases of distal colon obstruction. The overall mortality rate for colonic obstruction is 20%, with the rate being 40% in the event of cecal perforation. The higher mortality rate is likely associated with a completely obstructing cancer of the left or sigmoid colon causing a closed loop obstruction in combination with a competent ileocecal valve.

BIBLIOGRAPHY

Bauer AJ, Schwarz NT, Moore BA, et al. Ileus in critical illness: mechanisms and management [Review]. *Curr Opin Crit Care* 2002;47(5):1175–1181.

Dervenis C, Delis S, Filippou D, et al. Intestinal obstruction and perforation—the role of the surgeon [Review]. *Dig Dis* 2003;21(1):68–76.

11. **(D)** The Haggitt classification for colonic polyps is used to characterize polyps for treatment purposes (see Fig. 28-14). Level 0 polyps refer to carcinoma *in situ* and are considered noninvasive. They can be treated with excision only. Level I polyps contain carcinoma that invades the muscularis mucosa into the submucosa, but remains contained within the head of the polyp. Level II polyps contain carcinoma that invades the junction between the stalk and the adenoma itself. Both level I and level II polyps can generally be adequately treated with endoscopic excision. Level III polyps invade the stalk. These can occasionally be excised endoscopically depending on the margin obtained. The carcinoma in a level IV polyp invades the submucosa of the bowel but remains above the muscularis propria. Wide-based sessile polyps with any carcinoma are also considered level IV. All level IV polyps require segmental resection.

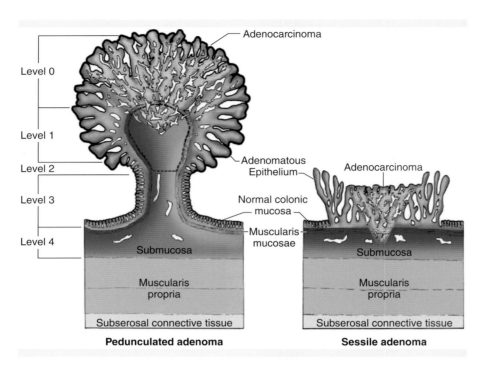

FIGURE 28-14. Haggitt classification of polyps. Reproduced with permission from Haggitt RC, Glotzbach RE, Soffer EE, Wruble LD. Prognostic factors in colorectal carcinomas arising in adenomas: Implications for lesions removed by endoscopic polypectomy. *Gastroenterology* 1985;89:328–336.

BIBLIOGRAPHY

Bullard Dunn KM, Rothenberger DA. Colon, rectum, and anus. In: Brunicardi F, Andersen DK, Billiar TR, et al. (eds.), *Schwartz's Principles of Surgery*, 10th ed. New York, NY: McGraw-Hill; 2014.

Inoue H. Endoscopic mucosal resection for the entire gastrointestinal mucosal lesions [Review]. *Gastrointest Endosc Clin North Am* 2001;11(3):459–478.

Steele SR, Johnson EK, Champagne B, et al. Endoscopy and polyps: diagnostic and therapeutic advances in management. *World J Gastroenterol* 2013;19(27):4277–4288.

Waye JD. Endoscopic mucosal resection of colon polyps [Review]. *Gastrointest Endosc Clin North Am* 2001;11(3):537–548.

12. **(E)** Colon cancer is the fourth most common type of cancer in the United States and accounts for the second most cancer deaths after lung cancer. Development of colon cancer is thought to involve malignant transformation of colonic polyps (adenoma to carcinoma sequence; see Fig. 28-15). There is a definite genetic predisposition to colon cancer. Although many persons are thought to have a heterozygous status for important cancer-related

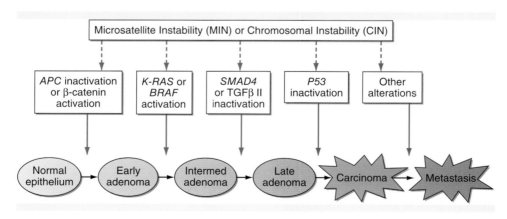

FIGURE 28-15. Genetic mutations in colorectal carcinoma. From Longo DL, Fauci AS, Kasper DL, Hauser SL, Jameson J, Loscalzo J (eds.). *Harrison's Principles of Internal Medicine*, 18th ed. New York, NY: McGraw-Hill; 2012:Fig. 83-2.

genes, loss of heterozygosity is related to both tumor-suppressor gene inactivation and oncogene activation. *Oncogenes* are genes that positively influence tumor formation. The activity of oncogenes is tightly regulated in normal cells, but mutational events in an allele of oncogenes lead to increased activity of the gene products. In contrast, *tumor-suppressor genes* negatively influence tumor formation through control of cell division (cell birth) or cell death (apoptosis). In cancer cells, this control function is lost through mutation in both alleles.

APC is a tumor-suppressor gene on chromosome 5. Loss of this gene is associated with familial adenomatous polyposis (FAP). This gene is autosomal dominant with 100% penetrance. *K-ras* and *BRAF* are oncogenes with increased activity in patients with colon cancer.

DCC is a tumor suppressor gene, and loss of both alleles is required for malignant degeneration. *DCC* mutations are present in more than 70% of colorectal carcinomas and may negatively impact prognosis.

SMAD4 functions in the signaling cascade of transforming growth factor-β and β-catenin. Loss of either of these genes is thought to promote cancer progression.

hMLH1/hMSH2 refers to a mismatch repair gene in which mutation leads to DNA instability. This gene is associated with hereditary nonpolyposis colorectal cancer (HNPCC).

CAG triplicate repeat sequence is related to certain neurodegenerative disorders but is not known to be related to colon cancer.

BIBLIOGRAPHY

Bullard Dunn KM, Rothenberger DA. Colon, rectum, and anus. In: Brunicardi F, Andersen DK, Billiar TR, et al. (eds.), *Schwartz's Principles of Surgery*, 10th ed. New York, NY: McGraw-Hill; 2014.

Grady WM. Genetic testing for high-risk colon cancer patients [Review]. *Gastroenterology* 2003;124(6):1574–1594.

Grady WM, Markowitz SD. Hereditary colon cancer genes [Review]. *Methods Mol Biol* 2003;222:59–83.

Lynch JP, Hoops TC. The genetic pathogenesis of colorectal cancer [Review]. *Hematol Oncol Clin North Am* 2002;16(4):775–810.

Shoup MC, Nissan A, Dangelica MI, et al. Randomized clinical trials in colon cancer [Review]. *Surg Oncol Clin North Am* 2002;11(1):133–148.

13. **(A)** According to the TNM staging system for colorectal cancer, T1 tumors invade the submucosa, T2 tumors invade the muscularis propria, T3 tumors invade into the subserosa or pericolic tissue, and T4 tumors perforate the visceral peritoneum or directly invade other organs or structures (Table 28-3). T5 tumors are not defined in the system. N0 classification refers to involvement of no regional lymph nodes, N1 involves one to three regional lymph nodes, N2 involves four or more regional lymph nodes, and N3 refers to any nodal involvement along a major, named vascular trunk. MX indicates that the

TABLE 28-3 TNM Staging of Colon Cancer (*AJCC Cancer Staging Manual*, 7th edition, 2010)

Stage	Definition
Primary tumor (T)	
TX	Primary tumor cannot be assessed
T0	No evidence of primary tumor
Tis	Carcinoma *in situ*: intraepithelial or invasion of lamina propria
T1	Tumor invades submucosa
T2	Tumor invades muscularis propria
T3	Tumor invades through muscularis propria into the subserosa or into nonperitonealized pericolic or perirectal tissues
T4a	Tumor perforates visceral peritoneum
T4b	Tumor directly invades other organs or structures
Regional lymph nodes (N)	
NX	Regional lymph nodes cannot be assessed
N0	No regional lymph node metastases
N1	Metastasis in 1–3 regional lymph nodes
N1a	1 positive lymph node
N1b	2–3 positive lymph nodes
N1c	Extranodal tumor deposits
N2	Metastasis in 4 or more regional lymph nodes
N2a	4–6 positive lymph nodes
N2b	≥7 positive lymph nodes
Distant metastasis (M)	
MX	Distant metastasis cannot be assessed
M0	No distant metastasis
M1	Distant metastasis
M1a	Metastases confined to 1 organ/site
M1b	Metastases in >1 organ/site
Extent of resection	
RX	Presence of residual tumor cannot be assessed
R0	No residual tumor
R1	Microscopic residual tumor
R2	Macroscopic residual tumor

presence of metastases cannot be adequately assessed. M0 refers to no distant metastases, and M1 refers to the presence of any distant metastases. Stage I colon cancer has a 5-year survival rate of greater than 90%.

BIBLIOGRAPHY

Benson AB 3rd, Bekaii-Saab T, Chan E, et al. Localized colon cancer, version 3.2013: featured updates to the NCCN Guidelines. *J Natl Compr Canc Netw* 2013;11(5):519–528.

Bullard Dunn KM, Rothenberger DA. Colon, rectum, and anus. In: Brunicardi F, Andersen DK, Billiar TR, et al. (eds.), *Schwartz's Principles of Surgery*, 10th ed. New York, NY: McGraw-Hill; 2014.

Fry RD, Mahmoud NN, Maron DJ, et al. Colon and rectum In: Townsend CM, Beauchamp RD, Evers BM, et al. (ed.), *Sabiston Textbook of Surgery*, 19th ed. Philadelphia, PA: W.B. Saunders; 2012:1294–1380.

Neuman HB, Park J, Weiser MR. Randomized clinical trials in colon cancer. *Surg Oncol Clin N Am* 2010;19(1):183–204.

14. **(A)** Gardner syndrome has a colonic manifestation similar to FAP with the addition of multiple extracolonic manifestations. FAP syndrome is categorized as Gardner syndrome when the intestinal findings are accompanied by certain benign extraintestinal growths, particularly osteomas, epidermoid cysts, desmoid tumors, and congenital hypertrophy of the retinal pigment epithelium. These growths may precede the development of the polyposis syndrome. Presentation with these signs, therefore, necessitates colonoscopy to evaluate for colonic polyposis. The presence of a retroperitoneal desmoid tumor may require biopsy, but this could likely be accomplished percutaneously. The other choices listed would not lead to an appropriate diagnosis.

Turcot syndrome is characterized by the presence of colonic polyps and brain tumors. The brain tumors in this population generally occur in the first two decades of life.

HNPCC is a genetic-linked autosomal dominant disorder with almost complete penetrance that accounts for approximately 5% of colorectal cancer cases annually in the United States. The associated genetic defect is a mutation in *hMLH1/hMSH2*, which is a mismatch repair gene. Mutation in this gene leads to DNA instability and predisposes to cancer. The diagnosis is clinical and made according to the Amsterdam criteria: at least three relatives with colorectal cancer (at least one must be first-degree relative), at least two successive generations affected, and colorectal cancer diagnosed before age 50 in at least one of the relatives (Table 28-4).

HNPCC patients also have a high risk of other cancers, and close surveillance is crucial in long-term management. Female patients are at particular risk of gynecologic malignancies and should be offered prophylactic hysterectomy and oophorectomy (Lynch syndrome type I includes all patients with HNPCC without

TABLE 28-4 Amsterdam Criteria I and II

Amsterdam Criteria I (1990)	Amsterdam Criteria II (1999)
At least three relatives with colorectal cancer, one of whom should be a first-degree relative of the other two.	There should be at least three relatives with HNPCC-associated cancer (colorectal cancer or cancer of the endometrium, small bowel, or ureter), one of whom should be a first-degree relative of the other two.
At least two successive generations should be affected.	At least two successive generations should be affected.
At least one colorectal cancer should be diagnosed before the age of 50 y.	At least one colorectal cancer should be diagnosed before the age of 50 y.
FAP should be excluded.	FAP should be excluded.
Tumors should be verified by a pathologist.	Tumors should be verified by a pathologist.
	Benign tumors, by definition, do not invade adjacent tissue borders, nor do they metastasize to distant sites. By contrast, malignant tumors have the added property of invading contiguous tissues and metastasizing to distant sites.
	A polyp is defined as a mass that protrudes into the lumen of the colon. They are subdivided according to the attachment to the bowel wall (e.g., sessile or pedunculated), their histologic appearance (e.g., hyperplastic or adenomas), and their neoplastic potential (i.e., benign or malignant).

FAP, familial polyposis syndromes; HNPCC, hereditary non-polyposis colorectal cancer.
Data from Vasen HFA. Clinical diagnosis and management of hereditary colorectal cancer syndromes. *J Clin Oncol* 2000; 18(21 suppl):81S–92S.

any additional diagnosis of cancer [no other noncolon site]). Lynch syndrome type II includes HNPCC patients with cancer diagnosed at an additional noncolon site. HNPCC patients are at high risk of colon cancer and should have close surveillance. Routine colonoscopy should begin in the second decade of life or 5 years earlier than the age of detection within the kindred. Definitive treatment for HNPCC includes subtotal colectomy given the high risk of synchronous colonic tumors. Cancers seen in Lynch syndrome type II, in addition to colon cancer, include noncolon GI tumors, urinary tract tumors, uterine and ovarian cancer, breast cancer, and pancreatic cancer.

Peutz-Jeghers syndrome manifests through an autosomal dominant transmission resulting in multiple hamartomas throughout the GI tract; melanin pigmentation of buccal mucosa, face, hands, and feet; and signs including GI hemorrhage, obstruction, and mucocutaneous hyperpigmentation.

Juvenile polyposis also has an autosomal dominant transmission and is a source of GI hemorrhage in the pediatric population. The peak age of symptoms in juvenile polyposis is 5–6 years when patients may experience abdominal pain, diarrhea, mucous discharge, and bleeding.

BIBLIOGRAPHY

Cao Y, Pieretti M, Marshall J, et al. Challenge in the differentiation between attenuated familial adenomatous polyposis and hereditary nonpolyposis colorectal cancer: case report with review of the literature [Review]. *Am J Gastroenterol* 2002;97(7):1822–1827.

Gala M, Chung DC. Hereditary colon cancer syndromes. *Semin Oncol* 2011;38(4):490–499.

Jasperson KW, Tuohy TM, Neklason DW, Burt RW. Hereditary and familial colon cancer. *Gastroenterology* 2010;138(6):2044–2058.

McGarrity TJ, Kulin HE, Zaino RJ. Peutz-Jeghers syndrome [Review]. *Am J Gastroenterol* 2000;95(3):596–604.

15. **(C)** Familial adenomatous polyposis (FAP) is related to the loss of the tumor-suppressor gene *APC* located on the long arm of chromosome 5. The *APC* gene mutation appears to be an early event in carcinogenesis and, in combination with other mutational events, leads to colon cancer. This genetic mutation is autosomal dominant with 100% penetrance, and all patients will develop colon cancer by the third decade of life, if not treated. FAP is characterized by the presence of hundreds to thousands of 5- to 10-mm polyps throughout the colon. Polyps more than 1 cm in diameter carry a 50% risk of carcinoma. By age 10, 15% of FAP patients will manifest colonic polyps, and this increases to 75% by age 20 and 90% by age 30. Extracolonic symptoms are frequently

seen and have been discussed previously as Gardner syndrome. Medical treatment of FAP is possible, and sulindac and celecoxib have been shown to decrease the number and size of colonic polyps. Sulindac and tamoxifen may also be effective in the treatment of desmoid growths. Surgical treatment of FAP includes total proctocolectomy with ileostomy or placement of an ileoanal or ileal pouch anastomosis.

BIBLIOGRAPHY

Bullard Dunn KM, Rothenberger DA. Colon, rectum, and anus. In: Brunicardi F, Andersen DK, Billiar TR, et al. (eds.), *Schwartz's Principles of Surgery*, 10th ed. New York, NY: McGraw-Hill; 2014.

Church J. Familial adenomatous polyposis. *Surg Oncol Clin N Am* 2009;18(4):585–598.

Kim B, Giardiello FM. Chemoprevention in familial adenomatous polyposis. *Best Pract Res Clin Gastroenterol* 2011;25(4–5):607–622.

16. **(C)** Carcinoma of the colon and rectum spreads by six modalities: intramucosal extension, direct invasion of adjacent structures, lymphatic spread, hematologic spread, intraperitoneal spread, and anastomotic implantation. Although the interest in lymphatic mapping and sentinel lymph nodes has been derived from favorable experiences in breast cancer and melanoma, most recent data do not support the value of this technique for colon cancer.

Surgical management of colon cancer is based on a number of factors, including tumor location and stage, the presence of synchronous colonic lesions or an underlying colonic disease, the risk for metachronous lesions, the patient's age and general condition, the extent of the local procedure, and the timing. Most colon cancers require resection, either for cure or for local control of the disease (see Fig. 28-16). Direct extension into adjacent fascia, vascular or nervous tissue, or solid organs requires *en bloc* resection of the colon with those involved structures because the adhesions usually contain tumor cells.

The length of bowel and mesentery resected is dictated by tumor location and distribution of the primary artery, but a radical resection of a colonic tumor should achieve at least a 5-cm clearance at the proximal and distal margin.

Approximately 20% of patients with colon cancer present as an emergency requiring an urgent operation for a tumor-related complication (e.g., bowel obstruction, perforation, or massive bleeding). Patients presenting with advanced stages of colorectal cancer have a significantly worse prognosis than patients with early diagnosis. Perioperative mortality in patients with perforated colon cancer approaches 30%, and those with obstructing colon cancer have in-hospital mortality

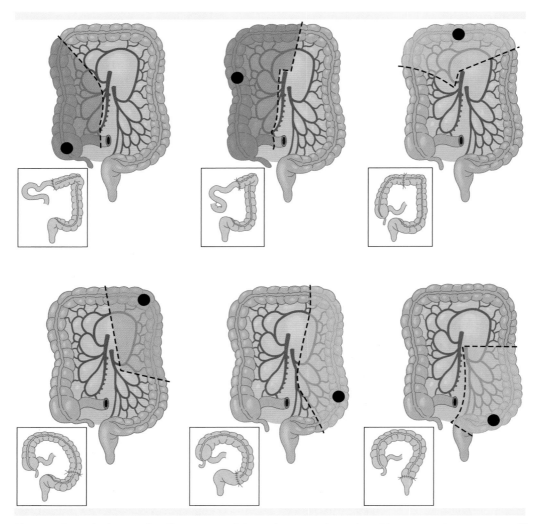

FIGURE 28-16. Extent of surgical resection for cancer of the colon at various sites. The cancer is represented by a black disk. Anastomosis of the bowel remaining after resection is shown in the small insets. From Chang GJ, Shelton AA, Welton ML. Large intestine. In: Doherty GM (ed.), *Current Diagnosis & Treatment: Surgery*, 13th ed. New York, NY: McGraw-Hill; 2010: Chapter 30, Fig. 30-10.

of 15% after initial presentation. Most patients do not require extensive resections for colon cancer.

Advances in minimally invasive technology have increased the popularity and capabilities of resection for colorectal malignancy, with large studies demonstrating equivalent outcomes for laparoscopic, hand-assisted laparoscopic, and open colorectal resections for cancer.

BIBLIOGRAPHY

Chang GJ, Shelton AA, Welton ML. Large intestine. In: Doherty GM (ed.), *Current Diagnosis & Treatment: Surgery*, 13th ed. New York, NY: McGraw-Hill; 2010:Chapter 30.

Kaiser AM, Etzioni D, Beart RW Jr. Tumors of the colon. In: Zinner MJ, Ashley SW (eds.), *Maingot's Abdominal Operations*, 12th ed. New York, NY: McGraw-Hill; 2013:Chapter 36.

17. **(A)** This patient has acute uncomplicated diverticulitis. This disease is characterized by localized diverticular inflammation without abscess formation, free perforation, or bleeding. The majority of patients present with left lower quadrant pain and fever, making diverticulitis principally a clinical diagnosis. Diagnostic dilemmas do occur, however, and a wide differential including bowel perforation or obstruction, appendicitis, inflammatory bowel disease, and ischemic colitis must be considered. An imaging study is indicated when the clinical picture is not clear or to help guide future therapy.

Endoscopy is contraindicated in the setting of acute diverticulitis because the insufflation required can disturb the tenuous seal containing the diverticular perforation and result in the conversion to free perforation and a need for more urgent surgical intervention with substantially higher morbidity and mortality. Endoscopy can be useful after the acute episode has resolved to evaluate for other distal pathologic processes.

Barium enema is also contraindicated in the acute setting for reasons similar to those described earlier. It is a very important part of the preparation for elective resection after recovery, because it accurately describes the extent of involvement and severity of disease, including strictures that may develop after acute diverticulitis.

Laparoscopy has been described as a highly sensitive diagnostic modality; however, its invasive nature precludes its routine use for this purpose.

Both CT and ultrasound can accurately diagnose diverticulitis. CT has a sensitivity of up to 95% and specificity of 72%. Both modalities can also identify abscesses, making it possible for patients to have early drainage of these collections. CT is generally more available in most institutions and is substantially less operator dependent. CT findings such as presence of an abscess, extraluminal contrast, or air strongly suggest that conservative treatment with antibiotics will not be successful.

In many cases, patients with uncomplicated diverticulitis can be successfully treated as an outpatient with oral antibiotics. Such a regimen would not be appropriate for this patient because of his inability to tolerate a diet. Appropriate antibiotic therapy provides for coverage of usual colonic flora and is successful in resolving the acute episode at least 70% of the time. As the patient improves, he can be rapidly transitioned to oral antibiotics and discharged to home. If improvement does not occur within 3–4 days and imaging does not reveal an abscess that is amenable to percutaneous drainage, immediate surgical treatment should be considered. Primary anastomosis can be considered in this situation, depending on the degree of local inflammation. Resection and Hartman's procedure is the preferred approach if any doubt exists as to the quality of the bowel or the degree of inflammation in the peritoneal cavity.

Overall, recurrent episodes of diverticulitis can be expected to occur in approximately 25% of patients, with the majority of those who develop a second episode continuing on to a third if elective resection is not performed. This has led to the recommendation that resection of the diseased segment of colon be considered after a second bout of uncomplicated diverticulitis. Preoperative preparation should include imaging to determine the extent of disease so that an appropriate resection and primary anastomosis can be planned. A laparoscopic approach to these resections has become increasingly popular.

This patient differs from the typical victim of acute diverticulitis by his young age. Diverticulitis in patients less than 40 years of age is characterized by a course that is typically more virulent than in the older population.

Recurrence rates after a single episode of uncomplicated diverticulitis are extremely high. Medical treatment of the initial episode is just as likely to be successful, but elective resection is recommended after a single episode of diverticulitis in these patients.

BIBLIOGRAPHY

Angenete E, Thornell A, Burcharth J, et al. Laparoscopic lavage is feasible and safe for the treatment of perforated diverticulitis with purulent peritonitis: the first results from the randomized controlled trial DILALA. *Ann Surg.* 2016 Jan;263(1):117-22.

Bullard Dunn KM, Rothenberger DA. Colon, rectum, and anus. In: Brunicardi F, Andersen DK, Billiar TR, et al. (eds.), *Schwartz's Principles of Surgery*, 10th ed. New York, NY: McGraw-Hill; 2014.

Gearhart SL. Diverticular disease and common anorectal disorders. In: Longo DL, Fauci AS, Kasper DL, Hauser SL, Jameson J, Loscalzo J (eds.), *Harrison's Principles of Internal Medicine*, 18th ed. New York, NY: McGraw-Hill; 2012:Chapter 297.

Humes DJ, Solaymani-Dodaran M, Fleming KM, Simpson J, Spiller RC, West J. A population-based study of perforated diverticular disease incidence and associated mortality. *Gastroenterology* 2009;136(4):1198–1205.

Simpson J, Scholefield JH, Spiller RC. Pathogenesis of colonic diverticula [Review]. *Br J Surg* 2002;89(5):546–554.

18. **(B)** This patient's findings and clinical scenario are most consistent with acute colonic pseudo-obstruction (ACPO), also known as Ogilvie syndrome. This condition is defined by signs, symptoms, and radiographic findings of colonic obstruction without a mechanical cause. It can be seen in a wide variety of medical conditions, but the postoperative state is perhaps the most common and most relevant to surgical practice. Autonomic imbalances, either sympathetic excess or parasympathetic deficiency, are believed to be responsible.

The clinical scenario described earlier is typical of ACPO. In addition, patients may complain of abdominal pain, nausea, and vomiting. A water-soluble contrast enema should be performed to rule out an actual distal colonic obstruction and can be therapeutic if the cause is simply postoperative constipation. Cecal diameters of greater than 12 cm are associated with a high risk of perforation, and diameters of 9 cm or greater merit close observation. Subject to LaPlace's law, the cecum—with its inherently larger diameter—is the site where perforation typically occurs if treatment is not promptly undertaken.

Surgical intervention is reserved for perforation or patients who fail to respond to less invasive treatments or if progression to ischemic necrosis and perforation has occurred. Perforation carries a mortality rate as high as 50%.

The initial approach is typically conservative management consisting of NG decompression, correction of any electrolyte disturbances, limitation of narcotic medications, and close monitoring of progress with serial abdominal radiographs. Many patients will improve with these measures only. If they fail to do so within 24–48 hours or if their cecal diameter continues to increase to 12 cm or greater, intervention should be pursued.

There are two viable approaches to intervention if conservative management fails. The first is colonoscopic decompression. This must be undertaken with great care and minimal insufflation of gas, and the endoscope should be passed at least to the hepatic flexure to ensure adequate decompression of the cecum. Rectal tubes can be placed at this time as well, but they are often ineffective. Colonoscopy is highly effective, but recurrence rates are up to 15%.

Another approach is pharmacologic in nature. Neostigmine, a powerful parasympathetic agonist, can produce a rapid and dramatic return of colonic motility. Results are usually dramatic and durable and begin from 30 seconds to 10 minutes after administration. Life-threatening bradycardia can result, however, so this drug should be administered with cardiac monitoring and with atropine available at the bedside.

This patient has not yet undergone a trial of conservative therapy and shows no signs of impending perforation.

BIBLIOGRAPHY

Bullard Dunn KM, Rothenberger DA. Colon, rectum, and anus. In: Brunicardi F, Andersen DK, Billiar TR, et al. (eds.), *Schwartz's Principles of Surgery*, 10th ed. New York, NY: McGraw-Hill; 2014.
De Giorgio R, Knowles CH. Acute colonic pseudo-obstruction. *Br J Surg* 2009;96(3):229–239.
Ehrenpreis ED. Gut and hepatobiliary dysfunction. In: Hall JB, Schmidt GA, Wood LH (eds.), *Principles of Critical Care*, 3rd ed. New York, NY: McGraw-Hill; 2005:Chapter 81.
Valle RG, Godoy FL. Neostigmine for acute colonic pseudo-obstruction: a meta-analysis. *Ann Med Surg (Lond)* 2014;3(3):60–64.

19. **(C)** This patient has sigmoid volvulus. This disease is typically found in elderly males who are often institutionalized or have chronic medical conditions. Abdominal radiographs reveal a large loop of colon pointing toward the right upper quadrant. A gastrografin enema will show a "bird's beak" deformity but is not usually required to make the diagnosis.

Indications for emergent surgery include hematochezia, peritonitis, or free intraperitoneal air. In the absence of these findings, sigmoidoscopy—either rigid or flexible—should be performed. This confirms the diagnosis and allows for an assessment of the viability of the colonic mucosa in the affected segment. It is also therapeutic in approximately 85% of cases, as the volvulus is reduced by the endoscope. If successful reduction is achieved and the colonic mucosa appears viable the patient can undergo bowel preparation prior to sigmoid resection at this hospital admission. Sigmoid-sparing procedures such as colopexy and mesosigmoidoplasty have a high rate of recurrence, and conservative management alone has a recurrence rate of 30–90%, making resection the only viable option.

If the volvulus cannot be reduced by sigmoidoscopy or if ischemia is encountered with the endoscope, emergent resection is required. In this setting, or the setting of hematochezia, peritonitis, or free air, a Hartman's procedure should be performed, because the risk of a primary anastomosis in this setting would be unacceptable.

This patient does not display any findings indicating a need for emergent surgery.

BIBLIOGRAPHY

Bullard Dunn KM, Rothenberger DA. Colon, rectum, and anus. In: Brunicardi F, Andersen DK, Billiar TR, et al. (eds.), *Schwartz's Principles of Surgery*, 10th ed. New York, NY: McGraw-Hill; 2014.
Cappell MS, Friedel D. The role of sigmoidoscopy and colonoscopy in the diagnosis and management of lower gastrointestinal disorders: endoscopic findings, therapy and complications. *Med Clin North Am* 2002;86(6):1253–1288.
Halabi WJ, Jafari MD, Kang CY, et al. Colonic volvulus in the United States: trends, outcomes, and predictors of mortality. *Ann Surg* 2014;259(2):293–301.
Sclabas GM, Sarosi GA, Khan S, Sarr MG, Behrns KE. Small bowel obstruction. In: Zinner MJ, Ashley SW (eds.), *Maingot's Abdominal Operations*, 12th ed. New York, NY: McGraw-Hill; 2013:Chapter 29.

20. **(B)** Colonic ischemia, also referred to as ischemic colitis, is the most frequent form of mesenteric ischemia, accounting for 75% of all intestinal ischemia and affecting primarily the elderly. Ischemic injury to the colon usually occurs as a consequence of a sudden and transient reduction in blood flow, resulting in a low-flow state. In the majority of cases, a specific occluding anatomic lesion cannot be identified.

In general, clinical factors that predispose to ischemic colitis fall into three major categories: arterial compromise, venous compromise, and vasospasm. The clinical presentations vary from transient abdominal pain indicative of mild ischemia after cardiopulmonary bypass to frank perforation as a result of transmural ischemia because of overdistension caused by obstruction or *C difficile* colitis.

Although it may occur anywhere, colonic ischemia most commonly affects the so-called watershed areas with a limited collateral blood supply, and the most common location is the splenic flexure (see Fig. 28-17).

The diagnosis of ischemic colitis is frequently clinical, and signs and symptoms range from diarrhea to frank peritonitis, reflecting the degree of bowel ischemia.

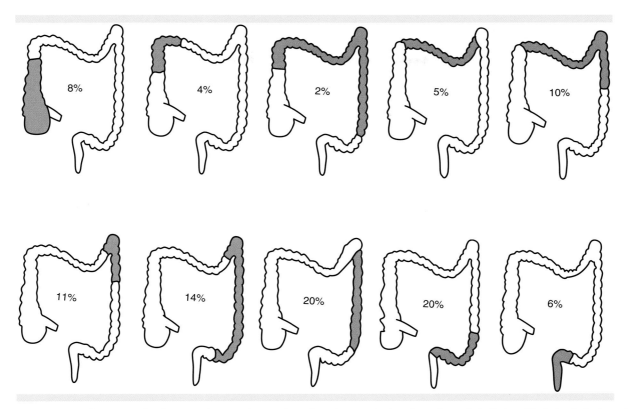

FIGURE 28-17. Distributions of colonic ischemia. Reproduced with permission from Brandt L, Boley SJ. Colonic ischemia. *Surg Clin North Am* 1992;72:212. Copyright Elsevier.

Initial management includes adequate resuscitation and optimization of hemodynamics with avoidance of vasopressors. Plain radiographs are typically obtained early in the evaluation and can provide valuable information, especially in excluding other potential etiologies. Findings of pneumatosis or of portal venous gas are indicative of gangrenous ischemia and suggest a poor prognosis. CT findings are nonspecific and include wall thickening and pericolic fat stranding. Sigmoidoscopy shows dark, hemorrhagic mucosa but carries a high risk of perforation and is therefore relatively contraindicated.

Patients with peritoneal signs or evidence of clinical instability that could be attributed to colonic ischemia should be taken urgently to the operating room for exploration. Long-term complications include stricture and chronic ischemia, and long-term follow up-with colonoscopy is advised.

BIBLIOGRAPHY

Bullard Dunn KM, Rothenberger DA. Colon, rectum, and anus. In: Brunicardi F, Andersen DK, Billiar TR, et al. (eds.), *Schwartz's Principles of Surgery*, 10th ed. New York, NY: McGraw-Hill; 2014.
Stoffel EM, Greenberger NJ. Mesenteric vascular disease. In: Greenberger NJ, Blumberg RS, Burakoff R (eds.), *Current Diagnosis &* *Treatment: Gastroenterology, Hepatology, & Endoscopy*, 2nd ed. New York, NY: McGraw-Hill; 2012:Chapter 6.

21. **(C)**

22. **(A)**

Explanation for questions 21 and 22

Figure 28-2 reveals an anal fissure. The history of an acute anal fissure is usually sudden anal pain after defecation that might be described as a tearing sensation and minimal bright red bleeding. Chronic anal fissures present with a variable degree of pain, frequently along with symptoms of pruritus, a lump in the anal area, and drainage. The pain may cease shortly after bowel movements but may persist for hours. If biopsied, the fissure will only show evidence of nonspecific inflammatory change and fibrosis through the internal sphincter; however, if a fissure appears atypical, is recurrent, or is persistent, then biopsy of the edge of the fissure is appropriate. Examination in the office should be visual observation with the buttocks gently spread, because anoscopy may cause severe pain. The fissure is a crack, or split, in the lining of the anal canal that extends to various degrees up to the dentate line. The fissure may be heralded by a classic

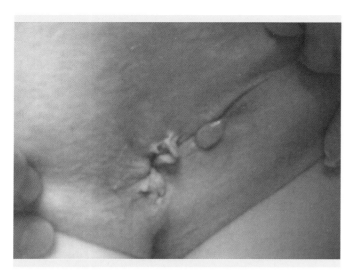

FIGURE 28-18. Posterior anal skin tag.

finding of a sentinel pile or skin tag (see Fig. 28-18) at the anal verge.

Eighty to ninety percent of fissures are located in the posterior midline, 10–15% are located in the anterior midline, and 1–2% are located elsewhere. Women might present with anterior fissures because of laxity of the anterior external sphincter secondary to child bearing. Acute anal fissures can be successfully treated with conservative measures such as a high-fiber diet with 25–35 g of fiber intake a day, increasing nonalcoholic, noncaffeinated fluids to 64 oz a day, and application of topical nitrites. Topical trinitrate in glycerin can provide pain relief and relaxation of the internal sphincter. The patient should be instructed to wear gloves because the topical nitrites can cause headache if systemically absorbed through the skin. Calcium channel blockers, such as nifedipine and diltiazem, offer an alternative in topical treatment of anal fissures. They have equivalent efficacy to nitrates with fewer associated side effects, particularly headaches. Stool softeners and sitz baths can also provide some relief. Botulinum toxin type A (Botox) is an additional method of chemical sphincterotomy. The cost is high; however, the injection acts by blocking the release of acetylcholine at the presynaptic membrane and allowing the sphincter to relax out of spasm. The effects may last up to 3 months, which may be enough time for the fissure to heal. It can be equivalent to pharmacologic methods, approaching 50% initial healing rates. It requires minimal effort by patients. Some transient incontinence has been reported.

If conservative measures fail, as with the patient in this case, the surgical procedure of choice is an open or closed lateral internal anal sphincterotomy. The internal sphincter has the involuntary action of maintaining the anal canal resting pressure. The internal sphincter may be partially divided without fear of significant incontinence if the external sphincter is spared. The open and closed methods are comparable and may be done under local anesthesia in an outpatient setting. The distal one-third to one-half of the internal sphincter is divided.

Complications are minimal, with anal fistula occurring in 1–2% and abscess in 2–3%. In the setting of refractory fissure or failure to heal, inflammatory bowel disease must be considered as well as adenocarcinoma causing atypical anal canal fissure and other malignancy such as basaloid or cloacogenic cancer. Biopsy would be appropriate with refractory of atypical fissures.

Anoscopy with dilation has no role in therapy because of the high rate of postoperative incontinence from 2 to 24% as the external fibers are also stretched. Incision and drainage with seton placement is indicated with a perirectal abscess with a transphincteric fistula. Fistulotomy with debridement should be considered in a superficial anal fistula.

BIBLIOGRAPHY

Cameron JL. *Current Surgical Therapy*, 10th ed. Baltimore, MD: Elsevier Saunders; 2011:230–233.

Corman ML. *Colon and Rectal Surgery*. Philadelphia, PA: Lippincott Williams & Wilkins; 2005:255–277.

Gordon PH, Nivatvongs S. *Principles and Practice of Surgery for the Colon, Rectum and Anus*, 3rd ed. St. Louis, MO: Quality Medical Publishing; 2006:167–187.

23. **(B)** The patient in Question 23 has pruritus ani. Pruritus ani is a very common malady. Itching and burning are often the presenting complaints with reddened, irritated anoderm and surrounding skin on examination. Most patients are not found to have an associated anorectal pathology, but contact dermatitis, yeast, diabetes, and pinworms (*Enterobius vermicularis*) have been associated with pruritus ani. Psoriasis of the anal verge must also be considered in the differential diagnosis. Certain foods such as cola, coffee, and tea have been suggested to promote pruritus. Reassurance of the patient that this is a manageable entity is paramount. Diphenhydramine may help with initial severe itching. A detailed history about toilet habits, bowel regiments, perianal hygiene, operations, medications, and diet should be asked. No special studies have been helpful in the diagnosis, although a lower threshold for internal sphincter relaxation has been observed in continence testing. Evaluation should consist of perineal exam, anoscopy, and proctosigmoidoscopy to evaluate for local cause, such as a draining fistula, if suspicion is high. Most diagnosis is based on visual inspection. Conservative therapy with daily gentle cleansing of plain water, drying lightly with

encouragement not to rub aggressively, and topical application of a mild- to moderate-potency corticosteroid alleviates symptoms in most cases. Remove all irritants including all soaps and harsh toilet paper. Control seepage and leakage by starting the patient on a bulking agent and high-fiber diet.

Biopsy will only reveal localized inflammation, although skin scrapings can be used with a potassium hydroxide prep to evaluate for yeast. Wide local excision and colonic diversion have no place in the therapy for pruritus ani.

BIBLIOGRAPHY

Cameron JL. *Current Surgical Therapy*, 10th ed. Baltimore, MD: Elsevier Saunders; 2011:243–246.

Corman ML. *Colon and Rectal Surgery*. Philadelphia, PA: Lippincott Williams & Wilkins; 2005:606–608.

Gordon PH, Nivatvongs S. *Principles and Practice of Surgery for the Colon, Rectum and Anus*, 3rd ed. St. Louis, MO: Quality Medical Publishing; 2006:247–258.

24. **(A)** Anal canal carcinoma is by definition located in the area bounded inferiorly by the anal verge and proximally by the puborectalis muscle that is located approximately 2 cm above the dentate line (see Fig. 28-19). The anal canal is lined distally by non–hair-bearing nonkeratanized, stratified squamous epithelium up to the dentate line. The 1.5- to 2-cm proximal anal canal above the dentate line is first lined with cloacal (transitional) and then glandular mucosal epithelium. Cephalad to the proximal margin of the anal canal is the rectum proper. The rectum is lined with columnar mucosa. Lateral and caudad to the anal verge is the anal margin that is covered by keratinized, hair-bearing, stratified squamous epithelium. Anal canal lesions are managed differently than anal margin lesions (see Question 28).

Anal canal cancer may present with nonspecific symptoms of difficulty with defecation, hematochezia, and different degrees of pain ranging from severe to minor discomfort. There frequently is a delay in diagnosis because of misdiagnosis with benign anal canal conditions such as hemorrhoids or fissures. Patients with persistent or unexplained complaints of pain, bleeding, tenesmus, or frequency should undergo a full perianal skin examination as well as anal canal, rectum, and perineum examination. The inguinal and femoral lymph nodes should be palpated for fullness or matting. A mass or fissure should be fully evaluated. A deep wedge biopsy or punch biopsy for more superficial lesions will be sufficient to make the diagnosis of cancer. Endoscopic ultrasound (EUS) is accurate for staging of anal canal carcinoma. Squamous cell carcinoma is the most common cancer of the anal canal.

Surgical therapy for anal canal carcinoma had historically been abdominal perineal resection with local recurrence rate of 50% and 5-year survival rates of approximately 40%. Dr. Norman Nigro from Wayne State University proposed a multimodality therapy for anal canal cancer, which is now considered standard of care with minimal modifications. Once the diagnosis of

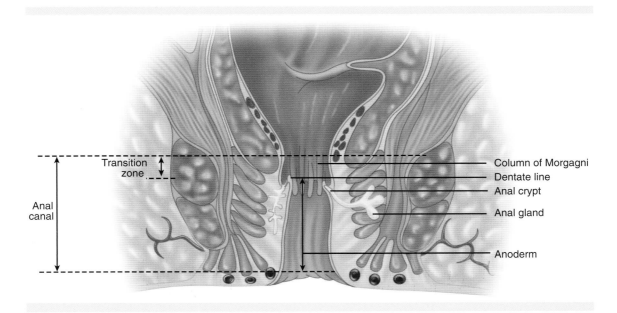

FIGURE 28-19. Layers of the rectum. Reproduced with permission from Goldberg SM, Gordon PH, Nivatvongs S (eds). In: *Essentials of Anorectal Surgery*. Philadelphia: J.B. Lippincott Company, 1980.

squamous cell carcinoma of the anal canal is made, the patient is treated with chemoradiation therapy using 5-fluorouracil, mitomycin C, and pelvic irradiation of 50 Gy. Follow-up anal biopsy 6–8 weeks after completion of therapy is frequently performed. If there is residual cancer, then second-line chemotherapy with completion radiation is initiated. Cisplatin is being evaluated as a second-line chemotherapeutic agent. A 90% complete response can be quoted with an 85% 5-year survival rate. Salvage abdominal perineal resection is offered only after second-line chemoradiation fails, with a long-term survival of 50%. Initial surgical resection might be adequate with very superficial well-differentiated squamous cell carcinoma that is confined above the submucosa.

BIBLIOGRAPHY

Brunicardi F, Andersen D, Billiar T, et al. (eds.). *Schwartz's Principles of Surgery*, 9th ed. New York, NY: McGraw-Hill; 2009:1053–1054.
Cameron JL. *Current Surgical Therapy*, 10th ed. Baltimore, MD: Elsevier Saunders; 2011:199–200.
Corman ML. *Colon and Rectal Surgery*. Philadelphia, PA: Lippincott Williams & Wilkins; 2005:1066–1079.
Gordon PH, Nivatvongs S. *Principles and Practice of Surgery for the Colon, Rectum and Anus*, 3rd ed. St. Louis, MO: Quality Medical Publishing; 2006:379–385.

25. **(A)** EUS provides an image of the sphincter mechanisms of the anus and the muscle and soft tissue of the rectum. The image is two dimensional and accurate. It can also be used in fecal continence evaluation and provides information with regard to complex fistulas, surveillance for anal cancers, and other congenital or acquired malformation of the rectum and anus. In a normal EUS, there are five distinct layers of the anal canal or rectum. The innermost hyperechoic region is the mucosal surface, followed by the hypoechoic mucosal/muscularis mucosa. The next hyperechoic region is the submucosa, followed by the hypoechoic muscularis propria. The most distant hyperechoic region is the serosa or perirectal fat. EUS is widely used for staging of rectal cancers. EUS can predict lymph node involvement with an accuracy of 62–85%. Most incorrect staging is because of overstaging of a cancer. Experience in interpretation can increase accuracy. Pelvic CT is a poor predictor of depth in rectal cancer. Endoluminal magnetic resonance imaging and EUS have similar accuracy, but EUS is far more cost-effective and accessible.

BIBLIOGRAPHY

Beck DE, Wexner SD. *Fundamentals of Anorectal Surgery*. London, United Kingdom: W.B. Saunders; 1998:286–290.

Cameron JL. *Current Surgical Therapy*, 10th ed. Baltimore, MD: Elsevier Saunders; 2011:189–190.
Corman ML. *Colon and Rectal Surgery*. Philadelphia, PA: Lippincott Williams & Wilkins; 2005:915–919.

26. **(C)** Hemorrhoids are formed at an embryonic level as highly vascular cushions in the anal canal that become engorged with blood during defecation, protecting the anal canal from trauma due to passage of stool. Hemorrhoids are usually referred to as pathologic once they prolapse or bleed. The pathophysiology of hemorrhoid development may occur secondarily to elevated anal sphincter pressures, abnormal dilation of the internal hemorrhoidal venous plexus, distention of the arteriovenous anastomosis, prolapse of the cushions and surrounding adjacent tissues, or a combination of these factors. Squamous epithelial change and darkened mucosa may form with chronic symptoms. Hemorrhoids are designated external or internal depending on whether they originate above or below the dentate line.

External hemorrhoids are located distal to the dentate line. They are sensitive to pain and heat sensation and are of ectodermal origin. Thrombosed external hemorrhoids may present with exquisite pain. Although conservative therapy is described, excision under local anesthesia may be indicated for acute thrombosed external hemorrhoids (Table 28-5).

Internal hemorrhoids are further broken down into stage, grade, or degree—all describing degree of prolapse from 1 to 4, depending on the amount of prolapse. Table 28-5 describes the four stages of hemorrhoids with options for management. In general, first- and second-degree hemorrhoids respond to medical management. Hemorrhoids that fail to respond to medical management may be treated with elastic rubber band ligation, sclerosis, or excisional hemorrhoidectomy. First-, second-, and select third degree hemorrhoids can be treated with rubber band ligation while third- and fourth-degree hemorrhoids are treated with hemorrhoidectomy. Stapled procedure or hemorrhoidopexy can be considered for third-degree circumferential hemorrhoids or mucosal prolapse.

All anal or rectal bleeding must be investigated to rule out cancer and other rectal and colonic lesions. Flexible sigmoidoscopy, colonoscopy, and barium enema are all methods of investigation of unanswered questions of etiology of lower gastrointestinal bleeding.

BIBLIOGRAPHY

Cameron JL. *Current Surgical Therapy*, 10th ed. Baltimore, MD: Elsevier Saunders; 2011:223–229.
Doherty GM. *Current Diagnosis and Treatment: Surgery*. New York, NY: McGraw-Hill; 2006:707–709.

TABLE 28-5 Four Stages of Internal Hemorrhoids and Thrombosed External Hemorrhoids With Options for Management

Stage/Grade/Degree	Signs and Symptoms	Management
One	Small amounts of painless bleeding No prolapse	Fully investigate other causes of bleeding Increase intake of fluids and dietary fiber to 20–25 g Infrared coagulation Rubber band ligation Electrocautery
Two	Protrusion noticed with defecation; spontaneous reduction Mild to moderate bleeding; blood streaked on stool	Increase intake of fluids and dietary fiber to 20–35 g Rubber band ligation Infrared coagulation Electrocautery
Three	Protrusion requiring manual reduction with defecation or straining	Rubber band ligation
	Mild to moderate bleeding; blood streaked on stool	Open or closed hemorrhoidectomy Stapled procedure for circumferential hemorrhoids or rectal mucosal prolapse
Four	Irreducible and permanently prolapsed hemorrhoid Mild to moderate bleeding; blood streaked on stool	Open or closed hemorrhoidectomy
Thrombosed external hemorrhoids	Exquisite tenderness Edematous, grapelike, irreducible hemorrhoid	Local anesthesia with lidocaine Excision or conservative therapy

Gordon PH, Nivatvongs S. *Principles and Practice of Surgery for the Colon, Rectum and Anus*, 3rd ed. St. Louis, MO: Quality Medical Publishing; 2006:143–166.

Schwartz SI. *Principles of Surgery*, 9th ed. New York, NY: McGraw-Hill; 2010:1057–1059.

27. **(E)** Anal canal tumors account for 1.5% of GI tract malignancies. Melanoma, carcinoid, and mucinous adenocarcinoma are often found incidentally with hemorrhoids on pathologic examination. Wide local excision is appropriate for most anal canal lesions. Aggressive initial surgical resection, such as abdominal perineal resection, has been found to have no survival benefit. The prognosis is often poor for melanoma and mucinous adenocarcinoma no matter what the surgical approach, so wide local excision is the surgical treatment of choice, after biopsy, for local control. Carcinoid of the anal canal is rare and can be adequately treated with wide local excision for lesions less than 2 cm. Squamous cell carcinoma is the most common cancer of the anal canal. These cancers are usually associated with chronic human papillomavirus. Squamous cell carcinoma of the anal canal should be treated in accordance to the Nigro protocol (see Question 24). Squamous cell carcinoma of the anal canal has over a 90% cure rate with initial chemoradiation treatment; abdominal perineal resection is only indicated for failure of second-line salvage chemotherapy. Condyloma of the anal canal should be fulgurated with electrocautery or bipolar cautery leaving the anoderm intact. Wide local excision of condyloma in the anal canal is unnecessary and carries a risk of anal stricture.

Figure 28-20 demonstrates a less than 3-cm anal canal mass biopsied as glandular carcinoma. Figure 28-21 is the wide local excision specimen.

BIBLIOGRAPHY

Cameron JL. *Current Surgical Therapy*, 10th ed. Baltimore, MD: Elsevier Saunders; 2011:196–200.

Corman ML. *Colon and Rectal Surgery*. Philadelphia, PA: Lippincott Williams & Wilkins; 2005:1063–1072.

Doherty GM. *Current Diagnosis and Treatment: Surgery*. New York, NY: McGraw-Hill; 2006:721–723.

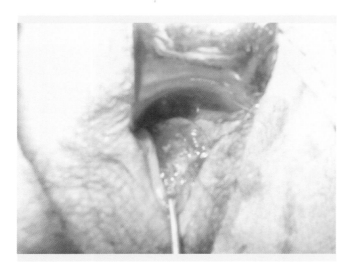

FIGURE 28-20. A 2.5-cm anal canal lesion.

28. **(E)** The anal margin lesions listed in this question have distinctly different pathologic findings, but wide local excision can be used for adequate surgical resection.

Melanoma of the anal margin is found on incidental hemorrhoidectomy at times. Bleeding is the overwhelming presenting complaint in 66% of patients with perianal melanoma. The anal margin melanoma may present as a small benign-looking grapelike growth. Because anal margin melanoma has a very poor prognosis with only a 10–20% survival at 5 years, abdominal perineal resection has not been found to improve survival; thus, wide local excision of perianal melanoma is the standard of care. Perianal Bowen disease is uncommon, with very few cases reported to date. Bowen disease is an intraepithelial squamous cell carcinoma *in situ*. Bowen perianal disease

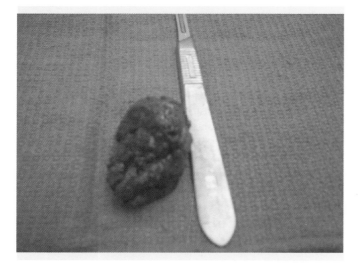

FIGURE 28-21. The excised 2.5-cm anal canal lesion from Fig. 28-20.

can present with symptoms such as burning, itching, and bleeding. The lesions appear eczematous with scaly and crusted plaques. Wide local excision is the surgical treatment of choice. Perianal Paget disease is a rare adenocarcinoma believed to come from apocrine cells. Noninvasive Paget disease can adequately be treated with wide local excision. Basal cell carcinoma of the anal margin is a very rare entity consisting of less than 0.2% of anal margin cancers and can be adequately treated with wide local excision.

BIBLIOGRAPHY

Cameron JL. *Current Surgical Therapy*, 10th ed. Baltimore, MD: Elsevier Saunders; 2011:196–200.
Corman ML. *Colon and Rectal Surgery*. Philadelphia, PA: Lippincott Williams & Wilkins; 2005:1063–1065.
Doherty GM. *Current Diagnosis and Treatment: Surgery*. New York, NY: McGraw-Hill; 2006:721–722.

29. **(C)** The anal canal and the rectum have very different embryologic origin, innervation, and lymphatic and venous drainage. Table 28-6 reviews the difference in the anal canal and the rectum. The anal canal is located below the dentate line and is ectodermal in origin. The anal canal is very sensitive to pain and accounts for complaints of pain with thrombosed external hemorrhoids. The lining of the anus is squamous epithelium. The venous drainage of the anal canal is systemic, and the primary lymphatic basin is inguinal. The most common neoplasm is squamous cell carcinoma. The distal rectum

TABLE 28-6 Physiologic and Embryonic Differences Between the Anal Canal and the Rectum

	Anal Canal	Rectum
Embryonic origin	Ectoderm	Endoderm
Pain/sensation	Sensitive to pain	Insensitive to pain
Cell type	Squamous epithelium	Glandular mucosa
Venous drainage	Systemic	Portal
Lymphatic drainage	Inguinal lymph nodes	Superior hemorrhoidal followed by para-aortic lymph nodes
Most common neoplasm	Squamous cell carcinoma	Adenocarcinoma

is located above the dentate line. There are no sharp pain receptors in the rectum, although stretch is felt. The rectum is lined with glandular mucosa. The venous drainage of the rectum is via the portal system. The rectal lymphatics drain into the superior hemorrhoidal lymph node basin and then to the para-aortic lymph nodes. Adenocarcinoma is the most common neoplasia of the rectum.

BIBLIOGRAPHY

Corman ML. *Colon and Rectal Surgery*. Philadelphia, PA: Lippincott Williams & Wilkins; 2005:10–30.

Doherty GM. *Current Diagnosis and Treatment: Surgery*. New York, NY: McGraw-Hill; 2006:698–700.

Gordon PH, Nivatvongs S. *Principles and Practice of Surgery for the Colon, Rectum and Anus*, 3rd ed. St. Louis, MO: Quality Medical Publishing; 2006:4–27.

30. **(A)** Perirectal (or perianal) abscess is the most common type of anorectal abscess accounting for 40–45% of cases reported. Figure 28-4 reveals chronic external fistula with surrounding erythema. Physical examination reveals fluctuance around the fistula in this case. The patient usually complains of pain and fevers, and examination can reveal fluctuance, erythema, and cellulitis. Erythema may also be present without fluctuance; however, more often than not, an abscess is still present, and incision and drainage is still required for treatment. If there is question of abscess, the erythematous or indurated area may be needle aspirated under local anesthesia. Etiology of perirectal abscess and fistula has been theorized to be related to infected anal crypts. Perirectal abscess is also seen with some frequency in patients with HIV and Crohn disease. Anorectal abscesses can be perirectal (perianal), ischiorectal, postanal, intersphincteric, and supralevator (see Fig. 28-22). Superficial perianal abscesses can usually be incised and drained under local anesthesia as an office procedure. Usually, minimal to no packing is required as long as incision is wide enough and skin edges are trimmed to prevent premature closure. Postprocedure care should include frequent sitz baths and good hygiene. Antibiotics are usually unnecessary unless there is excessive cellulitis with fevers and leukocytosis in an immunocompromised patient. More complex anorectal abscesses may require general or spinal anesthesia for patient comfort and adequate exposure. Perianal abscess is often seen in patients with leukemia, lymphoma, and granulocytopenia representing up to 8% of hematology admissions. The usual presenting complaint is that of pain, but fever, septicemia, and shock might also be present in a leukopenic patient. Fluctuance and pus may not be present. These patients are managed medically initially with antibiotic therapy and sitz baths until the hematologic disease can be better

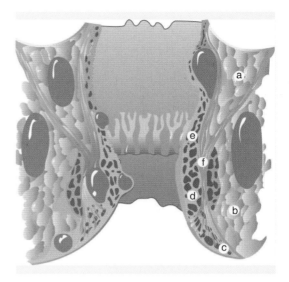

FIGURE 28-22. (*a*) Supralevator space. (*b*) Ischiorectal space. (*c*) Perianal/subcutaneous space. (*d*) Marginal/mucocutaneous space. (*e*) Submucous space. (*f*) Intramuscular space. From Doherty GM (ed.). *Current Diagnosis & Treatment: Surgery*, 13th ed. New York, NY: McGraw-Hill; 2010:Chapter 31, Fig. 31-5.

controlled. Fulminant sepsis, poor wound healing, and higher mortality rate can occur if operative intervention is undertaken without first initializing supportive therapy. However, operative intervention might be required for persistent abscess without resolution of symptoms with medical management.

BIBLIOGRAPHY

Cameron JL. *Current Surgical Therapy*, 10th ed. Baltimore, MD: Elsevier Saunders; 2011:233–236.

Corman MI, Allison SI, Kuehne JP. *Handbook of Colon and Rectal Surgery*. Philadelphia, PA: Lippincott Williams & Wilkins; 2002: 150–160.

Doherty GM. *Current Diagnosis and Treatment: Surgery*. New York, NY: McGraw-Hill; 2006:712–714.

31. **(B)**

32. **(A)**

Explanation for questions 31 and 32

Perianal abscess and fistula-in-ano can occur synchronously in many cases. Patients who return with recurrent abscess after frequent incision and drainage require an examination under anesthesia for possible fistula.

Figure 28-23 reveals a transphincteric fistula that extends radially from an opening just anterior to the transverse line. Goodsall's rule describes the common

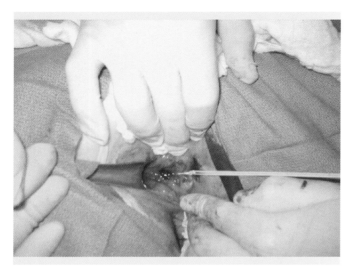

FIGURE 28-23. Deep transphincteric fistula involving a significant amount of internal and external sphincter muscle.

characteristics of the fistula-in-ano tract: when the external opening of the fistula tract lies anterior to the transverse plane, the opening tends to be located radially. When the external opening lies posterior to the transverse plane, the internal opening is usually located in the posterior midline (see Figs. 28-23 and 28-24). Exceptions to the rule can occur, so rigorous evaluation of the anal

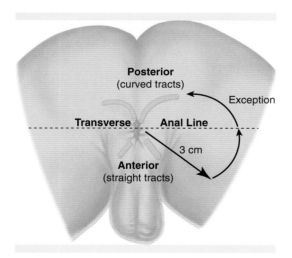

FIGURE 28-24. Goodsall's rule for fistula-in-ano tract: When external opening is anterior to transverse plane, internal opening is tends to be located radially. When external opening is posterior to transverse plane, internal opening tends to be located in posterior midline. From Brunicardi F, Andersen D, Billiar T, et al. (eds.). *Schwartz's Principles of Surgery*, 9th ed. New York, NY: McGraw-Hill; 2009:Fig. 29-39.

canal for the internal opening is paramount. Vigorous probing can create a fistula and should be discouraged.

The internal opening of the fistula tract can be difficult to identify and might require injection of hydrogen peroxide into the external tract to visualize the internal opening. A hypodermic syringe is filled with 3% hydrogen peroxide, and a 20-gauge soft angiocatheter without the needle trocar is attached to the syringe. The external opening of the fistula is cannulized with the angiocatheter, and the hypodermic needle is gently compressed while the retracted anal canal is being closely scrutinized for evidence of bubbling out of the internal opening. Other methods such as milk and dye have been used with less than optimal results. Fistula can be classified as intersphincteric, transphincteric, suprasphincteric, extrasphincteric (trauma), and horseshoe.

Intersphincteric fistula can usually be treated with fistulotomy if superficial. More complex fistula including transphincteric might require noncutting seton placement for preservation of the external and internal sphincter complex. Cutting setons are rarely used due to damage of the sphincter muscle and risk of incontinence. Figure 28-24 reveals a deep transphincteric fistula involving a significant amount of internal and external sphincter muscle. A vessel loop has been passed through the fistula tract after exposing the internal and external opening. The skin was opened and the superficial portion of the tract debrided. The seton will be tightened at weekly intervals until the fistula tract has healed with preservation of the muscle complex.

Other options for treatment of deep fistulas include usage of an anorectal advancement flap to close the internal opening. Figure 28-25 shows a completed

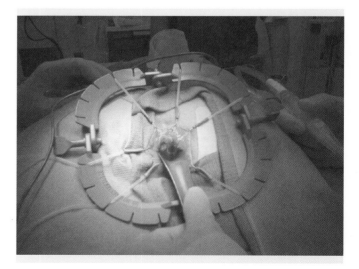

FIGURE 28-25. Completed anorectal advancement flap fully covering the internal opening of a chronic fistula.

anorectal advancement flap fully covering the internal opening of a chronic fistula. A lone-star retractor is ideal for exposure in reconstructive anal surgery.

Horseshoe fistulas tunnel through extensive soft tissue, most commonly the deep postanal space into the ischioanal fossa. A deep postanal abscess in association with the fistula must be opened, the granulation tissue must be debrided, and the area must be drained. In the Hanley procedure, the internal anal sphincter is divided in the posterior midline (or seton placed in the modified Hanley) in order to drain the infection. Counter incisions are also required over the ischioanal fossa. This approach will decrease the morbidity associated with a large perianal wound that would result if the entire fistula were opened in entirety.

BIBLIOGRAPHY

Cameron JL. *Current Surgical Therapy*, 10th ed. Baltimore, MD: Elsevier Saunders; 2011:235–250.

Corman ML. *Colon and Rectal Surgery*. Philadelphia, PA: Lippincott Williams & Wilkins; 2005:295–332.

Doherty GM. *Current Diagnosis and Treatment Surgery*. New York, NY: McGraw-Hill; 2006:712–714.

Gordon PH, Nivatvongs S. *Principles and Practice of Surgery for the Colon, Rectum and Anus*, 3rd ed. St. Louis, MO: Quality Medical Publishing; 2006:191–230.

33. **(A)** Rectovaginal fistula most often occurs following trauma, including obstetric injury with up to 5% third- and fourth-degree laceration. Inflammatory bowel disease is the second most common cause. Other well-known causes include foreign body, radiation, infectious processes, diverticulitis, carcinoma, congenital, or any type of pelvic, perineal, and rectal surgery. The fistula can be described as low or high rectal depending on the location of the rectal opening. Anovaginal fistulas can also be observed. Low rectovaginal fistulas usually are identified on physical examination. A midlevel or high rectovaginal fistula might be hard to identify. A barium enema could possibly assist with identification of the fistula if unable to readily see the internal vaginal opening. Other options include a methylene blue retention enema with endovaginal tampon in place. After an hour, the tampon is removed and inspected for blue coloring. A fistulogram might assist in identifying the segment of bowel involved. Inspection of the proximal colon should be strongly considered before deciding on therapy.

Repair of high rectovaginal fistulas is approached transabdominally. The bowel involved is resected or repaired (for obstetrical injury), and a piece of omentum or fascia is interposed between the repair and the vaginal wall.

TABLE 28-7 TNM Staging System for Anal Canal Cancers

T1	Tumor <2 cm
T2	Tumor 2–5 cm
T3	Tumor >5 cm
T4	Tumor of any size invading adjacent organs (vagina, urethra, bladder)
N0	Tumor not involved with regional lymph nodes
N1	Metastasis in perirectal lymph node(s)
N2	Metastasis in unilateral internal iliac and/or inguinal lymph node(s)
N3	Metastasis in perirectal and inguinal lymph nodes and/or bilateral internal iliac and/or inguinal lymph nodes
M0	No distant metastasis
M1	Distant metastasis

Low rectovaginal fistulas can be approached either transvaginally in layers with a vaginal flap, transanally with an endorectal advancement flap, or perineal. Fistulotomy alone should be avoided, because there is usually a degree of full-thickness muscle involved, which could cause some incontinence. Fibrin glue alone has not been effective in long-term treatment of rectovaginal fistula.

BIBLIOGRAPHY

Cameron JL. *Current Surgical Therapy*, 10th ed. Baltimore, MD: Elsevier Saunders; 2011:250–255.

Corman ML. *Colon and Rectal Surgery*. Philadelphia, PA: Lippincott Williams & Wilkins; 2005:333–345.

Gordon PH, Nivatvongs S. *Principles and Practice of Surgery for the Colon, Rectum and Anus*, 3rd ed. St. Louis, MO: Quality Medical Publishing; 2006:333–351.

34. **(B)** Anal canal cancer is staged differently than rectal cancer. The TNM classification is outlined in Table 28-7, and the stage groups are outlined in Table 28-8. Stage I anal canal cancer is a small lesion less than 2 cm without

TABLE 28-8 Staging Groups for Anal Canal Cancer

	TNM
Stage I	T1N0M0
Stage II	T2N0M0, T3N0M0
Stage III	Any T, N1, M0
Stage IV	Any T, any N, M1

regional nodal involvement or distant metastatic disease. Stage II anal canal cancer is any T2 or T3 lesion without nodal involvement or distant metastatic disease. Stage III anal canal is any size lesion with regional lymph node involvement and no distant metastasis. Stage IV disease is any size lesion with or without regional lymph node involvement in the presence of distant metastasis. The liver is the most common site of distant metastasis. The average survival for a patient who presents with liver metastasis is 9 months. Squamous cell (or epidermoid) carcinoma makes up the majority of the anal canal cancers followed by transitional (cloacogenic) cell and adenocarcinoma. Melanoma occurs in 0.5% of all tumors of the anorectum. Stage I–III squamous cell carcinoma has reported 5-year survival rates approaching 85% if treated with combination chemoradiation, even with locally advanced disease.

BIBLIOGRAPHY

Doherty GM. *Current Diagnosis and Treatment: Surgery*. New York, NY: McGraw-Hill; 2006:721–723.

Gordon PH, Nivatvongs S. *Principles and Practice of Surgery for the Colon, Rectum and Anus*, 3rd ed. St. Louis, MO: Quality Medical Publishing; 2006:371–373.

Schwartz SI. *Principles of Surgery*, 9th ed. New York, NY: McGraw-Hill; 2010:1053–1054.

35. **(E)** Anorectal manometry is a valuable tool in the complicated diagnosis and treatment of fecal incontinence. It is difficult to get an actual number measuring the extent of anal incontinence, but it appears to have an incidence of 2.2%. Most patients are women over the age of 65; however, etiology can include surgical, obstetrical, congenital anomalies, colorectal disease, and neurologic conditions. Fistula surgery and internal anal sphincterotomy can cause partial fecal incontinence as well as hemorrhoidal surgery. Understanding the mechanisms of the internal sphincter and the external sphincter is paramount to being able to diagnose and treat anal incontinence. The internal sphincter is composed of smooth muscle and is a continuation of the circular muscle of the rectum. The internal sphincter stays at near-maximal contraction at all times and relaxes in response to rectal distention. The external anal sphincter is composed of striated muscle and enables voluntary contraction. The response of the external sphincter to stimuli is contraction. The external sphincter must have voluntary inhibition of contraction. Anorectal manometry can be accomplished by any of the following methods: macro and micro balloons and open or closed catheters. There is no universally accepted method for collecting and analyzing data. Only a physician who has been trained to perform and interpret the results should evaluate the data obtained. Anorectal manometry, when used in conjunction with the balloon expulsion test or photodefecography, is useful in evaluation of anorectal dysfunction including anorectal sensation, rectal compliance, and assessment of anal muscle tone. Slow waves, ultraslow waves, and intermediate waveforms might be obtained during testing.

BIBLIOGRAPHY

Corman ML. *Colon and Rectal Surgery*. Philadelphia, PA: Lippincott Williams & Wilkins; 2005:357–359.

Doherty GM. *Current Diagnosis and Treatment: Surgery*. New York, NY: McGraw-Hill; 2006:701–703.

Gordon PH, Nivatvongs S. *Principles and Practice of Surgery for the Colon, Rectum and Anus*, 3rd ed. St. Louis, MO: Quality Medical Publishing; 2006:50–53.

36. **(B)** Colon and rectal cancer comprise 13% of all cancers in the United States. Rectal cancer is staged according to guidelines for colon cancer with the TNM staging. Table 28-9 is a review of the TNM staging system. Rectal cancer presents most commonly with bleeding (35–40%). Diarrhea, change in bowel habits, rectal mass, and abdominal pain have also been reported at presentation. Biopsy is mandatory and is usually done at diagnosis of the lesion. The histology of the cancer is primarily adenocarcinoma. Surgical treatment of carcinoma of the rectum could include abdominal perineal resection, low anterior resection, transanal excision, colostomy or ileostomy, and many other procedures depending on the stage of the lesion at diagnosis including presence of metastatic disease. Preoperative staging includes physical examination of the rectum and perineum, EUS or pelvic MRI to evaluate for regional lymphadenopathy and depth of tumor invasion, and CT of the abdomen and pelvis to evaluate for metastatic disease. Table 28-10 outlines the current guidelines for staging. Dukes classification is still used by some physicians and correlates closely to the TNM staging. Stage I rectal cancer has an 80–90% 5-year survival rate. Stage II rectal cancer has a 62–76% 5-year survival rate. Stage III rectal cancer has a 30–40% 5-year survival rate, and stage IV has a 4–7% 5-year survival rate. Stage IV rectal cancer can involve any T lesion with local lymph node involvement and distant metastasis.

BIBLIOGRAPHY

Cameron JL. *Current Surgical Therapy*, 10th ed. Baltimore, MD: Elsevier Saunders; 2011:188–196.

Gordon PH, Nivatvongs S. *Principles and Practice of Surgery for the Colon, Rectum and Anus*, 3rd ed. St. Louis, MO: Quality Medical Publishing; 2006:645–674.

Schwartz SI. *Principles of Surgery*, 9th ed. New York, NY: McGraw-Hill; 2010:1041–1052.

TABLE 28-9 TNM Classification for Rectal Cancer

Primary tumor (T)	T1	Tumor invades the submucosa
	T2	Tumor invades the muscularis propria
	T3	Tumor invades through the muscularis propria into the subserosa or nonperitonealized or perirectal tissues
	T4	Tumor perforates through the rectal wall and directly invades other structure
Lymph nodes (N)	N1	Metastasis in 1–3 perirectal lymph nodes
	N2	Metastasis in 4 or more perirectal lymph nodes
	N3	Metastasis in any lymph node along a named vascular trunk
Distant metastasis (M)	MX	Presence of metastasis cannot be assessed
	M0	No distant metastasis
	M1	Distant metastasis present

37. **(E)** Disorders of defecation present a source of social embarrassment and create hygiene issues for many patients. A fully functional colorectal physiology lab can perform anorectal manometry and endoanal ultrasound to document the presence of muscular and sensory deficits, document sphincter function, and assist with the evaluation of constipation and diarrhea. Defecography or voiding proctography is performed to evaluate pelvic floor dysfunction. Defecography is performed in the sitting position with a double contrast barium and barium paste to outline the anus under fluoroscopy. Bowel transit studies are used to evaluate for severe constipation. The patient is given a single capsule containing 24 radiopaque rings, and abdominal x-rays are taken on days 3 and 5 to evaluate transit time. If 80% of the markers are eliminated by the fifth day, the test is normal. EUS can identify sphincter anomalies that could be contributing to the incontinence. Biofeedback is also a very effective tool for patients with adequate but weak voluntary external sphincter squeeze.

BIBLIOGRAPHY

Corman ML. *Colon and Rectal Surgery*. Philadelphia, PA: Lippincott Williams & Wilkins; 2005:67–77, 130–162.

TABLE 28-10 Current for Rectal Cancer Staging Guidelines

Staging Rectal Cancer	TNM	Dukes
Stage I	T1-2, N0, M0	A
Stage II	T3-4, N0, M0	B
Stage III	Any T, N1-3, M0	C
Stage IV	Any T, Any N, M1	

Gordon PH, Nivatvongs S. *Principles and Practice of Surgery for the Colon, Rectum and Anus*, 3rd ed. St. Louis, MO: Quality Medical Publishing; 2006:50–59, 301–305, 1086–1091.

38. **(E)** The anorectal manifestations of Crohn disease and ulcerative colitis are used for definitive diagnosis in some cases. Seventy-five percent of patients with Crohn disease have associated anal disease including fissures and fistulas with sparing of the rectum. Bleeding is rare with Crohn disease. Biopsy of a recurrent fissure or fistula will show granulomas in up to 20% of patients with Crohn disease. Patients with ulcerative colitis always have rectal involvement from the anal verge cephalad to the proximal margin. Bleeding is very common with ulcerative colitis and may be refractory to steroid enemas and 5-aminosalicylic acid product. Fistula formation does not occur in association with ulcerative colitis.

BIBLIOGRAPHY

Corman ML. *Colon and Rectal Surgery*. Philadelphia, PA: Lippincott Williams & Wilkins; 2005:1323–1327.

Gordon PH, Nivatvongs S. *Principles and Practice of Surgery for the Colon, Rectum and Anus*, 3rd ed. St. Louis, MO: Quality Medical Publishing; 2006:758–761, 871–878, 898.

39. **(A)**

40. **(E)**

41. **(E)**

Explanations for 39 to 41

The patient in Question 39 is presenting with common symptoms found in rectal cancer. Bleeding is the most common complaint, followed by diarrhea or constipation and abdominal pain. Any patient who presents with unknown etiology of rectal bleeding should undergo a colonoscopy or flexible sigmoidoscopy with completion barium enema. If a lesion is too large to be completely removed by snaring, usually greater than 2 cm, a biopsy should be obtained. Tattooing the lesion with methylene blue should not be necessary in low-lying rectal carcinoma. A complete colonoscopy should always be performed, if possible, to evaluate for other polyps or masses.

Once the diagnosis of poorly differentiated adenocarcinoma has been made, staging of the cancer should take place. Local recurrence of aggressive poorly differentiated tumors is much greater than with well differentiated. Thorough physical examination with digital examination of the rectum, careful palpation of the perineum for nodal involvement, and complete cardiac and respiratory examinations should be performed. EUS is very sensitive and specific (>90%) for bowel wall involvement. Lymph node involvement is detected with EUS with a specificity of approximately 85%. CT of the abdomen and pelvis is useful in identifying metastatic disease; however, it is not especially useful in gauging depth of disease. Advances in MRI technology have shown more precise evaluation of nodal involvement and depth for tumor staging and can visualize the surrounding pelvic anatomy to assess the relationship of the tumor to the mesorectal fascia for a feasible total mesorectal excision. This is helpful when EUS is not readily available.

Low-lying carcinoma of the rectum has always been a point of discussion among surgeons. Low anterior resection (LAR) can often be safely performed with lesions approximately ≥8 cm. Newer data support the use of LAR for most rectal lesions except the ones invading or located at the internal and external sphincter where a 2-cm distal margin is unobtainable. Total mesorectal excision is paramount when performing an LAR because failure to excise the mesorectum can lead to local failure by leaving gross or microscopic residual disease.

Abdominal perineal resection is reserved for those cancers that are near the anal verge or is used at the surgeons discretion. Superficial T1 lesions may be adequately excised with transanal excision.

The presence of metastatic disease at diagnosis can lead to excision with colostomy or a Hartmann's resection or to simple transanal excision for low-lying rectal cancers for local control of bleeding.

Operative planning should include evaluation of body habitus, gender, and age. The narrow male pelvis may be difficult to maneuver with bulky tumors to perform a complete mesorectal excision.

Comorbidities such as severe coronary or lung disease might affect decision making regarding the extent of resection needed versus the operative time and blood loss encountered. Optimization of heart and lung function preoperatively should be accomplished.

Adjuvant therapy with 5-fluorouracil–based chemotherapy and radiotherapy to the pelvis is given with the goal of decreasing the chance of distant failure (metastatic disease) and improving local control. Neoadjuvant chemoradiation therapy improved 5-year local recurrence for patients with stage II or III disease. Surgical resection is usually performed 6–8 weeks after completion of neoadjuvant therapy with further adjuvant chemotherapy postoperatively.

BIBLIOGRAPHY

Cameron JL. *Current Surgical Therapy*, 10th ed. Baltimore, MD: Elsevier Saunders; 2011:188–196.

Corman ML. *Colon and Rectal Surgery*. Philadelphia, PA: Lippincott Williams & Wilkins; 2005:911–921, 1036–1042.

Klessen C, Rogalla P, Taupitz M. Local staging of rectal cancer: the current roll of MRI. *Eur Radiol* 2007;17:379–389.

Wexner SD, Rotholtz NA. Surgeon influenced variables in resectional cancer surgery. *Dis Colon Rectum* 2000;43(11):1606–1627.

42. **(E)** Dietary modification with increasing dietary fiber intake and water intake is useful in controlling symptoms of grade 1 and 2 hemorrhoids.

Rubber band ligation has been described with great success in grade 1 and 2 hemorrhoids and some select grade 3 hemorrhoids that have no external component. It is a relatively painless procedure that can be accomplished in an outpatient setting. Patients need to be cautioned about signs of impending pelvic sepsis such as urinary retention, fever, and worsening pain. If any of these symptoms occur, immediate follow-up in the emergency room needs to be undertaken. Figure 28-26 demonstrates two rubber banding devices with a long-handled fine-toothed grasper. The hemorrhoid is grasped with the long handled grasper and the rubber banding device is passed over the hemorrhoid and two or three

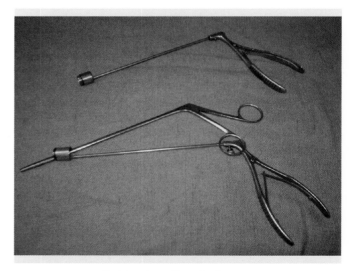

FIGURE 28-26. Rubber banding devices.

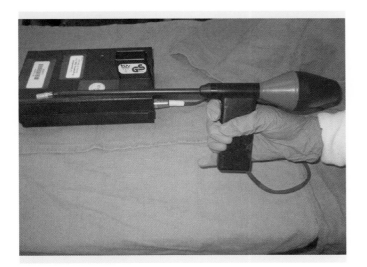

FIGURE 28-27. Infrared coagulation (IRC) device.

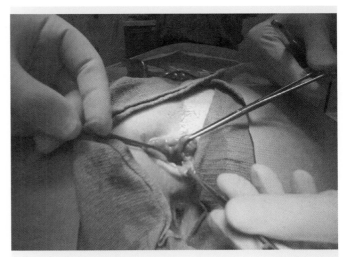

FIGURE 28-28. Patient in prone jackknife position with grade 3 hemorrhoids in the classical three quadrants: left lateral, right anterior, and right posterior.

rubber bands are placed at the neck of the hemorrhoid. The patient should not experience any pain, but may complain of some transient "pressure" or rectal fullness. If the band causes significant pain, the hemorrhoid is probably below the dentate line and should not be banded.

Infrared coagulation (IRC) with repeated applications up to three to four times per hemorrhoidal bundle has been reported successfully with grade 1 and 2 hemorrhoids. IRC has not been shown to be effective for large prolapsing circumferential hemorrhoids. The anoscope is inserted gently to better visualize the hemorrhoid. The IRC device is grasped, and the tip is gently touched to the base of hemorrhoid while depressing the trigger (see Fig. 28-27). The contact should be for 1–2 seconds.

Open or closed hemorrhoidectomy is indicated for grade 3 and 4 hemorrhoids. Grade 3 hemorrhoids with advanced mucosal prolapse might be better served with a stapled procedure to treat the prolapse and the hemorrhoids (see Figs. 28-29 to 28-32). There are commercially available stapling systems for the treatment of prolapse and hemorrhoids. Figure 28-28 demonstrates a patient in prone jackknife position with the surgeon and assistant holding out grade 3 hemorrhoids in the classical three quadrants of left lateral, right anterior, and right posterior.

These patients do well, and most go home after surgery as an outpatient.

BIBLIOGRAPHY

Cameron JL. *Current Surgical Therapy*, 10th ed. Baltimore, MD: Elsevier Saunders; 2011:223–229.

Chung CC, Ha JP, Li MK, et al. Double-blind, randomized trial comparing harmonic scalpel hemorrhoidectomy, bipolar scissors hemorrhoidectomy, and scissors excision: ligation technique. *Dis Colon Rectum* 2002;45(6):789–794.

Fleshman J. Advanced technology in the management of hemorrhoids: stapling, laser, harmonic scalpel, and ligature. 2001 Consensus conference on benign anorectal disease. *J Gastrointest Surg* 2002;6(3):299–301.

Schwartz SI. *Principles of Surgery*, 9th ed. New York, NY: McGraw-Hill; 2010:1057–1059.

43. (A) Anal canal melanoma is the most common alimentary tract melanoma but is extremely rare, accounting for 0.2% of all melanoma and 0.5% of all anorectal tumors. Rectal bleeding is the most common complaint.

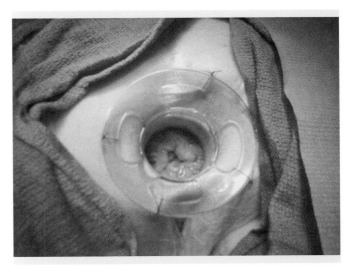

FIGURE 28-29. Anal dilator being sutured into place to attain stability. The redundant prolapsed anal tissue is evident.

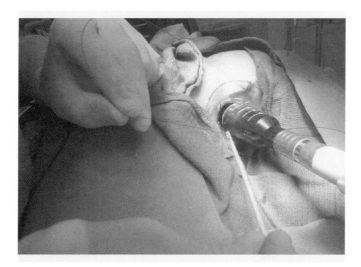

FIGURE 28-30. A nonabsorbable purse string suture being placed 4 cm from the dentate line.

One-tenth of patients with anorectal melanoma will have diagnosis on pathologic review of a hemorrhoid specimen. The melanoma may appear hemorrhoid-like or range from a deeply pigmented lesion to an amelanotic lesion. About 29% of anorectal melanomas are amelanotic.

Anorectal melanoma is rare but has a grim 5-year survival rate of less than 10%, with most patients presenting with systemic metastatic disease and/or deeply invasive tumors. Abdominal perineal resection has been the classic treatment for anorectal melanoma; however, no real survival benefit has been proven versus wide local excision. Chemotherapy, radiotherapy, and immunotherapy are still being evaluated but also offer no consistent benefit for survival.

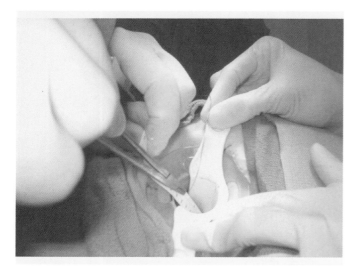

FIGURE 28-31. Stapling device being placed with the purse string pulled taut through the sides of the stapler.

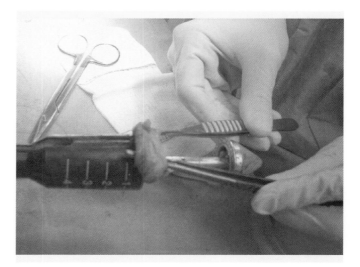

FIGURE 28-32. Tissue donuts being inspected for completion.

BIBLIOGRAPHY

Bullard KM, Tuttle TM, Spenser MP. Surgical therapy for anorectal melanoma. *J Am Coll Surg* 2003;96(2):206–208.

Corman ML. *Colon and Rectal Surgery*. Philadelphia, PA: Lippincott Williams & Wilkins; 2005:911–921, 1079–1081.

44. **(C)** This patient is suffering from a grade 3 left lateral prolapsed hemorrhoid and has an incidental skin tag found on examination. A single quadrant symptomatic prolapsed hemorrhoid is amendable to either open or closed hemorrhoidectomy. Open hemorrhoidectomy with the harmonic scalpel or traditional closed hemorrhoidectomy should effectively treat the grade 3 hemorrhoid. The skin tag should be resected because it may cause symptoms postoperatively that could be confusing to the patient and should be sent to pathology. A stapled procedure for prolapse and hemorrhoids would also be effective but is usually reserved for three quadrant prolapsed grade 3 or advancing grade 2 hemorrhoids and would not address the large redundant skin tag. Banding might also be an option, but this hemorrhoid appears to have an external component also, and banding would not address the skin tag. IRC is not appropriate for grade 3 prolapsed hemorrhoids. Lateral sphincterotomy would not be appropriate because there is no evidence of an anal fissure.

BIBLIOGRAPHY

Corman ML. *Colon and Rectal Surgery*. Philadelphia, PA: Lippincott Williams & Wilkins; 2005:911–921, 223–227.

Gordon PH, Nivatvongs S. *Principles and Practice of Surgery for the Colon, Rectum and Anus*, 3rd ed. St. Louis, MO: Quality Medical Publishing; 2006:148–158.

Khan S, Pawlak SE, Margolin DA, et al. Surgical treatment of hemorrhoids: prospective, randomized trial comparing closed excisional hemorrhoidectomy and the harmonic scalpel technique of excisional hemorrhoidectomy. *Dis Colon Rectum* 2001;44(6):845–849.

45. **(E)** The inverted prone jackknife position is extensively used in the United States for anorectal procedures. The exposure is unparalleled for many procedures such as hemorrhoidectomy, lateral internal sphincterotomy, and wide local excision of anal lesions. Both anterior and posterior anal and low rectal lesions can be exposed in the prone jackknife position; however, high lithotomy might be advantageous for posterior lesions, whereas prone jackknife position is excellent for anterior lesions. Of note, inverted jackknife position should not be used for patients in late pregnancy or who have had recent abdominal surgery, severe cardiac arrhythmias, or retinal detachment/severe glaucoma. General anesthesia is not mandatory because conscious sedation and local/regional anesthesia can be used in a prone jackknife position. Local anesthesia is an important part of anorectal surgery. A combination of 0.5% lidocaine and 0.25% bupivacaine is ideal and a 1:200,000 epinephrine dilution can be added to prolong the anesthesia and minimize absorption. Signs and symptoms of local anesthetic can range from mild, such as lightheadedness and dizziness, to severe, such as arrhythmia and cardiac arrest. The anesthesiologist should be alerted to the surgeon injecting the local anesthetic, and every possible reaction, either allergic or toxic should be investigated. Figure 28-33 demonstrates a perianal field block being administered. A subcutaneous perianal wheal is raised, and then deep injections are made into the intersphincteric groove

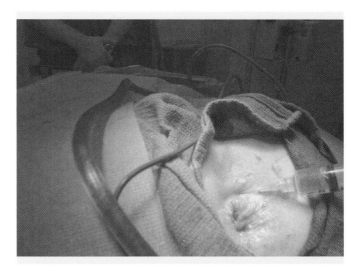

FIGURE 28-33. Perianal field block being placed with local anesthesia.

in each of the four quadrants to paralyze the sphincter mechanism and create total perianal anesthesia. Slow steady injection can minimize the pain of administration. Warming and buffering the local anesthesia have also been advocated to decrease pain of injection.

BIBLIOGRAPHY

Corman ML. *Colon and Rectal Surgery*. Philadelphia, PA: Lippincott Williams & Wilkins; 2005:212.

Gordon PH, Nivatvongs S. *Principles and Practice of Surgery for the Colon, Rectum and Anus*, 2nd ed. St. Louis, MO: Quality Medical Publishing; 1999:98, 117–123.

CHAPTER 29

VASCULAR-VENOUS AND LYMPHATIC DISEASE

RYAN KIM, ANAHITA DUA, SEPAN DESAI, AND RONALD BAYS

QUESTIONS

1. A 45-year-old woman presents for a preoperative evaluation. She relates a history of heavy bleeding during her menstrual cycles as well as easy bruising and bleeding gums. Bleeding time is 14 minutes. Which of the following is true?
   (A) The disease is X-linked recessive.
   (B) The most common variant is characterized by a functional abnormality.
   (C) Ristocetin cofactor assay will be normal.
   (D) Desmopressin is first-line treatment.
   (E) Epistaxis occurs in 90% of affected patients.

2. Which of the following is true regarding thoracic outlet syndrome (TOS)?
   (A) Patients may present with arterial, venous, or neurologic symptoms.
   (B) Paget-Schroetter syndrome is the most common presentation.
   (C) The Adson test is the most sensitive means of diagnosis.
   (D) Resection of the middle scalene muscle is curative.
   (E) Thrombolysis is contraindicated in venous TOS.

3. Which of the following patients is the best candidate for the device shown in Fig. 29-1?
   (A) 32-year-old woman with a pulmonary embolism and an international normalized ratio (INR) of 1.2
   (B) 45-year-old man with a history of gastroesophageal reflux disease (GERD) and a new finding of iliofemoral deep vein thrombosis (DVT)
   (C) 28-year-old man status post motor vehicle crash (MVC) with pelvic and femur fractures as well as a subdural hematoma
   (D) 52-year-old woman with left lower extremity swelling
   (E) 58-year-old man with a new diagnosis of a right upper extremity DVT and a history of heparin-induced thrombocytopenia

4. Indications for the device shown in Fig. 29-1 include all of the following *except*
   (A) Pulmonary embolism in a patient with an INR 2.2
   (B) Bleeding ulcer in a patient with an iliofemoral DVT on heparin therapy
   (C) Trauma patient with a spinal fracture as well as a subdural hematoma
   (D) Patient with a history of DVT with pulmonary embolism (PE) 1 year ago who develops left lower extremity swelling and has a duplex positive for DVT
   (E) Free-floating femoral DVT documented by duplex

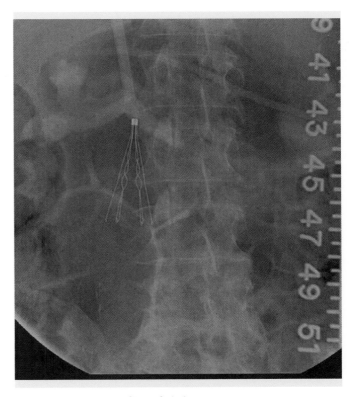

FIGURE 29-1. Plain film of abdomen.

5. Regarding the diagnosis and treatment of DVT, which of the following is true?
   (A) Diagnosis with ultrasound depends on augmentation of flow with proximal compression during the examination.
   (B) Development of proximal lower extremity DVT should be treated with heparin and conversion to 6 weeks of warfarin therapy.
   (C) Patients treated for DVT whose platelet counts drop below 100,000 should have all heparin products immediately stopped.
   (D) Perioperative warfarin use is the prophylactic measure of choice for patients at high risk for DVT.
   (E) Low-molecular-weight heparin (LMWH) exerts its effect through inhibition of activated factor VIII.

6. The initial dose of unfractionated heparin given to achieve anticoagulation is
   (A) 5000 units
   (B) 80 units/kg
   (C) 120 units/kg
   (D) 100 units/h
   (E) 1500 units

7. A 52-year-old man comes in with progressive swelling and discoloration of the left lower extremity (see Fig. 29-2).

   Which of the following is true regarding this condition?

   (A) It is rare.
   (B) Valve transplant is necessary for all patients with deep venous reflux.
   (C) Ablation of the great saphenous vein is associated with a 20% deep vein thrombosis risk.
   (D) Patients with venous insufficiency should wear support hose with 10-mmHg pressure.
   (E) A reflux time of 1.0 second for deep veins is significant.

8. A 52-year-old man presents with a 2-week history of progressive discoloration and pain in the right lower extremity (see Fig. 29-3).

   Which of the following is true regarding this condition?

   (A) Deep venous involvement is universal.
   (B) Treatment with warm compresses, anti-inflammatory agents, and elevation is curative.
   (C) Extended anticoagulation or ligation of the saphenous vein may be required for progressive disease.
   (D) Varicose veins are not risk factors.
   (E) Excision of the involved vein segment is mandatory.

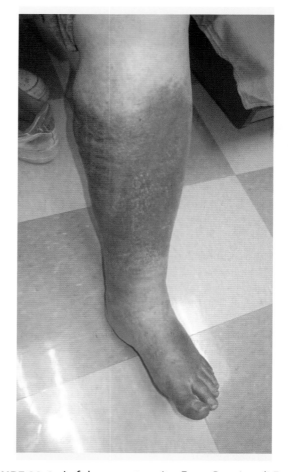

FIGURE 29-2. Left lower extremity. From Brunicardi F, Andersen DK, Billiar TR, et al. (eds.). *Schwartz's Principles of Surgery*, 10th ed. New York, NY: McGraw-Hill; 2014: Fig. 24-2.

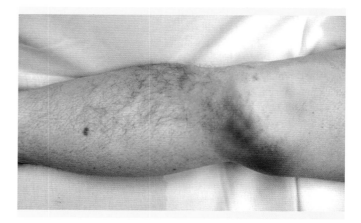

FIGURE 29-3. Right lower extremity. Used with permission of Steven Dean, DO.

9. Which of the following is true regarding lymphedema?
   (A) Lymphedema praecox is primary lymph-edema, whereas lymphedema tarda is secondary lymphedema.
   (B) Primary lymphedema has a marked male predominance.
   (C) It occurs as a result of buildup of protein-rich fluid in the interstitial space.
   (D) Lymphoscintigraphy has low sensitivity and specificity for lymphedema.
   (E) Congenital lymphedema is limited to the upper extremities.

10. Which of the following is the most common cause of secondary lymphedema?
    (A) *Wuchereria bancrofti*
    (B) DVT
    (C) Meige disease
    (D) Surgery
    (E) Milroy disease

11. Which of the following is the most common form of lymphedema?
    (A) Congenital lymphedema
    (B) Lymphedema praecox
    (C) Lymphedema tarda
    (D) Secondary lymphedema
    (E) Familial lymphedema

12. Which of the following is the most effective therapy for lymphedema?
    (A) Compression stockings
    (B) Surgical excision of the involved lymphatics
    (C) Surgical bypass of the obstructed lymphatics
    (D) Combined excision and bypass of the obstructed lymphatics
    (E) Benzopyrones and diuretics

13. A 62-year-old man with a history significant for diabetes, hypertension, and end-stage renal disease on hemodialysis presents with nonhealing ulcers (see Fig. 29-4). His dorsalis pedis and posterior tibial pulses are palpable bilaterally. Which of the following statements is correct regarding the role of arterial bypass?
    (A) His disease is not severe enough to warrant revascularization.
    (B) Peripheral arterial bypass is not indicated.
    (C) Hemodialysis is a contraindication to arterial bypass.
    (D) Because his ulcers are chronic, revascularization can be performed electively following appropriate cardiopulmonary optimization.
    (E) His disease is too far progressed and requires amputation.

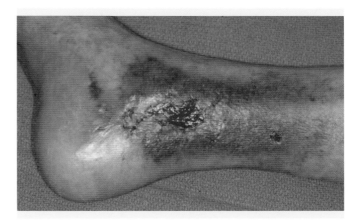

FIGURE 29-4. Right lower extremity. Used with permission of Thom Rooke, MD.

14. Which of the following correctly describes the mechanism of action of fibrinolytic agents?
    (A) Converting plasminogen to plasmin
    (B) Increasing the activity of plasmin
    (C) Converting thrombin to fibrin
    (D) Decreasing the activity of thrombin
    (E) Increasing the activity of antithrombin

15. Phlegmasia cerulea albans is caused by
    (A) Obliteration of the major deep venous channels of the leg
    (B) Obliteration of the collateral veins of the leg
    (C) Obliteration of the major deep venous channels and the collateral veins of the leg
    (D) Reperfusion injury following an isolated injury to the femoral vein
    (E) Infection of an edematous extremity

16. Which is the preferred surgical treatment in a patient with symptomatic varicose veins and an incompetent valve at the saphenofemoral junction?
    (A) Sclerotherapy
    (B) Radiofrequency ablation or laser ablation
    (C) Vein valvuloplasty
    (D) High ligation and stripping of the saphenous system
    (E) Leg elevation and compression therapy

17. Which of the following is true regarding duplex ultrasound imaging?
    (A) It is a combination of A-mode and D-mode ultrasound imaging.
    (B) Lower frequency transducers (e.g., 3 MHz) are better suited for deep structures, and higher frequencies (e.g., 7 MHz) are better for more superficial structures.
    (C) Dilated vein with <50% increase in diameter with Valsalva is diagnostic of DVT.
    (D) Color flow imaging is essential for the diagnosis of DVT.
    (E) Arterial wall calcium precludes an adequate vascular ultrasound examination.

18. A 72-year-old woman presents with a 12-week history of progressive swelling of the head, neck, and upper thorax. She has a 55 pack-year smoking history. Computed tomography angiogram is shown in Fig. 29-5.

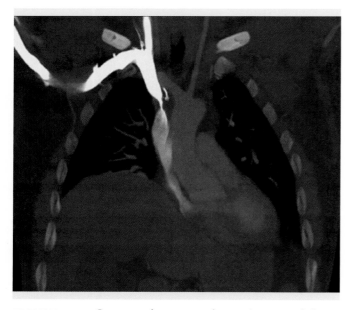

FIGURE 29-5. Computed tomography angiogram of chest. From Block J, Jordanov M, Stack L, Thurman RJ. *Atlas of Emergency Radiology.* New York, NY: McGraw-Hill; 2013: Fig. 5.93.

Which of the following is true of this condition?
    (A) Venous pressure is most likely 15 mmHg.
    (B) Small cell carcinoma is the most common cause.
    (C) Collateral venous channels are likely absent in this patient.
    (D) Obstruction between the azygos vein and the right atrium is less disabling than obstruction above the azygos vein.
    (E) Tumors with 30–50% involvement of the superior vena cava (SVC) are treated with resection and reconstruction.

19. Which of the following is true regarding venous circulation?
    (A) The perforating veins in the leg direct blood flow from deep to the superficial system.
    (B) The common iliac vein has no valves.
    (C) The superficial venous system of the leg consists of the greater saphenous, lesser saphenous, and popliteal veins.
    (D) In patients with obstructed deep veins, venous pressure increases with walking.
    (E) The superficial femoral and superficial circumflex veins join to form the common femoral vein.

20. Which of the following is an anatomic landmark associated with the saphenofemoral junction?
    (A) Boyd's perforator
    (B) Deep circumflex iliac vein
    (C) Internal pudendal vein
    (D) Hunter's perforator
    (E) Superficial epigastric vein

21. The most common electrocardiographic change after pulmonary embolism is
    (A) Atrial fibrillation
    (B) Sinus tachycardia
    (C) Right bundle branch block
    (D) S1, Q3, T3 pattern
    (E) Left bundle branch block

22. Which of the following is true of the lymphatic system?
    (A) The thoracic duct collects lymph from the entire body.
    (B) The right lymphatic duct is created by the union of the right jugular and right subclavian ducts.
    (C) The lymphatic system is valveless.
    (D) Lymph enters the venous system at the junction of the jugular and subclavian veins.
    (E) Approximately 500 mL of lymphatic fluid enters the cardiovascular system each day.

ANSWERS AND EXPLANATIONS

1. **(D)** von Willebrand factor (vWF) is produced by endothelial cells and megakaryocytes and is a necessary cofactor for platelet binding to vessel walls. This patient has von Willebrand disease (vWD), an autosomal dominant disorder of coagulation resulting from deficiency or defect in vWF. vWD is the most common inherited coagulopathy. The majority (75–80%) of patients with vWD have type 1, a quantitative deficiency of vWF characterized by reduced factor VIII activity, vWF antigen, and ristocetin cofactor activity. Patients with type 1 vWD usually have mild or moderate platelet-type bleeding. Type 2 vWD is heterogeneous and further divided into

TABLE 29-1 Laboratory Diagnosis of von Willebrand Disease

Type		vWF Activity	vWF Antigen	Factor VIII	RIPA	Multimer Analysis
1		↓	↓	Nl or ↓	↓	Normal pattern; uniform ↓ intensity of bands
2	A	↓↓	↓	↓	↓	Large and intermediate multimers decreased or absent
	B	↓↓	↓	↓	↑	Large multimers decreased or absent
	M	↓	↓	↓	↓	Normal pattern; uniform ↓ intensity of bands
	N	Nl	Nl	↓↓	Nl	Nl
3		↓↓↓	↓↓↓	↓↓↓	↓↓↓	Multimers absent

Nl, normal; RIPA, ristocetin-induced platelet aggregation; vWF, von Willebrand factor.

four subtypes (2A, 2B, 2M, and 2N); the common feature is a qualitative defect in the vWF molecule. Patients with type 2 vWD usually have moderate to severe bleeding that presents in childhood or adolescence.

The initial laboratory evaluation of patients suspected by history of having vWD includes the following tests: assay of factor VIII activity, vWF antigen, and vWF ristocetin cofactor (Table 29-1). Platelet counts are usually normal, because this is a qualitative rather than a quantitative platelet disorder. Bleeding times will be prolonged (>11 minutes) secondary to a defect in platelet function. Because vWF with factor VIII binds together to form a complex, factor VIII levels in vWD patients are generally coordinately decreased along with plasma vWF, thus altering the activated partial thromboplastin time (aPTT) as well.

The ristocetin-induced platelet aggregation (RIPA) assay measures platelet agglutination caused by ristocetin-mediated vWF binding to platelet membrane glycoprotein GPIbα.

First-line treatment is desmopressin, an analogue of antidiuretic hormone that acts through type 2 vasopressin receptors to induce secretion of factor VIII and vWF. Approximately 20–25% of patients with vWD do not respond adequately to desmopressin. Treatment with vWF-rich cryoprecipitate can correct bleeding dysfunction, as can administration of factor VIII concentrates.

BIBLIOGRAPHY

Desai SS, Shortell CK (ed.). *Clinical Review of Vascular Surgery.* New York, NY: Catalyst Publishers; 2010.

Iserson KV. Laboratory. In: Iserson KV (eds.), *Improvised Medicine: Providing Care in Extreme Environments.* New York, NY: McGraw-Hill; 2012:Chapter 19.

Johnson J, Ginsburg D. von Willebrand disease. In: Lichtman MA, Kipps TJ, Seligsohn U, Kaushansky K, Prchal JT (eds.), *Williams Hematology*, 8th ed. New York, NY: McGraw-Hill; 2010:Chapter 127.

Moore WS. *Vascular Surgery and Endovascular Surgery: A Comprehensive Review*, 8th ed. Philadelphia, PA: Saunders; 2013.

2. **(A)** Thoracic outlet syndrome (TOS) arises from compression of upper extremity neurovascular structures and can manifest with neurologic, arterial, or venous symptoms (see Figs. 29-6 and 29-7). The vast majority of patients present with neurologic symptoms (75%), whereas venous TOS accounts for about 20% of cases and arterial TOS accounts for about 5%.

Neurogenic TOS presents with weakness, paresthesia, and/or pain in the affected upper extremity. It is associated with repetitive stress injury of the affected limb, such as in painters and baseball players.

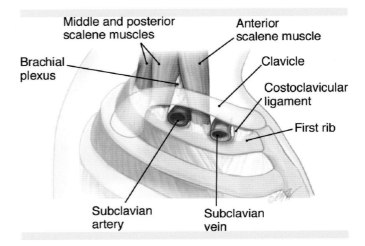

FIGURE 29-6. Normal thoracic outlet. From Sugarbaker DJ, Bueno R, Krasna MJ, Mentzer SJ, Zellos L (eds.). *Adult Chest Surgery*. New York, NY: McGraw-Hill; 2009:Fig. 143-9.

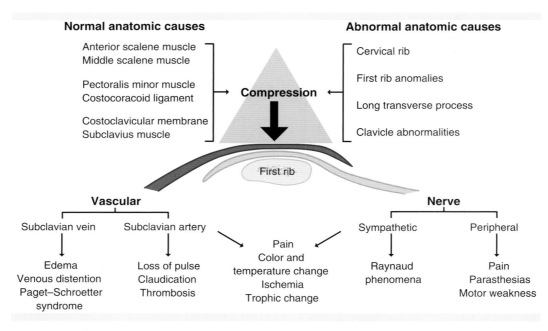

FIGURE 29-7. Mechanisms of compression in thoracic outlet syndrome. From Sugarbaker DJ, Bueno R, Krasna MJ, Mentzer SJ, Zellos L (eds.). *Adult Chest Surgery*. New York, NY: McGraw-Hill; 2009:Fig. 123-1.

Arterial TOS symptoms include the formation of a pseudoaneurysm that can lead to distal embolization and subsequent arm ischemia.

Venous TOS leads to severe stenosis and even occlusion of the subclavian vein, leading to arm edema and the formation of extensive collaterals within the chest. Effort thrombosis of the axillary-subclavian vein (Paget-Schroetter syndrome) is a hallmark of venous TOS.

Diagnosis of TOS is based on physical examination and diagnostic imaging. There are four basic maneuvers used to elicit the classical physical signs of thoracic outlet compression: the Adson test, the costoclavicular test, the Roos test, and the Wright test. However, these maneuvers are not specific for TOS, and 56% of normal patients may have at least one positive test. Patients with suspected arterial TOS should undergo angiography, with diagnostic subclavian artery stenosis seen when the arm is abducted above the head. Patients with venous TOS often have characteristic findings at the subclavian vein upon completion of venography. Failure of several months of physical therapy should prompt surgical management.

Although catheter-directed thrombolysis and even stent grafting can temporarily alleviate some symptoms, the accepted treatment for patients with TOS is resection of any cervical ribs, removal of the first rib, excision of all scar tissue, and repair/replacement of any affected vessels. A neurolysis of the brachial plexus should be undertaken in patients with neurogenic TOS. Patients with venous TOS may require patch angioplasty or interposition grafting of the subclavian vein. Patients with arterial TOS, thrombosis of the axillary-subclavian artery, or distal emboli secondary to TOS compression should be treated with first rib resection, thrombectomy, embolectomy, arterial repair or replacement, and dorsal sympathectomy.

BIBLIOGRAPHY

Cronenwett JL, Johnston KW. *Rutherford's Vascular Surgery*, 8th ed. Philadelphia, PA: Saunders; 2014.

Desai SS, Toliyat M, Dua A, et al. Outcomes of surgical paraclavicular thoracic outlet decompression. *Ann Vasc Surg* 2014;28(2):457–464.

Moore WS. *Vascular Surgery and Endovascular Surgery: A Comprehensive Review*, 8th ed. Philadelphia, PA: Saunders; 2013.

Stanley JC, Veith FJ, Wakefield TW. *Current Therapy in Vascular Surgery*, 5th ed. Philadelphia, PA: Saunders; 2014.

Urschel HC Jr, Mark PJ, Patel AN. Thoracic outlet syndromes. In: Sugarbaker DJ, Bueno R, Colson YL, et al. (eds.), *Adult Chest Surgery*, 2nd ed. New York, NY: McGraw-Hill; 2013.

3. **(C)**

4. **(D)**

Explanation for questions 3 and 4

Usually, patients with a DVT can be treated with anticoagulation to prevent propagation of clot or embolic complications. Heparinization and ultimate conversion to warfarin therapy with a target INR of 2–3 is desired.

There are, however, several instances when inferior vena cava (IVC) filter placement as protection against pulmonary embolism (PE) is warranted. Development of PE while adequately anticoagulated is one such indication.

There are, however, several clinical indications when vena caval filter placement is warranted:

1. Evidence-based guidelines
   - Documented venous thromboembolism (VTE) with contraindication to anticoagulation
   - Documented VTE with complications of anticoagulation
   - Recurrent PE despite therapeutic anticoagulation
   - Documented VTE with inability to achieve therapeutic anticoagulation
2. Relative expanded indications
   - Poor compliance with anticoagulation
   - Free-floating iliocaval thrombus
   - Renal cell carcinoma with renal vein extension
   - Venous thrombolysis/thromboembolectomy
   - Documented VTE and limited cardiopulmonary reserve
   - Documented VTE with high risk for anticoagulation complications
   - Recurrent PE complicated by pulmonary hypertension
   - Documented VTE: cancer patient, burn patient, pregnancy
   - VTE prophylaxis: high-risk surgical patient, trauma patient, high-risk medical condition

Patients who develop bleeding complications that require discontinuation of anticoagulation also may necessitate IVC filter placement.

Other indications for IVC filter include patients who have undergone pulmonary embolectomy or whose illness severity would likely make them intolerant to the effects of a PE. Septic emboli or propagating iliofemoral clots are also relative indications. A new use as a purely prophylactic device against PE in patients with massive trauma and a high risk of DVT/PE is also being considered as an indication, even in the absence of documented DVT.

Patients with contraindications to anticoagulation (such as neurologic or ocular injuries) or patients with large free-floating clots are at increased risk of embolization and may represent reasons to place a vena caval filter. Patients with DVT who are not currently anticoagulated do not require an IVC filter if no contraindications to anticoagulation exist. They may, however, require longer—even indefinite—anticoagulation secondary to the recurrent nature of the disease.

Contraindications to filter placement include the following:

- Chronically occluded vena cava
- Vena cava anomalies
- Inability to access the vena cava
- Vena cava compression
- No location in the vena cava available for placement

BIBLIOGRAPHY

Cronenwett JL, Johnston KW. *Rutherford's Vascular Surgery*, 8th ed. Philadelphia, PA: Saunders; 2014.

Dua A, Desai SS, Holcomb JB, Burgess A, Freischlag JA. *Clinical Review of Vascular Trauma*. New York, NY: Springer Verlag; 2013.

Moore WS. *Vascular Surgery and Endovascular Surgery: A Comprehensive Review*, 8th ed. Philadelphia, PA: Saunders; 2013.

Mowatt-Larssen E, Desai SS, Dua A, Shortell CEK (eds.). *Phlebology, Vein Surgery, and Ultrasonography*. New York, NY: Springer Verlag; 2014.

Rutherford RB (ed.). *Vascular Surgery*, 7th ed., vol. 1 and 2. St. Louis, MO: Mosby; 2010.

5. **(C)** Deep venous thrombosis (DVT) is a significant health concern with potentially fatal complications. Therefore, knowledge of diagnosis and treatment is very important. One of the mainstays of diagnosis is the duplex ultrasound. The Doppler probe is placed on the lower extremity to evaluate the venous signals. Flow with distal compression is augmented, while a proximal obstruction should cause dampened flow. Further information can be gained by duplex of the DVT, which uses the picture to evaluate presence of clot or compressibility of the vein.

Methods of prophylaxis are dependent on risk stratification of the patient. Low-risk patients require only early ambulation. Moderate-risk patients require either sequential compression devices (SCDs) or anticoagulation, often with LMWHs, which exert their effect via inhibition of factor X. High-risk patients, such as patients over 40, obese patients, patients with a history of cancer or major trauma, or those undergoing major joint replacement, often require anticoagulation with unfractionated heparin or LMWH.

Patients who develop DVT should be treated with anticoagulation if there are no contraindications. Either heparin or, in some cases, LMWH should be initiated with conversion to warfarin therapy to a target INR of 2–3. Duration of warfarin treatment is the subject of some debate; however, at least 3 months, and often 6 months, is recommended to minimize the risk of recurrence and to prevent PE. Recurrent DVT after completion of therapy often leads to indefinite anticoagulation secondary to an up to 20% risk of further recurrences if the patient is not anticoagulated.

Heparin therapy is not without its risks, however. Heparin-induced thrombocytopenia (HIT), secondary to formation of IgG antibodies against the heparin platelet factor (PF4), occurs in up to 10% of patients who receive heparin independent of the method of exposure (e.g., intravenous [IV], subcutaneous). Patients whose platelet count drops below 100,000 or who have a decrease in platelet count of 50% or more during heparin therapy should be suspected of suffering from HIT. Usually this occurs 4–5 days after initial exposure. Treatment is immediate cessation of all heparin products. Alternatives for anticoagulation, such as lepirudin or argatroban, can be used for IV anticoagulation, and warfarin can be used as an oral agent.

BIBLIOGRAPHY

Cronenwett JL, Johnston KW. *Rutherford's Vascular Surgery*, 8th ed. Philadelphia, PA: Saunders; 2014.

Moore WS. *Vascular Surgery and Endovascular Surgery: A Comprehensive Review*, 8th ed. Philadelphia, PA: Saunders; 2013.

Mowatt-Larssen E, Desai SS, Dua A, Shortell CEK (eds.). *Phlebology, Vein Surgery, and Ultrasonography.* New York, NY: Springer Verlag; 2014.

Stanley JC, Veith FJ, Wakefield TW. *Current Therapy in Vascular Surgery*, 5th ed. Philadelphia, PA: Saunders; 2014.

6. **(B)** Unfractionated heparin (UFH) binds and accelerates the activity of antithrombin (AT). AT inhibits thrombin and factor Xa, and the reaction is accelerated approximately 1000-fold in the presence of heparin. Factor Xa is additionally inhibited by binding heparin-AT complexes. UFH is initially dosed with a bolus of 80 units/kg. Although 5000 units is a common initial bolus dose, weight-based UFH dosages have been shown to be more effective than standard fixed boluses in rapidly achieving therapeutic levels.

The initial bolus is followed by a continuous infusion of 18 units/kg/h or 1000–1500 units/h, with the goal of achieving a target activated partial thromboplastin time (aPTT) 2–3 times the upper limit of normal (60–80 seconds).

The advantage of UFH is its half-life of 45–90 minutes, which is dose dependent. Disadvantages include the need to monitor heparin levels every 6 hours using the aPTT and the risk of HIT.

BIBLIOGRAPHY

Goldhaber SZ. Deep venous thrombosis and pulmonary thromboembolism. In: Longo DL, Fauci AS, Kasper DL, Hauser SL, Jameson J, Loscalzo J (eds.), *Harrison's Principles of Internal Medicine*, 18th ed. New York, NY: McGraw-Hill; 2012:Chapter 262.

7. **(E)** Chronic venous insufficiency (CVI) is a condition of the lower extremities characterized by persistent ambulatory venous hypertension. CVI affects 80 million Americans, and the incidence of venous disease continues to rise. The clinical presentation varies from pain and edema to skin changes and ulcerations, and definitive treatment is necessary to forestall clinically significant complications.

Dysfunction or incompetence of the valves in the superficial venous system also allows retrograde flow of blood, known as "reflux." Patients with CVI are most likely to have reflux within one of their superficial veins, such as the great saphenous vein and the small saphenous vein. Reflux of the deep system is most often a consequence of damage from previous DVT, but reflux may also occur in venous tributaries in the absence of any truncal superficial or deep vein or perforator vein reflux. Venous duplex imaging is currently the most common technique used to confirm the diagnosis of CVI. A reflux time of >0.5 seconds for superficial veins and 1.0 second for deep veins is typically used to diagnose the presence of reflux. Although longer durations imply more severe disease, there is no relationship between increased reflux time and worsening manifestations of CVI. The initial management of CVI is conservative and centers on use of 20–50 mmHg compressive stockings.

Venous sclerotherapy is a treatment modality for obliterating telangiectasias, varicose veins, and venous segments with reflux. Sclerotherapy may be used as a primary treatment or in conjunction with surgical procedures in the correction of CVI. Sclerotherapy is indicated for a variety of conditions, including spider veins (<1 mm), venous lakes, varicose veins of 1 to 4 mm in diameter, bleeding varicosities, and small cavernous hemangiomas (vascular malformation).

Radiofrequency or laser is used to ablate incompetent veins, frequently for great saphenous vein (GSV) reflux as an alternative to stripping. Endovenous ablation can also be applied to combined superficial and perforator reflux. A potential complication of ablation remains DVT and PE, although the reported incidence is <1%.

Abnormalities in venous outflow, involving iliac veins, contribute to symptoms in 10–30% of patients with severe CVI. Endovascular venous stenting has proven effective, and as a result, valve transplant and venous bypass are rarely necessary.

BIBLIOGRAPHY

Eberhardt RT, Raffetto JD. Chronic venous insufficiency. *Circulation* 2014;130(4):333–346.

Moore WS. *Vascular Surgery and Endovascular Surgery: A Comprehensive Review*, 8th ed. Philadelphia, PA: Saunders; 2013.

Mowatt-Larssen E, Desai SS, Dua A, Shortell CEK (eds.). *Phlebology, Vein Surgery, and Ultrasonography*. New York, NY: Springer Verlag; 2014.

8. **(C)** Superficial thrombophlebitis is a condition involving thrombosis of the superficial veins, usually of the lower extremity. Risk factors include trauma, varicose veins, pregnancy, hypercoagulable disorders, and malignancy. The most common vein affected is the GSV and its branches. In up to 20% of cases, a simultaneous DVT exists.

Patients typically present with localized extremity pain and hardened areas overlying the affected veins. Often, this is a self-limiting process that can be effectively treated with elevation, warm compresses, and anti-inflammatory agents. Duplex ultrasound can rule out an associated DVT, which may be asymptomatic.

Superficial thrombophlebitis is usually self-limited, and recovery may be accelerated by rest, elevation, warm compresses, and anti-inflammatory agents. Systemic anticoagulation is indicated if the phlebitis progresses despite conservative care or is located within 1–2 cm of the saphenofemoral junction.

Close follow-up is recommended, and progression of the thrombophlebitis toward the saphenofemoral junction (as noted by physical examination or serial duplex examinations) may warrant anticoagulation or ligation with or without stripping of the vein to ensure that progression into the deep system does not occur.

Suppurative thrombophlebitis is often related to IV cannulation, and prompt treatment is important. Removal of the IV, systemic antibiotics, and—if gross purulence is noted from the vein—excision of the offending vein segment may be required.

BIBLIOGRAPHY

Cronenwett JL, Johnston KW. *Rutherford's Vascular Surgery*, 8th ed. Philadelphia, PA: Saunders; 2014.

Moore WS. *Vascular Surgery and Endovascular Surgery: A Comprehensive Review*, 8th ed. Philadelphia, PA: Saunders; 2013.

Wennberg PW, Rooke TW. Diagnosis and management of diseases of the peripheral arteries and veins. In: Fuster V, Walsh RA, Harrington RA (eds.), *Hurst's the Heart*, 13th ed. New York, NY: McGraw-Hill; 2011:Chapter 109.

9. **(C)**

10. **(A)**

11. **(D)**

12. **(A)**

Explanation for questions 9 to 12

Lymphedema constitutes a condition in which an abnormality in the lymphatic channels causes a buildup of protein-rich fluid in the interstitial space. Lymphedema can be classified as primary or secondary.

Primary lymphedema has several classifications:

- Congenital lymphedema is clinically present at birth or by age 2.
- Lymphedema praecox is primary lymphedema that presents itself before age 35. The familial form of lymphedema praecox is Milroy disease. Lymphedema praecox is the most common form of primary lymphedema and has up to a 10:1 female predominance.
- Lymphedema tarda presents after age 35. The familial form is Meige disease.

Primary lymphedema is usually secondary to either a developmental abnormality in the lymphatics or a fibrotic obliteration of the lymph channels. Lymphedema congenita is present at birth and may involve a single lower extremity, multiple limbs, the genitalia, or the face. The edema typically develops before 2 years of age and may be associated with specific hereditary syndromes (Turner syndrome, Milroy syndrome, Klippel-Trenaunay-Weber syndrome).

Secondary lymphedema is far more common than primary lymphedema. Worldwide, the most common cause of secondary lymphedema is parasitic disease filariasis, caused by infection with roundworms such as *Wuchereria bancrofti*, *Brugia malayi*, and *Brugia timori*. Bacterial infections, tumors, surgery tuberculosis, contact dermatitis, lymphogranuloma venereum, rheumatoid arthritis, and pregnancy are other secondary causes.

Several diagnostic methods can be used to evaluate lower extremity swelling, including computed tomography (CT) scan and/or magnetic resonance imaging (MRI). CT findings can illustrate honeycomb appearance of the subcutaneous tissue, suspicious for lymphatic etiology, although it is not sensitive. Importantly, however, CT can help rule out tumor invasion as a cause for leg swelling. MRI is also useful and can be a good adjunct to lymphoscintigraphy.

Lymphoscintigraphy is an important diagnostic tool. Lymphoscintigraphy involves injection of radioactive tracer between the toes of the affected extremity. Uptake by the lymphatics occurs, and images track the tracer up the extremity. In this way, findings such as absence of lymph channels, delayed uptake, or absence of nodes can be seen.

The treatment of lymphedema has perplexed surgeons throughout history, and many different ideas and techniques have been developed. Basically, treatment can be divided into medical and surgical, with surgical involving drainage or excisional procedures. Currently, medical therapy is implemented first and consists of wearing compressive garments, massage, pneumatic compression devices, antibiotics, good hygiene, and limb elevation. Graded compression stockings reduce swelling by preventing edema while the extremity is dependent. Daily use is associated with long-term reduction in limb circumference. However, strict compliance is mandatory for efficacious medical therapy.

Four groups of drugs have been evaluated in the treatment of CVI, including coumarins (α-benzopyrenes), flavonoids (γ-benzopyrenes), saponosides (horse chestnut extracts), and other plant extracts. These venoactive drugs, which provide relief of pain and swelling or accelerate venous ulcer healing, carry a moderate recommendation in the clinical practice guidelines (grade 2B) when used in conjunction with compression therapy but are not approved by the US Food and Drug Administration (FDA). Diuretics are not therapeutic.

When medical treatment fails, surgery is indicated and usually only for severe cases. Surgical techniques aimed at lymphatic drainage include lymphatic to venous anastomoses, de-epithelialized dermal flaps, and the creation of fascial windows. Excisional procedures are more commonly performed and include removal of the affected tissue with skin grafts using the skin of the removed tissue. Unfortunately, surgery is mostly palliative instead of curative. A commonly performed procedure with a high rate of resultant lymphedema is mastectomy with axillary dissection. The rate of occurrence is anywhere from 6–30%, and the treatment is conservative, with surgery only for severe cases with failed medical therapy. Scrotal lymphedema is initially treated with elevation, but this only works for mild cases. Instead, this is one of the few instances where surgical therapy is initiated early and has reproducible results.

BIBLIOGRAPHY

Creager MA, Loscalzo J. Vascular diseases of the extremities. In: Longo DL, Fauci AS, Kasper DL, Hauser SL, Jameson J, Loscalzo J (eds.), *Harrison's Principles of Internal Medicine*, 18th ed. New York, NY: McGraw-Hill; 2012:Chapter 249.

Cronenwett JL, Johnston KW. *Rutherford's Vascular Surgery*, 8th ed. Philadelphia, PA: Saunders; 2014.

Moore WS. *Vascular Surgery and Endovascular Surgery: A Comprehensive Review*, 8th ed. Philadelphia, PA: Saunders; 2013.

Mowatt-Larssen E, Desai SS, Dua A, Shortell CEK (eds.). *Phlebology, Vein Surgery, and Ultrasonography*. New York, NY: Springer Verlag; 2014.

Stanley JC, Veith FJ, Wakefield TW. *Current Therapy in Vascular Surgery*, 5th ed. Philadelphia, PA: Saunders; 2014.

13. **(B)** Approximately 2.5 million people experience chronic venous insufficiency (CVI) in the United States, and of those, approximately 20% develop venous ulcers. One of the most serious consequence of CVI is ulceration. Venous stasis ulcers are large, painful, and irregular in outline with a shallow, moist granulation bed. They most commonly occur over the medial and lateral malleoli of the ankle and are often accompanied by stasis dermatitis and stasis pigmentation changes.

Duplex ultrasonography is helpful to evaluate for venous obstruction or venous incompetence. Air plethysmography has the ability to measure each potential component of the pathophysiologic mechanisms of CVI, including reflux, obstruction, and muscle pump dysfunction. CT and MRI are most useful to evaluate more proximal veins and their surrounding structures to assess for intrinsic obstruction or extrinsic compression.

Initial treatment recommendations should include limb elevation above heart level, compression garments, and weight loss with lifestyle changes. There is no role for arterial bypass in the setting of palpable pulses. In patients with venous ulcers, graded compression stockings and other compressive bandaging modalities are effective in both healing and preventing recurrences of ulceration. Common dressings include debriding agents, alginate, collagen, and hydrocolloids. With a structured regimen of compression therapy, complete ulcer healing can be achieved in >90% of patient with ulcers at a mean of 5.3 months. Venous valve reconstruction of the deep vein valves has been performed selectively in advanced CVI with recurrent ulceration and disabling symptoms.

BIBLIOGRAPHY

Cohoon KP, Rooke TW, Pfizenmaier DH II. Venous stasis ulceration. In: Dean SM, Satiani B, Abraham WT (eds.), *Color Atlas and Synopsis of Vascular Diseases*. New York, NY: McGraw-Hill; 2014.

Eberhardt RT, Raffetto JD. Chronic venous insufficiency. *Circulation* 2014;130:333–346.

14. **(A)** The goal of thrombolytic therapy is rapid restoration of flow in an occluded vessel achieved by accelerating fibrinolytic proteolysis of the thrombus. Several fibrinolytic agents are available (Table 29-2).

All of the agents in Table 29-2 share the ability to convert plasminogen to plasmin, which leads to the degradation of fibrin. They differ with regard to their half-lives, their potential for inducing fibrinogenolysis (generalized lytic state), their potential for antigenicity, and their FDA-approved indications for use.

BIBLIOGRAPHY

Wennberg PW, Rooke TW. Diagnosis and management of diseases of the peripheral arteries and veins. In: Fuster V, Walsh RA, Harrington RA (eds.), *Hurst's the Heart*, 13th ed. New York, NY: McGraw-Hill; 2011:Chapter 109.

TABLE 29-2 Comparison of Plasminogen Activators

Agent (Regimen)	Source (Approved/Available)	Antigenic	Half-Life (min)
Streptokinase (infusion)	*Streptococcus* (Y/Y)	Yes	20
This node is not processed by any templates: Urokinase (infusion)	Cell culture; recombinant (Y/N)	No	15
This node is not processed by any templates: Alteplase (t-PA) (infusion)	Recombinant (Y/Y)	No	5
Anistreplase (bolus)	*Streptococcus* + plasma product (Y/N)	No	70
This node is not processed by any templates: Reteplase (double bolus)	Recombinant (Y/Y)	No	15
Saruplase (scu-PA) (infusion)	Recombinant (N/N)	No	5
Staphylokinase (infusion)	Recombinant (N/N)	Yes	
This node is not processed by any templates: Tenecteplase (bolus)	Recombinant (Y/Y)	No	15

N, no; t-PA, tissue plasminogen activator; Y, yes.

15. **(A)** Phlegmasia dolens refers to the clinical manifestation of massive venous thrombosis. *Phlegmasia alba dolens* is caused by massive thrombosis of the iliofemoral veins that obliterates the major deep venous channel of the extremity with sparing of collateral veins. It is characterized by pitting edema of the entire lower extremity, tenderness in the inguinal area, and a pale extremity secondary to arterial occlusion (see Fig. 29-8). There is no associated cyanosis.

When the thrombosis extends to the collateral veins, massive fluid sequestration and more significant edema ensue, resulting in *phlegmasia cerulea dolens*. The affected extremity in phlegmasia cerulea dolens is extremely painful, edematous, and cyanotic, and arterial insufficiency or compartment syndrome may be present.

Phlegmasia dolens is seen in fewer than 10% of patients with venous thrombosis. Phlegmasia cerulea dolens is preceded by phlegmasia alba dolens in 50–60% of patients. Diagnosis is made via duplex ultrasonography, plethysmography, and venography. Treatment relies on systemic anticoagulation, systemic thrombolysis, or catheter-directed thrombolysis. If the condition is left untreated, venous gangrene can ensue, leading to amputation.

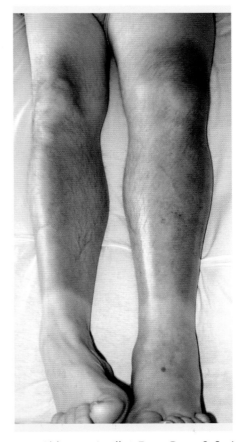

FIGURE 29-8. Phlegmasia alba. From Dean S, Satiani B, Abraham W (eds.). *Color Atlas and Synopsis of Vascular Diseases*. New York, NY: McGraw-Hill; 2013:Fig. 58-1.

BIBLIOGRAPHY

Tsekouras N, Comerota AJ. PHLEGMASIA CERULEA DOLENS. In: Dean SM, Satiani B, Abraham WT. eds. *Color Atlas and Synopsis of Vascular Diseases*. New York, NY: McGraw-Hill; 2015.

Chinsakchai K, Ten Duis K, Moll FL, de Borst GJ. Trends in management of phlegmasia cerulea dolens. *Vasc Endovascular Surg.* 2011 Jan;45(1):5–14. doi: 10.1177/1538574410388309. Review. PMID: 21193462

16. **(D)** Between 5 and 30% of the adult US population suffers from varicose veins, with a female predominance of 3:1. Risk factors found to be associated with CVI include age, sex, a family history of varicose veins, obesity, pregnancy, phlebitis, and previous leg injury. The clinical presentation is variable. Many patients are asymptomatic with only aesthetic concerns. More severe cases may present with pain, burning, edema, or ulceration. The triad of varicose veins, limb hypertrophy, and a cutaneous birthmark (port wine stain or venous malformation) in a young patient is suggestive of Klippel-Trenaunay syndrome.

The initial treatment for varicose veins is conservative, including leg elevation, avoidance of standing for prolonged periods, and compression stockings. Ablative procedures, using endovenous laser treatment and radiofrequency ablation (RFA), are effective in patients with persistent symptoms or who have recurrent superficial vein thrombosis or ulceration. Injection sclerotherapy is used for small veins (<3 mm in diameter) and in telangiectatic vessels. Saphenous vein ligation and stripping is the preferred therapy for patients with GSVs of very large diameter (>2 cm) (see Fig. 29-9).

BIBLIOGRAPHY

Creager MA, Loscalzo J. Vascular diseases of the extremities. In: Longo DL, Fauci AS, Kasper DL, Hauser SL, Jameson J, Loscalzo J (eds.), *Harrison's Principles of Internal Medicine*, 18th ed. New York, NY: McGraw-Hill; 2012:Chapter 249.

Desai SS, Mowatt-Larssen E. Overview of spider, reticular, and varicose veins. In: Dean SM, Satiani B, Abraham WT (eds.), *Color Atlas and Synopsis of Vascular Diseases*. New York, NY: McGraw-Hill; 2014.

17. **(B)** Ultrasound imaging modes include A-mode, B-mode, Doppler, M-mode, and duplex imaging. A-mode is a display of the raw radiofrequency signal over time. B-mode image is the two-dimensional reconstruction of the information obtained in the A-mode over a given space at a given time point, where the amplitude of the spikes on the A-mode image are now pixels whose brightness is governed by the amplitude of the received signal. M-mode, or motion mode, depicts movement of structures as a function of depth and time. Doppler image displays velocity (calculated from the frequency shift detected from moving objects) over time. In continuous-wave Doppler, an uninterrupted transmission of ultrasound is applied, and the return signal (sensed from a different piezoelectric element or array) is displayed as velocities detected at each time point on a time line.

Duplex ultrasound is a B-mode and uses Doppler images (see Fig. 29-10). The color flow map is useful in trying to distinguish moving structures from stationary structures or to get a sense of relative flow velocities.

High-frequency transducers (7–10 MHz) are used for superficial structures, with applications such as saphenous vein mapping and *in situ* vein bypasses or pedal bypasses, whereas lower frequency transducers (2.5,

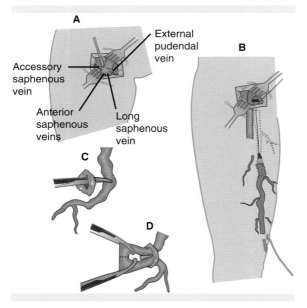

FIGURE 29-9. Saphenous vein stripping. Reproduced with permission from Bergan JJ, Kistner RL: *Atlas of Venous Surgery*. Saunders, 1992.

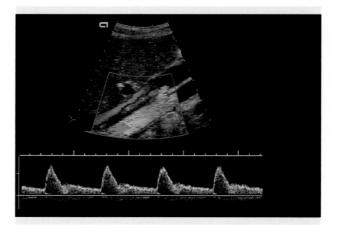

FIGURE 29-10. Duplex ultrasound. From Schrope B. *Surgical and Interventional Ultrasound*. New York, NY: McGraw-Hill; 2013:Fig. 1-11.

TABLE 29-3 Ultrasound Criteria for Acute DVT

Diagnostic Criteria	Adjunctive Criteria
Noncompressibility of veins Echogenic thrombus Diminished/absent venous flow Absence of respiratory phasicity Absent or incomplete color filling	Dilated vein <50% increase in diameter with Valsalva Nonvisualization of venous valves

3.5, or 5.0 MHz) are used for deeper structures. Because venous flow velocity is slower than arterial flow velocity, artifacts can more easily be introduced by transducer movement when performing a venous examination, especially to rule out DVT. For these reasons, a more accurate venous examination to look for DVT is one without color that demonstrates a dilated uncompressible vein. The black-and-white image allows better assessment of vein compressibility and is not confused by an artifact introduced by transducer movement. Diagnostic criteria for DVT include an evaluation of venous compressibility, intraluminal echoes, venous flow characteristics, and differential filling of the vessel in color Duplex (Table 29-3).

Arterial wall calcium occasionally interferes with vascular ultrasound scans by blocking transmission of the ultrasound wave, but it is unusual that one cannot perform an adequate vascular examination of the carotid artery or other structure.

Venography is the reference standard test for DVT, but it is rarely performed because it is invasive (painful), technically difficult, and exposes the patient to the risks of contrast dye (e.g., nephrotoxicity, anaphylaxis) and radiation. An intraluminal filling defect (i.e., section of a vein that remains dark when surrounded by white contrast dye) seen on at least two views is considered diagnostic for DVT.

BIBLIOGRAPHY

Linkins L, Kearon C. Diagnosis of venous thromboembolism. In: McKean SC, Ross JJ, Dressler DD, Brotman DJ, Ginsberg JS (eds.), *Principles and Practice of Hospital Medicine*. New York, NY: McGraw-Hill; 2012:Chapter 259.
Schrope B. Instrumentation, scanning techniques, and artifacts. In: Schrope B (ed.), *Surgical and Interventional Ultrasound*. New York, NY: McGraw-Hill; 2014:Chapter 2.

18. **(D)** Superior vena cava syndrome (SVCS) is a group of signs and symptoms that present after obstruction of the superior vena cava (SVC). More than 90% of SVC obstructions are caused by malignant tumors. More than 50% of cases result from mediastinal invasion by bronchogenic carcinoma, with lymphomas or germ cell cancers accounting for the remainder. When obstruction occurs, venous pressures rise to 20–50 mmHg.

The characteristic clinical picture of a patient with SVCS is facial swelling and dilation of the collateral veins of the head and neck, arms, and upper thoracic areas. Acute complete obstruction allows little time for the formation of collateral vessels and can therefore produce hypotension, orthostasis, significant edematous laryngeal obstruction, and even fatal cerebral edema. Obstruction between the azygos vein and the right atrium is less disabling because the azygos vein provides a large collateral venous channel for drainage of the SVC system into the IVC system. Obstruction above the azygos vein eliminates this collateral channel and is not as well tolerated.

For obstruction caused by malignancy, surgery is usually considered for non–small cell lung cancer, thymoma, thymic carcinoma, or a residual germ cell mass. Chemoradiotherapy is the mainstay of treatment for patients with small cell lung cancer, lymphoma, or germ cell tumor. Surgical management is based on location of the mass in question, involvement of associated structures besides the SVC, and degree of vascular exposure needed. Tumors with 30–50% involvement of the SVC may best be served by resection of the SVC and patch repair, whereas tumors with greater than 50% involvement of circumference of the SVC will require complete resection and reconstruction. In general, autologous grafts have performed better than prosthetic grafts. Balloon angioplasty and stenting can also be effective.

BIBLIOGRAPHY

Chmielewski GW, Liptay MJ. Resection of patients with superior vena cava syndrome. In: Sugarbaker DJ, Bueno R, Colson YL, et al. (eds.), *Adult Chest Surgery*, 2nd ed. New York, NY: McGraw-Hill; 2013.

19. **(B)**

20. **(E)**

Explanation for questions 19 and 20

The lower extremity veins are divided into superficial, perforating, and deep veins (see Fig. 29-11).

The superficial venous system of the lower extremity consists of the greater saphenous and lesser (great and small) saphenous veins. These veins contain many valves and show considerable variation in their location and branching points. The small saphenous vein begins behind the lateral malleolus and ascends the posterior calf to enter the popliteal vein behind the knee. The GSV emerges from the popliteal fossa and parallels the saphenous branch of the femoral nerve. The saphenofemoral

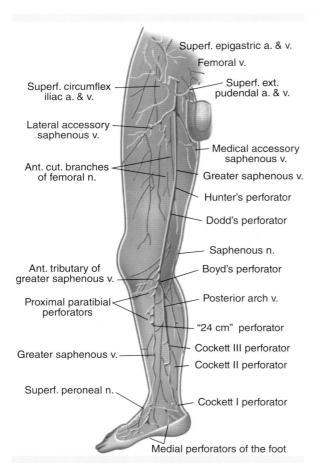

FIGURE 29-11. Veins of the lower extremity. Reproduced with permission from Mozes G, Gloviczki P, et al: Surgical anatomy for endoscopic subfascial division of perforating veins, *J Vasc Surg.* Nov;24(5):800–808, 1996.

junction is marked by five branches of the GSV: the superficial circumflex iliac vein, the external pudendal vein, the superficial epigastric vein, and the medial and lateral accessory saphenous veins.

The deep veins of the lower extremity follow the major arteries. Paired veins parallel the anterior and posterior tibial and peroneal arteries and join to form the popliteal vein. The popliteal vein becomes the superficial femoral vein as it passes through the adductor hiatus. In the proximal thigh, the superficial femoral vein joins with the deep femoral vein to form the common femoral vein.

Multiple perforating veins traverse the deep fascia to connect the superficial and deep venous systems of the lower extremity; blood flows from the superficial to the deep venous system. The Cockett perforators drain the lower part of the leg medially, whereas the Boyd perforators connect the GSV to the deep veins higher up in the medial lower leg. Incompetence of these perforators is a major contributor to the development of venous stasis and ulceration.

There are no valves in the portal vein, SVC or IVC, or common iliac vein. The calf muscles serve an important

function in augmenting venous return by acting as a pump to return blood to the heart. Venous pressure drops dramatically with walking due to the action of the calf muscles but increases in patients with venous obstruction.

At the inguinal ligament, the femoral and deep (profunda) femoral veins join medial to the femoral artery to form the common femoral vein. Proximal to the inguinal ligament, the common femoral vein becomes the external iliac vein. In the pelvis, external and internal iliac veins join to form common iliac veins that empty into the IVC. The right common iliac vein ascends almost vertically to the IVC, whereas the left common iliac vein takes a more transverse course.

BIBLIOGRAPHY

Chen H, Rectenwald JR, Wakefield TW. Veins & lymphatics. In: Doherty GM (ed.), *Current Diagnosis & Treatment: Surgery*, 14th ed. New York, NY: McGraw-Hill; 2014.

Cronenwett JL, Johnston KW. *Rutherford's Vascular Surgery*, 8th ed. Philadelphia, PA: Saunders; 2014.

21. **(B)** Approximately 200,000 patients in the United States die each year subsequent to pulmonary embolism (PE). The hemodynamic effects of PE are related to three factors: the degree of reduction of the cross-sectional area of the pulmonary vascular bed, the preexisting status of the cardiopulmonary system, and the physiologic consequences of pulmonary vasoconstriction. Obstruction of the pulmonary vascular bed by embolism acutely increases the workload on the right ventricle, leading to recruitment and distension of pulmonary vessels to maintain normal or near-normal pulmonary artery pressure and pulmonary vascular resistance. Similarly, increases in the right ventricular (RV) stroke volume and increases in the heart rate maintain cardiac output. At greater degrees of pulmonary artery obstruction, compensatory mechanisms are overcome. Cardiac output decreases and right atrial pressure increases, eventually leading to right heart dilation, increased RV wall tension, RV ischemia, decreased cardiac output, and systemic hypotension. Patients with prior cardiopulmonary disease may develop severe pulmonary hypertension in response to a relatively small reduction in pulmonary artery cross-sectional area.

Approximately 85% of patients with PE have changes on electrocardiography (ECG). ECG findings in acute PE are generally due to right heart dilation and include T-wave changes, ST-segment abnormalities, incomplete or complete right bundle branch block, right axis deviation in the extremity leads, and clockwise rotation of the QRS vector in the precordial leads. The "classic" S1, Q3, T3 pattern (a prominent S wave in lead I and a Q wave

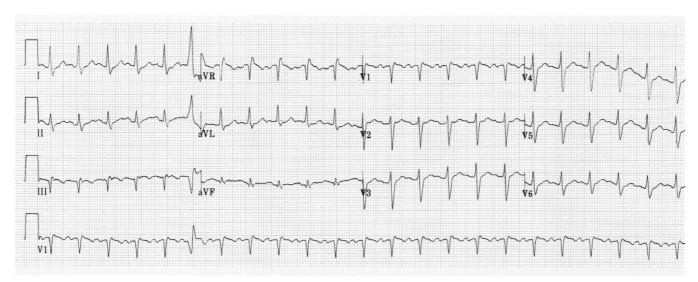

FIGURE 29-12. Sinus tachycardia and S1, Q3, T3 pattern in a patient with acute pulmonary embolism. From Knoop KJ, Stack LB, Storrow AB, Thurman RJ. *The Atlas of Emergency Medicine*, 3rd ed. New York, NY: McGraw-Hill; 2009:Fig. 23-47a.

and inverted T wave in lead III) is present in only 10% of PE cases, and approximately 20% of patients with PE have no ECG changes. The most common finding on ECG after a PE is sinus tachycardia (present in almost one half of patients) (see Fig. 29-12).

BIBLIOGRAPHY

Fedullo PF. Pulmonary embolism. In: Fuster V, Walsh RA, Harrington RA (eds.), *Hurst's the Heart*, 13th ed. New York, NY: McGraw-Hill; 2011:Chapter 72.

Fedullo PF, Yung GL. Pulmonary thromboembolic disease. In: Grippi MA, Elias JA, Fishman JA, et al. (eds.), *Fishman's Pulmonary Diseases and Disorders*, 5th ed. New York, NY: McGraw-Hill; 2014.

Hunt JM, Bull TM. Clinical review of pulmonary embolism: diagnosis, prognosis, and treatment. *Med Clin North Am* 2011;95(6):1203–1222.

22. **(D)** Flow of lymph from the tissues toward the entry point into the circulatory system is promoted by two factors: (1) increases in tissue interstitial pressure (due to fluid accumulation or due to movement of surrounding tissue) and (2) contractions of the lymphatic vessels themselves. Valves located in these vessels also prevent backward flow. Roughly 2.5 L of lymphatic fluid enters the cardiovascular system each day. In the steady state, this indicates a total body *net* transcapillary fluid filtration rate of 2.5 L/d. Thus, the lymphatics play a critical role in keeping the interstitial protein concentration low and in removing excess capillary filtrate from the tissues.

Lymphatic vessels associated with lymph nodes are of two types. Both contain valves to ensure unidirectional lymph flow through the node. Afferent lymphatic vessels deliver lymph by penetrating the capsule at several points on the convex surface. Efferent lymphatic vessels carry filtered lymph away from the node, exiting through the hilum on the concave surface.

The thoracic duct is the largest lymphatic channel in the body. It collects lymph from the entire body except the right hemithorax (thoracic wall, right lung, right side of the heart, part of the diaphragmatic surface of the liver, lower area of the right lower lobe of the liver), right head and neck, and right upper extremity.

The right lymphatic duct "typically" begins with the union of three lymphatic trunks: right jugular, right subclavian, and right bronchomediastinal ducts. It receives lymphatic drainage from the right lung, lower left lung, and right diaphragm, most of the drainage from the heart, and some drainage from the right lobe of the liver.

The lymphatic ducts deliver lymph to the venous system at the junction of the jugular and subclavian veins in the neck.

BIBLIOGRAPHY

Mohrman DE, Heller L. The peripheral vascular system. In: Mohrman DE, Heller L (eds.), *Cardiovascular Physiology*, 8th ed. New York, NY: McGraw-Hill; 2014:Chapter 6.

Paulsen DF. Lymphoid system. In: Paulsen DF (ed.), *Histology & Cell Biology: Examination & Board Review*, 5th ed. New York, NY: McGraw-Hill; 2010:Chapter 14.

Skandalakis JE, Colborn GL, Weidman TA, et al. Lymphatic system. In: Skandalakis JE, Colburn GL, Weidman TA, et al. (eds.), *Skandalakis' Surgical Anatomy*. New York, NY: McGraw-Hill; 2004:Chapter 29.

CHAPTER 30

ARTERIAL DISEASE

ANAHITA DUA, RYAN KIM, RONALD BAYS, AND SAPAN S. DESAI

QUESTIONS

1. A 62-year-old man who underwent the procedure shown in Figure 30-1 1 year ago presents with fever, abdominal pain, an ileus, and an elevated white blood cell (WBC) count. A WBC scan confirms graft infection. Which of the following is true?

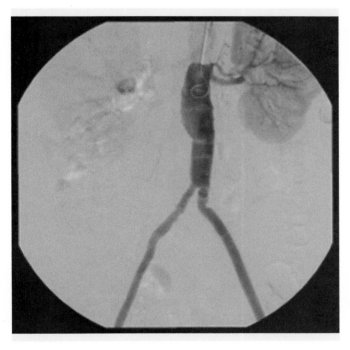

FIGURE 30-1. Endovascular aneurysm repair.

(A) The most common organism is *Bacteroides fragilis*.
(B) The risk of graft infection in this location is between 5 and 10%.
(C) Treatment consists of 6 weeks of broad-spectrum antibiotic coverage only.
(D) Implantation of a graft in an infected field is associated with 100% mortality.
(E) If surgery is performed, an axillobifemoral bypass should be constructed prior to graft excision if possible.

2. Figure 30-2 shows the aortogram of a 57-year-old male patient. Which of the following findings is this patient most likely to have on evaluation?

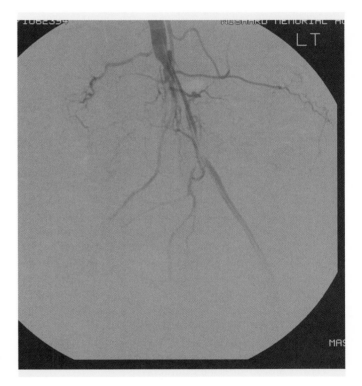

FIGURE 30-2. Aortogram.

(A) Buttock and thigh claudication
(B) Small bowel necrosis
(C) Phlegmasia cerulea dolens
(D) Ankle ulcer
(E) Lipodermatosclerosis

3. Which of the following is true regarding reconstruction for the disease present in the patient described in Question 2?
    (A) Aortobifemoral bypass patency rate is approximately 60% at 5 years.
    (B) Patients with smaller vessels have higher patency rates.
    (C) End-to-side proximal anastomosis may decrease risk of aortoenteric fistula.
    (D) Patients with a "hostile abdomen" may benefit from an axillobifemoral bypass.
    (E) Axillary-bifemoral bypasses have lower patency rates than do axillary-unifemoral bypasses.

4. A patient who required an aortobifemoral bypass graft for aortoiliac occlusive disease 3 years ago presents after an episode of severe hematemesis. His wife relates an episode of minor hematemesis 2 days prior. His hemoglobin is currently 7.2, and his systolic blood pressure (SBP) is 125. Nasogastric (NG) tube lavage illustrates profuse bright red blood. After appropriate resuscitation, the next step in management should be
    (A) Gastrointestinal (GI) consult for emergent esophagogastroduodenoscopy
    (B) Exploratory laparotomy
    (C) Computed tomography scan
    (D) Transfusion and admission to the intensive care unit
    (E) Angiography with embolization

5. A patient with a history of atrial fibrillation presents with a 6-hour history of acute right lower extremity pain. On examination, the lower extremity is cool to the touch and the patient has pain on attempts to move his foot. The femoral pulse is palpable but pulses are absent, as are Doppler signals below this level. The next step in management should be
    (A) Embolectomy and arteriogram
    (B) Echocardiogram
    (C) Anticoagulation and serial examinations
    (D) Common femoral to below knee popliteal bypass with vein
    (E) Catheter-directed thrombolysis

6. At the conclusion of the procedure mentioned in Question 5, fasciotomy is contemplated. Which of the following is true concerning compartment syndrome and the use of fasciotomy?
    (A) Compartment pressures below 30 mmHg essentially rule out the compartment syndrome.
    (B) More than 2 hours of acute ischemic time is an indication for fasciotomy.
    (C) Fasciotomy skin incisions should be closed after fascial release is completed.

    (D) Fluid resuscitation, diuretic use, and urine acidification are important measures to combat myoglobinuric renal failure.
    (E) Patients with myoglobinuric renal failure generally have favorable renal outcomes.

7. Which of the following is true regarding carotid artery stenosis?
    (A) The 5-year stroke rate for patients with a ≥60% asymptomatic lesion is 9% with surgery versus 26% with medical treatment.
    (B) The 2-year stroke rate for patients with a ≥70% symptomatic lesion is 5% with surgery versus 11% with medical treatment.
    (C) The 5-year stroke rate for patients with a ≥60% asymptomatic lesion is 5% with surgery versus 11% with medical treatment.
    (D) The 5-year stroke rate for patients with a ≥70% symptomatic lesion is 11% with surgery versus 26% with medical treatment.
    (E) Stroke rates for medical versus surgical treatment in patients with a ≥60% asymptomatic lesions are equivalent.

8. A patient presents to your office after an episode of left arm weakness. An arteriogram, shown in Figure 30-3, is obtained. Appropriate treatment would be

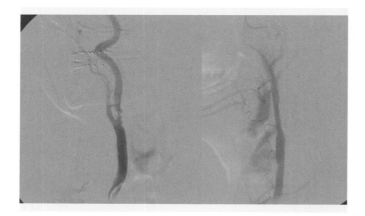

FIGURE 30-3. Arteriogram.

    (A) Medical treatment with acetylsalicylic acid 325 mg twice a day
    (B) Right carotid endarterectomy (CEA)
    (C) Left CEA followed by subsequent right CEA 2 weeks later
    (D) Right CEA followed by subsequent left CEA 2 weeks later
    (E) Heparinization and elective right CEA in 2 months

9. A 65-year-old woman is status post right-sided CEA. The procedure was complicated by injury to the right hypoglossal nerve. Which of the following would be found on physical examination?
   (A) No pinprick sensation on the right side of her tongue
   (B) Tongue deviation to the left when sticking out
   (C) Tongue deviation to the right when sticking out
   (D) No taste on the right side of the tongue
   (E) No taste on the left side of the tongue

10. The most common cranial nerve injured after CEA is
    (A) Vagus nerve
    (B) Hypoglossal nerve
    (C) Glossopharyngeal nerve
    (D) Spinal accessory nerve
    (E) Marginal mandibular nerve

11. A patient who presents for his 1-year follow-up appointment after undergoing a left CEA for stroke undergoes an arteriogram (see Fig. 30-4) after finding 50–69% recurrent stenosis on duplex ultrasound. Which of the following is true in this patient?

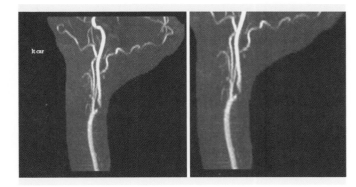

FIGURE 30-4. Arteriogram.

(A) The recurrent stenosis is most likely due to myointimal hyperplasia.
(B) The majority of these lesions are symptomatic.
(C) Treatment of the lesion is best performed by repeat endarterectomy with primary closure.
(D) Repeat operation carries a slightly lower risk of cranial nerve injury.
(E) Recurrent stenosis occurs more often with the use of a patch than during primary repairs.

12. Which of the following is true regarding the findings in Figure 30-5?

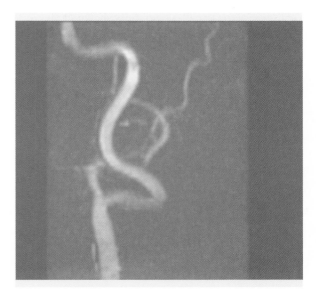

FIGURE 30-5. Arteriogram.

(A) Kinks and coils can be found in children as well as adults.
(B) Coils are more likely to be symptomatic than are kinks.
(C) Coils are usually the result of atherosclerotic disease.
(D) Definitive diagnosis can be made using duplex ultrasound.
(E) Treatment involves pexy of the redundant vessel to eliminate the kink or coil.

13. Anatomic considerations in the placement of an endoluminal abdominal aortic aneurysm stent include all of the following except
    (A) Proximal neck length
    (B) Proximal aortic diameter
    (C) Neck angulation
    (D) Aneurysm diameter
    (E) Iliac/femoral artery diameter

14. With regard to lower extremity arterial Doppler measurements, which of the following is true?
    (A) 0.94 is an abnormal ankle-brachial index (ABI).
    (B) Diabetic patients often have artificially elevated ABIs.
    (C) Segmental pressure gradients >5 mmHg signify significant disease in the intervening segment.
    (D) Most accurate pressure measurements are obtained with cuffs that are two times the diameter of the lower extremity being measured.
    (E) A change in ABI of >0.1 is clinically significant.

15. With regard to the pathologic entity shown in Figure 30-6, which of the following is true?

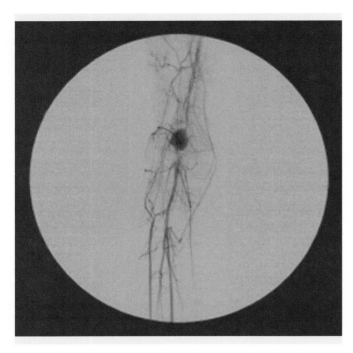

FIGURE 30-6. Angiogram.

(A) Presence in one leg is associated with up to a 10% incidence of bilaterality.
(B) Rupture is the most common complication.
(C) Embolic phenomena are rare.
(D) Asymptomatic lesions should be treated conservatively.
(E) Patients presenting with ischemia have up to a 30% primary amputation rate.

16. Which of the following is true in patients with subclavian steal?
(A) The right subclavian artery is affected significantly more often than the left.
(B) Clinical symptoms are secondary to vasospasm of the affected extremity.
(C) Bypass of the affected segment should be done using the great saphenous vein.
(D) Symptomatic lesions can be treated with median sternotomy and carotid-subclavian transposition.
(E) Transposition is contraindicated in patients with a left internal mammary artery coronary graft in place.

17. The treatment of choice for the lesion shown in Figure 30-7 is
(A) Embolectomy
(B) Replacement of the descending thoracic aorta
(C) Replacement of the aortic valve/aortic root
(D) Fenestration
(E) Endovascular repair

18. Which of the following is true regarding the lesion shown in Figure 30-7?

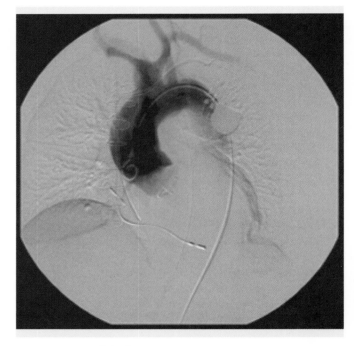

FIGURE 30-7. Arteriogram.

(A) Sudden hypotension may be due to retrograde dissection into the aortic root.
(B) Patients with abdominal pain may be observed for up to 24 hours.
(C) Malperfusion is a contraindication for endovascular repair.
(D) Intravascular ultrasound has poor sensitivity and specificity for diagnosis.
(E) A carotid-subclavian bypass should be completed in all cases.

19. A 54-year old woman undergoes abdominal computed tomography (CT) scan (see Fig. 30-8). Indications for follow-up CT arteriogram include all of the following *except*

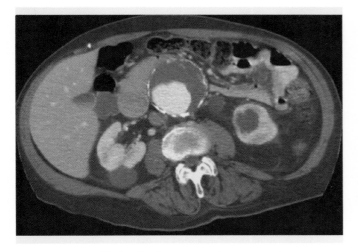

FIGURE 30-8. Abdominal computed tomography.

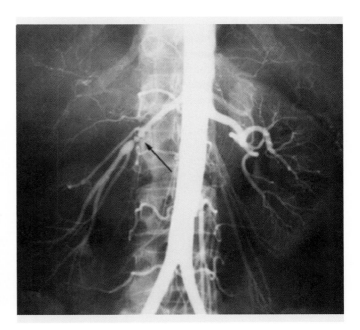

FIGURE 30-9. Arteriogram.

(A) Patient with a history of weight loss and postprandial epigastric pain
(B) Patient with calf pain after walking less than half a block
(C) Patient with blood pressure of 200/105 mmHg on three medications
(D) Patient with transient weakness of right arm and ultrasound evidence of left carotid stenosis of >80%
(E) Patient with a known horseshoe kidney and 6-cm abdominal aortic aneurysm on ultrasound

20. Embryologically, the pulmonary arteries develop from the
(A) First arch arteries
(B) Second arch arteries
(C) Third arch arteries
(D) Fourth arch arteries
(E) Sixth arch arteries

21. A 42-year-old woman undergoes an arteriogram for uncontrollable hypertension (see Fig. 30-9). What is the most likely diagnosis?
(A) Medial fibroplasia
(B) Intimal fibroplasia
(C) Perimedial fibroplasia
(D) Fibromuscular hyperplasia
(E) None of the above

22. A 76-year-old woman with hypertension, history of tobacco use, and peripheral vascular disease presents to her primary care physician complaining of intermittent epigastric abdominal pain and nausea. She states that her symptoms started 4 months ago and have been increasing in severity. The abdominal pain is dull and "gnawing," starts approximately 30 minutes after meals, and lasts 2–4 hours. The pain is sometimes accompanied by nausea. She denies vomiting, diarrhea, hematochezia, and melena. She has gotten to the point that she fears eating and has lost 18 lb since her symptoms began. She has no significant past surgical history except right carotid endarterectomy. Abdominal examination is unremarkable. Routine laboratory studies are normal except for hypoalbuminemia. Gallbladder ultrasound, esophagogastroduodenoscopy (EGD), and colonoscopy are normal. All of the following are true regarding the most likely diagnosis *except*
(A) Weight loss occurs because of severe malabsorption
(B) Greater than 95% of cases are secondary to atherosclerosis
(C) The incidence is higher in women than in men
(D) Mesenteric duplex ultrasound is a helpful screening tool in symptomatic patients
(E) This condition is a risk factor for acute mesenteric ischemia

23. Which of the following fulfills the imaging criteria for diagnosis of chronic mesenteric ischemia?
    (A) Celiac axis and superior mesenteric artery (SMA) without significant stenosis, 100% occlusion of inferior mesenteric artery (IMA)
    (B) 30% stenosis of celiac axis, 20% stenosis of both SMA and IMA
    (C) 75% stenosis of celiac axis and SMA, IMA without significant stenosis
    (D) 50% stenosis of celiac axis, SMA, and IMA
    (E) All of the above

24. Regarding the findings shown in Figure 30-10, which of the following is true?

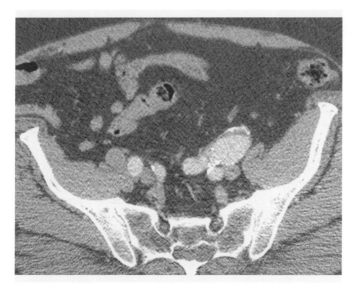

FIGURE 30-10. Computed tomography of pelvis.

    (A) The external iliac artery is most commonly involved.
    (B) It is associated with femoral artery aneurysms in 80% of cases.
    (C) It should be repaired at >2 cm in size.
    (D) Most are symptomatic.
    (E) Treatment of disease isolated to the hypogastric artery is ligation of the proximal vessel neck.

25. A patient undergoes an uncomplicated aortic aneurysm repair. The next morning, the patient is noted to have a large maroon liquid bowel movement. The patient is otherwise stable. The next step in evaluation and management should be
    (A) Immediate flexible sigmoidoscopy
    (B) Stool sample for *Clostridium difficile*
    (C) Intravenous fluid (IVF) hydration and observation
    (D) Reexploration
    (E) Abdominal x-ray with oral contrast

26. Which of the following patients with the condition seen in Figure 30-11 is the best candidate for an open repair?

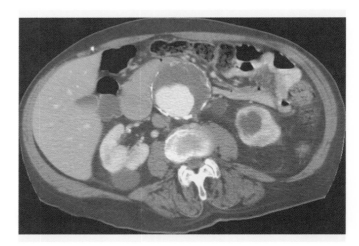

FIGURE 30-11. Computed tomography of abdomen.

    (A) 38-year-old man with a known horseshoe kidney
    (B) 36-year-old woman with 4-mm external iliac arteries bilaterally
    (C) 42-year-old woman with a preoperative creatinine of 1.2
    (D) 52-year-old man with a history of heparin-induced thrombocytopenia
    (E) 58-year-old woman with a proximal neck of 1.6 cm and a 50-degree angulated neck

27. Which of the following is true regarding aneurysmal disease of the aorta?
    (A) The aorta is considered aneurysmal when its size is twice that of the normal proximal aorta.
    (B) The incidence of aortic aneurysmal disease is greater in women than in men.
    (C) Aneurysm walls contain increased levels of collagen and elastin.
    (D) The most common presentation of abdominal aortic aneurysm (AAA) is back pain.
    (E) The 1-year risk of rupture is 80% in patients with a 7-cm AAA.

28. Which of the following patients is most likely to benefit from an endovascular intervention for renal hypertension?
    (A) 52-year-old man on two blood pressure medications with continuing hypertension
    (B) 56-year-old woman with a 7-cm-long kidney and 70% renal artery stenosis
    (C) 48-year-old woman on four blood pressure medications with severe decline in renal function
    (D) 38-year-old woman with fibromuscular dysplasia affecting the renal arteries
    (E) 61-year-old man on dialysis and four blood pressure medications

29. Which of the following is true regarding endoleaks?
    (A) They are defined as the inability to maintain blood flow around the endograft and into the lumbars or IMA.
    (B) They exist in three different types.
    (C) The main complication of an endoleak is graft thrombosis.
    (D) Type II endoleaks involve back-bleeding from persistently patent lumbar vessels.
    (E) Routing screening for endoleaks should be done with yearly angiography.

30. A 36-year-old woman with a body mass index of 23 presents with progressive abdominal pain over the past 4 years. She reports gradual weight loss over the past several years, but denies any pain with consuming food. Her physical exam is negative and contrast CT demonstrates satisfactory filling of her celiac and mesenteric arteries. What is the most likely diagnosis?
    (A) Cardiac emboli leading to intestinal ischemia
    (B) Thrombosis of a visceral artery
    (C) Renal artery stenosis
    (D) Celiac artery compression
    (E) Mesenteric venous thrombosis

31. Which of the following is true regarding the disease process pictured in Figure 30-12?

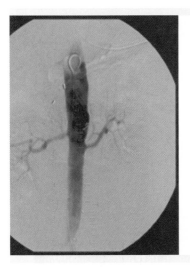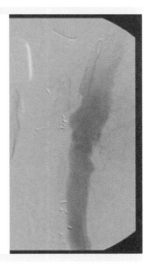

FIGURE 30-12. Mesenteric arteriogram.

    (A) Symptoms arise only when three-vessel disease is present.
    (B) Acute abdominal pain is a common presenting symptom.
    (C) Mesenteric angioplasty has replaced surgery as first-line treatment.

    (D) When surgery is performed, either the greater saphenous vein or prosthetic graft may be used as a bypass conduit.
    (E) Both the chronic and acute forms of this disease share atherosclerosis as the primary etiology.

32. Regarding cardiac risk assessment prior to peripheral vascular procedures, which of the following is the most significant independent predictor of postoperative myocardial infarction (MI)?
    (A) Angina
    (B) Age >70 years
    (C) Recent MI
    (D) Congestive heart failure (CHF)
    (E) Ectopy (>5 bpm)

33. Which of the following is true regarding the procedure shown in Figure 30-13?

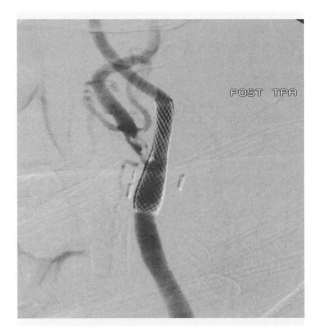

FIGURE 30-13. Arteriogram.

    (A) It should be considered an appropriate alternative to CEA for most patients with symptomatic lesions.
    (B) It is associated with a lower stroke rate compared to CEA.
    (C) It is less costly than CEA.
    (D) It is a viable alternative to CEA in high-risk patients.
    (E) It is contraindicated as treatment for carotid stenosis.

34. Regarding lower extremity amputations, which of the following is true?
    (A) Higher energy expenditure is required for ambulation after below-knee amputation (BKA) than after above-knee amputation (AKA).
    (B) Lower extremity digital amputations should be performed through the joint space to preserve smooth cartilaginous surfaces for granulation.
    (C) Dependent rubor at a proposed level of amputation is a contraindication to amputation at that level.
    (D) Guillotine amputation is inappropriate in the face of active infection.
    (E) Diabetic patients who undergo amputation have up to a 10% risk of contralateral amputation within 5 years.

35. Regarding renal artery aneurysms, which of the following is true?
    (A) Pregnancy is protective for rupture.
    (B) Etiology is almost exclusively atherosclerosis.
    (C) Risk of rupture is approximately 3%, with mortality of 10%.
    (D) Repair should be undertaken when size approaches 1 cm or greater.
    (E) Most are found intraparenchymally, making repair without nephrectomy difficult.

36. Which of the following is true regarding the group of diseases seen in Figure 30-14?
    (A) The most commonly involved vessel is the hepatic artery.
    (B) The most common complication is thrombosis and visceral ischemia.
    (C) Repair or resection is necessary in women of child-bearing age.
    (D) They are associated with abdominal aortic aneurysmal disease.
    (E) The vessel with the highest risk of rupture is the splenic artery.

37. A 35-year-old woman with hypertension is found to have a bruit on abdominal auscultation. An arteriogram was obtained and is shown in Figure 30-15. Which of the following predisposes this lesion to rupture?
    (A) Size greater than 1 cm
    (B) Pregnancy
    (C) Coexisting hypotension
    (D) Complete calcification
    (E) None of the above

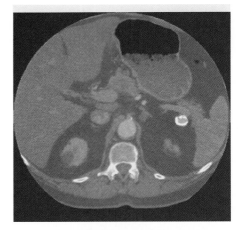

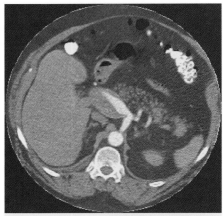

FIGURE 30-14. Visceral artery aneurysm.

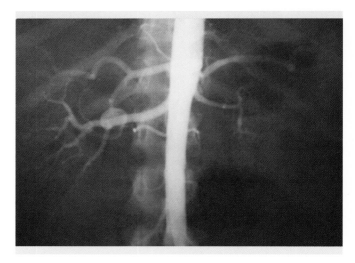

FIGURE 30-15. Abdominal arteriogram.

38. Which of the following is true regarding failing infrainguinal bypass grafts?
    (A) Early failures are usually the result of progressive atherosclerotic changes.
    (B) Critical stenoses are those that cause a 50% reduction in luminal area.
    (C) Revision of grafts should be performed only after the graft has occluded.
    (D) Grafts should be surveilled on a regular basis with duplex ultrasonography.
    (E) Percutaneous angioplasty is contraindicated in the face of a failing graft.

39. The patient with the arteriogram shown in Figure 30-16 most likely suffers from

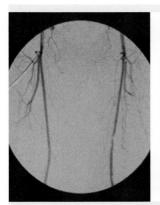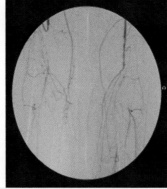

FIGURE 30-16. Arteriogram.

    (A) Diabetes
    (B) Hypertension
    (C) Tobacco abuse
    (D) Hypercholesterolemia
    (E) Hyperthyroidism

40. A healthy 24-year-old man presented with the following arteriogram after a posterior knee dislocation (see Fig. 30-17). Which of the following is true?

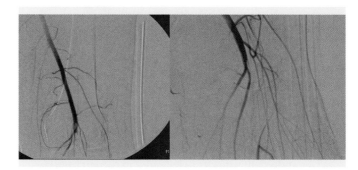

FIGURE 30-17. Arteriogram.

    (A) Presence of a pedal pulse reliably rules out significant arterial injury.
    (B) All patients with known posterior knee dislocations should undergo diagnostic arteriogram to rule out arterial injury.
    (C) Compartment syndrome is a rare complication of popliteal injury–associated knee dislocation.
    (D) In general, orthopedic repair should precede vascular repair in order to maintain lower extremity stability during arterial reconstruction.
    (E) Primary repair or bypass, usually with the contralateral saphenous vein, is indicated.

41. A 76-year-old woman with hypertension, history of tobacco use, and peripheral vascular disease presents to her primary care physician complaining of intermittent epigastric abdominal pain and nausea. The abdominal pain is dull and "gnawing," starts approximately 30 minutes after meals, and lasts 2–4 hours. The pain is sometimes accompanied by nausea. She has gotten to the point that she fears eating and has lost 18 lb since her symptoms began. She has no significant past surgical history except right CEA. Abdominal examination is unremarkable. The patient is found to have high-grade atherosclerotic lesions involving both her celiac artery and SMA. She is taken electively for antegrade prosthetic bypass grafting of both vessels. Which of the following is *not* considered to be a potential advantage of the antegrade approach versus the retrograde approach for this procedure?
    (A) Avoids direct contact with the bowel
    (B) Decreased possibility of graft kinking
    (C) Inflow comes from the less frequently diseased supraceliac aorta
    (D) Shorter graft length with direct in-line flow
    (E) Significantly better long-term patency rates

42. A 23-year-old woman in the first trimester of her pregnancy presents to the emergency department with complaints of acutely worsening left upper quadrant abdominal pain, nausea, and dizziness. She denies any fever, emesis, or any changes in bowel movements. She admits to a 5-month history of similar but milder pain in her midepigastrium and left upper abdomen, which was treated with antacids. Your evaluation reveals a well-nourished, well-developed woman who appears uncomfortable but is normotensive and only mildly tachycardic. Her abdomen is moderately tender in the left upper quadrant and epigastrium. Laboratory studies, including complete blood count, platelets, chemistries, and lipase, are appropriate. You obtain an acute abdominal series. The upright film is shown in Figure 30-18. Which of the following is true?

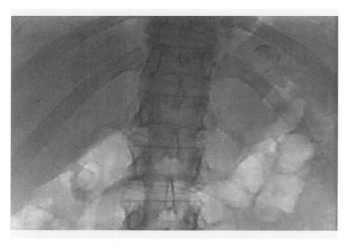

FIGURE 30-18. Splenic artery aneurysm.

(A) She should have splenectomy performed electively following delivery of her baby.
(B) Among patients with this problem, she is at relatively low risk for complications.
(C) The lesion poses a significant threat to the survival of the fetus.
(D) The most common time for complications to occur is at the time of labor and delivery.
(E) This lesion develops most commonly in patients with an alcohol abuse history or gallstones.

ANSWERS AND EXPLANATIONS

1. **(E)** Graft infections are a difficult problem for vascular surgeons; fortunately, the incidence of aortoiliac graft infection is fairly low at about 1.5%. Early graft infections (<4 months after bypass) are most often caused by *Staphylococcus aureus*, although later graft infections most often result from *Staphylococcus epidermidis*. Antibiotics alone are insufficient treatment for an aortic graft infection, but may occasionally be used in patients who are poor surgical candidates.

Aortic graft infections are best treated with graft excision and extra-anatomic bypass, such as an axillobifemoral bypass. A staged procedure is completed with extra-anatomic bypass first, followed by explantation of the infected graft several days later. Patients who present in extremis may require immediate explantation of the graft followed by a limb salvage procedure.

Szilagyi's classification

- Grade I: cellulitis involving the wound
- Grade II: infection involving subcutaneous tissue
- Grade III: infection involving the vascular prosthesis

Bunt's classification modified:
- Peripheral graft infection:
  - P0 graft infection: infection of a cavitary graft
  - P1 graft infection: infection of a graft whose entire anatomic course is noncavitary
  - P2 graft infection: infection of the extracavitary portion of a graft whose origin is cavitary
  - P3 graft infection: infection involving a prosthetic patch angioplasty
- Graft-enteric erosion
- Graft-enteric fistula
- Aortic stump sepsis after excision of an infected aortic graft

BIBLIOGRAPHY

Cronenwett JL, Johnston KW. *Rutherford's Vascular Surgery*, 8th ed. Philadelphia, PA: Saunders; 2014.
Desai SS, Shortell CK (ed.). *Clinical Review of Vascular Surgery*. New York, NY: Catalyst Publishers; 2010.

2. **(A)**

3. **(D)**

Explanation for questions 2 and 3

Leriche syndrome is a specific triad of symptoms that can affect male patients with aortoiliac occlusive disease. This triad includes thigh and buttock claudication resulting from insufficient collateralization to compensate for the increased oxygen requirements needed during activity.

Sexual dysfunction (impotence) can be a result of decreased arterial inflow. Femoral pulses will also be diminished as a result of the inflow disease. Pathology such as this can often be suggested by arterial Doppler studies. Abnormal arterial waveforms at the groin level, diminished thigh pulse volume recordings, and a decreased segmental pressure at the thigh level would signify disease at the aortoiliac level.

Small bowel necrosis and intestinal angina would not be a symptom of distal aortoiliac disease, but rather would signify mesenteric arterial disease. Phlegmasia, cerulea dolens, ankle ulcers, and lipodermatosclerosis are findings in venous disease. Lower extremity ulcers are uncommon in aortoiliac occlusive disease unless there is concomitant multilevel disease.

Revascularization of aortoiliac disease most often entails an aortobifemoral bypass. This repair is a very durable repair, with 5-year patency rates of up to 85%. Incorporating the profunda origin in the distal anastomosis has been noted to influence these increased patency rates by ensuring an adequate outflow, especially in patients who may have more distal (superficial femoral artery) disease. Other factors influencing patency of an aortobifemoral bypass include size of the aorta and age. Patients with small aortas, especially those aortas smaller than 1.8 cm, and patients younger than 50 years have significantly decreased patency rates compared with their older counterparts and those with aortas of larger diameter.

The proximal anastomosis of the bypass can be performed in an end-to-end or an end-to-side manner. Proponents of the end-to-end anastomosis cite easier ability to perform aortic endarterectomy, less chance of distal embolization from dislodgement of plaque from distal clamping, and less competitive flow down the native iliac vessels as benefits. Further, it is felt that end-to-end anastomosis may decrease the incidence of aortoenteric fistula, as the graft sits in a more anatomic position and there may be less protrusion of the graft anteriorly where the duodenum can lie against it.

However, certain situations may benefit from an end-to-side anastomosis. Patients with patent inferior mesenteric arteries may warrant this type of anastomosis to preserve flow to the IMA. In a similar manner, patients with distal iliac disease may preferentially undergo end-to-side anastomosis, as an end-to-end anastomosis may prevent any flow into the internal iliacs (prograde flow interrupted by the end-to-end nature of the anastomosis and retrograde flow prohibited by external iliac stenoses/occlusions).

If aortobifemoral bypass is not an ideal option, other alternatives exist. Axillofemoral bypasses are good options in high-risk patients. It should be noted, however, that axillobifemoral bypass has a higher patency rate than does axillounifemoral bypass. This is likely secondary to higher flow rates through the axillary limb in a bifemoral as opposed to a unifemoral graft. Patients with severely calcified aortas or multiple prior abdominal procedures may also benefit from a bypass using the descending thoracic aorta as the inflow vessel. Long-term patency rates for this bypass approach 85%.

BIBLIOGRAPHY

Cronenwett JL, Johnston KW. *Rutherford's Vascular Surgery*, 8th ed. Philadelphia, PA: Saunders; 2014.

Moore WS. *Vascular Surgery and Endovascular Surgery: A Comprehensive Review*, 8th ed. Philadelphia, PA: Saunders; 2013.

Stanley JC, Veith FJ, Wakefield TW. *Current Therapy in Vascular Surgery*, 5th ed. Philadelphia, PA: Saunders; 2014.

4. **(A)** This patient's presentation should raise concern for an aortoduodenal fistula. Patients with a known AAA or history of aortic graft placement who present with evidence of a GI bleed should be considered to have an aortoenteric fistula until proven otherwise. Aortoenteric fistulas are indeed a rather rare entity (approximately 2% of those with a GI bleed and aortic graft actually suffer from this entity); however, a misdiagnosis is often fatal. Therefore, vigilant attempts to rule out this diagnosis should be undertaken. Patients with aortoenteric fistulas usually present with a "herald bleed"—mild GI bleeding (such as hematemesis, hematochezia, or melena) that does not cause instability. If undiagnosed, however, further devastating, often fatal, hemorrhage can ensue. Thus, once presentation occurs, that window of opportunity should be taken to identify an aortoenteric fistula if present. In stable patients, prompt EGD with investigation of the third and fourth portions of the duodenum should be the first step. Findings such as extrinsic mass effect, duodenal wall bleeding, or a visible graft suture line are red flags for the diagnosis.

An exploratory laparotomy should be considered for any unstable patients or who have evidence for ongoing bleeding. In such patients, vascular control, repair of the GI fistula, removal of the graft, and revascularization if necessary (usually via extra-anatomic bypass) are often warranted. Patients who are stable and are diagnosed with an aortoenteric fistula can often undergo extra-anatomic bypass first, with graft excision under more controlled circumstances a day or two later.

CT scan can complement endoscopy, with such findings as perigraft fluid, gas bubbles, or pseudoaneurysm helping to add weight to the diagnosis of aortoenteric fistula. Aortography can illustrate anastomotic aneurysms or kinks in grafts, which can heighten suspicion of the entity and can give further anatomic information; however, this diagnostic modality generally does not demonstrate the fistula itself.

Simple conservative management in the intensive care unit without further investigation is a gross management error.

BIBLIOGRAPHY

Cronenwett JL, Johnston KW. *Rutherford's Vascular Surgery*, 8th ed. Philadelphia, PA: Saunders; 2014.
Desai SS, Shortell CK (ed.). *Clinical Review of Vascular Surgery*. New York, NY: Catalyst Publishers; 2010.
Moore WS. *Vascular Surgery and Endovascular Surgery: A Comprehensive Review*, 8th ed. Philadelphia, PA: Saunders; 2013.
Stanley JC, Veith FJ, Wakefield TW. *Current Therapy in Vascular Surgery*, 5th ed. Philadelphia, PA: Saunders; 2014.

5. **(A)** This patient has most likely developed thromboembolism of his right lower extremity due to atrial fibrillation. When emboli occur, they most often affect the lower extremities at bifurcations, such as the origin of the superficial femoral artery or tibioperoneal trunk, which tends to block all collateral channels of distal flow. These patients should be heparinized while further intervention decisions are being made.

Acute arterial occlusion of the lower extremity often presents with the six "P"s: pulselessness, pallor, pain, paralysis, paresthesia, and poikilothermia. Sensorimotor changes are usually late manifestations of the disease. Patients who present with signs and symptoms of acute arterial occlusion should be treated as vascular emergencies, as timely diagnosis and treatment are important to potential limb salvage. Patients who present with sensorimotor impingement should be taken to the operating room for a mechanical embolectomy of the affected extremity. Patients who present relatively early in the course of acute limb ischemia and who do not have sensorimotor deficits may be candidates for anticoagulation, catheter-directed thrombolytics, and serial examinations. Any progression of symptoms or failure to successfully treat the embolism requires an operative intervention. Peripheral bypass may be necessary if inline flow cannot be achieved through mechanical thrombectomy.

Identification of the embolic source via an echocardiogram is indicated once the acute limb ischemia has been resolved. Long-term anticoagulation may be necessary.

BIBLIOGRAPHY

Cronenwett JL, Johnston KW. *Rutherford's Vascular Surgery*, 8th ed. Philadelphia, PA: Saunders; 2014.
Desai SS, Shortell CK (ed.). *Clinical Review of Vascular Surgery*. New York, NY: Catalyst Publishers; 2010.
Moore WS. *Vascular Surgery and Endovascular Surgery: A Comprehensive Review*, 8th ed. Philadelphia, PA: Saunders; 2013.
Stanley JC, Veith FJ, Wakefield TW. *Current Therapy in Vascular Surgery*, 5th ed. Philadelphia, PA: Saunders; 2014.

6. **(E)** Compartment syndrome and its sequelae are potentially life-threatening complications of acute limb ischemia. Acute ischemia causes depletion of cellular energy stores, which, once repleted by reperfusion, can release toxic oxygen radicals. This can cause calcium influx and cellular disruption, releasing toxins such as potassium and myoglobin, as well as causing interstitial and cellular edema. Failure to recognize this syndrome of increased tissue pressure and release the affected compartments can cause further ischemia as the compartment pressure equalizes with the capillary pressure (as net blood flow approaches zero). The longer this condition goes untreated, the more tissue damage occurs.

Therefore, a high index of suspicion is necessary. Patients who have experienced approximately 6 hours or more of acute ischemic time have a very high likelihood of suffering from compartment syndrome and potentially irreversible tissue damage.

Thus, fasciotomy to release compartments is an important step in treatment in high-risk patients. In those cases that are questionable, compartment pressures can be measured. It used to be felt that pressures above 30–40 mmHg indicated compartment syndrome, and pressures below this were safe; however, it is now understood that perfusion pressure—rather than only an absolute pressure—is important. Patients whose compartment pressures are within 20 mmHg of their diastolic blood pressure or who are within 30 mmHg of the mean arterial pressure are at risk and should undergo fasciotomy.

Once fasciotomy is performed, skin incisions should be left open, because closure can compromise the pressures even if the fascia is released. Wounds should be carefully tended and allowed to gradually reapproximate. Skin grafts are sometimes required to close the wounds if significant swelling is seen.

Patients with reperfusion injury are at risk for acute renal failure (ARF) secondary to precipitation of myoglobin in the renal tubules. Careful attention to this is imperative, and creatine phosphokinase levels, urine myoglobin levels, and urine pH should be monitored. Fluid resuscitation, as well as diuretic use to keep urine output high (60–100 mL/h), in addition to bicarbonate for urine alkalinization, are often necessary to prevent renal damage. Mannitol is often recommended as a diuretic of choice secondary to its antioxidant effects. Patients who ultimately do suffer ARF in this setting, however, generally do well long term.

BIBLIOGRAPHY

Cronenwett JL, Johnston KW. *Rutherford's Vascular Surgery*, 8th ed. Philadelphia, PA: Saunders; 2014.

Dua A, Desai SS, Holcomb JB, Burgess AR, Freischlag, JA. *Clinical Review of Vascular Trauma*. New York, NY: Springer Verlag; 2013.

Moore WS. *Vascular Surgery and Endovascular Surgery: A Comprehensive Review*, 8th ed. Philadelphia, PA: Saunders; 2013.

Stanley JC, Veith FJ, Wakefield TW. *Current Therapy in Vascular Surgery*, 5th ed. Philadelphia, PA: Saunders; 2014.

7. **(C)** Treatment of patients with carotid stenosis has been the subject of multiple investigations over the years. The Asymptomatic Carotid Atherosclerosis Study (ACAS) investigated patients with asymptomatic lesions. This large study shows definitive benefit of surgical treatment over medical management of patients with asymptomatic lesions ≥60%. The 5-year stroke rate for patients undergoing surgical treatment (endarterectomy) was 5%, whereas those in the medical arm had a stroke rate at 5 years of 11% (an absolute risk reduction of 6% and a relative risk reduction of 53%).

Patients with symptomatic lesions have also been the subject of numerous studies, the most significant of which may be the North American Symptomatic Carotid Endarterectomy Trial (NASCET). This randomized trial illustrated a significant benefit to surgical treatment of patients with a ≥70% symptomatic stenosis of the internal carotid artery. Patients undergoing medical treatment had a 2-year stroke rate of 26%, whereas those in the surgical arm had a 2-year stroke rate of 9%. This illustrates an absolute risk reduction of 17% and relative risk reduction of 65%. In point of fact, more recent information has been published as an extension of this initial NASCET trial, indicating a statistically significant benefit to repairing symptomatic lesions ≥50%, whereas lower grade stenoses showed no statistically significant benefit from surgical treatment versus medical treatment with aspirin.

BIBLIOGRAPHY

Cronenwett JL, Johnston KW. *Rutherford's Vascular Surgery*, 8th ed. Philadelphia, PA: Saunders; 2014.

Ferguson GG, Eliasziw M, Barr HW, et al. The North American Symptomatic Carotid Endarterectomy Trial: Surgical results in 1415 patients. *Stroke* 1999;30:1751–1758.

Moore WS. *Vascular Surgery and Endovascular Surgery: A Comprehensive Review*, 8th ed. Philadelphia, PA: Saunders; 2013.

Stanley JC, Veith FJ, Wakefield TW. *Current Therapy in Vascular Surgery*, 5th ed. Philadelphia, PA: Saunders; 2014.

Executive Committee for the Asymptomatic Carotid Atherosclerosis Study. Endarterectomy for asymptomatic carotid artery stenosis. *JAMA* 1995;273(18):142–1428.

8. **(B)** Determining surgical treatment of carotid disease involves many factors, including symptoms, clinical stability of the patient, and the degree of stenosis. This patient illustrates a symptomatic right-sided lesion with complete chronic occlusion of the contralateral carotid artery. Because the left carotid is occluded and asymptomatic, surgical intervention is not warranted. The right side, however, is tightly stenotic and symptomatic. Therefore, surgical repair is advisable (2-year stroke rate for medical management of 26% vs 9% with surgical treatment). Elective repair in patients who have a recent history of transient ischemic attack or stroke is associated with recurrent stroke, and CEA should be completed within 2 weeks.

There are two main options to monitor cerebral perfusion while under general anesthesia: the measurement of internal carotid artery backpressure and the intraoperative use of electroencephalogram. The current literature supports either selective shunting based on clinical finding or routine shunting.

Intraoperatively, the decision to shunt a patient is very important, because up to 15% of patients without contralateral occlusion will have inadequate collateral circulation to supply the brain during carotid occlusion during surgery. Awake patients can be "tested" by occluding the common carotid artery and external and internal carotid arteries for 3 minutes. If no neurologic changes occur during this time, shunting can be safely forgone.

Patients who are under general anesthetic, however, should be investigated to determine if a shunt is indeed required. The most common method is measurement of "stump" or "back" pressures from the internal carotid artery after ipsilateral common carotid artery occlusion. A 22-gauge needle can be introduced into the common carotid artery distal to its clamp, and backpressures can be measured. Alternatively, some shunts are made to allow measurement of backpressures once the shunt is in place. Pressures of >30–50 mmHg have been used as a cutoff for performance of the endarterectomy without shunting. Pressures lower than this indicate the need for shunt placement. Other options include cerebral oximetry and electroencephalogram monitoring.

BIBLIOGRAPHY

Cronenwett JL, Johnston KW. *Rutherford's Vascular Surgery*, 8th ed. Philadelphia, PA: Saunders; 2014.

Moore WS. *Vascular Surgery and Endovascular Surgery: A Comprehensive Review*, 8th ed. Philadelphia, PA: Saunders; 2013.

Stanley JC, Veith FJ, Wakefield TW. *Current Therapy in Vascular Surgery*, 5th ed. Philadelphia, PA: Saunders; 2014.

9. **(C)** The hypoglossal nerve travels in a plane between the jugular vein and internal carotid artery (see Fig. 30-19).

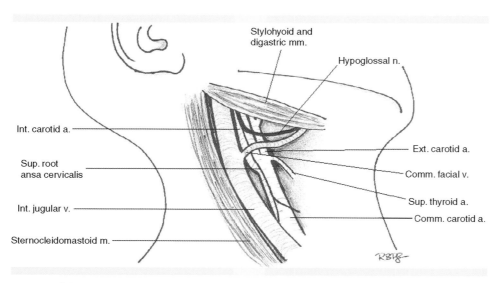

FIGURE 30-19. Anatomy of the neck.

It passes medially over the carotid usually distal to the bifurcation and proximal to the posterior belly of the digastric muscle. It is identified by following the superior root of the ansa cervicalis (often referred to as the descending hypoglossal nerve) superiorly to the point where it meets the hypoglossal nerve crossing the internal carotid. It can be mobilized superomedially to allow adequate exposure for CEA, and this may require transection of the superior root of the ansa cervicalis (this usually causes no noticeable loss of strap muscle function). Occasionally the hypoglossal nerve is not easily identified at surgery, as it can be hidden under the facial vein or digastric muscle. Accidental transection of the nerve is a rare complication. More often, it is injured by prolonged retraction. Retraction injury will usually recover relatively quickly.

The hypoglossal is a pure motor nerve, responsible for the innervation of the intrinsic and extrinsic muscles of the tongue (except palatoglossus, which is innervated by the vagus nerve). When injured, there is weakness of ipsilateral tongue muscles, causing the tongue to protrude toward the side of injury.

Sensation of the anterior two-thirds of the tongue is mediated by the lingual nerve (a branch of the mandibular division of the trigeminal nerve). The posterior one-third is supplied by the glossopharyngeal nerve. Taste is a special sensation mediated by the facial, glossopharyngeal, and vagus nerves.

The hypoglossal nerve descends in the neck in a plane between the internal jugular vein and internal carotid artery before swinging medially toward the tongue. It will cross the internal and external carotid between the bifurcation and the digastric muscle. The superior root

of the ansa cervicalis can be mobilized off the common carotid and retracted medially or even sacrificed to allow superomedial retraction of the hypoglossal nerve. Occasionally the nerve is difficult to identify, because it may be fixed to the underside of the common facial vein or the digastric muscle.

BIBLIOGRAPHY

Ballotta E, Da Giau G, Renon L, et al. Cranial and cervical nerve injuries after carotid endarterectomy: a prospective study. *Surgery* 1999;125:85–91.

Hayashi N, Hori E, Ohtani Y, Ohtani O, Kuwayama N, Endo S. Surgical anatomy of the cervical carotid artery for carotid endarterectomy. *Neurol Med Chir (Tokyo)* 2005;45:25–30.

Kim GE, Cho YP, Lim SM. The anatomy of the circle of Willis as a predictive factor for intra-operative cerebral ischemia (shunt need) during carotid endarterectomy. *Neurol Res* 2002;24:237–240.

10. **(B)** Nerve injuries are a significant risk during CEA, because several important nerves run in very close proximity to the carotid artery (see Table 30-1 and Fig. 30-20). The overall incidence of cranial nerve injuries can be up to 20% based on close clinical examination and has been found to be up to 39% if more detained investigation by ear, nose, and throat (ENT)/speech pathology is undertaken. The vast majority are asymptomatic and/or temporary, resolving over the next 6 weeks. In CREST, there was no significant impact of cranial nerve injury after 1 year.

The most commonly injured nerve after CEA is the hypoglossal nerve. The hypoglossal nerve runs at the superior extent of the incision just above the bifurcation

TABLE 30-1 Incidence of Cranial Nerve Dysfunction
TABLE 30-1 Incidence of Cranial Nerve Dysfunction Following Carotid Endarterectomy

Hypoglossal nerve	4.4–17.5%
Recurrent laryngeal nerve	1.5–15%
Superior laryngeal nerve	1.8–4.5%
Marginal mandibular nerve	1.1–3.1%
Glossopharyngeal nerve	0.2–1.5%
Spinal accessory nerve	<1.0%

of the common carotid artery. It is in close relation to the posterior belly of the digastric muscle and is injured in up to 17.5% of cases secondary to excess traction.

Injury to the hypoglossal nerve manifests as ipsilateral deviation of the tongue upon extension; most cases are temporary and resolve within a few months.

Injury to branches of the vagus nerve are less common, occurring in between 1.5 and 15% of cases. These injuries tend to be subclinical in most cases but can be detected with careful examination by an experienced otolaryngologist or neurologist.

Injury to the spinal accessory nerve is rare because this nerve is not commonly seen in the operative field.

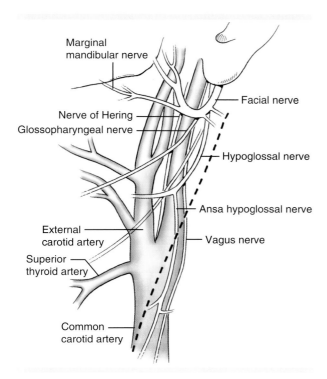

FIGURE 30-20. Nerves encountered during carotid endarterectomy. From Minter R, Doherty G. *Current Procedures Surgery*. New York, NY: McGraw-Hill; 2010:Figure 35-2.

Injury to the marginal mandibular nerve occurs in up to 3.1% of cases and is commonly secondary to vigorous retraction along the inferior border of the mandible. This presents with ipsilateral lip drooping; contralateral drooping of the lip is concerning for an intraoperative or postoperative stroke.

BIBLIOGRAPHY

Cronenwett JL, Johnston KW. *Rutherford's Vascular Surgery*, 8th ed. Philadelphia, PA: Saunders; 2014.

Desai SS, Shortell CK (ed.). *Clinical Review of Vascular Surgery*. New York, NY: Catalyst Publishers; 2010.

Ferguson GG, Eliasziw M, Barr HW, et al. The North American Symptomatic Carotid Endarterectomy Trial: surgical results in 1415 patients. *Stroke* 1999;30:1751–1758.

Moore WS. *Vascular Surgery and Endovascular Surgery: A Comprehensive Review*, 8th ed. Philadelphia, PA: Saunders; 2013.

11. **(A)** Recurrent carotid stenosis is believed to occur in anywhere from 1 to 21% of endarterectomized carotid arteries. The etiology of the disease differs depending on the time interval between operation and restenosis. In patients with restenosis within the first 2 years after operation, the etiology is most often myointimal hyperplasia (collagen proliferation in the arterial wall). This is more common in women. Those developing recurrent stenosis after 2 years are more likely to suffer from recurrent atherosclerotic disease.

Patients who present with myointimal hyperplasia are most often asymptomatic, because there usually is a smooth surface that tends to preclude plaque formation, ulceration, and embolization. This is usually discovered on routine surveillance, and treatment of the asymptomatic lesion is usually preempted until the stenosis is ≥80%.

Those who suffer from recurrent atherosclerotic disease should be treated under the same guidelines as are those with primary carotid stenosis. Regardless of the etiology, recurrent stenosis should be treated with the use of patch angioplasty. The risk of restenosis after initial CEA has been shown to be significantly greater after primary arterial closure—especially of small vessels—than with patch (up to 21% vs 7% in ACAS trials). Thus, on reoperation, the use of a patch is extremely important. One difference in the operative treatment of myointimal hyperplasia as opposed to recurrent atherosclerotic disease is the fact that myointimal hyperplasia rarely is amenable to repeat endarterectomy. The smooth surface usually makes it difficult to find a dissection plane. Patching the artery is usually sufficient. Atherosclerotic lesions, on the other hand, require repeat endarterectomy to remove the plaque from the diseased vessel.

Due to the increased technical difficulty and higher complication rate of repeat CEA, carotid stenting with distal filter protection may be an alternative option. Although this is usually a lower risk procedure, the studies from AbuRahma and colleagues and Bowser and colleagues reported lower perioperative stroke rates with repeat CEA than with carotid artery stenting for recurrent stenosis.

BIBLIOGRAPHY

Cronenwett JL, Johnston KW. *Rutherford's Vascular Surgery*, 8th ed. Philadelphia, PA: Saunders; 2014.
Moore WS. *Vascular Surgery and Endovascular Surgery: A Comprehensive Review*, 8th ed. Philadelphia, PA: Saunders; 2013.
Stanley JC, Veith FJ, Wakefield TW. *Current Therapy in Vascular Surgery*, 5th ed. Philadelphia, PA: Saunders; 2014.

12. **(A)** Kinks and coils can be found in both children and adults, as they can be primary or acquired. Those found in children are often coils and are the result of incomplete straightening of the carotid artery (from the third aortic arch/dorsal aorta) as the heart descends into the mediastinum during development. In adults, coils often result from progressive elongation of the vessel as a person ages. Kinks are usually secondary to atherosclerosis and therefore are more commonly symptomatic.

Kinks and coils are often initially found after examination notes a pulsatile mass in the neck suspicious for aneurysm. Noninvasive studies can be suggestive, but primary diagnosis requires angiogram.

Once symptomatic lesions are diagnosed, surgical treatment should be undertaken. Unfortunately, simply pexying of the elongated artery is insufficient. Treatment entails removal of the redundant segment of the vessel, which can be done via resection of the segment with

reanastomosis, interposition, or reimplantation of the internal carotid artery to the common carotid artery.

BIBLIOGRAPHY

Cronenwett JL, Johnston KW. *Rutherford's Vascular Surgery*, 8th ed. Philadelphia, PA: Saunders; 2014.
Moore WS. *Vascular Surgery and Endovascular Surgery: A Comprehensive Review*, 8th ed. Philadelphia, PA: Saunders; 2013.
Stanley JC, Veith FJ, Wakefield TW. *Current Therapy in Vascular Surgery*, 5th ed. Philadelphia, PA: Saunders; 2014.

13. **(D)** When considering placing an endoluminal stent graft for aortic aneurysm repair, several anatomic considerations must be addressed. The neck of the aneurysm (the area between the renal arteries and the start of the aneurysmal dilatation) should ideally be at least 10 mm in length to prevent the graft from crossing the renal artery orifices and yet have a solid docking purchase. Endograft diameter is a maximum of 36 mm; therefore, a neck diameter in excess of 32 mm precludes this type of repair. Aortic angulation in excess of 60 degrees also prevents proper deployment of the graft. And because the femoral route is used to deploy the devices, femoral and iliac artery diameter and tortuosity are important in that arteries that are too tortuous or too small to accommodate the 12- to 24-French diameter devices are contraindications to graft placement.

Once grafts are in place, close follow-up is required to identify endoleaks should they occur. The purpose of the stent graft is to exclude the aneurysm from the arterial system, thus preventing further enlargement. If for some reason the aneurysm sees arterial flow and, therefore, pressure (an endoleak), enlargement and eventual rupture could occur. There are four types of endoleaks (see Fig. 30-21).

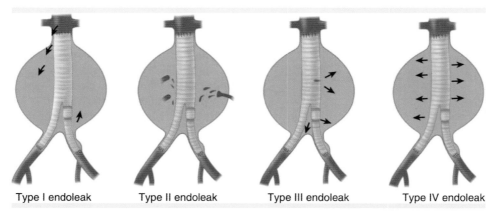

FIGURE 30-21. Types of endoleak. From Brunicardi F, Andersen DK, Billiar TR, et al. (eds.), *Schwartz's Principles of Surgery*, 10th ed. New York, NY: McGraw-Hill; 2014:Figure 23-34.

Type I: Inadequate seal of proximal or distal end of endograft or inadequate seal of iliac occluder plug

Type II: Flow from patent lumbar, middle sacral, or IMA, hypogastric, accessory renal, or other visceral vessel

Type III: Fabric disruption or tear or module disconnection

Type IV: Flow from fabric porosity, suture holes

Endoleaks can occur at any time throughout the life of the graft; therefore yearly, ultrasound or contrast-enhanced CT scans are required to evaluate for any such leak or expansion of the aneurysm with subsequent intervention if necessary.

BIBLIOGRAPHY

Cronenwett JL, Johnston KW. *Rutherford's Vascular Surgery*, 8th ed. Philadelphia, PA: Saunders; 2014.
Moore WS. *Vascular Surgery and Endovascular Surgery: A Comprehensive Review*, 8th ed. Philadelphia, PA: Saunders; 2013.

14. **(B)** Ankle-brachial index (ABI) is often used as a noninvasive screening tool for lower extremity arterial disease. The highest upper extremity SBP measurements from each arm are obtained and compared with SBP measurements obtained at the posterior tibial and dorsalis pedis arteries. Normal ABIs are approximately 1, and anything below 0.90 is considered abnormal, indicating lower extremity arterial disease; however, medial wall calcification seen with diabetic patients can cause an inability to compress the vessels of the calf, leading to an artificially elevated ABI. Waveform analysis and toe-brachial indices are helpful in these patients.

Inappropriate cuff size can also be the cause of erroneous measurements. Cuffs that are too small can lead to erroneously elevated pressures. Therefore, cuff size should be at least 1.5 times the diameter of the vessel to ensure more accurate measurements.

Serial ABIs can be used to follow progression of disease. There is inherent variability, however, from one measurement to the next, even with a single person doing the measurements. Variability of up to 0.15 has been reported; therefore, anything greater than that should be considered clinically significant for disease progression.

In addition to ABIs, segmental pressures at different levels in the lower extremities can be measured to better delineate the level of disease. Measurements are sequentially taken at the thigh, upper calf, and ankle levels. Pressure differences of 10 mmHg or more indicate significant disease in the intervening segment. The larger the gradient, the more significant is the disease.

BIBLIOGRAPHY

Cronenwett JL, Johnston KW. *Rutherford's Vascular Surgery*, 8th ed. Philadelphia, PA: Saunders; 2014.
Moore WS. *Vascular Surgery and Endovascular Surgery: A Comprehensive Review*, 8th ed. Philadelphia, PA: Saunders; 2013.

15. **(E)** Popliteal artery aneurysms are primarily associated with atherosclerosis. The presence of an aneurysm in one leg should precipitate an investigation for the presence of an aneurysm in the other popliteal artery because bilaterality is common. Up to 50% of patients have bilateral popliteal aneurysms, and 30–50% of patients may have AAA. Patients with popliteal aneurysms can present in several ways. The usual presentation is secondary to ischemic complications from thrombosis of the aneurysm or embolism of clot distally. Compression of venous or nervous structures adjacent to a large aneurysm can also lead to pain or swelling of the lower extremity. Rarely, aneurysms present as rupture (see Fig. 30-22).

Because patients who present with ischemic complications tend to ultimately do much worse (up to 30% primary amputation rate) than do patients who undergo elective repair (up to a 95% limb salvage rate), early repair of popliteal aneurysms is important.

Symptomatic aneurysms should be repaired regardless of size. Treatment of asymptomatic aneurysms is a bit more controversial. Aneurysms 2 cm or greater in size, even if asymptomatic, are recommended for surgical repair, whereas some advocate repair of smaller

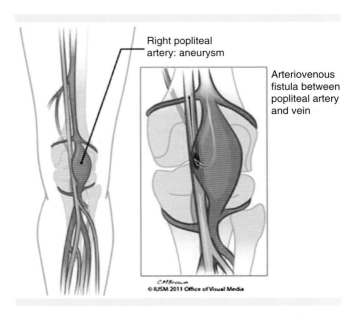

Right popliteal artery: aneurysm

Arteriovenous fistula between popliteal artery and vein

© IUSM 2011 Office of Visual Media

FIGURE 30-22. Popliteal artery aneurysm rupture. Used with permission of Thom Rooke, MD.

asymptomatic aneurysms with thrombus precisely because the complications can be so devastating.

Options for elective repair are endovascular approach with an intraluminal stent graft and open surgical bypass of the aneurysmal segment with ligation above and below the aneurysm to prevent collateral flow and subsequent continued flow into the aneurysmal segment. Although endovascular repair of popliteal artery aneurysms is widely performed and successful, the US Food and Drug Administration has not yet approved the use of stent graft for this particular procedure. Contraindications for endovascular repair are lack of proximal and/or distal landing zones, lack of adequate inflow and outflow, a marked discrepancy in the diameter of the proximal and distal landing zones, and a marked stenosis at the edge of the aneurysm.

BIBLIOGRAPHY

Cronenwett JL, Johnston KW. *Rutherford's Vascular Surgery*, 8th ed. Philadelphia, PA: Saunders; 2014.
Moore WS. *Vascular Surgery and Endovascular Surgery: A Comprehensive Review*, 8th ed. Philadelphia, PA: Saunders; 2013.
Stanley JC, Veith FJ, Wakefield TW. *Current Therapy in Vascular Surgery*, 5th ed. Philadelphia, PA: Saunders; 2014.

16. **(A)** Subclavian artery disease, although not common, can present with symptom constellations that require surgical correction. The left subclavian artery is more often affected than the right. Symptoms can develop in the form of upper extremity ischemia. Upper extremity "claudication" or rest pain can be the result of significant proximal stenosis. In addition, proximal subclavian stenotic lesions can embolize, leading initially to significant ischemia at the digital level and progressing proximally if diagnosis is delayed. This can lead to potential limb-threatening ischemia.

In addition to upper extremity ischemia, the clinical subclavian "steal" syndrome can be the first manifestation of proximal subclavian stenosis. In this situation, the patient, although asymptomatic at rest, cannot compensate for the increased blood flow requirements with use of the arm. Flow is then "stolen" from the ipsilateral vertebral artery. Vertebral artery flow reverses to supply the arm. As a result of the decreased vertebrobasilar perfusion, clinical symptoms of dizziness, drop attacks, vertigo, syncope, or ataxia may arise.

When clinical symptoms arise, surgical treatment is indicated. Aortography with views of the arch and extremity run-off is necessary to identify the location of the lesion and any affected distal vessels. Once decision to treat surgically is made, options include

carotid-subclavian bypass, carotid-subclavian artery transposition, or stenting. Both bypass and transposition have excellent patency rates of >90–95%. Bypass with prosthetic materials—polytetrafluoroethylene (PTFE) or Dacron—have a higher patency rate than vein (85–95% with prosthetic vs approximately 65% with vein). Transposition (division of the subclavian artery proximally with anastomosis to the common carotid artery) is also a viable option but is contraindicated in patients with left internal mammary artery (LIMA) coronary bypass grafts secondary to the coronary ischemia that would result from occlusion of the subclavian proximal to the take-off of the internal mammary artery vessel.

In selected patients with focal narrowing, angioplasty and stenting can also be a successful means of treatment. In experienced hands, initial success rates can approach 100%, with up to a 70% 2-year continued patency.

BIBLIOGRAPHY

Cronenwett JL, Johnston KW. *Rutherford's Vascular Surgery*, 8th ed. Philadelphia, PA: Saunders; 2014.
Moore WS. *Vascular Surgery and Endovascular Surgery: A Comprehensive Review*, 8th ed. Philadelphia, PA: Saunders; 2013.
Stanley JC, Veith FJ, Wakefield TW. *Current Therapy in Vascular Surgery*, 5th ed. Philadelphia, PA: Saunders; 2014.

17. **(E)**

18. **(A)**

Explanation for questions 17 and 18

Figure 30-7 illustrates a type B aortic dissection. Aortic dissections are classified according to the site of the intimal tear. The DeBakey classification separates aortic dissections into types I, II, and III (see Fig. 30-23): type I aortic dissections involve the ascending aorta and extend into the descending aorta; type II aortic dissections are limited to just the ascending aorta; and type III aortic dissections are limited to just the descending aorta.

The Stanford classification separates aortic dissections into types A and B: type A aortic dissections involve the ascending aorta and may involve the descending aorta; and type B aortic dissections involve exclusively the descending aorta.

Diagnosis of aortic dissection is often initially made by a CT of the chest, abdomen, and pelvis with intravenous (IV) contrast. Confirmatory studies include transesophageal echocardiography, which can visualize the proximal tear for patients with type A aortic dissection. Intraoperative studies that can confirm the diagnosis, identify the site of the tear, and assist with proper placement of the stent graft for type B aortic dissection include arteriography and

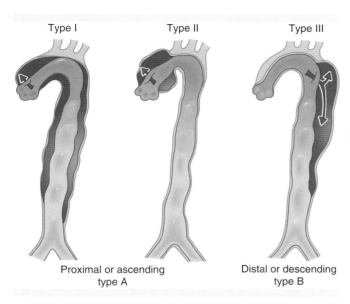

FIGURE 30-23. DeBakey and Stanford classifications of aortic dissection. From Doherty GM (ed.). *Current Diagnosis & Treatment: Surgery*, 13th ed. New York, NY: McGraw-Hill; 2010:Figure 19-16.

intravascular ultrasound (IVUS). All of these are relatively sensitive and specific tests for aortic dissection.

Patients who present with a type A aortic dissection often require emergent or urgent operative repair due to the risk of rupture, retrograde dissection into the aortic root (leading to subsequent myocardial ischemia and hypotension), and progression of disease. Many of these patients will require circulatory bypass and replacement of their ascending aorta. Depending on the extent of disease, replacement of the aortic root, reimplantation of the coronary arteries, and replacement of the aortic arch may also be necessary.

Patients with type B aortic dissection who present with intestinal malperfusion, limb ischemia, severe pain, or uncontrollable hypertension (i.e., failure with two or more agents) should undergo a thoracic endovascular aneurysm repair (TEVAR) using a stent-graft. Depending upon the site of the intimal tear, coverage of the left subclavian artery may be necessary to ensure a satisfactory proximal landing zone for the stent-graft. In emergency situations, most patients do not require a carotid-subclavian bypass, and subsequent arm ischemia tends to be negligible due to the rich collaterals present. For patients with a LIMA to left anterior descending (LAD) bypass from a prior coronary artery bypass graft (CABG) and for most elective cases, an initial carotid to subclavian bypass may be necessary prior to completion of the TEVAR.

BIBLIOGRAPHY

Cronenwett JL, Johnston KW. *Rutherford's Vascular Surgery*, 8th ed. Philadelphia, PA: Saunders; 2014.

Estrera AL, Miller CC, Goodrick J, et al. Update on outcomes of acute type B aortic dissection. *Ann Thorac Surg* 2007;83(2): S842–S845.

Moore WS. *Vascular Surgery and Endovascular Surgery: A Comprehensive Review*, 8th ed. Philadelphia, PA: Saunders; 2013.

Stanley JC, Veith FJ, Wakefield TW. *Current Therapy in Vascular Surgery*, 5th ed. Philadelphia, PA: Saunders; 2014.

19. **(D)** Current technology has increased the available imaging modalities for evaluation of vascular disease. The easiest and least invasive screening tool is abdominal ultrasonography. Ultrasound is considered the study of choice for evaluation of suspected aneurysmal disease and for routine follow-up of asymptomatic, known aneurysms. There are drawbacks to ultrasound, however. Skill of the operator and overlying bowel gas or significant obesity can limit accuracy of ultrasound. Therefore, alternate imaging techniques are required. Modalities such as CT scanning with three-dimensional reconstructions can demonstrate not only the size of an aneurysm, but also the extent of involvement of the aorta itself (e.g., thoracic or iliac involvement) as well as the aneurysm's relationship to other structures such as the renal or mesenteric arteries. CT angiography (CTA) with maximum-intensity projection (MIP) three-dimensional reconstructions has become the best minimally invasive tool of choice for evaluation of most vascular conditions prior to treatment.

Patients who present with symptoms of intestinal ischemia, such as weight loss, postprandial pain, or food fear, should be investigated with CTA to rule out mesenteric occlusive disease. Patients with evidence of iliac or infrainguinal occlusive disease likewise may benefit from optimal evaluation of their arterial tree. Patients with evidence of renovascular hypertension or renal anomalies such as horseshoe kidney also should undergo CTA. In this way, surgical correction of symptomatic renal artery stenosis may be planned or identification of important renal artery anomalies can be made and surgery planned accordingly.

A patient with transient ischemic attack and ultrasound evidence of high-grade stenosis in an accredited lab is an indication for surgery to prevent stroke. Further imaging studies are not necessary unless other complications exist.

BIBLIOGRAPHY

Cronenwett JL, Johnston KW. *Rutherford's Vascular Surgery*, 8th ed. Philadelphia, PA: Saunders; 2014.

Moore WS. *Vascular Surgery and Endovascular Surgery: A Comprehensive Review*, 8th ed. Philadelphia, PA: Saunders; 2013.

Stanley JC, Veith FJ, Wakefield TW. *Current Therapy in Vascular Surgery*, 5th ed. Philadelphia, PA: Saunders; 2014.

20. **(E)** The embryology of the vascular system is complex and is especially so for the aortic arch and its branches. There are embryologically six paired aortic arch arteries, which undergo development, regression, or alteration to become ultimately the aortic arch and its branches (see Fig. 30-24).

Early in gestation, the embryo develops paired dorsal aortas, which continue to about the C7–T1 level, where the heart is beginning to form. Below this, the aorta fuses. The paired arch arteries form from the paired dorsal aortae and ultimately fuse into the arch and its branch arteries.

The first arches develop into a part of the internal carotid arteries, whereas the second and fifth arches are essentially obliterated.

The third aortic arches form the common carotid arteries, whereas the fourth arches ultimately form the

roots of the right and left subclavian arteries. The left fourth arch artery also forms the aortic arch. The sixth arch arteries form the pulmonary arteries after the left sixth artery helps form the ductus arteriosus.

BIBLIOGRAPHY

Cronenwett JL, Johnston KW. *Rutherford's Vascular Surgery*, 8th ed. Philadelphia, PA: Saunders; 2014.

Moore WS. *Vascular Surgery and Endovascular Surgery: A Comprehensive Review*, 8th ed. Philadelphia, PA: Saunders; 2013.

Stanley JC, Veith FJ, Wakefield TW. *Current Therapy in Vascular Surgery*, 5th ed. Philadelphia, PA: Saunders; 2014.

21. **(A)** The arteriogram reveals fibromuscular dysplasia (FMD), also known as fibrodysplasia, involving the main renal artery with the characteristic "string of beads" appearance (see Fig. 30-25). Medial fibroplasia is the most common fibrous lesion, accounting for 68–91% of

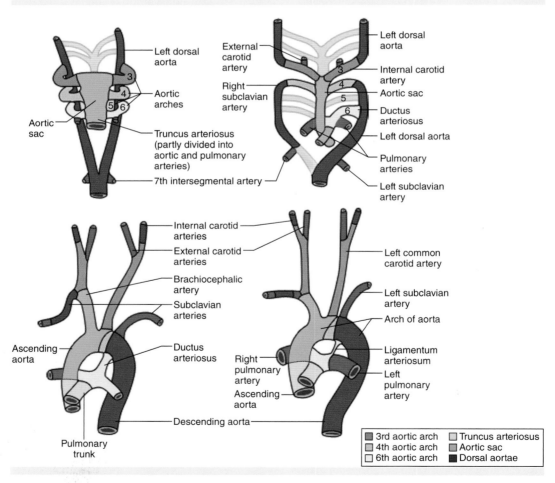

FIGURE 30-24. Arch development. Reproduced with permission from Moore KL. *The Developing Human: Clinically Oriented Embryology*. Philadelphia: WB Saunders Co., 1982.

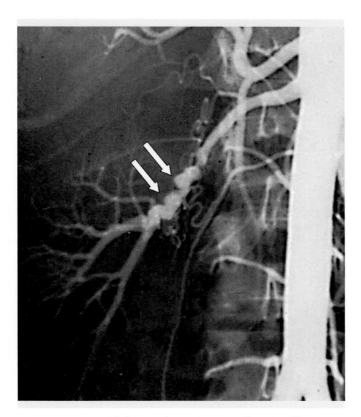

FIGURE 30-25. Abdominal arteriogram showing fibromuscular dysplasia (*arrows*). From Brunicardi F, Andersen DK, Billiar TR, et al. (eds.), *Schwartz's Principles of Surgery*, 9th ed. New York, NY: McGraw-Hill; 2009.

the fibromuscular dysplasias. The string of beads appearance results from the presence of collagenous rings alternating with aneurysmal dilations. These involve the media of the distal main renal artery and often extend into smaller branches.

These lesions tend to occur more frequently in Caucasians and females. The patients usually presents with treatment-resistant or malignant hypertension. The lesion may cause aneurysms and dissection; however, complete vessel occlusion, renal infarction, and severe renal insufficiency are infrequent.

Percutaneous transluminal renal angioplasty (PTRA) has become the treatment of choice over open surgical procedure for renovascular hypertension due to FMD. PTRA provides good results, and stenting is usually not required. The indications of stent placement in FMD are severe procedural complications, persistent pressure gradient after multiple angioplasty attempts, or aneurysms in the renal artery.

BIBLIOGRAPHY

Cronenwett JL, Johnston KW. *Rutherford's Vascular Surgery*, 8th ed. Philadelphia, PA: Saunders; 2014.

Stanley JC, Veith FJ, Wakefield TW. *Current Therapy in Vascular Surgery*, 5th ed. Philadelphia, PA: Saunders; 2014.

22. **(A)**

23. **(C)**

Chronic mesenteric ischemia is caused by atherosclerosis in more than 90% of cases. Other causes include thrombosis associated with thoracoabdominal aneurysm, aortic coarctation, aortic dissection, mesenteric arteritis, fibromuscular dysplasia, neurofibromatosis, middle aortic syndrome, Buerger disease, and extrinsic celiac artery compression by the median arcuate ligament. Although atherosclerosis of the mesenteric vessels is common, the chronic mesenteric ischemia is uncommon due to the development of collateral vessels and slow progression of arterial stenosis.

The median age of diagnosis is 65 years, and there is a higher incidence in women than men. The most common risk factor for chronic mesenteric ischemia is smoking, and most patients with chronic mesenteric ischemia have evidence of vascular disease elsewhere as well. It has similar risk factors as atherosclerosis anywhere in the body; however, hypercholesterolemia may be absent in these patients secondary to malnutrition.

Symptoms of chronic mesenteric ischemia commonly include postprandial abdominal pain, fear of eating, and weight loss. Diarrhea, nausea and vomiting, and constipation are less common symptoms. Abdominal pain is the most consistent symptom and typically occurs 15 to 45 minutes after a meal and lasts several hours. It is generally described as midabdominal, achy or crampy in quality, and worsening in severity as the disease progresses. Some patients will naturally reduce the size of their meals, which may at least initially decrease their symptoms. In most cases, abdominal pain eventually leads the patient to avoid eating and lose weight. This unintentional weight loss correlates well with the severity of symptoms. Although some degree of malabsorption occurs with chronic mesenteric ischemia, malabsorption does not account for the majority of weight loss in these patients. On physical examination, abdominal tenderness is nonlocalized and mild, an abdominal bruit may be appreciated in 50–70% of patients, and evidence of peripheral vascular disease is often present.

Diagnosis of chronic mesenteric ischemia requires ruling out other causes for abdominal pain and documenting significant mesenteric stenosis in a symptomatic patient. Mesenteric duplex ultrasound is a good screening test for symptomatic patients before progressing to CTA. It is inexpensive, noninvasive, and has a sensitivity of 87% for celiac stenosis and 92% for SMA stenosis for >70% stenosis. Disadvantages are that it requires expertise to both perform and interpret, and the inferior mesenteric artery is visualized less than 50% of the time. The diagnosis of chronic mesenteric ischemia requires at least two-vessel stenosis, and most patients with chronic mesenteric ischemia have significant stenosis involving the celiac axis and/or SMA. Therefore, patients without disease visualized on ultrasound can usually be ruled out for chronic mesenteric ischemia, and patients with significant disease on ultrasound should be followed up with CTA.

Diagnosis of chronic mesenteric ischemia has three requirements. The patient must have symptoms consistent with the disease, other causes of abdominal pain and weight loss must be excluded, and moderate- to high-grade stenosis must be demonstrated in at least two mesenteric arteries.

First, the patient must have a clinical presentation consistent with the disease. Symptoms of chronic mesenteric ischemia commonly include postprandial abdominal pain, fear of eating, and weight loss. Diarrhea, nausea and vomiting, and constipation are less common symptoms. Abdominal pain is the most consistent symptom and typically occurs 15–60 minutes after a meal and lasts several hours. It is generally described as midabdominal, achy or crampy in quality, and worsening in severity as the disease progresses. Some patients will naturally reduce the size of their meals, which may at least initially decrease their symptoms. In most cases, abdominal pain eventually leads the patient to avoid eating and lose weight. Average weight loss is around 10 kg. This weight loss correlates well with the severity of symptoms. Although some degree of malabsorption occurs with chronic mesenteric ischemia, malabsorption does not account for the majority of weight loss in these patients. On physical examination, abdominal tenderness is nonlocalized and mild, an abdominal bruit may be appreciated, and evidence of peripheral vascular disease is often present. Occasionally an asymptomatic patient will incidentally be found to have significant mesenteric artery stenosis on aortogram. Those patients who go on to require aortic reconstruction generally have their mesenteric stenosis corrected at the time of aortic surgery; however, optimal management of the subgroup of asymptomatic patients who have mesenteric stenosis and do not require aortic surgery is not known.

The second criterion for diagnosis of chronic mesenteric ischemia is exclusion of other causes of abdominal pain and weight loss. Patients typically undergo an extensive workup before the diagnosis is made. Laboratory studies tend to be nonspecific and may include anemia, hypoalbuminemia, hypoproteinemia, and leukopenia. Malabsorption tests including fecal fat and D-xylose may also be abnormal. Common diagnostic tests performed include abdominal ultrasound and EGD. These exclude other causes of upper abdominal pain originating from gastroduodenal, hepatic, or biliary sources. EGD may on occasion demonstrate gastroduodenal ischemic ulcers. Colonoscopy should also be performed if there are symptoms concerning for lower tract disease, but is rarely helpful in diagnosis of chronic mesenteric ischemia. CT is also a good choice for further evaluation of causes for abdominal pain; however, it is not the best choice for demonstrating mesenteric artery disease.

Last, demonstration of significant two-vessel mesenteric stenosis must be made to complete the diagnosis. Often symptomatic patients are now screened for mesenteric stenosis with duplex ultrasound. If stenosis of one or more arteries is suspected on ultrasound, the patient should next undergo mesenteric CTA to demonstrate the extent of the disease and possibly confirm the diagnosis. A diagnosis of chronic mesenteric ischemia can be made if angiography shows moderate-grade (50–74%) to high-grade (75–99%) stenosis or occlusion in at least two mesenteric arteries. In up to 90% of cases, significant disease of both the celiac axis and SMA will be discovered. Half of these patients will also have IMA disease. Rarely a patient may be found to have symptomatic single-vessel occlusion because of poor development of collaterals. This is only seen in occlusion of the celiac axis or SMA. The clinician should be cautious in the diagnosis of chronic mesenteric ischemia in patients with only single-vessel occlusion because of the rarity of its occurrence.

There is no role for a conservative management in symptomatic patients. Chronic mesenteric ischemia puts a patient at risk for acute mesenteric ischemia. Up to 80% of patients presenting with acute mesenteric ischemia from thrombosis may have had previous symptoms consistent with chronic ischemia. It has also been estimated that 20–50% of acute mesenteric ischemia secondary to thrombosis occurs in the setting of preexisting mesenteric stenosis. Therefore, the treatment for the patient who has documented symptomatic mesenteric stenosis is a revascularization procedure (open or endovascular).

BIBLIOGRAPHY

Brandt LJ, Boley SJ. AGA technical review on intestinal ischemia. *Gastroenterology* 2000;118:954–968.

Cronenwett JL, Johnston KW. *Rutherford's Vascular Surgery*, 8th ed. Philadelphia, PA: Saunders; 2014.

Laissy J, Trillaud H, Douek P. MR angiography: noninvasive vascular imaging of the abdomen. *Abdom Imaging* 2002;27(5):488–506.

Moore WS. *Vascular Surgery and Endovascular Surgery: A Comprehensive Review*, 8th ed. Philadelphia, PA: Saunders; 2013.

Sreenarasimhaiah J. Chronic mesenteric ischemia. *Best Pract Res Clin Gastroenterol* 2005;19:283–295.

Stanley JC, Veith FJ, Wakefield TW. *Current Therapy in Vascular Surgery*, 5th ed. Philadelphia, PA: Saunders; 2014.

24. **(E)** Iliac artery aneurysms are, as isolated entities, rare, accounting for less than 2% of all aneurysms. Most often they are seen in combination with aortic aneurysmal disease, and they most often involve the common iliac artery (70%), the internal iliac artery (20%), or both. Approximately one-third of patients with iliac aneurysmal disease will have bilateral lesions. Although difficult to diagnose with certainty from history and physical examination, most iliac aneurysms are symptomatic, even when unruptured. Most commonly, abdominal, flank, or groin pain is the presenting complaint and is often attributed to some other etiology. The aneurysm itself is often diagnosed during imaging studies for that other presumed pathology.

The larger the aneurysm, the higher is the risk of rupture, and ruptured iliac artery aneurysms carry an extremely high mortality rate (approximately 40%). Thus, early detection and appropriate intervention are key. Isolated iliac artery aneurysms should be fixed if symptomatic or if asymptomatic at a diameter of 3 cm or greater. Lesser aneurysms should be addressed if in conjunction with repair of an AAA.

Treatment of iliac artery aneurysms is dependent on location. If isolated to the common iliac artery, it can often be treated transabdominally by graft replacement. Internal iliac disease can be addressed via catheter-based coil embolization or endoaneurysmorrhaphy; however, simple ligation of the neck of the aneurysm is not adequate treatment because collateral flow will still allow expansion of an internal iliac artery aneurysm.

BIBLIOGRAPHY

Cronenwett JL, Johnston KW. *Rutherford's Vascular Surgery*, 8th ed. Philadelphia, PA: Saunders; 2014.

Desai SS, Shortell CK (ed.). *Clinical Review of Vascular Surgery*. New York, NY: Catalyst Publishers; 2010.

Moore WS. *Vascular Surgery and Endovascular Surgery: A Comprehensive Review*, 8th ed. Philadelphia, PA: Saunders; 2013.

25. **(A)** One of the most devastating complications that can arise from AAA repair is colonic ischemia. Several factors can influence the development of ischemia. Ligation of the IMA or interruption of both hypogastric arteries in a patient with inadequate collateralization of the colon from the SMA, embolization during aneurysm manipulation, intraoperative hypotension, and direct compression from retractors can all have an effect.

Certain measures can be taken intraoperatively to help prevent ischemia. Minimal manipulation of the aortic neck and prevention of hypotension or compression can help. Measurement of the backpressures within the IMA can usually be done from inside the opened aneurysm sac. Mean pressure >40 mmHg can be an indication for safe ligation of the IMA. Pressures lower than this would require reimplantation of the IMA.

Postoperatively, early diagnosis of colonic ischemia requires a high index of suspicion. Acidosis, elevated WBC, and increased fluid requirements can be early warning signs. Diarrhea, especially bloody or watery and especially in the first day or two after surgery, should also be aggressively investigated.

Patients with obvious peritoneal signs or evidence of hemodynamic instability should be taken emergently to the operating room; however, stable patients suspected of having colonic ischemia should undergo immediate flexible sigmoidoscopy because the left colon and rectum are most often involved. Patients with full-thickness necrosis should be taken to the operating room for resection, whereas patients with ischemia limited to the mucosa should be treated supportively with nothing by mouth status, NG tube decompression, broad-spectrum antibiotics, and fluid resuscitation. Repeat endoscopy should be performed to document resolution or progression of the ischemia, and appropriate subsequent action should be taken.

BIBLIOGRAPHY

Cronenwett JL, Johnston KW. *Rutherford's Vascular Surgery*, 8th ed. Philadelphia, PA: Saunders; 2014.

Moore WS. *Vascular Surgery and Endovascular Surgery: A Comprehensive Review*, 8th ed. Philadelphia, PA: Saunders; 2013.

Stanley JC, Veith FJ, Wakefield TW. *Current Therapy in Vascular Surgery*, 5th ed. Philadelphia, PA: Saunders; 2014.

26. **(B)** This patient has an abdominal aortic aneurysm (AAA). Patients who have an AAA greater than 5.0–5.5 cm are candidates for operative intervention. Patients who undergo endovascular aneurysm repair (EVAR) require at least a 1.5-cm proximal landing zone and neck angulation of less than 60 degrees; furthermore, the size of their iliac vessels must be large enough to tolerate the placement of 18- to 24-French sheaths (at least 6–8 mm in size).

Patients who have some element of renal dysfunction may undergo EVAR using intravascular ultrasound and limited contrast; preoperative hydration is necessary in these patients. Patients with a history of heparin-induced thrombocytopenia can undergo anticoagulation using argatroban or bivalirudin. The presence of a horseshoe kidney is not an absolute contraindication to EVAR. Careful examination of the preoperative and intraoperative imaging is required to ensure that accidental coverage of a main renal artery does not occur.

BIBLIOGRAPHY

Cronenwett JL, Johnston KW. *Rutherford's Vascular Surgery*, 8th ed. Philadelphia, PA: Saunders; 2014.
Moore WS. *Vascular Surgery and Endovascular Surgery: A Comprehensive Review*, 8th ed. Philadelphia, PA: Saunders; 2013.
Stanley JC, Veith FJ, Wakefield TW. *Current Therapy in Vascular Surgery*, 5th ed. Philadelphia, PA: Saunders; 2014.

27. **(E)** Aneurysmal disease is a fairly common disease. The aorta is considered aneurysmal when the diameter of the diseased aorta is dilated to a diameter 50% greater than that of the proximal, normal aorta. In a male, the average normal diameter of the abdominal aorta is approximately 2 cm, whereas in a female, it measures about 1.8 cm. Therefore, an aorta that measures approximately 3 cm in a male and 2.7 cm in a female would be considered aneurysmal. Once again, however, these "averages" are subject to some variability based on the normal aorta above the aneurysmal dilation.

AAA affects both men and women, although males are affected much more frequently, with a male-to-female ratio of about 4–5:1. White ethnicity, increased age, positive family history, smoking, and hypertension are also associated with aneurysmal disease, with smoking being one of the most strongly associated factors.

Collagen and elastin are substances found in the aortic wall but are significantly decreased in AAA formation. Aneurysmal aortas are noted to have increased levels of metalloproteases such as collagenase and elastase in relation to their inhibitors, such as α_1-antitrypsin. This imbalance leads to weakening of the aortic wall and aneurysmal changes.

Although back or abdominal pain is the most common symptom of aortic aneurysmal disease, most AAAs are asymptomatic at presentation. In fact, 70% of patients with aneurysms are diagnosed as an incidental finding on physical examination or imaging studies performed for unrelated issues. Other symptoms include embolic phenomena, dissection, and rupture.

Indeed, rupture of an AAA is the most significant and indeed life-threatening sequela of aneurysmal disease. The risk of rupture of an AAA increases with increasing size of the aneurysm, with about a 5-year rupture rate of 25% for aneurysms 5–6 cm. This risk increases to approximately 50% for aneurysms 6–7 cm and 80–100% for aneurysms ≥7 cm. Sudden, acute back, flank, or abdominal pain, especially when coupled with shock and/or pulsatile abdominal mass, should alert one to the presence of ruptured AAA.

Chronic obstructive pulmonary disease (COPD) and hypertension also have been found to be independent risk factors for aneurysm expansion and risk of rupture.

BIBLIOGRAPHY

Cronenwett JL, Johnston KW. *Rutherford's Vascular Surgery*, 8th ed. Philadelphia, PA: Saunders; 2014.
Moore WS. *Vascular Surgery and Endovascular Surgery: A Comprehensive Review*, 8th ed. Philadelphia, PA: Saunders; 2013.
Stanley JC, Veith FJ, Wakefield TW. *Current Therapy in Vascular Surgery*, 5th ed. Philadelphia, PA: Saunders; 2014.

28. **(D)** Patients with renal artery stenosis may develop severe hypertension. Renal artery stenosis leads to a decrease in afferent arteriole pressure in the affected kidney, leading to a decrease in glomerular filtration rate. This is interpreted as a drop in blood pressure by the affected kidney, leading to activation of the renin-angiotensin-aldosterone axis. The net result is an increase in sodium absorption, vasoconstriction, and increase in intravascular volume, resulting in hypertension. Severe hypertension and stenosis can lead to renal atrophy and a subsequent decline in renal function. The success of endovascular management declines significantly in these patients.

The best candidates for endovascular management are patients who continue to have hypertension refractory to medical management after maximizing the use of at least three agents. Success from endovascular management is maximized in patients with at least a 10-cm kidney and no significant decline in renal function. Other candidates for endovascular stent placement for renal artery stenosis are patients with fibromuscular dysplasia.

BIBLIOGRAPHY

Cronenwett JL, Johnston KW. *Rutherford's Vascular Surgery*, 8th ed. Philadelphia, PA: Saunders; 2014.
Moore WS. *Vascular Surgery and Endovascular Surgery: A Comprehensive Review*, 8th ed. Philadelphia, PA: Saunders; 2013.

29. **(D)** When considering placing an endoluminal stent graft for aortic aneurysm repair, several anatomic considerations must be addressed. The neck of the aneurysm (the area between the renal arteries and the start of the aneurysmal dilatation) should ideally be at least 15 mm in length to prevent the graft from crossing the renal artery orifices and yet have a solid docking purchase. Endograft diameter is a maximum of 30 mm; therefore, a neck diameter in excess of 28 mm

precludes this type of repair. Aortic angulation in excess of 60 degrees also prevents proper deployment of the graft. In addition, because the femoral route is used to deploy the devices, femoral and iliac artery diameter and tortuosity are important in that arteries that are too tortuous or too small to accommodate the 18- to 23-French diameter devices are contraindications to graft placement.

Once grafts are in place, close follow-up is required to identify endoleaks should they occur. The purpose of the stent graft is to exclude the aneurysm from the arterial system, thus preventing further enlargement. If, for some reason, the aneurysm sees arterial flow and, therefore, pressure (an endoleak), enlargement and eventual rupture could occur. There are several types of endoleaks described.

A type I leak is an inability of the proximal or distal end of the device to completely seal, thus allowing blood flow into the aneurysm sac.

A type II leak occurs when lumbar vessels or the IMA remain patent, allowing continued pressure to be exposed to the aneurysm sac.

A type III leak occurs when component pieces of the endograft (such as an iliac extension) break apart, whereas type IV leaks occur secondary to graft porosity.

Endoleaks can occur at any time throughout the life of the graft; therefore, yearly contrast-enhanced CT scans are required to evaluate for any such leak or expansion of the aneurysm with subsequent intervention if necessary.

BIBLIOGRAPHY

Cronenwett JL, Johnston KW. *Rutherford's Vascular Surgery*, 8th ed. Philadelphia, PA: Saunders; 2014.

Desai SS, Shortell CK (ed.). *Clinical Review of Vascular Surgery*. New York, NY: Catalyst Publishers; 2010.

Moore WS. *Vascular Surgery and Endovascular Surgery: A Comprehensive Review*, 8th ed. Philadelphia, PA: Saunders; 2013.

30. **(D)** Patients with a gradual weight loss and no evidence of food fear should be ruled out for occult tumors, mesenteric ischemia, and feeding disorders. In this relatively young patient with gradual weight loss over several years and no evidence of food fear and negative diagnostic imaging, the most likely diagnosis is celiac artery compression. This disorder is also known as median arcuate ligament syndrome and occurs when the median arcuate ligament compresses upon the celiac artery during expiration. Diagnostic arteriography during expiration is diagnostic. Treatment for this condition is laparotomy and resection of the median arcuate ligament.

Acute intestinal ischemia is a surgical emergency and, as such, requires a high index of suspicion when circumstances are consistent with its possibility. Of the options listed in the question, all except celiac artery compression are common etiologies of acute ischemic changes.

Arterial embolism is the most common cause of acute mesenteric ischemia. Embolic phenomena (as shown in Fig. 30-6) are usually cardiac in origin and tend to occlude the SMA secondary to its relatively parallel course with the aorta. Preexisting atherosclerotic disease can also serve as a nidus for thrombus formation, causing acute occlusion of the vessel. Low-flow states, often termed nonocclusive mesenteric ischemia (NOMI), are seen most commonly in situations that present with hypotension, such as sepsis or heart failure. Use of high doses of α-agonists can compound this phenomena because vasoconstriction in the face of already compromised blood supply can further risk ischemic damage to the bowel.

Mesenteric venous thrombosis causes ischemia secondary to the high backpressures caused by obstruction of venous outflow. The bowel subsequently becomes edematous and distended, and hemorrhagic infarction can occur.

Celiac artery compression (median arcuate ligament syndrome) does not usually cause acute ischemic events but can be an uncommon contributing factor in chronic mesenteric ischemia.

BIBLIOGRAPHY

Cronenwett JL, Johnston KW. *Rutherford's Vascular Surgery*, 8th ed. Philadelphia, PA: Saunders; 2014.

Moore WS. *Vascular Surgery and Endovascular Surgery: A Comprehensive Review*, 8th ed. Philadelphia, PA: Saunders; 2013.

Stanley JC, Veith FJ, Wakefield TW. *Current Therapy in Vascular Surgery*, 5th ed. Philadelphia, PA: Saunders; 2014.

31. **(D)** Unlike acute mesenteric ischemia, chronic mesenteric ischemia is caused by atherosclerotic progression in the vast majority of cases. As a result, the process is often insidious, usually not becoming symptomatic until two of the three mesenteric vessels become significantly stenotic. Often, large fully developed collateral vessels to the bowel can be seen as a result. The most common complaint of patients with chronic mesenteric ischemia is crampy, postprandial pain, often called "intestinal angina." In fact, the pain associated with food intake often leads to "food fear," and weight loss develops, with significant malnutrition, as the patient avoids food.

Duplex ultrasound can sometimes be used to aid in diagnosis, using elevated visceral artery peak systolic flow velocities as an indication of disease; however, this is operator dependent, and therefore, mesenteric angiography is still the study of choice for diagnosis.

Once diagnosed, treatment is planned. Angioplasty with or without stenting has been proposed as an alternative to surgical revascularization; however, the ostial location of many of the lesions and a relatively high restenosis rate have prevented endoluminal treatment from becoming more widespread. Further studies and longer follow-up are required to determine its place in the treatment of this condition.

Surgery in the form of aortomesenteric bypass is still the treatment of choice. Greater saphenous vein or prosthetic grafts may be used, although kinking of the greater saphenous vein from the weight of the intestine can be an issue if improperly positioned during surgery.

BIBLIOGRAPHY

Cronenwett JL, Johnston KW. *Rutherford's Vascular Surgery*, 8th ed. Philadelphia, PA: Saunders; 2014.
Moore WS. *Vascular Surgery and Endovascular Surgery: A Comprehensive Review*, 8th ed. Philadelphia, PA: Saunders; 2013.
Mowatt-Larssen E, Desai SS, Dua A, Shortell CEK (eds.). *Phlebology, Vein Surgery, and Ultrasonography*. New York, NY: Springer Verlag; 2014.
Stanley JC, Veith FJ, Wakefield TW. *Current Therapy in Vascular Surgery*, 5th ed. Philadelphia, PA: Saunders; 2014.

32. **(C)** Patients with peripheral vascular disease have a high likelihood of having concomitant coronary disease (up to 50%). In fact, MI is the most common cause of perioperative morbidity and mortality in the vascular patient. Therefore, identifying patients at risk is of extreme importance.

Elderly patients (>70 years), patients who have suffered an MI within the previous 6 months, and those who have mitral regurgitation, ventricular ectopy, or severe CHF are at statistically significantly increased risk of perioperative MI than are their counterparts who do not suffer these symptoms. However, patients with stable angina pectoris without evidence of the other risk factors mentioned earlier are not at significantly higher risk for perioperative MI.

Of the factors listed, recent MI is the most important risk factor for perioperative cardiac events. Risk is up to 30% within 3 months of an MI and finally levels off at 5% after 6 months.

Selective coronary angiography may be beneficial in identifying patients at higher risk who would require further cardiac treatment prior to vascular interventions.

BIBLIOGRAPHY

Cronenwett JL, Johnston KW. *Rutherford's Vascular Surgery*, 8th ed. Philadelphia, PA: Saunders; 2014.

Moore WS. *Vascular Surgery and Endovascular Surgery: A Comprehensive Review*, 8th ed. Philadelphia, PA: Saunders; 2013.

33. **(D)** The procedure demonstrated is a carotid angioplasty and stent placement for carotid artery stenosis. The Carotid Revascularization Endarterectomy Versus Stent Trial (CREST; 2010) reported no significant difference between carotid artery stenting (CAS) and CEA in regard to the perioperative morbidity and mortality.

Several recent studies have demonstrated that patients who undergo carotid artery stenting have a higher risk of stroke compared to patients who undergo CEA. However, patients who undergo CEA are more likely to develop a postoperative myocardial infarction (Table 30-2).

TABLE 30-2 Centers for Medicare and Medicaid Services Criteria: Patients at High Risk for Carotid Endarterectomy

Age >80 y Recent (<30 d) MI LVEF <30% Contralateral carotid occlusion New York Heart Association class III or IV CHF Unstable angina: Canadian Cardiovascular Society Class III/IV Renal failure: ESRD on dialysis	Common carotid artery lesions below clavicle Severe chronic lung disease Previous neck radiation High cervical ICA lesion Restenosis of prior CEA Tracheostomy Contralateral laryngeal nerve palsy

CEA, carotid endarterectomy; CHF, congestive heart failure; ESRD, end-stage renal disease; ICA, internal carotid artery; LVEF, left ventricular ejection fraction; MI, myocardial infarction.

When considering the composite end point of stroke, MI, and death, there is no difference between CEA and stenting. However, subgroup analysis demonstrated that patients who developed an MI following CEA were far less likely to be debilitated compared to patients who had a stroke. When comparing carotid artery stenting to CEA with regard to quality of life, patients who undergo CEA tend to fare better. The national trend over the past 5 years has been a severe decline in carotid stenting.

The best candidates for carotid angioplasty and stent placement are patients who have had multiple prior neck operations, who have an anatomically inaccessible lesion, or who would not tolerate open surgery.

BIBLIOGRAPHY

Centers for Medicare and Medicaid Services. National coverage determination (NCD) for percutaneous transluminal angioplasty (PTA). https://www.cms.gov/medicare-coverage-database/details/ncd-details.aspx?NCDId=201&bc=AgAAQAAAAAAA&ncdver=9. Accessed November 25, 2015.

Cronenwett JL, Johnston KW. *Rutherford's Vascular Surgery*, 8th ed. Philadelphia, PA: Saunders; 2014.

Moore WS. *Vascular and Endovascular Surgery: A Comprehensive Review*, 8th ed. Philadelphia, PA: Saunders; 2013.

Vilain KR, Magnuson EA, Li H, et al. Costs and cost-effectiveness of carotid stenting versus endarterectomy for patients at standard surgical risk: results from the Carotid Revascularization Endarterectomy Versus Stenting Trial (CREST). *Stroke* 2012;43(9):2408–2416.

34. **(C)** Decisions regarding site of amputation can be difficult for the vascular surgeon, especially when differentiating between a BKA and an AKA. When amputation is required, it is important to remove all necrotic or infected tissue while providing enough blood flow to heal. If ambulation is a goal, BKA is preferable to AKA because the energy expenditure required to ambulate on a below-knee prosthesis is lower than that of an above-knee prosthesis (approximately a 40% increase for BKA vs 70% increase for AKA).

It can be difficult to determine by clinical examination alone which level is appropriate for amputation. Often, further testing such as Doppler studies or transcutaneous oximetry ($TCPO_2$) levels are obtained. One physical finding that can be useful, however, is presence of dependent rubor. This redness that occurs with the leg in the dependent position is an indication of tissue ischemia, and any amputation through this level should be avoided. Further testing, such as Doppler studies or $TCPO_2$ levels, is often obtained. Skin temperature measurements and arteriography have been found to be not reliable and do not correlate well with the healing potential.

Patients with active infection or gangrene can also pose special problems. Often formal amputation with skin closure is not optimal in patients with active infection or hemodynamic instability. In these instances, guillotine amputation can remove offending tissue, allowing stability of the patient and control of infection with definitive amputation several days later.

Technique and clinical judgment regarding amputations are not just important for major amputations. Toe amputations also require forethought. Amputation should be performed just distal or proximal to a joint space because cartilage is avascular and does not allow for adequate granulation or healing.

Unfortunately for diabetics, the need for amputation of one lower extremity is a fairly significant risk factor for the loss of the other lower extremity, with a 5-year cumulative incidence of second amputation of up to 33%.

BIBLIOGRAPHY

Cronenwett JL, Johnston KW. *Rutherford's Vascular Surgery*, 8th ed. Philadelphia, PA: Saunders; 2014.

Moore WS. *Vascular Surgery and Endovascular Surgery: A Comprehensive Review*, 8th ed. Philadelphia, PA: Saunders; 2013.

Stanley JC, Veith FJ, Wakefield TW. *Current Therapy in Vascular Surgery*, 5th ed. Philadelphia, PA: Saunders; 2014.

35. **(C)** Renal artery aneurysms are rare entities. The incidence in the general population is approximately 0.1%. Several etiologic factors play a role in the development of these aneurysms, including medial degeneration (as with other visceral artery aneurysms), hypertension, and even trauma. Atherosclerosis can be an etiologic factor but is often a secondary result. The vast majority of these aneurysms are saccular aneurysms that are found outside the parenchyma at first- or second-order branch points.

Despite the aneurysmal dilation, rupture is not common. Only approximately 3% of renal artery aneurysms rupture, and rupture carries a mortality rate of approximately 10%. One exception to this general rule is the pregnant patient. Pregnant women have a much higher mortality rate than do other patients with renal artery aneurysms. Mortality in these patients approached 40–50% for the mother and 80% for the fetus. Therefore, it is imperative that women of child-bearing age who plan on conceiving or are pregnant undergo repair of these aneurysms when diagnosed.

Other indications for repair include symptomatic aneurysms. Symptoms include rupture, embolization to the renal parenchyma (with worsening renal failure), renovascular hypertension, pain, or dissection. Increasing size of the aneurysm is also an indication for surgery. In the absence of these symptoms, however, size at which a renal artery aneurysm should be fixed has been somewhat controversial, but most now recommend repair at a size of 2 cm or greater.

Repair of these aneurysms often can be accomplished with simple resection of the aneurysm and primary patch angioplasty of the renal vessel (if the vessel is large enough; e.g., main renal artery) or renal artery bypass, usually with saphenous vein. The internal iliac artery can also be used. Stent grafting or coil embolization may be an alternative for the high-risk patient or as a bridge procedure until after pregnancy; however, radiation must be avoided to a fetus. Nephrectomy is not usually necessary in these cases but may be the only recourse for ruptured aneurysms. Rare intraparenchymal aneurysms may also require resection, but partial nephrectomy will usually suffice.

BIBLIOGRAPHY

Cronenwett JL, Johnston KW. *Rutherford's Vascular Surgery*, 8th ed. Philadelphia, PA: Saunders; 2014.
Moore WS. *Vascular Surgery and Endovascular Surgery: A Comprehensive Review*, 8th ed. Philadelphia, PA: Saunders; 2013.
Stanley JC, Veith FJ, Wakefield TW. *Current Therapy in Vascular Surgery*, 5th ed. Philadelphia, PA: Saunders; 2014.

36. **(C)** Visceral artery aneurysms can affect just about any intra-abdominal vessel, from the splenic artery, as shown in Figure 30-14 (the most commonly involved, at 60%), to the pancreaticoduodenal and pancreatic arteries (at 1.5%). Other visceral vessels are variably involved with aneurysmal disease: hepatic (20%), SMA (5.5%), celiac (4%), gastric/gastroepiploic (4%), and intestinal (jejunal/ileal/colic, 3%). The vast majority are the result of medial degeneration; atherosclerosis is usually a secondary event. Pancreaticoduodenal artery aneurysms are often the result of pancreatitis and its associated arterial necrosis.

　　Just as the incidence of these aneurysms is variable, so too is their rate of rupture. Although splenic artery aneurysms are the most common visceral artery aneurysms, their rate of rupture is one of the lowest (at approximately 2%), whereas gastric and gastroepiploic artery aneurysms, although much more rare, have a rupture rate of up to 90%. Mortality from rupture of visceral artery aneurysms is about 50% for most aneurysms. A definite exception is the splenic artery aneurysm in the pregnant female, which carries a 70% maternal mortality and 75% fetal mortality. Repair of visceral aneurysms should be undertaken in women of child-bearing age who desire pregnancy.

　　Most aneurysms should be fixed when they are found. Coil embolization or covered stents may be possible via endovascular approach. Surgical treatment usually involves resection of the aneurysm with arterial reconstruction. Gastric and intestinal aneurysms often require resection of a portion of the stomach or intestine along with the aneurysm if the aneurysm is intramural, and splenectomy may be required. Pancreatitis-related false aneurysms can often be ligated because dissection in inflamed areas previously affected by pancreatitis may be difficult. Distal pancreatectomy may sometimes be required. Some mesenteric aneurysms may be treatable with stent grafting.

BIBLIOGRAPHY

Cronenwett JL, Johnston KW. *Rutherford's Vascular Surgery*, 8th ed. Philadelphia, PA: Saunders; 2014.
Moore WS. *Vascular Surgery and Endovascular Surgery: A Comprehensive Review*, 8th ed. Philadelphia, PA: Saunders; 2013.
Stanley JC, Veith FJ, Wakefield TW. *Current Therapy in Vascular Surgery*, 5th ed. Philadelphia, PA: Saunders; 2014.

37. **(B)** The arteriogram reveals an aneurysm of the main renal artery at its bifurcation. The overall incidence of renal artery aneurysms is between 0.09 and 0.3%. They occur with equal frequency in both sexes and have been reported in all age groups (1 month to 82 years). Renal artery aneurysms can be categorized into four basic types: true (saccular or fusiform), false, dissecting, and intrarenal.

　　The image illustrates a saccular aneurysm, which is a localized outpouching that communicates with the arterial lumen by either a narrow or wide opening. Extraparenchymal aneurysms are the most common type of renal artery aneurysm, accounting for more than 90%. They typically occur at the bifurcation possibly because of an inherent weakness in this region. These lesions often become involved with atherosclerotic degeneration or intramural calcification. Incompletely calcified aneurysms may become thin and ulcerated between areas of calcification, predisposing them to rupture.

　　Most renal artery aneurysms are small and asymptomatic. Well-calcified, small (<2 cm) aneurysms in an asymptomatic normotensive patient can be followed with serial radiographs. However, surgical intervention is indicated for: (1) aneurysms associated with local symptoms such as flank pain or hematuria, (2) dissecting aneurysms, (3) aneurysms occurring in a woman of child-bearing age who is likely to conceive, (4) aneurysms causing renal ischemia, (5) aneurysms occurring with functionally significant renal artery stenosis, (6) aneurysms with radiographic evidence of expansion on serial radiographs, and (7) aneurysms containing a thrombus with evidence of distal embolization.

　　The risk of rupture is significantly increased with pregnancy due to the hyperdynamic state, increased blood volume and cardiac output, hormonal influence on the aneurysm, and increased intra-abdominal pressure.

BIBLIOGRAPHY

Cronenwett JL, Johnston KW. *Rutherford's Vascular Surgery*, 8th ed. Philadelphia, PA: Saunders; 2014.
Moore WS. *Vascular Surgery and Endovascular Surgery: A Comprehensive Review*, 8th ed. Philadelphia, PA: Saunders; 2013.
Stanley JC, Veith FJ, Wakefield TW. *Current Therapy in Vascular Surgery*, 5th ed. Philadelphia, PA: Saunders; 2014.

38. **(D)** Infrainguinal vein grafts should be carefully and closely monitored to ensure continued patency. Grafts that are "failing" are those that are affected by a defect that causes hemodynamically significant changes in the graft and ultimately put the graft at risk of occlusion if not corrected. Grafts can fail in the early or late postoperative period. Perioperatively (within 30 days), graft failure is usually secondary to a technical error or poor outflow vessels. Early failures (within 2 years) are usually secondary to intimal hyperplasia, whereas late failures (after 2 years) are usually secondary to progressive atherosclerotic changes.

Narrowing of the graft to a point where it becomes hemodynamically significant is termed a "critical stenosis." This usually occurs at a diameter reduction of 50%, which corresponds to a cross-sectional area reduction of approximately 75%. At this level, grafts are in danger of occluding if intervention is not undertaken. To ensure identification of these lesions, grafts should be surveilled on a regular basis with duplex studies to identify these lesions. Duplex can visually identify these areas, and velocity changes can also be used to localize areas of stenosis. Finding these lesions prior to graft occlusion is especially important, because grafts that are revised prior to progressing to total occlusion have much better assisted patency rates than do grafts that occlude.

Once the stenosis is identified, revision should be undertaken. Depending on the lesion, this can be accomplished by vein patch angioplasty, segmental bypass, or in some cases, angioplasty of the lesion. Lesions at the proximal or distal segment of the bypass are more amenable to angioplasty than are those in the midgraft, and short-segment stenoses are better candidates for angioplasty than are longer lesions.

BIBLIOGRAPHY

Cronenwett JL, Johnston KW. *Rutherford's Vascular Surgery*, 8th ed. Philadelphia, PA: Saunders; 2014.
Moore WS. *Vascular Surgery and Endovascular Surgery: A Comprehensive Review*, 8th ed. Philadelphia, PA: Saunders; 2013.
Mowatt-Larssen E, Desai SS, Dua A, Shortell CEK (eds.). *Phlebology, Vein Surgery, and Ultrasonography*. New York, NY: Springer Verlag; 2014.

39. **(A)** Many risk factors exist for peripheral arterial occlusive disease. The most significant risk factors include advanced age, hypertension, cigarette smoking, diabetes, hyperlipidemia, and homocysteinemia. Other factors that can be involved in the development of peripheral occlusive disease include male sex, high-fat diet, alcoholism, and hypercoagulability.

Patients with diabetes often see a different pattern of peripheral arterial disease than do patients with other risk factors such as hypertension or tobacco use. Patients with these risk factors tend to develop aortoiliac and femoral occlusive disease; however, patients with diabetes tend to develop disease in the tibial vessels while the aortoiliac and femoral-popliteal segments remain relatively free of disease. If the femoral and popliteal arteries are involved, the lesions tend not to advance to occlusion; however, the tibial vessels become severely diseased, often throughout their course. This is likely secondary to increased calcification of the intima and thickening of capillary basement membranes. Hyperthyroidism is not a risk factor for peripheral occlusive disease.

BIBLIOGRAPHY

Cronenwett JL, Johnston KW. *Rutherford's Vascular Surgery*, 8th ed. Philadelphia, PA: Saunders; 2014.
Moore WS. *Vascular Surgery and Endovascular Surgery: A Comprehensive Review*, 8th ed. Philadelphia, PA: Saunders; 2013.
Stanley JC, Veith FJ, Wakefield TW. *Current Therapy in Vascular Surgery*, 5th ed. Philadelphia, PA: Saunders; 2014.

40. **(E)** Popliteal artery injury is a serious complication of knee dislocation. It is the second most frequently injured artery of the lower extremity. Injury can occur with both anterior and posterior dislocations (approximately 35% incidence) but is more common after posterior dislocation. Therefore, diagnosis and appropriate management are of the utmost importance because undetected injury can lead to significant lower extremity ischemia and even amputation.

A high index of suspicion is necessary. "Hard signs," such as lack of pulse, bruit, distal ischemia, or expanding hematomas, are clearly indicative of arterial injury; however, subtler examination findings cannot be overlooked. Pulse examination, both before and after reduction, is important, and the presence of a *normal* pedal pulse can be a reliable indication of arterial integrity. Often, however, a palpable, but diminished, pulse may be present in the face of significant injury and should lead to suspicion of possible arterial injury.

Contrary to previous beliefs, not every patient with a knee dislocation requires an arteriogram. Patients with a normal ABI and a normal examination can safely be observed with serial examinations. Likewise, patients with clear evidence of acute ischemia should not have repair delayed by arteriogram, but rather, should be taken directly to the operating room. Patients with suspected—but not proven—ischemia may benefit most from preoperative arteriography.

If arterial injury is identified, repair should be undertaken expeditiously. Primary repair may be selectively applied, but in the setting of more extensive arterial injury, vein bypass may be more appropriate. Most often, the contralateral saphenous vein is used secondary to the high incidence of concomitant deep venous injury associated with knee dislocation.

In most instances, arterial repair should be undertaken first to minimize ischemia time. Orthopedic repair, often in the form of external fixation, can then be undertaken with close attention to pulse examination during reduction and fixation. If orthopedic injury must be done first, often arterial shunting may be employed to prevent or minimize further ischemia time.

Compartment syndrome is common, secondary to acute edema/ischemia and associated reperfusion, and increased index of suspicion is required. If there is any doubt, four-compartment fasciotomy should be performed.

BIBLIOGRAPHY

Cronenwett JL, Johnston KW. *Rutherford's Vascular Surgery*, 8th ed. Philadelphia, PA: Saunders; 2014.

Dua A, Desai SS, Holcomb JB, Burgess AR, Freischlag, JA. *Clinical Review of Vascular Trauma*. New York, NY: Springer Verlag; 2013.

Moore WS. *Vascular Surgery and Endovascular Surgery: A Comprehensive Review*, 8th ed. Philadelphia, PA: Saunders; 2013.

Stanley JC, Veith FJ, Wakefield TW. *Current Therapy in Vascular Surgery*, 5th ed. Philadelphia, PA: Saunders; 2014.

41. **(E)** The treatment goals of chronic mesenteric ischemia are to resolve symptoms, regain weight loss, and prevent bowel infarction. Endovascular approach with transluminal angioplasty and stenting has become the initial treatment in high-risk patients and has been shown to have a lower morbidity and mortality. However, open surgical revascularization for chronic mesenteric ischemia remains the standard because of its durable long-term patency and freedom from recurrent symptoms requiring reinterventions.

Antegrade bypass is best performed using a left retroperitoneal approach. The descending thoracic aorta, supraceliac aorta, and mesenteric arteries are exposed. The distal thoracic aorta is usually spared from atherosclerosis and offers a great aortic inflow source.

Although the retrograde bypass offers the advantages of limited dissection and avoids the supraceliac aortic occlusion, it has been used less frequently. Studies suggest (but have not proven) that retrograde bypass is less durable than antegrade bypass. This is thought to be due to the tendency for SMA grafts to kink or twist with the viscera when they return to the normal anatomic position.

Currently retrograde bypass is reserved for when an endovascular approach and antegrade bypass and aortomesenteric endarterectomy are not feasible. Specific indications are:

- Emergency revascularization in patients undergoing laparotomy for acute mesenteric ischemia
- Inaccessible supraceliac aorta due to previous surgery or subphrenic inflammation
- Severe cardiac disease with contraindications to supraceliac aortic occlusion
- The need for simultaneous infrarenal aortic and mesenteric revascularization

BIBLIOGRAPHY

Cronenwett JL, Johnston KW. *Rutherford's Vascular Surgery*, 8th ed. Philadelphia, PA: Saunders; 2014.

Moore WS. *Vascular Surgery and Endovascular Surgery: A Comprehensive Review*, 8th ed. Philadelphia, PA: Saunders; 2013.

Stanley JC, Veith FJ, Wakefield TW. *Current Therapy in Vascular Surgery*, 5th ed. Philadelphia, PA: Saunders; 2014.

42. **(C)** Aneurysms of the splenic artery are the most prevalent splanchnic artery aneurysm, accounting for 60% of cases. Although rare, improvements in radiologic imaging have resulted in an increased awareness of their significance. They are four times more common among women but occur in almost 10% of patients with portal hypertension with equal distribution among genders. Rarely, they may occur as a result of congenital anomalies of the foregut circulation. They occur most often external to the pancreatic parenchyma except when induced by periarterial chronic pancreatitis.

Three factors have been identified as fundamental to the development of these lesions: arterial fibrodysplasia, pregnancy with its hemodynamic changes and estrogen-related effects on elastic vascular tissue, and cirrhosis with portal hypertension. Pregnancy, especially with multiparity, is a major risk factor for both the development and rupture of aneurysms, with a rate of rupture approaching 95% in lesions identified during pregnancy. Aneurysms less commonly result from penetrating trauma, periarterial inflammation as in the case of chronic pancreatitis, or a systemic vasculitic process.

The aneurysms are predominantly saccular, occur at vessel bifurcations, and are multiple in 20% of cases. Pancreatic lesions tend to be solitary and occur proximally. Aneurysms are usually found incidentally during studies performed for other reasons and can be diagnosed with arteriography, magnetic resonance imaging, color flow Doppler ultrasound, and CT scan. When seen on plain abdominal films, they classically appear as signet ring calcifications in the left upper quadrant.

Patients may be asymptomatic, or they may present with midepigastric or left upper quadrant pain. On rupture, patients may remain hemodynamically stable if the bleeding remains confined to the lesser sac, or they may present in extremis with free intraperitoneal rupture. Less commonly, GI bleeding may be the presentation, resulting either from rupture of a pancreatitis-induced aneurysm into adjacent hollow viscera or from esophageal varices that form after rupture of the aneurysm into the neighboring splenic vein, producing an arteriovenous fistula. Pregnancy-related lesions have a much higher rate of rupture compared to the 2% risk in other populations. Rupture typically occurs during the third trimester with a very high mortality rate for both the mother and fetus, and thus, it mandates operative intervention.

Percutaneous transcatheter embolization is the preferred treatment of choice. Open ligation of the aneurysm or exclusion with vascular reconstruction is an alternative option. Distal pancreatectomy may be needed for the aneurysm imbedded within the pancreas. Splenectomy is another alternative; however, although formerly the standard of care, given the risks of overwhelming postsplenectomy infection, it should be avoided when possible. The vaccination in splenic artery embolization is still debated.

BIBLIOGRAPHY

Cronenwett JL, Johnston KW. *Rutherford's Vascular Surgery*, 8th ed. Philadelphia, PA: Saunders; 2014.

Moore WS. *Vascular Surgery and Endovascular Surgery: A Comprehensive Review*, 8th ed. Philadelphia, PA: Saunders; 2013.

Stanley JC, Veith FJ, Wakefield TW. *Current Therapy in Vascular Surgery*, 5th ed. Philadelphia, PA: Saunders; 2014.

CHAPTER 31

TRANSPLANTATION AND IMMUNOLOGY

KELLY M. COLLINS AND JASON R. WELLEN

QUESTIONS

1. Which of the following is an indication for pancreas transplantation?
   (A) Poor glycemic control caused by lack of compliance with the prescribed insulin regimen
   (B) New-onset type 1 diabetes in a 10-year-old child
   (C) Body mass index (BMI) greater than 35 with poor glycemic control
   (D) Type 1 diabetes with diabetic nephropathy
   (E) Poor glycemic control in a 17-year-old on subcutaneous insulin injections

2. Which of the following is true regarding potential cadaveric organ donors?
   (A) Brain death is a clinical diagnosis that can be determined by a single physician.
   (B) Nuclear scintigraphic determination of brain blood flow must be accompanied by electroencephalographic (EEG) electrocerebral silence to be considered confirmatory.
   (C) Consent for organ donation is best obtained by the transplant surgery team.
   (D) After the period of preoxygenation, hypocarbia with an arterial carbon dioxide tension ($PaCO_2$) less than 60 mmHg should be documented.
   (E) Reversible causes of comatose state must be excluded (i.e., hypothermia, neuromuscular blockade, shock).

3. Which of the following statements is true concerning techniques for multiple-organ procurement and preservation?
   (A) Preservation solutions are designed to prevent cellular swelling and minimize potassium loss.
   (B) Previous chest surgery with sternal wires in place is a contraindication to organ donation.
   (C) In a standard pancreas procurement, the distal duodenum is divided with a stapler near the ligament of Treitz.
   (D) In the presence of a replaced left hepatic artery arising from the left gastric, the pars flaccida of the lesser omentum may be divided.
   (E) Heparin is given immediately following infusion of preservation solution.

4. Which of the following statements about split-liver transplantation (SLT) is true?
   (A) The approach for living donors is the same as for deceased donors.
   (B) The SLT is now routinely used for two adult recipients.
   (C) A replaced left hepatic artery arising from the left gastric precludes splitting of the liver.
   (D) Graft failure is higher with split grafts than with whole-organ grafts.
   (E) The left graft is smaller.

5. Which of the following is *not* a complication associated with a pancreas allograft that has its exocrine function drained to the bladder?
   (A) Cystitis
   (B) Reflux pancreatitis
   (C) Metabolic acidosis
   (D) Volume overload
   (E) Graft thrombosis

6. Which of the following neoplasms are increased in patients undergoing transplantation?
   (A) Neuroendocrine tumors
   (B) Squamous cell skin cancer
   (C) T-cell lymphoma
   (D) Ovarian cancer
   (E) Pancreatic cancer

7. Which of the following is true regarding clinical rejection after organ transplant?
   (A) Hyperacute rejection results from donor antibodies against recipient major histocompatibility complex (MHC).
   (B) Chronic rejection is characterized by a thrombosed, darkened graft.
   (C) Acute rejection is the most common type of rejection.
   (D) Acute rejection is characterized by atrophy and fibrosis.
   (E) Acute rejection is predominantly cell mediated.

8. Which of the following is true regarding the Major Compatibility Complex (MHC)?
   (A) Class I molecules are expressed by antigen-presenting cells (APCs).
   (B) Class II molecules are named *human leukocyte antigen* (HLA) A, B, and C.
   (C) It is known as the HLA system in humans.
   (D) Cellular rejection occurs if the recipient has circulating antibodies specific to the donor's HLA.
   (E) MHC molecules play no role in cellular rejection.

9. Which of the following is *not* an indication for liver transplant?
   (A) Cirrhosis complicated by ascites and esophageal varices
   (B) Acute liver failure secondary to acetaminophen overdose
   (C) NASH (nonalcoholic steatohepatitis) complicated by hepatic encephalopathy
   (D) Hepatocellular carcinoma with underlying cirrhosis
   (E) Hepatocellular carcinoma with biopsy-proven lymph node metastasis

10. Which of the following statements is correct concerning postoperative complications after hepatic transplantation?
    (A) Biliary leak is a rare complication of liver transplantation.
    (B) Portal venous thrombosis occurs more commonly than does hepatic arterial thrombosis.
    (C) Seizure is a common complication of calcineurin inhibitors after liver transplantation.
    (D) If postoperative bleeding is encountered, immediate return to the operating room is indicated.

11. Which of the following is true regarding cytokines?
    (A) Interleukin (IL) 8 functions to downregulate the inflammatory response.
    (B) IL-10 increases hepatic acute-phase proteins.
    (C) IL-15 activates natural killer (NK) cells.

   (D) IL-6 stimulates the release of IL-1 and tumor necrosis factor alpha (TNF-α).
   (E) IL-18 induces fever.

12. Which of the following is true regarding cytokines?
    (A) IL-1 is released by T lymphocytes.
    (B) IL-2 has a long half-life.
    (C) IL-4 induces class switching.
    (D) IL-12 release is stimulated by IL-10.
    (E) IL-13 affects thymocytes.

13. Tumor necrosis factor alpha
    (A) Is mainly produced by the endothelium
    (B) Decreases cell adhesion molecules
    (C) Is an anticoagulant
    (D) Secretion leads to increase growth factors
    (E) Downregulates macrophages and polymorphonuclear leukocytes (PMNs)

14. Hepatic acute-phase proteins
    (A) Are most strongly stimulated by IL-1
    (B) Decrease haptoglobin
    (C) Lead to complement activation
    (D) Increase production of transferrin
    (E) Decrease IL-3 production

15. Which of the following is true regarding cells of the innate immune system?
    (A) Macrophages attack host cells infected by viruses.
    (B) NK cells attack microbes directly.
    (C) Eosinophils bridge innate and adaptive immune responses.
    (D) Mast cells are involved in the type III hypersensitivity response.
    (E) NK cells attack cells with low expression of MHC.

16. Which of the following is true regarding T cells?
    (A) They are not presented by APCs.
    (B) CD4 lymphocytes attack cells that are damaged or dysfunctional.
    (C) CD8 lymphocytes increase antibody production.
    (D) CD8 lymphocytes are activated by IL-2.
    (E) CD4 lymphocytes suppress autoimmunity.

17. Which of the following is true regarding immunoglobulin (Ig)?
    (A) IgM is most common antibody overall.
    (B) IgG is responsible for primary immune response.
    (C) IgD has a critical role in mucosal immunity.
    (D) IgA is released by plasma cells.
    (E) IgE mediates allergic response.

18. Which of the following is true regarding hypersensitivity reactions?
    (A) Type I involves antibody-dependent cell cytotoxicity (ADCC).
    (B) Type III is IgE mediated.
    (C) Type IV includes serum sickness.
    (D) Type II includes graft-versus-host disease.
    (E) Type I involves both local and systemic effects.

19. Which of the following is true regarding crossmatching?
    (A) It detects recipient antigen to donor antibody.
    (B) A positive crossmatch results in a type IV reaction.
    (C) Liver, kidney, and pancreas transplantation require preoperative crossmatching.
    (D) Donor lymphocytes are responsible for a positive reaction.

20. Which of the following is *false* regarding panel reactive antibodies (PRAs)?
    (A) It is positive in patients who have previously been sensitized.
    (B) Patients with a high PRA are more likely to have a positive crossmatch.
    (C) It is a component of acquired immunity.
    (D) Treatments include plasmapheresis.
    (E) It detects preformed antibodies in the donor.

21. Which of the following describes the mechanism of action of cyclosporine?
    (A) It binds FK binding protein.
    (B) It inhibits de novo purine synthesis.
    (C) It blocks activation of T cells only.
    (D) It is cleared by hepatic metabolism.

22. Which of the following is a polyclonal antibody against T-cell antigen?
    (A) OKT3
    (B) Sirolimus
    (C) Azathioprine
    (D) Mycophenolate
    (E) Thymoglobulin

23. The most common cause of mortality after kidney transplant is
    (A) Sepsis
    (B) Vascular thrombosis
    (C) Hemorrhage
    (D) Rejection
    (E) Cardiac arrest

24. Which of the following are used to calculate the model for end-stage liver disease (MELD)?
    (A) International normalized ratio (INR), bilirubin, creatinine
    (B) INR, ammonia, creatinine
    (C) Bilirubin, aspartase aminotransferase (AST), creatinine
    (D) Bilirubin, AST, alkaline phosphatase
    (E) AST, INR, creatinine

25. Which of the following is true regarding cardiac transplantation?
    (A) Cardiac transplantation is the last resort for patients with end-stage cardiac disease and severe functional limitation.
    (B) The most common primary indications for heart transplant is congenital defect.
    (C) Contraindications include age greater than 60 years old and pulmonary artery (PA) systolic pressure greater than 30 mmHg.
    (D) Crossmatching is mandatory prior to donor recipient matching.
    (E) Body size within 20% of body weight is considered compatible.

26. Which of the following is true regarding lung transplantation?
    (A) Donor-to-recipient lung volume matching is based on the vertical apex to diaphragm along the midaxillary line.
    (B) Oversize donor lungs may be downsized by lobectomy prior to transplantation.
    (C) HLA matching is mandatory prior to donor-recipient matching.
    (D) Cigarette smokers must quit smoking 2 weeks before transplantation.
    (E) All of the above.

27. A 62-year-old male presents 2 weeks postrenal transplantation with elevated creatinine and decreased urine output. His postoperative course was uneventful, and a surgical drain was removed on day of discharge. He is afebrile, and vital signs are within normal limits. A ureteral stent remains in place. Ultrasound of the iliac fossa reveals a $10 \times 8 \times 3$ cm fluid collection; duplex flow and velocity are normal. What is the most likely diagnosis?
    (A) Lymphocele
    (B) Hematoma
    (C) Urinoma
    (D) Abscess

28. A 53-year-old woman is at postoperative day 3 from a liver transplant for cirrhosis associated with hepatitis C. Her laboratory values are within normal limits with the exception of increasing hepatic enzymes (AST, alanine aminotransferase [ALT]) and a bilirubin of 2. On examination, her vitals are within normal limits. Her abdomen is slightly distended but soft, and her surgical drain has bilious colored fluid. She has moderate volume ascites. The most likely diagnosis is
    (A) Acute cellular rejection
    (B) Recurrent hepatitis C with early fibrosis
    (C) Antibody-mediated rejection
    (D) Biliary anastomotic leak
    (E) Biliary anastomotic stricture

29. A 55-year-old man is 8 h after a zero-antigen HLA mismatch standard criteria deceased donor kidney transplantation for hypertension-associated stage 5 chronic kidney disease (CKD-V). His intraoperative course was uncomplicated, and he received steroids and antthymocyte globulin induction therapy. A ureteral stent was placed. Postoperatively, his urine output is initially 100 mL/h; however, 6 h postoperatively, it abruptly drops to zero. His urine output does not respond to a 500-mL bolus of 0.9% saline solution. He made minimal urine at baseline. Which of the following is the most likely cause of the drop in output?
    (A) Hyperacute rejection
    (B) Catheter obstruction
    (C) Hypovolemia
    (D) Urine leak

30. A 35-year-old woman presents for a clinic follow-up 1 week after kidney transplantation for end-stage renal disease (ESRD) secondary to diabetic nephropathy. Her postoperative course was uncomplicated. Her laboratory results are as follows: serum creatinine 0.89 mg/dL (0.70–1.30), white blood cell count 4000/cumm (3.8–9.8), hematocrit 30% (40.7–50.3%). Her only complaint is diarrhea. Which of the following is the most likely culprit?
    (A) *Clostridium difficile* as a result of antibiotic prophylaxis with Bactrim
    (B) Mycophenolate mofetil
    (C) Uremia
    (D) Tacrolimus
    (E) Prednisone

31. Which of the following is the mechanism of action of mycophenolate mofetil?
    (A) Poorly understood mechanism; also has anti-inflammatory properties
    (B) Inhibits the guanosine synthesis de novo pathway, producing a selective, reversible antiproliferative effect on T and B lymphocytes

    (C) Binds FK binding protein, resulting in inhibition of T-cell activation
    (D) Inhibits DNA and RNA synthesis through the non-specific suppression of de novo purine synthesis

32. A 40-year-old man with ESRD secondary to diabetic nephropathy is in the operating room as a recipient of a cadaveric kidney transplant. When the graft is reperfused, the kidney parenchyma becomes mottled, purple, and cyanotic in appearance. There is a pulse at the level of the renal-to-iliac arterial anastomosis. What is the most likely explanation for the kidney's appearance?
    (A) Hyperacute rejection
    (B) Acute T cell–mediated rejection
    (C) Calcineurin inhibitor toxicity
    (D) Heparin-induced thrombocytopenia and thrombosis

ANSWERS AND EXPLANATIONS

1. **(D)** The first human pancreas transplant was performed in 1966. Since that time, the pancreas transplant has been used to establish normoglycemia and insulin independence, as well as prevent end-organ damage in diabetic recipients. Indications for pancreas transplantation are previous total pancreatectomy, disabling or life-threatening hypoglycemic unawareness, and presence or high risk of secondary complications of diabetes.

BIBLIOGRAPHY

Humar A, Dunn DL. Transplantation. In: Brunicardi F, Andersen DK, Billiar TR, et al., (eds.), *Schwartz's Principles of Surgery*. 9th ed. New York, NY: McGraw-Hill; 2010: Chapter 11.
White SA, Shaw JA, Sutherland DER. Pancreas transplantation. *Lancet* 2009;373(9677):1808–1817.

2. **(E)** Prior to organ donation, the diagnosis of brain death must be made by two physicians at a given interval depending on the patient's age. The diagnosis of brain death is a clinical one. Criteria include normothermia, absence of drug intoxication, coma, absence of motor reflexes, absence of pupillary responses to light, absence of corneal reflexes, absence of caloric responses, absence of gag, absence of coughing in response to tracheal suctioning, absence of sucking or rooting reflex, and absence of respiratory drive at aPaCO$_2$ that is 60 mmHg or 20 mmHg above normal baseline values.

    In addition to clinical diagnosis, confirmatory testing can be performed, including cerebral angiography, nuclear imaging, transcranial Doppler ultrasonography, and EEG. Confirmatory testing in adults is optional, but at least one confirmatory test is required in pediatric populations.

When a potential organ donor is identified, the treating physician should notify the organ procurement organization (OPO) that serves the region. OPOs are specialized coordination teams that help coordinate the logistics of organ donation, including contacting the family for consent, assessing the donor physiologic status, and contacting local and regional transplant centers about their organ needs. Local transplant teams are forbidden from contacting potential donors within their hospital, although the treating physician may do so. Family consent should be solicited regardless of organ donation status. Obtaining consent for organ donation from families is enhanced by allowing time for families to accept death, having someone who is an expert in donation consent approach the family, and approaching the family in a private, quiet area in an unhurried manner.

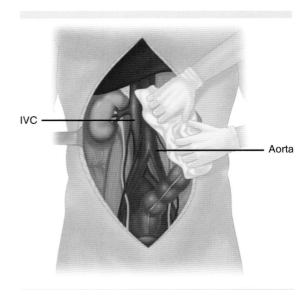

FIGURE 31-1. Midline incision for multiorgan procurement (from Brunicardi FC, Andersen DK, Billiar TR, et al., (eds.), *Schwartz's Principles of Surgery*. 9th ed. New York, NY: McGraw-Hill; 2010: Fig. 11-4. Copyright © The McGraw-Hill Companies, Inc. All rights reserved).

BIBLIOGRAPHY

Baker TB, Skaro AI, Alvord P, Chaudhury P. Organ procurement. In: Ashley S, Cance W, Chen H, et al., (eds.), *ACS Surgery: Principles and Practice*. 7th ed. Philadelphia, PA: Decker; 2014: Section 10, Chapter 6.

D'Ovidio FF, McRitchie DD, Keshavjie SS. Care of the multiorgan donor. In: Hall JB, Schmidt GA, Wood LH, eds. *Principles of Critical Care*. 3rd ed. New York, NY: McGraw-Hill; 2005: Chapter 91.

Merion RM Organ preservation. In: Mulholland MW, Lillemoe KD, Doherty GM, Maier RV, Upchurch GR Jr, eds. *Greenfield's Surgery: Scientific Principles and Practice*. 5th ed. Philadelphia, PA: Lippincott Williams & Wilkin; 2011: Chapter 34.

3. **(A)** Multiorgan procurement begins with a midline incision from the sternal notch to the pubis (Fig. 31-1) to expose all of the intra-abdominal and thoracic organs. The sternum and pericardium are opened to allow for inspection of the heart and exposure of the right atrium. The right colon and duodenum are mobilized (Kocher maneuver) to expose the distal aorta, inferior vena cava (IVC), and iliac bifurcation, and the distal aorta is encircled with a large silk suture. The liver is mobilized by division of the left triangular and gastrohepatic ligaments. The gastrohepatic ligament should be inspected for an accessory or replaced left hepatic artery prior to division and must be preserved if either is present. The common hepatic artery and porta hepatis are exposed, and the common bile duct is divided just proximal to the entry into the pancreas. The gallbladder contents are suctioned, and the common bile duct is flushed with a bulb syringe. The supraceliac abdominal aorta is exposed by dividing the arcuate ligaments of the diaphragm. Heparin is infused prior to cross-clamping. Cross-clamping proceeds with tying of the silk suture around the distal aorta, placement of a perfusion cannula into the aortic lumen proximal to the tie, cross-clamping

of the supraceliac aorta using a large aortic clamp and opening the right atrium to allow infusion of the preservation solution through the vasculature. At this time, ice is placed around the organs to allow cooling. The most common preservation solutions are University of Wisconsin (UW) solution and Histidine-tryptophan-ketoglutarate (HTK). These are low-viscosity solutions designed to prevent hypothermia-induced cellular swelling and minimize potassium loss from the cell.

BIBLIOGRAPHY

Baker TB, Skaro AI, Alvord P, Chaudhury P. Organ procurement. In: Ashley S, Cance W, Chen H, et al., (eds.), *ACS Surgery: Principles and Practice*. 7th ed. Philadelphia, PA: Decker; 2014: Section 10, Chapter 6.

Humar A, Dunn DL. Transplantation. In: Brunicardi F, Andersen DK, Billiar TR, et al., (eds.), *Schwartz's Principles of Surgery*. 9th ed. New York, NY: McGraw-Hill; 2010: Chapter 11.

Merion RM Organ preservation. In: Mulholland MW, Lillemoe KD, Doherty GM, Maier RV, Upchurch GR Jr, eds. *Greenfield's Surgery: Scientific Principles and Practice*. 5th ed. Philadelphia, PA: Lippincott Williams & Wilkin; 2011: Chapter 34.

4. **(E)** Split Liver Transplantation (SLT) involves division of a whole liver from a cadaveric donor into two sections, which are then transplanted into two recipients (Fig. 31-2). The left lateral segment is significantly smaller than the

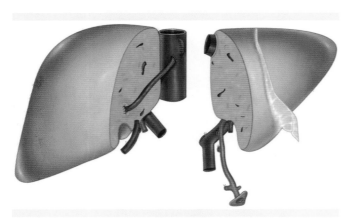

FIGURE 31-2. Cadaveric split-liver graft (from Brunicardi FC, Andersen DK, Billiar TR, et al., (eds.), *Schwartz's Principles of Surgery*. 9th ed. New York, NY: McGraw-Hill; 2010: Fig. 11-32. Copyright © The McGraw-Hill Companies, Inc. All rights reserved).

extended-right lobe; therefore the majority of these procedures are performed on one adult and one pediatric recipient. Two types of SLT, *ex vivo* and *in situ*, have been described. *Ex vivo* SLT involves standard rapid en bloc multiorgan procurement, followed by parenchymal and vessel dissection of the allograft on the back table. In contrast, *in situ* splitting involves hilar dissection and parenchymal transection before procurement, similar to a living donor liver operation. To date, no large national studies have been performed. However, single-center studies have shown graft and patient survival rates comparable to whole-liver and living donation, although there were significantly higher rates of complications.

BIBLIOGRAPHY

Humar A, Dunn DL. Transplantation. In: Brunicardi F, Andersen DK, Billiar TR, et al., (eds.), *Schwartz's Principles of Surgery*. 9th ed. New York, NY: McGraw-Hill; 2010: Chapter 11.

Majella Doyle MB, Maynard E, Lin Y, et al. Outcomes with split liver transplantation are equivalent to those with whole organ transplantation. *J Am Coll Surg* 2013;217(1):102–112.

Vagefi PA, Parekh J, Ascher NL, Roberts JP, Freise CE. Outcomes with split liver transplantation in 106 recipients: the University of California, San Francisco, experience from 1993 to 2010. *Arch Surg* 2011;146(9):1052–1059.

5. **(D)** There are two options for enteric drainage of the exocrine pancreas. Historically, the bladder had been used for drainage, with one of the major advantages being the ability to monitor urinary amylase, which, if low, can signal rejection. However, due to complications associated with bladder drainage (recurrent urinary

tract infections, hematuria, chemical urethritis, severe bicarbonate wasting resulting in metabolic acidosis, and dehydration), many centers now use enteric drainage, creating an enteroenterostomy using donor duodenum and recipient jejunum.

Thrombosis of the pancreas graft is the most common cause of early graft loss (regardless of type of enteric drainage). It is probably due to a combination of factors, including the procoagulant state of diabetic patients, ischemia reperfusion injury of the pancreas graft, and the low flow through the venous outflow. Thrombosis is often detected by a rising glucose and confirmed with duplex ultrasound or contrasted computed tomographic (CT) scan. Treatment ranges from graft thrombectomy to removal of the graft (in cases of complete graft thrombosis/necrosis).

BIBLIOGRAPHY

Baker TB, Skaro AI, Alvord P, Chaudhury P. Organ procurement. In: Ashley S, Cance W, Chen H, et al., (eds.), *ACS Surgery: Principles and Practice*. 7th ed. Philadelphia, PA: Decker; 2014: Section 10, Chapter 6.

Sung R. Pancreas and islet transplantation. In: Mulholland MW, Lillemoe KD, Doherty GM, Maier RV, Simeone DM, Upchurch GR Jr, eds. *Greenfield's Surgery: Scientific Principles and Practice*. 5th ed. Philadelphia, PA: Lippincott Williams & Wilkins; 2011: Chapter 39.

6. **(B)** The most common posttransplant malignancies are skin cancers, usually squamous or basal cell carcinomas located on sun-exposed areas. Malignant melanomas are also commonly seen. Posttransplant lymphoproliferative disorder (PTLD) is a spectrum of B-cell proliferation disorders associated with Epstein-Barr virus. Manifestations vary widely, and symptoms include fever, weight loss, and fatigue.

BIBLIOGRAPHY

Azzi J, Lee BT, Chandraker A. Kidney transplantation 2: care of the kidney transplant recipient. In: Ashley S, Cance W, Chen H, et al., (eds.), *ACS Surgery: Principles and Practice*. Philadelphia, PA: Decker; 2014: Chapter 195.

Humar A, Dunn DL. Transplantation. In: Brunicardi F, Andersen DK, Billiar TR, et al., (eds.), *Schwartz's Principles of Surgery*. 9th ed. New York, NY: McGraw-Hill; 2010: Chapter 11.

7. **(E)** Rejection can be classified into four types based on timing and pathogenesis: hyperacute, accelerated acute, acute, and chronic.

Hyperacute rejection, which usually results from preformed antibodies in the recipient, occurs within minutes after the transplanted organ is reperfused. Recipient antibodies may be directed against the donor's HLA antigens, or they may be anti-ABO blood group antibodies. These antibodies bind to the vascular endothelium in the graft and activate the complement cascade, leading to platelet activation and to diffuse intravascular coagulation. Clinically, this results in ischemic necrosis and a swollen, darkened graft.

Accelerated acute rejection involves both cellular and antibody-mediated injury and is seen within the first few days posttransplant. It is more common when a recipient has been sensitized by previous exposure to antigens present in the donor.

Acute rejection is predominantly a cell-mediated process and is becoming less frequent as methods of immunosuppression improve. It usually occurs within days to months after transplant. Histologically, it is characterized by cellular infiltrate, membrane damage, and apoptosis of graft cells. Systemic symptoms such as fever, chills, malaise, and arthralgias are common. Acute rejection episodes may also be mediated by a humoral response, secondary to B-cell generation of anti donor antibodies.

Chronic rejection occurs months to years posttransplant and is characterized by slow deterioration of graft function. Histologically, the process is characterized by atrophy, fibrosis, and arteriosclerosis. Both immune and nonimmune mechanisms are likely involved.

8. **(C)** The main antigens involved in triggering rejection are coded for by a group of genes known as the *major histocompatibility complex* (MHC). In humans, the MHC is known as the *human leukocyte antigen* (HLA) system. It comprises a series of genes located on chromosome 6. The HLA antigens are grouped into two classes, which differ in their structure and cellular distribution. Class I molecules (named HLA-A, -B, and -C) are found on the membrane of all nucleated cells. Class II molecules (named HLA-DR, -DP, and -DQ) generally are expressed by APCs, such as B lymphocytes, monocytes, and dendritic cells. In a nontransplant setting, the main function is antigen presentation to T lymphocytes. In the transplant setting, HLA molecules can initiate rejection and graft damage via either humoral or cellular mechanisms.

Humoral rejection occurs if the recipient has circulating antibodies specific to the donor's HLA. These antibodies may be from prior exposure (i.e., blood transfusion, previous transplant, or pregnancy), or posttransplant, the recipient may develop antibodies specific to the donor's HLA. The antibodies then bind to the donor's recognized foreign antigens, activating the complement cascade and leading to cell lysis. The blood group antigens of the ABO system, although not part of the HLA system, may also trigger this form of humoral rejection.

Cellular rejection is the more common type of rejection after organ transplants. Mediated by T lymphocytes,

it results from their activation and proliferation after exposure to donor MHC molecules.

BIBLIOGRAPHY

Humar A, Dunn DL. Transplantation. In: Brunicardi F, Andersen DK, Billiar TR, et al., (eds.), *Schwartz's Principles of Surgery*. 9th ed. New York, NY: McGraw-Hill; 2010: Chapter 11.

9. **(E)** Cirrhosis in the setting of chronic liver disease is not by itself an indication for liver transplant. However, cirrhosis with signs of decompensation warrants evaluation for transplant.

A statistical MELD is used to identify patients with end-stage liver disease who were at greatest risk for mortality within 3 months. The MELD score is based on three laboratory values: total bilirubin, INR, and creatinine value.

Criteria for transplantation in the setting of acute liver failure are as follows:

In the setting of acetaminophen toxicity: pH < 7.30, prothrombin time > 100 s (INR > 6.5), serum creatinine > 300 μmol/L (>3.4 mg/dL).
In the absence of acetaminophen toxicity: prothrombin time > 100 s (INR > 6.5); age < 10 or > 40 years; non-A, non-B hepatitis; duration of jaundice before onset of encephalopathy > 7 days; serum creatinine > 300 μmol/L (>3.4 mg/dL).

In the setting of hepatocellular carcinoma, the *Milan criteria* are used to predict disease-free survival rate and require the presence of a single tumor lesion less than 5 cm or no more than three lesions, each no more than 3 cm in diameter, without evidence of vascular invasion or distant metastases. *In patients who satisfy these criteria,* a 5-year disease-free survival rate of 83% is observed.

BIBLIOGRAPHY

Markmann JF, Yeh H, Naji A, Olthoff KM, Shaked A, Barker CF. Transplantation of abdominal organs. In: Townsend CM Jr, ed. *Sabiston Textbook of Surgery*. 18th ed. Philadelphia, PA: Saunders; 2008;(28):692–707.

10. **(C)** Bile leak after liver transplantation is usually secondary to a technical error or ischemia of the donor bile duct. Early leakage can be diagnosed by the appearance of bile in the drains and is confirmed by T-tube cholangiography, hepatic iminodiacetic acid (HIDA) scanning, or endoscopic retrograde cholangiopancreatography (ERCP). Surgical exploration and revision of the anastomosis or stenting of the anastomosis by ERCP are mandatory and will solve the problem in most cases. However, a leak secondary to ischemic bile duct injury

as a result of early hepatic artery thrombosis (HAT) is an indication for urgent retransplantation.

The incidence of vascular complications after liver transplantation ranges from 8–12%. Thrombosis is the most common early event, and Doppler ultrasound evaluation is the initial investigative method of choice. HAT has a reported incidence of about 3–5% in adults, with slightly higher rates in partial liver transplant recipients. Symptoms range from absent to severe, including ischemia-induced bile leak or late diffuse biliary stricture.

Thrombosis of the portal vein is less common than HAT. Signs include liver dysfunction, tense ascites, and variceal bleeding. Operative thrombectomy and revision of the anastomosis may be successful in early cases. If thrombosis occurs late, liver function is usually preserved due to the presence of collaterals, but left-sided portal hypertension must be treated.

Primary nonfunction of the transplanted liver occurs in 2–5% of liver grafts. Laboratory findings demonstrate worsening acidosis, coagulopathy, and extremely elevated liver enzymes (lactate dehydrogenase, aspartate aminotransferase, and alanine aminotransferase). The development of primary nonfunction is a surgical emergency that can be successfully treated by early retransplantation. Failure to find a suitable graft within 7 days is associated with higher morbidity and mortality.

Persistence of immediate posttransplant coagulopathy, fibrinolysis, and the presence of multiple vascular anastomoses place these patients at high risk for postoperative bleeding. A persistent drop in hemoglobin and a need for transfusion of more than 6 units of packed red blood cells are usually indications for reexploration and evacuation of the hematoma. In most cases, removal of the clot will be sufficient to arrest further fibrinolysis and will stop the bleeding. Occasionally, it will be necessary to repair the bleeding sites.

BIBLIOGRAPHY

Humar A, Dunn DL. Transplantation. In: Brunicardi F, Andersen DK, Billiar TR, et al., (eds.), *Schwartz's Principles of Surgery*. 9th ed. New York, NY: McGraw-Hill; 2010: Chapter 11.

Markmann JF, Yeh H, Naji A, Olthoff KM, Shaked A, Barker CF. Transplantation of abdominal organs. In: Townsend CM Jr, ed. *Sabiston Textbook of Surgery*. 18th ed. Philadelphia, PA: Saunders; 2008;(28):692–707.

11. (C)

12. (C)

Explanation for questions 11 and 12

Cytokines are a class of protein signaling compounds that play prominent roles in the innate and adaptive immune responses. Cytokines mediate a broad sequence of cellular responses, mediate the eradication of microorganisms, and promote wound healing.

Interleukin 1 is primarily synthesized by monocytes, macrophages, endothelial cells, fibroblasts, and epidermal cells. IL-1 is released in response to inflammatory stimuli, including cytokines (TNF, IL-2, interferon gamma [IFN-γ]) and foreign pathogens, and acts on the hypothalamus by stimulating prostaglandin activity and thereby mediates a febrile response. High doses of either IL-1 or TNF are associated with profound hemodynamic compromise.

Interleukin 2 is primarily a promoter of T-lymphocyte proliferation and differentiation, immunoglobulin production, and gut barrier integrity and is upregulated in response to IL-1. It has a half-life of less than 10 min; therefore, it is not readily detectable after acute injury. IL-2 receptor blockade induces immunosuppressive effects and is a pharmacological target of immunosuppression after organ transplantation.

Interleukin 4 is released by activated helper T cells and stimulates the differentiation of T cells; it also stimulates T-cell proliferation and B-cell activation. It is also important in antibody-mediated immunity and in antigen presentation. IL-4 induces class switching of differentiating B lymphocytes to produce predominantly immunoglobulin G4 and immunoglobulin E, which are important immunoglobulins in allergic and antihelmintic responses. IL-4 has anti-inflammatory effects on macrophages, exhibited by an attenuated response to proinflammatory mediators such as IL-1, TNF, IL-6, and IL-8.

Interleukin 6 release by macrophages is stimulated by inflammatory mediators such as endotoxin, TNF, and IL-1. IL-6 is increasingly expressed during times of stress, as in septic shock. Plasma levels of IL-6 are proportional to the degree of injury during surgery. Interestingly, IL-6 has counterregulatory effects on the inflammatory cascade through the inhibition of TNF and IL-1. IL-6 also promotes the release of soluble TNF receptors (TNFRs) and IL-1 receptor antagonists and stimulates the release of cortisol. High plasma IL-6 levels have been associated with mortality during intra-abdominal sepsis.

Interleukin 8 is synthesized by macrophages as well as other cell lines, such as endothelial cells. Critical illness as manifested during sepsis is a potent stimulus for IL-8 expression. IL-8 stimulates the release of IFN-γ and functions as a potent chemoattractant for neutrophils. Elevated plasma IL-8 also has been associated with disease severity and end-organ dysfunction during sepsis.

Interleukin-10 (IL-10) is an anti-inflammatory cytokine synthesized primarily by monocytes. IL-10 is expressed during times of systemic inflammation, and its release is enhanced by TNF and IL-1. IL-10 inhibits the secretion of proinflammatory cytokines, including TNF and IL-1, partly through the downregulation of nuclear factor kappa B (NF-κB) and thereby functions as a negative-feedback regulator of the inflammatory cascade. Increased plasma levels of IL-10 also have been associated with mortality and disease severity after traumatic injury.

Interleukin-12 is a regulator of cell-mediated immunity. IL-12 is released by activated phagocytes, including monocytes, macrophages, neutrophils, and dendritic cells, and is increasingly expressed during endotoxemia and sepsis. IL-12 stimulates lymphocytes to increase secretion of IFN-γ with the costimulus of IL-18 and stimulates NK cell cytotoxicity and helper T-cell differentiation. IL-12 release is inhibited by IL-10. IL-12 deficiency inhibits phagocytosis in neutrophils.

Interleukin-13 inhibits monocyte release of TNF, IL-1, IL-6, and IL-8, while increasing the secretion of IL-1 receptor antagonist. Similar to IL-4 and IL-10, IL-13 has a net anti-inflammatory effect. However, unlike IL-4, IL-13 has no identifiable effect on T lymphocytes and only has influence on selected B-lymphocyte populations. Increased IL-13 expression is observed during septic shock and mediates neutropenia, monocytopenia, and leukopenia.

Interleukin-15 is synthesized in many cell types, including macrophages and skeletal muscle after endotoxin administration. IL-15 stimulates NK cell activation as well as B-cell and T-cell proliferation and thus functions as a regulator of cellular immunity. In addition, IL-15 acts as a potent inhibitor of lymphocyte apoptosis by enhancing the expression of antiapoptotic molecules such as Bcl-2.

Interleukin-18 is synthesized primarily by macrophages in response to inflammatory stimuli, including endotoxin, TNF, IL-1, and IL-6. The IL-18 level also is elevated during sepsis. IL-18 activates NF-κB. This molecule also mediates hepatotoxicity associated with Fas ligand and TNF. IL-18 and IL-12 act synergistically to release IFN-γ from T cells.

BIBLIOGRAPHY

Jan BV, Lowry SF. Systemic response to injury and metabolic support. In: Brunicardi F, Andersen DK, Billiar TR, et al., (eds.), *Schwartz's Principles of Surgery*. 9th ed. New York, NY: McGraw-Hill; 2010: Chapter 2.

13. **(D)** Tumor necrosis factor alpha is a cytokine that is a potent mediator of the inflammatory response, being rapidly mobilized in response to stressors such as injury and infection. TNF is primarily synthesized by macrophages, monocytes, and T cells, and the circulating half-life of TNF is brief. TNF stimulates muscle breakdown and cachexia through increased catabolism, insulin resistance, and redistribution of amino acids to hepatic circulation as fuel substrates. It also mediates coagulation activation, cell migration, and macrophage phagocytosis and enhances the expression of adhesion molecules, prostaglandin E_2, platelet-activating factor, glucocorticoids, and eicosanoids.

BIBLIOGRAPHY

Jan BV, Lowry SF. Systemic response to injury and metabolic support. In: Brunicardi F, Andersen DK, Billiar TR, et al., (eds.), *Schwartz's Principles of Surgery*. 9th ed. New York, NY: McGraw-Hill; 2010: Chapter 2.

14. **(C)** The liver acute-phase response is a protein synthetic response by the liver to trauma or infection. The purpose of the response is to restrict organ damage, maintain vital hepatic function, and control defense mechanisms. Proinflammatory cytokines such as IL-1, IL-6, and TNF, induce acute-phase protein gene expression in the liver, including $α_1$-, $α_2$-, and β-globulin; C-reactive protein; and serum amyloid A. The acute-phase response is usually over in 24–48 h, but in the context of ongoing injury, it can be prolonged (Fig. 31-3).

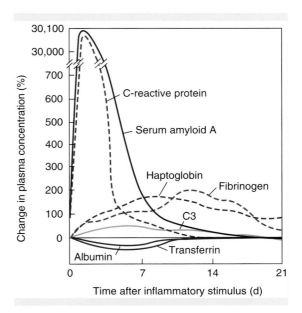

FIGURE 31-3. Time course of acute-phase proteins. Modified from McAdam KP, Elin RJ, Sipe JD, Wolff SM: *Changes in human serum amyloid A and C-reactive protein after etiocholanolone-induced inflammation. J Clin Invest,* 1978 Feb;61(2):390-394.

BIBLIOGRAPHY

Sicklick JK, D'Angelica M, Fong Y. Ch 54: The liver. In: *Sabiston Textbook of Surgery*. Courtney M. Townsend Jr, R. Daniel Beauchamp (Eds). 19th ed. Elseiver Saunders Philadelphia PA.

15. **(E)** Natural killer cells do not require recognition of MHC molecules or antigen processing. They produce IFN-α, IFN-γ, and B cells. NK cells are a critical component of innate immunity. NK cells express cell receptors that are distinct from the T Cell Receptor (TCR) complex. NK cells lyse cell targets that lack expression of self-MHC class I by incorporating lipophilic protein into target cell membrane to increase cell wall permeability, cell swelling, and destruction. NK cells produce the cytokine IFN-γ, which in turn activates macrophages to kill host cells infected by intracellular microbes. NK cells also play an important role in immune defenses, especially after hematopoietic stem cell and organ transplantation. In addition, they contribute to the defense against virus-infected cells, graft rejection, and neoplasia and participate in the regulation of hematopoiesis through cytokine production and cell-to-cell interaction. NK cells also mediate rejection in xenotransplantation (Fig. 31-4).

Macrophages are the main effector cells of the immune response to infection and injury, primarily

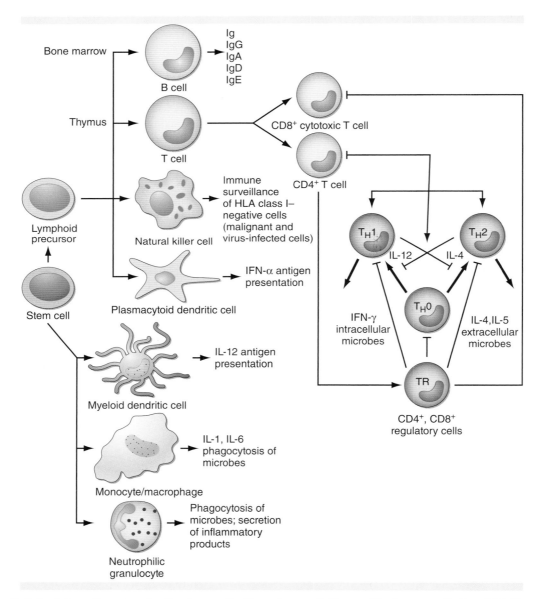

FIGURE 31-4. Cellular interactions in adaptive immunity (from Longo D, Kasper DL, Jameson JL, Fauci AS, Hauser SL, Loscalzo J, eds. *Harrison's Principles of Internal Medicine*. 18th ed. New York, NY: McGraw-Hill; 2012: Fig. 314-2. Copyright © The McGraw-Hill Companies, Inc. All rights reserved).

through mechanisms that include phagocytosis of microbial pathogens, release of inflammatory mediators, and clearance of apoptotic cells. In humans, downregulation of monocyte and neutrophil TNFR expression has been demonstrated experimentally and clinically during systemic inflammation. In clinical sepsis, nonsurviving patients with severe sepsis had an immediate reduction in monocyte surface TNFR expression with failure to recover, whereas surviving patients had normal or near-normal receptor levels from the onset of clinically defined sepsis. In patients with congestive heart failure (CHF), there is also a significant decrease in the amount of monocyte surface TNFR expression compared with control patients. In experimental models, endotoxin has been shown to differentially regulate over 1000 genes in murine macrophages, with approximately 25% of these corresponding to cytokines and chemokines. During sepsis, macrophages undergo phenotypic reprogramming highlighted by decreased surface HLA DR (a critical receptor in antigen presentation), which also may contribute to host immunocompromise during sepsis. Macrophages express class I MHC on their surface (nucleated) as well as class II MHC (specialized immune cells).

Eosinophils are immunocytes whose primary functions are antihelmintic. Eosinophils are found mostly in tissues such as the lung and gastrointestinal tract, which may suggest a role in immune surveillance. Eosinophils can be activated by IL-3, IL-5, granulocyte-macrophage colony-stimulating factor (GM-CSF), chemoattractants, and platelet-activating factor. Eosinophil activation can lead to subsequent release of toxic mediators, including reactive oxygen species, histamine, and peroxidase.

Mast cells are important in the primary response to injury because they are located in tissues. TNF release from mast cells has been found to be crucial for neutrophil recruitment and pathogen clearance. Mast cells are also known to play an important role in the anaphylactic response to allergens. On activation from stimuli, including allergen binding, infection, and trauma, mast cells produce histamine, cytokines, eicosanoids, proteases, and chemokines, which leads to vasodilation, capillary leakage, and immunocyte recruitment. Mast cells are thought to be important cosignaling effector cells of the immune system via the release of IL-3, IL-4, IL-5, IL-6, IL-10, IL-13, and IL-14, as well as macrophage migration–inhibiting factor.

BIBLIOGRAPHY

Jan BV, Lowry SF. Systemic response to injury and metabolic support. In: Brunicardi F, Andersen DK, Billiar TR, et al., (eds.), *Schwartz's Principles of Surgery.* 9th ed. New York, NY: McGraw-Hill; 2010: Chapter 2.

J. Patrick O'Leary MD FACS, Arnold Tabuenca MD, Wolters Kluwer/ Lippincott Williams and Wilkins Rohrer RJ. Basic immunology for surgeons. In: *The Physiologic Basis of Surgery.* 4th ed.; 2008: Chapter 7.

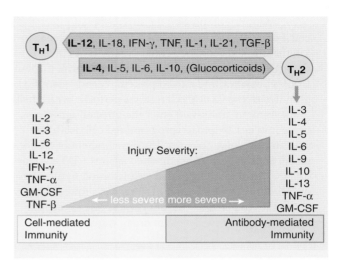

FIGURE 31-5. T cell–mediated immunity. Adapted with permission from Lin E, Calvano SE, Lowry SF: Inflammatory cytokines and cell response in surgery. *Surgery* 127:117, 2000. Copyright Elsevier.

16. **(D)** Fundamental properties of a mature T-cell repertoire include (1) restriction to self-MHC and (2) tolerance to self-antigens (Fig. 31-5). MHC-antigen recognition by T cells is the initiating stimulus for their activation and proliferation, cytokine production, and performance of regulatory or cytolytic effector functions. Activated T cells produce and secrete IL-2, thereby exerting an *autocrine* (acting on self) and *paracrine* (acting on cells nearby) response.

The CD4 and CD8 molecules that differentiate the two major functional classes of T cells function as coreceptor molecules on the T-cell surface. During recognition of antigen, the CD4 and CD8 molecules interact with the T-cell receptor complex and with MHC molecules on the APC. CD4 binds to MHC class II molecules, and CD8 binds to MHC class I molecules.

Proliferating CD4 T cells can become one of four main categories of effector T cells: Th1 cells, Th2 cells, Th17 cells, or regulatory T (Treg) cells. In an environment of IFN-γ, Th1 cells dominate and either activate macrophages or cause B cells to switch to produce different subclasses of IgG. In either case, this can promote bacterial clearance either by direct destruction in the IFN-γ-activated macrophage or by destruction after phagocytosis of opsonized particles. These Th1 cells also produce IL-2 and IFN-γ. In an environment where IL-4 is being produced, Th2 cells predominate, activate mast cells and eosinophils, and cause B cells to synthesize IgE. This aids in the response to helminths. The Th2 cells secrete IL-4, IL-5, IL-9, and IL-13.

CD8 cells differentiate into effector cytotoxic cells by engagement of their TCR and recognition of class I

MHC–peptide complex on the surface on an infected cell. Following recognition, the CD8 T cell proceeds to kill the infected cell. The primary method of killing is through cytotoxic granules containing perforin, the family of granzymes, and a third protein recently identified, granulysin. The CD8 T cell releases perforin, which helps granzyme and granulysin enter the infected cell. Granzyme initiates apoptosis (programmed cell death) by activating cellular caspases. The development of monoclonal antibodies (mAbs) directed against CD3, such as OKT3, which interfere with T-cell function by altering or inhibiting intracellular signaling, has allowed these antibodies to play a significant clinical role as focused immunosuppressive agents in organ transplantation.

BIBLIOGRAPHY

Detrick B. Immunology. In: Carroll KC, Brooks GF, Butel JS, Morse SA, Mietzner TA, eds. *Jawetz, Melnick, & Adelberg's Medical Microbiology*. 26th ed. New York, NY: McGraw-Hill; 2013: Chapter 8.

17. **(D)** B cells are derived from pluripotent bone marrow stem cells and express immunoglobulin (antibody) on their cell surface. These membrane-bound immunoglobulins are the B-cell antigen receptors and allow specific antigen recognition. Only one antigen-specific antibody is produced by each mature B cell. Each antibody is composed of two heavy chains and two light chains. Both heavy and light chains have a constant region (Fc), as well as a variable, antigen-binding region (Fab). The antibody-binding site is composed of both the heavy- and light-chain variable regions. Resting naïve B cells express IgD and IgM on their cell surface. On antigen stimulation and with the help of CD4$^+$ T cells, B cells undergo isotype switching. Distinct immune effector functions are assigned to each isotype.

    IgM and IgG antibodies provide a pivotal role in the endogenous or intravascular immune response.

    IgM is the first isotype produced in response to a foreign and is the initial type of antibody made by neonates.

    IgG constitutes about 75–85% of total serum immunoglobulin.

    IgA constitutes only 7–15% of total serum immunoglobulin but is the predominant class of immunoglobulin in secretions. IgA is secreted into the lumen of the gastrointestinal and respiratory tracts and is responsible for *mucosal immunity*.

    IgD is found in minute quantities in serum and, together with IgM, is a major receptor for antigen on the B-cell surface. IgE, which is present in serum in very low concentrations, is the major class of immunoglobulin involved in arming mast cells and basophils by binding to these cells via the Fc region. Antigen crosslinking of IgE molecules on basophil and mast cell surfaces results in release of mediators of the immediate hypersensitivity (allergic) response.

BIBLIOGRAPHY

Adams AB, Kirk AD and Larsen CP. Transplantation immunology and immunosuppression. In: *Sabiston Basic Immunology for Surgeons*. In: *The Physiologic Basis of Surgery*. (Courtney M. Townsend Jr, R. Daniel Beauchamp.) 19th ed; 2012: Chapter 26.

Haynes BF, Soderberg KA, Fauci AS. Introduction to the immune system. In: Longo DL, Fauci AS, Kasper DL, Hauser SL, Jameson J, Loscalzo J, eds. *Harrison's Principles of Internal Medicine*. 18th ed. New York, NY: McGraw-Hill; 2012: Chapter 314.

18. **(E)** Type I hypersensitivity reaction involves the formation of IgE after exposure to an antigen. The IgE binds to mast cells, with the consequence of degranulation of the mast cells and release of mediators (e.g., histamine, bradykinin), leading to increased vascular permeability, edema, and increased smooth muscle contraction and eventually to bronchoconstriction (early phase). Type I hypersensitivity reactions also have a late phase, characterized by infiltration by neutrophils, eosinophils, basophils, and monocytes, and results in mucosal damage due to release of mediators by these recruited inflammatory cells. Clinical manifestations of type I hypersensitivity reactions may be local (urticaria) or systemic (anaphylaxis).

    Type II hypersensitivity reaction involves antibodies directed against target antigens on cells or in extracellular matrix. The target antigens may be endogenous or absorbed exogenous antigens. The three mechanisms by which the reaction occurs are complement-dependent reactions, antibody-dependent cell-mediated cytotoxicity, and antibody-mediated cellular dysfunction.

    Type III hypersensitivity reactions involve formation of an immune complex after antigen-antibody binding. The immune complex causes activation of the complement cascade, and under certain circumstances, they do elicit an immune reaction.

    Type IV hypersensitivity reactions are mediated by sensitized T cells rather than by antibodies. Specific mechanisms include activation of macrophages by CD4$^+$ helper T cells (T$_H$1 type), sensitized from previous exposure to an antigen; these cells secrete IFN-γ. Cell-mediated cytotoxicity can also occur, by which sensitized CD8$^+$ cells kill antigen-bearing class I MHC molecules, either via the perforin-granzyme system or the FAS-FAS ligand system.

BIBLIOGRAPHY

Kemp WL, Burns DK, Brown TG. Pathology of the immune system. In: *Pathology: The Big Picture*. New York, NY: McGraw-Hill; 2008: Chapter 3.

19. **(D)**

20. **(E)**

Explanation for questions 19 and 20

The crossmatch is an *in vitro* test that involves mixing the donor's cells with the recipient's serum to look for evidence of donor cell destruction by recipient antibodies. A positive crossmatch indicates the presence of preformed antibodies in the recipient that are specific to the donor and is associated with a high risk of hyperacute rejection (if the transplant is performed). The crossmatch is required in kidney, pancreas, and lung transplantation, and a positive crossmatch is a contraindication to renal transplantation because of its strong association with hyperacute rejection (type II hypersensitivity reaction).

The PRA is a quantitation of how much antibody is present in a candidate against a panel of cells representing the distribution of antigens in the donor pool. In addition to typing for HLA antigens, most laboratories use technology to detect antibodies to HLA antigens. This is important for solid-organ transplantation, for which the presence of anti-HLA antibodies can cause irreversible rejection on transplantation. The serologic test involves a patient's serum reacted with a panel of lymphocytes of defined HLA type. Analysis of the reaction patterns yields information about the breadth of alloimmunization, or PRA (percentage reactive antibody), and the specificity of the reactions.

BIBLIOGRAPHY

Coppage M, Stroncek D, McFarland J, Blumberg N. Human leukocyte and platelet antigens. In: Lichtman MA, Kipps TJ, Seligsohn U, Kaushansky K, Prchal JT, eds. *Williams Hematology*. 8th ed. New York, NY: McGraw-Hill; 2010: Chapter 138.
Markmann JF, Yeh H, Naji A, Olthoff KM, Shaked A, Barker CF. Transplantation of abdominal organs. In: Townsend CM Jr, ed. *Sabiston Textbook of Surgery*. 18th ed. Philadelphia, PA: Saunders; 2008;(28):692–707.

21. **(D)** Cyclosporin plays a central role in maintenance immunosuppression in many types of organ transplants. Cyclosporine binds with its cytoplasmic receptor protein, cyclophilin, which subsequently inhibits the activity of calcineurin and impairs expression of several critical T-cell activation genes, the most important being for IL-2, and the result is suppression of T-cell activation. Cyclosporine also suppresses some humoral immunity but is more effective against T cell–dependent immune mechanisms, such as those underlying transplant rejection and some forms of autoimmunity. The metabolism of cyclosporine is via the cytochrome P-450 system, and nephrotoxicity is the most important and troubling adverse effect. Hirsutism, gingival hyperplasia, hyperlipidemia, hepatotoxicity, and hyperuricemia are other common side effects.

BIBLIOGRAPHY

Humar A, Dunn DL. Transplantation. In: Brunicardi F, Andersen DK, Billiar TR, et al., (eds.), *Schwartz's Principles of Surgery*. 9th ed. New York, NY: McGraw-Hill; 2010: Chapter 11.

22. **(E)** A number of different mAbs are currently under development or have entered the phase of clinical testing for use in transplantation. Polyclonal antibodies are produced by immunizing animals, such as horses or rabbits, with human lymphoid tissue, allowing for an immune response, removing the resultant immune sera, and purifying the sera in an effort to remove unwanted antibodies. These lymphocyte-depleting antibodies are potent suppressors of the T cell–mediated immune response and selectively prevent the activation of B cells by a range of stimuli. Polyclonal antibodies have been successfully used as induction agents to prevent rejection and to treat acute rejection episodes.

Antithymocyte globulin (ATGAM) is a purified gamma globulin solution obtained by immunization of horses with human thymocytes. It contains antibodies to a wide variety of human T-cell surface antigens, including the MHC antigens.

Antithymocyte immunoglobulin (Thymoglobulin) is a polyclonal antibody obtained by immunizing rabbits with human thymocytes. It has been approved by the Food and Drug Administration to prevent and treat rejection in solid-organ transplant recipients.

Monoclonal Antibodies

Monoclonal antibodies have emerged as a new class of immunosuppressive agents that appear to be effective in both the treatment and prevention of acute rejection and are well tolerated in renal transplant recipients. These mAbs are produced by the hybridization of murine antibody-secreting B lymphocytes with a nonsecreting myeloma cell line. The highly specific nature of these drugs makes them less toxic than the oral, long-term maintenance agents, such as corticosteroids and calcineurin inhibitors.

Muromonab-CD3 is directed against the CD3 antigen complex found on all mature human T cells. Inactivation of CD3 by muromonab-CD3 causes the TCR to be lost from the cell surface. The T cells are then ineffective and are rapidly cleared from the circulation and deposited into the reticuloendothelial system. The serious side effect is a rapidly developing, noncardiogenic pulmonary edema. The risk of this side effect significantly increases if the patient is fluid overloaded before beginning muromonab-CD3 treatment. Other serious side effects include encephalopathy, aseptic meningitis, and nephrotoxicity.

Anti-CD25 Monoclonal Antibodies (Basiliximab and Daclizumab).

The alpha subunit of the IL-2 receptor, also known as Tac or *CD25*, is found exclusively on activated T cells. Blockade of this component by mAbs selectively prevents T-cell activation induced by IL-2. Basiliximab (Simulect) and daclizumab (Zenapax) are currently the two anti-CD25 mAbs approved for clinical use. They are used as part of induction immunosuppression in renal transplantation, in association with calcineurin inhibitors, corticosteroids, and Mycophenolate Mofetil (MMF).

BIBLIOGRAPHY

Humar A, Dunn DL. Transplantation. In: Brunicardi F, Andersen DK, Billiar TR, et al., (eds.), *Schwartz's Principles of Surgery*. 9th ed. New York, NY: McGraw-Hill; 2010: Chapter 11.

23. **(E)** Cardiovascular disease (CVD) is common among the kidney transplant population and is the leading cause of death (30–50%) in patients who die with a functioning allograft. In addition to traditional risk factors for CVD, renal transplant recipients have the associative cardiovascular (CV) risk of many years of chronic kidney disease (CKD) and end-stage kidney disease (ESKD), compounded by the unwanted CV side effects of immunosuppressive medication. Tobacco use, diabetes mellitus (DM), elevated BMI, hypertension, and dyslipidemia have been found to be independent risk factors of CVD in kidney transplant recipients. The cumulative incidence of CV events approaches 40% at 3 years after kidney transplantation, with CHF the number one cause of CV hospitalizations. The incidence of myocardial infarction after kidney transplantation has been reported to be as high as 4.3, 5.6, and 11.1% at 6, 12, and 36 months, respectively.

BIBLIOGRAPHY

Azzi J, Lee BT, Chandraker A. Kidney transplantation 2: care of the kidney transplant recipient. In: Ashley S, Cance W, Chen H, et al., (eds.), *ACS Surgery: Principles and Practice*. Philadelphia, PA: Decker; 2014: Chapter 195.

24. **(A)** MELD is a linear regression model based on objective laboratory values (INR, bilirubin level, and creatinine level). It was originally developed as a tool to predict mortality after transjugular intrahepatic portosystemic shunt (TIPS) but has been validated and has been used as the sole method of liver transplant allocation in the United States since 2002. The MELD formula is as follows:

MELD score = $10 [0.957 \text{ Ln}(\text{SCr}) + 0.378 \text{ Ln}(\text{Tbil}) + 1.12 \text{ Ln}(\text{INR}) + 0.643]$.

where SCr is serum creatinine level, and Tbil is serum bilirubin level.

Northup and colleagues demonstrated that the MELD score was the only statistically significant predictor of 30-day mortality, with mortality rate increasing by approximately 1% for each MELD point up to a score of 20 and by 2% for each MELD point above 20.

BIBLIOGRAPHY

Geller DA, Goss JA, Tsung A. Liver. In: Brunicardi F, Andersen DK, Billiar TR, et al., (eds.), *Schwartz's Principles of Surgery*. 9th ed. New York, NY: McGraw-Hill; 2010: Chapter 31.

25. **(E)** Cardiac transplantation remains the treatment of choice for patients with end-stage cardiac disease with severe functional limitation, usually New York Heart Association (NYHA) functional class III or IV, whose symptoms are refractory to management with medications; electrophysiological device therapy such as cardiac resynchronization; and, in some cases, surgical intervention. The primary indications for adult heart transplantation today continue to be divided between nonischemic cardiomyopathy (44%) and coronary artery disease (35%). Congenital (3%) and valvular (2%) disease are also indications.

Contraindications include irreversible severe PA hypertension (pulmonary vascular resistance [PVR] > 5 Wood units, pulmonary vascular resistance index [PVRI] > 6, transpulmonary gradient > 16–20 mmHg, PA systolic pressure > 50–60 mmHg or > 50% of systemic pressures), advanced age (>70 years), active systemic infection, active malignancy or recent malignancy with high risk of recurrence or progression, and DM with end-organ damage, poor glycemic control, or marked obesity.

Donor-recipient matching is performed on the basis of ABO blood group compatibility and overall body size comparability within 20% of body weight. Although the benefit of matching donor organs and recipients with respect to HLA has been well established in renal transplantation, HLA prospective crossmatching is reserved for presensitized heart transplant recipients or those with more than 10–20% reactivity to a standard panel of common donor antigens. More recently, the use of flow cytometry with recombinant single HLA antigen bead technology has facilitated the prediction of incompatible organs by comparing the recipient's HLA antibodies with the donor's HLA type. This "virtual crossmatch" can eliminate the need for a prospective crossmatch and therefore increase the availability of potential organs, particularly in patients who are sensitized with preformed HLA antibodies as a result of previous pregnancy, transplant, or blood transfusions.

26. **(B)** Lung transplant is prioritized based on a lung allocation score (LAS): age, height, weight, lung diagnosis code, functional status, diabetes, assisted ventilation, supplemental O_2 requirement, percentage predicted forced vital capacity, pulmonary artery systemic pressure, mean pulmonary artery pressure, pulmonary capillary wedge pressure, current Pco_2, highest Pco_2, lowest Pco_2, change in Pco_2, 6-min walk distance, and serum creatinine.

ABO compatibilities are strictly adhered to because isolated cases of hyperacute rejection have been reported in transplants performed across ABO barriers. Donor-to-recipient lung volume matching is based on the vertical (apex to diaphragm along the midclavicular line) and transverse (level of diaphragmatic dome) radiologic dimensions on chest x-ray, as well as body weight, height, and chest circumference. Matching donor and recipient height seems the most reproducible method for selection of appropriate donor lung size, and donor lung dimensions should not be greater than 4 cm over those of the recipient. If need be, donor lungs may be downsized by lobectomy or wedge resection.

In contrast to renal transplantation, HLA matching is not a criterion for thoracic organ allocation. Because only short ischemic times are tolerated by lung and heart-lung blocs, it is not possible to perform this tissue typing preoperatively.

Absolute contraindications include renal dysfunction, malignancy (bronchoalveolar carcinoma is a contraindication but not nonmelanoma skin cancer), infection with human immunodeficiency virus (HIV), hepatitis B antigen positivity or hepatitis C infection with biopsy-proven liver disease, infection with panresistant respiratory flora, active or recent cigarette smoking, drug abuse, alcohol abuse, severe psychiatric illness, noncompliance with medical care, extreme obesity, progressive unintentional weight loss, malnutrition, and absence of a consistent and reliable social support network. Relative contraindications include active extrapulmonary infection, symptomatic osteoporosis, and recent history of active peptic ulcer disease. Cigarette smokers must quit smoking and remain abstinent for several months before transplantation.

BIBLIOGRAPHY

Sheikh AY, Joyce DL, Mallidi HR, Robbins RC. Lung transplantation and heart-lung transplantation. In: Cohn LH, ed. *Cardiac Surgery in the Adult*. 4th ed. New York, NY: McGraw-Hill; 2012: Chapter 65.

27. **(A)** A Lymphocele is a fluid collection of lymph that generally results from cut lymphatic vessels in the recipient. The reported incidence of lymphoceles is 0.6–18%, and they usually do not occur until at least 2 weeks post-transplant. Symptoms are generally related to the mass effect and compression of nearby structures (e.g., ureter, iliac vein, allograft renal artery), and patients develop hypertension, unilateral leg swelling on the side of the transplant, and elevated serum creatinine. Ultrasound is used to confirm a fluid collection, although percutaneous aspiration may be necessary to exclude the presence of other collections, such as urinomas, hematomas, or abscesses. The standard surgical treatment is creation of a peritoneal window to allow for drainage of the lymphatic fluid into the peritoneal cavity, where it can be absorbed. Either a laparoscopic or an open approach may be used.

BIBLIOGRAPHY

Humar A, Dunn DL. Transplantation. In: Brunicardi F, Andersen DK, Billiar TR, et al., (eds.), *Schwartz's Principles of Surgery*. 9th ed. New York, NY: McGraw-Hill; 2010: Chapter 11.

28. **(D)** While all of the choices are potential causes of transaminitis posttransplant, most of them will not cause bilious fluid in the surgical drain when the serum bilirubin is only 2 mg/dL. Biliary complications after liver transplant are common, occurring in 6–30% of patients. They manifest as leak, stricture, or obstruction. They are associated with hepatic arterial thrombosis 70–80% of the time. Options for treatment include surgical revision to Roux-en-Y hepaticojejunostomy, nasobiliary drainage, endoscopic stenting or balloon dilation, or percutaneous dilation or stenting. Early diagnosis and intervention are key to preventing arterial pseudoaneurysm and arterial rupture as a result of the bile contamination.

BIBLIOGRAPHY

Gastaca M. Biliary complications after orthotopic liver transplantation: a review of incidence and risk factors. *Transplant Proc* 2012;44(6):1545–1549.

Welling TH, Heidt DG, Englesbe MJ, et al. Biliary complications following liver transplantation in the model for end-stage liver disease era: effect of donor, recipient, and technical factors. *Liver Transpl* 2008;14(1):73–80.

29. **(C)** Low urine output after kidney transplant is a common occurrence. The most common causes of low urine output are hypovolemia, hypotension, obstruction, acute tubular necrosis, bleeding, and medication effect. Hyperacute rejection occurs immediately on reperfusion,

not early in the postoperative period. Hypovolemia is common but typically results in a decrease of urine output, not complete cessation, and should respond to fluid bolus. Urine leak is an uncommon complication, occurring in 1–3% of transplants. Urine leak secondary to technical failure is most likely to occur in the first 24 h postoperatively. Urine leak due to ischemia or necrosis will occur within the first 14 days. If cessation of urine output is abrupt, the first step should be to gently flush the catheter to flush any blood clots or debris. If urine output does not immediately resume, an alternative diagnosis must be considered.

Other causes of cessation of urine output (UOP) include arterial thrombosis or ureteral obstruction. A duplex ultrasound of the transplant should be obtained to assess for flow in the graft or hydronephrosis. A nuclear medicine scan can alternatively be obtained to evaluate for vascular perfusion, excretion, and urine leak.

BIBLIOGRAPHY

Farris A, Cornell L, Colvin R. Pathology of kidney transplantation. In: Morris P, Knetchtle S, eds. *Kidney Transplantation*. 7th ed. New York, NY: Elsevier; 2014: Chapter 26.

Shoskes D, Jimenez JA. Urological complications after kidney transplantation. In: Morris P, Knetchtle S, eds. *Kidney Transplantation*. 7th ed. New York, NY: Elsevier; 2014: Chapter 29.

30. **(B)**

31. **(B)**

Explanation for questions 30 and 31

Mycophenolate mofetil is isolated from the mold *Penicillium glaucum*. It works by inhibiting inosine monophosphate dehydrogenase, which is a crucial, rate-limiting enzyme in de novo synthesis of purines. Specifically, this enzyme catalyzes the formation of guanosine nucleotides from inosine. Many cells have a salvage pathway and therefore can bypass this need for guanosine nucleotide synthesis by the de novo pathway. Activated lymphocytes, however, do not possess this salvage pathway and require de novo synthesis for clonal expansion. The net result is a selective, reversible antiproliferative effect on T and B lymphocytes. The most common gastrointestinal side effects are diarrhea, gastritis, and vomiting. Significant leukopenia also is common, affecting about one-third of recipients. Glucocorticoids have a poorly understood mechanism in immunosuppression. Side effects include poor wound healing, cushingoid facies, growth retardation, diabetes, hyperlipidemia, bone disease, peptic ulcers, cataracts. Tacrolimus binds FK binding protein, which forms a complex with calcineurin that inhibits the phosphatase activity of calcineurin. This results in an inhibition of NF-AT and ultimately IL-2, leading to inhibition of T-cell activation. Cyclosporin has a similar mechanism; however, tacrolimus is 10–100 times more potent. Side effects of tacrolimus include nephrotoxicity, neurotoxicity, hypertension, and metabolic disturbances. Azathioprine prevents interconversion of the precursors of purine synthesis, thereby blocking purine synthesis and lymphocyte proliferation. The most common side effect is leukopenia (reflective of bone marrow aplasia).

BIBLIOGRAPHY

Gaston, R. Mycophenolates. In: Morris P, Knetchtle S, eds. *Kidney Transplantation*. 7th ed. New York, NY: Elsevier; 2014: Chapter 18.

Humar A, Dunn DL. Transplantation. In: Brunicardi F, Andersen DK, Billiar TR, et al., (eds.), *Schwartz's Principles of Surgery*. 9th ed. New York, NY: McGraw-Hill; 2010: Chapter 11.

Mejia J, Basu A, Shapiro R. Calcineurin inhibitors. In: Morris P, Knetchtle S, eds. *Kidney Transplantation*. 7th ed. New York, NY: Elsevier; 2014: Chapter 17.

Morris P. Azathioprine. In: Morris P, Knetchtle S, eds. *Kidney Transplantation*. 7th ed. New York, NY: Elsevier; 2014: Chapter 15.

32. **(A)** Hyperacute rejection results from preformed antibodies against the donor organ. The classic form of hyperacute rejection is rare because crossmatching is fairly reliable at identifying recipients with such antibodies. Within minutes of revascularization, the kidney turns blue and soon undergoes vascular thrombosis. Histologically, extensive intravascular deposits of fibrin and platelets and intraglomerular accumulation of PMNs, fibrin, platelets, and red blood cells occur along with accumulation of leukocytes in the peritubular and glomerular capillaries.

CHAPTER 32

SOFT TISSUE SARCOMA AND SKIN

JESSICA ROSE AND JAMES WARNEKE

QUESTIONS

1. Which of the following is the appropriate surgical management of a 1.5-mm melanoma?
   (A) Excision with 1.0-cm margins
   (B) Excision with 2.0-cm margins
   (C) Excision with 2.0-cm margins and sentinel lymph node (SLN) biopsy
   (D) Excision with 2.0-cm margins and lymph node dissection
   (E) Excision with 3.0-cm margins

2. Which of the following is true of biopsy for suspected melanoma?
   (A) Melanoma is a clinical diagnosis, and biopsy is unnecessary.
   (B) A punch biopsy is necessary to confirm diagnosis.
   (C) Shave biopsy should be performed for lesions in cosmetically sensitive locations.
   (D) Incisions on the extremities should be horizontally oriented.

3. A 60-year-old, otherwise-healthy, male presents 6 months after wide local excision (WLE) of a melanoma from his ankle with 30 in-transit lesions scattered on his lower leg (Fig. 32-1). Which of the following is the best treatment?
   (A) Amputation
   (B) WLE of all lesions
   (C) Isolated limb perfusion with melphalan
   (D) Systemic therapy
   (E) None of the above

4. Which of the following is true about groin dissection for melanoma?
   (A) It is indicated when patients have a positive SLN biopsy.
   (B) Regional lymph node disease is not predictive of survival or local recurrence.

(C) Cloquet's node marks the most inferior lymph node.
(D) Borders of the lymph node dissection are the femoral vein, adductor longus muscle, Poupart's ligament, and the abdominal wall.
(E) Deep iliac nodes should be taken routinely.

5. Which of the following lesions are correctly matched with the TNM stage?
   (A) Melanoma with a depth of 1 mm and two positive lymph nodes: stage IIc
   (B) Melanoma with a depth of 4 mm with ulceration: stage IIIa
   (C) Melanoma with a depth of 2 mm with one positive lymph node: stage II
   (D) Melanoma with a depth of 1.5 mm and two positive lymph nodes: stage IIIa
   (E) Melanoma with a depth of 1 mm and a lung lesion: stage IIIc

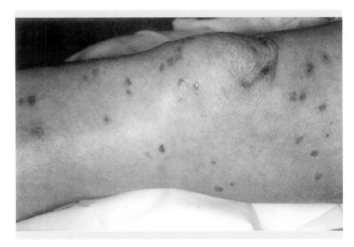

FIGURE 32-1. In-transit metastasis from melanoma on the leg of an elderly male.

6. Which of the following is true of melanoma prognosis?
   (A) The most important prognostic feature of localized melanoma is tumor diameter.
   (B) Younger age, female gender, and site of disease on the trunk are all favorable prognostic indicators.
   (C) The number of metastatic nodes, tumor burden (microscopic vs. macroscopically positive nodes), and primary tumor ulceration are the most sensitive predictors of survival in node-positive disease.
   (D) Patients with lung metastases have a worse prognosis than those with metastases to other visceral sites.

7. Which of the following is true of retroperitoneal soft tissue sarcomas?
   (A) The most common histologic cellular type is malignant fibrous histiosarcoma.
   (B) Preoperative biopsy is contraindicated because of the risk of tumor seeding.
   (C) It is often necessary to resect contiguous organs en bloc to obtain clear margins.
   (D) Death usually results from distant metastases.
   (E) Lung is the most common site of distant metastases.

8. Which of the following is true of soft tissue sarcoma staging?
   (A) Location of the sarcoma (extremity vs. retroperitoneal) is included in the American Joint Committee on Cancer (AJCC) classification.
   (B) The components of soft tissue sarcoma stage grouping are primary tumor, regional lymph nodes, distant metastasis, and histologic grade.
   (C) Retroperitoneal, mediastinal, and pelvic sarcomas are staged by a different scheme than extremity sarcomas.
   (D) A malignant fibrous histiocytoma of the calf, 2 cm in diameter, superficial to the fascia, without regional node or distant metastasis, histologic grade 3 is stage I disease.
   (E) Only 10% of soft tissue sarcomas are node positive.

9. Which of the following is true of extremity soft tissue sarcoma?
   (A) Amputation provides better local control than WLE plus radiation.
   (B) At least 95% of patients presenting with soft tissue sarcomas of the extremities are effectively treated with limb-preserving surgery.
   (C) The most common site of metastases is the liver.
   (D) There is no role for surgery in the treatment of distant recurrences.
   (E) Repeat excision of an incompletely excised sarcoma is futile and should rarely be attempted.

10. Which of the following is true of gastrointestinal stromal tumors (GISTs)?
    (A) They arise from smooth muscle cells of the gastrointestinal tract.
    (B) They are immunohistochemically positive for CD117 and often CD34.
    (C) The small intestine is the most common primary site.
    (E) Primary therapy for unresectable tumors is doxorubicin-based cytotoxic chemotherapy.

11. A 45-year-old lady has a biopsy-proven, ill-defined morpheaform basal cell carcinoma (BCC) on the tip of the nose (Fig. 32-2). The best therapeutic option for this patient is

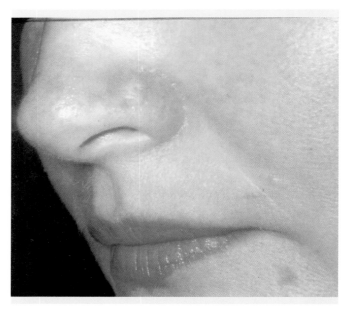

FIGURE 32-2. Morpheaform basal cell carcinoma on nasal tip.

    (A) Radiation therapy
    (B) Surgical excision
    (C) Electrodesiccation and curettage
    (D) Cryosurgery
    (E) Mohs micrographic surgery

12. Which of the following is true of immunotherapy for melanoma?
    (A) Vaccine therapies have been demonstrated to induce regression of established metastatic melanoma.
    (B) Treatment with high-dose interleukin 2 (IL-2) results in more durable responses than treatment with combination chemotherapy.

(C) Experimental treatment with adoptive cell transfer of tumor-specific lymphocytes in combination with high-dose IL-2 has shown objective response rates of 35%.

(D) High-dose interferon lacks efficacy in the treatment of high-risk melanoma.

13. Which of the following is considered to be a poor prognostic variable of subcutaneous squamous cell carcinoma (SCC)?
(A) Underlying immunosuppression
(B) Perineural invasion
(C) Arising in a chronic wound
(D) Induction by radiation
(E) All of the above

14. Which of the following statements is true regarding treatment of cutaneous SCC?
(A) Achieving histological negative margins completely eliminates the risk of local recurrence.
(B) Local in-transit metastases are always removed during surgical resection.
(C) Clinically well-defined low-risk tumors less than 2 cm require a minimum of 2-cm surgical margins.
(D) Adjuvant radiotherapy may be beneficial for high-risk SCC.

15. A 69-year-old male with a previous history of skin cancer presented to his dermatologist with a new, enlarging erythematous nodule on his nose (Fig. 32-3). A biopsy was performed and revealed Merkel cell carcinoma. What percentage of patients with a similar presentation will have regional lymph node disease?
(A) 0%
(B) 10%
(C) 30%
(D) 50%
(E) 75%

16. A 35-year-old male presented with a 5-year history of a scar-like lesion on his anterior shoulder (Fig. 32-4). Histopathology revealed a dermatofibrosarcoma protuberans (DFSP). What would be your initial management?
(A) Local resection followed by Radiation Therapy (XRT)
(B) WLE and lymph node dissection
(C) Radiation therapy, then surgical resection
(D) Local resection and SLN biopsy
(E) WLE with 2- to 3-cm margins alone

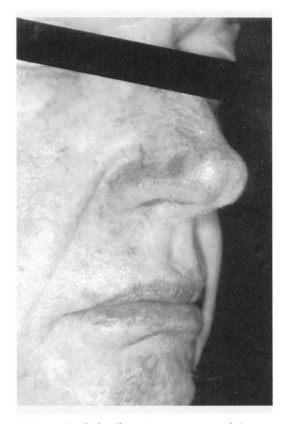

FIGURE 32-3. Merkel cell carcinoma on nasal tip.

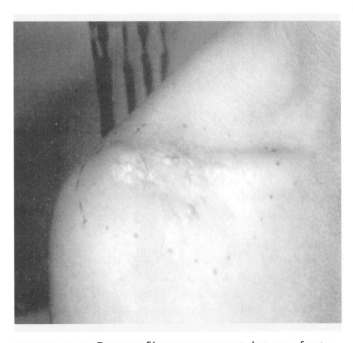

FIGURE 32-4. Dermatofibrosarcoma protuberans of anterior shoulder.

17. A 74-year-old female with a history of early-stage breast cancer was treated with lumpectomy and radiotherapy 5 years ago. She now presents with ill-defined bruise-like patches, ulcerated nodules, and edema over her treated breast. What is the most likely diagnosis?
    (A) Kaposi's sarcoma
    (B) Steward-Treves' syndrome
    (C) Metastatic melanoma
    (D) Recurrent breast cancer
    (E) Radiation-induced angiosarcoma

18. What is the most important prognostic indicator for sarcoma?
    (A) Size
    (B) Location
    (C) Lymph node status
    (D) Grade
    (E) Depth

19. What primary skin cancer is the most common cause of intussusception?
    (A) Merkel cell
    (B) Melanoma
    (C) Squamous cell
    (D) Basal cell

20. Which of the following are the A, B, C, Ds of melanoma?
    (A) Airway, breathing, circulation, disability
    (B) Asymmetry, border irregularity, color, diameter
    (C) Asymmetry, border irregularity, clarity, depth
    (D) Asymmetry, bleaching pattern, color, depth
    (E) Absence of color, border irregularity, color, diameter

21. Which of the following is the most aggressive type of melanoma?
    (A) Nodular
    (B) Superficial spreading
    (C) Lentigo maligna
    (D) Acral lentiginous
    (E) They all are equally aggressive

ANSWERS AND EXPLANATIONS

1. **(C)** The National Comprehensive Cancer Network (NCCN) Guidelines in Oncology has a set of recommended guidelines for treating malignant melanoma based on depth of the lesion. The current standard is a 1-cm margin for lesions 1 mm or less in depth. For lesions 1–2 mm in depth, a 2-cm margin is appropriate, but a smaller margin is accepted in a cosmetically sensitive area. A smaller margin is also appropriate when a limited resection can help preserve function, such as when crossing a joint. A depth of 2 mm or greater requires a 2-cm margin, and some advocate for a 3-cm margin for lesions greater than 4 mm deep. The tissue

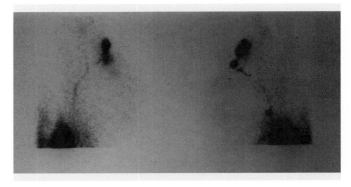

FIGURE 32-5. Lymphoscintigraphy using sulfur colloid labeled with technetium-99.

should be excised down to the level of the fascia to include all subcutaneous lymphatic channels.

To provide adequate staging and treatment, lymph node assessment is necessary. The SLN biopsy has become the standard of care and should be performed routinely for melanomas with a depth of 1 mm or greater. It should also be considered for lesions between 0.75 and 1 mm with high-grade features (ulceration, lymphovascular invasion, and high mitotic rate). Lesions less than 0.75 mm are unlikely to have regional lymph-adenopathy and do not require biopsy.

Sentinel lymph node biopsy is a sampling of the first draining lymph node(s) from the lesion and the most likely to have metastasis if any is present. For melanoma, lymphatic mapping (Fig. 32-5) is performed to identify the draining nodal basin. Lymphatic mapping is performed by injecting either isosulfan blue dye (Fig. 32-6) or technetium-labeled sulfur colloid at the site of the lesion and then identifying the "hot" or blue nodes. The hot or blue nodes are the sentinel nodes. They are identified with a gamma probe and exploration of the lymph node basin.

If micrometastases are seen in the SLN biopsy, then a regional lymphadenectomy is required.

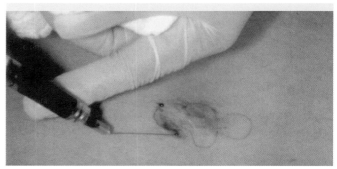

A

FIGURE 32-6A. Blue dye injected intradermally around the tumor.

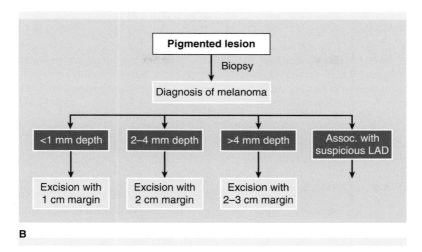

FIGURE 32-6B. Chart of options for melanoma treatment (from Brunicardi F, Andersen DK, Billiar TR, et al., (eds.), *Schwartz's Principles of Surgery*. 9th ed. New York, NY: McGraw-Hill; 2010: Chapter 16: Image 16-13).

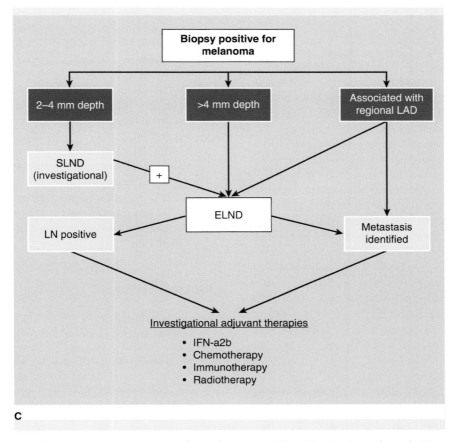

FIGURE 32-6C. Flow chart of steps from positive biopsy for melanoma; ELND = Elective Lymph Node Dissection; SLND = Sentinel lymph node dissection; LAD = Lymphadenopathy; IFN = interferon (from Brunicardi F, Andersen DK, Billiar TR, et al., (eds.), *Schwartz's Principles of Surgery*. 9th ed. New York, NY: McGraw-Hill; 2010: Chapter 16: Image 16-14).

BIBLIOGRAPHY

Cole P, Heller L, Bullocks J, Hollier LH, Stal S. The skin and subcutaneous tissue. In: Brunicardi F, Andersen DK, Billiar TR, et al., (eds.), *Schwartz's Principles of Surgery*. 9th ed. New York, NY: McGraw-Hill; 2010: Chapter 16. http://accesssurgery.mhmedical.com.ezproxy2.library.arizona.edu/content.aspx?bookid=352&Sectionid=40039758. Accessed April 06, 2014.

Meric-Bernstam F, Pollock RE. Oncology. Brunicardi F, Andersen DK, Billiar TR, et al., (eds.), *Schwartz's Principles of Surgery*. 9th ed. New York, NY: McGraw-Hill; 2010: Chapter 10. http://accesssurgery.mhmedical.com.ezproxy1.library.arizona.edu/content.aspx?bookid=352&Sectionid=40039751. Accessed May 12, 2014.

National Comprehensive Cancer Network (NCCN). *NCCN Clinical Practice Guidelines in Oncology. Melanoma Version 3.2014*. Fort Washington, PA: National Comprehensive Cancer Network; February 10, 2014. http://www.nccn.org/professionals/physician_gls/pdf/melanoma.pdf.

Sabel MS. Oncology. In: Doherty GM, ed. *Current Diagnosis & Treatment: Surgery*. 13th ed. New York, NY: McGraw-Hill; 2010: Chapter 44. http://accesssurgery.mhmedical.com.ezproxy2.library.arizona.edu/content.aspx?bookid=343&Sectionid=39702832. Accessed April 06, 2014.

2. **(B)** The approach to skin lesions suspected to be melanoma should address diagnosis and treatment in two separate processes. The diagnosis should be established first and the histopathologic features and tumor thickness determined. After this information has been obtained, staging and definitive treatment may be accomplished. The biopsy technique must provide tissue that includes the full thickness of the tumor and skin at the thickest part of the tumor. Shave biopsies are not acceptable. Smaller lesions may be excised with 1- to 2-mm margins. Wider margins result in unnecessarily large incisions and may interfere with subsequent lymphatic mapping. Biopsy incisions should be planned to allow for subsequent WLE. On the extremities, they should be oriented longitudinally. Large lesions and those in cosmetically sensitive areas, such as the palm of the hand, sole of the foot, digits, and face or ears, should be approached with incisional biopsy. A punch or a knife may be used, but the biopsy must be full thickness. Multiple biopsies of a single lesion may be required to ensure adequate sampling.

Specimens should be examined by an experienced dermatopathologist. Depth of invasion (Breslow staging), Clarks's level, ulceration, regression, mitotic rate, tumor-infiltrating lymphocytes (TILs), vertical growth phase, angiolymphatic invasion, satellitosis, neurotropism, and histologic subtype should be reported. These characteristics have prognostic significance and influence decisions about excision margins, staging with SLN biopsy, and surveillance.

BIBLIOGRAPHY

Houghton AN, Coit DG. Melanoma. 8-29-0001. In: *The Complete Library of Practice Guidelines in Oncology*. Vol. 1. Fort Washington, PA: National Comprehensive Cancer Network; 2002.

Kanzler MH, Mraz-Gernhard S. Treatment of primary cutaneous melanoma. *JAMA* 2001;285(14):1819–1821.

3. **(C)** Five to eight percent of patients with a high-risk lesion will develop in-transit lesions. Most of these lesions are on the lower extremity. When there are only a few small lesions, surgical resection is indicated. Amputation is a consideration in patients who have impaired function of that limb. When patients do not fall into either of these situations, they require treatment with hyperthermic isolated limb perfusion (HILP) with a chemotherapeutic agent, most commonly melphalan. Isolated limb perfusion is a form of regional therapy, and it provides the benefits of systemic chemotherapy with less overall toxicity. Patients with melanoma in transit do not have a good regional response with systemic chemotherapy, and amputation does not increase disease-free survival. Of these patients, 50% have a complete response. However, there are side effects and complications. HILP can cause neutropenia, ischemia or necrosis requiring amputation, and death. Limb perfusion has shown a benefit for local recurrence but does not decrease overall mortality. When interferon gamma or tumor necrosis factor alpha are added, 90% of patients will have tumor regression.

The HILP procedure is performed by directly cannulating the major artery supplying the tumor and placing a tourniquet over that extremity to prevent venous return. The heated chemotherapy solution is infused with a setup similar to a cardiopulmonary bypass. Melphalan is heated and perfused in the operating room for 60–90 min.

BIBLIOGRAPHY

Cole P, Heller L, Bullocks J, Hollier LH, Stal S. The skin and subcutaneous tissue. In: Brunicardi F, Andersen DK, Billiar TR, et al., (eds.), *Schwartz's Principles of Surgery*. 9th ed. New York, NY: McGraw-Hill; 2010: Chapter 16. http://accesssurgery.mhmedical.com.ezproxy2.library.arizona.edu/content.aspx?bookid=352&Sectionid=40039758. Accessed April 06, 2014.

Rossi CR, Foletto M, Mocellin S, Pilati P, Lise M. Hyperthermic isolated limb perfusion with low-dose tumor necrosis factor-α and melphalan for bulky in-transit melanoma metastases. *Ann Surg Oncol* 2004;11(2):173–177.

Sabel MS. Oncology. In: Doherty GM, ed. *Current Diagnosis & Treatment: Surgery*. 13th ed. New York, NY: McGraw-Hill; 2010: Chapter 44. http://accesssurgery.mhmedical.com.ezproxy2.library.arizona.edu/content.aspx?bookid=343&Sectionid=39702832. Accessed April 06, 2014.

4. **(A)** Regional lymphadenectomy is indicated when nodes are either microscopically positive (diagnosed by SLN biopsy) or clinically positive in patients who do not have metastatic disease. Excluding distant metastasis, nodal disease is the most important prognostic factor for melanoma, in terms of both survival and local recurrence. Performing the node dissection allows for better prognostication and helps with disease control and potential cure.

   A groin dissection begins with a lazy S incision, from the medial border of the anterior superior iliac spine to the apex of the femoral triangle. The borders of the superficial dissection include Sartorius laterally, adductor longus medially, and the inguinal (Poupart's) ligament superiorly. Prior biopsy sites and palpable nodes need to be excised with the specimen. Skin flaps to the Sartorius laterally and to the adductor longus medially are fashioned. The suprainguinal lymph node tissue is taken off the external oblique fascia, and the dissection continues inferiorly. The tissue is dissected free laterally to Sartorius and medially to adductor longus. The saphenous vein is encountered during the medial dissection and can be taken if grossly involved. Cloquet's node is found underneath the inguinal ligament. If Cloquet's node is positive or preoperative imaging shows iliac node involvement, a deep dissection is warranted. This can be done by splitting the external oblique and inguinal ligament medial to the femoral artery to expose the iliac vessels. Then, the nodal tissue is dissected free from the iliac vessels. During the deep dissection, care has to be taken to prevent injuring the ureter and obturator nerve. Once the nodes are removed, the inguinal ligament has to be repaired and the femoral canal has to be closed.

   Complications of a groin dissection can include wound infection, wound dehiscence, hematoma, lymphocele, and lymphedema.

   Some surgeons advocate for routine deep dissection (to include iliac and obturator nodes), as 30% can be positive on pathologic specimen. Because studies have failed to show a survival benefit for doing the deep dissection, some surgeons advocate performing only the superficial node dissection, decreasing the overall morbidity of the operation.

BIBLIOGRAPHY

Cole P, Heller L, Bullocks J, Hollier LH, Stal S. The skin and subcutaneous tissue. In: Brunicardi F, Andersen DK, Billiar TR, et al., (eds.), *Schwartz's Principles of Surgery*. 9th ed. New York, NY: McGraw-Hill; 2010: Chapter 16. http://accesssurgery.mhmedical.com.ezproxy2.library.arizona.edu/content.aspx?bookid=352&Sectionid=40039758. Accessed April 06, 2014.

Ghaferi AA, Sabel MS. Operative management of melanoma. In: Minter RM, Doherty GM, eds. *Current Procedures: Surgery*. New York, NY: McGraw-Hill; 2010: Chapter 28. http://accesssurgery.mhmedical.com.ezproxy1.library.arizona.edu/content.aspx?bookid=429&Sectionid=40112042. Accessed April 22, 2014.

Kretschmer L, Neumann C, Preuber KP, Marsch WC. Superficial inguinal and radical ilioinguinal lymph node dissection in patients with palpable melanoma metastases to the groin: an analysis of survival and local recurrence. Acta Oncol 2001;40(1):72–78.

Meyer T, Merkel S, Gohl J, Hohenberger W. Lymph node dissection for clinically evident lymph node metastases of malignant melanoma. *Eur J Surg Oncol* 2002;28:424–430.

Wallack MK, Degliuomini JJ, Joh JE, Berenji M. Cutaneous melanoma. In Cameron JL, Cameron AM, eds. *Current Surgical Therapy*. Philadelphia, PA: Elsevier; 2011:625–631.

5. **(D)** Staging in melanoma is important to predict the prognosis of these patients. Clinical staging is determined by preoperative exam, biopsy, and imaging. After definitive operation, final pathologic staging can be determined. The TNM stage is based on tumor, nodes, and metastasis as described next.

Tumor:

   Tx: Primary tumor cannot be assessed

   Tis: Melanoma in situ

   T1: Melanoma with a depth of 1 mm or less

   T2: Melanoma with a depth of 1.01–2.0 mm

   T3: Melanoma with a depth of 2.01–4.0 mm

   T4: Melanomas more than 4.0 mm deep

   a: Without ulceration and mitosis $<1/mm^2$

   b: With ulceration or mitoses $\geq 1/mm^2$

Lymph nodes:

   N0: No nodes

   N1: 1 positive lymph node

   N2: 2–3 positive lymph nodes

   N3: 4 or more positive lymph nodes

   a: Micrometastasis

   b: Macrometastasis

   c: In-transit metastases without metastatic nodes

Distant metastasis:

   M0: No metastatic disease

   M1a: Metastasis to skin, subcutaneous tissue, or distant lymph nodes

   M1b: Metastasis to lungs

   M1c: Metastasis to all other visceral sites or anywhere with an elevated lactate dehydrogenase (LDH) value

   Once these are combined, the final stage can be determined.

Stages:

   0: Carcinoma in situ

   1A: T1a

   1B: T1b, N0, M0

      T2a N0, M0

   IIA: T2b, N0, M0

      T3a, N0, M0

   IIB: T3b, N0, M0

      T4a, N0, M0

   IIC: T4b, N0, M0

   IIIA: T1-4a, N1a, M0

      T1-4a, N2a, M0

   IIIB: T1-4b, N1a, M0

      T1-4b, N2a, M0

      T1-4a, N1b, M0

      T1-4a, N2b, M0

      T1-4a, N2c, M0

   IV: Any T, Any N, M1

BIBLIOGRAPHY

Wallack MK, Degliuomini JJ, Joh JE, Berenji M. Cutaneous melanoma. In Cameron JL, Cameron AM, eds. *Current Surgical Therapy*. Philadelphia, PA: Elsevier; 2011:625–631.

Melanoma of the skin. In: Edge SB, Byrd DR, Compton CC, Fritz AG, Greene FL, Trotti A, eds. *AJCC Cancer Staging Manual*. New York, NY: Springer-Verlag; 2010: Chapter 31. STAT!Ref Online Electronic Medical Library. http://online.statref.com/Document.aspx?fxId=73&docId=149. Accessed April 23, 2014.

6. **(C)** Many things affect the prognosis of melanoma. However, the TMN staging system, as recommended by the AJCC (see the staging in Table 32-1) influences

TABLE 32-1

T classification	Thickness (mm)	Ulceration Status/Mitoses
T1	≤1.0	a: without ulceration and mitosis <1/mm^2
		b: with ulceration or mitoses ≥1/mm^2
T2	1.01–2.0	a: without ulceration
		b: with ulceration
T3	2.01–4.0	a: without ulceration
		b: with ulceration
T4	>4.0	a: without ulceration
		b: with ulceration
N Classification	**No. of Metastatic Nodes**	**Nodal Metastatic Mass**
N1	1 node	a: Micrometastasis[a]
		b: Macrometastasis[b]
N2	2–3 nodes	a: Micrometastasis[a]
		b: Macrometastasis[b]
		c: In-transit metastase(s)/satellite(s) without metastatic nodes
N3	4 or more metastatic nodes, or matted nodes, or in-transit metastase(s)/satellite(s) with metastatic node(s)	

[a]Micrometastases are diagnosed after sentinel lymph node biopsy and completion of lymphadenectomy (if performed).
[b]Macrometastases are defined as clinically detectable nodal metastases confirmed by therapeutic lymphadenectomy or when nodal metastasis exhibits gross extracapsular extension.

(Continued)

TABLE 32-1 (*Continued*)

M Classification	Site	Serum LDH					
M1a	Distant skin, subcutaneous, or nodal metastases	Normal					
M1b	Lung metastases	Normal					
M1c	All other visceral metastases Any distant metastasis	Normal Elevated					

Anatomic Stage/Prognostic Groups							
Clinical Staging[a]				Pathologic Staging[b]			
Stage 0	Tis	N0	M0	0	Tis	N0	M0
Stage IA	T1a	N0	M0	IA	T1a	N0	M0
Stage IB	T1b	N0	M0	1B	T1b	N0	M0
	T2a	N0	M0		T2a	N0	M0
Stage IIA	T2b	N0	M0	IIA	T2b	N0	M0
	T3a	N0	M0		T3a	N0	M0
Stage IIB	T3b	N0	M0	IIB	T3b	N0	M0
	T4a	N0	M0		T4a	N0	M0
Stage IIC	T4b	N0	M0	IIC	T4b	N0	M0
Stage III	Any T	≥N1	M0	IIIA	T1-4a	N1a	M0
					T1-4a	N2a	M0
				IIIB	T1-4b	N1a	M0
					T1-4b	N2a	M0
					T1-4a	N1b	M0
					T1-4a	N2b	M0
					T1-4a	N2c	M0
				IIIC	T1-4b	N1b	M0
					T1-4b	N2b	M0
					T1-4b	N2c	M0
					Any T	N3	M0
Stage IV	Any T	Any N	M1	IV	Any T	Any N	M1

[a]Clinical staging includes microstaging of the primary melanoma and clinical/radiologic evaluation for metastases. By convention, it should be used after complete excision of the primary melanoma with clinical assessment for regional and distant metastases.

[b]Pathologic staging includes microstaging of the primary melanoma and pathologic information about the regional lymph nodes after partial or complete lymphadenectomy. Patients with pathologic stage 0 or stage IA are the exception; they do not require pathologic evaluation of their lymph nodes.

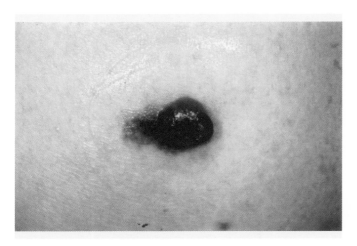

FIGURE 32-7. Clinically ulcerated melanoma.

BIBLIOGRAPHY

Buzaid AC, Gershenwald JE. Tumor node metastasis (TNM) staging system and other prognostic factors in cutaneous melanoma. In: Ross ME, ed. *UpToDate.* Waltham, MA: UpToDate. Accessed April 28, 2014.

Cole P, Heller L, Bullocks J, Hollier LH, Stal S. The skin and subcutaneous tissue. In: Brunicardi F, Andersen DK, Billiar TR, et al., (eds.), *Schwartz's Principles of Surgery.* 9th ed. New York, NY: McGraw-Hill; 2010: Chapter 16. http://accesssurgery.mhmedical.com.ezproxy2.library.arizona.edu/content.aspx?bookid=352&Sectionid=40039758. Accessed April 06, 2014.

Melanoma of the skin. In: Edge SB, Byrd DR, Compton CC, Fritz AG, Greene FL, Trotti A, eds. *AJCC Cancer Staging Manual.* New York, NY: Springer-Verlag; 2010: Chapter 31. STAT!Ref Online Electronic Medical Library. http://online.statref.com/Document.aspx?fxId=73&docId=149. Accessed April 23, 2014.

Wallack MK, Degliuomini JJ, Joh JE, Berenji M. Cutaneous melanoma. In Cameron JL, Cameron AM, eds. *Current Surgical Therapy.* Philadelphia, PA: Elsevier; 2011:625–631.

the prognosis of melanoma. When dealing with a focal lesion, without lymphadenopathy or metastasis, depth of invasion is more predictive; deeper lesions and higher T stages portend a worse prognosis. Mitotic rate is another important prognostic factor, as increasing mitotic rates indicate a more aggressive lesion. The 10-year survival rate decreased progressively from 93% for those with less than 1 mitosis/mm^2 to 48% for those with more than 20 mitoses/mm^2. Lesions with ulceration also have a worse prognosis when compared to nonulcerated lesions (Fig. 32-7). The 10-year survival rate for patients with local disease (stage I) and an ulcerated melanoma was 50%, compared to 78% for the same stage lesion without ulceration. Also, location of the primary lesion should be taken into account. Those with extremity melanomas do better than those with head and neck or trunk lesions. Females also tend to have a better survival rate than males.

With the exception of metastatic disease, positive lymph nodes are the most important prognostic feature. Patients who have more positive nodes and patients who have macrometastasis have a worse outcome. Metastatic disease is obviously the worst feature, but prognosis does vary by site of metastasis. Disease in the skin, in-transit lesions, and distant lymph node metastasis are more favorable than disease in the lung or other locations.

In summary, overall poor prognostic factors include thick tumors, ulceration, high mitotic rate, age over 60 years, truncal lesions, male gender, higher Clark level, macrometastases, increased number of positive nodes, and an elevated LDH.

7. **(C)** Sarcomas are uncommon tumors and account for only about 1% of adult malignancies annually. About 12,020 patients are diagnosed annually, and sarcoma accounts for 4740 annual deaths. Sarcomas can develop from essentially all organs and has more than 50 different histologic subtypes. Almost half of sarcomas are in the extremities, and another third occur in the abdomen and pelvis (retroperitoneal and intraperitoneal). The most common subtype overall is malignant fibrous histiocytoma, but the most common subtype in the retroperitoneum is liposarcoma.

Sarcomas are diagnosed by finding a painless mass on physical examination or incidentally with imaging. If not previously imaged, computed tomography (CT) or magnetic resonance imaging (MRI) should be obtained to determine the extent of disease. These lesions may be biopsied with incisional biopsy, excisional biopsy, and core needle biopsy. In most cases, a biopsy is not necessary before considering surgical resection. However, if carcinoma, lymphoma, or germ cell tumor is suspected, tissue diagnosis is imperative. Once the disease is diagnosed, chest imaging (x-ray or CT) should be obtained to rule out metastatic disease.

Primary treatment for all sarcomas is surgical resection. Given the rarity of these tumors, they should be treated at a specialized center with a multidisciplinary approach. The most important factor in overall survival is complete surgical resection at the time of diagnosis. To have negative margins free of microscopic disease, 1- to 2-cm margins should be obtained when possible. If necessary, contiguous organs should be resected en bloc to achieve local disease control. The prior biopsy site needs to be included in the resection. In retroperitoneal sarcoma, the most common cause of death is local recurrence. In contrast, it is from metastatic disease in extremity sarcoma.

Adjuvant and neoadjuvant chemotherapy and radiation therapy can be considered on an individual basis. Those with concerning features, large tumors with difficult-to-obtain margins, high-grade lesions, incompletely resected lesions, and recurrent disease are commonly considered for additional therapy, again necessitating the multidisciplinary approach. When disease recurs, it should be reresected when possible. Eventually, these tumors metastasize, and extremity lesions most commonly go to lung, while retroperitoneal lesions metastasize to liver and lung equally. In some instances, pulmonary metastatectomy may be considered if the primary disease is controlled.

BIBLIOGRAPHY

Mullen JT, DeLaney TF. Clinical features, evaluation, and treatment of retroperitoneal soft tissue sarcoma. In: Savarese DMF, ed. *UpToDate*. Waltham, MA: UpToDate. Accessed April 28, 2014.

Ryan CW, Meyer J. Clinical presentation, histopathology, diagnostic evaluation, and staging of soft tissue sarcoma. In: Savarese DMF, ed. *UpToDate*. Waltham, MA: UpToDate. Accessed April 28, 2014.

Singer S. Soft tissue sarcoma. In: Townsend CM, Beauchamp RD, Evers BM, Mattox KL, eds. *Sabiston Textbook of Surgery: The Biological Basis of Modern Surgical Practice*. Philadelphia, PA: Elsevier; 2012:768–782.

Yoon SS, Hornieck FJ. Management of soft tissue sarcomas. In: Cameron JL, Cameron AM, eds. *Current Surgical Therapy*. Philadelphia, PA: Elsevier; 2011:631–637.

8. **(B)** Staging in sarcoma can be a complicated process. Staging is done initially by the workup of the disease with imaging (CT or MRI for the initial lesion and chest imaging for metastatic disease). Biopsies or operative specimens are used to determine the histology and grade of the tumor. Fine-needle aspiration (FNA) is not useful to diagnose sarcoma. Superficial, small (less than 3 cm) sarcomas can be diagnosed with excisional biopsy. Larger tumors require incisional biopsy or core needle biopsy for diagnosis. It is important to perform a biopsy in the center of the mass so that the biopsy site can be removed during formal excision.

The AJCC staging system is the most widely accepted system for staging sarcoma (Table 32-2). It uses the TNM system but adds tumor grade to the overall stage. Thus, the major features of staging in sarcoma are grade of the tumor, size of the tumor, and presence of metastatic disease. Size of the tumor and grade are the most important for prognosis. Grading is determined by differentiation, mitotic activity, and necrosis. Grade is defined in a three-tier manner: well differentiated/low grade, moderately differentiated/intermediate grade, or poorly

TABLE 32-2 AJCC Staging System for Soft Tissue Sarcoma

Primary Tumor (T)	
T1	Tumor 5 cm or less
T1a	Superficial tumor
T1b	Deep tumor
T2	Tumor more than 5 cm
T2a	Superficial tumor
T2b	Deep tumor
Regional Lymph Nodes (N)	
N0	No regional lymph node metastasis
N1	Regional lymph node metastasis
Distant Metastasis (M)	
M0	No distant metastasis
M1	Distant metastasis
Histopathologic Grade (G)	
G1	Well differentiated
G2	Moderately differentiated
G3	Poorly differentiated
G4	Undifferentiated
Stage Grouping	
Stage IA	G1-2, T1a-1b, N0, M0
Stage IB	G1-2, T2a, N0, M0
Stage IIA	G1-2, T2b, N0, M0
Stage IIB	G3-4, T1a-1b, N0, M0
Stage IIC	G3-4, T2a, N0, M0
Stage III	G3-4, T2b, N0, M0
Stage IV	Any G, any T, either N1 or M1

differentiated/high grade. Grade is indicative of degree of malignancy and likelihood of distant disease.

Sarcomas tend to metastasize hematogenously and rarely have associated lymphadenopathy. Most tumors go to the lung, while retroperitoneal sarcomas tend to go to the liver as well as the lung.

Location has important implications for prognosis, but it is not included in the staging system. Patients with retroperitoneal sarcomas tend to do worse than those with extremity sarcomas. Other prognostic factors are size, age, and histologic subtype.

BIBLIOGRAPHY

Ryan CW, Meyer J. Clinical presentation, histopathology, diagnostic evaluation, and staging of soft tissue sarcoma. In: Savarese DMF, ed. *UpToDate*. Waltham, MA: UpToDate. Accessed April 28, 2014.

Sabel MS. Oncology. In: Doherty GM, ed. *Current Diagnosis & Treatment: Surgery*. 13th ed. New York, NY: McGraw-Hill; 2010: Chapter 44. http://accesssurgery.mhmedical.com.ezproxy2.library.arizona.edu/content.aspx?bookid=343&Sectionid=39702832. Accessed April 06, 2014.

Singer S. Soft tissue sarcoma. In: Townsend CM, Beauchamp RD, Evers BM, Mattox KL, eds. *Sabiston Textbook of Surgery: The Biological Basis of Modern Surgical Practice*. Philadelphia, PA: Elsevier; 2012:768–782.

Soft tissue sarcoma. In: Edge SB, Byrd DR, Compton CC, Fritz AG, Greene FL, Trotti A, eds. *AJCC Cancer Staging Manual*. New York, NY: Springer-Verlag; 2010: Chapter 31. STAT!Ref Online Electronic Medical Library. http://online.statref.com/Document.aspx?fxId=73&docId=137. Accessed April 23, 2014.

9. **(B)** Soft tissue sarcomas are rare tumors, only representing about 1% of new cancer diagnoses. About 60% of sarcomas arise in the extremities, the most common location for them to present. Other locations include the retroperitoneum, trunk, and head/neck. When tumors arise in the extremity, treatment can be problematic as the goals are maximizing survival and decreasing local control while preserving limb function and preventing morbidity. Treatment is surgical resection with 1- to 2-cm margins, and less than 5% of patients require amputation to achieve this.

For low-grade, superficial, small sarcomas (T1 lesions, <5 cm), excision is the only treatment required. However, most lesions benefit from radiation therapy 4–8 weeks after excision. This can be done with either traditional radiotherapy or brachytherapy. Adding radiation therapy is especially important in patients who have a close or microscopically positive margin, as it reduces the risk of local recurrence by 20–25%. Using this combination, local recurrence is less than 10%, and 95% of patients are able to receive limb-sparing treatment. Despite better local control, survival is not improved by the addition of radiation therapy.

Tumors that were incompletely resected should undergo re-resection. This can take place either before or after radiation therapy.

Chemotherapy after sarcoma excision is a controversial topic. The most common agents are doxorubicin, dacarbazine (DTIC), and ifosfamide. There is also some efficacy in giving neoadjuvant chemotherapy to be able to perform limb-sparing surgery.

Once treatment has commenced, surveillance should be performed to find recurrences. This is done with history and physical with lesion site and chest imaging every 3–6 months initially. After 2 years, 6-month follow-ups are advised for 3 more years. It is important to obtain a chest x-ray, as the lungs are the most common site of metastasis.

BIBLIOGRAPHY

Cormier JN, Pollock RE. Soft tissue sarcomas. In: Brunicardi F, Andersen DK, Billiar TR, et al., (eds.), *Schwartz's Principles of Surgery*. 9th ed. New York, NY: McGraw-Hill; 2010: Chapter 36. http://accesssurgery.mhmedical.com.ezproxy2.library.arizona.edu/content.aspx?bookid=352&Sectionid=40039778. Accessed May 11, 2014.

DeLaney TF, Harmon DC, Gebhardt MC. Local treatment for primary soft tissue sarcoma of the extremities and chest wall. In: Savarese DMF, Duda RB, eds. *UpToDate*. Waltham, MA: UpToDate. Accessed May 11, 2014.

Sabel MS. Oncology. In: Doherty GM, ed. *Current Diagnosis & Treatment: Surgery*. 13th ed. New York, NY: McGraw-Hill; 2010: Chapter 44. http://accesssurgery.mhmedical.com.ezproxy2.library.arizona.edu/content.aspx?bookid=343&Sectionid=39702832. Accessed April 06, 2014.

10. **(B)** Gastrointestinal stromal tumors are the most common mesenchymal-derived tumor of the intestinal tract. They are rare in frequency, with about 5000 cases annually in the United States. GISTs are usually found in patients who are about 60 years old, and more frequently in men. Historically, these tumors were thought to be leiomyomas, as they were thought to be of smooth muscle origin. They frequently cause gastrointestinal bleeding, but they can also obstruct or be found incidentally on imaging. The most frequent location for a GIST is the stomach (60%), followed by the small intestine (30%), and then the esophagus and rectum (10%).

The GISTs arise from the interstitial cells of Cajal, part of the autonomic nervous system and acting as the pacemaker cells of the gastrointestinal tract. They are characterized histologically by expression of tyrosine kinase KIT (*c-KIT* proto-oncogene). Histologically, they stain for CD117 (KIT) and CD34 (Fig. 32-8), and they can sometimes stain for actin, S-100, desmin, and keratin. GISTs can be benign or malignant, and although there are no standard criteria, size larger than 10 cm and more than five mitoses per high-power field are likely malignant.

Treatment for GIST is primarily by surgical resection. Because this tumor expresses a tyrosine kinase, imatinib mesylate (Gleevec), a tyrosine kinase inhibitor, can be used as adjuvant therapy. Imatinib mesylate is indicated for those with tumors at high risk of recurrence. There are newer tyrosine kinase inhibitors currently being tested for similar use.

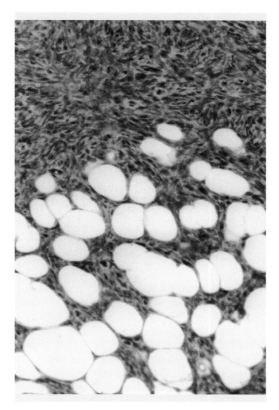

FIGURE 32-8. Biopsy permanent section CD34 positive showing tumor excision into fat.

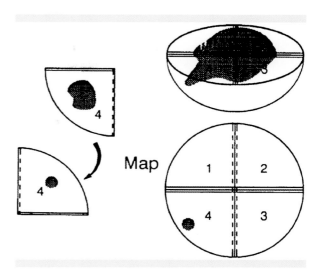

FIGURE. 32-9. Diagram of Mohs map.

BIBLIOGRAPHY

Demetri GD, Morgan J, Raut CP. Epidemiology, classification, clinical presentation, prognostic features, and diagnostic work-up of gastrointestinal mesenchymal neoplasms including GIST. In: Savarese DMF, ed. *UpToDate*. Waltham, MA: UpToDate. Accessed May 11, 2014.

Karakousis GC, DeMatteo RP. Gastrointestinal stromal tumors. In: Cameron JL, Cameron AM, eds. *Current Surgical Therapy*. Philadelphia, PA: Elsevier; 2011:85–88.

Mahvi DM, Krantz SB. Stomach (GIST). In: Townsend CM, Beauchamp RD, Evers BM, Mattox KL, eds. *Sabiston Textbook of Surgery: The Biological Basis of Modern Surgical Practice*. Philadelphia, PA: Elsevier; 2012:1220–1221.

Raut CP. Gastrointestinal stromal tumors. In: Zinner MJ, Ashley SW, eds. *Maingot's Abdominal Operations*. 12th ed. New York, NY: McGraw-Hill; 2013: Chapter 24. http://accesssurgery.mhmedical.com.ezproxy2.library.arizona.edu/content.aspx?bookid=531&Sectionid=41808804. Accessed May 11, 2014.

11. **(E)** Basal cell carcinoma is the most common form of skin cancer. It arises from the basal layer of the epidermis and is typically slow growing. It can be difficult to diagnose clinically, and a biopsy is warranted. However, the lesions can look nodular, or they can look like a chronic nonhealing wound; nodular lesions frequently have central umbilication.

Treatment of BCC is by excision with 0.5- to 1-cm margins, although, lesions smaller than 2 mm can be treated with curettage, electrodesiccation, or laser vaporization. In areas where a cosmetically pleasing approach is necessary (the face), Mohs surgery may be beneficial. Mohs surgery incorporates microscopic analysis during excision so that the smallest amount of tissue can be taken without compromising surgical margins. It is performed by taking excisions, obtaining biopsies, and mapping the location of the lesion (Fig. 32-9). The defect can be closed primarily or may require flap reconstruction (Fig. 32-10). Thus, a BCC lesion on the nose is best treated with Mohs surgery.

BIBLIOGRAPHY

Cole P, Heller L, Bullocks J, Hollier LH, Stal S. The skin and subcutaneous tissue. In: Brunicardi F, Andersen DK, Billiar TR, et al., (eds.), *Schwartz's Principles of Surgery*. 9th ed. New York, NY: McGraw-Hill; 2010: Chapter 16. http://accesssurgery.mhmedical.com.ezproxy2.library.arizona.edu/content.aspx?bookid=352&Sectionid=40039758. Accessed April 06, 2014.

McMasters KM, Urist MM. Melanoma and cutaneous malignancies. In: Townsend CM, Beauchamp RD, Evers BM, Mattox KL, eds. *Sabiston Textbook of Surgery: The Biological Basis of Modern Surgical Practice*. Philadelphia, PA: Elsevier; 2012:742–767.

12. **(C)** The first clear evidence that immunotherapy can cause regression of established metastatic tumors came from the administration of high-dose IL-2 for the treatment of melanoma and kidney cancer. IL-2 is a cytokine

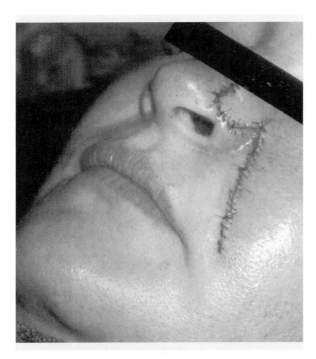

FIGURE 32-10. Nasal labial flap reconstruction.

secreted by T-helper lymphocytes that has profound effects on lymphocytes, including induction of expansion and activation. High-dose IL-2 for the treatment of metastatic melanoma has an objective response rate of about 15%, with a complete, and usually durable, response seen in about 50% of responders.

By comparison, chemotherapy with single-agent dacarbazine (DTIC) or temozolomide (TMZ), both prodrugs of the active alkylating agent imidazole-4-carboximide (MTIC), is associated with response rates of around 20%. Unfortunately, durable complete responses with these drugs are rare. Treatment with combination chemotherapy also remains disappointing. Despite initial reports of increased efficacy with the Dartmouth regimen (combination [DTIC], carmustine [BCNU], cisplatin [DDP], and tamoxifen [TAM]), randomized trials have not consistently shown improved responses compared to single-agent chemotherapy.

The ineffectiveness of chemotherapy has led to several experimental immunotherapies. These treatments can be classified as either active vaccine immunization or passive transfer of immune cells. Active immunotherapy by vaccination with peptides derived from tumor antigens sometimes results in high numbers of circulating T cells directed against cancer antigens but does not induce tumor regression. Passive immunotherapy by adoptive transfer of TILs recovered from resected

tumors, expanded in vitro, and transferred with IL-2 back into the patient results in response rates of 35%. Lymphodepletion of the patient with nonmyeloablative chemotherapy prior to cell transfer results in improved response rates (>40%).

Immunotherapy has also been employed in the adjuvant setting. High-dose interferon alfa-2b is approved by the Food and Drug Administration for the adjuvant treatment of resected high-risk melanoma. Studies examining the ability of interferon to prolong survival have yielded conflicting results, and the therapy is associated with significant morbidity, which may limit its use.

BIBLIOGRAPHY

Bajetta E, Del Vecchio M, Bernard-Marty C, et al. Metastatic melanoma: chemotherapy. *Semin Oncol* 2002;29(5):427–445.

Dudley ME, Rosenberg SA. Adoptive-cell-transfer therapy for the treatment of patients with cancer. *Nat Rev Cancer* 2003;3(9):666–675.

Rosenberg SA. Progress in human tumour immunology and immunotherapy. *Nature* 2001;411(6835):380–384.

Sabel MS, Sondak VK. Pros and cons of adjuvant interferon in the treatment of melanoma. *Oncologist* 2003;8(5):451–458.

Yang JC, Sherry RM, Steinberg SM, et al. Randomized study of high-dose and low-dose interleukin-2 in patients with metastatic renal cancer. *J Clin Oncol* 2003;21(16):3127–3132.

13. **(E)** SCC is the second-most-common skin cancer. It frequently arises on the head and neck, as sunlight is a major risk factor. Other risk factors are burns, chronic wounds, chronic inflammatory states, and radiation exposure. It arises from malignant proliferation of epidermal keratinocytes. SCC is known to be an aggressive cancer, and around 2–5% of patients will have nodal disease or distant metastasis. Small, indolent lesions can be treated with electrodesiccation, but most SCCs require surgical excision.

For the most part, SCCs that developed from actinic keratosis (sun exposure) are more indolent, while those that develop from radiation, ulcers, burns, and scars are more aggressive. Figure 32-11 shows an SCC of the lip. Certain features make these lesions more high risk. These include size greater than 20 mm on the trunk or extremities, size greater than 10 mm on the head and neck, tumors with poorly defined borders, tumors on immunosuppressed patients, tumors in prior radiation beds or chronic wounds, tumors that are moderately or poorly differentiated, those more than 2 mm deep, those that are rapidly growing, and those with perineural and vascular involvement.

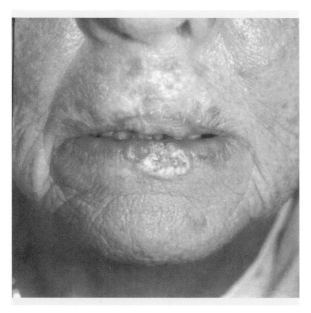

FIGURE 32-11. Squamous cell carcinoma of the lower lip in 70-year-old female.

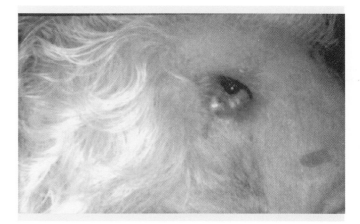

FIGURE 32-12. Large SCC located on temple of 60-year-old male.

BIBLIOGRAPHY

Chartier TK, Aasi SZ. Treatment and prognosis of cutaneous squamous cell carcinoma. In: Corona R, ed. *UpToDate*. Waltham, MA: UpToDate. Accessed on May 11, 2014.

Cole P, Heller L, Bullocks J, Hollier LH, Stal S. The skin and subcutaneous tissue. In: Brunicardi F, Andersen DK, Billiar TR, et al., (eds.), *Schwartz's Principles of Surgery*. 9th ed. New York, NY: McGraw-Hill; 2010: Chapter 16. http://accesssurgery.mhmedical.com.ezproxy2.library.arizona.edu/content.aspx?bookid=352&Sectionid=40039758. Accessed April 06, 2014.

Vasconez HC, Habash A. Plastic and reconstructive surgery. In: Doherty GM, ed. *Current Diagnosis & Treatment: Surgery*. 13th ed. New York, NY: McGraw-Hill; 2010: Chapter 41. http://accesssurgery.mhmedical.com.ezproxy2.library.arizona.edu/content.aspx?bookid=343&Sectionid=39702829. Accessed May 11, 2014.

14. **(D)** SCC is treated with surgical excision. The size of the lesion and the presence of concerning features determine margins and other treatments. Figure 32-12 shows a large SCC on the scalp.

Low-risk lesions do not have the high-risk features listed in this answer. These lesions can be treated with smaller margins; 0.4 cm should be adequate, although there is also some evidence that these lesions can be treated nonsurgically with cryotherapy, electrodesiccation, 5-fluorouracil, imiquimod, radiation therapy, and photodynamic therapy.

High-risk lesions are large lesions, lesions from chronic inflammation, or those in high-risk individuals. These include trunk and extremity lesions larger than 2 cm, head and neck lesions larger than 1 cm, lesions in immunosuppressed individuals, lesions arising in burn scars, lesions arising in radiation beds, lesions with poor differentiation, and lesions with perineural invasions. These lesions should be excised with 1-cm margins. Some consideration should be made for performing SLN biopsies, although there are no clear guidelines for determining who should undergo SLN biopsy.

For both groups, Mohs surgery is an option for treatment, especially in areas where obtaining a margin may be difficult (the face, genitalia). This technique incorporates microscopic evaluation at the time of excision to ensure adequate margins without removing unnecessary tissue.

In-transit lesions are more frequently associated with malignant melanoma. However, they do occur in some patients with SCC and most commonly in patients with high-risk features, especially immunosuppressed patients. These lesions essentially represent metastases and are not usually removed with the initial surgery. Although excision is recommended, margin control with these lesions is difficult; therefore, radiation is important in eradicating the lesions and treating the surrounding area.

Radiotherapy can be used as both sole treatment and as adjuvant treatment for SCC. For low-risk lesions, especially in patients who have contraindications for operative excisions, radiation can be used as the only treatment modality. It may be beneficial for lesions in cosmetically sensitive areas, as it spares the nearby healthy tissue and does not require removal of a large amount of skin, necessitating reconstruction. In high-risk lesions, it is used in addition to surgery to decrease the risk of local recurrence. It can also be used as an adjunct for incompletely excised lesions.

BIBLIOGRAPHY

Carucci JA, Martinez JC, Zeitouni NC, et al. In-transit metastasis from primary cutaneous squamous cell carcinoma in organ transplant recipients and nonimmunosuppressed patients: clinical characteristics, management, and outcome in a series of 21 patients. *Dermatol Surg* 2004;30:651–655.

Chartier TK, Aasi SZ. Treatment and prognosis of cutaneous squamous cell carcinoma. In: Corona R, ed. *UpToDate*. Waltham, MA: UpToDate. Accessed on May 11, 2014.

DeSimone JA, Karia PS, Schumlts CD. Recognition and management of high-risk (aggressive) cutaneous squamous cell carcinoma. In: Corona R, ed. *UpToDate*. Waltham, MA: UpToDate. Accessed on May 11, 2014.

Wargo JA, Tenabe K. Surgical management of melanoma and other skin cancers. Ashley S, Cance W, Chen H, et al., (eds.), *ACS Surgery: Principles and Practice*. 7th ed. Philadelphia, PA: Decker; 2014. STAT!Ref Online Electronic Medical Library. http://online.statref.com/Document.aspx?fxId=61&docId=417. Accessed May 12, 2014.

15. **(C)** Merkel cell carcinoma is a rare neuroendocrine tumor of the skin. It typically affects patients in their 50s, with a male-to-female ratio of 3:1. It is an aggressive lesion, as it grows rapidly, usually on sun-exposed surfaces. Risk factors include radiation, UV light, and immunosuppression. It has a tendency to spread quickly, and once diagnosed by biopsy, additional imaging via CT or positron emission tomographic (PET) CT is necessary to evaluate for lymphadenopathy or metastatic disease. At diagnosis, 12–31% of patients will have regional nodal disease; within 2 years, 50–70% of patients will develop lymph node metastasis. Disseminated disease will occur in 30% of patients, frequently to lung, liver, bone, and brain. The overall 5-year survival rate is between 50 and 68%.

Treatment consists of WLE of the primary lesion, down to the level of the fascia with a minimum of 1- to 2-cm margins. Mohs surgery can be used in cosmetically sensitive areas to ensure negative margins while decreasing the amount of excised tissue. Patients who present with palpable lymphadenopathy in the draining lymph node basin should undergo a CT scan and a FNA of the node to confirm the diagnosis. Full lymph node dissection followed by adjuvant radiation therapy are indicated.

Patients who have clinically negative nodes should be considered candidates for lymphoscintigraphy and SLN biopsy (Figs. 32-13 and 32-14).

If the biopsy is positive, then regional lymph node dissection and radiotherapy are warranted. If the biopsy is negative, then only radiotherapy is recommended. If the SLN biopsy is not available, then formal lymph node dissection and radiotherapy may be justified. According to several publications, SLN biopsy may be a strong predictor of disease recurrence.

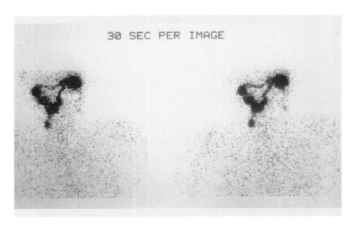

FIGURE 32-13. Lymphoscintigraphy showing draining lymph node basin.

Adjuvant therapy consists of radiation and chemotherapy, frequently with etoposide and cisplatin.

BIBLIOGRAPHY

Iseli TA, Rosenthal EL. Skin lesions: evaluation, management, and treatment. In: Cameron JL, Cameron AM, eds. *Current Surgical Therapy*. Philadelphia, PA: Elsevier; 2011:621–615.

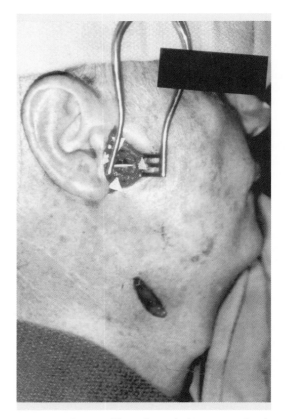

FIGURE 32-14. Sentinel lymph node biopsies of right parotid and right neck.

Mehrany K, Otley CC, Weenig RH, et al. A meta-analysis of the prognostic significance of sentinel lymph node status in Merkel cell carcinoma. *Dermatol Surg* 2002;28(2):113–117.

Zeitouni NC, Cheney R, DeLacure MD. Lymphoscintigraphy, sentinel lymph node biopsy and Mohs micrographic surgery in the treatment of Merkel cell carcinoma. *Dermatol Surg* 2000;26:12–18.

16. **(E)** DFSP is a slow-growing, low-grade spindle cell tumor. It is characterized by local invasion and a propensity to recur after surgical resection. It is typically seen in young to middle-aged adults, with an equal male-to-female ratio. The trunk is the most common location, followed by the proximal extremities and the head and neck region. The rate of metastasis is between 1 and 5%, seen especially with recurrent tumors and tumors with fibrosarcomatous change.

Treatment of DFSP is by surgery. Local excision is associated with a high rate of local recurrence. Therefore, WLE with margins of 2–3 cm down to and including fascia is recommended. Confirmation of histologic-free margins is necessary for local control of this tumor. For tumors located on the head and neck region, where tissue sparing is important, many authors recommend the use of Mohs micrographic surgery. Mohs surgery has also been advocated for tumors elsewhere on the body, given the very local recurrence rate (1.6%) seen with this procedure.

The use of radiation therapy for DFSP is controversial because of reports of high-grade malignant transformation after radiation treatment. Chemotherapy does not appear to alter the prognosis of DFSP and is therefore not a management option.

BIBLIOGRAPHY

Ah-Weng A, Marsden JR, Sanders DS, Waters R. Dermatofibrosarcoma protuberans treated by micrographic surgery. *Br J Cancer* 2002;87(12):1386–1389.

Minter RM, Reith JD, Hochwald SN. Metastatic potential of dermatofibrosarcoma protuberans with fibrosarcomatous change. *J Surg Oncol* 2003;82(3):201–208.

Nouri K, Lodha R, Jimenez G, Robins P. Mohs micrographic surgery for dermatofibrosarcoma protuberans: University of Miami and NYU experience. *Dermatol Surg* 2002;28(11):1060–1064.

Oliveira-Soares R, Viana I, Vale E, et al. Dermatofibrosarcoma protuberans: a clinicopathological study of 20 cases. *J Eur Acad Dermatol Venereol* 2002;16(5):441–446.

Vandeweyer E, De Saint Aubain Somerhausen N, Gebhart M. Dermatofibrosarcoma protuberans: how wide is wide in surgical excision? *Acta Chir Belg* 2002;102(6):455–458.

17. **(E)** Angiosarcomas are rare, aggressive sarcomas from the endothelium of blood vessels and lymphatic channels. They most commonly present on the face or scalp of elderly white males. They can also arise as a consequence of chronic lymphedema after axillary dissection

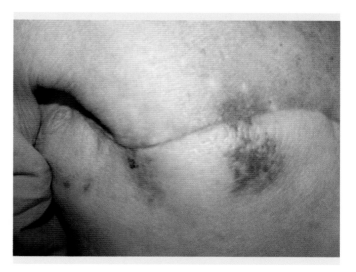

FIGURE 32-15. Angiosarcoma of a mastectomy scar of a 90-year-old female (from Yen TF, Lorek JD, Basir Z. Nonepithelial neoplasms of the breast. In: Kuerer HM, ed. *Kuerer's Breast Surgical Oncology*. New York, NY: McGraw-Hill; 2010: Chapter 23, Fig. 23-3.

(Stewart-Treves syndrome) (Fig. 32-15). They arise in the breast more than any other tissue. Other than lymphedema, radiation is another important risk factor, and angiosarcoma usually arises 10–20 years after treatment.

The lesion is a flat, painless, red/blue/purple mass that may ulcerate. They have high-grade characteristics on histology. They also have a high rate of lymph node involvement on presentation. Figure 32-15 shows a 90-year-old female with angiosarcoma in her prior mastectomy site.

Angiosarcomas are more aggressive than other sarcomas, and 15% have lymph node metastasis at presentation. They are treated with wide excision with radiation. If adenopathy is present, they should undergo a lymph node dissection. There are no current guidelines regarding adjuvant chemotherapy. The 5-year survival rate is less than 40%.

BIBLIOGRAPHY

McMasters KM, Urist MM. Melanoma and cutaneous malignancies. In: Townsend CM, Beauchamp RD, Evers BM, Mattox KL, eds. *Sabiston Textbook of Surgery: The Biological Basis of Modern Surgical Practice*. Philadelphia, PA: Elsevier; 2012:742–767.

Yen TF, Lorek JD, Basir Z. Nonepithelial neoplasms of the breast. In: Kuerer HM, ed. *Kuerer's Breast Surgical Oncology*. New York, NY: McGraw-Hill; 2010: Chapter 23.

18 **(D)** Sarcomas encompass a wide variety of tumors that are mesodermal in origin. Sarcomas are relatively uncommon, with an incidence of around 10,000 new

cases annually. They can occur at any age, but the average age is in the 50s. There are over 100 different histologic subtypes. These tumors are staged using the TNM system (described in previous questions) with the addition of grade; meaning that the tumor size, grade, lymph node status, and distant metastasis determine the stage. There are many prognostic factors at the time of diagnosis, the most important being stage and within that the most significant is tumor grade. Other important prognostic features include size (>5 cm), anatomic site (retroperitoneal worse than extremity), patient age, and histologic subtype.

BIBLIOGRAPHY

Ryan CW, Meyer J. Clinical presentation, histopathology, diagnostic evaluation, and staging of soft tissue sarcoma. In Savarese DMF, ed. *UpToDate*. Waltham, MA: UpToDate. Accessed April 28, 2014.

Singer S. Soft tissue sarcoma. In: Townsend CM, Beauchamp RD, Evers BM, Mattox KL, eds. *Sabiston Textbook of Surgery: The Biological Basis of Modern Surgical Practice*. Philadelphia, PA: Elsevier; 2012:768–782.

Yoon SS, Hornieck FJ. Management of soft tissue sarcomas. In: Cameron JL, Cameron AM, eds. *Current Surgical Therapy*. Philadelphia, PA: Elsevier; 2011:631–637.

19. **(B)** Metastatic disease to the small bowel is a rate entity; however, metastatic disease is more common than primary small bowel neoplasms. Disease can spread by direct invasion, hematogenous spread, or intraperitoneal seeding. Pancreatic and colon cancers frequently invade directly, while lung, breast, and melanoma spread hematogenously. Peritoneal seeding can come from a gastrointestinal disease, such as gastric, ovarian, and appendiceal tumors. The small bowel is the most common site of gastrointestinal metastases from malignant melanoma. Tumors of the small bowel can start to occlude the lumen of the bowel, leading to obstruction, or function as the lead point in intussusception.

BIBLIOGRAPHY

Cusack JC, Overman MJ. Epidemiology, clinical features, and types of small bowel neoplasms. In: Savarese DMF, ed. *UpToDate*. Waltham, MA: UpToDate. Accessed May 12, 2014.

Fischer C, Bass B. Tumors of the small intestine. In: Zinner MJ, Ashley SW, eds. *Maingot's Abdominal Operations*. 12th ed. New York, NY: McGraw-Hill; 2013: Chapter 30. http://accesssurgery.mhmedical.com.ezproxy2.library.arizona.edu/content.aspx?bookid=531&Sectionid=41808811. Accessed May 12, 2014.

Shelton AA, Chang G, Welton ML. Small intestine. In: Doherty GM, ed. *Current Diagnosis & Treatment: Surgery*. 13th ed. New York, NY: McGraw-Hill; 2010: Chapter 29. http://accesssurgery.

mhmedical.com.ezproxy2.library.arizona.edu/content.aspx?bookid=343&Sectionid=39702817. Accessed May 12, 2014.

20. **(B)** Melanoma is one of the more frequent malignancies, with an incidence of 62,000 cases a year. It is the most common malignancy of young adults (25–29 years old). The incidence is rising, likely the result of increasing sun exposure. Risk factors for malignant melanoma include xeroderma pigmentosa, fair skin, UV light exposure (sunlight), blistering sunburns, family history of melanoma, and the presence of multiple or dysplastic nevi. The best treatment is prevention. However, when prevention is not possible, early diagnosis can lead to surgical cure with excision. Patients with thicker lesions, and those who present with regional or metastatic disease have a poor prognosis. Therefore, early diagnosis is key. Melanoma can be identified clinically, and definitively diagnosed via full-thickness biopsy (excisional, incisional, or punch biopsy). An easy mnemonic to help identify melanoma clinically is ABCD:

A: Asymmetry—asymmetric shape, color, or contour

B: Borders—irregular or poorly defined borders

C: Color—black, brown, blue, red, gray, white, or irregular coloration

D: Diameter—larger than 5 mm or growing

BIBLIOGRAPHY

Sabel MS. Oncology. In: Doherty GM, ed. *Current Diagnosis & Treatment: Surgery*. 13th ed. New York, NY: McGraw-Hill; 2010: Chapter 44. http://accesssurgery.mhmedical.com.ezproxy2.library.arizona.edu/content.aspx?bookid=343&Sectionid=39702832. Accessed April 06, 2014.

Wallack MK, Degliuomini JJ, Joh JE, Berenji M. Cutaneous melanoma. In Cameron JL, Cameron AM, eds. *Current Surgical Therapy*. Philadelphia, PA: Elsevier; 2011:625–631.

21. **(A)** Melanoma either arises de novo or develops from dysplasia and malignant degeneration of an existing lesion. Melanomas have clinical patterns that allow them to be subclassified into four distinct categories.

Superficial spreading is the most common type of melanoma and accounts for 70% of lesions. They occur on sun-exposed surfaces and frequently arise in preexisting nevi. They are usually brown or black lesions and typically are on the back or legs. They grow in a radial pattern and frequently present at an early stage.

Nodular melanomas are the next most frequent, representing around 20% of lesions. They are more common in men and occur anywhere on the body. They usually develop de novo. They are difficult to diagnose as there are many color patterns, and they can also be amelanotic and can sometimes be misdiagnosed as a blood blister or hemangioma. They have an early vertical growth phase, are usually deep at time of diagnosis, and are very invasive. Because tumor thickness (depth) portends a worse prognosis, these are the most aggressive subtype.

Lentigo maligna have the most favorable prognosis of all subtypes. They tend to present on the face of older patients. They develop in sun-exposed areas and are locally aggressive with high recurrence rates. However, they have a long horizontal growth phase and rarely develop a vertical growth face, making them more indolent than other categories.

Acral lentiginous are the most common melanomas in black, Asian, and Hispanic patients, although they do also develop in Caucasians. They do not occur in sun-exposed areas but are found on the sole of the foot, palm, and underneath nail beds. They behave very aggressively, frequently develop rapidly, and metastasize early.

BIBLIOGRAPHY

Demierre MF, Chung C, Miller DR, Geller AC. Early detection of thick melanomas in the United States: beware of the nodular subtype. *Arch Dermatol* 2005;141:745–750.

Habif TP. Nevi and malignant melanoma. In: Habif TP. *Clinical Dermatology: A Color Guide to Diagnosis and Therapy*. 5th ed. New York, NY: Elsevier/Mosby; 2010:847–890.

Sabel MS. Oncology. In: Doherty GM, ed. *Current Diagnosis & Treatment: Surgery*. 13th ed. New York, NY: McGraw-Hill; 2010: Chapter 44. http://accesssurgery.mhmedical.com.ezproxy2.library.arizona.edu/content.aspx?bookid=343&Sectionid=39702832. Accessed April 06, 2014.

CHAPTER 33

PLASTIC AND RECONSTRUCTIVE SURGERY

KRISTEN A. KLEMENT, KARRI A. KLUESNER, AND JOHN LOGIUDICE

QUESTIONS

1. A 42-year-old female is seen in clinic with swelling of her left breast 3 years after undergoing augmentation mammoplasty. She reports the swelling has been persistent for a few weeks, and she has no recent history of trauma. Mammogram is negative. Ultrasound and magnetic resonance imaging (MRI) demonstrate a fluid collection around the implant. What is the most likely diagnosis?
   (A) Hematoma
   (B) Breast cancer
   (C) Autoimmune disorder
   (D) Anaplastic large cell lymphoma (ALCL)

2. A 62-year-old female is seen in clinic for her postoperative visit following a lumpectomy for ductal carcinoma *in situ* (DCIS). Her daughter accompanies her and recently had an augmentation mammoplasty with silicone implants. What are the appropriate screening tests for the daughter for breast cancer and silicone leaks?
   (A) Standard mammography views (craniocaudal [CC], mediolateral-oblique [MLO])
   (B) Standard mammography views (CC, MLO) plus Eklund technique
   (C) CC, MLO, Eklund mammography technique, and MRI at 3 years and every 2 years thereafter
   (D) CC, MLO, Eklund mammography technique, and ultrasound at 3 years and every 2 years thereafter

3. What is the blood supply for a free muscle-sparing transverse rectus abdominus muscle (TRAM) flap?
   (A) Superior epigastric artery
   (B) Inferior epigastric artery
   (C) Internal iliac artery
   (D) Intercostal artery

4. After performing a bilateral reduction mammoplasty, the recovery room nurse calls to tell you that the patient's right nipple is turning blue. What is the most appropriate next step?
   (A) Remove more breast tissue
   (B) Convert to a free nipple graft
   (C) Release the sutures
   (D) Start intravenous heparin

5. What is the central zone of a burn called?
   (A) Zone of stasis
   (B) Zone of hyperemia
   (C) Zone of coagulation
   (D) Zone of dermolysis

6. Which of the following is typically used as the criterion regarding timing of cleft lip repair?
   (A) Age greater than 7 weeks
   (B) Weight about 10 lb
   (C) Hemoglobin of at least 8 g/dL
   (D) Cleft lip defect greater than 10 mm

7. What is the incidence of cleft lip with or with out palate?
   (A) 1 in 500 live births
   (B) 2 in 1000 live births
   (C) 1 in 10,000 live births
   (D) 1 in 1000 live births
   (E) 1 in 750 live births

8. A wrestler from a local high school visits you in clinic complaining of swelling in his right ear after practice that afternoon. You notice that he has a large, doughy mass with overlying ecchymosis on his ear. What is the current treatment?
   (A) Observe only
   (B) Drainage with a 16-gauge needle
   (C) Compression bandage only
   (D) Drainage with a 16-gauge needle, followed by a compression bandage
   (E) Drainage through a small incision, followed by a compression bandage

9. In the orbit, which fissure or foramen does the oculomotor nerve (cranial nerve III) travel through?
   (A) Infraorbital notch
   (B) Superior orbital fissure
   (C) Supraorbital notch
   (D) Optic canal
   (E) Inferior orbital fissure

10. While you are obtaining consent from a patient to excise and graft a third-degree burn injury to his leg, you explain to him that he will eventually need a skin graft to cover the defect. He asks you how a piece of skin could possibly survive once it has been totally detached from the body. Which of the following is the first stage of skin graft survival?
    (A) Imbibition
    (B) Inosculation
    (C) Revascularization
    (D) Reepithelialization
    (E) None of the above

11. When a hair follicle is in the telogen stage of the growth cycle, what is it doing?
    (A) Growing
    (B) Turning gray
    (C) Resting
    (D) Dividing

12. A concerned mother brings in her 7-month-old infant for a red "tumor" on her cheek. This lesion appeared a few weeks after birth, and it is rapidly growing. What is the most likely diagnosis?
    (A) Vascular malformation
    (B) Spitz nevus
    (C) Hemangioma
    (D) Congenital melanocytic nevus
    (E) Squamous cell carcinoma

13. A patient comes to you for keloid resection and wants it permanently removed. Her lesion has been present for many years and recurred after a previous excision. What option gives the patient the best opportunity to avoid recurrence?
    (A) Re-excision with margins
    (B) Steroids
    (C) Silicone sheeting
    (D) Excision with radiation

14. A 30-year-old man presents to your clinic for recommendations regarding tattoo removal. He has multiple tattoos all over his body. He asks you if you are able to remove his purple and yellow tattoos. Which laser is the most appropriate to use for this patient?
    (A) Q-switched ruby
    (B) Carbon dioxide
    (C) Argon
    (D) Frequency-doubled Q-switched Nd:YAG
    (E) Copper vapor

15. Lidocaine is used commonly as a local anesthetic. Which cell membrane channel does it block?
    (A) Bicarbonate (HCO^-_3)
    (B) Chloride (Cl^-)
    (C) Calcium (Ca^{2+})
    (D) Magnesium (Mg^{2+})
    (E) Sodium (Na^{2+})

16. A patient presents to the emergency department (ED) with an open tibia fracture after motorcycle collision. A 10×5 cm soft tissue avulsion of the middle of the leg at the anterior aspect is evident, with loss of periosteum over the tibia. The patient's foot is well perfused. What is the Gustilo and Anderson classification of this open fracture?
    (A) I
    (B) II
    (C) IIIA
    (D) IIIB
    (E) IIIC

17. What is the most common cause of lymphedema worldwide?
    (A) *Wuchereria bancrofti*
    (B) *Entamoeba histolytica*
    (C) *Clonorchis sinensis*
    (D) *Cyclospora cayetanensis*
    (E) *Ixodes scapularis*

18. A patient presents to you with a brownish-black lesion on his arm that is 7 mm in diameter and has been bleeding occasionally. What is the most appropriate therapy for this patient?
    (A) Fine-needle aspiration (FNA)
    (B) Incisional biopsy
    (C) Excisional biopsy
    (D) Laser
    (E) Cryotherapy

19. The dominant pedicle of the latissimus dorsi flap consists of which artery and vein?
    (A) Thoracodorsal
    (B) Internal mammary
    (C) Transverse cervical
    (D) Suprascapular
    (E) Axillary

20. In the operating room, your assistant accidentally cuts the main pedicle of your patient's forehead flap. What vessels did he cut?
    (A) Supratrochlear and superficial temporal
    (B) Occipital and supraorbital
    (C) Posterior auricular and superficial temporal
    (D) Supratrochlear and supraorbital
    (E) Angular and infratrochlear

21. Which structure may be affected by Fournier gangrene?
    (A) Forearm
    (B) Axilla
    (C) Face
    (D) Scrotum

22. During tissue expansion, what happens to the tissues histologically over the expander?
    (A) Epidermis thins
    (B) Dermis thins
    (C) Muscle thickens
    (D) Vascularity decreases between the capsule and dermis

23. What is the most common type of collagen in the body?
    (A) I
    (B) II
    (C) III
    (D) IV
    (E) V

24. A components separation involves division of which layer of the abdominal wall?
    (A) Rectus abdominus fascia and muscle
    (B) Transversalis fascia
    (C) External oblique fascia and muscle
    (D) Internal oblique fascia and muscle

25. A 12 year-old presents with recent development of bilateral gynecomastia. In addition to a careful history and physical, the following should be recommended:
    (A) Liposuction
    (B) Needle biopsy
    (C) Observation
    (D) Direct excision

26. A panniculectomy in a high-risk patient may be considered when
    (A) The patient is unsatisfied with the way he or she looks
    (B) The patient refuses bariatric surgery
    (C) The pannus interferes with ambulation and activities of daily living
    (D) The patient has never had panniculitis

27. A patient is to undergo breast reconstruction at the time of mastectomy. The chest wall has been radiated, and her abdomen is chosen for flap harvest. Which of the following is an absolute contraindication to the use of the abdominal donor site for breast reconstruction?
    (A) Abdominal liposuction
    (B) Hernia
    (C) Normal body mass index (BMI)
    (D) None of the above

28. Which of the following is true regarding breast reduction surgery?
    (A) All patients are unable to breastfeed after surgery.
    (B) Most patients have a permanent lack of sensation in their nipples after surgery.
    (C) Most patients are dissatisfied with the results.
    (D) Scarring is the primary reason for patient dissatisfaction.

29. After healing of acute facial burns, resurfacing for improved functional and cosmetic outcomes can be best accomplished by which of the following?
    (A) Split-thickness skin graft
    (B) Full-thickness skin graft
    (C) Debridement and granulation
    (D) Cultured epithelial autografts

30. Which of the following is required for addressing any pressure sore?
    (A) Antibiotics
    (B) Pressure reduction
    (C) Hyperbaric oxygen
    (D) Flap coverage

31. A 32-year-old man comes into the ED after a motor vehicle crash. He has a large scalp laceration and neck pain with good strength in all extremities. He is hypotensive with a blood pressure of 80/40 mmHg and a pulse of 145. His chest x-ray (CXR), focused assessment with sonography (FAST) exam, and pelvic x-rays are normal. The most likely cause of his hypotension is
    (A) Hypovolemic shock
    (B) Neurogenic shock
    (C) Hypothermic shock
    (D) Cardiogenic shock

32. After routine three-vessel coronary artery bypass grafting (CABG) with use of the left internal mammary artery, a 72-year-old type II diabetic female develops hypotension and a fever. On examination, she is found to have a small area of wound dehiscence with thick drainage. On computed tomographic (CT) scan, she has a substernal fluid collection and is diagnosed with fulminant mediastinitis. Previously, this woman had undergone a gastrectomy for gastric cancer. Following debridement, which of the following flaps is most appropriate?
    (A) Omental flap
    (B) Right pectoralis major turnover flap
    (C) Left pectoralis major turnover flap
    (D) Left rectus abdominis flap

33. A 52-year-old patient with hypertension and vasculopathy undergoes left leg revascularization with an aorto-bifemoral bypass using a polytetrafluoro-ethylene (PTFE) graft. On postoperative day 5, he is noted to have wound dehiscence of his left groin with cloudy drainage. After incision and drainage, cultures reveal *Staphylococcus aureus* in the wound, and antibiotics are initiated. The most appropriate management is
    (A) Wet-to-dry dressings
    (B) Primary closure
    (C) Sartorius muscle flap
    (D) Bedside application of a V.A.C.® (vacuum-assisted closure) sponge

34. An 18-year-old male was struck in the left eye with a baseball. He complains of double vision, nausea, and tenderness in his left cheek. He has periorbital ecchymosis and edema, and his upward gaze is restricted. The most likely injury is
    (A) Orbital floor fracture
    (B) Intracranial hemorrhage
    (C) Retinal detachment
    (D) LeFort III fracture

35. Which one of the following is associated with carpal tunnel syndrome?
    (A) Numbness of the long finger
    (B) Numbness of the base of palm
    (C) Symptom relief with sleep
    (D) Symptom relief with wrist flexion

36. Which bacterium is the most common pathogen when an infection develops after a hand bite from a human?
    (A) *Pasteurella multocida*
    (B) *Neisseria gonorrhoeae*
    (C) *Staphylococcus aureus*
    (D) *Eikenella corrodens*

37. After multiple attempts followed by successful insertion of an arterial line at the distal forearm, the patient's hand is found to be cool and pale. Which of the following physical exam findings should have been considered when deciding to place the arterial line?
    (A) Doppler signal in the radial artery
    (B) Palpable ulnar artery pulse
    (C) Normal capillary refill
    (D) Abnormal Allen test
    (E) Anatomic snuffbox tenderness

38. What is the most common complication of a rhytidectomy?
    (A) Skin necrosis
    (B) Hematoma
    (C) Facial nerve injury
    (D) Hypertrophic scarring

39. A patient presents to the ED with an amputation through the proximal phalanx of his left index finger. What is the treatment of choice?
    (A) Replantation
    (B) Revision amputation
    (C) Toe-to-finger transfer
    (D) Local flap

ANSWERS AND EXPLANATIONS

1. **(D)** There is no evidence that breast implants cause breast cancer or autoimmune disorders. ALCL is a rare form of non-Hodgkin lymphoma that has been reported rarely in women after breast augmentation. The typical presenting symptom is a late-onset, persistent seroma. When there is a suspicion, fresh seroma fluid and representative portions of the capsule should be collected and sent for pathology tests to rule out ALCL. ALCL associated with an implant typically has an indolent clinical course with favorable prognosis.

BIBLIOGRAPHY

Bengtson B, Brody GS, Brown MH, Glicksman C, Hammond D, Kaplan H, et al., and Late Periprosthetic Fluid Collection After Breast Implant Working Group. Managing late periprosthetic fluid collections (seroma) in patients with breast implants: a consensus panel recommendation and review of the literature. *Plast Reconstr Surg* 2011;128(1):1–7.

Jewell M, Spear SL, Largent J, et al. Anaplastic large T-cell lymphoma and breast implants: a review of the literature. *Plast Reconstr Surg* 2011 Sep;128(3):651–661.

2. **(C)** Breast implants can interfere with visualization of breast tissue on mammography. The interference is

higher for subglandular versus submuscular implants. In addition to the standard views, the Eklund technique can be used for improved visualization and increased sensitivity. This technique compresses the breast tissue anteriorly and displaces the implant posteriorly.

Patients with silicone implants should undergo additional screening to detect a silent rupture. The Food and Drug Administration (FDA) recommends MRI at 3 years postimplantation and every 2 years afterward. MRI has improved sensitivity and specificity for detecting ruptures compared to other imaging modalities.

BIBLIOGRAPHY

Grady I, Hansen P. Mammography. In: Kuerer HM, ed. *Kuerer's Breast Surgical Oncology*. New York, NY: McGraw-Hill; 2010: Chapter 28.

Gorczyca DP, Gorczyca SM, Gorczyca KL. The diagnosis of silicone breast implant rupture. *Plast Reconstr Surg* 2007;120(7 Suppl 1):49S–61S.

Handel N, Silverstein MJ. Breast cancer diagnosis and prognosis in augmented women. *Plast Reconstr Surg.* 2006 Sep;118(3):587–593.

McIntosh SA, Horgan K. Augmentation mammoplasty: effect on diagnosis of breast cancer. *J Plast Reconstr Aesthet Surg* 2008;61(2):124–129. Epub 2007 Nov 26.

Ojeda-Fournier H, Comstock CE. Breast cancer screening. In: Kuerer HM, eds. *Kuerer's Breast Surgical Oncology*. New York, NY: McGraw-Hill; 2010: Chapter 5.

Uematsu T. Screening and diagnosis of breast cancer in augmented women. *Breast Cancer.* 2008;15(2):159–164. Epub 2008 Feb 22.

US Food and Drug Administration. Silicone Gel-Filled Breast Implants. September 20, 2013. Retrieved from http://www.fda.gov/MedicalDevices/ProductsandMedicalProcedures/ImplantsandProsthetics/BreastImplants/ucm063871.htm.

3. **(B)** A pedicled TRAM flap is based off the blood supply from the superior epigastric artery, while the deep inferior epigastric artery supplies the free TRAM flap once it is anastomosed to the donor artery. Donor arteries can be either the thoracodorsal or internal mammary. Free TRAMs have demonstrated less partial flap loss and fat necrosis compared to pedicled TRAMs but require microsurgical skills. Less donor site morbidity is seen with newer muscle-sparing techniques or perforator flaps (which do not transfer any muscle with the flap).

Other flaps used include the latissimus, superior gluteal, inferior gluteal, and transverse upper gracilis flaps. Implants may also be used for breast reconstruction following mastectomy for breast cancer, but they carry the normal implant risks (infection, rupture, contracture, and so on) and have higher complication rates in the setting of radiation.

BIBLIOGRAPHY

Losee JE, Gimbel M, Rubin J, Wallace CG, Wei F. Plastic and reconstructive surgery. In: Brunicardi F, Andersen DK, Billiar TR, et al., (eds.), *Schwartz's Principles of Surgery*. 9th ed. New York, NY: McGraw-Hill; 2010: Chapter 45.

Nahabedian MY, Patel K. Total breast reconstruction using autologous tissue: TRAM, DIEP, and SIEA flaps. In: Kuerer HM, ed. *Kuerer's Breast Surgical Oncology*. New York, NY: McGraw-Hill; 2010: Chapter 81.

4. **(C)** The most likely cause is kinking of the pedicle, and the first thing you should do is release the sutures. If the pedicle is not kinked, then more breast tissue might need to be removed to inset the pedicle without tension. However, if removing more breast tissue does not help, free nipple grafts should be your next consideration. Other complications include tissue necrosis, hematoma, asymmetry, hypertrophic scarring, decreased nipple-areola complex sensation, and altered mammography.

The blood supply to the breast is derived from the following arteries: internal mammary, lateral thoracic, thoracodorsal, thoracoacromial, and intercostal artery perforators. The nipple receives its blood supply from the subdermal plexus and is innervated by the lateral cutaneous branch of T4. The rest of the breast is innervated by the anteromedial and anterolateral branches of the thoracic intercostal nerves T3–T5. Also, the supraclavicular nerves from the cervical plexus innervate the superior and lateral breast.

BIBLIOGRAPHY

Danikas D, Theodorou S, Kokkalis G, Vasiou K, Kyriakopoulou K. Mammographic findings following reduction mammoplasty. *Aesth Plast Surg* 2001;25(4):283–285.

Harris L, Morris S, Freiberg A. Is breast feeding possible after reduction mammoplasty? *Plast Reconstr Surg* 2001;89(5):836–839.

Hunt KK, Newman LA, Copeland EM III, Bland KI. The breast. In: Brunicardi F, Andersen DK, Billiar TR, et al., (eds.), *Schwartz's Principles of Surgery*. 9th ed. New York, NY: McGraw-Hill; 2010: Chapter 17.

Kerrigan CL, Slezak SS. Evidence-based medicine: reduction mammaplasty. *Plast Reconstr Surg* 2013;132(6):1670–1683.

Losee JE, Gimbel M, Rubin J, Wallace CG, Wei F. Plastic and reconstructive surgery. In: Brunicardi F, Andersen DK, Billiar TR, et al., (eds.), *Schwartz's Principles of Surgery*. 9th ed. New York, NY: McGraw-Hill; 2010: Chapter 45.

5. **(C)** Following a burn injury, three different zones of tissue injury develop: zone of coagulation, zone of stasis, and zone of hyperemia (Fig. 33-1). The zone of coagulation is the most severe, central, and necrotic. The zone of stasis responded to injury with vasoconstriction and

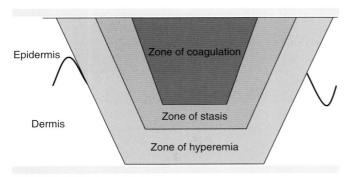

FIGURE 33-1. Zones of burn injury (from Mattox KL, Moore EE, Feliciano DV, eds. *Trauma*. 7th ed. New York, NY: McGraw-Hill; 2013: Fig. 48-1. Copyright © The McGraw-Hill Companies, Inc. All rights reserved).

ischemia. Adequate resuscitation can allow maintenance of perfusion to prevent conversion to a deeper wound. The outer zone is the zone of hyperemia, and this heals with minimal or no scaring. Burns can also be classified as superficial (painful, no blisters), partial (dermal involvement with blisters), or full thickness (painless, firm, leathery eschar).

Burn resuscitation is determined by the Parkland's formula: 4 mL/kg × % total body surface area (TBSA) burned. TBSA is calculated using only partial- and full-thickness burns and not superficial areas (Fig. 33-2). Half is given within the first 8 h after injury, and the other half is given over the following 16 h. It is paramount to maintain a urinary output of at least 30 mL/h or 0.5 mL/kg/h.

Topical burn care is standard treatment using silver sulfadiazine, silver nitrate, or mafenide acetate (sulfamylon). Silver sulfadiazine (Silvadene) is the most commonly used and inhibits growth of gram-positive and gram-negative organisms, *Candida albicans*, and possibly herpesviruses. Application is minimally painful, penetrates intermediately (toxicity is rare), but may cause leukopenia, which reverses with discontinuation. Silver nitrate is widely antimicrobial, but only penetrates minimally, making its use prophylactic only instead of in the face of established infection. Its concentration (0.5%) is in distilled water, making it hypotonic. This may sequester serum electrolytes and mandates careful monitoring of them. Silver nitrate stains everything it touches black, is painless on application, but must be kept wet at all times to prevent

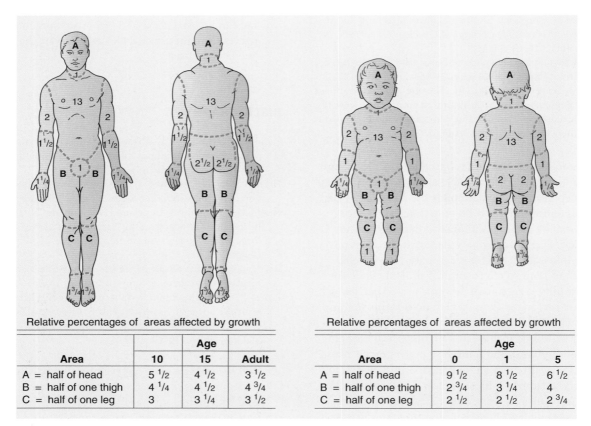

		Age	
Area	**10**	**15**	**Adult**
A = half of head	5 1/2	4 1/2	3 1/2
B = half of one thigh	4 1/4	4 1/2	4 3/4
C = half of one leg	3	3 1/4	3 1/2

		Age	
Area	**0**	**1**	**5**
A = half of head	9 1/2	8 1/2	6 1/2
B = half of one thigh	2 3/4	3 1/4	4
C = half of one leg	2 1/2	2 1/2	2 3/4

FIGURE 33-2. TBSA estimates, the "rule of 9s" (from Doherty GM, ed. *Current Diagnosis & Treatment: Surgery*. 13th ed. New York, NY: McGraw-Hill; 2010: Fig. 14-2. Copyright © The McGraw-Hill Companies, Inc. All rights reserved).

cytotoxic concentrations from occurring (>2%). Mafenide acetate is also broadly antimicrobial and penetrates deeply, making it ideal for eschars and cartilage (burned noses and ears). Caution must be exercised with judicious use because of the fact that mafenide acetate is a carbonic anhydrase inhibitor and may cause an alkaline diuresis. If polyuria develops, a hyperchloremic metabolic acidosis may ensue, leading to hyperventilation and pulmonary compromise in an already critically ill patient.

Most chemical burns must be washed thoroughly regardless of acid/base status. Lime is one exception to this because it reacts with water to produce a burn. Therefore, lime powder should be brushed off, and solid pieces of lime should be removed before flushing with water. Oral and intravenous antibiotics in the burn setting should only be used for documented infection, not prophylactically.

BIBLIOGRAPHY

Endorf FW, Gibran NS. Burns. In: Brunicardi F, Andersen DK, Billiar TR, et al., (eds.), *Schwartz's Principles of Surgery*. 9th ed. New York, NY: McGraw-Hill; 2010: Chapter 8.

Watts AM, Tyler MP, Perry ME, et al. Burn depth and its histological measurement. *Burns* 2001;27:154.

6. **(B)** The rule of tens is typically used to determine the timing of repair. This includes age greater than 10 weeks, weight is about 10 lb, and a hemoglobin of at least 10 g/dL. The following are several characteristics of a cleft lip: a shortened columella on the cleft side; the medial crus of the cleft side alar cartilage is moved posteriorly; the lateral crus is widened and spans the width of the cleft; the cleft side nostril has a horizontal axis compared to the vertical axis of the noncleft nostril; the cleft side philtrum is shortened; the Cupid's bow peak is too high; and the dome of the nose is pulled down on the cleft side (Fig. 33-3).

Cleft lip occurs at a rate of 1 in 1000 live births in whites, with the highest rate being 1 in 500 births in Asians and the lowest at 1 in 2000 births in blacks. The only known cause of cleft lip is the use of phenytoin during pregnancy (10-fold increase). Smoking may be associated with double the incidence of cleft lip compared to nonsmoking mothers.

Historically, Chinese physicians first reported surgical correction of a cleft lip, but it was not until 1955 that Ralph Millard described the most frequently used technique today. He described the rotation-advancement technique where the Cupid's bow rotates downward into a normal position via release of the medial lip while the lateral lip is advanced into the space left by the previous rotation. Repair of the orbicularis oris muscle is also

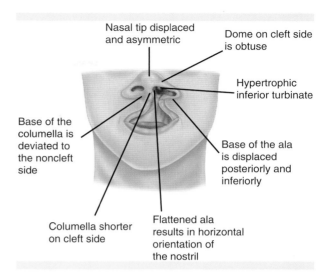

FIGURE 33-3. Characteristics of cleft lip (from Brunicardi FC, Andersen DK, Billiar TR, et al., (eds.), *Schwartz's Principles of Surgery*. 9th ed. New York, NY: McGraw-Hill; 2010: Fig. 45-14. Copyright © The McGraw-Hill Companies, Inc. All rights reserved).

performed to allow for normal lip function and eversion of the lip border.

Intrauterine repair of a cleft lip has been done in animals, but the risk of fetal loss is still too high to attempt this in humans. Along the same lines, neonatal cleft lip repair poses too many perioperative risks for a purely psychologic benefit to the parents.

BIBLIOGRAPHY

Burt JD, Byrd HS. Cleft lip: unilateral primary deformities. *Plast Reconstr Surg* 2000;105(3):1043–1055.

Losee JE, Gimbel M, Rubin J, Wallace CG, Wei F. Plastic and reconstructive surgery. In: Brunicardi F, Andersen DK, Billiar TR, et al., (eds.), *Schwartz's Principles of Surgery*. 9th ed. New York, NY: McGraw-Hill; 2010: Chapter 45.

7. **(D)** Cleft lip with or without cleft palate occurs at a rate of 1 in 1000 live births in whites, with the higher incidence in Asians (1/500) and lower incidence in African Americans (1/2000). Genetics can play a role. The cause of clefting is thought to be multifactorial; however, some factors may be increased parental age, drug use, infections during pregnancy, smoking during pregnancy, and family history. A parent with a cleft increases the risk to 4% in the fetus.

Clefting of the lip occurs during the fifth to sixth week of embryogenesis from failure of fusion of the medial nasal process and maxillary prominence.

Clefting of the palate occurs later, around the seventh to eighth week, from failure of the lateral palatine process to descend and fuse. The primary palate is anterior to the incisive foramen (lip, nose, alveolus, and anterior hard palate or premaxilla). Posterior to the incisive foramen is the secondary palate, which includes both hard and soft palate.

The anatomy of a cleft palate varies with severity of the cleft. Yet, the basic concept is that the barrier between the nasal and oral cavities is incomplete. The palate is divided into the hard palate anteriorly and the soft palate posteriorly, with its blood supply coming from the internal maxillary artery. The internal maxillary artery divides into the greater palatine artery to supply the hard palate via the greater palatine foramen and the lesser palatine artery to supply the soft palate via the lesser palatine foramen. The nerve supply to the palatal muscles is from the maxillary branches of the trigeminal nerve. Cranial nerves VII and IX are also present. The soft palate (velum) is muscular, while the hard palate is not. It is these muscles that play vital roles in speech, facial growth, and dentition. The muscles are the tensor veli palatini, palatoglossal, palatophyarngeal, uvular, superior constrictors, palatothyroideus, and salpingopharyngeus. The soft palate provides an anchoring point for these muscles, and when a cleft is present, their positions are incorrect, which leads to problems.

Today, most major cleft palates are repaired before 1 year of age to avoid any problems with speech development.

BIBLIOGRAPHY

Burt JD, Byrd HS. Cleft lip: unilateral primary deformities. *Plast Reconstr Surg* 2000;105(3):1043–1055.
Losee JE, Gimbel M, Rubin J, Wallace CG, Wei F. Plastic and reconstructive surgery. In: Brunicardi F, Andersen DK, Billiar TR, et al., (eds.), *Schwartz's Principles of Surgery*. 9th ed. New York, NY: McGraw-Hill; 2010: Chapter 45.

8. **(E)** Blunt trauma to the ear, especially around the helix, results in a hematoma that requires drainage. Symptoms include a history of trauma with an edematous, fluctuant, and ecchymotic pinna with loss of normal landmarks. If the hematoma is subperichondrial and is not adequately drained, it may calcify or fibrose, causing a permanent mass to form, which is known as "cauliflower ear." Cartilage is dependent on adjacent soft tissue for blood supply, and separation from the perichondrium increases the risk of necrosis.

Drainage is performed through small incisions, followed by a compression dressing against the ear, which is secured with a bandage placed around the head. Ear reconstruction following trauma is greatly facilitated by the excellent blood supply to the ear. The posterior auricular artery off the external carotid is the main source, with the superficial temporal, deep auricular, and occipital arteries as additional sources.

BIBLIOGRAPHY

Kellman RM. Face. In: Mattox KL, Moore EE, Feliciano DV, eds. *Trauma*. 7th ed. New York, NY: McGraw-Hill; 2013: Chapter 21.
Mueller RV. Facial trauma: soft tissue injuries. In: Neligan PC, ed. *Plastic Surgery*. 3rd ed. St. Louis, MO: Elsevier Saunders; 2013: Chapter 2.

9. **(B)** The following seven bones make up the orbit: frontal, zygoma, maxilla, palatine, greater and lesser wings of the sphenoid, lacrimal, and ethmoid bones (Fig. 33-4). Of note, the nasal and temporal bones do not contribute. Orbital anatomy is intricate, and surgery on or around the eye requires thorough knowledge of it. The optic nerve passes through the optic foramen. The superior orbital fissure, located between the greater and lesser wings of the sphenoid, permits passage of cranial nerves III, IV, V_1, and VI (Fig. 33-5).

The greater wing of the sphenoid is separated from the orbital floor by the inferior orbital fissure, which provides passage of the infraorbital artery, V_2, branches of the inferior ophthalmic vein to the

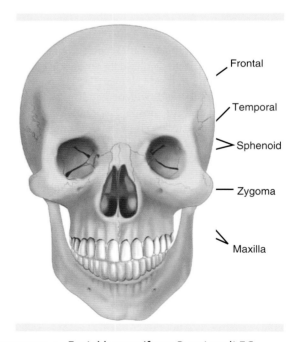

FIGURE 33-4. Facial bones (from Brunicardi FC, Andersen DK, Billiar TR, et al., (eds.), *Schwartz's Principles of Surgery*. 9th ed. New York, NY: McGraw-Hill; 2010: Fig. 45-28. Copyright © The McGraw-Hill Companies, Inc. All rights reserved).

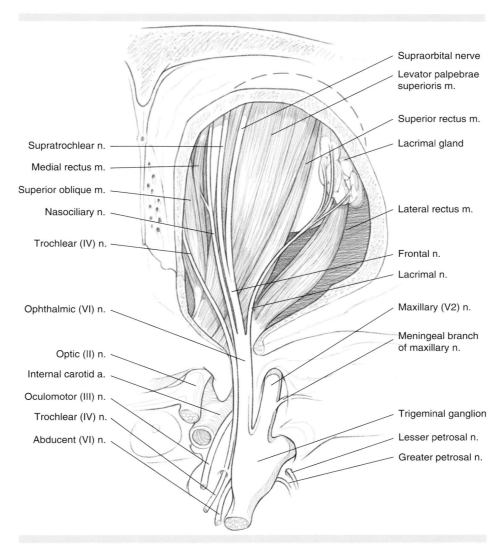

FIGURE 33-5. Contents of orbital cavity. Lalwaniak. Current Diagnosis and Treatment of Otolaryngology—Head and Neck Surgery, 3rd Ed. New York, NY: McGraw-Hill; 2012: Fig. 1-25.

pterygoid plexus, and branches of the sphenopalatine ganglion. The supraorbital vessels and nerve are transmitted through the supraorbital notch/foramen, while the infraorbital vessels and nerve travel via the infraorbital notch (Fig. 33-6).

Compression of the structures contained in the superior orbital fissure leads to symptoms of eyelid ptosis, globe proptosis, paralysis of the extraocular muscles, and anesthesia in the cranial nerve V_1 distribution. Orbital apex syndrome involves these symptoms plus blindness, indicating compression of the optic nerve as well. Both of these syndromes are medical emergencies.

Five orbital fat compartments exist in the eyelids: two in the upper lid and three in the lower lid. These

are manipulated or removed during blepharoplasty, but excessive removal may cause a hollowed-out appearance. Hemostasis is key during a blepharoplasty as blindness may ensue following an untreated hematoma. You may be called into the recovery room after a blepharoplasty because the patient is complaining of excessive pain around the eye or lack of the ability to see light or the nurse notices excessive edema. It is imperative to release the sutures and take the patient back to the operating room and remove any hematoma. Further, if no hematoma is found and all possible bleeding points are stable, then a lateral canthotomy is indicated to relieve any retrobulbar pressure. The incidence of blindness following blepharoplasty is very small (<0.1%), but its prevention is still paramount.

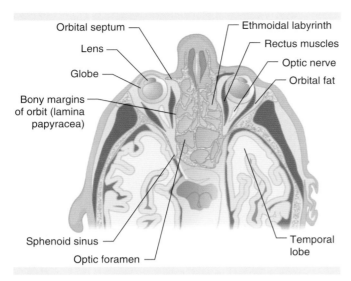

FIGURE 33-6. Orbital anatomy (from Tintinalli JE, Stapc-zynski JS, Ma OJ, Cline DM, Cydulka RK, Meckler GD, American College of Emergency Physicians, eds. *Tintinalli's Emergency Medicine: A Comprehensive Study Guide*. 7th ed. New York, NY: McGraw-Hill; 2011: Fig. 115-1. Copyright © The McGraw-Hill Companies, Inc. All rights reserved).

Another complication following blepharoplasty, although not as severe as blindness, is ectropion. This is defined by an outward turning or eversion of the eyelid and, in the case of blepharoplasty, is usually caused by excessive removal of skin, fat, or muscle; damage to the orbicularis oculi muscle; lid edema; hematoma; proptosis; or scar contracture. Treatment includes massage of the lower eyelid and application of cool compresses; if persistent, it may require full-thickness skin grafting or tightening or shortening of the lateral canthus.

Lacerations of the eyelid require meticulous repair to prevent any cosmetic or functional problems. Three layers of the eyelid exist: the anterior lamella (skin, orbicularis), septum, and posterior lamella (tarsus and conjunctiva). Repair of a laceration should start with a suture at the end through the skin and tarsus that, with gentle traction, aligns the wound edges. Next, the pretarsal muscle is repaired with an absorbable suture, followed by a nylon suture for skin approximation. To prevent scarring, suture removal should occur after 3–5 days.

BIBLIOGRAPHY

Losee JE, Gimbel M, Rubin J, Wallace CG, Wei F. Plastic and reconstructive surgery. In: Brunicardi F, Andersen DK, Billiar TR, et al., (eds.), *Schwartz's Principles of Surgery*. 9th ed. New York, NY: McGraw-Hill; 2010: Chapter 45.

Norton, NS. Eye and orbit. In: *Netter's Head and Neck Anatomy for Dentistry*. St. Louis, MO: Elsevier Saunders; 2013: Chapter 19.

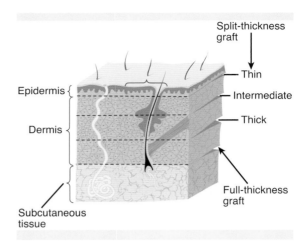

FIGURE 33-7. Skin graft types (from Doherty GM, ed. *Current Diagnosis & Treatment: Surgery*. 13th ed. New York, NY: McGraw-Hill; 2010: Fig. 41-1. Copyright © The McGraw-Hill Companies, Inc. All rights reserved).

10. **(A)** Skin grafts survive by three mechanisms: plasmatic imbibition, inosculation, and revascularization. During the first 1–2 days, the graft undergoes imbibition; a thin layer of fibrin and plasma separates the graft from the wound bed to provide nutrients. Following this, a period of inosculation occurs; the blood vessels in the wound bed and the graft make contact to establish blood flow. Last, new blood vessels actually grow into the skin graft by day 6 or 7 during a process of revascularization (Fig. 33-7).

Harvest of a split-thickness skin graft results in shrinkage of the graft. This is because of the elastin present in the dermis and is called primary contracture. Several weeks after application, secondary contracture may occur from the action of myofibroblasts. Full-thickness skin grafts have more dermis than split-thickness grafts, resulting in greater primary contracture; however, there is less secondary contracture.

Failure of skin grafts can be multifactorial. The most common causes include hematoma, seroma, inadequate vascularity (lack of paratenon or periosteum), infection, and shear. A bolster dressing is typically applied to maximize graft adherence, minimize shearing, and prevent hematoma or seroma formation. This can be completed using either a bolster dressing (Xeroform and cotton soaked with mineral oil) or negative-pressure therapy.

BIBLIOGRAPHY

Losee JE, Gimbel M, Rubin J, Wallace CG, Wei F. Plastic and reconstructive surgery. In: Brunicardi F, Andersen DK, Billiar TR, et al., (eds.), *Schwartz's Principles of Surgery*. 9th ed. New York, NY: McGraw-Hill; 2010: Chapter 45.

Zollinger RM Jr, Ellison E, Bitans M, Smith J. In: Zollinger RM Jr, Ellison E, Bitans M, Smith J, eds. *Zollinger's Atlas of Surgical Operations*. New York, NY: McGraw-Hill; 2011: Plate 235.

11. **(C)** Each hair follicle goes through three phases during its growth cycle: anagen, catagen, and telogen. Anagen is the phase of active follicular growth. About 90% of all hair follicles are in this stage, which lasts approximately 2–5 years. Catagen is the next stage and represents regression. Affecting about 1–2% of the follicles, it lasts 2–3 weeks, during which the base of the follicle becomes keratinized, the melanocytes stop producing melanin, and the follicular bulb is eventually destroyed. Finally, the telogen phase lasts 3–4 months and represents approximately 10% of the follicles. This phase is the resting phase; the follicle is inactive, and the dermal papilla releases from the epidermal attachment. The old hair is shed, and the hair enters the anagen phase of the cycle. Every hair follicle is divided into three parts: the infundibulum (upper), isthmus (middle), and bulb (lower) (Fig. 33-8).

Hair loss is common among men and women and affects more than half of them in the United States. The percentage of women who lose hair is the same as men, but hormones allow them the benefit of not losing as much volume. Forms of hair loss include traumatic alopecia, alopecia areata (patchy reversible hair loss), drug-induced alopecia (warfarin, allopurinol),

and the most common form, androgenic alopecia or male-pattern baldness. Androgenic alopecia can affect females as well and is defined by increased sensitivity to dihydrotestosterone (DHT), which shortens the anagen phase, causing the hair follicles to become progressively thinner. Other causes of alopecia include lupus, syphilis, cancers, liver and kidney failure, poor nutrition, and stress. 5-Alpha reductase converts testosterone to DHT, and male-pattern baldness may be treated with synthetic 5-alpha reductase inhibitors (finasteride).

Male-pattern baldness is categorized by the Hamilton-Norwood classification, with type I being minimal hairline recession, progressing to type VII, the most severe form with only a small horseshoe-shaped band of hair posterior to the ears and around the occiput. Before the late 1980s and early 1990s, physicians were rotating flaps of hair around the scalp, using tissue expanders, excising pieces of scalp, or transplanting strips or plugs of hair to treat hair loss. These techniques frequently resulted in donor site defects or flap necrosis and were aesthetically unattractive. Now, the technique of hair grafting involves placing small grafts with 1–2 hair follicles per graft in a pattern on the scalp that appears natural. This procedure does not involve flaps, has little donor site defect, and is the way most hair transplantation is performed today.

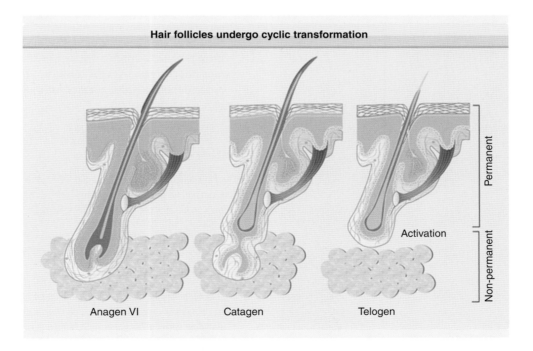

FIGURE 33-8. Hair follicles and hair loss (from Goldsmith LA, Katz SI, Gilchrest BA, Paller AS, Leffell DJ, Wolff K, eds. *Fitzpatrick's Dermatology in General Medicine*. 8th ed. New York, NY: McGraw-Hill; 2012: Fig. 88-0.1. Copyright © The McGraw-Hill Companies, Inc. All rights reserved).

BIBLIOGRAPHY

Fisher J. Hair restoration. In: Neligan PC. *Plastic Surgery*. 3rd ed. St. Louis, MO: Elsevier Saunders; 2013: Chapter 23.
Price VH. Treatment of hair loss. *N Engl J Med* 1999;341(13):964–973.

12. **(C)** Hemangiomas are the most common birthmark (Fig. 33-9). They are typically noted shortly after birth as a small pink spot. Hemangiomas have three stages of growth: rapid or proliferating, involuting phase (where they grow at the same rate as the child), and involuted phase. By 5 years of age, 50% of hemangiomas involute completely, followed by 70% at age 7. Further involution occurs until the ages of 10–12. Although the typical management of a hemangioma is observation, around 10% will require treatment due to airway obstruction, visual or hearing disturbances, or bleeding/ulceration. Treatment for these hemangiomas includes intralesional or systemic steroids, propranolol, vincristine, interferon, laser, or surgery.

Hemangiomas are commonly confused with vascular malformations. Hemangiomas are tumors, and vascular malformations are aberrations of embryonic development. Vascular malformations are present at birth and grow proportionately with the child. They are subclassified by vessel type (arterial, venous, capillary, or lymphatic) or by flow characteristics (slow or fast).

Slow-flow lesions include capillary malformations (CMs) and telangiectasias, lymphatic malformations (LMs), and venous malformations (VMs). Fast-flow lesions include arterial malformations (AMs) and arteriovenous malformations (AVMs). In addition, there are combined malformations.

The AVMs can cause ischemic pain, ulceration, bleeding, and high-output cardiac failure. Treatment typically is arterial embolization 24–48 h prior to surgical resection. Ligation of the arterial feeding vessels should never be done. This prevents access for further therapeutic embolization as well as recruits more vessels to the nidus.

Certain syndromes include hemangiomas or vascular malformations as one of their main characteristics. For example, Sturge-Weber's syndrome involves vascular lesions of the upper facial dermis, choroid plexus, and ipsilateral leptomeninges. Kasabach-Merritt describes thrombocytopenia in the face of a large hemangioma; Maffucci syndrome is low-flow vascular malformations with multiple enchondromas.

Congenital melanocytic nevi are brown lesions present at birth. Over time, they have an increase in texture and hypertrichosis. They are classified according to size: small, large, and giant. There is concern that these lesions can transform into melanoma. Any changes in the lesion require biopsy. The rate of melanoma is highest in the giant lesions, at approximately 5–10%. Giant congenital melanocytic nevi over the posterior trunk midline also raise concerns of neurocutaneous melanocytosis and require screening.

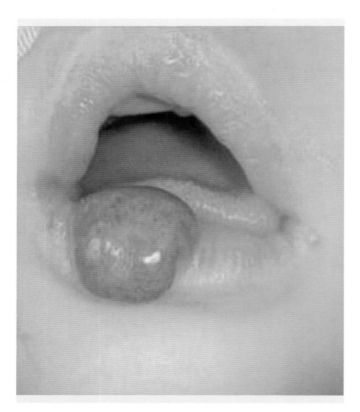

FIGURE 33-9. Hemangioma (from Brunicardi FC, Andersen DK, Billiar TR, et al., (eds.), *Schwartz's Principles of Surgery*. 9th ed. New York, NY: McGraw-Hill; 2010: Fig. 16-7. Copyright © The McGraw-Hill Companies, Inc. All rights reserved).

BIBLIOGRAPHY

Losee JE, Gimbel M, Rubin J, Wallace CG, Wei F. Plastic and reconstructive surgery. In: Brunicardi F, Andersen DK, Billiar TR, et al., (eds.), *Schwartz's Principles of Surgery*. 9th ed. New York, NY: McGraw-Hill; 2010: Chapter 45.
Mulliken J. Vascular anomalies. In: Thorne CHM, eds. *Grabb and Smith Plastic Surgery*. 6th ed. New York, NY: Lippincott-Raven; 2006: Chapter 22.

13. **(D)** Keloids are an excessive form of healing, as are hypertrophic scars. They occur in about 10% of wounds and are more common in African Americans and Asians. The difference between keloids and hypertrophic scars is that keloids grow beyond the original scar margin, and hypertrophic scars do not. The time interval for appearance can be as early as 1 week for hypertrophic

scars, while keloids can develop up to 1 year later. Both keloids and hypertrophic scars have thickened epidermal layers and rich vasculature. The composition of keloids includes excessive mucinous ground substance and irregular and malaligned collagen fibers with 20 times the amount of collagen synthesis compared to normal skin. Hypertrophic scars also have abnormal collagen fibers, with three times the amount of collagen synthesis compared to normal skin.

A keloid can be resected, but one cannot guarantee that it will be permanently removed. In fact, it may recur and be worse, which is why conservative therapy is usually initiated before surgery. Therefore, indications for surgery include failure of conservative therapy, cosmetic deformity, and functional impairment. Examples of conservative therapy include topical silicone sheeting, intralesional steroids, and pressure garments.

The mechanism of action of silicone sheeting involves the occlusive hydration effect; pressure devices act by producing local tissue hypoxia. Scar massage as well as intralesional steroids decrease the amount of connective tissue.

Multiple studies suggested the most effective treatment for recurrent keloids involves using postoperative radiation therapy. This has been proven safe, with minimal risk of carcinogenesis and high rates of success.

BIBLIOGRAPHY

Gurtner GC. Wound healing: normal and abnormal. In: Thorne CHM, ed. *Grabb and Smith Plastic Surgery*. 6th ed. New York, NY: Lippincott-Raven; 2006: Chapter 2.

Ogawa R, Yoshitatsu S, Yoshida K, Miyashita T. Is radiation therapy for keloids acceptable? The risk of radiation-induced carcinogenesis. *Plast Reconstr Surg* 2009;124.4:1196–1201.

Park TH, Park JH, Chang CH. Analysis of surgical treatments for earlobe keloids: analysis of 174 lesions in 145 patients. *Plast Reconstr Surg* 2014;133.5:724e–726e.

van Leeuwen MCE, Stokmans SC, Bulstra AEJ, Meijer OW, van Leeuwen PA, Niessen FB. High-dose-rate brachytherapy for the treatment of recalcitrant keloids: a unique, effective treatment protocol. *Plast Reconstr Surg* 2014;134.3:527–534.

14. **(D)** The word *laser* stands for "light amplification by stimulated emission of radiation," and the laser was developed based on Einstein's quantum theory of radiation. Use of lasers in plastic surgery is relatively recent, but many different conditions are amenable to laser therapy. For tattoos, lasers are chosen based on the pigments used. Blue, green, and black amateur tattoos are removed with the Q-switched ruby laser because all of the energy is absorbed by the pigments, sparing the epidermis. The frequency-doubled, Q-switched Nd: YAG laser can remove red, orange, purple, yellow, and brown tattoo inks.

Tattoo removal usually requires multiple visits for completion. Other uses for lasers include treatment of rhytids, hemangiomas, CMs, telangiectasias, scars, and warts. A CO_2 laser targets water and can be used for facial resurfacing. The intense pulsed light is the most popular laser for vascular lesions and targets oxyhemoglobin.

BIBLIOGRAPHY

Low DW. Lasers in plastic surgery. In: Thorne CHM, eds. *Grabb and Smith Plastic Surgery*. 6th ed. New York, NY: Lippincott-Raven, 2006: Chapter 20.

15. **(E)** Local anesthetics are divided into two groups: the amides and the esters. The esters have a higher allergic potential and are metabolized by plasma cholinesterase. The amides are more commonly used and are metabolized by the liver. Local anesthetics work by blocking the sodium channels in the cell membrane, thus inhibiting nerve conduction. The total amount of lidocaine one can give is 5 or 7 mg/kg if epinephrine is added. Lidocaine should not be taken lightly, and toxicity can lead to death. Symptoms of lidocaine toxicity are initially related to the central nervous system (CNS) (headache, lips and tongue effects, tinnitus, lightheadedness, and facial twitching). As severity progresses, one may see loss of consciousness, seizures, apnea, cardiovascular collapse, or even ventricular fibrillation (V-fib) arrest. If your patient begins to seize, secure an airway, hyperventilate with 100% oxygen, and administer diazepam. Other signs or symptoms require supportive care as needed. A tourniquet may be used to delay further lidocaine absorption.

EMLA cream is helpful for superficial anesthesia. It is a mixture of lidocaine and prilocaine. It has to be applied copiously and covered with a semiocclusive dressing. Typically, it takes an hour for anesthesia, which can reach to a depth of 5 mm. Caution must be exercised with use of EMLA cream as lidocaine toxicity can occur. The usual adult dose is 1.5 g/10 cm^2.

In the ED, suturing an extensive laceration in a child can best be done under conscious sedation. Fentanyl with midazolam and ketamine are the anesthetics best suited for this. You may inject marcaine into the surgical site to provide local anesthesia (4–6 h), with dosage at 3 mg/kg, 200 mg maximum.

The major risk with the use of local anesthetic such as marcaine is reentrant tachycardia or V-fib. Epinephrine is helpful to prevent bleeding during laceration repair. A concentration of 1:100,000 provides excellent vasoconstriction (greater concentrations do not improve duration or amount of bleeding); a minimum of 7 min is required for its onset of action. Studies have disproven the avoidance of epinephrine in ears, nose, fingers, and toes.

Bicarbonate can also be added to the injection, typically as 1 mL to 9 mL local anesthesia. This increases the pH and decreases burning with injection.

BIBLIOGRAPHY

Dorian RS. Anesthesia of the surgical patient. In: Brunicardi F, Andersen DK, Billiar TR, et al., (eds.), *Schwartz's Principles of Surgery*. 9th ed. New York, NY: McGraw-Hill; 2010: Chapter 47.

Thomson CJ, Lalonde DH, Denkler KA, Feicht AJ. A critical look at the evidence for and against elective epinephrine use in the finger. *Plast Reconstr Surg* 2007;119(1):260–266.

Thorne A. Local anesthetics. In: Thorne CHM, eds. *Grabb and Smith Plastic Surgery*. 6th ed. New York, NY: Lippincott-Raven, 2006: Chapter 11.

16. **(D)** Open tibial fractures have a wide range of severity, and lower limb injuries commonly require plastic surgical intervention because of the limited skin and muscle availability in that area. The Gustilo classification is as follows:

I: Open fracture with a wound less than 1 cm

II: Open fracture with a wound larger than 1 cm without extensive soft tissue damage

III: Open fracture with extensive soft tissue damage

IIIA: III with adequate soft tissue coverage

IIIB: III with soft tissue loss with periosteal stripping and bone exposure

IIIC: III with arterial injury requiring repair

Consultation with a plastic surgeon concerning coverage of the fracture should occur with classifications IIIB and IIIC. Options for coverage vary widely, but mainly depend on what skin, muscle, arteries, and veins are available; the location of the defect; and whether or not the nerves have been damaged. Nerve disruption to the foot can be a relative contraindication to reconstruction. For instance, if the tibial nerve is destroyed, the patient will lose plantar flexion of the foot as well as sensation on the plantar aspect of the foot, leading to a step-off in ambulation, a loss of position sense, and an increased risk of chronic wounds on the bottom of the foot. In the proximal two-thirds of the lower leg, local flaps may be available for coverage. Most commonly, this is a muscle flap, such as the lateral and medial gastrocnemius flap (proximal one-third and knee) and soleus flap (middle one-third of leg). The lower one-third of the leg or foot or very large wounds typically require free tissue transfer.

BIBLIOGRAPHY

Gustilo R, Anderson J. Prevention of infection in the treatment of one thousand and twenty-five open fractures of long bones: retrospective and prospective analysis. *J Bone Joint Surg* 1976;58:453.

Kasabian A, Karp N. Lower extremity reconstruction. In: Thorne CHM, eds. *Grabb and Smith Plastic Surgery*. 6th ed. New York, NY: Lippincott-Raven; 2006: Chapter 70.

17. **(A)** Worldwide, the most common cause is infection, with the parasite *W. bancrofti* causing filariasis. In the United States, tumor invasion, radiation, and surgery are the leading causes. Lymphedema is either primary or secondary, with the primary form divided into three subtypes: congenita, praecox, and tarda. Lymphedema congenita is present at birth; lymphedema praecox is the most common of the primary types (94%) and occurs during adolescence; and the onset of lymphedema tarda is after the age of 35. A familial form of lymphedema praecox is known as Milroy's disease and is X-linked dominant. Secondary lymphedema is much more common in the United States. This is typically due to lymphatic obstruction or disruption. The most common cause is axillary node dissection. Other causes include radiation therapy, trauma, infection, malignancy, and parasites (Fig. 33-10).

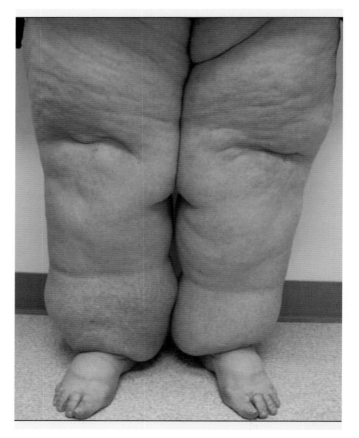

FIGURE 33-10. Lymphedema (from Brunicardi FC, Andersen DK, Billiar TR, et al., (eds.), *Schwartz's Principles of Surgery*. 10th ed. New York, NY: McGraw-Hill; 2014: Fig. 24-21. Copyright © The McGraw-Hill Companies, Inc. All rights reserved).

The treatment of lymphedema has perplexed surgeons throughout history, and many different ideas and techniques have been developed. Basically, treatment can be divided into medical and surgical, with surgical involving physiologic or excisional procedures. Currently, medical therapy is implemented first and consists of wearing compressive garments, massage, pneumatic compression devices, antibiotics, good hygiene, and limb elevation. Strict compliance is mandatory for efficacious medical therapy. Diuretics are not therapeutic. Surgery may complement patients optimized with medical therapy. Physiologic techniques aimed at lymphatic drainage include lymphatic-to-venous or lymphaticolymphatic anastomosis, lymph node transfer, or flap transfer. These techniques have demonstrated improvement in lymphedema of the extremities. Excisional procedures (Charles procedure) include removal of the affected tissue with skin grafting for coverage. Other options include liposuction.

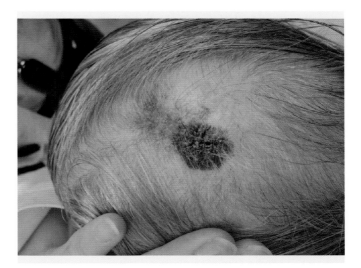

FIGURE 33-11. Melanoma (from Brunicardi FC, Andersen DK, Billiar TR, et al., (eds.), *Schwartz's Principles of Surgery*. 10th ed. New York, NY: McGraw-Hill; 2014: Fig. 16-10. Copyright © The McGraw-Hill Companies, Inc. All rights reserved).

BIBLIOGRAPHY

Liem TK, Moneta GL. Venous and lymphatic disease. In: Brunicardi F, Andersen DK, Billiar TR, et al., (eds.), *Schwartz's Principles of Surgery*. 9th ed. New York, NY: McGraw-Hill; 2010: Chapter 24.

Losee JE, Gimbel M, Rubin J, Wallace CG, Wei F. Plastic and reconstructive surgery. In: Brunicardi F, Andersen DK, Billiar TR, et al., (eds.), *Schwartz's Principles of Surgery*. 9th ed. New York, NY: McGraw-Hill; 2010: Chapter 45.

18. **(C)** A punch or excisional biopsy will provide the necessary information for diagnosis and further therapy. If the lesion is melanoma, further workup is indicated. A shave biopsy typically does not obtain the entire depth of the lesion, which limits treatment guidelines.

Melanoma incidence is rapidly increasing, faster than any other cancer, with a lifetime risk of 1 in 40. Concerning characteristics for melanoma are the ABCDE criteria, these are asymmetry, border irregularity, color changes, diameter greater than 0.6 cm, and evolving changes (Fig. 33-11).

Four types of melanoma exist: superficial spreading, nodular, acral lentiginous, and lentigo maligna. Each type has certain unique characteristics. The most common type is superficial spreading (70%). Nodular has a rapid vertical growth pattern. Acral lentiginous typically occurs on the palm and soles, and this subtype is more common in African Americans and Asians. Lentigo maligna grows slowly over many years and is most commonly found on the head and neck.

Important prognostic factors include nodal status, Breslow thickness (millimeter depth of the lesion), ulceration, and more than 1 mitotic figure per high-power field. Overall, stage I melanoma has a high 5-year survival rate (89–100%) depending on the subtype, but stage IV melanoma usually indicates fatal disease (5-year survival rate 7–9%).

Margins of resection are determined by the Breslow thickness of the biopsy. The current recommendations are as follows: melanoma *in situ* = 0.5 cm, < 1 mm = 1 cm, > 1 mm = 2 cm. Sentinel lymph node biopsy should be performed for a patient without palpable disease and a lesion more than 0.76 mm thick, ulceration present, or any mitotic figures (Fig. 33-11). Complete lymph node dissections are performed if there is a positive sentinel lymph node or clinically palpable disease. There are new exciting targeted treatments for melanoma that have demonstrated improved survival for those with metastatic disease. These include ipilimumab (antibody directed against cytotoxic T lymphocytic–associated antigen CTLA-4) and vemurafenib or dabrafenib (selective BRAF kinase inhibitor for lesions positive for BRAF V600E mutation).

BIBLIOGRAPHY

Coit DG et al. Melanoma. *J Natl Compr Canc Netw* 2012;10:366–400.

Cole P, Heller L, Bullocks J, Hollier LH, Stal S. The skin and subcutaneous tissue. In: Brunicardi F, Andersen DK, Billiar TR, et al., (eds.), *Schwartz's Principles of Surgery*. 9th ed. New York, NY: McGraw-Hill; 2010: Chapter 16.

19. **(A)** An array of free flaps has been described, but a certain group of them is worth mentioning because of their versatility, durability, ease of harvest, and

common use. First, the rectus abdominis flap, supplied by the deep inferior and superior epigastric arteries and veins, provides a large muscle mass with the option of a skin paddle. Second, the radial forearm flap, supplied by the radial artery, venae comitantes, and cephalic vein, has a long, useful vascular pedicle with thin, pliable skin. Third, the gracilis flap, supplied by the ascending branch of the medial circumflex femoral artery and vein, may assist with facial paralysis or extremity muscle function as it has both motor (obturator) and sensory (femoral cutaneous) innervation. Fourth, the great toe flap, supplied by the first dorsal metatarsal artery and vein, can be used for thumb replacement. Last, the latissimus dorsi flap, supplied by the thoracodorsal artery and vein, is a reliable flap with a large muscle mass and a long vascular pedicle. In fact, it can be made even larger if the serratus anterior or scapular muscles are included as a "chimeric" flap.

Free flaps may be designated as muscular, musculocutaneous, fasciocutaneous, or osteofasciocutaneous flaps depending on their composition. For example, the fibula flap is an osteofasciocutaneous flap with its blood supply from the peroneal artery.

BIBLIOGRAPHY

Vasconez HC, Habash A. Plastic and reconstructive surgery. In: Doherty GM, ed. *Current Diagnosis & Treatment: Surgery.* 13th ed. New York, NY: McGraw-Hill; 2010: Chapter 41.

20. **(D)** The dominant pedicle is the supratrochlear artery, with the minor pedicle being the supraorbital artery. The flap may survive via connections from the angular, infratrochlear, and dorsal nasal arteries as flap survival has been reported after division of the supratrochlear and supraorbital arteries.

The history of nasal reconstruction dates to 600–700 BC, with Sushruta in India having performed the first recorded plastic surgery procedure. Tagliacozzi also made contributions to nasal reconstruction in 1597 with his description of staged transfer of skin from the arm to the nose. Historically, efforts were encouraged by the results of hand-to-hand combat and by the cutting off of one's nose as criminal punishment. Today, however, nasal reconstruction is most commonly undertaken after removal of nasal skin cancer.

The anatomy of the nose is intricate, involving an internal layer of mucosa and an external layer of skin supported by bone and cartilage. The nose can be divided into nine subunits based on shadows produced by normal lighting. The subunit borders allow for excellent concealment of scars, and the subunits are as follows: the dorsum, two nasal side walls, the tip, two ala, two soft tissue triangles, and the columella (Fig. 33-12).

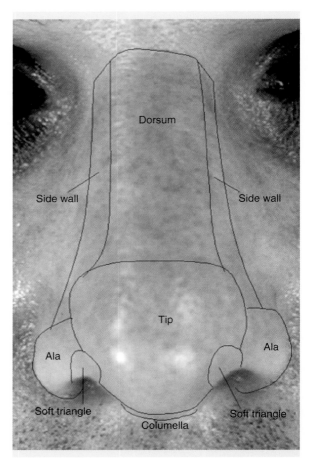

FIGURE 33-12. Nasal subunits (from Brunicardi FC, Andersen DK, Billiar TR, et al., (eds.), *Schwartz's Principles of Surgery.* 10th ed. New York, NY: McGraw-Hill; 2014: Fig. 45-31. Copyright © The McGraw-Hill Companies, Inc. All rights reserved).

For defects greater than 50% of the corresponding nasal subunit, a general rule dictates that the defect should be enlarged to include the entire subunit for the best cosmetic result. Anything less than 50% should be treated without making it larger.

Nasal reconstruction can be done with a variety of flaps and grafts. The forehead flap is the ultimate flap for nasal reconstruction as it can be used to replace any or all of the nasal subunits. However, the patient must be stable enough to tolerate the two-stage procedure. Reconstructing the nasal lining is performed with a septal mucosal flap using vascular inflow coming from the superior labial artery. Grafts from the rib and concha can be used for dorsal nasal and alar lobule support. Defects located near the medial canthus are best treated with healing by secondary intention. Defects on the nasal dorsum or side walls can be treated with a bilobed, nasolabial flap or Reiger flap (dorsal nasal) flap (Fig. 33-13).

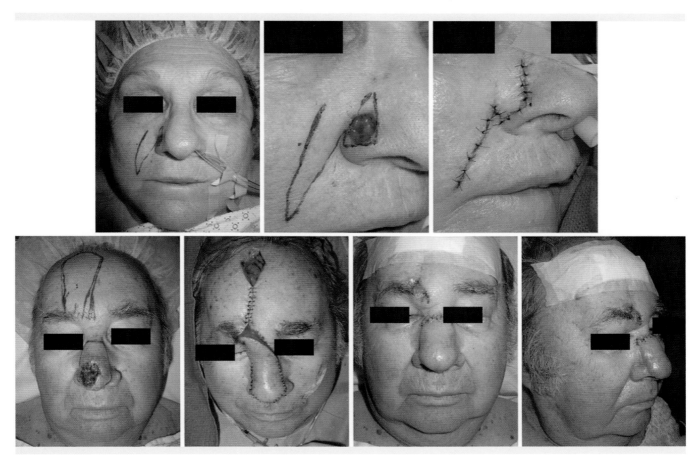

FIGURE 33-13. Nasal reconstruction (from Brunicardi FC, Andersen DK, Billiar TR, et al., (eds.), *Schwartz's Principles of Surgery*. 10th ed. New York, NY: McGraw-Hill; 2014: Fig. 45-32. Copyright © The McGraw-Hill Companies, Inc. All rights reserved).

BIBLIOGRAPHY

Burget G, Menick F. The subunit principle in nasal reconstruction. *Plast Reconstr Surg* 1985;76(2):239–247.

Menick F. Nasal reconstruction In: Thorne CHM, ed. *Grabb and Smith Plastic Surgery*. 6th ed. New York, NY: Lippincott-Raven, 2006: Chapter 38.

21. **(D)** Fournier gangrene is necrotizing fasciitis of the genital, perianal, or perineal areas. Like other types of necrotizing soft tissue infections, it is rapidly progressive and life threatening (Fig. 33-14). Patients often have a history of diabetes mellitus, and they present with erythema, edema, and pain out of proportion at the affected site. If allowed to progress, the skin begins to blister and necrose, and there may be crepitus. The diagnosis should be made clinically; however, patients will have leukocytosis and may have air on imaging or enhancing fascia on CT. Organisms known to cause necrotizing soft tissue infections include classically group A *Streptococcus*, but also *Bacteroides*, *Escherichia coli*, *Staphylococcus*, and *Enterococcus*. *Clostridium*

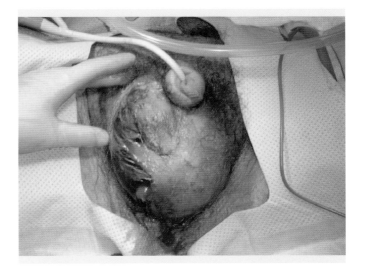

FIGURE 33-14. Fournier's gangrene (from Brunicardi FC, Andersen DK, Billiar TR, et al., (eds.), *Schwartz's Principles of Surgery*. 10th ed. New York, NY: McGraw-Hill; 2014: Fig. 40-9. Copyright © The McGraw-Hill Companies, Inc. All rights reserved).

perfringens is most commonly found in gas gangrene infections. If a necrotizing soft tissue infection is suspected, rapid resuscitation and emergent surgical debridement, as well as broad-spectrum antibiosis, should be initiated.

BIBLIOGRAPHY

Parrett BM, Winer J, Orgill DP. Surgical management of soft tissue infections. In: Guyuron B, Eriksson E, Persing JA, eds. *Plastic Surgery*. Edinburgh, Scotland: Saunders/Elsevier; 2009:175.

22. **(B)** Tissue expansion stretches cells and then leads to cell proliferation, returning the tissue to its baseline tension. Important properties include creep (the skin stretches in response to a constant load) and stress relaxation (the amount of force necessary to stretch the skin decreases over time). In this process, the epidermis thickens and the dermis thins. The capsule that forms around the expander is highly vascular, making the expanded tissue essentially a delayed skin flap. If an expander is placed under muscles, the muscle thins.

    Tissue expanders come in different shapes and sizes, with integrated or remote ports. The expander is placed over an area with skeletal support and is intermittently filled with saline, being careful not to fill to the point of skin compromise. Tissue expansion can be used for reconstruction of the scalp, face, trunk, breast, and extremities. Complications are not uncommon and include infection, exposure, and skin flap ischemia.

BIBLIOGRAPHY

Bauer BS. Tissue expansion. In: Thorne CH, Beasley RW, Aston SJ, Bartlett SP, Gurtner GC, Spear SL, eds. *Grabb and Smith's Plastic Surgery*. Philadelphia, PA: Lippincott-Raven; 2007:84–90; 2006: Chapter 10.
Fang RC, Mustoe TA. Structure and function of the skin. In: Guyuron B, Eriksson E, Persing JA, eds. *Plastic Surgery*. Edinburgh, Scotland: Saunders/Elsevier; 2009:109.

23. **(A)** Collagen comprises 25% of proteins in the body. Type I collagen is the most common type and is present in skin, bones, tendons, and ligaments. Up to 90% of collagen in the skin is type I collagen. Increased levels of type III collagen are present in embryos and in early wound healing. Types II and XI are present in cartilage, and type IV composes basement membranes.

    Wound healing consists of three phases: inflammatory, proliferative, and remodeling. The inflammatory phase begins at the time of injury, with vasoconstriction and hemostasis by the clotting cascade. A provisional fibrin matrix is produced, and inflammatory cells are activated. Neutrophils are present during the first few days but are not imperative for wound healing. Macrophages are involved within 48–72 h and are critical for wound healing by phagocytosis of bacteria and by stimulating growth factor production. The proliferative phase occurs from days 4–21 and consists of replacement of the provisional matrix with granulation tissue. Fibroblasts predominate. Finally, the remodeling phase takes place from 21 days to up to 1 year. Wound contraction is mediated by myofibroblasts, and type III collagen is replaced by type I. The wound has approximately 20% the strength of normal skin at week 3. By week 6, the wound has at least 80% of its eventual strength, which will only be 70–80% that of normal skin.

    Major factors that inhibit wound healing include infection, foreign body, hypoxia (including smoking), radiation, malnutrition, cancer, advanced age, diabetes, immunosuppression (including steroid use), and chemotherapy.

BIBLIOGRAPHY

Gupta S, Lawrence WT. Wound healing: normal and abnormal mechanisms and closure techniques. In: O'Leary JP, ed. *The Physiologic Basis of Surgery*. Philadelphia, PA: Lippincott Williams & Wilkins; 2008:150–158.
Gurtner GC. Wound healing: normal and abnormal. In: Thorne CH, Beasley RW, Aston SJ, Bartlett SP, Gurtner GC, Spear SL, eds. *Grabb and Smith's Plastic Surgery*. Philadelphia, PA: Lippincott-Raven; 2006: Chapter 2.

24. **(C)** Component separation is a procedure involving division of the external oblique fascia and muscle to mobilize the rectus muscle medially to close an abdominal wall defect. The intercostal neurovascular bundles are protected, as they course deep to the internal obliques. The blood supply to the skin should also be respected. This release allows each rectus muscle to be moved up to 9 cm medially.

    Separation of components can be used in conjunction with prosthetic or biologic mesh repair and has also been described as an adjunct to abdominal wall repair with tensor fascia lata (Fig. 33-15).

BIBLIOGRAPHY

Dumanian GA. Abdominal wall reconstruction. In: Thorne CH, Beasley RW, Aston SJ, Bartlett SP, Gurtner GC, Spear SL, eds. *Grabb and Smith's Plastic Surgery*. Philadelphia, PA: Lippincott-Raven; 2007:670–674.

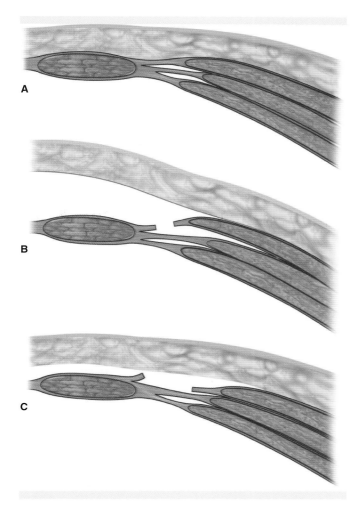

FIGURE 33-15. Separation of components. This demonstrates the division of the external oblique fascia and muscle to allow mobilization of the rectus. (from Zinner MJ, Ashley SW, eds. *Maingot's Abdominal Operations*. 12th ed. New York, NY: McGraw-Hill; 2013: Fig. 7-17. Copyright © The McGraw-Hill Companies, Inc. All rights reserved.)

Seymour NE, Bell RL. Abdominal wall, omentum, mesentery, and retroperitoneum. In: Brunicardi F, Andersen DK, Billiar TR, et al., (eds.), *Schwartz's Principles of Surgery*. 10th ed. New York, NY: McGraw-Hill; 2014: Chapter 35.

25. **(C)** Gynecomastia is an increase in male breast tissue (Fig. 33-16). Incidence is trimodal, occurring in infants, adolescents, and the elderly. While some cases are attributed to hormonal imbalances, medication (antiandrogens, anabolic steroids, highly active antiretroviral therapy [HAART], cimetidine, digoxin), illicit drugs (marijuana), adrenal, liver, pituitary, thyroid, renal, lung, or testicular disease, the most common cause is idiopathic. Patients with gynecomastia do not have an increased risk of breast cancer unless they also have Klinefelter syndrome.

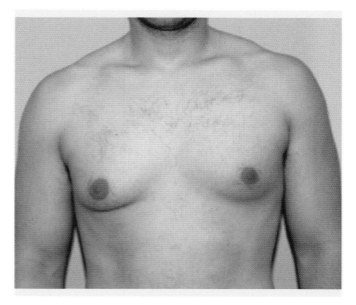

FIGURE 33-16. Gynecomastia (from Kuerer HM, ed. *Kuerer's Breast Surgical Oncology*. New York, NY: McGraw-Hill; 2010: Fig. 70-3. Copyright © The McGraw-Hill Companies, Inc. All rights reserved).

A detailed history and physical is necessary to rule out the causes of gynecomastia mentioned and, if found, to treat them. Patients with new gynecomastia and a normal history and physical should be observed for up to a year, as many patients have spontaneous resolution. After this period, surgical treatment, including liposuction, direct excision, or a combination, can be pursued.

BIBLIOGRAPHY

Karp NS. Gynecomastia. In: Thorne CH, Beasley RW, Aston SJ, Bartlett SP, Gurtner GC, Spear SL, eds. *Grabb and Smith's Plastic Surgery*. Philadelphia, PA: Lippincott-Raven; 2007:616–620.

26. **(C)** A panniculectomy is performed in high-risk patients when the pannus becomes so large that it inhibits ambulation and activities of daily living. In this case, the procedure is strictly functional. The umbilicus is often excised, and rectus plication is not performed. A large pannus often results in lymphedema, which can increase risk of infections. The large pannus contributes to recurrent panniculitis, or intertrigo. These are also indications for panniculectomy.

During panniculectomy, the pannus may be suspended, allowing venous drainage and preventing the weight on the chest and abdomen from impairing ventilation. Large vessels should be expected and swiftly ligated. Postoperatively, there is a high risk of wound-healing complications as well as a risk of deep vein thrombosis.

BIBLIOGRAPHY

Rubin JP, Gusenoff J. Bodylifts and post massive weight loss body contouring. In: Guyuron B, Eriksson E, Persing JA, eds. *Plastic Surgery*. Edinburgh, Scotland: Saunders/Elsevier; 2009:1627–1654.

27. **(D)** The most common donor site for autologous breast reconstruction is the abdomen, as the donor site is well hidden and donor tissue may be plentiful. Newer techniques such as the Deep inferior epigastric perforator (DIEP) flap spare the morbidity of abdominal muscle harvest. The patient does not need to be repositioned after her mastectomy. Abdominal flaps may be pedicled or free and may harvest muscle (as in the TRAM flap) or skin and subcutaneous tissue only (as in the DIEP flap). Relative contraindications include central abdominal liposuction and abdominal scars, indicating the epigastric vessels may be compromised. Most women with normal BMI have adequate donor tissue, especially if they have had children.

    While abdominal flap reconstruction is often desirable, many autologous alternatives exist. These include reconstruction with the latissimus dorsi, the gluteal flap, anterior lateral thigh flap, and Ruben's flap over the iliac crest.

BIBLIOGRAPHY

Elliott LF. Breast reconstruction-free flap techniques. In: Thorne CH, Beasley RW, Aston SJ, Bartlett SP, Gurtner GC, Spear SL, eds. *Grabb and Smith's Plastic Surgery*. Philadelphia, PA: Lippincott-Raven; 2007:648–656.

28. **(D)** Indications for breast reduction include chronic neck, back, and shoulder pain and recurrent skin maceration or infections. The most common techniques of breast reduction include the vertical approach and inverted T technique, leaving scars around the nipple areolar complex, vertically, and also horizontally in the inverted T procedure (Fig. 33-17). Patients should be aware that they may have significant scarring. Most patients, however, report excellent physical and psychological outcomes.

    Patients should be counseled about the risk of decreased nipple sensation and inability to breastfeed, although about 85% of patients recover near-normal sensation, and about 50% of patients are able to breastfeed after breast reduction. Other complications include hematoma, seroma, infection, and nipple-areolar necrosis. Careful attention to the nipple blood supply is important to prevent nipple-areolar necrosis. In patients with very large breasts, consideration should be made to excise and graft the nipple in its new location.

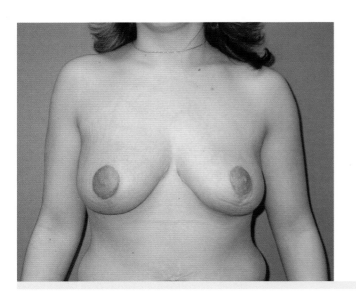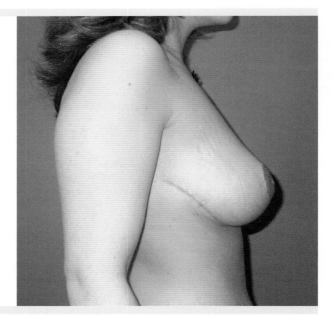

FIGURE 33-17. Inverted T-shaped scars after breast reduction (from Brunicardi FC, Andersen DK, Billiar TR, et al., (eds.), *Schwartz's Principles of Surgery*. 10th ed. New York, NY: McGraw-Hill; 2014: Figs. 45-61C, 45-61D. Copyright © The McGraw-Hill Companies, Inc. All rights reserved).

BIBLIOGRAPHY

Hall-Findlay EJ. Breast reduction. In: Guyuron B, Eriksson E, Persing JA, eds. *Plastic Surgery*. Edinburgh, Scotland: Saunders/Elsevier; 2009:1575–1590.

Hall-Findlay EJ. Vertical reduction mammoplasty. In: Thorne CH, Beasley RW, Aston SJ, Bartlett SP, Gurtner GC, Spear SL, eds. *Grabb and Smith's Plastic Surgery*. Philadelphia, PA: Lippincott-Raven; 2007:604–615.

Spear SL. Breast reduction: inverted-T technique. In: Thorne CH, Beasley RW, Aston SJ, Bartlett SP, Gurtner GC, Spear SL, eds. *Grabb and Smith's Plastic Surgery*. Philadelphia, PA: Lippincott-Raven; 2007:593–603.

29. **(B)** Full-thickness grafts are a good option for facial burn reconstruction. Although they have greater primary (immediate) contraction compared to split-thickness grafts, they have less secondary contracture. Granulating wounds healing by secondary intention have the greatest amount of contracture and increased hypertrophic scarring.

   Compared to split-thickness skin grafts, full-thickness grafts are less shiny, have fewer pigmentation changes, and retain epithelial appendages. They also have improved sensation. Full-thickness grafts require a well-vascularized bed, however, and donor sites are limited.

BIBLIOGRAPHY

Donelan MB. Principles of burn reconstruction. In: Thorne CH, Beasley RW, Aston SJ, Bartlett SP, Gurtner GC, Spear SL, eds. *Grabb and Smith's Plastic Surgery*. Philadelphia, PA: Lippincott-Raven; 2007:150–157.

Thorne CH. Techniques and principles in plastic surgery. In: Thorne CH, Beasley RW, Aston SJ, Bartlett SP, Gurtner GC, Spear SL, eds. *Grabb and Smith's Plastic Surgery*. Philadelphia, PA: Lippincott-Raven; 2007:7–8.

30. **(B)** Pressure ulcers develop from "unrelieved pressure over a bony prominence." These are staged as follows: I with erythema, II with dermal injury, III with subcutaneous tissue injury, and IV with muscle or bone involvement.

   Pressure relief is necessary in the treatment of pressure sores, with even 5 min of relief every 2 h preventing injury in animal models. Important adjuncts include proper nutrition, decolonization by debridement or frequent dressing changes, and control of spasm and contractures. Most wounds are contaminated but not infected and do not require chronic antibiotics. Definitive treatment consists of surgical debridement, ostectomy (removal of the bony prominence), and closure, often with a musculocutaneous or fasciocutaneous flap. Recurrence rates are high; therefore, surgery should not be performed unless predisposing conditions and social issues have been rectified.

BIBLIOGRAPHY

Bauer JD, Mancoll JS, Phillips LG. Pressure sores. In: Thorne CH, Beasley RW, Aston SJ, Bartlett SP, Gurtner GC, Spear SL, eds. *Grabb and Smith's Plastic Surgery*. Philadelphia, PA: Lippincott-Raven; 2007:150–157.

31. **(A)** Patients can lose large volumes of blood at the scene from a large scalp laceration and may even exsanguinate due to the high density of vessels in the scalp. Although scalp laceration bleeding frequently stops spontaneously or with the application of pressure, if bleeding does not stop immediately, prompt surgical attention must be directed to the wound. Typically, this involves suture ligation of bleeding vessels from the occipital artery or the temporal artery. Closure facilitates hemostasis. In a patient with any traumatic injury, hypovolemic shock must be anticipated and treated immediately if it occurs. Intracranial trauma may also occur concomitantly and therefore should be on the list of differential diagnoses.

BIBLIOGRAPHY

Turnage B, Maull K. Scalp laceration: an obvious "occult" cause of shock. *South Med J* 2000;93(3):265–266.

Yap LH, Langstein HN. Reconstruction of the scalp, calvarium, and forehead. In: Thorne CH, Beasley RW, Aston SJ, Bartlett SP, Gurtner GC, Spear SL, eds. *Grabb and Smith's Plastic Surgery*. Philadelphia, PA: Lippincott-Raven; 2007:358–364.

32. **(B)** Pectoralis major flaps are the most common flaps for reconstruction of sternal defects. The dominant blood supply is the thoracoacromial artery and venae comitantes, with segmental pedicles from the intercostals branching from the internal mammary artery (Fig. 33-18). The muscle may be advanced, or the dominant pedicle may be divided and the flap turned over on itself, relying on the segmental blood supply. A history of left internal mammary artery harvest would preclude a left-sided pectoralis turnover flap.

   The rectus abdominus pedicled flap would be based on the superior epigastric vessels, which originate from the internal mammaries. The left rectus flap would therefore not be an option in this patient.

   The omental flap is also a well-described option for chest wall reconstruction, but because this patient has a history of gastrectomy, the gastroepiploic vessels may not be intact.

   Sternal infections should be treated with wide debridement prior to reconstruction.

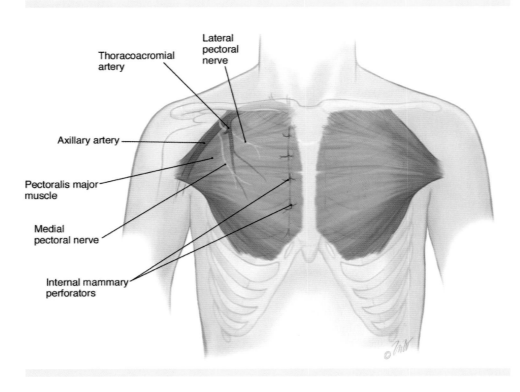

FIGURE 33-18. Pectoral anatomy and vasculature (from Sugarbaker DJ, Bueno R, Krasna MJ, Mentzer SJ, Zellos L, eds. *Adult Chest Surgery*. New York, NY: McGraw-Hill; 2009: Fig. 117-2A. Copyright © The McGraw-Hill Companies, Inc. All rights reserved).

BIBLIOGRAPHY

Chang RR. Thoracic reconstruction. In: Thorne CH, Beasley RW, Aston SJ, Bartlett SP, Gurtner GC, Spear SL, eds. *Grabb and Smith's Plastic Surgery*. Philadelphia, PA: Lippincott-Raven; 2007:150–157.

33. **(C)** The sartorius flap is first line for coverage of exposed femoral vessels or grafts. It is an expendable muscle and often is available and present within the wound. Its blood supply is segmental, and its skin paddle is unreliable, so skin should not be carried with the muscle. The sartorius muscle flap may be difficult to transfer reliably after groin surgery due to scarring in the region as well as unreliable blood supply. In that case, other local or regional flaps are available.

Application of wet-to-dry dressings would not be sufficient to protect the femoral vessels. Extreme caution should be used when placing a V.A.C. dressing over vessels, as a patient can rapidly exsanguinate if the anastomosis is disrupted. Furthermore, significant infection is a contraindication to V.A.C. therapy.

BIBLIOGRAPHY

Galiano RD, Mustoe TA. Wound care. In: Thorne CH, Beasley RW, Aston SJ, Bartlett SP, Gurtner GC, Spear SL, eds. *Grabb and Smith's Plastic Surgery*. Philadelphia, PA: Lippincott-Raven; 2007:27.
Zenn MR, Jones G. *Reconstructive Surgery*. St. Louis, MO: Quality Medical; 2012:1468–1481, 1554–1582.

34. **(A)** This most likely represents an orbital floor fracture or "blowout fracture," which occurs following trauma involving the orbit (Figs. 33-19 and 33-20). A complete visual exam should be performed, and an ophthalmology consultation may be necessary. A CT scan of the face should be obtained. Mechanical entrapment of the inferior rectus muscle causing diplopia is an indication for surgical repair.

A LeFort III fracture is a fracture of the maxilla, involving the zygomatic arch, lateral orbital wall, and nasofrontal region.

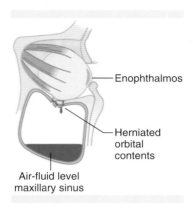

FIGURE 33-19. Orbital floor fracture schematic (from Tintinalli JE, Stapczynski JS, Ma OJ, Cline DM, Cydulka RK, Meckler GD, American College of Emergency Physicians, eds. *Tintinalli's Emergency Medicine: A Comprehensive Study Guide.* 7th ed. New York, NY: McGraw-Hill; 2011: Fig. 256-9. Copyright © The McGraw-Hill Companies, Inc. All rights reserved).

BIBLIOGRAPHY

Hollier L, Kelley P. Soft tissue and skeletal injuries of the face. In: Thorne CH, Beasley RW, Aston SJ, Bartlett SP, Gurtner GC, Spear SL, eds. *Grabb and Smith's Plastic Surgery.* Philadelphia, PA: Lippincott-Raven; 2007:316–323.

35. **(A)** Ten structures are present in the carpal tunnel: the median nerve, four flexor digitorum superficialis tendons, four flexor digitorum profundus tendons, and the

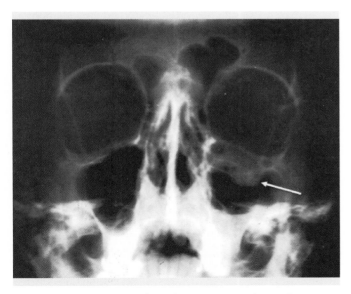

FIGURE 33-20. Orbital floor fracture x-ray (from Blowout fracture. In *Exploring Essential Radiology: Head.* Copyright © The McGraw-Hill Companies, Inc. All rights reserved).

flexor pollicis longus tendon. Patients typically present with numbness in the distribution of the median nerve (thumb, index, long, and radial ring fingers), sparing the base of the palm because the palmar cutaneous branch is subcutaneous and does not pass through the carpal tunnel. Symptoms are often worse at night, awakening patients from sleep, and may progress to involve weakness of the thumb.

Provocative maneuvers include carpal compression and passive wrist flexion (Phalen test). Electrodiagnostic studies usually correspond with the examination and can rule out other sites of median nerve compression. Treatment consists of transection of the transverse carpal ligament (carpal tunnel release) and antebrachial fascia (Fig. 33-21).

BIBLIOGRAPHY

Effron CR, Beasley RW. Compression Neuropathies in the Upper Limb and Electrophysiologic Studies. In: Thorne CH, Beasley RW, Aston SJ, Bartlett SP, Gurtner GC, Spear SL, eds. *Grabb and Smith's Plastic Surgery.* Philadelphia, PA: Lippincott-Raven; 2007:830–831.

36. **(C)** Human bites to the hand are common when punching a person in the mouth. These wounds occur over the metacarpophalangeal joints, and radiographs should be obtained to confirm that a fracture or foreign body (tooth) is not also present.

These wounds should be irrigated and debrided, and broad-spectrum antibiotic therapy should be started prophylactically. Coverage should include *Eikenella corrodens*, a common anaerobe in human saliva, as well as S. aureus and *Streptococcus viridans*.

Cat and dog bites also have a high risk of infection, and antibiotic therapy should cover *Staphylococcus, Streptococcus, Bacteroides,* and *Pasteurella multocida*.

Other common hand infections include paronychia, an infection of the soft tissues around the nail; felon, a fingertip pulp abscess; and suppurative flexor tenosynovitis. Kanavel signs (fusiform swelling, flexed finger posture, flexor tendon sheath tenderness, and pain with passive extension) are often present in patients with suppurative flexor tenosynovitis; these patients usually require operative drainage.

BIBLIOGRAPHY

Chao JJ, Morrison BA. Infections of the upper limb. In: Thorne CH, Beasley RW, Aston SJ, Bartlett SP, Gurtner GC, Spear SL, eds. *Grabb and Smith's Plastic Surgery.* Philadelphia, PA: Lippincott-Raven; 2007:817–825.

37. **(D)** Arterial lines may cause injury to the radial artery by causing arterial laceration, intimal flaps,

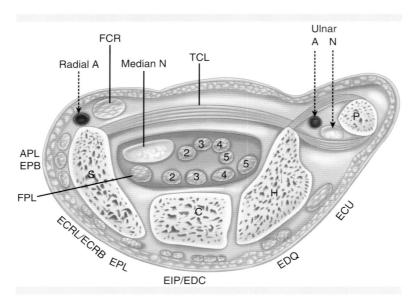

FIGURE 33-21. Anatomy of the wrist, FCR = flexor carpi radialis; TCL = transverse carpal ligament; APL = abductor pollicis longus; FPL = flexor pollicis longus; ECRL = extensor carpi radialis longus; ECRB = extensor carpi radialis brevis; EPL = extensor pollicis longus; EIP = extensor indicis proprius; EDC = extensor digitorum comminus; EDQ = extensor digitorum quinti; ECU = extensor carpi ulnaris (from Brunicardi FC, Andersen DK, Billiar TR, et al., (eds.), *Schwartz's Principles of Surgery*. 10th ed. New York, NY: McGraw-Hill; 2014: Fig. 44-3. Copyright © The McGraw-Hill Companies, Inc. All rights reserved).

hematoma, pseudoaneurysm, arteriovenous fistula, or thrombosis. An Allen test should be performed prior to radial arterial line placement to confirm whether the palmar arch is intact. This test consists of compressing the radial and ulnar arteries, having the patient clench the hand several times, and releasing pressure on one of the arteries, watching for quick return of blood flow to the hand. The examination is then repeated, releasing pressure on the opposite artery. An abnormal exam suggests that the collateral circulation may be inadequate.

Acute ischemia of the hand usually presents with pain, cool temperature, and pallor or petechiae. A palpable pulse does not rule out a diagnosis of ischemia. Acute ischemia in this setting is treated with thrombolysis or exploration in the operating room with thrombectomy and repair or reconstruction of injured vessels. Results after repair, whether primary, with vein patch, or graft, are excellent.

Snuffbox tenderness is classically associated with scaphoid fractures and would not contribute to vascular compromise.

BIBLIOGRAPHY

Koman LA, Smith BP, Smith TL, Ruch DS, Li Z. Vascular disorders. In: Wolfe SW, Hotchkiss RN, Pederson WC, Kozin SH, eds. *Green's Operative Hand Surgery*. Philadelphia, PA: Elsevier; 2011:2207–2218.

38. **(B)** The most common complication of a rhytidectomy, or facelift (Fig. 33-22), is hematoma (3–4% of all cases), which often presents as anxiety and increasing pain unilaterally. The dressing should be removed, and the hematoma should be evacuated. Other complications include skin slough, most often in the retroauricular area; hypertrophic scarring, which is more common with high-tension closures; and rarely, facial nerve injury. The facial nerve is more at risk when dissection of the superficial musculoaponeurotic system (SMAS) is performed.

BIBLIOGRAPHY

Thorne CH. Facelift. In: Thorne CH, Beasley RW, Aston SJ, Bartlett SP, Gurtner GC, Spear SL, eds. *Grabb and Smith's Plastic Surgery*. Philadelphia, PA: Lippincott-Raven; 2007:498–508.

39. **(B)** Replantation is generally indicated in patients with sharp amputations of the thumb, multiple digits, and the hand/wrist/forearm. Absolute contraindications include other life-threatening injuries or comorbidities making the patient unfit for prolonged surgery. Relative contraindications include

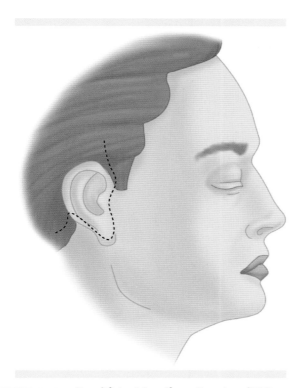

FIGURE 33-22. Facelift incision (from Brunicardi FC, Andersen DK, Billiar TR, et al., (eds.), *Schwartz's Principles of Surgery*. 9th ed. New York, NY: McGraw-Hill; 2010: Fig. 45-54. Copyright © The McGraw-Hill Companies, Inc. All rights reserved).

multiple-level amputations, avulsion of the digital arteries, prolonged warm ischemia time (over 6 h), massive contamination, and single-digit amputation in an adult (except for the thumb).

The index finger is particularly expendable, as the middle finger is intuitively substituted for pinch, giving a functional result with revision amputation. Replantation may yield satisfactory results when the injury is distal to the insertion of the flexor digitorum superficialis (FDS) tendon on the middle phalanx, while injuries proximal to this will be less functional due to complications associated with tendon repair at this level.

Local flaps can be used in tip amputations with exposed bone. These include advancements within the injured finger (V-Y or Moberg), as well as cross-finger flaps and thenar flaps.

Vascularized wounds can be treated with skin grafts.

BIBLIOGRAPHY

Jones NF. Replantation in the upper extremity. In: Thorne CH, Beasley RW, Aston SJ, Bartlett SP, Gurtner GC, Spear SL, eds. *Grabb and Smith's Plastic Surgery*. Philadelphia, PA: Lippincott-Raven; 2007:868–869.

Tymchak J. Soft-tissue reconstruction of the hand. In: Thorne CH, Beasley RW, Aston SJ, Bartlett SP, Gurtner GC, Spear SL, eds. *Grabb and Smith's Plastic Surgery*. Philadelphia, PA: Lippincott-Raven; 2007:771–780.

CHAPTER 34

PEDIATRIC SURGERY

MARIA MICHAILIDOU AND CATHERINE M. COSENTINO

QUESTIONS

1. Which of the following statements regarding fetal physiology is correct?
   (A) The circulatory pattern of the fetus is two ventricles working in series, rather than in parallel as in an adult.
   (B) The right ventricle ejects highly oxygenated blood to the most metabolically active tissues.
   (C) There are three components of venous return in the fetus: superior vena cava (SVC), inferior vena cava (IVC), and pulmonary veins.
   (D) Renal blood flow is 3–5% of fetal cardiac output.
   (E) Fetal water homeostasis relies primarily on fluid generated by the fetal lung.

2. A full-term 2-month-old presents with failure to thrive, tachypnea, and recurrent pulmonary infections. A holosystolic machine-like murmur is auscultated on physical exam. An echocardiogram is shown in Fig. 34-1. Which of the following is true about this condition?
   (A) It presents most commonly in full-term neonates.
   (B) Surgical closure should be reserved for symptomatic patients.
   (C) The patent ductus arteriosus (PDA) connects the main pulmonary trunk with the descending aorta just proximal to the origin of the left subclavian artery.
   (D) The most common cause of death in premature infants with PDA is pulmonary hypertension.
   (E) In full-term newborns and older children, the ductus arteriosus is divided rather than ligated.

3. Which of the statements regarding nutrition best applies to an infant/child?
   (A) A neonate requires approximately 90 kcal/kg/d and 1 g of protein/kg per day for growth.
   (B) Newborns lose weight during the first 1–2 weeks of life.
   (C) The preferred enteral diet for the full-term infant is formula milk, which provides more calories and minerals than human milk.

   (D) Enteral feedings are appropriate in patients with sepsis, hypotension, apnea, or bradycardia.
   (E) Substitution of omega-3 fatty acids for omega-6 lipid emulsions can prevent or reverse cholestasis associated with total parenteral nutrition (TPN) in children.

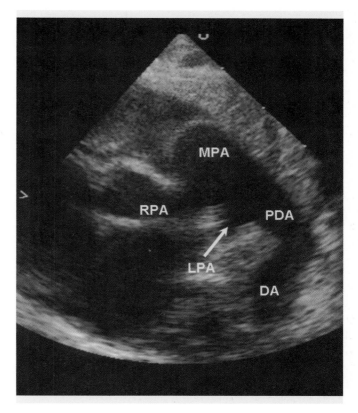

FIGURE 34-1. Echocardiogram high parasternal view; AI = aortic isthmus; DAO = descending aorta; LPA = left pulmonary artery; MPA = middle pulmonary artery; RPA = right pulmonary artery. Used with permission from William Ravekes, MD, Division of Pediatric Cardiology, The Johns Hopkins Hospital.

4. In a newborn baby with type E tracheoesophageal fistula, what surgical approach is indicated?
   (A) Right thoracotomy
   (B) Left thoracotomy
   (C) Right cervical incision
   (D) Midline laparotomy
   (E) Endoscopic (endobronchial)

5. A 5-day-old, 26-week premature baby develops sudden-onset feeding intolerance and bloody stools. Over the following 12 h, abdominal distension ensues; the abdominal radiograph is shown in Fig. 34-2. Which of the following is true regarding this condition?

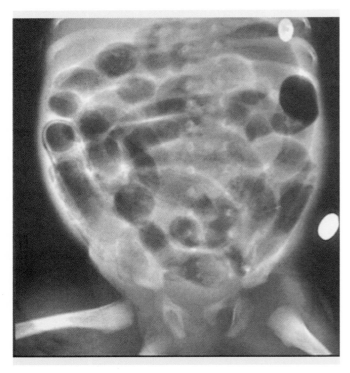

FIGURE 34-2. Abdominal x-ray in a premature baby.

   (A) The jejunum is the most common site of stricture formation.
   (B) Surgical intervention is mandated in all cases.
   (C) Surgical treatment includes resection of the diseased bowel with primary anastomosis.
   (D) Of these cases, 90% have been reported after the initiation of enteral feedings.
   (E) The disease is inherited in an autosomal recessive pattern.

6. A 6-week-old child presents with bilious emesis. Which of the following is the appropriate next step?
   (A) Operative management
   (B) Computed tomography (CT) of the abdomen/pelvis
   (C) Upper gastrointestinal (UGI) series with small bowel follow-through
   (D) Nutrition/dietician consultation
   (E) Intravenous fluid bolus

7. In counseling parents concerning abdominal wall defects, which of the following characteristics distinguishes an omphalocele from gastroschisis?
   (A) The abdominal wall defect is to the right of an intact umbilical cord.
   (B) There is no sac.
   (C) The liver and spleen rarely herniate through the defect.
   (D) The mesentery of the herniated bowel may be compromised as it passes through the umbilical ring.
   (E) Major associations with congenital malformations.

8. The chest radiograph (Fig. 34-3) demonstrates a surgically correctable cause of respiratory distress. Which is true regarding the possible differential diagnosis?

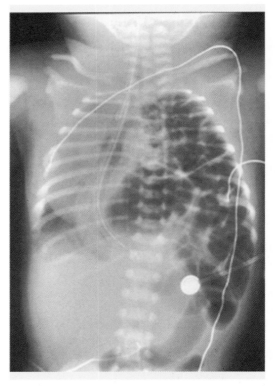

FIGURE 34-3. Chest radiograph in a newborn with respiratory distress.

(A) A diaphragmatic eventration generally refers to the attenuation of the lateral portion of the diaphragm.

(B) Congenital diaphragmatic hernia (CDH) can be diagnosed prenatally by ultrasound as early as 12 weeks' gestation.

(C) CDH is a surgical emergency.

(D) Morgagni hernias account for the majority of CDHs.

(E) Decreasing pulmonary hypertension and decompressing the gastrointestinal (GI) tract are the first lines of treatment in a newborn with CDH.

9. A 3-week-old, full-term, firstborn male develops forceful, nonbilious emesis. An ultrasound of the abdomen is shown in Fig. 34-4. Which of the following is true?

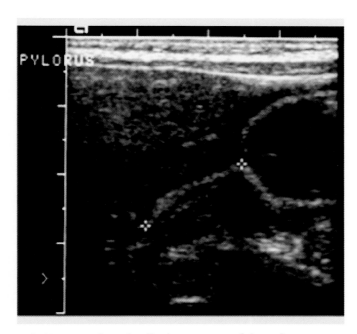

FIGURE 34-4. Longitudinal sonogram of the pylorus.

(A) Laboratory studies will reveal metabolic acidosis.

(B) Correction of metabolic abnormalities must precede surgical intervention.

(C) Pyloric channel length of 8 mm confirms the diagnosis.

(D) A UGI series will show a classic "double-bubble" sign.

(E) Patients commonly suffer from delayed gastric emptying in adulthood.

10. A 30-week-old infant presents with persistent symptoms consistent with irritability, frequent vomiting, apnea, history of aspiration pneumonia, and failure to thrive.

Despite medical therapy, these symptoms continue. Which statement is correct?

(A) Transient lower esophageal sphincter relaxation is the predominant mechanism, and surgical therapy is indicated once intestinal malrotation has been ruled out.

(B) The majority of infants and children with this problem do not respond to medical management due to the hypertonicity of the esophageal sphincter mechanism.

(C) The etiology of this disease is related to pharyngogastric incompetence, and treatment is related to bypassing this mechanism with insertion of a feeding gastrostomy tube.

(D) Most infants and children are not neurologically impaired, and treatment is based on changing feeding volume and using feed thickeners to reduce liquid reflux.

(E) Promoting factors include a bout of viral gastroenteritis or upper respiratory infection, and treatment is based on eradicating these infectious agents.

11. A mother brings her 9-month-old infant to a small-town emergency department; she describes a 4-h period when the infant developed cycles of abdominal discomfort that occurred every 5–10 min. She notes that during the episodes of pain, the infant screams and draws up her legs. What is true about this condition?

(A) The majority of patients present with the triad of intermittent abdominal pain, currant jelly stool, and palpable abdominal mass.

(B) Surgical intervention is mandated after one recurrent manual reduction.

(C) Most pediatric cases are idiopathic.

(D) Abdominal x-ray confirms the diagnosis.

(E) The most common site of occurrence is at the ligament of Trietz.

12. An otherwise-healthy 2-year-old male presents to the emergency department with bright red blood in the stool, and laboratory studies indicate anemia. A technetium-99m pertechnetate radionuclide study is performed (Fig. 34-5). Which of the following is true about this condition?

(A) The majority of patients will become symptomatic by 2 years of age.

(B) Most ectopic mucosa is made of pancreatic tissue.

(C) Most patients present with obstruction.

(D) This results from failure of the omphalomesenteric duct to regress.

(E) This is most commonly found on the mesenteric border of the small intestine.

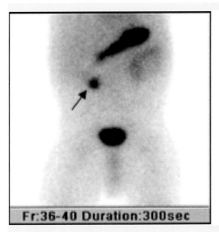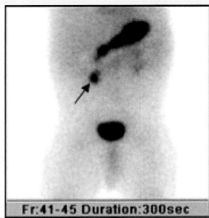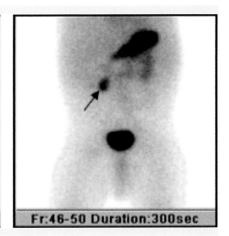

| Fr:36-40 Duration:300sec | Fr:41-45 Duration:300sec | Fr:46-50 Duration:300sec |

FIGURE 34-5. Nuclear medicine study of the abdomen (from Hill WP, ed. *Pediatric Practice: Gastroenterology.* New York, NY: McGraw-Hill; 2010: Fig. 9-5. Copyright © The McGraw-Hill Companies, Inc. All rights reserved).

13. A full-term newborn infant presents with abdominal distention and absence of meconium passage in the first 24 h after birth. A contrast enema is obtained (Fig. 34-6). Which of the following is true about this condition?

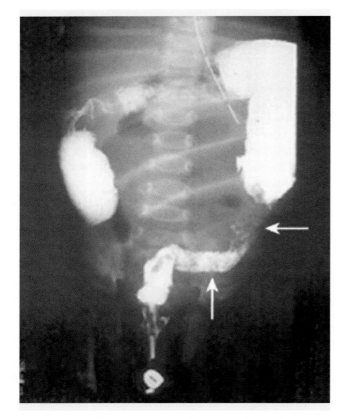

FIGURE 34-6. Contrast enema. Arrows indicate decompressed bowel.

(A) A contrast enema is the best study to confirm the diagnosis.
(B) Emergent exploratory laparotomy and colostomy creation are warranted.
(C) Initial treatment involves fluid resuscitation, nasogastric decompression, and rectal irrigation.
(D) This condition results from viscid, protein-rich meconium causing an intraluminal obstruction in the distal colon.
(E) Levelling colostomy should be performed.

14. A 3-week-old infant has had persistent jaundice since birth. The physical examination reveals an active infant with obvious jaundice, mild hepatomegaly, and the presence of acholic stools. Abdominal ultrasound shows absent gallbladder. The HIDA (hepatic iminodiacetic acid) scan (Fig. 34-7) suggests what abnormality?
(A) Choledochal cyst
(B) Biliary dyskinesia
(C) Choledocholithiasis
(D) Biliary fistula
(E) Biliary atresia

15. What is the most appropriate treatment for the condition described in question 14?
(A) Hepatic transplantation on availability of a donor liver
(B) A hepaticoportoenterostomy (Roux-en-Y portoenterostomy) at approximately 4 months of age
(C) A Roux-en-Y portoenterostomy prior to 2 months of age
(D) A Roux-en-Y hepaticojejunostomy prior to 2 months of age
(E) An emergent cholecystectomy

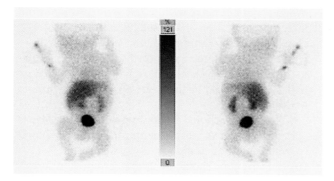

FIGURE 34-7. Hepatobiliary nuclear scintigram shows images taken at 1 min (A), 15 min (B), 30 min (C), 60 min (D), 4 h (E), and 24 h (F) after tracer injection. There was excretion into the bladder (small arrow) via the kidneys from backup of tracer in the blood pool. Large arrow shows excretion of radiotracer into the liver. (from Eng K, Alkhouri N. Neonatal cholestasis. In: Usatine RP, Sabella C, Smith M, Mayeaux EJ Jr, Chumley HS, Appachi E, eds. *The Color Atlas of Pediatrics*. New York, NY: McGraw-Hill; 2015: Fig. 61-1. Copyright © The McGraw-Hill Companies, Inc. All rights reserved).

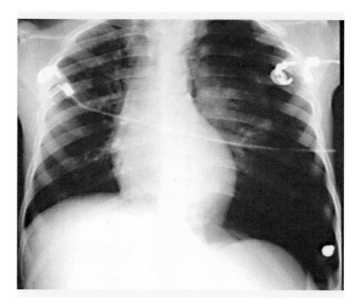

FIGURE 34-8. Chest x-ray.

16. A 2-month-old male presents with persistent jaundice. An ultrasound of the abdomen is obtained that shows a choledochal cyst. Which of the following is true regarding this condition?
    (A) Serial ultrasound examinations are a safe alternative to surgical intervention.
    (B) It mandates surgical excision of the cyst with bilioenteric anastomosis.
    (C) Internal drainage with cystoduodenostomy or cystojejunostomy is the preferred surgical approach.
    (D) Type V involves intrahepatic and extrahepatic duct disease.
    (E) Ultrasound is the most sensitive imaging study for diagnosis.

17. A 5-year-old presents after a fall off a second-story apartment building. The patient is hypotensive and the trauma team is experiencing difficulty obtaining peripheral venous access. What should be done next?
    (A) Place a femoral central venous catheter
    (B) Continue attempts at peripheral access
    (C) Venous surgical cutdown of the saphenous vein
    (D) Umbilical vascular access
    (E) Proximal tibia intraosseous (IO) catheter placement

18. An 8-year-old female is thrown off her horse onto the ground, striking her face and upper torso. Examination reveals an arousable child complaining of

diffuse chest pain and shortness of breath. The chest radiograph is shown in Fig. 34-8. Regarding thoracic trauma in children, which of the following statements is correct?
    (A) Children have a less-compliant chest wall; therefore, they are more susceptible to rib fractures.
    (B) Pulmonary contusions account for the majority of thoracic injuries.
    (C) Immediate blood return of 10 mL/kg after tube thoracostomy in a pediatric patient with hemothorax mandates surgical exploration.
    (D) Hemodynamically stable patients with high suspicion of blunt cardiac injury and abnormal electrocardiogram (ECG) should have an echocardiogram and serial troponin evaluation.
    (E) Blunt diaphragmatic rupture in children usually involves the right hemidiaphragm.

19. An 11-year-old boy is brought to the emergency department with a 6-h history of abdominal pain. He apparently was a restrained backseat passenger involved in a motor vehicle crash earlier that day. No one was injured in the crash, and he did not voice any complaints at the time of the crash. He is hemodynamically normal on arrival, with a mildly distended abdomen and a "seatbelt sign" over his lower abdomen. An abdominal CT demonstrates a grade II spleen injury with moderate free fluid. Concerning diagnostic modalities in pediatric blunt abdominal trauma, which statement is true?

(A) The focused abdominal sonogram for trauma
(FAST) examination in children is poor at identifying organ-specific injury.
(B) The use of intravenous contrast during a CT scan to
evaluate intrathoracic or intra-abdominal trauma is
required.
(C) Laparoscopy has not been shown to be a viable
treatment option in selected pediatric patients with
blunt abdominal trauma.
(D) A CT scan of the abdomen is reliable for the diagnosis of lumbar spine and intestinal injuries.
(E) Diagnostic peritoneal lavage is contraindicated in
children.

20. An 18-month-old girl falls while her right hand is being
held by her mother. She immediately screams and then
refuses to use the right upper extremity. Musculoskeletal
trauma in children is unique in that the growing bone
has remarkable healing potential. Which of the following
statements is correct?
(A) Only the endosteum (inner lining of the bone) is
responsible for new bone formation during fracture
healing.
(B) Plastic deformation of bone must be surgically corrected in children.
(C) Nursemaid's elbow (radial head subluxation)
requires surgical intervention.
(D) The most common site of fracture in children is the
humerus.
(E) Shoulder dislocations in children commonly are
associated with neurologic and vascular injury.

21. A 12-month-old, full-term male is diagnosed with an
inguinal and an umbilical hernia (ring diameter > 2 cm).
During the discussion of pediatric hernias with parents,
select the correct statement from the following:
(A) The most common cause of indirect hernia in this
age group is a connective tissue disorder.
(B) Laparoscopy has aided in evaluation of the
contralateral inguinal area for hernias; routine
laparoscopic evaluation for a patent contralateral
processus vaginalis (PV) should be advocated for all
patients.
(C) The inguinal hernia should be repaired, and the
umbilical defect left alone.
(D) Repair of both inguinal and umbilical hernias
should be made.
(E) Femoral hernias in children are easier to detect
compared to an adult.

22. Worried parents bring in their full-term 18-month-old
infant for evaluation of a unilateral undescended testicle (UDT). On examination, normal male genitalia
with scrotal asymmetry are noted. Despite maneuvers
to detect a retractile testicle, a right testis is not palpable. What should be the next step in this patient's
management?
(A) The patient should be reexamined prior to 2 years
of age because most patients undergo spontaneous
descent of the testicle by 2 years of age.
(B) Laparoscopy should be used to examine for presence and localization of the testicle.
(C) Hormonal therapy with human chorionic gonadotropin (HCG) is necessary.
(D) The testicle should be examined by ultrasound.
(E) Scrotal exploration should be performed.

23. A 5-year-old female presents with bilateral ecchymotic
periorbital areas (see Fig. 34-9). Child abuse has been
suspected, and the primary team consults a pediatric
surgeon as part of the workup. On physical examination,
an abdominal mass is appreciated. The abdominal CT is
shown in Fig. 34-10. Concerning the diagnosis, which
statement is correct?
(A) The tumor originates from the kidney.
(B) The cause of this malignancy has been directly
linked to the tumor suppressor p53 gene product.
(C) Children older than 1 year of age usually experience
more favorable outcomes than children less than 1
year of age.
(D) Management and prognosis can vary significantly
in each scenario and depend on age and stage at
diagnosis, histopathologic classification, and MYCN
amplification status.
(E) It is usually detected at early stages.

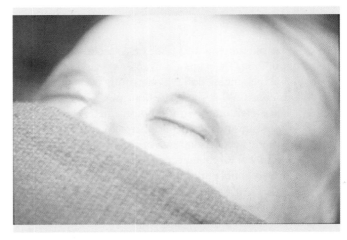

FIGURE 34-9. Periorbital ecchymosis.

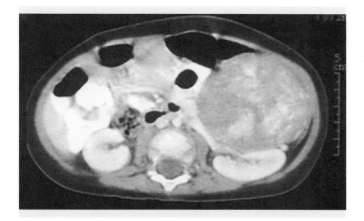

FIGURE 34-10. Abdominal CT in a child obtained with concern for non-accidental trauma.

24. A 3-year-old child presents for evaluation of an abdominal mass that was detected during a bath. The abdominal CT is shown in Fig. 34-11. After determining that the primary tumor is resectable, the following applies during operative management:
    (A) The renal arteries lie anterior to the renal vein, and the left renal vein is posterior to the origin of the inferior mesenteric artery.
    (B) Preresection percutaneous biopsy is superior to open operative exploration and biopsy.
    (C) Neoadjuvant chemotherapy can obscure the post-staging and inadequately define the risk of relapse or recurrence.
    (D) The reliability of imaging contralateral tumors is firmly established in these tumors.
    (E) Partial nephrectomy is never advocated in patients with unilateral Wilms tumor (WT).

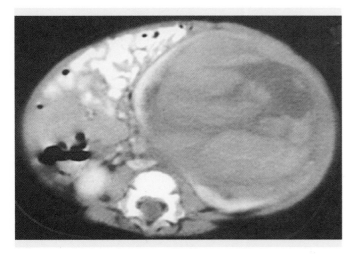

FIGURE 34-11. Abdominal CT in a patient with an abdominal mass.

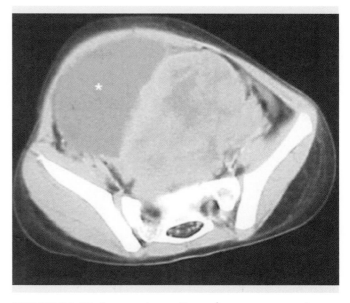

FIGURE 34-12. Large retroperitoneal mass compressing the bladder.

25. A 4-year-old female presented to her primary care physician with fatigue and anorexia over a 2-week period. An abdominal mass was appreciated, and CT confirmed a solid, retroperitoneal lesion causing a mass effect to the bladder (Fig. 34-12; bladder indicated by asterisk).

    Incisional biopsy confirmed the diagnosis of rhabdomyosarcoma (RMS). Which of the following statements is correct?
    (A) The alveolar histologic type accounts for the majority of cases in infants.
    (B) Surgical excision alone offers excellent survival outcomes.
    (C) Around one-third of RMS cases arise in the head and neck area.
    (D) During primary resection of RMS, extent of lymph node dissection affects survival.

26. A 2.5-year-old male is referred to a pediatric surgeon for progressive abdominal enlargement. Physical examination reveals a large intra-abdominal mass within the right upper quadrant. The CT scan is shown in Fig. 34-13. The lesion crosses the midline and extends toward the pelvis. Alpha fetoprotein (AFP) levels are markedly elevated. This lesion most likely represents
    (A) A benign liver tumor
    (B) Metastatic disease
    (C) Teratoma
    (D) Hepatoblastoma
    (E) Hepatocellular carcinoma (HCC)

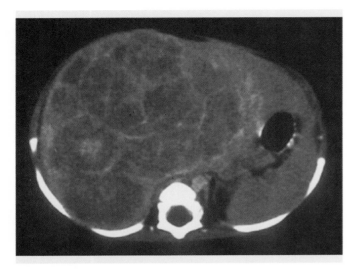

FIGURE 34-13. Abdominal CT in a patient with a right upper quadrant mass.

27. A 16-year-old female presents with increased abdominal girth and now pain. In the past, she has been treated with enemas and laxatives for constipation. Unfortunately, her symptoms have progressed over the last 7 days. AFP, β-HCG, and CA-125 levels are normal. Plain abdominal radiographs reveal laterally displaced small and large bowel and areas of calcification within the central area of the abdomen and lower pelvis. A CT scan of the abdomen and pelvis confirms the diagnosis (Fig. 34-14).

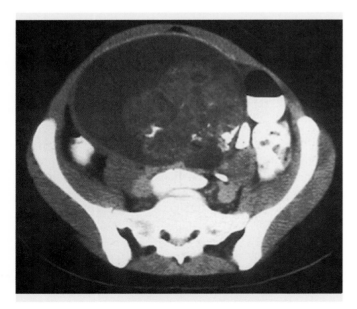

FIGURE 34-14. Abdominal CT in a patient with increased abdominal girth.

Which of the following options should be *avoided* in this patient?
(A) Laparotomy via midline or Pfannenstiel incision
(B) Laparoscopic excision of lesion
(C) Pelvic/retroperitoneal lymph node dissection with lymph node sampling
(D) Inspection of the contralateral ovary
(E) Ultrasound-guided drainage of the lesion

28. The care of pediatric trauma patients differs from the care of adult trauma patients for many reasons. Which of these statements accurately describes the differences between these two patient populations?
(A) Children have a lower ratio of body surface area to weight and therefore are less susceptible to hypothermia.
(B) The pediatric skeletal system has areas of growth and remodeling that make bones less susceptible to injury.
(C) Children have greater physiologic reserve than adults and do not manifest signs of shock until they have lost more than 45% of their blood volume.
(D) Children's torsos are broad and shallow, providing greater protection of solid organs.
(E) The body of a child is very elastic, and energy can be transferred, creating internal injuries without significant external signs.

29. The signs of hypovolemia in children differ from those of an adult because
(A) A child will have minimal signs of shock with a blood loss of 20%
(B) The presence of hypotension in a child suggests a blood loss of 30%
(C) Poor skin perfusion is not a reliable indicator of blood loss in children
(D) A child's circulating blood volume is more than 100 mL/kg
(E) A systolic blood pressure of 40 mmHg is appropriate in children less than 6 months of age

30. A 10-month-old female presents after involvement in a motor vehicle crash. On initial examination, her heart rate is 220 bpm, her systolic blood pressure is 80 mmHg, she is difficult to arouse, and her skin is cyanotic. The appropriate steps for resuscitation include
(A) 10 mL/kg bolus of warm saline solution
(B) Saline administration until her urine output is greater than 3 mL/kg/h

(C) A 20-mL/kg bolus of packed red blood cells (PRBCs) if her vital signs do not normalize after one saline bolus

(D) Continued resuscitation until her heart rate is less than 100 bpm and her systolic blood pressure is greater than 110 mmHg

(E) Consideration of operative intervention if she does not stabilize after receiving three saline boluses and two boluses of PRBCs

31. A 12-year-old female presents to the emergency department after being involved in a motor vehicle crash. She was a restrained front seat passenger in a vehicle struck on the passenger side. On arrival, she is alert and hemodynamically stable. She complains of pain in her left shoulder and left lower chest. She demonstrates tenderness on palpation inferior to her left costal margin. A CT scan of her abdomen was obtained (see Fig. 34-15). This is her only injury. What is the next best step in her management?

(A) Admit her to the intensive care unit (ICU).

(B) Proceed to the operating room for splenectomy.

(C) Take her to the operating room for splenectomy if she requires transfusion of greater than 10 mL/kg of PRBCs in the trauma bay.

(D) Follow her as an inpatient for at least 7 days to be certain this injury will not bleed.

(E) Perform a repeat CT scan of the abdomen before she is released to home.

32. The child in question 31 becomes hemodynamically unstable while being observed in the ICU. Her blood pressure was only transiently responsive to fluid boluses, and she required transfusion of PRBCs. After receiving 4 units of PRBCs, she is taken to the operating room. Which of the following is true regarding overwhelming postsplenectomy sepsis?

(A) It occurs in greater than 10% of children who have undergone splenectomy for trauma.

(B) It has greater than 60% mortality.

(C) It occurs most often greater than 5 years after splenectomy.

(D) It can be prevented by the administration of vaccines against pneumococcus and *Haemophilus influenzae*.

(E) It can initially present as a simple febrile illness.

33. A 14-year-old child presents after a bicycle crash. The finding in Fig. 34-16 is noted on physical examination. The child was noted to have a large filling defect on a UGI series (see Fig. 34-17).
Which statement is correct?

(A) Blunt trauma to the pelvis is the most common mechanism for this injury.

(B) This injury rarely is associated with pancreatic injury.

(C) MRI is required to confirm the diagnosis.

(D) This injury usually responds to nonoperative management.

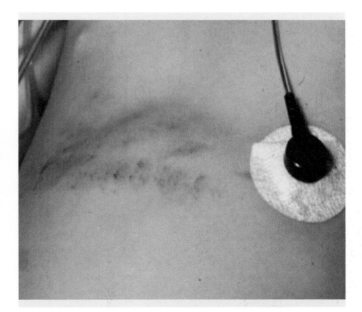

FIGURE 34-16. Clinical finding on the abdomen of a 14-year-old after a bicycle crash.

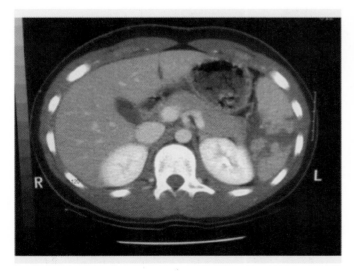

FIGURE 34-15. Abdominal CT of 12-year-old female after motor vehicle crash.

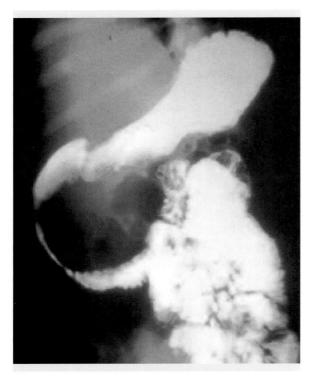

FIGURE 34-17. Upper GI findings after a bicycle crash.

34. A CT of the abdomen and pelvis is obtained on the patient in question 33 after the UGI series and shows a large duodenal hematoma. Which statement is true regarding the management of duodenal injuries?

(A) Regardless of the presence of other injuries requiring operative intervention, duodenal hematomas need to be treated operatively with drainage.
(B) Duodenal hematomas usually resolve within 3 weeks. If resolution has not occurred by this point, consideration must be given to operative evacuation of the clot.
(C) Grade I injuries requiring surgical intervention require pyloric exclusion.
(D) Lacerations less than 50% of the duodenal circumference are best managed with Roux-en-Y reconstruction.

35. A 5-year-old female was pinned between the bumpers of two cars. The abdominal CT of the abdomen and pelvis in Fig. 34-18A obtained as part of her trauma evaluation was highly suspicious of proximal pancreatic duct injury and was confirmed by endoscopic retrograde cholangio-pancreatography (ERCP) (see Fig. 34-18B).
What is the next best step in her management?
(A) Nothing by mouth, TPN, placement of interventional radiology (IR) drains
(B) Pancreaticoduodenectomy
(C) ERCP with placement of pancreatic stent
(D) Distal pancreatectomy
(E) Roux-en-Y pancreaticojejunostomy

36. Which of the following is true regarding pancreatic trauma and its complications?
(A) Complications of pancreatic trauma include pancreatic pseudocyst, abscess, hemorrhage, and fistula.
(B) Asymptomatic pseudocysts should undergo drainage, as only 10% will spontaneously resolve.

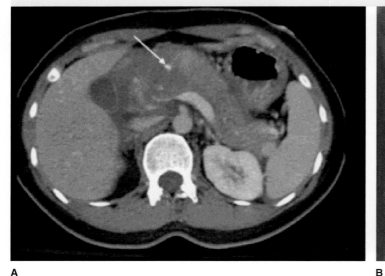
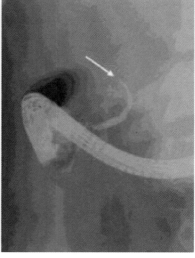

A   B

FIGURE 34-18. A. Abdominal CT and **B.** ERCP of 5-year-old female after she was pinned between the bumpers of two cars.

(C) Pseudocysts that do not resolve spontaneously can be managed with percutaneous drainage if ductal disruption is identified.

(D) If a pancreatic fistula is secondary to a major ductal disruption, it will not respond to sphincterotomy and pancreatic duct stenting via ERCP.

(E) Overall mortality from pancreatic injuries is approximately 45%.

37. What findings on history or physical examination should raise suspicions for child abuse?
    (A) Inconsistencies between the reported mechanism of injury and the injuries sustained
    (B) A significant delay in presentation for medical evaluation
    (C) A history of frequent injury
    (D) A long-bone fracture in a child under age 3
    (E) All of the above

38. A 2-year-old child was found outside at 2 a.m. The ambient temperature was 10°F. The child was lying in a snowdrift and was wearing a cotton tee shirt and diaper only. It is unclear how long the child had been outside. On arrival to the emergency department, the child is unresponsive and apneic. What initial evaluations and treatments should be performed?
    (A) Measurement of oral temperature
    (B) Face mask oxygen supplementation
    (C) Boluses of room temperature fluids
    (D) Cardiopulmonary resuscitation (CPR)
    (E) Preparations for active rewarming

ANSWERS AND EXPLANATIONS

1. **(D)** Neonatal and infant physiology is considerably different from an adult. The circulatory pattern of the fetus is unique in that the lungs are bypassed, and intracardiac/extracardiac shunts enable blood to be oxygenated (Fig. 34-19). Shunts (foramen ovale, ductus arteriosus, and ductus venosus) allow the fetus to receive blood from both ventricles, commonly referred to as parallel circulation. Adults experience a circulatory pattern in series that allows for an equal but separate output for each ventricle.

   The right ventricle receives relatively deoxygenated blood and ejects the majority of its output to the placenta. The left ventricle receives relatively highly oxygenated blood and ejects the majority of its output to the most metabolically active tissues. There are five components of venous return in the fetus: the upper body systemic venous return via the SVC; the lower body systemic venous return via the IVC; the placental return, also via the IVC; the coronary venous return, primarily

via the coronary sinus (CS); and the pulmonary venous return via the pulmonary veins.

Renal blood flow is 3–5% of fetal cardiac output during the last trimester of gestation and increases to 12–16% during the first year of life. This is due to the relatively high vascular resistance of the fetal kidney, which decreases within the first 48 h after birth as a result of increase perfusion of the renal glomeruli. The decrease in vascular resistance is also responsible for increasing renal blood flow and glomerular filtration rate (GFR; full-term infant at birth GFR is 2–4 mL/min; this increases to 8–20 mL/min within a few days postnatally).

During gestation, the placenta serves as the principal regulator of fetal fluid homeostasis. Amniotic fluid volumes increase progressively until around 28 to 39 weeks' gestation. The ability to excrete water and solute relies on the concentrating capacity of the immature kidney. The primary source of amniotic fluid during the latter half of gestation is fetal urine production, with secretion of fluid generated by the fetal lung accounting for up to 25% in the term infant. Major routes of fluid reabsorption include fetal swallowing (approximately 500–1000 mL/d) and intramembranous flow of fluid across the fetal amniotic membranes into the fetal circulation (approximately 200–500 mL/d).

BIBLIOGRAPHY

Piscione TD. Development of renal function. In: Rudolph CD, Rudolph AM, Lister GE, First LR, Gershon AA, eds. *Rudolph's Pediatrics*. 22nd ed. New York, NY: McGraw-Hill; 2011: Chapter 465.

Teitel DF. Neonate and Infant with Cardiovascular Disease. In: Rudolph CD, Rudolph AM, Lister GE, First LR, Gershon AA, eds. *Rudolph's Pediatrics*. 22nd ed. New York, NY: McGraw-Hill; 2011: Chapter 483.

2. **(E)** The ductus arteriosus is a normal fetal vascular structure, connecting the main pulmonary arterial trunk with the descending aorta just distal to the origin of the left subclavian artery. During fetal development, the ductus arteriosus allows right-to-left shunting of oxygenated placental blood to the systemic circulation. Approximately 10–15 h after birth, the ductus arteriosus contracts in response to increased oxygen tension, and it completes its closure via fibrosis by 2–3 weeks in the majority of patients. Final closure is uncommon beyond 6 months of age, and persistence of the ductus arteriosus as a vascular structure rather than a ligamentous one is referred to as *patent ductus arteriosus*.

   Patent ductus arteriosus occurs in 1/2500–3000 births. Etiologic factors of PDA include maternal rubella and living in high altitudes, prematurity,

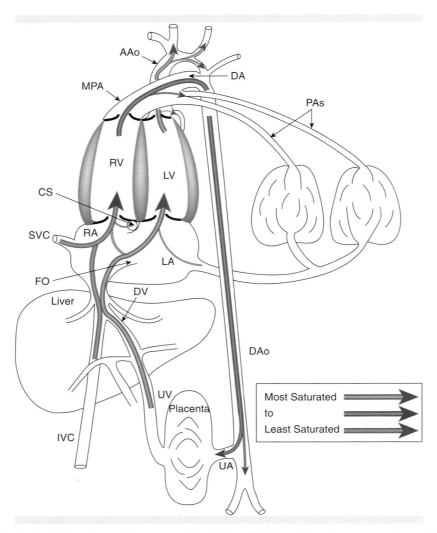

FIGURE 34-19. Fetal circulation AAo = Ascending aorta; CS = Crista dividens; DA = Ductus arteriosus; DAo = Descending aorta; DV = Ductus venosus; FO = Foramen ovale; IVC = Inferior vena cava; LA = Left atrium; LV = Left ventricle; MPA = Main pulmonary artery; PAs = Pulmonary arteries; RA = Right atrium; RV = Right ventricle; SVC = Superior vena cava; UA = Umbilical artery; UV = Umbilical vein; (from Rudolph CD, Rudolph AM, Lister GE, First LR, Gershon AA, eds. *Rudolph's Pediatrics.* 22nd ed. New York, NY: McGraw-Hill; 2011: Fig. 483-3. Copyright © The McGraw-Hill Companies, Inc. All rights reserved).

neonatal hypoxia, and respiratory distress of the newborn. The prevalence is higher in girls by a ratio of 2:1. PDA is more common in preterm infants. This high incidence is related to decreased smooth muscle in the ductal wall, diminished response of the muscle to oxygen, and increasing levels of E series prostaglandins. In these cases, the presence of a left-to-right shunt aggravates any associated conditions of prematurity, such as such as bronchopulmonary dysplasia, necrotizing enterocolitis, and intraventricular hemorrhage, and therefore causes higher mortality rates.

Congestive heart failure (CHF) symptoms are typically present within the first 6 months and include tachypnea, tachycardia, failure to thrive, and recurrent pulmonary

infections. A physical exam may reveal a continuous murmur, enlarged liver, dilated jugular veins, and bounding peripheral pulses. Echocardiogram confirms the diagnosis. Untreated PDA leads to high mortality rates. Infants with large PDAs die from left CHF, whereas older patients die from right CHF secondary to chronic pulmonary hypertension. Small and hemodynamically insignificant PDAs can be observed but are high-risk sites for development of bacterial endocarditis.

Treatment strategies include pharmacologic closure, percutaneous closure in the catheterization laboratory, video-assisted thoracoscopic (VATS) hemoclip occlusion and conventional posterolateral thoracotomy with ligation or division. Typically, the first attempt at closure is with indomethacin unless clinically contraindicated (hyperbilirubinemia, sepsis, coagulopathy, GI bleeding, and renal insufficiency), and pharmacologic closure is successful in 60% of premature infants. Percutaneous closure is reserved for full-term infants and adults. Ductal division avoids the risk of recanalization or aneurysm formation following ligation and is the preferred approach in full-term newborns and all older children whenever possible. Ductal ligation is reserved for preterm infants and small newborns and should be performed early to reduce the need for mechanical ventilation and oxygen supplementation. It shortens hospital stay and decreases the incidence of retrolental fibroplasia and necrotizing enterocolitis when compared to pharmacologic closure.

BIBLIOGRAPHY

Clyman RI. Patent ductus arteriosus and ductus venosus. In: Rudolph CD, Rudolph AM, Lister GE, First LR, Gershon AA, eds. *Rudolph's Pediatrics*. 22nd ed. New York, NY: McGraw-Hill; 2011: Chapter 55.

Fiore AC, Hines M, Pennington D. The surgical treatment of patent ductus arteriosus and aortic coarctation. In: Ziegler MM, Azizkhan RG, Allmen D, Weber TR, eds. *Operative Pediatric Surgery*. 2nd ed. New York, NY: McGraw-Hill; 2014: Chapter 72.

Hsia T, Wu JJ, Ringel R. Patent ductus arteriosus. In: Yuh DD, Vricella LA, Yang SC, Doty JR, eds. *Johns Hopkins Textbook of Cardiothoracic Surgery*. 2nd ed. New York, NY: McGraw-Hill; 2014: Chapter 63.

3. **(B)** A neonate has higher growth and energy requirements compared to an adult. After approximately 3 months of age, growth rates gradually decline. Nevertheless, all newborns lose weight during the first 1–2 weeks of life as a result of postnatal diuresis. A similar trend occurs with caloric requirements in infants and children; the recommended dietary allowance (RDA) in the pediatric population decreases with age. Preterm infants require 120–130 kcal/kg per day and 3.0–4.0 g protein/kg per day; full-term infants require 110–120 kcal/kg per day and 2.0–2.5 g protein/kg per day; from 6 months to 3 years, 100 kcal/kg per day and 1.2–1.6 g protein/kg per day; by 7–10 years of age, 70 kcal/kg per day and 1.0 g protein/kg per day. The final diet composition should provide 35–65% of calories as carbohydrates, 7–16% as protein, and 30–50% as fat.

   Enteral formula selection depends on many patient-specific factors, such as age, intestinal function, and underlying disease. The preferred enteral diet for the full-term newborn is human milk (20 kcal/oz), which provides sufficient macronutrients, minerals, and water for normal growth. The preterm infant may not grow as fast with human milk alone because of higher nutritional requirements. Using human milk fortifiers, 4 kcal/oz are added to provide 24 kcal/oz of fortified breast milk.

   The enteral route of nutrition delivery has certain advantages over parenteral nutrition. Some of these include better maintenance/structural integrity of the GI tract, decreased risk of bacterial translocation, and more efficient use of nutrient substrates. However, timing of initial enteral feedings should be optimized to improve chances for feeding tolerance. Clinical signs of acute sepsis, hypotension, significant apnea, and bradycardia should be absent. In addition, enteral nutrition should be avoided in necrotizing enterocolitis, bowel obstruction, intestinal atresia, severe inflammatory bowel disease (IBD), intestinal side effects of cancer therapy, and acute pancreatitis. Pediatric patients who will withstand a period greater than 5–7 days without nutrition due to a dysfunctional GI tract will necessitate institution of parenteral nutrition. Neonates may require initiation of TPN after 1-2 days. When highly concentrated carbohydrate solutions (>12.5 g/dL) are required, TPN must be administered to avoid thrombophlebitis in peripheral veins.

   Complications related to TPN can be categorized as mechanical, metabolic, or infectious. While the field of parenteral nutrition continues to evolve in prevention of complications and refining nutritional needs, cholestasis remains a challenge, particularly in premature infants of very low birth weight. The etiology of cholestasis is multifactorial, involving lack of enteral intake, toxicity of TPN constituents or contaminants, and interaction with underlying disease processes requiring intravenous nutrition. Substitution of omega-3 fatty acids for omega-6 lipid emulsions can prevent or reverse TPN-associated cholestasis in children. Initiating even minimal enteral feedings as soon as feasible, avoiding sepsis by meticulous line care, avoiding overfeeding, using cysteine- and taurine-containing amino acid formulations, preventing or treating small bowel bacterial overgrowth, protecting TPN solutions from light, and avoiding hepatotoxic medications are accepted measures to minimize cholestasis.

BIBLIOGRAPHY

Athalye-Jape G, Deshpande G, Rao S, Patole S. Benefits of probiotics on enteral nutrition in preterm neonates: a systematic review. *Am J Clin Nutr* 2014 Dec;100(6):1508–1519. doi:10.3945/ajcn.114.092551. Epub 2014 Nov 5.

Haemer MA, Primak LE, Krebs NF. Normal childhood nutrition and its disorders. In: Hay WW Jr, Levin MJ, Deterding RR, Abzug MJ, eds. *Current Diagnosis & Treatment: Pediatrics*. 22 ed. New York, NY: McGraw-Hill; 2013: Chapter 11.

4. **(C)** The incidence of esophageal atresia (EA) with or without tracheoesophageal fistula (TEF) remains 1:2500

to 1:3000 live births, with a slight male predominance. Prenatally, these cases are linked to polyhydramnios, which is present in 95% of isolated EA and 35% of EA with TEF. Associated anomalies have been described including VACTERL (*v*ertebral, *a*norectal, *c*ardiac, *t*racheo*e*sophageal, *r*enal, and *l*imb abnormalities) and CHARGE (*c*oloboma, *h*eart defects, *a*tresia of the choanae, developmental *r*etardation, *g*enital hypoplasia, and *e*ar deformities). Therefore, infants with newly diagnosed EA/TEF require thorough physical examination and should undergo additional diagnostic imaging to rule out other anomalies.

Five types of EA with or without TEF have been described (Fig. 34-20), with type C (EA with distal fistula) accounting for the majority of cases.

A chest x ray showing a curved nasogastric tube ending in the upper pouch confirms the diagnosis. In addition, presence of stomach bubble indicates distal fistulous connection between the esophagus and the trachea. Initial management includes placement of a Replogle tube to decrease oral secretions, respiratory support, and diagnosis of any linked anomalies.

Surgical repair is most commonly approached from a right posterolateral thoracotomy through the fourth intercostal space or approximately 1 cm below the tip of the scapula. In rare cases of right descending arch, a left thoracotomy may also be used. An extrapleural approach is favored. Initially, the fistula is ligated, and the two ends of the esophagus are approximated with an end-to-end anastomosis with 5-0 absorbable sutures over a nasogastric tube. A contrast study should be obtained in the early postoperative period to rule out anastomotic leak. Patients who lack a fistula initially require a gastrostomy tube and laryngotracheobronchoscopy.

In cases of TEF without atresia (type E, isolated TEF), examination of the back wall of the trachea with a 30° bronchoscope frequently reveals the tracheal fistulous opening. Surgical repair is approached via a cervical incision just superior to the clavicle.

BIBLIOGRAPHY

Hendren W III, Weldon CB. Congenital disorders of the esophagus in infants and children. In: Sugarbaker DJ, Bueno R, Krasna MJ, Mentzer SJ, Zellos L, eds. *Adult Chest Surgery*. New York, NY: McGraw-Hill; 2009: Chapter 38.

Lal DR. Anatomic disorders of the esophagus. In: Rudolph CD, Rudolph AM, Lister GE, First LR, Gershon AA, eds. *Rudolph's Pediatrics*. 22nd ed. New York, NY: McGraw-Hill; 2011: Chapter 392.

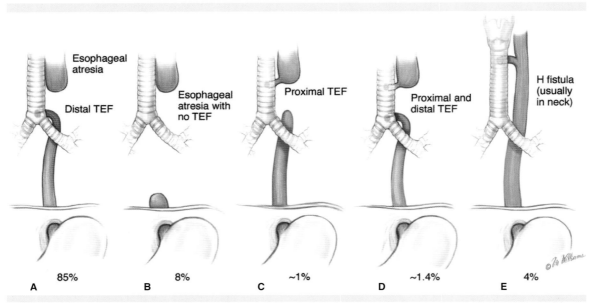

FIGURE 34-20. The five varieties of esophageal atresia and tracheoesophageal fistula. **A.** Isolated esophageal atresia. **B.** Esophageal atresia with tracheoesophageal fistula between proximal segment of esophagus and trachea. **C.** Esophageal atresia with tracheoesophageal fistula between distal esophagus and trachea. **D.** Esophageal atresia with fistula between both proximal and distal ends of esophagus and trachea. **E.** Tracheoesophageal fistula without esophageal atresia (H-type fistula). In David J. Hackam; Tracy Grikscheit; Kasper Wang; Jeffrey S. Upperman; Henri R. Ford. Schwart'z Principles of Surgery. New York, NY: McGraw-Hill; 2010: Fig. 39-8. Copyright © The McGraw-Hill Companies, Inc. All rights reserved.

Rothenberg S. Esophageal atresia and tracheoesophageal fistula malformations. In: Holcomb WG, Murphy JP, Ostlie JD, eds. *Ashcraft's Pediatric Surgery*. 6th ed. New York, NY: Elsevier; 2014:365–379.

5. **(D)** In this scenario, the appearance of pneumatosis in the abdominal radiograph (see Fig. 34-2) along with the clinical symptoms suggests the diagnosis of necrotizing enterocolitis (NEC). Despite medical advances, NEC remains the most common surgical emergency and major cause of death in the newborn period. NEC is an acquired neonatal GI disease process that afflicts premature, low birth weight infants in the majority of cases. The etiology is likely multifactorial and involves a combination of mucosal compromise, impaired gut barrier, pathogenic bacteria, and enteral feedings that in a susceptible host results in bowel injury and an inflammatory cascade. Ninety percent of NEC presents after initiation of enteral feedings.

Necrotizing enterocolitis should be suspected in a preterm infant who develops physiologic derangement, abdominal distention, and feeding intolerance after the initiation of enteral feedings. The most common GI symptoms include abdominal distention, high gastric residuals, emesis, and bloody stools. Laboratory studies will reveal neutropenia, thrombocytopenia, and metabolic acidosis. Leukopenia is common, especially in severe cases, and thrombocytopenia is associated with worse outcomes. Anteroposterior (AP) and left lateral decubitus abdominal films remain the gold standard imaging studies in the diagnosis of NEC. Early findings include dilated loops of small bowel and air-fluid levels. Pneumatosis intestinalis is the hallmark of NEC and is frequently accompanied by portal venous gas and free intraperitoneal air.

Management of mild NEC includes bowel rest with nasogastric decompression, aggressive fluid resuscitation, and broad-spectrum antibiotics. While the x-ray finding of pneumatosis by itself is not an indication for surgery, the presence of pneumoperitoneum is the only absolute indication for surgery. Most infants who require surgery will manifest indications within 24 h from the onset of disease. Relative indications include a positive paracentesis, palpable abdominal mass, abdominal wall erythema, portal venous gas, fixed intestinal loop, and clinical deterioration despite maximal medical therapy.

Ultimate goals of surgical intervention include resection of the gangrenous bowel and preservation of intestinal length to avoid short-bowel syndrome in the future. Currently, the safest surgical management in a single involved gangrenous small bowel segment includes resection with creation of ostomy and mucous fistula. Patients with multifocal disease and more than 50%

intestinal viability may require a single proximal enterostomy and multiple primary anastomoses to avoid the morbidity of multiple stomas.

Hospital survival for surgically treated patients with NEC averages 70%. Complications are common and include recurrent NEC, sepsis, disseminated intravascular coagulation (DIC), wound infection, stomal complications, enteric fistulas, and cholestasis. Long-term complications include intestinal strictures, malabsorption, short-gut syndrome, and neurodevelopmental complications. Intestinal strictures, one of the most frequent long-term complications, are observed after nonoperative treatment of NEC. They are a result of fibrotic healing in an ischemic area. The majority of intestinal strictures affect the colon (80%).

BIBLIOGRAPHY

Castle SL, Speer AL, Grikscheit TC, Ford H. Necrotizing enterocolitis. In: Ziegler MM, Azizkhan RG, Allmen D, Weber TR, eds. *Operative Pediatric Surgery*. 2nd ed. New York, NY: McGraw-Hill; 2014: Chapter 46.

Sylvester KG, Liu GY, Albanese CT. Necrotizing enterocolitis. In: Coran AG, Caldamone A, Adzick NS, Krummel TM, Laberge J-M, Shamberger R, eds. *Pediatric Surgery*. New York, NY: Elsevier; 2012:1187–1207.

6. **(C)** Malrotation with midgut volvulus most commonly occurs in the first month of life or before 1 year of age. Bilious vomiting in a child under 1 year of age is assumed to be due to malrotation with volvulus until proven otherwise. Normal rotation of the midgut, which occurs during the 6th–12th week of embryonic development, is a process characterized by the herniation of the midgut into the body stalk, returning, and undergoing a counterclockwise rotation of the ligament of Treitz (duodenojejunal junction) 270° around the superior mesenteric artery (SMA) such that the final position of the ligament of Treitz is to the left of the spine and at or above the pylorus. The ileocolic junction rotates 270° counterclockwise around the SMA to lie in the right lower quadrant. The major cause of midgut volvulus is nonrotation of the ligament of Treitz or cecocolic limb.

Radiologic evaluation is indicated when one suspects malrotation, and several imaging studies are necessary in sequence to determine the position of the ligament of Treitz and its distance to the ileocecal junction. Plain abdominal radiographs are mostly nonspecific in patients with malrotation. However, when obstruction is determined by x-rays or peritonitis is present, further studies are contraindicated, and the patient should undergo emergent exploration. The UGI series with small bowel follow-through is the gold standard test to make the diagnosis of malrotation. Principle diagnostic findings on UGI include an abnormal right-sided position of the ligament of Treitz, obstruction of the duodenum, and right-sided filling of jejunal loops. The abnormal UGI in Fig. 34-21 demonstrates a spiral course ("corkscrew deformity") of the midgut loops in the right side of the abdomen, which is pathognomic for malrotation.

Ultrasonography can be used to give anatomic details of the mesenteric vessels. The superior mesenteric vein (SMV) is normally to the right of the SMA. If malrotation is suspected, ultrasound can be helpful in that if the SMV lies anterior or to the left of the SMA, malrotation may be present.

The operative approach for the management of malrotation with midgut volvulus involves the Ladd procedure: assessment of bowel and counterclockwise detorsion of the volvulus, division of Ladd's bands, widening of the mesenteric base to allow the colon to be placed on the left side of the patient and the small bowel with a straightened duodenum on the right, and performing an incidental appendectomy.

BIBLIOGRAPHY

Christison-Lagay EC, Langer JC. Intestinal rotation abnormalities. In: Ziegler MM, Azizkhan RG, Allmen D, Weber TR, eds. *Operative Pediatric Surgery*. 2nd ed. New York, NY: McGraw-Hill; 2014: Chapter 41.

Okada PJ, Minkes RK. Gastrointestinal emergencies. In: Stone C, Humphries RL, Drigalla D, Stephan M, eds. *Current Diagnosis & Treatment: Pediatric Emergency Medicine*. New York, NY: McGraw-Hill; 2014: Chapter 36.

7. **(E)** Congenital abdominal wall defects (omphalocele and gastroschisis) refer to an abnormal process by which the abdominal wall fails to develop properly. Omphalocele develops due to a failure of the viscera to return to the abdominal cavity during the 6th–10th week of gestation; the omphalocele can contain liver, bladder, stomach, ovary, and testis in addition to the intestines. The sac consists of the covering layers of the umbilical cord and includes amnion, Wharton's jelly, and peritoneum. They are characterized by a central defect that can vary from 4 to 12 cm at the site of the umbilical ring. Omphaloceles have a high incidence of associated conditions that can involve the cardiovascular, GI, musculoskeletal, or genitourinary systems, as well as chromosomal anomalies (trisomies 13–15, 18, and 21). All neonates should undergo an echocardiographic evaluation as well as abdominal ultrasound to rule out renal abnormalities.

Gastroschisis is noted by a small defect, which is to the right of the umbilicus with no sac. Currently, the ventral body folds theory suggests failure of migration of the lateral folds (more frequent on the right side). In-utero vascular injury leading to ischemia of the embryonic vessels between 4 and 6 weeks has also been implicated in the pathogenesis. Concomitant bowel atresia is the most common associated anomaly in patients with gastroschisis, with rates ranging from 6.9 to 28% in several series. Management of both of these abdominal wall defects mandates operative intervention to close the abdomen. While the operative options for omphaloceles and gastroschisis differ, one of the most important issues in surgical management for the abdominal wall defect is related to whether to close the abdomen primarily or proceed with a staged silo closure. As a general rule, timing of closure depends on the patient's gestational age and birth weight, size of the defect, and associated congenital abnormalities (Figs. 34-22 and 34-23).

BIBLIOGRAPHY

Islam S. Congenital abdominal wall defects. In: Holcomb WG, Murphy JP, Ostlie JD, eds. *Ashcraft's Pediatric Surgery*. 6th edition. New York, NY: Elsevier; 2014:660–668.

Islam S. Abdominal wall defects: omphalocele and gastroschisis. In *Operative Pediatric Surgery*. 7th edition. New York, NY: McGraw-Hill, 2014: Chapter 34.

8. **(E)** The spectrum of congenital lung and diaphragm ailments amenable to surgical therapy is diverse. Congenital lung anomalies include lobar emphysema, Congenital Pulmonary Airway (cystic adenomatoid) Malformation (CPAM), bronchopulmonary sequestration (BPS), and bronchogenic cysts (BCs).

Congenital diaphragm disorders consist of eventration and diaphragmatic hernia. The formation of the diaphragm, during the fourth and eighth week of gestation, results from the fusion of three embryologic elements: (1) the septum transversum, which forms the central tendon; (2) bilateral pleuroperitoneal membranes or folds, which are reinforced by striated muscle components; and (3) the mesentery of the esophagus, which forms crural and dorsal structures. CDHs result from incomplete fusion of pleuroperitoneal folds and are categorized by the location of herniation (Fig. 34-24) or by their etiology, with posterolateral hernias through the foramen of Bochdalek the most common at 90% of cases.

Development of the diaphragm is complete by 10 to 11 weeks of gestation. While diagnosis is therefore theoretically possible by 12 weeks of gestation, current ultrasonographic limitations restrict diagnosis to 14–15 weeks' gestational age. Fetal ultrasound features include polyhydramnios, bowel loops within the chest, an echogenic chest mass, or an intrathoracic stomach. In most neonates, CDH manifests as varying degrees of respiratory distress. The diagnosis is usually confirmed during the neonatal period with a chest radiograph, demonstrating intrathoracic intestinal loops, a

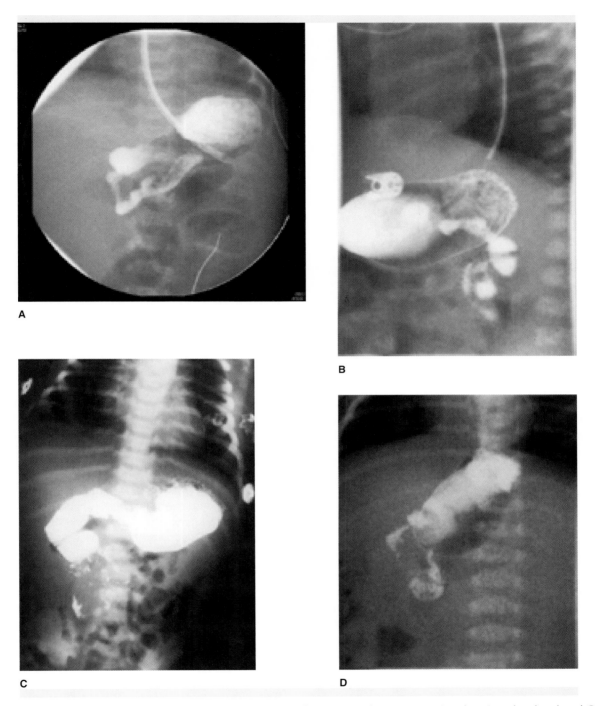

FIGURE 34-21. Upper GI series with small bowel follow-through. **A.** Normal contrast series showing the duodenal C-loop crossing the midline; **B.** lateral view of malrotation demonstrating "corkscrew" appearance of jejunum; **C.** lateral view suggestive of duodenal obstruction secondary to Ladd bands or volvulus; and **D.** false-positive study with Duodenojejunal (DJ) flexure pushed rightward by a large multicystic kidney (from Ziegler MM, Azizkhan RG, Weber TR, eds. *Operative Pediatric Surgery*. New York, NY: McGraw-Hill; 2014: Fig. 41-4. Copyright © The McGraw-Hill Companies, Inc. All rights reserved).

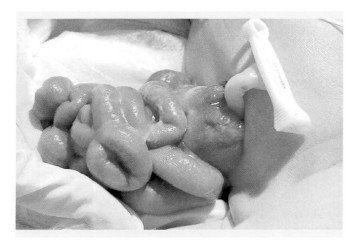

FIGURE 34-22. Infant with gastroschisis (from Brunicardi F, Andersen DK, Billiar TR, et al., (eds.), *Schwartz's Principles of Surgery*. 10th ed. New York, NY: McGraw-Hill; 2014: Fig. 39-31. Copyright © The McGraw-Hill Companies, Inc. All rights reserved).

nasogastric tube curled up in the chest, absence of a diaphragmatic shadow on the affected side, mediastinal and cardiac shift to the contralateral side, and occasionally intrathoracic location of the left lobe of the liver. As CDH is associated with abnormal intestinal rotation and fixation, some children may present with intestinal obstruction or volvulus.

The two most critical elements of CDH are pulmonary hypertension and hypoplasia. Initial postnatal therapy aims at resuscitation of the infant with cardiopulmonary distress, which mainly aims at decreasing pulmonary hypertension, as well as decompression of the GI tract with a nasogastric tube. Surgical repair of a CDH should be performed after cardiopulmonary stability has been achieved. Currently, minimally invasive techniques have evolved; these involve either a thoracoscopic or laparoscopic approach. Large defects mandate use of a prosthetic patch to achieve tension-free repair.

Eventration refers to the abnormal elevation of the diaphragm, which results in paradoxical motion during respiration. The central portion of the diaphragm is most affected and allows the abdominal contents to push the diaphragm upward. Eventration is of either a congenital or an acquired origin. While the congenital form is rare, the acquired form is due to injury to the phrenic nerve during intrathoracic surgery or trauma during birth. Although often first detected on chest X-Ray, ultrasound or fluoroscopy confirms the diagnosis with abnormal movement of the diaphragm. Treatment of choice is plication of the eventrated diaphragm.

Congenital lobar emphysema (CLE) is abnormal inflammation of an anatomically normal lung. Babies are

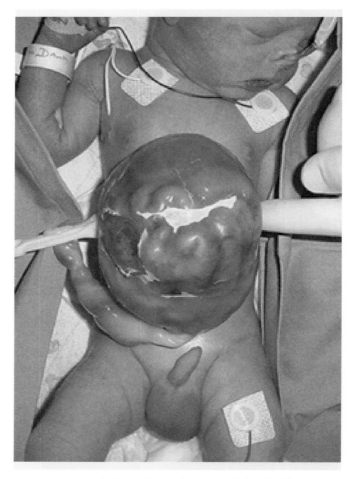

FIGURE 34-23. Infant with a giant omphalocele (from Brunicardi F, Andersen DK, Billiar TR, et al., (eds.), *Schwartz's Principles of Surgery*. 10th ed. New York, NY: McGraw-Hill; 2014: Fig. 39-30. Copyright © The McGraw-Hill Companies, Inc. All rights reserved).

usually asymptomatic at birth but develop respiratory distress and tachypnea within the first few days of life. Treatment of choice for CLE is lobectomy of the afflicted lung.

Bronchopulmonary sequestration refers to nonfunctioning lung tissue that does not communicate with the normal tracheobronchial tree and contains its own anomalous blood supply. Two types of sequestration exist: extralobar and intralobar. If the lung mass has its own pleural covering, then an extralobar pulmonary defect exists. A sequestrum that lies within the normal lung parenchyma is classified as an intralobar defect. Surgical resection is mandated. It is important to establish blood supply because vascular supply differs to these lesions. The most common origin of the arterial supply is the thoracic aorta. Venous drainage to these lesions is usually to the azygous veins for extralobar pathology and to the pulmonary veins for intralobar sequestrations.

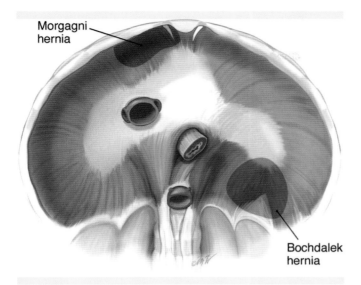

FIGURE 34-24. Locations of congenital diaphragmatic hernias (from Sugarbaker DJ, Bueno R, Krasna MJ, Mentzer SJ, Zellos L, eds. *Adult Chest Surgery.* New York, NY: McGraw-Hill; 2009: Fig. 153-1. Copyright © The McGraw-Hill Companies, Inc. All rights reserved).

Congenital cystic adenomatoid malformation (CCAM) refers to intercommunicating cysts within the lung that develop as a consequence of increases/overgrowth of the terminal bronchioles in one lobe of the lung. Surgical excision manages CCAMs. There is some question regarding whether to proceed with surgery in an asymptomatic patient with a CCAM. Yet, when definitive diagnosis is confirmed, studies suggest that surgical intervention in the asymptomatic infant is associated with shorter length of stay, fewer complications, and decreased medical cost as compared with intervening after symptoms have developed. There is also the rare risk of malignant degeneration with CCAM.

Bronchogenic cysts originate from the foregut, as do most congenital lung anomalies. BCs are mucus-filled cysts that arise from the tracheobronchial tree. Clinical presentation of BCs varies from respiratory distress at birth to infection (secondary to abnormal drainage of secretions) later in life. Main symptoms in infants and children are due to intrathoracic compression, while cough, infection, and hemoptysis occur later in adulthood. Treatment involves excision of the cyst by segmentectomy or lobectomy. Asymptomatic cases warrant excision due to the high risk of complications, including infection and malignant degeneration.

BIBLIOGRAPHY

Linden BC. Long-term outcomes after a congenital diaphragmatic hernia repair: implications for adult thoracic surgeons. In: Sugarbaker DJ, Bueno R, Colson YL, et al., (eds.), *Adult Chest Surgery.* 2nd ed. New York, NY: McGraw-Hill; 2015: Chapter 153.

Tracy T Jr, Luks FI. Diaphragmatic hernias and eventration. In: Ziegler MM, Azizkhan RG, Weber TR, eds. *Operative Pediatric Surgery.* New York, NY: McGraw-Hill; 2014:445–454.

9. **(B)** Hypertrophic pyloric stenosis (HPS) is one of the most common surgical conditions of infancy. It occurs in 1–3 of every 1000 live births. Boys are affected four times more often than girls. Pathogenesis involves pyloric muscle fiber hypertrophy causing a mechanical obstruction of the gastric outlet. The etiology of HPS remains elusive, but family history, sex, birth order, and maternal feeding patterns all have been implicated. HPS most commonly develops from 2 to 12 weeks (peak incidence of 3–6 weeks) of age in an otherwise-healthy infant who feeds normally at birth. A pattern of vomiting ensues that varies but classically progresses to projectile, nonbilious emesis.

Diagnosis of HPS is made by history and physical and confirmed by ultrasound findings (Fig. 34-25). The absence of these findings with a strong history of HPS should prompt an ultrasound or UGI contrast study. Ultrasound criteria include a pyloric muscle thickness of 4 mm or greater, pyloric muscle diameter greater than

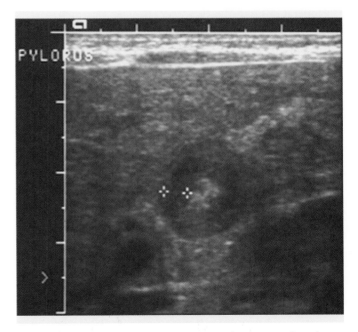

FIGURE 34-25. Transverse sonogram demonstrating the target sign and heterogeneous echoic texture of the muscle layer in a patient with HPS.

14 mm, and a channel length greater than 15 mm. If ultrasound is nondiagnostic, a UGI contrast study can aid in ruling out reflux, malrotation, or obstruction. UGI findings consistent with HPS include a "string" sign, a "double-track" sign, or "shoulders" at the proximal end of the pylorus.

Patients with HPS have a hypochloremic, hypokalemic, metabolic alkalosis from repeated emesis. Once the fluid and electrolyte status has been corrected, operative intervention is undertaken. The Ramstedt pyloromyotomy is the procedure of choice and can be performed via an open or laparoscopic approach. Failure to correct metabolic abnormalities can result in postanesthetic apnea. Most patients will have a rapid and complete resolution of vomiting by 1 week following their procedure. The hypertrophied muscle returns to normal caliber at about 3 to 4 weeks after surgery. There appear to be no major long-term residua in patients who have had surgery for HPS.

BIBLIOGRAPHY

Barksdale EM Jr, Ponsky TA. Pyloric stenosis. In: Ziegler MM, Azizkhan RG, Allmen D, Weber TR, eds. *Operative Pediatric Surgery*. 2nd ed. New York, NY: McGraw-Hill; 2014: Chapter 40.

Murphy SG. Hypertrophic pyloric stenosis. In: Mattei P, ed. *Surgical Directives Pediatric Surgery*. Philadelphia, PA: Lippincott, Williams & Wilkins; 2002:269–272.

10. **(A)** Antireflux procedures are commonly performed operations in pediatric surgery centers. Gastroesophageal reflux disease (GERD) occurs when antireflux barriers fail to prevent passage of gastric contents into the esophagus. These include low esophageal sphincter (LES), short length of LES, and increased intra-abdominal pressure. Neurologic retching, obesity, ascites, and certain congenital disorders (e.g., CDH, omphalocele, gastroschisis, and TEF) can cause GERD. Infant/childhood clinical manifestations are irritability, frequent vomiting, apnea, aspiration, pneumonia, a failure to thrive, and even some cases of apparent life-threatening event (ALTE) spells.

The diagnostic preoperative workup should include a UGI series to rule out anatomic abnormalities and obstruction of the esophagus, stomach, and duodenum. Occasionally, 24-h pH monitoring is used to quantitate the frequency and duration of acid reflux over time. An esophagogastroduodenoscopy (EGD)/biopsy may be valuable in some cases for visualizing mucosal areas of injury. Nonoperative management of GERD should be attempted first and includes upright positioning, small-volume feedings or continuous tube feedings, thickened formula, and H_2 antagonists/proton pump inhibitors. The majority of neurologically intact children will respond to medical therapy.

When medical therapy fails to control GERD symptoms or complications arise (strictures, chronic pulmonary disease, worsening reactive airway disease, or failure to thrive), surgery is indicated. In select circumstances, operative management should be used as first-line treatment. These include neurologically impaired children with need for gastrostomy and concern for aspiration, infants with ALTE spells and GERD, as well as patients with documented Barrett's esophagus or esophageal stricture. Surgery for GERD is aimed toward reestablishing the antireflux barrier while not obstructing food passage. Laparoscopic Nissen fundoplication (360° wrap) is the most commonly used procedure.

BIBLIOGRAPHY

Iqbal CW, Holcomb GW III. Gastroesophageal reflux. In: Holcomb WG, Murphy JP, Ostlie JD, eds. *Ashcraft's Pediatric Surgery*. 6th ed. New York, NY: Elsevier; 2014:387–399.

Jolley SG, Roaten JB. Gastroesophageal reflux disease. In: Ziegler MM, Azizkhan RG, Allmen D, Weber TR, eds. *Operative Pediatric Surgery*. 2nd ed. New York, NY: McGraw-Hill; 2014: Chapter 27.

11. **(C)** Intussusception generally refers to a part of bowel invaginating into an adjacent section of bowel and causing intestinal obstruction and venous compression, which ultimately result in venous, then arterial, insufficiency and necrosis if left untreated. The condition is a common abdominal emergency between 3 months and 2 years of age, with a peak incidence between 6 and 9 months. While most cases are idiopathic with a lead point due to an enlarged Peyer's patch (reported due to a viral infection), 5% are due to a polyp, Meckel's diverticulum (MD), duplication cyst, or tumor. The most common site of occurrence is the ileocecal junction.

Clinically, a history of crampy, intermittent abdominal pain in an otherwise-healthy infant should prompt the diagnosis of intussusception. A classical triad of acute abdominal pain, currant jelly stools, and a palpable abdominal mass is present in less than 50% of children with intussusception. In addition, intussusception may manifest solely with diarrhea or changes in mentation. Because of its many presentations, intussusception may avoid detection. Studies showed that delay in diagnosis of greater than 12 h from initial medical contact is associated with increased mortality.

Radiologic studies should confirm the diagnosis of intussusception. Plain abdominal films may show paucity of gas in the right iliac fossa, an abdominal mass in the right upper quadrant, or air-fluid levels suggesting small bowel obstruction. In experienced operators, ultrasound provides excellent sensitivity and specificity for intussusception and therefore has been adopted as the initial screening tool in the majority of institutions. The findings of a "target" sign on transverse imaging and a "pseudokidney" sign on longitudinal imaging effectively confirm the diagnosis.

Once the diagnosis is made, intravenous fluid resuscitation should be started and radiologic reduction with hydrostatic (fluid) or pneumatic (air) should be performed. Contraindications to nonoperative management include perforation, peritonitis, and persistent hypotension. Nonoperative treatment is successful in approximately 80% of cases. Patients with recurrent intussusception should proceed with repeat enema reduction. Chung and colleagues found that risk factors leading to surgical reduction were long-standing duration of illness (>12 h); clinical triad of vomiting, colicky abdominal pain, and bloody stools; positive pathologic lead point; and radiologic finding of bowel obstruction. Generally, the surgical procedure is followed by making a transverse right lower quadrant incision and manually reducing the intussusception with retrograde milking of the intussuscipiens. Bowel resection is necessary when the intussusception cannot be reduced or bowel shows evidence of gangrene or perforation.

BIBLIOGRAPHY

Feltis AB, Schmeling JD. Intussusception. In: Ziegler MM, Azizkhan RG, Allmen D, Weber TR, eds. *Operative Pediatric Surgery.* 2nd ed. New York, NY: McGraw-Hill; 2014: Chapter 45.

Maki CA, Fallat EM. Intussusception. In: Holcomb WG, Murphy JP, Ostlie JD, eds. *Ashcraft's Pediatric Surgery.* 6th ed. New York, NY: Elsevier; 2014:531–538.

12. **(D)** Meckel's diverticulum is the most common congenital abnormality of the small intestine (2% of population) and is also the most common vitelline duct (VD) abnormality. The VD or omphalomesenteric duct is the *in utero* connection between the fetal gut and the yolk sac, which involutes during the seventh to eighth week of gestation.

The majority of MDs are asymptomatic and found incidentally, but they may cause complications in children, such as inflammation, bleeding, intestinal obstruction, perforation, volvulus, and intussusception. Bleeding accounts for the majority of presentations. The commonly cited "rule of twos" regarding the diverticulum is that it occurs in 2% of the population, has a 2:1 male/female ratio, usually is discovered by 2 years of age, is located 2 ft (60 cm) from the ileocecal valve, commonly is 2 cm in diameter and 2 in. (5 cm) long, and can contain two types of heterotopic mucosa. Most MDs

are found along the antimesenteric border of the ileum within 100 cm of the ileocecal junction.

The diagnosis of a symptomatic MD may be difficult, and more than 75% of symptomatic MDs occur in children younger than 10 years of age. Moreover, children less than 2 years represent 50% of those having symptomatic MDs. Ectopic mucosa (gastric mucosal tissue is the most prevalent) within the diverticulum is often the causative factor in 50–80% of symptomatic patients. Bleeding due to mucosal irritation in cases of MD represents the most common cause of significant lower GI hemorrhage in children. A ^{99m}Tc (technetium pertechnetate) Meckel's scan can be used to detect ectopic gastric mucosa, and if negative, laparoscopy may be needed for diagnostic and therapeutic means of managing an MD. A positive ^{99m}Tc Meckel's scan (Fig. 34-5) completed prior to surgery confirms the presence of an MD as ectopic tissue present in the lower abdomen.

Intestinal obstruction due to MD may occur and is caused by the diverticulum itself or by fibrous bands that develop between the MD and the umbilicus that allow an extrinsic bowel obstruction to occur. Surgical intervention is needed to prevent late complications of strangulation and infarction of bowel. Inflammation of an MD is a condition that presents similarly to appendicitis, although inflammation of the diverticulum presents with a shifting tenderness as well as a shorter time course for development of diffuse peritonitis. Nevertheless, an operation for a suspected appendicitis would reveal a normal appendix and on further exploration an inflamed diverticulum in cases of Meckel's diverticulitis. The decision to perform a diverticulectomy versus a bowel resection for Meckel's diverticulitis is based on the following intraoperative factors: a wide-based diverticulum or a densely inflamed, adherent ileum. Completing an incidental appendectomy concludes the case.

The definitive treatment strategy for an asymptomatic MD is controversial. Some surgeons resect an asymptomatic diverticulum based on the presence of ectopic mucosa, male gender, preadolescent age, or a narrow base because these factors have higher risks of complications. More important, however, are the indications for not removing an incidental MD. These would include patients undergoing surgery for life-threatening emergencies, elective procedures for which the bowel is not opened, and in the presence of peritonitis.

BIBLIOGRAPHY

Emil SGS, Laberge JM. Meckel's diverticulum. In: Mattei P, ed. *Surgical Directives Pediatric Surgery.* Philadelphia, PA: Lippincott, Williams & Wilkins; 2002:327–330.

Leys MC. Meckel diverticulum. In: Holcomb WG, Murphy JP, Ost-lie JD, eds. *Ashcraft's Pediatric Surgery*. 6th ed. New York, NY: Elsevier; 2014:548–552.

Onen A, Cigdem MK, Ozturk H, Otcu S, Dokucu AI. When to resect and when not to resect an asymptomatic Meckel's diverticulum: an ongoing challenge. *Pediatr Surg Int* 2003;19:57–61.

13. **(C)** Hirschprung disease occurs in 1:5000 live births and usually presents with abdominal distention, feeding intolerance, bilious emesis, and absence of passage of meconium in the first 24 h. It is characterized by the absence of ganglion cells in the myenteric and submucosal enteric plexus, typically located in the rectum or rectosigmoid area in the majority of cases (80%). The remainder of cases have more proximal colonic involvement, whereas 5–10% have total colonic aganglionosis with variable involvement of the distal small bowel.

Although suggested by contrast enema showing the transition zone from normal to aganglionic colon, the gold standard of diagnosis is suction rectal biopsy, which will reveal absence of ganglion cells. A full-thickness biopsy is indicated for the child in whom there has been more than one indeterminate suction rectal biopsy.

Initial management includes gastric decompression with a nasogastric tube, initiation of broad-spectrum antibiotics, and rectal irrigations. Universal creation of a right transverse or leveling colostomy is controversial but is indicated in infants presenting with severe enterocolitis, perforation, malnutrition, or massively dilated proximal bowel and when it is not possible to reliably identify the transition zone on frozen section. The goals of surgical management are to remove the aganglionic bowel and reconstruct the intestinal tract by bringing the normally innervated bowel down to the anus while preserving normal sphincter function. The most commonly performed operations are the Swenson, Duhamel, and Soave (endorectal pull-through) procedures. Most involve a combined abdominal and perineal approach; however, a pure transanal pull-through technique can be utilized, with the advantages of short hospital stay, minimal risk of damage to pelvic structures, and low incidence of intra-peritoneal bleeding and adhesion formation.

BIBLIOGRAPHY

Langer CG. Hirschsprung disease. In: Holcomb WG, Murphy JP, Ostlie JD, eds. *Ashcraft's Pediatric Surgery*. 6th ed. New York, NY: Elsevier; 2014:474–484.

Teitelbaum HD, Wulkan LM, Georgeson EK, Langer CG. Hirschsprung disease. In: Ziegler MM, Azizkhan RG, Allmen D, Weber TR, eds. *Operative Pediatric Surgery*. 2nd ed. New York, NY: McGraw-Hill; 2014: Chapter 44.

14. **(E)**

15. **(C)**

Explanations 14 and 15

Newborn infants have a rate of bilirubin formation that is two to three times higher than that of adults due both to the higher hematocrit and to the shorter life span of the red blood cells in the newborn. The limited ability of the newborn liver to conjugate bilirubin and increased enterohepatic circulation can result in decreased elimination relative to production, resulting in jaundice. Although jaundice can result from an increase in either unconjugated (indirect) or conjugated (direct) bilirubin, a rise in the indirect fraction is the most common cause of newborn jaundice.

In healthy infants, jaundice usually resolves by 2 weeks of age. Persistence of neonatal jaundice beyond 2 weeks of age or once biochemical tests have confirmed pathologic jaundice (conjugated bilirubin greater than 2 mg/dL or over 15% of the total bilirubin concentration) warrants radiologic evaluation. Ultrasound is usually the first modality used to evaluate pathologic jaundice, as it can easily examine the liver, bile ducts, gallbladder, pancreas, spleen, and portal vein. In biliary atresia, ultrasound may show increasing echogenicity, a small or absent gallbladder, and nonvisible biliary ducts. The presence of polyspenia also supports the diagnosis. The triangular cord sign is an abnormal hyperechogenic triangular area seen in the porta hepatitis that corresponds to the fibrous remnant of the bile duct seen in biliary atresia. This sign has 80% sensitivity and 98% specificity for biliary atresia.

In many centers, a nuclear medicine scan is performed after pretreatment with phenobarbital. If the nucleotide is excreted into the bowel, the diagnosis of biliary atresia is excluded. In hepatocellular jaundice, isotope uptake is delayed due to parenchymal disease, and excretion into the intestine may or may not be seen. Failure to show gut excretion is nondiagnostic in that it cannot distinguish biliary atresia from other causes of cholestasis. Figure 34-7 shows images taken at 1 min (A), 15 min (B), 30 min (C), 60 min (D), 4 h (E), and 24 h (F) after tracer injection. There was excretion into the bladder (small arrow) via the kidneys from backup of tracer in the blood pool. Lack of bowel visualization on 24-h images is suggestive of biliary atresia.

Biliary atresia remains the most common cause of neonatal jaundice requiring surgery and has become the most common indication of liver transplantation in children. It is characterized by an obliteration or discontinuation of the biliary system that results in obstruction of bile flow. The etiology seems to involve a viral or nonviral toxic insult to the bile duct epithelium that induces the expression of new antigens on bile duct epithelial cells and causes a T cell–mediated fibrosclerosing response. Infants appear well and active, presenting with

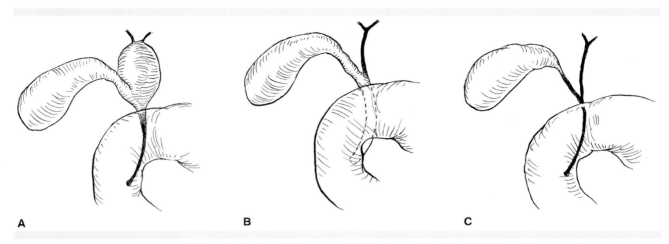

FIGURE 34-26. Variants of biliary atresia. Type I **A.** Distal obliteration with hilar bile cysts (formerly "correctable" type). Type II **B.** Patency of the distal biliary tree with proximal obliteration. Type III **C.** Complete obliteration of the extrahepatic ducts (from Ziegler MM, Azizkhan RG, Weber TR, eds. *Operative Pediatric Surgery*. New York, NY: McGraw-Hill; 2014: Fig. 56-1. Copyright © The McGraw-Hill Companies, Inc. All rights reserved).

jaundice, clay-colored stools, and hepatomegaly. Conjugated levels of bilirubin are elevated and greater than 15% of the total bilirubin. Early diagnosis is essential in biliary atresia because successful treatment depends on critical timing of surgical biliary reconstruction. There are three types of biliary atresia described: type I, atresia of the common bile duct (CBD); type II, atresia of the common hepatic duct with or without atresia of the CBD; type III, atresia of all extrahepatic bile ducts up to porta hepatis (Fig. 34-26).

Type III remains the most common type. Treatment options for biliary atresia are limited to surgery and include hepaticoportoenterostomy (Kasai procedure) and liver transplantation, both of which have been shown to provide long-term success for biliary atresia. The results for the Kasai procedure are best when the operation is performed before 2 months of age. Transplantation should be reserved for those infants greater than 4 months of age and those who fail to drain bile after portoenterostomy. The rationale for performing the Kasai procedure within 2 months of age is that in the first 2 months of life, histologic changes of the liver show preservation of the basic hepatic architecture with bile duct proliferation, bile plugs, and mild periportal fibrosis in infants with biliary atresia. As the infant ages, the fibrosis extends into the hepatic lobule, resulting in cirrhosis.

Once the decision has been made to proceed with surgical intervention, diagnostic confirmation is the initial goal of surgery. In biliary atresia, gross involvement of the extrahepatic bile ducts is noted, and cholangiography shows CBD occlusion. On inspection, the visualization

of a fibrotic gallbladder with obliterated cystic duct mandates a Roux-en-Y hepaticoportoenterostomy (Kasai procedure). The general concept in the Kasai procedure is to remove the extrahepatic bile ducts *en bloc*, and the exposed transected surface at the liver hilus is anastomosed to the intestine. Autoapproximation of the intestine and biliary ductal epithelial elements occurs, and this attempts to provide biliary drainage for the liver. The major postoperative complication is cholangitis secondary to bile stasis and intestinal conduit bacterial contamination. Approximately one-third of patients with the Kasai procedure can be considered cured. Another one-third of patients will develop biliary cirrhosis due to minimal bile flow after reconstruction, and the final third will develop bile cirrhosis with moderate drainage. Children who fail reconstruction will ultimately require liver transplantation.

BIBLIOGRAPHY

Yamataka A, Cazares J, Miyano T. Biliary atresia. In: Holcomb WG, Murphy JP, Ostlie JD, eds. *Ashcraft's Pediatric Surgery*. 6th ed. New York, NY: Elsevier; 2014:580–592.

Eng K, Alkhouri N. Neonatal cholestasis. In: Usatine RP, Sabella C, Smith M, Mayeaux EJ Jr, Chumley HS, Appachi E, eds. *The Color Atlas of Pediatrics*. New York, NY: McGraw-Hill; 2015: Chapter 61.

Hackam DJ, Grikscheit T, Wang K, Upperman JS, Ford HR. Pediatric surgery. In: Brunicardi F, Andersen DK, Billiar TR, et al., (eds.), *Schwartz's Principles of Surgery*. 10th ed. New York, NY: McGraw-Hill; 2014: Chapter 39.

Jones SA, Karrer FM. Biliary atresia and choledochal cyst. In: Ziegler MM, Azizkhan RG, Allmen D, Weber TR, eds. *Operative Pediatric Surgery*. 2nd ed. New York, NY: McGraw-Hill; 2014: Chapter 56.

16. **(B)** A choledochal cyst can produce symptoms at any age, but they usually present within the first decade of life. The classic triad of pain, jaundice, and a palpable mass is noted in less than one-third of afflicted individuals. Infants present with persistent asymptomatic jaundice, while children can present with advanced disease, including cholangitis, pancreatitis, or portal hypertension. Congenital choledochal cysts arise from a structural defect in the bile ducts, whereas the acquired type is thought to be caused by abnormal reflux of pancreatic juice into the bile ducts. Any patient with persistent jaundice or abdominal mass should be evaluated with an ultrasound first. However, magnetic resonance cholangiopancreatography (MRCP) offers high sensitivity in detecting choledochal cysts and has been widely used as the preoperative guide. Five types of choledochal cyst have been described, with type I accounting for the majority of cases (Fig. 34-27). Untreated choledochal cyst leads to hepatic fibrosis and possible malignant degeneration; therefore, surgical excision with reconstruction is mandated Treatment depends on the type of cystic malformation, and surgical therapy is aimed at total cyst excision via a Roux-en-Y hepaticojejunostomy (types I, II, IVb [multicystic disease that extends into the intrahepatic bilary ducts]). Type III (choledochoceles) and type IVa (intraductal cysts) variants may require a lateral hilar dissection and fillet of the intrahepatic cyst. Type V, known as Caroli disease, affects only the intrahepatic ducts and should be treated with partial hepatectomy in localized disease or liver transplantation in cases of diffuse disease.

BIBLIOGRAPHY

Karrer FM, Jones AS. Biliary atresia and choledochal cyst. Ziegler MM, Azizkhan RG, Allmen D, Weber TR, eds. *Operative Pediatric Surgery*. 2nd ed. New York, NY: McGraw-Hill; 2014: Chapter 56.

Liem TN, Holcomb WG. Choledochal cyst and gallbladder disease. In: Holcomb WG, Murphy JP, Ostlie JD, eds. *Ashcraft's Pediatric Surgery*. 6th ed. New York, NY: Elsevier; 2014:593–598.

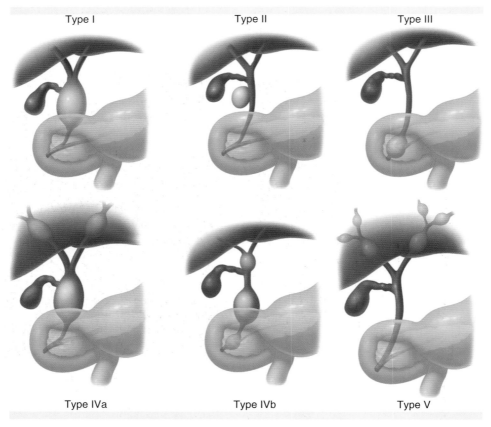

FIGURE 34-27. Classification of choledochal cysts (from Brunicardi F, Andersen DK, Billiar TR, et al., (eds.), *Schwartz's Principles of Surgery*. 10th ed. New York, NY: McGraw-Hill; 2014: Fig. 32-22. Copyright © The McGraw-Hill Companies, Inc. All rights reserved).

Pham TH, Hunter JG. Gallbladder and the extrahepatic biliary system. In: Brunicardi F, Andersen DK, Billiar TR, et al., (eds.), *Schwartz's Principles of Surgery*. 10th ed. New York, NY: McGraw-Hill; 2014: Chapter 32.

17. **(E)** Seriously injured children who are hypotensive and have decreased circulating volume may have obscured venous landmarks that make placement of peripheral intravenous catheters difficult. Some advocate a "60-s rule" when placing intravenous access; if intravenous access cannot be cannulated within 1 min, other routes are recommended. Advanced Trauma Life Support (ATLS) guidelines support IO catheter placement in children under 6 years of age when rapid venous access cannot be achieved after two attempts in a critically injured child. In children older than 6 years of age, either a venous cutdown may be performed at the ankle or a percutaneous femoral line should be placed. The IO route for vascular access is based on the presence of noncollapsible veins that drain the medullary sinuses in the bone marrow. The vascular network empties into the central venous circulation via nutrient and emissary veins. As a result, drugs, crystalloid solutions, and blood products may be given by the IO route with almost immediate absorption.

A 16- to 18-gauge bone aspiration needle is inserted through the skin 1–3 cm below and medial to the tibial tuberosity and advanced through the bone into the bone marrow. Contraindications to IO placement include lower extremity or pelvic fractures or if access to the tibia is not possible; other bones adequate for IO vascular access include the distal femur and the distal humerus. The IO line is considered a temporary maneuver; the child should have IO access discontinued once an appropriate intravenous line has been obtained. Complications related to IO access occur infrequently, yet rates increase with long-term use and include osteomyelitis, local cellulitis, infiltration of fluid into the subperiosteal and subcutaneous tissues, and leakage at the insertion site. Of note, only newborns with an attached umbilicus are candidates for an umbilical venous catheter.

BIBLIOGRAPHY

Luck RP, Haines C, Mull CC. Intraosseous access. *J Emerg Med* 2010 Oct;39(4):468–475. doi:10.1016/j.jemermed.2009.04.054. Epub 2009 Jul 9.

Noah Z. Intraosseous line insertion. In: Goodman DM, Green TP, Unti SM, Powell EC, eds. *Current Procedures: Pediatrics*. New York, NY: McGraw-Hill; 2007: Chapter 9.

18. **(B)** Thoracic injury occurs in 4.5% of injured children. Because of a pliable skeleton that is surrounded by less fat and elastic connective tissues, rib fractures are uncommon in younger children and indicate a significant amount of energy transfer to the chest and thoracic contents. The presence of rib fractures should focus a clinician's attention to the risk of multiple serious injuries in a child with a history of trauma. Moreover, the identification of three or more fractured ribs is a sensitive marker of injury severity and multisystem injuries and fulfills criteria for transfer to a trauma center.

Pulmonary contusions are the most common thoracic injury in traumatized children. While initial chest radiographs may not reveal demonstrable pulmonary injury, a repeat chest film 48–72 h after the injury is diagnostic. A chest CT frequently may show evidence of pulmonary contusion and hemopneumothorax that are sometimes not apparent on chest radiography. However, a chest CT for the sole purpose of evaluating lung contusions seen on chest x-ray should be done only in patients with serious respiratory compromise. A study by Wagner and colleagues showed that when greater than 28% of lung is involved, mechanical ventilation was required, but it was not needed when less than 18% was involved. Management of lung contusions is largely supportive (fluid administration, pain control, and pulmonary toilet) but may require more nontraditional modes of ventilation in more severe cases.

Mediastinal injuries, which involve the great vessels and the heart, are uncommon in children. The most common great vessel injury is aortic disruption, and it is seen in older adolescents as a result of a high-impact motor vehicle crash. Mechanisms of aortic disruption include sheer forces, compression of the aorta over the vertebral column, and intraluminal hyperextension. Diagnosis may be suggested by radiographic chest film demonstrating a widened mediastinum and abnormal aortic knob contour (these two signs are the most reliable radiographic markers). Yet, a prominent thymic shadow in young children can make mediastinal shape interpretation difficult.

Blunt cardiac injury should be suspected in a patient with direct blunt trauma to the chest who is complaining of chest pain. Initially, an ECG should be obtained to identify any arrhythmias. The right ventricle is most frequently affected given its most anterior location. In hemodynamically unstable patients with abnormal ECG findings, an echocardiogram is mandated to further assess the extent of injury. Nevertheless, stable patients with abnormal ECG findings can be safely monitored. Troponins have not been proven useful in the diagnosis of blunt cardiac injury.

In situations involving multisystem trauma, it may be difficult to differentiate causes of hypoxia and hypotension. Hemorrhage, cardiac tamponade, pulmonary embolism, and tension pneumothorax may all show similar clinical presentations, and further diagnostic modalities (chest radiography, CT, echo, FAST) are needed if the child is stable. In a hemodynamically unstable child, a chest tube should be inserted to treat cases of tension pneumothorax and hemothorax. Immediate drainage of 15 mL/kg or more than 2–3 mL/kg/h for three consecutive hours are indications for thoracotomy. Beck's triad (hypotension, jugular venous distension, and muffled heart sounds) is infrequently present in children in cases of suspected cardiac tamponade. Pericardiocentesis should be performed in the trauma bay. If the patient is deteriorating rapidly, a left lateral thoracotomy must be performed. Echocardiogram is both sensitive and specific for tamponade. In addition, pericardial fluid may be detected in a FAST examination of an injured child. An operating room thoracotomy should be the next step in cases of positive pericardiocentesis or FAST examination.

Diaphragm injuries from blunt trauma are often difficult to diagnose, and as a consequence, management may be delayed. Reports indicate that 40–50% are not diagnosed in the initial phase of trauma. The left hemidiaphragm is involved in two-thirds of cases (usually in the posterolateral location). When diaphragmatic rupture is suspected (visceral herniation, nasogastric tube within the hemithorax, or abnormal diaphragm contour), operative exploration is indicated.

In the chest radiograph shown in Fig. 34-8, a tension pneumothorax is responsible for the patient's clinical presentation.

BIBLIOGRAPHY

Beaudin M, Falcone AR Jr. Thoracic injuries. In: Ziegler MM, Azizkhan RG, Allmen D, Weber TR, eds. *Operative Pediatric Surgery.* 2nd ed. New York, NY: McGraw-Hill; 2014: Chapter 80.

Kenefake ME, Swarm M, Walthall J. Nuances in pediatric trauma. *Emerg Med Clin North Am* 2013 Aug;31(3):627–652. doi:10.1016/j.emc.2013.04.004. Epub 2013 Jun 27.

Ruiz-Elizalde, RA, Tuggle WD. Thoracic trauma. In: Holcomb WG, Murphy JP, Ostlie JD, eds. *Ashcraft's Pediatric Surgery.* 6th ed. New York, NY: Elsevier; 2014:190–197.

19. **(A)** Evaluation of a child with a history of intra-abdominal trauma begins with a primary survey and a thorough secondary survey. Physical examination signs that are suspicious for intra-abdominal injury include abdominal wall abrasions and contusions, abdominal distension, and abdominal pain. The spleen and liver are the most commonly injured intra-abdominal organs in children.

Several diagnostic approaches are available for the stable patient. CT scanning of the abdomen/pelvis with intravenous contrast can reveal injury to the many solid organs (spleen, liver, kidneys, pancreas, adrenals, and the retroperitoneum). Given the concerns of radiation

exposure, several algorithms have been developed that include laboratory values and physical exam findings that predict clinically significant intra-abdominal injuries and therefore the need for CT scans of the abdomen and pelvis. Contrast can also be omitted during the initial scan depending on the experience and protocols of the trauma center. Identification of bowel injury can be difficult on CT scan. Extravasation of oral contrast, free intraperitoneal air, free fluid in the abdomen without solid-organ injury, bowel wall thickening, and multiple loops of fluid-filled bowel are indicative of intestinal injury.

FAST has emerged as an effective and inexpensive approach to identify intra-abdominal fluid in adults. Many children sustain intra-abdominal injuries that do not demonstrate any free fluid. Therefore, a negative FAST does not rule out intra-abdominal injury. In addition, FAST is poor at identifying organ-specific injury and cannot detect retroperitoneal injuries. Nevertheless, a positive FAST in a hemodynamically unstable patient supports the decision for operative exploration.

Diagnostic laparoscopy should be used in patients with free fluid seen on CT but absence of solid-organ injuries, or in patients with abdominal pain and negative imaging studies. Advocates of diagnostic laparoscopy support the use of this tool not only for diagnostic purposes but also for therapeutic means.

Diagnostic peritoneal lavage can be performed in the operating or emergency room, particularly if other imaging modalities are unavailable or the child is going to the operating room for another reason. The usefulness of diagnostic peritoneal lavage remains in debate.

BIBLIOGRAPHY

Atabaki SM, Lucid W, Taylor T. Abdominal trauma. In: Strange GR, Ahrens WR, Schafermeyer RW, Wiebe RA, eds. *Pediatric Emergency Medicine.* 3rd ed. New York, NY: McGraw-Hill; 2009: Chapter 32.

Gaines AB, Austin MK. Abdominal and renal trauma. In: Holcomb WG, Murphy JP, Ostlie JD, eds. *Ashcraft's Pediatric Surgery.* 6th ed. New York, NY: Elsevier; 2014:200–202.

Tuggle DW, Kreykes NS. The pediatric patient. In: Mattox KL, Moore EE, Feliciano DV, eds. *Trauma.* 7th ed. New York, NY: McGraw-Hill; 2013: Chapter 43.

20. **(B)** In a growing child, the bony skeleton is one organ system that is characterized with persistent growth, remodeling potential, elasticity, open physes, thick periosteum, and smaller anatomic structure. The basic anatomy of bone consists of several components that participate in fracture healing when bony disruption (fracture) occurs. The outer layer (periosteum) is thick and flexible and plays a major role in fracture healing

due to the vascularity and bone-forming capabilities associated with this layer. Under the periosteum, the hard cortex gives bone its shape and strength. A Haversian system (vascular passages running the length of the bone) and cellular elements such as osteocytes, osteoblasts, and osteoclasts are present within this bony component. The inner lining of the bone (endosteum) also plays a role in new bone formation during fracture healing. The innermost structure, the medullary canal, contributes to the fracture-healing cascade and progresses most rapidly. Finally, marrow elements within the cancellous bony canal are another factor in the healing potential of bone.

Different fracture patterns may result in children due to the varying amounts of cartilage residing in their immature bones. In pediatric skeletal trauma, plastic deformation of bone is a common finding. Persistent bony deformity results as the bone is bent beyond its elastic recoil potential; thus, this type of bone deformity must be straightened or broken to effect reduction. Other types of fractures include torus or buckle fractures and greenstick fractures.

In terms of select injury fractures, the forearm is the most common site of fracture in children. The distal one-third of the radius or ulna is involved in 55% of all childhood fractures; 75% occur in the distal one-third of the radius, thereby making it the single most common fracture. Supracondylar humeral fractures make up approximately 60% of elbow fractures in children. The importance in identifying and immobilizing this type of injury in children is essential because of the high incidence of associated neurovascular injury. In addition, particular attention should be directed toward the forearm compartments as forearm and elbow fractures can lead to compartment syndromes. Radial head subluxation (nursemaid's elbow) usually occurs in children less than 6 years of age. Typically, a history of a vigorous pull on the arm by a caretaker is elicited. The child usually holds the arm pronated and partially flexed, refusing to use the arm voluntarily. Treatment is geared toward reducing the trapped annular ligament, which is trapped between the radial head and the capitellum. This can usually be achieved by reducing the elbow through a series of nonsurgical maneuvers that allow that annular ligament to slide over the radial head to its normal position around the radial neck. While trauma is the cause of most anterior shoulder dislocations (posterior dislocations usually due to anatomic instability or epileptic seizure), brachial plexus and vascular injuries can occur but are rare.

Growth plate (physeal) injuries are a concern in the pediatric arena in that the injured area involves a functioning growth plate; if the open growth plate is sufficiently damaged, premature physeal arrest may occur leading to extremity deformity or shortening. For example, injury to the distal femoral physis can lead to partial or near-complete growth arrest and is more common than in any other similarly injured physis. Overall management of pediatric orthopedic trauma includes considering future growth and bone-remodeling potential, recognizing and minimizing physeal plate injury, and aggressive treatment of compartment syndromes.

BIBLIOGRAPHY

Rab GT. Pediatric orthopedic surgery. In: Skinner HB, McMahon PJ, eds. *Current Diagnosis & Treatment in Orthopedics.* 5th ed. New York, NY: McGraw-Hill; 2014: Chapter 10.

Thomas BJ, Fu FH, Muller B, et al. Orthopedic surgery. In: Brunicardi F, Andersen DK, Billiar TR, et al., (eds.), *Schwartz's Principles of Surgery.* 10th ed. New York, NY: McGraw-Hill; 2014: Chapter 43.

21. **(D)** The repair of pediatric hernias constitutes one of the most common congenital anomalies that confront pediatric surgeons. The majority of inguinal hernias in infants and children are indirect and are a result of the failure of the PV (a diverticulum of peritoneum) to involute as the process of gonad descent proceeds into the scrotum in males and the lower pelvis in females. The PV is an anteromedial structure that appears to aid in testicular descent into the scrotum; it later regresses and thereby obliterates the entrance of the peritoneal cavity into the inguinal canal. A patent processus vaginalis (PPV) is a potential inguinal hernia, only becoming an actual, clinically detectable, symptomatic hernia when it contains an abdominal viscus. The incidence of inguinal hernias is around 2–5% in full-term neonates but is significantly higher in preterm infants. Inguinal hernias occur more frequently in boys and affect the right side 60% of the time. The left testis reaches a final intrascrotal position before that of its right counterpart, leading to an earlier onset of the gradual obliteration of the PPV, explaining the higher incidence of right inguinal hernias. It also accounts for the increased incidence of UDT on the right.

Various conditions are associated with inguinal hernias and include a positive family history, UDT, prematurity, ascites, hypospadias or epispadias, presence of a ventriculoperitoneal shunt, use of continuous peritoneal dialysis, ambiguous genitalia, and children with connective tissue disorders (Ehlers-Danlos and Hunter-Hurler syndrome). Because this type of hernia will not close spontaneously and because of the high risk of incarceration (especially in infants under 1 year of age), inguinal hernias should be repaired within 4 weeks of diagnosis. While repair of inguinal hernias involves high suture ligation of the sac at the level of the internal ring, the issue of contralateral exploration continues to be a subject of debate. There seems to have evolved a selective approach to managing the opposite groin based on age, gender, and PPVs. In children less than 2 years of age, the patency of the PV is high, and some advocate contralateral exploration because of the frequent occurrence of unsuspected hernias.

Recent studies have not shown significant differences in determining the presence of a contralateral PPV in cases of unilateral inguinal hernia. Laparoscopy has aided in detection of a contralateral PPV. Yet, the issue of a PPV is that it is a potential factor for inguinal hernia development; it does not represent a true hernia. Spontaneous closure occurs in the majority of cases (60% by 2 years of age), and it appears that not all PPVs develop into inguinal hernias. Nevertheless, some justify a contralateral exploration in children who are at high anesthetic risk, when distance and transportation issues may impede the return of an infant to the hospital, and if the child is at risk for subsequent development for an inguinal hernia (children with Ventriculoperitoneal (VP) shunts, connective tissue disorders, family history of bilateral inguinal hernias). Currently, three different approaches are used in clinical practice: open through a groin incision with high ligation of the hernia; fully laparoscopic "closed," occluding the internal ring with an intracorporeally placed suture from "above" or "inside," usually without excision of the sac; and "laparoscopic guided/assisted," a hybrid in which the tying of the suture placed around the sac at the internal ring is done extracorporeally.

Umbilical hernias are a result of intestinal protrusion through an incompletely closed, contracting umbilical ring. Some conditions that predispose an infant to umbilical hernias include low birth weight, Beckwith-Weidemann's syndrome (BWS), Down's syndrome, and ascites. Most umbilical hernias close after birth, and the risk of strangulation or incarceration is extremely low. Most pediatric surgeons defer treatment until 4 or 5 years of age before operating on asymptomatic patients. A relative surgical indication is related to size of the defect: A defect greater than 2 cm is not likely to close spontaneously.

Femoral hernias in infants and children are rare. Because of the similarity in clinical presentation to an indirect inguinal hernia, femoral hernia is easily misdiagnosed. Furthermore, the diagnosis may not be made until the patient returns to the clinic with a recurrent inguinal hernia. Thus, any child with recurrence after an adequate inguinal herniorrhaphy should be considered to have a femoral hernia. A high index of suspicion is needed especially when the absence of an expected indirect inguinal hernia is encountered in the operating room. Management consists of approaching the hernia

that occupies the femoral canal just medial to the femoral vein; infrainguinal, transinguinal, suprainguinal open approaches are described, and laparoscopic repair has been described.

In this case, the repair of the inguinal hernia should be undertaken in addition to the umbilical hernia due to the size of the umbilical hernia.

BIBLIOGRAPHY

Gauderer WLM, Cina AR. Hernias of the inguinal region. In: Ziegler MM, Azizkhan RG, Allmen D, Weber TR, eds. *Operative Pediatric Surgery*. 2nd ed. New York, NY: McGraw-Hill; 2014: Chapter 36.

Kokoska ER, Weber TR. Umbilical and supraumbilical disease. In: Ziegler MM, Azizkhan RG, Allmen D, Weber TR, eds. *Operative Pediatric Surgery*. 2nd ed. New York, NY: McGraw-Hill; 2014: Chapter 35.

Pini Prato A, Rossi V, Mosconi M, et al. Inguinal hernia in neonates and ex-preterm: complications, timing and need for routine contralateral exploration. *Pediatr Surg Int* 2015 Feb;31(2):131–136. doi:10.1007/s00383-014-3638-z. Epub 2014 Nov 9.

22. **(B)** An UDT, or cryptorchidism, describes the failure of a testis to descend into the scrotum and is located at any point along the normal path of descent or at an ectopic site. The reported incidence is from 2 to 5% of all full-term newborn males, whereas the rate increases to 25% in premature and small-for-gestational-age neonates. The mechanisms of normal testicular descent are multifactorial and include an intact hypothalamic-pituitary-testicular axis along with functional, mechanical, and neural components. The process of testicular descent has been proposed to occur in two steps; the first step is the movement of the testis from the retroperitoneum to the internal inguinal ring (controlled by Mullerian inhibiting substance from Sertoli cells). The secondary phase involves the migration of the testis from the internal inguinal ring to the scrotum (androgen-dependent phase and mediated by genitofemoral nerve release of calcitonin gene-related peptide). Disorders that are associated with cryptorchidism include chromosomal syndromes, anterior abdominal wall abnormalities, cerebral or neuromuscular disorders, and endocrine dysfunction.

If unrecognized, an UDT will undergo degenerative changes, and about one-third of UDTs lack germ cells by the age of 2. Spermatic cord torsion and incarcerated inguinal hernias are also potential problems if the testicle is left untreated. The most important long-term complications of cryptorchidism are infertility and testicular germ cell cancer (the risk is highest in men who have had an intra-abdominal testis). The malignancy risk does not lessen with orchiopexy in cases of delayed treatment.

The goal of diagnosis is to identify the presence or absence of a testis. The physical examination should evaluate the genitalia and the presence of scrotal asymmetry, which is suggestive of an UDT. Because a retractile testis can be confused with cryptorchidism secondary to cremasteric muscle hyperactivity, the patient should be positioned to inhibit the reflex (upright, cross-legged). Additional methods to reduce the cremasteric reflex include a warm environment, warm hands, and distracting the patient. An UDT is one that does not stay within the scrotal sac without overstretching the spermatic cord. UDTs can be further classified in terms of whether they arrested in the normal line of descent (superficial inguinal pouch, canalicular, or intra-abdominal), are ectopic, or are absent. Ectopic sites such as prepenile, femoral, and perineal locations should be examined in cases of a nonpalpable testicle. As spontaneous testicular descent remains unlikely after 6 months of life, current recommendation is to perform orchiopexy shortly after the child reaches 6 months.

Some argue that preoperative localization of the nonpalpable testis is difficult and an unneeded tool. Specifically, scrotal ultrasound is appealing in that it is noninvasive, and radiation exposure is negligible. Yet, in the evaluation of an UDT, ultrasound has been demonstrated to lack benefit in most boys because it rarely localizes a true nonpalpable testis, and when it is located, the testis is palpable in the clinician's office. Nevertheless, ultrasound is useful for documenting testicular size in secondary or recurrent cryptorchidism and in evaluating obese males with nonpalpable testes. An alternative that has received attention is gadolinium-infusion magnetic resonance angiogram (Gd-infusion MRA). Lam and colleagues have shown the usefulness of Gd-infusion MRA in the preoperative localization of nonpalpable undescended testes; when compared to conventional MRI, detection rates were 82% (MRI) versus 100% for MRA. Regardless of imaging, the most efficacious tool for locating a nonpalpable testis is laparoscopy.

The treatment for an UDT is surgical. The use of hormonal treatment has fallen out of favor because of a low success rate, in the 20% range; the significant patient/parent discomfort of daily injections; and the possible side effect of androgen hormone administration. However, in patients with bilateral nonpalpable testes, a human chorionic gonadotropin (hCG) stimulation test can be performed to determine the presence of testicular tissue. If there is no corresponding rise of testosterone with stimulation by hCG and if the basal level of FSH is high, it indicates absence of testicular tissue, and surgical exploration may not be necessary. Surgical therapy consists of inguinal orchiopexy for a palpable UDT, while a laparoscopic approach may be used to confirm the presence or absence of a testis in nonpalpable cases. Then,

an orchiopexy is performed if a testicle is visualized. The basic principles of an orchiopexy include identification of a testicle, mobilization of the spermatic vessels and vas deferens, isolation and high ligation of the PV, and fixation of the testis in the subdartos pouch. Patients with intra-abdominal testis detected on laparoscopy and short cord should undergo a two-step orchiopexy (Fowler-Stephens).

BIBLIOGRAPHY

Kolon TF, Herndon CD, Baker LA, et al. Evaluation and treatment of cryptorchidism: AUA guideline. *J Urol* 2014 Aug;192(2):337–345. doi:10.1016/j.juro.2014.05.005. Epub 2014 May 20.

Stehr W, Betts JM. Cryptorchidism. In: Ziegler MM, Azizkhan RG, Allmen D, Weber TR, eds. *Operative Pediatric Surgery*. 2nd ed. New York, NY: McGraw-Hill; 2014: Chapter 62.

Walsh TJ, Smith JF. Male infertility. In: McAninch JW, Lue TF, eds. *Smith and Tanagho's General Urology*. 18th ed. New York, NY: McGraw-Hill; 2013: Chapter 44.

23. **(D)** Neuroblastoma (NB) is known as the most common solid extracranial malignancy in children, accounting for 10–15% of pediatric neoplasms. The tumor originates from embryonal neural crest cells that can occur anywhere along the sympathetic nervous system from the neck to the pelvis. While the site of the tumor dictates clinical symptoms, in 50% of cases children present with an abdominal mass as the tumor arises from the adrenal gland. At the time of diagnosis, 50% of patients will have a metastatic lesion, with regional lymph node involvement occurring in nearly 35%. NB most commonly metastasizes to the bony skeleton, particularly the long bones, spine, skull, pelvis, and ribs. Periorbital ecchymosis or "raccoon eyes" and proptosis are classic signs of metastatic disease and are related to the propensity of NB to metastasize to the bony orbit. Excessive catecholamine or vasoactive intestinal peptide (VIP) secretion can cause flushing, hypertension, and watery diarrhea. Acute cerebellar ataxia with opsoclonus-myoclonus syndrome has been also observed as a result of paraneoplasmatic syndrome. A combination of imaging, laboratory studies, and bone marrow biopsy confirmed by histopathology provides the diagnosis and staging of NB. Traditionally, CT would have been obtained that would show a calcified mass in 85% of cases. However, recently MRI has become the most sensitive imaging modality in diagnosis and staging of NB.

Diverse clinical variability is a hallmark of this malignancy; in children younger than 1 year of age, the tumor shows lower-stage disease (1, 2, and 4S) and in a majority of cases spontaneously regresses, whereas in children diagnosed older than 1 year of age NB presents as progressive, advanced-stage disease (3 and 4) with poor prognosis. Specific biologic and genetic factors associated with NB have been identified and aid not only in determining clinical behavior but also directing therapy regimens, which may include surgery, chemotherapy, or radiotherapy, depending on stage and age of presentation. Biologic factors associated with NB include serum ferritin, lactate dehydrogenase, nerve growth factor receptor TRK-A/B, and CD44. Genetic analysis has provided important chromosomal aberrations correlating to NB; the most common include DNA ploidy changes, deletions of chromosomal arms 1 p and 11q, amplification of MYCN oncogene, and gains of chromosome 17q.

Treatment of NB requires a multimodality approach that may include surgery, chemotherapy, or radiation, depending on classification and staging of the disease. The operative goal is complete tumor removal of both the primary tumor and its adjacent involved lymph nodes (for stage I and II disease). In contrast, patients with stage 4S disease do not benefit from surgical intervention, given the disseminated disease.

BIBLIOGRAPHY

Long E, Chang DH. Neuroblastoma. In: Ziegler MM, Azizkhan RG, Allmen D, Weber TR, eds. *Operative Pediatric Surgery*. 2nd ed. New York, NY: McGraw-Hill; 2014: Chapter 89.

Shaikh R, Prabhu SJ, Voss DS. Imaging in the evaluation and management of childhood cancer. In: Orkin HK, Fisher DE, Ginsburg D, Look AT, Lux ES, Nathan GD. *Nathan and Oski's Hematology and Oncology of Infancy and Childhood*. New York, NY: Elsevier; 2015:2146–2254.

24. **(C)** The CT scan demonstrates a large, spherical intrarenal mass with a well-defined rim of compressed renal parenchyma consistent with WT or nephroblastoma. WT is the most common malignant primary renal tumor of childhood and makes up approximately 6% of all pediatric cancers.

The genetic evaluation of WT has revealed that there are two main loci that are responsible for both hereditary and sporadic forms of WT. Deletions in the band 13 on the short arm of chromosome 11 (WT1 gene) or the band 15 on chromosome 11 (WT2 gene) have been shown to be involved in not only the predisposition of WT but also some of the congenital syndromes associated with WT. Additional genes for WT include 16q, 1p, and 17p (p53).

The peak incidence of WT is between 2 and 3 years of age, with typical presentation of an abdominal mass appreciated by a parent while the child is being bathed or dressed. Other presenting signs and symptoms may include hypertension, hematuria, malaise, pain, weight loss, and left-sided varicocele (secondary to tumor extension into the left renal vein and subsequent obstruction of the spermatic vein). Several congenital disorders are often seen with WT. Conditions known to have an association with WT include WAGR (WT, aniridia, genitourinary malformations, and mental retardation) syndrome; Beckwith–Wiedemann syndrome (omphalocele, visceromegaly, macroglossia, and gigantism); Denys-Drash's syndrome (WT, intersex disorders, and nephropathy); sporadic aniridia; isolated hemihypertrophy; and nephropathy with a female genotype/phenotype.

Evaluation of a child with a suspected WT should begin with an ultrasound to determine if the mass is intrarenal or extrarenal and evaluation of the IVC for flow and tumor thrombus. A CT should follow to evaluate the contralateral kidney and function of the kidneys and for planning surgical and radiation therapy.

Therapy is based on the stage of disease; factors guiding staging are disease extent, primary tumor respectability, lymph node status, adjacent organ involvement, presence of metastatic disease, and contralateral kidney involvement. The two most important factors continue to be the histology and the stage of the tumor. Other factors affecting prognosis are histology, stage, age, tumor weight, response to therapy, and loss of heterozygocity at 1p and 16q. The main responsibility of the surgeon is to remove the primary tumor completely, without spillage; to accurately assess the extent to which the tumor has spread; and to provide adequate lymph node sampling to accurately stage the disease.

Controversial areas in the management of WT are related to different therapeutic protocols; such issues include preresection biopsy, preoperative chemotherapy, preoperative imaging of the contralateral kidney, and partial nephrectomy. With regard to preresection biopsy, current protocols forgo preoperative biopsy and proceed with either primary surgical therapy (National Wilms Tumor Study Group, NWTSG) or preresection chemotherapy (International Society of Pediatric Oncology, SIOP). Preoperative, as well as intraoperative, biopsies are generally contraindicated and should only be performed when a tumor is deemed inoperable or the patient is unable to tolerate a laparotomy.

Indications for neoadjuvant chemotherapy include bilateral disease; disease in a solitary kidney; unilateral disease in a patient with a WT predisposition syndrome (such as WAGR, Beckwith-Weidmann, and Denys-Drash); pulmonary insufficiency from a heavy metastatic burden in the lungs; extensive intravascular thrombus above the level of the hepatic veins; clear evidence of preoperative rupture (a circumstance unreliably determined by preoperative imaging); unresectable disease, in the surgeon's judgment, without resection of adjacent organs (an assessment generally made at laparotomy).

In addition, the benefits of neoadjuvant chemotherapy include decreasing the incidence of tumor rupture and tumor debulking and avoiding radiotherapy in the presence of metastatic disease. However, one of the major concerns with routine use of preoperative chemotherapy is the accuracy of posttherapy staging; unfavorable histology may result, which could potentially lead to unnecessary intensification of therapy. Of importance is that the surgical complication rate for this malignancy has been shown to increase when preoperative imaging fails to provide the correct diagnosis.

Partial nephrectomy in WT is most commonly used for bilateral disease. In addition, it is advocated for cases of WT complicated by a solitary kidney or renal insufficiency. The issue of parenchymal sparing procedures for unilateral WT is questionable. The incidence of renal dysfunction in patients with unilateral WT is low; however, one reason for pursuing renal-preserving surgery is the concern for later developing renal dysfunction secondary to hyperfiltration damage to remaining nephrons. One dilemma for the subject of partial nephrectomy and unilateral disease is the potential for residual disease and higher rates of local reoccurrence compared with radical nephrectomy. Some advocate the role of preoperative chemotherapy as an integral component in achieving successful outcomes with unilateral WT and renal-sparing surgery. Nevertheless, while the issues of WT protocols continue to be further defined, the outcomes achieved from cooperative groups place WT among pediatric malignancies for which survival rates are high.

Anatomically, the kidneys are supplied by renal arteries, which branch directly from the abdominal aorta slightly inferior to the branching point of the SMA. The renal arteries travel to each kidney, each one *posterior* to its respective renal vein, which drain directly into the IVC. Of interest, the "nutcracker phenomenon" or left renal vein entrapment syndrome occurs with compression of the left renal vein between the abdominal aorta and the SMA as it passes medially to join the IVC.

BIBLIOGRAPHY

Davidoff AM. Nephroblastoma (Wilms' tumor). In: Ziegler MM, Azizkhan RG, Allmen D, Weber TR, eds. *Operative Pediatric Surgery*. 2nd ed. New York, NY: McGraw-Hill; 2014: Chapter 88.

Ko EY, Ritchey ML. Current management of Wilms' tumor in children. *J Pediatr Urol* 2009 Feb;5(1):56–65. doi:10.1016/j.jpurol.2008.08.007. Epub 2008 Oct 9.

25. **(C)** Rhabdomyosarcoma accounts for over 50% of all soft tissue sarcomas in children and is the third most common solid malignancy in children after NB and WT. The most common sites are the head and neck or the genitourinary system. Biologically, RMS is one of the small, round, blue-cell neoplasms that arises from the embryonal mesenchyme (NBs, Ewing's sarcoma, peripheral neural ectodermal tumors, non-Hodgkin's lymphoma, and soft tissue sarcomas are other small cell tumors). Five major subtypes of RMS exist (embryonal, alveolar, botryoid, spindle cell, and pleomorphic), yet embryonal and alveolar are the two major subtypes. The embryonal type usually presents in younger children and has more favorable outcomes. RMS has a bimodal distribution, with approximately 65% of cases occurring in children younger than 6 years and the remaining cases developing in children aged 10–18 years.

As with most solid tumors, the site of RMS presentation usually reflects clinical symptoms. Nevertheless, diagnosis requires tissue examination, which may be attained by a variety of methods, which include fine-needle, core biopsy, incisional biopsy, or endoscopic techniques. Specifically, extremity/truncal RMS lesions should be excised or biopsied through an incision in line with the anticipated incision for future resection. Therefore, a longitudinal biopsy incision should be made in a mass presenting on an extremity such that future resection is not hindered. In addition, the regional lymph node status in patients with extremity RMS has important impact on survival; thus, lymph nodes may be evaluated by lymphatic mapping with sentinel node biopsy, although limited information exists on sentinel node biopsy for children.

Staging depends on the location, histologic type, size, lymph node involvement, and presence of distal metastasis. Preoperative workup includes standard laboratory work; imaging of primary lesion with CT or MRI; and metastatic workup that involves bone scan, bone marrow biopsy, CT of the brain, lungs, and liver, and lumbar puncture for cerebrospinal fluid sampling. While surgical intervention plays a key role in the management of this disease, surgery alone has been shown to have poor survival rates. Nevertheless, complete tumor resection with absence of microscopic residual disease offers the best survival outcomes. The present management of RMS is multimodal, which includes surgery, radiation, and chemotherapy. All patients with RMS receive chemotherapy. Standard therapeutic regimens consist of a combination of vincristine, actinomycin-D, and cyclophosphamide (VAC). Survival rates are greater than 70% with multimodal therapy, and operative procedures for RMS are less disfiguring and more conservative organ-sparing procedures. Lymph node sampling is necessary for adequate staging of the disease that will determine further adjuvant therapy; however, it does not offer therapeutic purposes.

Little is known regarding the etiology of RMS, yet genetic evaluation has demonstrated that certain pathways are altered in this malignancy. For example, central regulatory components for RMS are *c-Met* (tyrosine kinase oncogene), *pRB* (retinoblastoma), and *p53*. Simultaneous disruption of these component pathways aggravates the regulation of myogenic growth and differentiation and promotes tumor formation. In addition, RMS may be associated with Li-Fraumeni's syndrome and neurofibromatosis type 1.

BIBLIOGRAPHY

De Corti F, Dall'Igna P, Bisogno G, et al. Sentinel node biopsy in pediatric soft tissue sarcomas of extremities. *Pediatr Blood Cancer* 2009 Jan;52(1):51–54. doi:10.1002/pbc.21777.

Malkin D. Cancer genetics and biology. In: Rudolph CD, Rudolph AM, Lister GE, First LR, Gershon AA, eds. *Rudolph's Pediatrics.* 22nd ed. New York, NY: McGraw-Hill; 2011: Chapter 443.

Williams NF, Rodeberg AD. Diagnosis and treatment of rhabdomyosarcoma. In: Ziegler MM, Azizkhan RG, Allmen D, Weber TR, eds. *Operative Pediatric Surgery.* 2nd ed. New York, NY: McGraw-Hill; 2014: Chapter 91.

26. **(D)** The age of this patient combined with the findings on CT scan, which show a large intrahepatic mass with heterogeneous attenuation and well-defined margins with multiple areas of reduced echogenicity, are suggestive of a hepatoblastoma. Primary pediatric hepatic tumors in the United States are rare (approximately 120 cases per year); more than two-thirds of cases account for malignant disease. Hepatoblastoma and HCC make up greater than 90% of hepatic neoplasms in children. Both of these malignancies have distinct features.

Hepatoblastoma is an embryonal tumor that occurs in children less than 3 years of age (average 1 year). A male predominance is seen with hepatoblastoma, usually twice as many males as females. Presentation is typically with asymptomatic progressive abdominal growth within the right upper quadrant that is incidentally noted. Because these tumors present with few symptoms, greater than 60% of hepatoblastomas are diagnosed with advanced-stage large, unresectable masses. The patient may present with anemia and thrombocytosis; however, the majority (90%) will present with elevated AFP levels. AFP is a sensitive marker for the presence of hepatoblastoma that can be used clinically to monitor the effectiveness of treatment or disease progression or to detect tumor recurrence. Associated anomalies are not uncommon with hepatoblastoma. The risk of hepatoblastoma is elevated with FAP and BWS, suggesting that the genes responsible (chromosomes 5 and 11, respectively) may play a role in the pathogenesis for this malignancy. Patients with Beckwith–Wiedemann syndrome must be monitored with serial AFP levels every 3 months until the age of 4 years and with an abdominal ultrasound every 3 months until they reach age 8 years. Screening studies for hepatoblastoma are also recommended in patients with FAP. These patients should be screened for the Adenomatous polyposis coli (APC) tumor/suppressor gene. Initial radiographic evaluation for suspected hepatic malignancies includes an ultrasound, followed by CT or MRI, which will aid not only in the diagnosis but also in staging and treatment protocols. Once malignancy has been suspected, accurate diagnosis is confirmed with an open, laparoscopic, or percutaneous needle biopsy.

Two staging systems are currently used: one used by the Children's Oncology Group (COG), a combined histologic and surgical staging system; and the Pretreatment Extent of Disease (PRETEXT) staging system, which is being used by the SIOP and is based on the radiologic location of the tumor before treatment. Treatment is based on complete resection of the tumor with employment of neoadjuvant or adjuvant chemotherapy in selected patients with advanced disease. Approximately 75% of children with hepatoblastoma can be cured completely; nevertheless, large tumor burden, multifocal tumors, and metastatic disease lead to poor prognosis. Additional prognostic factors include histologic type, complete resection of tumor, tumor response to chemotherapy, and AFP levels.

In contrast to hepatoblastoma, HCC is more common in older children (between 12 and 15 years old) and often develops in the presence of underlying liver disease and cirrhosis; this includes viral diseases (especially hepatitis B); metabolic disorders (e.g., chronic cholestasis, tyrosinemia, hemochromatosis, and α-1 antitrypsin); and children with biliary obstructive processes (e.g., BA, primary biliary cirrhosis, and primary sclerosing cholangitis). Clinical signs include hepatomegaly, which is occasionally associated with dull epigastric pain. Molecular evidence underlying HCC is limited and includes mutations in p53 and other cell cycle proteins, such as pRB, p16, p21, and p27. As with hepatoblastoma, imaging and diagnostic approaches are similar, yet treatment outcomes for these patients contrast sharply with patients with hepatoblastoma. Laboratory studies will reveal elevated aspartate aminotransferase, lactate dehydrogenase, and AFP levels. Unfortunately, the overall cure rate is low (15%). Treatment for HCC is complete tumor excision, followed by adjuvant chemotherapy. Alternative therapies include transarterial chemoembolization, cryosurgery, thermotherapy, radio-frequency ablation, and liver transplantation.

Infantile hepatic hemangioma (IHH) is the most common benign solid hepatic tumor in children, and the majority present in the first 6 months of age. Infants with IHH can present with significant symptoms, including hepatomegaly, high-output CHF, respiratory distress, and anemia. Occasionally, these infants present with Kasabach-Merritt syndrome, which is characterized by acute thrombocytopenia, microangiopathic hemolytic anemia, and a consumptive coagulopathy. This syndrome can be life threatening and requires aggressive supportive treatment, as well as treatment of the hemangioma itself. All asymptomatic lesions should be monitored with ultrasound until resolution. Patients with multifocal disease should be screened for hypothyroidism. Symptomatic lesions should be treated with steroids or propranolol. If there is no response, then the hemangioma should be embolized. Other benign tumors that may undergo operative management due to symptoms or to establish diagnosis include mesenchymal hamartomas, adenomas, focal nodular hyperplasia, and cysts.

Hepatic metastasis in children is uncommon, yet liver resection is warranted for hepatic tumor extension or for isolated tumor deposits. Nephroblastomas, adrenal cortical carcinomas, pheochromocytomas, and germ cell tumors (GCTs) are malignancies that have a tendency for rare hepatic involvement and may require operative resection.

BIBLIOGRAPHY

Andrews SW, Hendrickson JR. Benign hepatic tumors. In: Holcomb WG, Murphy JP, Ostlie JD, eds. *Ashcraft's Pediatric Surgery*. 6th ed. New York, NY: Elsevier; 2014:906–909.
Meyers LR, Tiao MG. Hepatic tumors. In: Ziegler MM, Azizkhan RG, Allmen D, Weber TR, eds. *Operative Pediatric Surgery*. 2nd ed. New York, NY: McGraw-Hill; 2014: Chapter 93.

27. **(E)** Ovarian tumors in children originate from one of three cell types: germinal epithelium of the urogenital ridge, stromal cell components of the urogenital ridge, or germ cells from the yolk sac. Of importance is age of presentation because the frequency of tumor type is age dependent. Age distribution of various ovarian tumors includes the following: Girls under 4 years typically have sex cord-stromal tumors (granulosa-theca cell and Sertoli-Leydig cell); older teenage females have epithelial tumors (serous or mucinous cystadenoma); and adenocarcinoma tends to occur more in adult females. Regardless, GCTs make up from 60 to 74% of all ovarian tumors in females under 18 years of age and are the most common type of tumor in children.

Plain abdominal radiography may show coarse calcification, teeth, or bone consistent with a teratoma. Ultrasound can also be used to visualize a mass or inspect for ovarian torsion. CT better characterizes a mass and aids in tumor extension. Laboratory studies should include the tumor serum markers AFP, β-HCG, and CA-125. GCT subtypes exist that are based on degree

TABLE 34-1 Ovarian Tumor Markers and Incidence of Bilateral Involvement

Tumor	Markers	Bilateral
Teratoma	±AFP	10%
Dysgerminoma	LDH-1	15%
Endodermal sinus tumor	AFP	Low
Choriocarcinoma	β-HCG	Low
Epithelial tumors	CA-125	15%

Abbreviations: AFP, α-fetoprotein; LDH, lactate dehydrogenase; β-HCG, β-human chorionic gonadotropin.

of differentiation: dysgerminomas, endodermal sinus tumors, embryonal carcinomas, choriocarcinoma, and teratomas (Table 34-1). Teratomas are the most common GCT and maybe immature, mature, or malignant. In children, the mature teratoma is the predominant type.

Usually, surgery alone is adequate therapy. Surgical principles regarding ovarian lesions are based on adequately removing tumorous tissue and staging while preserving ovarian tissue if possible. Because it may not be possible to distinguish between benign versus malignant, it is important to recognize that a cancer operation may be necessary (salpingo-oophorectomy and contralateral ovary inspection/biopsy, lymph node sampling [both iliac and retroperitoneal], ascitic fluid cytology or peritoneal washings, peritoneal/diaphragm surface inspection, and infracolic omentectomy). Entering the abdomen may be achieved by a midline approach or a Pfannenstiel incision, and some advocate the benefits of laparoscopy. Laparoscopic removal of benign ovarian masses is safe and without long-term sequelae, even in the presence of rupture and spillage (see Fig. 34-28). When malignancy is suspected, oophorectomy through a midline laparotomy incision allows proper staging with careful exploration, collection of pelvic cytology, and pelvic and periaortic lymph node sampling. Aspiration of an ovarian mass with cystic features should never be done because of the uncertainty of malignancy. Parents should be carefully counseled about the risks of future fertility of their child, risks of laparotomy/laparoscopy (tumor spillage and adhesions), and recurrence/malignant transformation.

BIBLIOGRAPHY

Breech L, Weber A. Pediatric and adolescent gynecology. In: Ziegler MM, Azizkhan RG, Allmen D, Weber TR, eds. *Operative Pediatric Surgery*. 2nd ed. New York, NY: McGraw-Hill; 2014: Chapter 70.

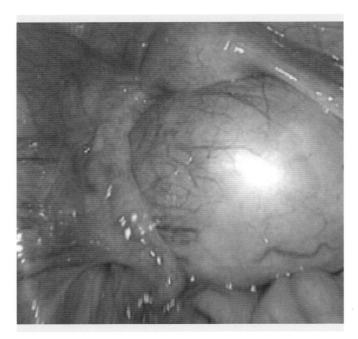

FIGURE 34-28. A benign cystic teratoma of the ovary.

Paradis J, Koltai PJ. Pediatric teratoma and dermoid cysts. *Otolaryngol Clin North Am* 2015 Feb;48(1):121–136. doi:10.1016/j.otc.2014.09.009.

Strickland LJ. Adnexal disease. In: Holcomb WG, Murphy JP, Ostlie JD, eds. *Ashcraft's Pediatric Surgery*. 6th ed. New York, NY: Elsevier; 2014:1053–1054.

28. **(E)** There are many significant differences in anatomy of pediatric patients and their physiologic response to injury when compared to adults. Children have a larger ratio of surface area to weight. This, in combination with a lack of subcutaneous fat and increased metabolism, makes them more susceptible to hypothermia. The pediatric skeletal system is incompletely ossified, and the body is therefore very elastic. The areas of growth and remodeling make bones more susceptible to injury, while significant energy can be transferred, creating internal injuries without significant external signs. A child's blood volume is approximately 70–80 mL/kg. Children have greater physiologic reserve than adults and do not manifest signs of shock until they have lost more than 25% of their blood volume. A loss of more than 45% of their blood volume is required to see hypotension. Children have a smaller body mass, which means that any traumatic force will result in more damage per unit of body area. Multisystem injury occurs in more than 50% of cases of pediatric trauma.

Mechanism of injury differs significantly between adults and children. Penetrating trauma is less common, and most injuries result from falls or the blunt force of a motor vehicle crash. Children's head sizes are proportionally larger; thus, head injuries are more common in children than adults. Conversely, children's torsos are broad and shallow, leaving solid organs and the bladder less protected.

BIBLIOGRAPHY

Cooper A. Early assessment and management of trauma. In: Holcomb WG, Murphy JP, Ostlie JD, eds. *Ashcraft's Pediatric Surgery*. 6th ed. New York, NY: Elsevier; 2014:177–183.

Tuggle DW, Kreykes NS. The pediatric patient. In: Mattox KL, Moore EE, Feliciano DV, eds. *Trauma*. 7th ed. New York, NY: McGraw-Hill; 2013: Chapter 43.

29. **(A)**

30. **(E)**

Explanations 29 and 30

The signs of hypovolemia in a child may be subtle. A child has a greater physiologic reserve than an adult and therefore demonstrates only minimal signs of shock until more than 25% of his or her blood volume is lost. Given that a child's circulating blood volume is 80 mL/kg, this magnitude of blood loss is approximately 20 mL/kg. Tachycardia is the child's primary response to hypovolemia. Other signs include a narrowed pulse pressure, cool or mottled skin, decreased level of consciousness, or decreased urine output. See Tables 34-2 and 34-3 for age-specific normal vital functions and systemic responses to blood loss. Table 34-4 provides a pediatric trauma scoring matrix. The presence of hypotension or bradycardia signals blood loss in excess of 45% of the child's circulating volume and severe shock for which the child is no longer able to compensate. Initial volume resuscitation is given as a bolus of 20 mL/kg (based on the goal of replacing 25% of the child's circulating volume) of warmed crystalloid solution. This may be repeated two times if appropriate hemodynamic response is not demonstrated or maintained. Response to fluid resuscitation is demonstrated by a decrease in heart rate, return of skin warmth and color, improving mental status, increased systolic blood pressure, and adequate urine output (1–2 mL/kg/h). If a third bolus is required, a 10- to 20-mL/kg bolus of PRBCs should be used as the next bolus. If type-specific blood is not available, the child may initially be given O-negative blood. Efforts should be ongoing to identify the source of blood loss and control that hemorrhage. Any child who cannot be stabilized after infusion of 40–60 mL/kg of lactated Ringer's solution and 10–20 mL/kg of PRBCs likely has internal bleeding and needs an operation (Tables 34-2 and 34-3).

TABLE 34-2 Systemic Responses to Blood Loss in the Pediatric Patient

System	<25% Blood Volume Loss	25–45% Blood Volume Loss	>45% Blood Volume Loss
Cardiac	Weak pulse; increased heart rate	Increased heart rate	Hypotension, tachycardia to bradycardia
CNS	Lethargic, irritable, confused	Change in level of consciousness, dulled response to pain	Comatose
Skin	Cool, clammy	Cyanotic, decreased capillary refill, cold extremities	Pale, cold
Kidneys	Minimal decrease in urinary output; increased specific gravity	Minimal urine output	No urinary output

CNS, central nervous system.

BIBLIOGRAPHY

American College of Surgeons Committee on Trauma. *Advanced Trauma Life Support® ATLS® Student Course Manual.* 9th ed. Chicago, IL: American College of Surgeons; 2012.

Cooper A. Early assessment and management of trauma. In: Holcomb WG, Murphy JP, Ostlie JD, eds. *Ashcraft's Pediatric Surgery.* 6th ed. New York, NY: Elsevier; 2014:177–183.

31. **(A)**

32. **(E)**

Explanations 31 and 32

The spleen is a commonly injured organ after blunt trauma. The child may complain of pain in the abdomen or referred pain in the left shoulder (Kehr's sign).

TABLE 34-3 Vital Functions

Age Group	Weight (kg)	Heart Rate (bpm)	Blood Pressure (mmHg)	Respiratory Rate	Urinary Output (mL/kg/h)
Birth to 6 months	3–6	180–160	60–80	60	2
Infant	12	160	80	40	1.5
Preschool	16	120	90	30	1
Adolescent	35	100	100	20	0.5

Source: Reproduced with permission from American College of Surgeons Committee on Trauma. *Advanced Trauma Life Support for Doctors, Student Course Manual.* 6th ed. Chicago, IL: American College of Surgeons; 1997:297.

TABLE 34-4 Pediatric Trauma Score

Component	+2	+1	−1
Size	>20 kg	10–20 kg	<10 kg
Airway	Normal	Maintainable	Unmaintainable
Systolic BP	>90 mmHg	50–90 mmHg	<50 mmHg
CNS	Awake	Obtunded/LOC	Coma/decerebrate
Skeletal	None	Closed fracture	Open/multiple fractures
Cutaneous	None	Minor	Major/penetrating

LOC, loss of consciousness.
Source: Reproduced with permission from Tepas JJ 3rd, Ramenofsky ML, Mollitt DL, Gans BM, DiScala C. The pediatric trauma score as a predictor of injury severity: an objective assessment. *J Trauma* 1988;28:425–429.

TABLE 34-5 American Association for the Surgery of Trauma Splenic Organ Injury Scale, 1994 Revision

Grade[a]			Injury Description
I		Hematoma	Subcapsular, <10% surface area
		Laceration	Capsular tear, <1 cm parenchymal depth
II		Hematoma	Subcapsular, 10–50% surface area; intraparenchyma, <5 cm in diameter
		Laceration	1–3 cm parenchymal depth, which does not involve a trabecular vessel
III		Hematoma	Subcapsular, >50% surface area or expanding; ruptured subcapsular or parenchymal hematoma; intraparenchymal hematoma >5 cm or expanding
		Laceration	>3 cm parenchymal depth or involving trabecular vessels
IV		Laceration	Laceration involving segmental or hilar vessels production major devascularization (>25% of spleen)
V		Laceration	Completely shattered spleen
		Vascular	Hilar injury which devascularizes the spleen

[a]Advance one grade for multiple injuries, up to grade III.
Source: Reproduced with permission from Moore EE, Cogbill TH, Jurkovich GJ, et al. Organ injury scaling: spleen and liver (1994 revision). *J Trauma* 1995;38:323–324.

Inspection of the abdomen may demonstrate bruising or abrasions in the left upper quadrant. Palpation may elicit localized or generalized abdominal tenderness. CT scan of the abdomen is the imaging test of choice in the evaluation of intra-abdominal injuries. CT scan allows grading of splenic injuries, which in turn guides management. Splenic injuries are divided into five grades (see Table 34-5).

The majority of splenic injuries in children can be successfully managed nonoperatively. The decision for laparotomy for splenic injury is based on the child's hemodynamic status, not the grade of injury. Nonoperative management is appropriate in a child who is hemodynamically stable, has no concomitant intra-abdominal injuries, and has not required more than 40 mL/kg volume of blood replacement in 24 h. Nonoperative management has been standardized and prospectively evaluated in the pediatric trauma population. The data

from two papers outline guidelines for the nonoperative management of splenic injuries (see Table 34-6). Recent prospective data have shown that one night of bed rest for grade I and II injuries and two nights for grade III and above injuries can be safely implemented. ICU admission is limited to those children with grade IV injuries secondary to their increased rate of transfusion and operation as compared to other injury grades. Total hospital stay and time to resumption of normal activities are adjusted according to injury grade. No follow-up imaging is recommended. Follow up studies evaluating compliance with these new guidelines found no compromise in patient safety.

The large majority of splenic injuries resolve with nonoperative management. Operative management is undertaken when the child is hemodynamically unstable, has required more than 40 mL/kg blood replacement, or has other intra-abdominal injuries that require exploratory

TABLE 34-6 Guidelines for Resources Used in Children With Isolated Spleen or Liver Injury

	Grade I	Grade II	Grade III	Grade IV
ICU stay (days)	None	None	None	1
Hospital stay (days)	2	3	4	5
Predischarge imaging	None	None	None	None
Postdischarge imaging	None	None	None	None
Activity restriction (weeks)	3	4	5	6

laparotomy. Mobilization of the spleen by releasing all splenic attachments is necessary for adequate inspection. The type of procedure to be performed on the injured spleen is dependent on the patient's hemodynamic status and his or her ability to withstand a longer operative period. Splenorrhaphy may be undertaken in the hemodynamically stabilized, resuscitated patient. Techniques used include horizontal or vertical mattress sutures, omental buttressing, argon beam coagulation, use of hemostatic agents, and the use of a mesh "bag" or "sling." Dissection of the hilar vessels may allow for selective ligation or subsequent partial splenectomy. Total splenectomy should be performed in those children with physiologic compromise or excessive hemorrhage in whom prolongation of operative time would be life threatening.

During splenectomy, care must be taken to avoid injury to the stomach and tail of the pancreas. As always, a thorough exploration of the abdomen must be undertaken to assess for any associated injuries. Once a child has undergone a total splenectomy, measures should be taken to prevent overwhelming postsplenectomy sepsis syndrome (OPSI). OPSI following splenectomy after trauma occurs in 1.5% of splenectomized children. The mortality of OPSI is almost 50%.

This risk of OPSI after splenectomy occurs most frequently in the first 5 years of life. The reported incidence is around 0.23% a year, with an increased incidence in children less than 2 years of age and those that underwent splenectomy for hematologic reasons. To help prevent this, all splenectomized patients should receive vaccines against pneumococcus, *H. influenzae*, and meningococcus. It is recommended that splenectomized children under the age of 5 should receive antibiotic prophylaxis with penicillin or ampicillin. The need for continued prophylaxis in all splenectomized children is controversial. Decisions regarding prophylaxis beyond the age of 5 should be made on an individual basis. Both the patient and the parents should be educated about OPSI. They should be instructed for the child to be evaluated by a physician should the child experience a febrile illness. Medic alert tags may also be helpful.

BIBLIOGRAPHY

Murphy EE, Murphy SG, Cipolle MD, Tinkoff GH. The pediatric trauma center and the inclusive trauma system: impact on splenectomy rates. *J Trauma Acute Care Surg.* 2015 May;78(5):930–934. doi:10.1097/TA.0000000000000610.

St. Peter SD, Sharp SW, Snyder CL, et al. Follow-up of prospective validation of an abbreviated bedrest protocol in the management of blunt spleen and liver injury in children. *J Pediatr Surg* 2013;48(12):2437–2441.

Stylianos S, Egorova N, Guice KS, Arons RR, Oldham KT. Variation in treatment of pediatric spleen injury at trauma centers versus nontrauma centers: a call for dissemination of American Pediatric Surgical Association benchmarks and guidelines. *J Am Coll Surg* 2006 Feb;202(2):247–251. Epub 2005 Dec 19.

33. **(D)**

34. **(B)**

Explanations 33 and 34

Blunt trauma to the upper abdomen is the most common mechanism for injury to both the duodenum and the pancreas in children. Both are susceptible to injury from compression against the vertebral column. Figure 34-16 demonstrates upper abdominal bruising, which should raise suspicions for a duodenal or pancreatic injury. Diagnosis of blunt duodenal injury is difficult. Loss of the right psoas shadow (retroperitoneal fluid) or right perinephric air is suggestive of this injury. Figure 34-29 demonstrates duodenal wall thickening and pneumatosis. The use of water-soluble oral contrast during CT scan can aid in identification of this injury.

Injuries can range from intramural hematoma to rupture. Intramural duodenal hematomas are caused by shearing force between the submucosa and muscularis. The hematoma may be large enough to cause narrowing of the duodenal lumen and subsequent gastric outlet obstruction. The finding of a "coiled spring" sign on UGI radiographic studies is suggestive of a duodenal hematoma. CT scan of the abdomen and pelvis is the test of choice to evaluate for duodenal injury.

In the absence of other injuries requiring operative intervention, these hematomas can be managed nonoperatively with supportive care, including total parenteral nutrition. They usually resolve within 3 weeks. If resolution has not occurred by this point, consideration must be given to operative evacuation of the clot. If the

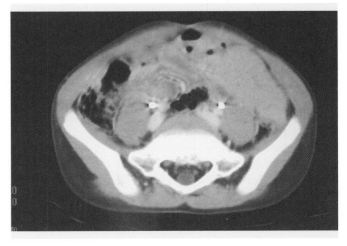

FIGURE 34-29. Abdominal CT demonstrating duodenal wall thickening and pneumatosis.

abdomen is being explored and a duodenal hematoma is encountered, evacuation of the hematoma may be considered. Incising of the serosa and muscularis allows for clot evacuation and inspection of the submucosa. If the submucosa is intact, the seromuscular layer may be reapproximated.

Surgical repair of duodenal injuries depends on the grade and extent of injury. Grade I and II injuries can be repaired, primarily covered by an omental or serosal jejunal patch. Grade III injuries (>50% of duodenal circumference) that cannot be primarily repaired tension free can be managed with Roux-en-Y reconstruction; the three-tube technique (decompressive gastrostomy, retrograde duodenostomy, and feeding jejunostomy); or pyloric exclusion and gastrojejunostomy. The pylorus will reopen within 2–3 weeks. Grade IV and V injuries that involve the ampulla or the distal CBD require pancreaticoduodenectomy.

BIBLIOGRAPHY

Cooper Z, Jurkovich JG. Duodenal injury repairs. In: Cioffi WG, Asensio JA, Adams JA Jr, Connolly MD, Britt LD, eds. *Atlas of Trauma/Emergency Surgical Techniques*. New York, NY: Elsevier; 2014:143–154.

Gaines AB, Austin MK. Abdominal and renal trauma. In: Holcomb WG, Murphy JP, Ostlie JD, eds. *Pediatric Surgery*. 6th ed. New York, NY: Elsevier; 2014:207–209.

35. **(E)**

36. **(A)**

Explanations 35 and 36

Pancreatic injuries in children are uncommon, occurring in less than 5% of all blunt traumas. Blunt trauma is the most common cause of pancreatic injury in children. This injury may result from motor vehicle crash, handlebar injury, or other direct blow to the upper abdomen. Associated injuries are common. Patients may present with upper abdominal abrasions or contusion, or they may demonstrate few external signs of injury.

The mechanism of injury should raise the index of suspicion for pancreatic injury. CT scan is the most accurate radiologic test to evaluate for this injury. CT scans with 3-mm cut are preferred. Radiologic signs of an injury range from obvious (visible pancreatic transection), to subtle (a small amount of fluid in the lesser sac), to no signs of injury at all. Figure 34-18 demonstrates the CT finding of proximal pancreatic transection, confirmed by ERCP, which shows free contrast extravasation. Serial abdominal examinations are required to diagnose those injuries that are not readily apparent on initial evaluation. Initial amylase or lipase levels may be misleading. Looking at these levels over time (24–48 h) is more accurate in diagnosing significant injuries.

The keys to decreased morbidity and mortality from this injury are prompt diagnosis and treatment. Nonoperative management may be used in those patients who are found to have no major ductal disruption, no clinical deterioration, and no additional injuries requiring operative intervention. Minor injuries such as contusions and minor lacerations make up more than 75% of pediatric pancreatic injuries. Operative management should be undertaken when pancreatic transection is seen or clinical deterioration occurs during a period of observation. Operative management must include inspection and palpation of the entirety of the pancreas, adequate debridement of devitalized tissue, closure of any ductal injuries, and drainage.

Pancreatic transections to the left of the superior mesenteric vessels should be managed with spleen-preserving distal pancreatectomy, via an open or laparoscopic approach. Injuries to the head of the pancreas often are associated with duodenal injuries. In these severe injuries, efforts should be made to conserve as much pancreatic tissue as possible. Combined repairs with duodenal exclusion or Roux-en-Y drainage may be employed. Major resections are rarely needed. Children can tolerate resection of 75% of the pancreas and still progress normally in growth and development. Recently, nonoperative approaches with IR drainage and stent placement through the pancreatic duct have been advocated in pediatric patients with pancreatic duct disruption. However, a recent multi-institutional study comparing operative versus nonoperative management of grade II and III pancreatic injuries reported superior outcomes in the operative study group.

Complications of pancreatic trauma include pancreatic pseudocyst, abscess, hemorrhage, and fistula. Asymptomatic pseudocysts may be managed conservatively. Pancreatic pseudocysts will spontaneously resolve in approximately 50% of cases. Of those that become symptomatic, the majority can be treated with percutaneous or internal drainage. Pseudocysts that do not spontaneously resolve can be managed with percutaneous drainage if no ductal disruption is identified. If the duct does communicate to the cyst, internal drainage should be used. Pancreatic fistulas that are not secondary to major ductal disruption will most often close with supportive care. If the fistula is secondary to a major ductal disruption, it may respond to sphincterotomy and pancreatic duct stenting via ERCP, or it may require operative intervention. Overall mortality from pancreatic injuries is approximately 5–10% and is usually secondary to associated injuries.

BIBLIOGRAPHY

Iqbal CW, St. Peter SD, Tsao K, et al. Operative versus nonoperative management for blunt pancreatic transection in children: multi-institutional outcomes. *J Am Coll Surg* 2014 Feb;218(2):157–162.

Melamud K, LeBedis AC, Soto AJ. Imaging of pancreatic and duodenal trauma. *Radiol Clin North Am* 2015;53(4):757–771.

37. **(E)** The syndrome of the abused child describes a child who has sustained multiple injuries and has bruises of varying ages, injury marks consistent with being caused by a specific object, subdural hematomas, and poor growth or development. These injuries or the failure to thrive were caused by the acts of a parent, guardian, or acquaintance of the child. Inconsistencies between the described mechanism of injury and the injuries themselves or a significant delay between the time of injury and the presentation for evaluation should raise suspicions that abuse has occurred. Injury patterns that include multiple subdural hematomas without associated external signs of trauma, retinal hemorrhages, perioral injuries, perforated viscera without preceding major blunt trauma, genital or perineal trauma, evidence of frequent injuries, long-bone fractures in children under the age of 3, or burns of unusual shape or in unusual locations are suspicious and warrant extensive investigation.

BIBLIOGRAPHY

Advanced Trauma Life Support for Physicians. Chicago, IL: American College of Surgeons; 1997:291–310.

Harris BH, Stylianos S. Special considerations in trauma: child abuse and birth injuries. In: O'Neill JA, Rowe MI, Grosfeld JL, et al., (eds.), *Pediatric Surgery*. 5th ed. St. Louis, MO: Mosby Year Book; 1998:359–365.

38. **(E)** Hypothermia is defined as a core temperature below 35°C in a patient with an otherwise-normal thermoregulatory system. Children are more susceptible to hypothermia because of their high ratio of body surface area to weight. These patients may experience many cardiac, respiratory, renal, and metabolic complications related to the magnitude of their hypothermia. Cardiac complications include an initial tachycardia, which is followed by progressive bradycardia as the core temperature approaches 28°C. Osborn (J) waves become evident on ECG at a core temperature below 30°C. Dysrhythmias are common as the core temperature decreases, with ventricular fibrillation (VF) and asystole occurring when the core temperature falls below 25°C. VF rarely responds to defibrillation below a core temperature of 30°C.

Hypothermia causes diuresis. This diuresis is more pronounced in intoxicated individuals and those who suffer cold water immersion. Respiratory drive is stimulated by decreasing core temperature initially. As hypothermia progresses, respiratory drive decreases, carbon dioxide is retained, secretions pool, pulmonary edema occurs, and respiratory arrest follows. For those patients with severe hypothermia (core temperature < 30°C), some of these complications do not become apparent until rewarming is initiated. A further drop in core temperature, called the afterdrop, can be observed despite the initiation of external warming.

Initial assessment of the hypothermic patient should include a core temperature measurement. Care should be taken to use a measuring device capable of reading low temperatures. Oral temperatures are unreliable, and while tympanic membrane temperatures equalize with core temperature most rapidly, the reliability of these measuring devices at low temperatures is uncertain. Therefore, rectal or esophageal temperatures should be followed.

Endotracheal intubation is warranted unless the degree of hypothermia is minimal enough to allow for spontaneous airway protection. Patients should have intravenous or IO access established. Boluses of warm (40–42°C) fluid should be given to initiate treatment of both the hypothermia and the associated dehydration.

Cardiac monitoring should be followed. If the patient has no organized electrical activity, CPR should be initiated. Any organized electrical activity is presumed to provide sufficient flow in the hypothermic patient. The initiation of CPR could convert the organized rhythm into VF. CPR should be continued until organized electrical activity returns, cardiopulmonary bypass (CPB) has been initiated, or a core temperature of at least 35°C has been achieved with failure of all resuscitative measures. As arrhythmias are not responsive to defibrillation until a core temperature of 30°C, defibrillation should be attempted to a maximum of three times until sufficient warming has occurred.

Active rewarming is indicated in those patients with cardiac instability or core temperature below 32°C. Active rewarming can be done externally or internally (core rewarming). Techniques included in active external warming are forced air heating systems, hot water bottle application, and radiant heating sources. Active core rewarming techniques include administration of heated, humidified oxygen; peritoneal lavage; gastric or bladder lavage; thoracic lavage; and CPB. These techniques warm at rates from 2°C/h with heated oxygen administration to 1°C/min on CPB. Outcome after severe hypothermia is difficult to predict. The rapidity of onset of hypothermia, the overall length of time spent hypothermic, and any preexisting medical problems all affect the patient's ability to recover from this insult.

BIBLIOGRAPHY

American Heart Association in collaboration with International Liaison Committee on Resuscitation. Guidelines 2000 for cardiopulmonary resuscitation and emergency cardiovascular care: International Consensus on Science. Part 3. Adult basic life support. *Circulation* 2000;102(Suppl I):1-22-1-59.

Corneli HM. Accidental hypothermia. *Pediatr Emerg Care* 2012 May;28(5):475–480; quiz 481–482. doi:10.1097/PEC.0b013e3182539098.

Fox SM. Heat and cold illness. In: Schafermeyer R, Tenenbein M, Macias CG, Sharieff GQ, Yamamoto LG, eds. *Strange and Schafermeyer's Pediatric Emergency Medicine*. 4th ed. New York, NY: McGraw-Hill; 2015: Chapter 139.

CHAPTER 35

NEUROSURGERY

JOSH ABECASSIS AND AMY LEE

1. An 18-year-old man presents to the emergency department (ED) by ambulance after a motor vehicle crash. He was unconscious at the scene with a Glasgow Coma Scale (GCS) score of 3. He was intubated and received 1 L of normal saline en route. On exam, he has obvious head trauma. With deep painful stimuli, he briefly opens his eyes, extends his right upper extremity, and reaches for the painful stimulus with his left upper extremity. His lower extremities are flaccid and do not move with any stimulation. He does not follow commands. His GCS now is
   (A) 5T
   (B) 6T
   (C) 7T
   (D) 8T

2. A 21-year-old college student is admitted to the intensive care unit (ICU) with a GCS of 5 after a motor vehicle crash. A computed tomography (CT) scan (see Fig. 35-1) shows loss of cisterns. An intracranial pressure (ICP) monitor reveals a pressure of 35 mmHg. He is treated with ventricular drainage, mannitol, and high-dose barbiturate-induced coma. On day 3, his pupils are large and fixed, and the ICP monitor reads 60 mmHg. Brain death is suspected, and organ donation is being considered. The best method of declaring brain death is
   (A) Isotope flow study
   (B) Isotope flow study after normalization of barbiturate level
   (C) Normalization of barbiturate level and check for brainstem reflexes and absence of spontaneous respiration and then make clinical decision
   (D) Normalization of barbiturate level and check for brainstem reflexes and absence of respiration, and then perform electroencephalogram (EEG)

Questions 3 and 4 refer to the following scenario.
A 35-year-old man is involved in a high-speed motor vehicle crash. There was a prolonged extrication, and

he was intubated at the scene. On arrival to the ED, he is given a GCS of 4T. Head CT scan is consistent with diffuse injury without hematoma and basilar skull fracture. CT of the abdomen and pelvis reveals a grade 2 liver laceration. He is hemodynamically normal after a large-volume resuscitation including two units of packed red blood cells. An ICP monitor is placed, and he is admitted to the ICU with intravenous fluids 0.9% NaCl with 20 mEq KCl/L at 11/2 times maintenance. His ICPs range from 15–18 mmHg. Eighteen hours after admission, the patient's urine output increases to 350 mL/h. Serum Na is 150, and urine specific gravity is 1.004. Central venous pressure by subclavian catheter is 7 mmHg.

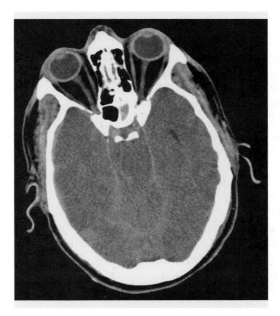

FIGURE 35-1. Noncontrast computed tomography of the head, revealing absence of cerebrospinal fluid cisterns and loss of the normal gray matter–white matter interface.

3. The most likely explanation for the patient's current status is
   (A) Syndrome of inappropriate antidiuretic hormone (SIADH)
   (B) Neurogenic diabetes insipidus (DI)
   (C) Normal diuresis after large-volume resuscitation
   (D) Cerebral salt wasting

4. The most appropriate treatment for this patient at this time is
   (A) Continue 0.9% NaCl with 20 mEq KCl/L and decrease rate to maintenance
   (B) Replace urinary water losses and treat polyuria as needed with aqueous vasopressin
   (C) Change intravenous fluids (IVF) to 5% dextrose (D_5) and 0.45% NaCl with 20 mEq KCl/L at maintenance rate
   (D) Continue current management and recheck electrolytes in 8 hours

5. A 16-year-old boy is seen in the ED after falling out of a tree. He is awake and alert with a GCS of 15, but he has a blood collection behind his right tympanic membrane. There is swelling of the scalp in the right temporal area and a laceration over the occiput. He is neurologically intact. After several hours, it is apparent that he is having cerebrospinal fluid (CSF) otorrhea. A CT scan of the head without contrast demonstrates a basilar skull fracture but no acute intracranial processes. The decision is made to *not* start antibiotics. The following morning, he is wide awake, but his exam is notable for a new left-sided hemiplegia. There is also ptosis of the right eyelid. The right pupil is slightly smaller than the left, and the extraocular muscles are normal. The most likely diagnosis is
   (A) Right epidural hematoma
   (B) Right subdural hematoma
   (C) Evolving right temporal lobe contusion
   (D) Stroke of the right hemisphere

6. Appropriate treatment is begun in the patient in Question 5. Two days later, his hemiplegia has not improved, and he is now comatose. The right ptosis is worse, and the right pupil is large, oval, and poorly reactive. A repeat CT scan (see Fig. 35-2) shows massive intraparenchymal hemorrhage with associated midline shift and evidence of herniation.
   The best treatment for this patient is
   (A) Mannitol
   (B) Placement of an external ventricular drain (EVD)
   (C) High-dose dexamethasone
   (D) Decompressive hemicraniectomy

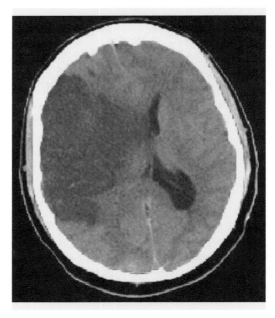

FIGURE 35-2. Noncontrast CT scan of the head.

Questions 7 through 9 refer to the following scenario.
An 18-year-old woman is an unrestrained driver in a motor vehicle crash and strikes her head and face on the windshield. She is neurologically intact after a brief loss of consciousness at the scene. A CT scan of the head reveals no evidence of brain injury, but there are nasal and facial fractures. She is admitted for observation. The following morning, she complains of bloody fluid leaking from her nose. You suspect the fluid is blood mixed with CSF.

7. The *most specific* test to confirm CSF rhinorrhea in this situation is
   (A) Clear halo around bloody drop on a gauze pad
   (B) Fluid glucose level
   (C) Fluid β-transferrin level
   (D) CT cisternogram

8. The most appropriate treatment for CSF rhinorrhea is
   (A) Lumbar CSF drainage for 5 days
   (B) Craniotomy for intradural repair of CSF fistula
   (C) Transnasal repair of CSF fistula
   (D) Observation with head of bed elevation

9. The plastic surgeon would like to repair her facial fractures. Which of the following is most appropriate?
   (A) Proceed with facial fracture repair
   (B) Wait for the CSF fistula to spontaneously resolve before operative repair of fractures
   (C) Wait 2 weeks for repair of fractures due to increased risk of meningitis
   (D) Combined procedure with facial fracture repair and repair of CSF fistula

10. A 32-year-old man presents to the ED complaining of redness and swelling of his right eye, right-sided headache, and double vision. He sustained a mild concussion and basilar skull fracture in a motor vehicle crash 2 months ago. On physical examination, his right eye has 7 mm of proptosis, edema, hyperemia of the conjunctiva, and complete external ophthalmoplegia. The most likely diagnosis is
   (A) Carotid-cavernous sinus fistula
   (B) Orbital pseudotumor
   (C) Ethmoid sinusitis
   (D) Traumatic aneurysm in the cavernous sinus

11. A 30-year-old woman presents with right-sided facial pain, transient loss of vision in the right eye, paralysis of the right side of the tongue, and a right Horner syndrome. Results of CT of the head prompted cerebral angiography, which is shown in Fig. 35-3.

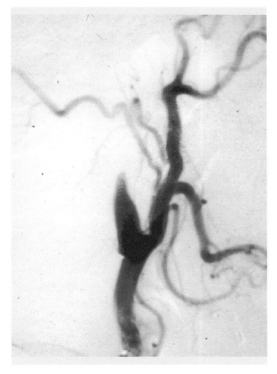

FIGURE 35-3. Right common carotid arteriogram.

The appropriate treatment for this patient is
   (A) Heparin
   (B) Endarterectomy
   (C) Stent placement
   (D) Aspirin

12. A very anxious 25-year-old male patient is 21 days status post complete C6 spinal cord injury. He is on multiple medications for anxiety. He develops sudden hypertension, sweating of the face, piloerection, and bradycardia. He is awake and alert and complaining of headache. The most appropriate intervention at this point would be to
   (A) Insert urinary catheter
   (B) Stop haloperidol and treat neuroleptic malignant syndrome
   (C) Order pulmonary ventilation/perfusion scan to check for pulmonary embolus
   (D) Stop anticholinergic medications

13. A 65-year-old woman is status post right-sided carotid endarterectomy. The procedure was complicated by injury to the right hypoglossal nerve. Which of the following would be found on physical examination?
   (A) No pinprick sensation on the right side of her tongue
   (B) Tongue deviation to the left on protrusion
   (C) Tongue deviation to the right on protrusion
   (D) Loss of taste on the right side of her tongue

Questions 14 and 15 refer to the following scenario.
A 17-year-old male patient undergoes a cervical lymph node biopsy. A diagnosis of Hodgkin disease is made. When seen for suture removal, he complains of severe pain in his shoulder and he is unable to elevate the shoulder and abduct the right arm.

14. The most likely diagnosis is
   (A) Injury to the upper trunk of the brachial plexus
   (B) Injury to the axillary nerve
   (C) Injury to the spinal accessory nerve
   (D) Injury to the suprascapular nerve

15. After 3 months, there is no clinical evidence of recovery. Which of the following statements is most appropriate?
   (A) Prescribe physical therapy with no attempt to repair the nerve because such a nerve injury causes minimal disability.
   (B) Perform baseline electromyogram and observe for 3 more months.
   (C) Explore the wound and do a primary repair if at all possible.
   (D) Explore the wound and be prepared to do a nerve graft if there is any tension on the anastomosis.

16. During exploration of a gunshot wound to the elbow, the ulnar nerve is found to be transected. Both severed ends are identifiable. The most appropriate treatment would be
(A) Primary nerve repair after extensive mobilization of proximal and distal ends to avoid any tension on suture line
(B) Primary nerve repair and immobilization of extremity in marked flexion to prevent tension on suture line
(C) No repair, even though the proximal and distal stumps can be easily approximated in this fresh wound
(D) Nerve graft with sural nerve and transposition away from the damaged tissue

Questions 17 and 18 refer to the following scenario.
A 19-year-old college student serves as a pallbearer at the funeral of a friend who was killed in a motor vehicle accident. Shortly after the funeral, he develops numbness in his fingers of the right hand. That night, he has difficulty sleeping because of discomfort in the entire right upper extremity and worsening paresthesias of all of his fingers. He comes to the ED 6 days later because of weakness in his right hand and aching of the upper extremity. Paresthesias waken him at night and are accentuated by driving a car and holding up a book. He frequently shakes his hand for relief.

17. The most likely diagnosis is
(A) Median nerve neuropathy at the wrist
(B) Ulnar nerve neuropathy at the elbow
(C) C7 radiculopathy
(D) C8 radiculopathy

18. The best way to make this diagnosis would be
(A) Careful neurologic examination
(B) Electromyography (EMG) of the upper extremity
(C) Magnetic resonance imaging (MRI) of the cervical spine
(D) X-rays of the right wrist

Questions 19 and 20 refer to the following scenario.
A 32-year-old woman slips on a wet floor in a supermarket and falls on her outstretched right arm. She has the immediate onset of pain in her wrist. When seen in the local ED, examination reveals that all of her peripheral nerves are intact and the injury appears trivial. The patient's pain continues, and early and delayed x-rays of the wrist show no fracture. When seen in the pain clinic 8 weeks later, her symptoms seem out of proportion to the injury. She complains of burning pain in the right hand and discomfort of the entire upper extremity. Even a mild sensory stimulus to the hand produces severe pain (allodynia), and a mildly painful stimulus results

in horrible discomfort (hyperpathia). She is anxious, depressed, and has difficulty sleeping. Repeat examination reveals all of the peripheral nerves remain intact. The forearm and hand are cool and dry, there is loss of hair, and the fingernails are long and uncut. Her joints are stiff, and she refuses to use her hand. In fact, there appears to be spasms of the involved limb—the fourth and fifth fingers are flexed and the arm is held in adduction with the elbow flexed. She is considering litigation.

19. The most likely diagnosis is
(A) Conversion reaction
(B) Causalgia
(C) Complex regional pain syndrome 1
(D) Complex regional pain syndrome 2

20. Which of the following would probably have the *least* value to treating this patient?
(A) Psychotherapy
(B) Surgical sympathectomy
(C) Dorsal column stimulation
(D) Intrathecal baclofen

21. A 64-year-old diabetic man develops pain in the right back and hip followed several days later by severe sciatica. On examination, he has weakness of the right quadriceps muscle and absence of the right knee and both ankle reflexes. The rest of his leg muscles have good strength. An MRI scan is obtained (see Fig. 35-4). The most likely diagnosis is
(A) A herniated disk at L5–S1 with S1 nerve root compression
(B) A herniated disk at L4–5 with L4 nerve root compression
(C) A herniated disk at L3–4 with L4 nerve root compression
(D) Proximal diabetic neuropathy

22. A 72-year-old man has severe discomfort in both lower extremities when he attempts to walk more than half a city block. His symptoms are relieved by rest. He has no back pain. His neurologic examination is normal. His pedal pulses are very difficult to palpate, but Doppler vascular studies suggest only moderate vascular insufficiency. An MRI of the lumbar spine (see Fig. 35-5) reveals spinal stenosis at L3–4 and L4–5.

Which of the following tests is most useful to distinguish between vascular and neurogenic claudication?
(A) Myelogram followed by CT of lumbar spine
(B) Aortogram with run off
(C) A more detailed history
(D) EMG and nerve conduction studies of the lower extremities

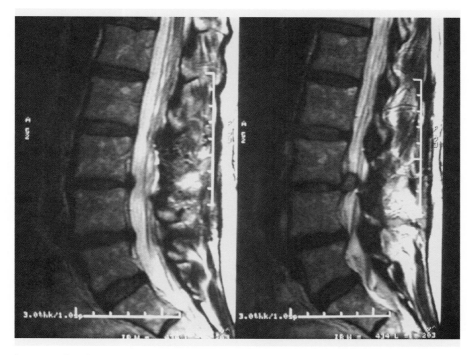

FIGURE 35-4. Sagittal T2-weighted magnetic resonance imaging of the lumbosacral spine in a patient with back pain.

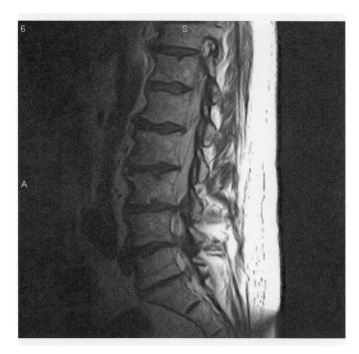

FIGURE 35-5. Sagittal T2-weighted magnetic resonance imaging of the lumbosacral spine in a patient with leg pain.

23. A 26-year-old man undergoes a routine microlumbar discectomy at left L4–5. He is obese, and there is considerable epidural bleeding. When he arrives in the recovery room, his blood pressure is 70/30 mmHg, and his pulse is 140. Emergency management should consist of
   (A) Treatment for sepsis after drawing blood for cultures
   (B) Immediate exploration of the wound
   (C) Intense fluid resuscitation and observation
   (D) Immediate laparotomy

24. A 37-year-old man with insulin-dependent diabetes mellitus has sudden onset of low back pain radiating down both legs and urinary incontinence. He has been feeling tired and ill for several days. On physical examination, he has a left-sided foot drop and loss of bilateral Achilles reflexes. He has hypalgesia on the bottoms of his feet and in his perineum. MRI of the lumbar spine is obtained (see Fig. 35-6).

   The most likely diagnosis is
   (A) Ependymoma of the filum terminale
   (B) Epidural abscess
   (C) Herniated L4–5 intervertebral disk
   (D) Infarct of the conus medullaris

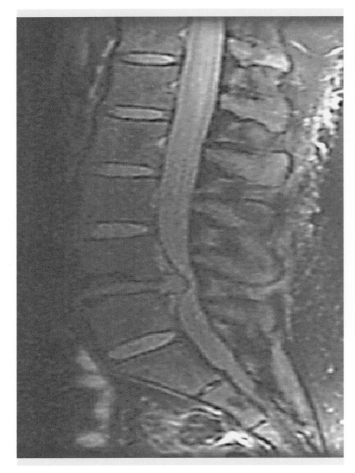

FIGURE 35-6. Sagittal magnetic resonance imaging of the lumbosacral spine in a patient with back pain and urinary incontinence.

25. A 47-year-old man with insulin-dependent diabetes mellitus and chronic renal failure on hemodialysis presents with fever, malaise, and localized signs of infection of his left forearm arteriovenous fistula. He is admitted and placed on intravenous antibiotics. Throughout his hospitalization, he has complained of neck pain requiring opioids. On the fourth hospital morning, he is found to be quadriparetic. MRI is obtained (see Fig. 35-7). The most appropriate next step in this patient's management is
    (A) Steroids and high-dose antibiotics
    (B) Anterior decompression of infected vertebral body
    (C) Percutaneous aspiration
    (D) Laminectomy

26. A 67-year-old man presents with occasional incontinence of urine. He also reports that he has been having trouble walking for a few weeks, stating his feet feel like they are "glued to the ground." His family physician has found no evidence of paresis or spinal cord dysfunction on examination of his lower extremities. He denies any

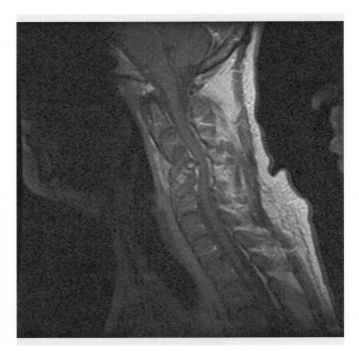

FIGURE 35-7. Sagittal T1-weighted magnetic resonance imaging with contrast of the cervical spine.

headaches. His urologist said his prostate and bladder are normal. His wife tells you that during the past several months, he has fallen once or twice a week, and he has trouble remembering recent events. This patient's history is most consistent with
    (A) Brain tumor
    (B) Chronic subdural hematoma
    (C) Alzheimer disease
    (D) Normal pressure hydrocephalus (NPH)

27. A 46-year-old woman presents to the ED with the worst headache of her life. She has a 40-pack-year history of smoking, migraine headaches, and mitral valve prolapse, and is 4 years status post right-sided modified radical mastectomy followed by appropriate adjuncts for breast cancer. She has photophobia and also complains of neck pain and nausea. She is also short of breath. On physical examination, she is drowsy but otherwise neurologically intact. There is a heart murmur, and electrocardiogram (ECG) shows diffuse ST segment changes throughout the inferior leads with an associated elevation in cardiac enzymes. Additionally, chest x-ray shows increase vascular markings and pulmonary edema. CT scan of the head is obtained (see Fig. 35-8). The most likely diagnosis for this patient is
    (A) Ruptured intracranial aneurysm
    (B) Carcinomatous meningitis from metastatic breast cancer
    (C) Migraine headache
    (D) Septic thromboemboli from valvular heart disease

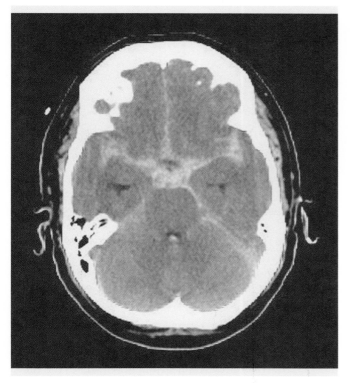

FIGURE 35-8. Noncontrast computed tomography scan of the head in a patient with a headache.

28. A 29-year-old woman who is 5 days postpartum presents with headache, confusion, and lethargy. She becomes unresponsive and has a generalized seizure. Noncontrast head CT and MRI are shown in Figs. 35-9 and 35-10, respectively.
    The most appropriate management of this patient includes
    (A) Anticoagulation
    (B) Steroids
    (C) Ventriculostomy
    (D) Fresh frozen plasma

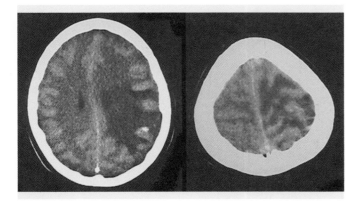

FIGURE 35-9. Noncontrast computed tomography scan of the head, with hypodensity (left greater than right) with small focal hyperdensities in the left cortex.

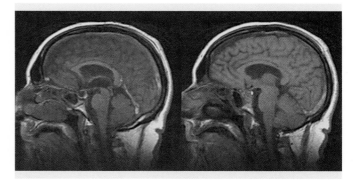

FIGURE 35-10. Sagittal T1-weighted magnetic resonance imaging without contrast of the brain (midline cuts).

Questions 29 and 30 refer to the following scenario.
A 52-year-old man who was previously in good health presents with complaints of severe paroxysms of facial pain when talking, chewing, brushing his right upper teeth, and eating. An imaging study is performed.

29. The most likely diagnosis is
    (A) A multiple sclerosis (MS) plaque in the pons
    (B) An arteriovenous malformation around the brainstem
    (C) A cerebellopontine angle tumor
    (D) Compression of the trigeminal nerve by a normal blood vessel

30. The best treatment option for this patient would be
    (A) Immunotherapy
    (B) Carbamazepine
    (C) Posterior fossa microvascular decompression
    (D) Gamma knife radiosurgery

Questions 31 and 32 refer to the following scenario.
A 36-year-old woman presents with pain and loss of vision in her right eye, worsening over 3 days. Her past medical history is significant for left trigeminal neuralgia treated with carbamazepine for 4 years and depression controlled with sertraline. On neurologic examination, her right eye vision is 20/400, and left eye vision is 20/40. She has a Marcus-Gunn pupil (afferent pupillary defect) on the right. Her extraocular movements are intact, although testing causes increased pain in the eye. Funduscopic examination reveals no abnormality in either eye.

31. The most likely diagnosis for this patient is
    (A) Hysteria
    (B) Carbamazepine toxicity
    (C) Optic neuritis
    (D) Amaurosis fugax

32. The most appropriate next step in this patient's management is
    (A) Psychological evaluation
    (B) Serum carbamazepine level and liver function testing
    (C) MRI of the brain and possible lumbar puncture
    (D) Carotid duplex imaging

33. A 19-year-old woman presents to the ED via ambulance after having a 5-minute long generalized tonic-clonic seizure. She has not yet recovered from the postictal state when she has another generalized seizure of 3 minutes in duration. Her friend tells you that the patient recently immigrated to the United States from Iraq, has had epilepsy since childhood, and takes seizure medicine. You realize this patient is in status epilepticus (SE). All of the following should be instituted immediately *except*
    (A) Lorazepam intravenous (IV)
    (B) Phenytoin IV
    (C) Intubation
    (D) Draw glucose and anticonvulsant levels

34. A 22-year-old woman presents with complaints of intermittent bilateral hand tingling, "funny feeling" in her legs, and occasional loss of balance. Her mother says that she stumbles around and bumps into things. On physical examination, she has intact strength in upper and lower extremities. Sensation is intact to light touch, pinprick, and proprioception on your testing. She has brisk reflexes at the knees and ankles, bilateral Hoffman signs, and equivocal Babinski signs. T2-weighted MRI is shown in Fig. 35-11.
    The most appropriate surgical intervention for this patient would be
    (A) Resection of spinal cord tumor
    (B) Syringosubarachnoid shunt
    (C) Syringopleural shunt
    (D) Posterior fossa and upper cervical decompression

35. A 6-year-old boy with hydrocephalus treated with ventriculoperitoneal (VP) shunt since birth presents to the ED with acute onset of right lower quadrant abdominal pain, anorexia, nausea, and vomiting. His temperature is 38°C, and peripheral white blood cell (WBC) count is 13,000/mL. Abdominal ultrasound reveals an inflamed appendix with thickened mucosa and fecalith. There is no obvious peritoneal fluid collection. The most appropriate treatment would be
    (A) Appendectomy with externalization of the peritoneal portion of the shunt
    (B) Appendectomy without manipulation of the shunt
    (C) Appendectomy with conversion to ventriculogallbladder shunt
    (D) Appendectomy with conversion to ventriculoatrial shunt

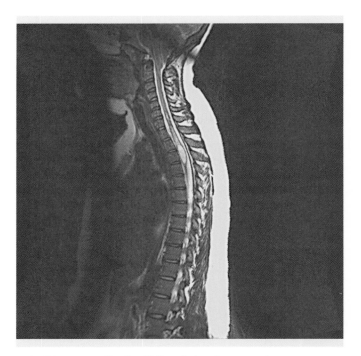

FIGURE 35-11. Sagittal T2-weighted magnetic resonance imaging from the craniocervical junction through the thoracic spine.

36. A 10-month-old child is admitted to the hospital for lethargy, emesis, and failure to thrive. His height and weight are below the 10th percentile for his age. A thorough examination by the pediatrician reveals bilateral retinal hemorrhages, and these are documented by the ophthalmologist (see Fig. 35-12).

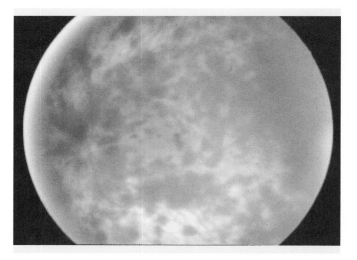

FIGURE 35-12. Diffuse retinal hemorrhages; photograph taken with retinal camera.

His fontanelle is slightly full. On laboratory evaluation, he is anemic, and baseline coagulation studies are normal. A CT scan of the head is performed (see Fig. 35-13). The most appropriate consultation to assist in this patient's management is

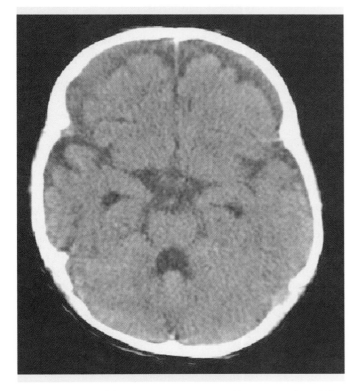

FIGURE 35-13. Noncontrast computed tomography of the head, revealing bilateral subdural hypodense collections, right greater than left.

(A) Pediatric gastroenterology
(B) Pediatric hematology/oncology
(C) Medical genetics
(D) Social worker and child protective services

37. A 5-year-old boy is brought to the office by his parents who tell you that he wakes with headache on most mornings and sometimes in the middle of the night. After he is up for a while, he is able to pursue his normal playful activities. On examination, he is neurologically intact. MRI of his brain is shown in Fig. 35-14.
All of the following diagnoses are likely *except*
(A) Medulloblastoma
(B) Ependymoma
(C) Astrocytoma
(D) Choroid plexus papilloma

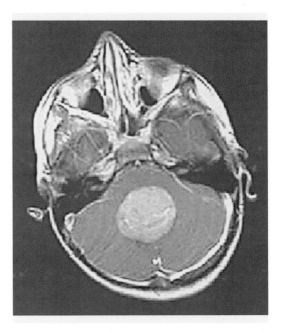

FIGURE 35-14. Magnetic resonance imaging of brain.

Questions 38 and 39 refer to the following scenario.
A 34-year-old man presents with a 3-week history of headaches, lethargy, and vomiting. On examination, his optic discs are flat. He has a mild left hemiparesis and a left extensor toe sign. An MRI scan of the brain is performed with and without contrast enhancement (see Fig. 35-15). The patient improves after starting high-dose dexamethasone.

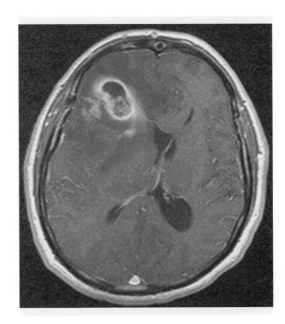

FIGURE 35-15. Axial T1-weighted magnetic resonance imaging with contrast of the brain, revealing a ring-enhancing lesion in the right frontal lobe, with considerable vasogenic edema and middle shift.

38. The next step in the patient's management should be
    (A) Craniotomy with resection of the lesion
    (B) Stereotactic needle biopsy and possible delayed craniotomy
    (C) Open biopsy with neuronavigation
    (D) Metastatic workup followed by an appropriate procedure

39. The patient's condition has stabilized after undergoing appropriate initial and definitive treatment, and he is ready to be released from the hospital. A repeat MRI scan done 24 hours after the procedure shows no contrast enhancement and complete excision of the lesion. All of the following statements are correct *except*
    (A) Tumor cells have infiltrated beyond the area of previous enhancement and resection.
    (B) Radiation therapy is the most important next treatment that will prolong life.
    (C) Chemotherapy with temozolomide should be administered
    (D) The patient's young age makes the prognosis worse, even though the tumor appears to have been completely excised.

40. A 57-year-old man with a 60-pack-year smoking history presents with a seizure. His contrast-enhanced head CT is shown in Fig. 35-16.

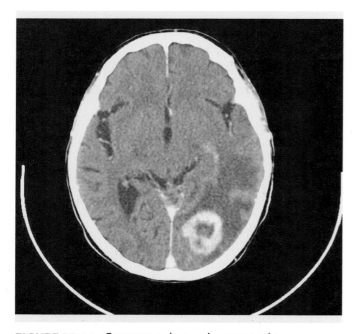

FIGURE 35-16. Contrast-enhanced computed tomography of the head, revealing enhancing lesion in the left occipital lobe, with surrounding vasogenic edema.

His past medical history is only significant for mild chronic obstructive pulmonary disease (COPD). Complete workup reveals a right middle lobe lung lesion. Bronchoscopic biopsy is consistent with adenocarcinoma. The lung lesion is felt to be completely respectable by the thoracic surgeon. There is no further evidence of metastases. The most appropriate management for this patient is
    (A) Resection of brain lesion followed by resection of lung lesion, then appropriate adjuvant therapies
    (B) Resection of lung lesion and radiation therapy for brain lesion
    (C) Resection of lung lesion and radiosurgery for brain lesion
    (D) Resection of brain lesion and radiation and chemotherapy for lung lesion

41. A 52-year-old woman with a long history of cigarette smoking presents with a cough and hilar mass. Workup reveals a nonresectable adenocarcinoma of the lung. She is treated with radiation therapy and chemotherapy. Eighteen months later, she presents to the ED with a 4-week history of progressive painless paraparesis and dysesthesias in the lower extremities. On examination, she is unable to lift her legs off the bed. The knee and ankle reflexes are hyperactive, clonus is present, and there is hypalgesia to pinprick in the lower extremities extending up to the level of the midabdomen. There is sphincter dysfunction. An MRI scan shows swelling of the spinal cord in the midthoracic level with high signal intensity on T2-weighted images. There is ring-enhancing intrathecal contrast enhancement. The most likely diagnosis is
    (A) Spinal cord tumor
    (B) Paraneoplastic necrotizing myelopathy
    (C) Radiation myelopathy
    (D) Metastasis to the spinal cord

42. A 34-year-old homosexual man presents to the ED with a 1-week history of headache, vomiting, and lethargy. A CT scan obtained in the emergency shows multiple low-density lesions in the basal ganglia and white matter (see Fig. 35-17).
    All of the following should be considered in the differential diagnosis *except*
    (A) Toxoplasmosis
    (B) Lymphoma
    (C) Diffuse glioma
    (D) Progressive multifocal leukoencephalopathy (PML)

43. A patient is brought to the ED 3 months following liver transplantation. The patient had been doing well until

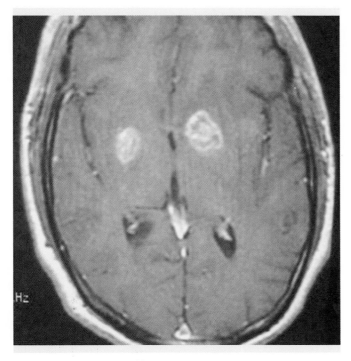

FIGURE 35-17. Axial T1-weighted magnetic resonance imaging with contrast of the brain, revealing multiple bilateral enhancing lesions of the deep white matter and basal ganglia.

about 1 week prior to admission when he became confused and tremulous and complained of unsteadiness and difficulty with vision. An MRI scan showed T2 hyperintense lesions in both occipital lobes (see Fig. 35-18).

The most likely diagnosis is

(A) Creutzfeldt-Jakob disease (prion disease)
(B) Cyclosporin toxicity
(C) PML
(D) Posttransplantation lymphoma

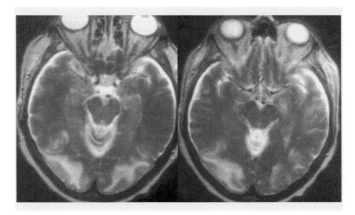

FIGURE 35-18. Axial T2-weighted magnetic resonance imaging of the brain, revealing white matter hyperintensity in both occipital lobes.

ANSWERS AND EXPLANATIONS

1. **(D)** The GCS was developed as a means to quantify and communicate a patient's overall neurologic status. It is generally used in trauma situations but also applies to medical illnesses affecting the nervous system. By no means does a documented GCS obviate the need for a thorough neurologic examination. Scoring is based on eye opening (4 possible total points), verbal response (5 possible total points), and motor response (6 possible total points) (Table 35-1). The best exam within each category is used. Generally, a GCS score of 8 or less is considered "comatose" and an indication for intubation.

Following the table, the minimum score is 3 and maximum score is 15. Head injuries are often classified according to the GCS, with the postresuscitation GCS being more accurate than the GCS at the scene. GCS of 13–15 is a mild head injury, 9–12 is moderate, and 3–8 is severe. Importantly, if a patient is intubated, they have no verbal exam and so receive a score of 1 (minimum), although with the designation of "T" at the end of the score.

TABLE 35-1 Glasgow Coma Scale (GCS) Score

GCS	Eye Opening	Verbal Response	Motor Response
1	None	None (or intubated)	None
2	To pain	Incomprehensible	Decerebrate posture
3	To voice	Inappropriate words	Decorticate posture
4	Spontaneous	Confused	Withdraws to pain
5		Normal, oriented	Localizes pain
6			Follows commands

The score is designated by the best responses from the patient. This patient opens his eyes to pain (2 points out of a potential 4), is intubated (assumed nonverbal, so 1 point, but designated with "T"), and localizes to pain (5 points out a potential 6). Therefore, his GCS score is 8T.

BIBLIOGRAPHY

Greenberg M, Greenberg MS. *Handbook of Neurosurgery*, 7th ed. New York, NY: Thieme; 2010:279.

Teasdale G, Jennett B. Assessment of coma and impaired consciousness: a practical scale. *Lancet* 1974;2:81–84.

2. **(A)** Brain death is suspected in this case because the patient has had a severe head injury with radiographic evidence of diffuse brain injury alongside elevated ICPs that have not responded to aggressive treatment. The pupils are dilated and fixed presumably as a result of bilateral uncal herniation with resultant compression of both third cranial nerves (which supply the parasympathetic innervation of the pupil that enables constriction).

The diagnosis of "brain death" varies from country to country. In the United States, it requires evidence of irreversible damage to both the cerebrum and brainstem. This diagnosis can generally be made clinically from the history, radiology, and certain well-established criteria, including unresponsiveness, flaccidity, apnea with an appropriate level of carbon dioxide (CO_2) to drive respiration, and loss of all brainstem reflexes including pupillary (no response of pupils to bright light), corneal (no response to touching cornea), oculocephalic, oculovestibular, cough, and gag. Importantly, there cannot be any sedating drugs, shock, or significant hypothermia. Withdrawing barbiturates from this patient would risk further brain damage if he were not brain dead. Also it would take at least several days for the barbiturates to reach nonsedating levels (this can be tracked via known half-lives). In all cases of brain death, there is definite loss of significant cerebral blood flow. There are three acceptable tests to demonstrate this, including invasive angiography, transcranial Doppler flow studies, or a nuclear flow study. Angiograms are significantly invasive and time consuming. If performed (though rarely done so for brain death diagnosis), this study would show contrast in the carotid and vertebral arteries stopping at the base of the skull and failing to perfuse the brain. The same phenomenon can be more safely and economically demonstrated by radioactive isotope scans or Doppler ultrasound.

The technique most widely used is a nuclear flow study. Most studies now are performed with technetium (Tc)-99m injected at the bedside with a scintillation camera. This isotope is normally taken up by the cerebral hemispheres and cerebellum. In brain death, neither of these structures have uptake, and the skull interior appears empty, producing a classic "hollow skull" sign. In early brain death, occasionally there will be some uptake in the cerebellum. Invariably, a repeat scan will show no uptake. If ^{99m}Tc-hexamethylpropyleneamineoxime (HMPAO) is not available, the flow study with ^{99m}Tc-labeled human serum albumin may be used. In brain death, using this isotope, there is no intracranial arterial circulation. There may be some venous sinus visualization. Occasionally (2%) patients with clinical brain death will have arterial flow. If brain death is present, a repeat scan in 12–24 hours will be confirmatory.

In the event of a cardiac arrest, where there can be persistent blood flow to the brain despite a poor neurologic exam and incomplete radiographic evidence of diffuse irreversible damage, a combination of negative bilateral somatosensory evoked potentials (SSEPs) and an elevated creatinine kinase BB (CK-BB; brain equivalent of CK-MB) in the CSF can definitely rule out neurological recovery.

BIBLIOGRAPHY

Goodman J, Heck L, Moore B. Confirmation of brain death with portable isotope angiography. A review of 204 consecutive cases. *Neurosurgery* 1985;16:492–497.

Greenberg MS. *Handbook of Neurosurgery*, 7th ed. New York, NY: Thieme; 2010:289–292.

Sherman AL, Tirschwell DL, Micklesen PJ, Longstreth WT, Robinson LR. Somatosensory potentials, CSF creatinine kinase BB activity, and awakening after cardiac arrest. *Neurology* 2000;54:889–894.

3. **(B)**

4. **(B)**

Explanations for questions 3 and 4

This patient has developed DI, a well-known complication of severe traumatic brain injury. It is caused by injury to the hypothalamus and hypothalamic-pituitary axis secondary to diffuse axonal injury and is heralded by polyuria (>30 mL/kg/h or >200 mL/h in adults), decreased urine specific gravity/osmolarity, and increased serum sodium (Na)/osmolarity.

Injury to the hypothalamus results in a *lack* of antidiuretic hormone (ADH), causing the patient to make large volumes of dilute urine independent of the current hemodynamic status. Onset after injury is usually delayed at least 6–8 hours by circulating endogenous ADH. Due to large losses of free water, serum Na and osmolarity increase. Serum Na and osmolarity, along with urine specific gravity or osmolarity should, be assessed with any large-volume urine output in a head-injured patient.

TABLE 35-2 Disorders of Sodium Metabolism

	DI	SIADH	CSW
Volume status	Hypovolemia	Nl or hypervolemia	Hypovolemia
Serum Na	High	Low	Low
Urine volume	High	Low, Nl or high	High early, then low
Urine osmolarity	Low	High	High
Treatment	Water replacement, vasopressin	Fluid restriction	Sodium and fluids

CSW, cerebral salt wasting; DI, diabetes insipidus; Nl, normal; SIADH, syndrome of inappropriate antidiuretic hormone.

Any administration of mannitol or diuretics should be taken into account, as they will alter these parameters. Treatment should be instituted quickly to avoid systemic complications from hypovolemia and hypernatremia, and includes replacement of calculated free water deficit and ongoing urinary losses with D_5 0.225% NaCl or dextrose 5% in water (D_5W). Urine output needs to be monitored hourly, and serum electrolytes should be checked every 4–6 hours. Patients with complete DI will require administration of desmopressin (DDAVP, oral [PO] or nasal spray) or vasopressin (subcutaneous [SC], IV, or intramuscular [IM]) to control urine output. Quick correction or overcorrection of Na levels can worsen brain swelling, and often, elevated sodium levels are desirable when there is concern for herniation, so "goal sodium levels" must be discussed with the neurosurgical team and a treatment plan developed accordingly.

In the severely brain-injured patient, early development of DI is indicative of profound and diffuse injury and is highly predictive of mortality. It can also be seen in brain death.

SIADH and cerebral salt wasting (CSW) are both disorders that can also occur with brain injury and similarly result in increased urine output but are associated with hyponatremia. The best way to clinically distinguish between SIADH and CSW is to check volume status via a central venous pressure (CVP) monitor. CVP is normal or elevated in SIADH and low in CSW. A test for serum ADH is available but rarely practical. The important parameters of each process are shown in Table 35-2. SIADH is extremely common, whereas CSW is relatively rare. SIADH is treated via fluid restriction, whereas CSW requires fluid replacement.

BIBLIOGRAPHY

Andrews BT. Fluid and electrolyte management in the head-injured patient. In: Narayan RK, Wilberger JR, Povlishock JT (eds.), *Neurotrauma*. New York, NY: McGraw-Hill; 1996:335–339.

Diringer M, Ladenson PW, Borel C, et al. Sodium and water regulation in a patient with cerebral salt wasting. *Arch Neurol* 1989;46:928–930.

Ellison DH, Berl T. Clinical practice. The syndrome of inappropriate antidiuresis. *N Engl J Med* 2007;356:2064–2072.

Nelson PB, Seif SM, Maroon JC, et al. Hyponatremia in intracranial disease. Perhaps not the syndrome of inappropriate secretion of antidiuretic hormone (SIADH). *J Neurosurg* 1981;55:938–941.

Wolf AL, Salcman M. Complications of head injuries in adults. In: Post KD, Friedman E, McCormack P (eds.), *Post-operative Complications in Intracranial Neurosurgery*. New York, NY: Thieme; 1993:140.

5. **(D)**

6. **(D)**

Explanations for questions 5 and 6

The patient suddenly developed unilateral hemiplegia 1 day after a head injury secondary to an infarction of the left cerebral hemisphere. The factors in the history that suggest this diagnosis include the presence of a basilar skull fracture (which predisposes to vascular injuries), the acute onset of hemiplegia, and the fact that he remains awake and alert. Most patients who develop hemiplegia secondary to a mass lesion are obtunded or comatose secondary to associated hydrocephalus. The mild ptosis is secondary to a partial Horner syndrome, which is often seen with injuries to the carotid vessels where the sympathetic nerve plexuses sit. The other manifestations of a third nerve palsy are absent. The patient had dissection of the right carotid artery secondary to the basilar skull fracture in the area of the carotid canal (see Fig. 35-19); however, the most common location of carotid injury and dissection associated with trauma is in the cervical neck, with the dissection beginning several centimeters above the bifurcation. The mechanism can be direct blunt trauma or stretching. In most patients, symptoms develop within 1–24 hours after trauma; however, some patients may not have symptoms of cerebral ischemia for several or more

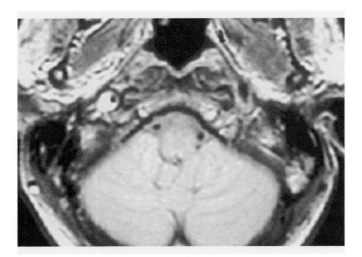

FIGURE 35-19. Axial T1-weighted magnetic resonance image without contrast, revealing bright crescent sign in the right internal carotid artery at the skull base.

days after injury. The sympathetic nerves, except those that cause sweating of the face, travel around the carotid artery and are injured as the carotid is distended by the false lumen, resulting in Horner syndrome. Although cerebral angiography is the gold standard in diagnosing carotid dissection, the lesion can often be suspected on CT or MRI scan, particularly the latter. Often when a basilar skull fracture is diagnosed, imaging of the vessels (like CT angiogram) is obtained. On axial images the bright crescent signal in the wall of the carotid may be seen (see Fig. 35-19). If this patient were obtunded or comatose when the hemiplegia developed, an acute epidural, subdural, or temporal lobe contusion would be suspected.

It was elected not to treat the otorrhea with antibiotics, because the incidence of meningitis is very low, resistant meningitic organisms can emerge on prophylactic antibiotics, and a recent Cochrane Review found there to be no benefit in treating basilar skull fractures prophylactically with antibiotics. Broad-spectrum antibiotics may be employed if a skull fracture extends into nasal sinus cavities or extends through the dura and into the outside environment. Spinal fluid otorrhea usually stops spontaneously after a couple days. If a persistent CSF fistula develops, it can be treated with placement of a lumbar drain to divert CSF away from the site of injury to allow for healing.

The patient's level of consciousness decreased several days after his stroke because of swelling in the infarcted brain due to reperfusion of the ischemic tissue and hemorrhagic conversion, resulting in a marked right to left shift. Although there are conservative ICP management options available including mannitol, hyperosmolar therapy, hyperventilation, and elevation of the head,

ultimately a decompressive hemicraniectomy may be necessary to acutely intervene on herniation syndrome. The bone flap must be huge, the dura is left opened, and the scalp is closed. The bone flap can be frozen or buried in the anterior abdominal wall until the brain swelling resolves. Most neurosurgeons would not consider decompressive craniotomy with a massive infarct of the dominant hemisphere.

BIBLIOGRAPHY

Ahmadi J, Levy M, Aarabi B. Vascular lesions resulting from head injury. In: Wilkins R, Rengachary S (eds.), *Neurosurgery*, 2nd ed. New York, NY: McGraw Hill; 1996:2821–2840.

Dalgic A, Okay HO, Gezici AR, Daglioglu E, Akdag R, Ergungor MF. An effective and less invasive treatment of post traumatic cerebrospinal fluid fistula: closed lumbar drainage system. *Minim Invasive Neurosurg* 2008;51:154–157.

El Ahmadieh TY, Adel JG, El Tecle NE, et al. Surgical treatment of elevated intracranial pressure: decompressive craniectomy and intracranial pressure monitoring. *Neurosurg Clin N Am* 2013;24:375–391.

Morki B, Piepgras D, Houser O. Traumatic dissections of the extracranial internal carotid artery. *J Neurosurg* 1988;68:189–197.

Ratital BO, Costa J, Sampaio C, Pappamikail L. Antibiotic prophylaxis for preventing meningitis in patients with basilar skull fractures. *Cochrane Database Syst Rev* 2011;8:CD004884.

7. **(C)**

8. **(D)**

9. **(A)**

Explanations for questions 7 to 9

Confirmation that rhinorrhea is CSF can be difficult, especially when the amount is small and mixed with blood. Most commonly and conveniently, staff can try to appreciate a "ring sign" of CSF surrounding a blood droplet when transferred to a piece of tissue or gauze, although this is often unreliable. Common clinical features associated with a CSF fistula include a positional worsening with leaning forward, a salty taste in the back of the mouth, and obviously a history of head injury or cranial surgery, particularly endonasal transsphenoidal approaches. However, there are tests available at the bedside and in the laboratory to assist with diagnosis. CSF contains glucose, but if there is contamination with blood (which there often is with trauma), the results of a glucose swab or lab test may be falsely positive. High-resolution CT scan can reveal skull fractures near the site of a leak. This can be helpful in the late presentation of a CSF leak when there is fluid density in a sinus adjacent to the fracture. The most specific and sensitive test is for β-transferrin (which is only physiologically located in CSF and the vitreous fluid of the eye), and the results are not compromised by the presence of blood in the fluid. At some institutions, however, this test may require outside lab analysis.

Treatment of posttraumatic CSF fistula is initially conservative because the majority will spontaneously resolve in 7 days or less. The head of the bed is elevated to approximately 45 degrees or higher, and the patient is instructed to avoid straining or coughing. If the leak persists after 4–7 days, lumbar spinal fluid drainage can be used to divert CSF until the fistula resolves. The major risks associated with placement of a lumbar drain include pneumocephalus due to negative pressure and meningitis. It is contraindicated in patients with intracranial mass lesions due to the risk of herniation from mass effect and a pressure gradient. Occasionally surgery is required for persistent leaks; the approach is based on the location and characteristics of the leak. Repair of facial fractures can take place at the convenience of the surgeons involved and should not be altered by the presence of CSF rhinorrhea. Indeed, repair of facial fractures may even cause the fistula to close due to postoperative edema of the soft tissues. Patients with a CSF fistula are at increased risk for meningitis, but prophylactic antibiotics have not been shown to decrease this risk.

BIBLIOGRAPHY

Geisler FH. Skull fractures. In: Wilkins RH, Rengachary SS (eds.), *Neurosurgery*, 2nd ed. New York, NY: McGraw-Hill; 1996:2753–2754.

McCormack B, Cooper PR. Traumatic cerebrospinal fluid fistulas. In: Narayan RK, Wilberger JR, Povlishock JT (eds.), *Neurotrauma*. New York, NY: McGraw-Hill; 1996:639–653.

Ratilal BO, Costa J, Sampaio C, Pappamikail L. Antibiotic prophylaxis for preventing meningitis in patients with basilar skull fractures. *Cochrane Database Syst Rev* 2011;8:CD004884.

Ryall RG, Peacock MK, Simpson DA. Usefulness of B2-transferrin assay in the detection of cerebrospinal fluid leaks following head injury. *J Neurosurg* 1992;77:737–739.

10. **(A)** The carotid-cavernous fistula (CCF) is an abnormal connection from the internal carotid artery to the cavernous sinus. It is a rare but well-documented complication of head trauma and basilar skull fracture, but can also develop from spontaneous rupture of a cavernous carotid artery aneurysm. Symptoms of traumatic CCF can develop acutely or more often over weeks to months. Pulsatile proptosis, chemosis, ophthalmoplegia (partial or complete), and ocular bruit are the cardinal features. Often patients complain of retro-orbital pain or ipsilateral headache. Ocular hypoxia from decreased ocular perfusion pressure and increased venous pressure may threaten vision. Diagnosis is confirmed with cerebral angiography, and endovascular treatment with detachable coils or balloons is the treatment of choice. An aneurysm of the cavernous carotid artery can result from trauma, and cranial neuropathies are more prominent signs than proptosis or chemosis. It is often associated with blindness at the time of injury secondary to ophthalmic artery injury or fracture in the area of the optic canal.

Orbital pseudotumor is a rare inflammatory process of unknown etiology. It is extremely painful. There is edema of the lids and conjunctiva. The inflammation is very steroid sensitive. Ethmoid sinusitis usually will cause lateral displacement of the globe, lid swelling, fever, and other usual symptoms of sinusitis, and is less often associated with chemosis.

BIBLIOGRAPHY

Gianotta SL, Gruen P. Vascular complications of head injury. In: Barrow DL (ed.), *Neurosurgical Topics: Complications and Sequelae of Head Injury*. Park Ridge, IL: American Association of Neurological Surgeons; 1992:44.

Harris ME, Barrow DL. Traumatic carotid-cavernous fistulas. In: Barrow DL (ed.), *Neurosurgical Topics: Complications and Sequelae of Head Injury*. Park Ridge, IL: American Association of Neurological Surgeons; 1992:13–29.

Lewis AI, Tomsick TA, Tew JM. Carotid-cavernous fistula and intracavernous aneurysms. In: Wilkins RH, Rengachary SS (eds.), *Neurosurgery*, 2nd ed. New York, NY: McGraw-Hill; 1996:2529–2535.

Yee RD. Evaluation and treatment of vision loss, diplopia, and orbitopathies. In: Batjer HH, Loftus CM (eds.), *Textbook of Neurological Surgery*. New York, NY: Lippincott Williams & Wilkins; 2003:482–490.

11. **(A)** The clinical symptoms suggest a right carotid artery dissection, and the CT scan confirms the diagnosis by showing a clot in the wall of the carotid artery at the base of the skull. Most cases of carotid dissection are spontaneous, but they have been associated with fibromuscular dysplasia, Marfan syndrome, and strenuous activity. Dissection is sometimes precipitated by minor trauma and occasionally occurs following chiropractic manipulation. The dissection may occur intracranially or extracranially. The hallmark is extraluminal extravasation of blood. This patient's dissection took place in the neck, and the extravasation was between the media and adventitia. The amaurosis fugax was caused by emboli, the pain by distention of the carotid, and the tongue paralysis and partial Horner syndrome by stretching of nerves adjacent to the suddenly enlarged carotid.

Most patients with carotid dissections are treated with heparin for several weeks and then oral anticoagulants. About 75% will do well with resolution of symptoms. An occasional patient will throw emboli from a pseudoaneurysm that form on the carotid when blood causes outpouching of the adventitia. Transcranial Dopplers can be employed on a daily basis to evaluate for microembolic events. If emboli or symptoms continue with anticoagulation, options include adding an additional antiplatelet agent, ligation of the cervical carotid with or without an extracranial-intracranial bypass, very occasionally a direct repair in the neck, or endovascular intervention with or without stent placement.

BIBLIOGRAPHY

Anson J, Crowell R. Cervicocranial arterial dissection. *Neurosurgery* 1991;29:89–96.

Bouzat P, Francony G, Brun J, et al. Detecting traumatic internal carotid artery dissection using transcranial Doppler in head-injured patients. *Intensive Care Med* 2010;36:1514–1520.

Morki B, Sundt T, Houser O. Spontaneous internal carotid artery dissection, hemicrania, and Horner's syndrome. *Arch Neurol* 1979;36:677–680.

12. **(A)** Autonomic dysreflexia (aka autonomic hyperreflexia, autonomic storm) is a syndrome of sympathetic overactivity that can occur in up to 85% of patients with spinal cord injury at the T6 level or above, usually after the acute phase of injury (approximately 2 weeks). Symptoms occur when a noxious stimulus to an organ innervated by spinal nerves below the level of injury (e.g., distended urinary bladder) causes a spinal reflex to the adrenal glands. Due to interruption of descending inhibitory control from the injured spinal cord, there is massive sympathetic discharge resulting in hypertension, perspiration, and piloerection. The hypertension can be extreme, and fatal intracranial hemorrhage has been reported. The bradycardia is a reflex response to severe hypertension mediated by carotid baroreceptors, and its presence is not necessary to make the diagnosis. Patients are often tachycardic in the early stages.

Autonomic dysreflexia is a *medical emergency*. Treatment involves immediate removal of the stimulus, which is by far most commonly a distended urinary bladder. Other common causes include fecal impaction, gastrointestinal (GI) or genitourinary (GU) procedures, and urinary tract infection (UTI). It has also been reported with testicular torsion and birth labor. Care must be taken not to increase stimulation in attempt to remove the causative factor. For example, an anesthetic ointment or gel should be used when breaking up a fecal impaction.

Removal of the stimulus nearly always immediately resolves the hypertension; however, if it does not, pharmacologic therapy is indicated with such drugs as nitroprusside, nitroglycerine, or hydralazine. Patients with recurrent episodes may require prophylaxis with α-blockers such as phenoxybenzamine or clonidine.

Neuroleptic malignant syndrome is an idiosyncratic reaction to phenothiazine medications such as haloperidol. It is characterized by autonomic dysfunction, hyperthermia, and extrapyramidal effects such as dystonia, muscle rigidity, and even catatonia. It can be treated with dopamine agonists (e.g., bromocriptine) and dantrolene sodium. An anticholinergic crisis presents as tachyarrhythmias, hypertension, mydriasis, and altered level of consciousness, and is usually the result of overdose of medication (e.g., tricyclic antidepressants, antihistamines). Deep venous thrombosis and pulmonary embolism occur more frequently in the spinal cord–injured patient but do not present with a hypertensive crisis.

BIBLIOGRAPHY

Cahill DW, Rechtire GR. The acute complications of spinal cord injury. In: Narayan RK, Wilberger JR, Povlishock JT (eds.), *Neurotrauma*. New York, NY: McGraw-Hill; 1996:1210.

Lovejoy FH, Linden CH. Acute poisoning and drug over-dosage. In: Isselbacher KJ, Braunwald E, Wilson JD, et al. (eds.), *Harrison's Principles of Internal Medicine*, 13th ed. New York, NY: McGraw-Hill; 1994:2442.

Owens GF, Addonizio JC. Urologic evaluation and management of the spinal cord injured patient. In: Lee BY, Ostrander LE, Cochran GVB, et al. (eds.), *The Spinal Cord Injured Patient: Comprehensive Management*. Philadelphia, PA: W.B. Saunders; 1991:130–131.

Petersdorf RG. Hypothermia and hyperthermia. In: Isselbacher KJ, Braunwald E, Wilson JD, et al. (eds.), *Harrison's Principles of Internal Medicine*, 13th ed. New York, NY: McGraw-Hill; 1994:2476–2477.

13. **(C)** The hypoglossal nerve travels in a plane between the jugular vein and internal carotid artery (see Fig. 35-20). It passes medially over the carotid usually distal to the bifurcation and proximal to the posterior belly of the digastric muscle. It is identified by following the superior root of the ansa cervicalis (often referred to as the descending hypoglossal nerve) superiorly to the point where it meets the hypoglossal nerve crossing the internal carotid.

The hypoglossal nerve can be mobilized superomedially to allow adequate exposure for carotid endarterectomy, and this may require transection of the superior root of the ansa cervicalis (this usually causes no noticeable loss of strap muscle function). Occasionally the hypoglossal nerve is not easily identified at surgery, because it can be hidden under the facial vein or digastric muscle. Accidental transection of the nerve is a rare complication. More often, it is injured by prolonged retraction. Retraction injury will usually recover relatively quickly.

The hypoglossal is a pure motor nerve, responsible for the innervation of the intrinsic and extrinsic muscles of the tongue (except palatoglossus, innervated by the

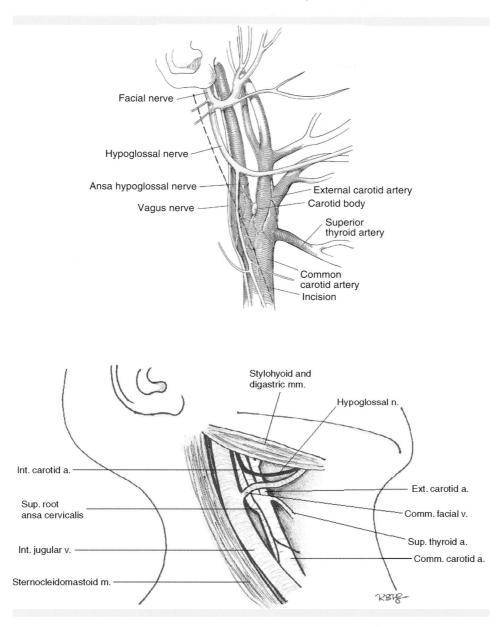

FIGURE 35-20. A and B. The hypoglossal nerve in relation to carotid endarterectomy. **A.** From Zollinger R Jr, Ellison E. *Zollinger's Atlas of Surgical Operations*, 9th ed. New York, NY: McGraw-Hill; 2010:Plate 159.

vagus nerve). When injured, there is weakness of ipsilateral tongue muscles, causing the tongue to protrude toward the side of injury.

Sensation of the anterior two-thirds of the tongue is mediated by the lingual nerve (a branch of the mandibular division of the trigeminal nerve, cranial nerve [CN] V). The posterior one-third is supplied by the glossopharyngeal nerve (CN IX). Taste is a special sensation mediated by the facial (anterior two-thirds), glossopharyngeal (posterior one-third), and vagus (epiglottis) nerves.

The hypoglossal nerve descends in the neck in a plane between the internal jugular vein and internal carotid artery before swinging medially toward the tongue. It will cross the internal and external carotid between the bifurcation and the digastric muscle. The superior root of the ansa cervicalis can be mobilized off the common carotid and retracted medially or even sacrificed to allow superomedial retraction of the hypoglossal nerve. Occasionally the nerve is difficult to identify, because it may be fixed to the underside of the common facial vein or the digastric muscle.

BIBLIOGRAPHY

Crowell RM, Ogilvy CS, Ojemann RG. Extracranial carotid artery atherosclerosis; carotid endarterectomy. In: Wilkins RH, Rengachary SS (eds.), *Neurosurgery*, 2nd ed. New York, NY: McGraw-Hill; 1996:2107.

Pansky B. *Review of Gross Anatomy*, 5th ed. New York, NY: Macmillan; 1984:62–63, 74–75.

14. **(C)**

15. **(D)**

Explanations for questions 14 and 15

Injury to the spinal accessory nerve is one of the most common iatrogenic nerve injuries during a surgical procedure. Lymph node biopsy in the posterior triangle of the neck is the usual culprit. The injury often goes unrecognized until the patient complains of pain, difficulty abducting the shoulder, and noticeable drooping of the shoulder. The injury is very serious and disabling. Prevention is critical when working in the posterior triangle of the neck for the well-being of the patient as well as for the surgeon; injury to the spinal accessory nerve often has legal consequences. Although each patient must be individualized, some surgeons suggest doing lymph node biopsies in this area under general anesthesia without muscle paralysis, use of a nerve stimulator, magnification, and bipolar coagulation.

This patient can be followed for several months to see if there is spontaneous recovery. EMG by a very experienced clinician can show signs of voluntary muscle contraction in all three portions of the trapezius, but if function is not evident clinically at 3 months, exploration of the wound should be undertaken because the EMG findings do not necessarily predict a good clinical outcome. The results of surgical repair may be excellent when performed within 3 months. At the time of reexploration, if the nerve appears to be in continuity, the nerve should be stimulated distal to the site of injury. If there is muscle contraction, then a neurolysis without repair should be considered. If the nerve had been divided, a primary anastomosis should be performed if there is no tension. Otherwise, a nerve graft is preferable. Finding the proximal and distal stumps can be difficult, and confusion of the accessory nerve with sensory nerves in the area must be avoided. Knowledge of the anatomy is critical (see Fig. 35-21).

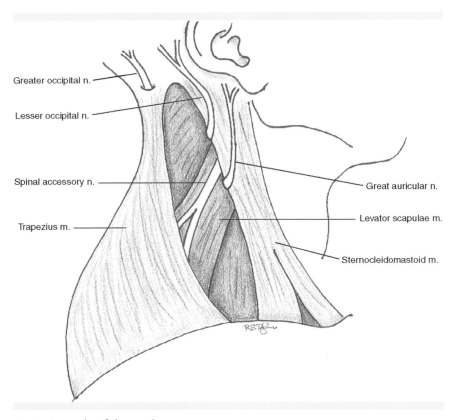

FIGURE 35-21. The posterior triangle of the neck.

The sternocleidomastoid, trapezius, and clavicle define the posterior triangle of the neck. The spinal accessory nerve runs superficially through the triangle. Lymph nodes can be found along the border of the sternocleidomastoid and along the course of the nerve. The great auricular and lesser occipital nerves are sensory, and injury may not be as noticeable as injury to the spinal accessory nerve.

BIBLIOGRAPHY

Nakamichi K, Shintaro T. Iatrogenic injury of the spinal accessory nerve. *J Bone Joint Surg* 1998;80-A:1616–1621.

Nason R, Abdurlrauf B, Stranc M. The anatomy of the accessory nerve and cervical lymph node biopsy. *Am J Surg* 2000;180:241–243.

Novak C, MacKinnon S. Patient outcome after surgical management of an accessory nerve injury. *Otolaryngol Head Neck Surg* 2002;127:221–224.

16. **(C)** With a gunshot wound (GSW) to an extremity, tissue injury is determined by the projectile's direct course and by shock waves from its trajectory ("blast" injury). They frequently will require operative management. Immediate operative treatment consists of debridement of devitalized tissues, restoration of distal circulation, and stabilization of fractures.

Primary repair of transected nerves is not performed for GSW due to inability to determine the extent of the blast injury to the severed ends in the acute phase. The most appropriate treatment is to suture the proximal and distal stump to nearby clean tissue beds and marking them with suture that can be identified at delayed repair. Care should be taken to avoid extensive mobilization, especially of the proximal stump (at debridement and at delayed surgery), because this may interrupt the vascular supply of the nerve and inhibit the axonal regeneration, which occurs from proximal to distal. Recovery of function with delayed surgical repair can be as high as 50%, but may take months or even years to return, and is dependent on many factors such as location and nature of nerve injury, need for nerve graft, and tension on the nerve. Nerves with primarily motor function (e.g., axillary and radial nerves) have better recovery rates than those with a large sensory component (e.g., median and ulnar nerves). In a GSW with neurologic deficit and no direct nerve injury at surgical exploration (or that which is treated nonoperatively), recovery is as high as 69%. This is likely due to axonotmesis, which is injury to the axon of the nerve without disruption of the nerve sheath, leaving a good path for axonal regeneration.

This management differs from laceration injury, in which primary repair is indicated.

BIBLIOGRAPHY

Awasthi D, Hudson AR, Kline DG. Treatment strategies for the patient suffering from peripheral nerve injury. In: Benzel EC (ed.), *Neurosurgical Topics: Practical Approaches to Peripheral Nerve Surgery*. Park Ridge, IL: American Association of Neurological Surgeons; 1992:35–36.

Friedman A. Restoration of extremity function. In: Benzel EC (ed.), *Neurosurgical Topics: Practical Approaches to Peripheral Nerve Surgery*. Park Ridge, IL: American Association of Neurological Surgeons; 1992:214–220.

Omer GE. Peripheral nerve injuries and gunshot wounds. In: Omer GE, Spinner M, VanBeek AL (eds.), *Management of Peripheral Nerve Problems*, 2nd ed. Philadelphia, PA: W.B. Saunders; 1998:398–404.

Omer GE. The prognosis for untreated traumatic injuries. In: Omer GE, Spinner M, VanBeek AL (eds.), *Management of Peripheral Nerve Problems*, 2nd ed. Philadelphia, PA: W.B. Saunders; 1998:365–369.

17. **(A)**

18. **(A)**

Explanations for questions 17 and 18

This patient's symptoms are classical for carpal tunnel syndrome except for the acute onset and rapid progression, which will be discussed later. Patients with carpal tunnel syndrome frequently complain of numbness in all of their fingers, even though the median nerve supplies sensation to the lateral four and a half fingers. Nocturnal paresthesias, paresthesias while driving or holding a book, and discomfort in the entire extremity are very common. Of the choices given, the best way to arrive at the diagnosis is by clinical examination. When examining for involvement of a peripheral nerve or nerve root, motor examination is usually more reliable then sensory examination. The median nerve supplies four intrinsic muscles of the hand—lateral two lumbricals, opponens pollicis, abductor pollicis brevis, and half the flexor pollicis brevis (LOAF muscles—mnemonic device). All the other intrinsic muscles of the hand are supplied by the ulnar nerve. The radial nerve does not supply any of the intrinsic muscles of the hand. The best muscle to test for carpal tunnel is the abductor pollicis brevis. The patient is asked to maintain abduction of the thumb at right angles to the palm against pressure by the examiner. Subtle weakness of the median nerve can be demonstrated in this way. When testing sensation, two-point discrimination is much better than pinprick.

Phalen's sign, also characteristic of carpal tunnel, is elicited by wrist flexion. Paresthesias are reproduced in less than a minute. Tinel's sign, paresthesias elicited by tapping over the median nerve at the wrist, may also be present. EMG changes in the hand muscles would not appear for about 3 weeks after the onset of symptoms and therefore would not be helpful in this patient; however, the patient might have delayed sensory conduction (latency) across the wrist that could be demonstrated by electrophysiologic studies.

Ordinarily carpal tunnel surgery would not be undertaken with only a week of symptoms, but this young man's history suggests an acute process. He was explored and had a hematoma under the transverse carpal ligament secondary to an undiagnosed inherited coagulopathy. Aside from fractures, another cause of acute carpal tunnel syndrome is thrombosis of a persistent median artery.

BIBLIOGRAPHY

Greenberg M. *Handbook of Neurosurgery*, 7th ed. New York, NY: Thieme; 2010:804–810.

Rengachary S. Entrapment neuropathies. In: Wilkins Rengachary S (eds.), *Neurosurgery*, 2nd ed. New York, NY: McGraw-Hill; 1996:3073–3098.

19. **(C)**

20. **(A)**

Explanations for questions 19 and 20

Causalgia was a term introduced by Weir Mitchell during the Civil War to describe burning pain that occasionally appeared after partial nerve injuries. Autonomic symptoms and trophic changes were also part of the clinical picture. Causalgia major referred to high-velocity missile injuries that involved a peripheral nerve, and causalgia minor referred to less severe or nonpenetrating soft tissue injury. Early in the last century, the pain was thought to be sympathetically mediated, and the term reflex sympathetic dystrophy (RSD) was introduced. Today, most theories of this group of painful disorders do not involve the autonomic nervous system, and consequently, the term complex regional pain syndrome (CRPS) is used to encompass a variety of clinical entities with somewhat similar symptoms with perhaps diverse etiologies. In CRPS 1, there is no nerve injury, and in CRPS 2, there is a definable nerve injury.

CRPS 1 occurred in the patient in this scenario without a peripheral nerve injury after minor trauma. A similar symptom complex can be produced by mere immobilization of an extremity or by psychologic disuse and guarding.

It was initially thought that symptoms were produced by ephaptic transmission between afferent pain fibers and efferent sympathetic fibers, but this theory is no longer accepted. Most contemporary theories do not involve the direct involvement of the sympathetic nervous system; the autonomic manifestation may merely be an epiphenomenon.

Symptoms of CRPS may begin within 24 hours or days to weeks after injury. If there is a specific nerve injury, the median, ulnar, and sciatic nerves are most frequently implicated. The patient will have burning pain and allodynia and may resist having his or her hand or foot examined, particularly the palmar and plantar surfaces. The vasomotor tone can vary from a pink and warm to a cold and mottled extremity. The skin may be dry and scaly and the joints stiff. There may be hair loss or excess hair. There may be edema of the soft tissue and eventually atrophy. The attitude of this patient's extremity is probably secondary to a dystonic component of the syndrome.

There is no evidence that psychiatric support and physical therapy can cure CRPS, but most clinicians will use these modalities in managing such patients. There is controversy about the value of sympathetic blocks and peripheral sympathectomy in the treatment of CRPS. There is some literature claiming cure rates of 80–95%, but some authors claim that these results result from bias in defining the condition as RSD if they get benefit from sympathectomy. Other data claim that only 7% of patients are cured with treatment directed toward the sympathetic nervous system. There is a very high response rate to placebo. Recently there has been evidence that dorsal column stimulation in carefully selected patients can reduce pain and improve quality of life when other treatments have failed. When there is a dystonic component, intrathecal baclofen may be useful in ameliorating some symptoms of CRPS.

BIBLIOGRAPHY

Arguelles J, Burcdhiel K. Causalgia and reflex sympathetic dystrophy. In: Wilkins R, Rengachary S (eds.), *Neurosurgery*, 2nd ed. New York, NY: McGraw-Hill; 1996:3209–3215.

Kelmer M, Barendse G, van Kleef M, et al. Spinal cord stimulation in patients with chronic reflex sympathetic dystrophy. *N Engl J Med* 2000;343:618–624.

Schwartzman R. New treatments for reflex sympathetic dystrophy. *N Engl J Med* 2000;343:654–656.

Van Hilten B, van d Beek W, Hoff J, et al. Intrathecal baclofen for the treatment of dystonia in patients with reflex sympathetic dystrophy. *N Engl J Med* 2000;343:625–630.

21. **(C)** The MRI scan shows a herniated disk at L3–4 with compression of the L4 nerve root. The L4 nerve root supplies the quadriceps muscle and, along with L3 nerve root, is responsible for the knee reflex. Weakness of the quadriceps muscle is best demonstrated by having the patient step up on a platform about 15 in. high, first with the normal side and then with the involved side. Weakness not apparent on manual testing may be demonstrated by this maneuver. This patient's disk herniation is

in a posterior lateral position. The L4 nerve root passes the L3–4 disk space and exits at the L4–5 neural foramen. A far lateral disk at L4–5 could also cause L4 nerve root compression. If the MRI scan were normal, one would have to consider the diagnosis of diabetic proximal neuropathy, which might be the first manifestation of diabetes mellitus. In this disorder, it is likely that, if an EMG were performed, the paraspinal muscles would not be involved, whereas the paraspinal muscles ordinarily would be involved in nerve root compression by a herniated disk. Proximal diabetic neuropathy causes hip and leg pain for 6–9 months and then usually subsides spontaneously, but the opposite side may become involved.

A herniated disk at L5–S1 usually compresses the S1 nerve root, which exits through the S1–2 intervertebral foramen. With S1 nerve root compression, the ankle reflex is usually lost. In this case, both ankle reflexes are absent because the patient is a diabetic. In the adult, the two most common causes of absent ankle reflexes are diabetes and chronic alcoholism. A herniated disk at L4–5 usually compresses the L5 nerve root, which exits through the L5–S1 intervertebral foramen. There is no reflex to test for the L5 nerve root, but the extensor hallucis longus muscle is supplied almost exclusively by L5, and weakness of this muscle can usually be demonstrated.

BIBLIOGRAPHY

Jorge A, Przybylski G. Herniated lumbar disc. In: Batjer H, Loftus C (eds.), *Textbook of Neurological Surgery*. Philadelphia, PA: Lippincott Williams & Wilkins; 2003:1657–1661.
Naftulin S, Fast A, Thomas M. Diabetic lumbar radiculopathy: sciatica without disc herniation. *Spine* 1993;18:2419–2422.

22. **(C)** An elderly patient may have structural evidence of both lumbar spinal stenosis and vascular insufficiency of the lower extremities. In fact, 30% of elderly individuals have spinal stenosis on imaging studies but have no clinical symptoms. Both disorders can cause claudication-type pain in one or both lower extremities with walking. Sorting out the etiology may be difficult when these conditions coexist, but the subtle aspects of the clinical history can be helpful. The neurologic examination in symptomatic spinal stenosis is often normal, and patients with symptomatic spinal stenosis may have poor pedal pulses. In vascular claudication, cramping symptoms can usually be reproduced by a specific amount of exercise, like walking 25 ft. The claudication-type symptoms in spinal stenosis vary from day to day as does the distance required to bring on the symptoms. Spinal stenosis symptoms are more apt to appear with just standing. Vascular claudication is not posture related. The pain elicited in both disorders can be relieved by

rest. Vascular claudication is relieved almost immediately when ambulation is stopped. Relief is slower in neurogenic claudication, and the patient usually has to sit down. Patients with stenosis may also find relief with bending forward, and they will occasionally walk this way. The anterior-posterior diameter of the spinal canal increases with flexion. Also in spinal stenosis, back or leg discomfort can occur with bending or lifting. When spinal stenosis is severe, there may be some curling up of the nerve roots in the spinal canal, giving the appearance of spaghetti. When present, this imaging picture is supportive of neurogenic claudication.

Treatment of spinal stenosis is by laminectomy, which involves removal of lamina and a portion of the facets. When there is evidence of spinal instability, such as degenerative spondylolisthesis due to disease of the facet joints, spinal stabilization at the time of laminectomy may be recommended.

BIBLIOGRAPHY

Ciric I, Salehi S, Gravely L. Lumbar spinal stenosis and laminectomy. In: Batjer H, Loftus C (eds.), *Textbook of Neurological Surgery*. Philadelphia, PA: Lippincott Williams & Wilkins; 2003:1777–1684.
Epstein N. Symptomatic lumbar spinal stenosis. *Surg Neurol* 1998;50:3–10.

23. **(D)** This patient is in hypotensive shock. The wound is obviously too small for the profound blood loss required to produce shock after the incision is closed. Even if there is considerable epidural bleeding during a single-level disk operation under the microscope, the volume of blood lost is actually small, and very rarely would transfusion be necessary. During lumbar discectomy, it is possible to injure the aorta or iliac artery with the bite of a rongeur that goes through the anterior annulus. In about 50% of cases, there is no back bleeding from the disk space and the surgeon is unaware that a vascular injury has occurred. When examined in the recovery room, the hypotensive patient's flanks may become discolored and the abdomen distended. If there is some stability during fluid resuscitation, a CT scan of the abdomen could be obtained to confirm the diagnosis; however, more often the patient is *in extremis* and it is life-saving to return the patient to the operating room, open the abdomen, and secure the bleeding site. The vessel involved is usually the iliac artery, and the injury is usually more common with left-sided discectomy. It is good practice when doing disk surgery to palpate the anterior aspect of the disk space with an instrument to be sure there has been no perforation.

An occasional patient may present with anemia and tachycardia several days to weeks after lumbar disk surgery secondary to an accidental fistula created between an iliac artery and vein.

BIBLIOGRAPHY

Anda S, Askhus S, Skaanes K, et al. Anterior perforation in lumbar diskectomies: a report of four cases of vascular complications and a CT study of the prevertebral lumbar anatomy. *Spine* 1991;16:54–60.

Lange M, Fink U, Philipp A, et al. Emergency diagnosis with spiral CT angiography in case of suspected ventral perforation following lumbar disc surgery. *Surg Neurol* 2002;57:15–19.

Pappas C, Harrington T, Sonntag V. Outcome analysis in 654 surgically treated lumbar disc herniations. *Neurosurgery* 1992;30:862–866.

24. **(C)** Cauda equina syndrome (CES) is an acute or chronic condition caused by compression of the nerve roots of the cauda equina (by ruptured intervertebral disk, tumor, trauma, postoperative hematoma, or other mass lesions) and consists of a usually asymmetric distribution of pain, sensory, and motor loss in the lower extremities. There is often an acute worsening (herniated disk) on top of a chronic, longstanding process (spinal stenosis). Saddle anesthesia and urinary sphincter problems are very common. The level of involvement can often be localized on physical examination. Rectal tone and sensation in the sacral dermatomes must be documented in any patient with suspected CES. There is urinary retention with resultant overflow incontinence in acute cases. Checking a postvoid residual is helpful in determining bladder function. The imaging modality of choice for the spine is the MRI, which can assist in surgical planning. Most agree that decompression for acute CES should take place as soon as possible, and usually within 24 hours. Expeditious decompression gives the best chance for recovery of function, which is better for lower extremity function than for bladder function.

    Acute epidural abscess in the lumbosacral area would typically present with excruciating low back pain, fever, and malaise and then progress to neurologic deficit over the course of hours or days. This can occur commonly in patients predisposed to bacteremia, such as IV drug users. Injury or infarct of the conus medullaris typically causes a symmetric syndrome of sensory and motor loss with sphincter dysfunction, and there is usually a predisposing condition (e.g., hypercoagulable state, angiogram with shower emboli). Pain is less severe if present, and the motor findings are less prominent than with cauda equina lesions.

BIBLIOGRAPHY

Greenberg MS. *Handbook of Neurosurgery*, 7th ed. New York, NY: Thieme; 2010:442–447.

Rengachary SS. Examination of motor and sensory systems and reflexes. In: Wilkins RH, Rengachary SS (eds.), *Neurosurgery*, 2nd ed. New York, NY: McGraw-Hill; 1996:155–156.

Shapiro S. Cauda equina syndrome secondary to lumbar disc herniation. *Neurosurgery* 1993;32:743–747.

25. **(B)** The most likely diagnosis based on this patient's current complaints, medical history, and imaging studies is spinal epidural abscess. Well-documented risk factors are diabetes mellitus, chronic renal failure, and IV drug abuse. Over half of abscesses are from hematogenous spread. The clinical picture usually begins with localized pain (which may be excruciating) in the affected area of the spine, fever, malaise, and occasionally symptoms of meningeal irritation. Nerve root and then spinal cord symptoms (in lesions of the cervical and thoracic spine) ensue and may progress to paralysis. Timing of progression varies according to organism from hours (acute bacterial infections) to months (mycobacterial and fungal infections). *Staphylococcus aureus* is the most commonly isolated organism in acute abscesses, with *Mycobacterium tuberculosis* common in chronic cases. There is often associated discitis and osteomyelitis, and the presence of these may alter the surgical therapy. Erythrocyte sedimentation rate (ESR) is usually elevated but not specific. MRI with gadolinium contrast is the imaging modality of choice and usually will reveal a fluid intensity enhancing mass in the epidural space. Straightforward spinal epidural abscesses are usually located dorsally and removed via laminectomy. Those associated with discitis and/or osteomyelitis, as in this case, are usually anterior, and treatment often involves removal of infected disk and vertebral bodies with reconstruction and fusion. Percutaneous aspiration may reveal the causative organism but will not relieve or prevent further neurologic injury. The pathophysiology of spinal cord injury involves direct compression of the nervous structures and, more importantly, thrombophlebitis of epidural and spinal veins causing venous infarction. Rates of recovery of deficits are very low, even with expeditious surgery, and mortality is as high as 23%. Early diagnosis is extremely important. Any patient with risk factors, fever, and local spine tenderness warrants investigation.

BIBLIOGRAPHY

Allen MB, Flannery AM, Fisher J. Spinal epidural and subdural abscesses. In: Wilkins RH, Rengachary SS (eds.), *Neurosurgery*, 2nd ed. New York, NY: McGraw-Hill; 1996:3327–3330.

Baker AS, Ojemann RG, Swartz MN, et al. Spinal epidural abscesses. *N Engl J Med* 1975;293:463–468.

Greenberg MS. *Handbook of Neurosurgery*, 7th ed. New York, NY: Thieme; 2010:376–380.

Hlavin ML, Kaminski HJ, Ross JS, et al. Spinal epidural abscesses: a 10-year perspective. *Neurosurgery* 1990;27:177–184.

26. **(D)** NPH is described as a classic triad of gait disturbance, urinary incontinence, and dementia (or in other more memorable words, "wet, wobbly, and weird"). It is usually idiopathic but may also be a long-term sequela of head injury or subarachnoid hemorrhage (SAH). The pathophysiology is not well understood but is related to altered CSF dynamics. It is one of the few treatable causes of dementia. The onset usually begins with gait problems, progressing to a slow, unsteady wide-based shuffle, often described as "magnetic." Urinary incontinence from lack of awareness and frontal lobe–type dementia later ensue. There is usually no fecal incontinence. The diagnosis is made by history and physical examination, and other possible causes for the patient's condition are ruled out with CT and/or MRI. Further evidence of NPH can be obtained with a large-volume lumbar puncture followed by assessment for improvement in gait, but this is not a very sensitive test. An improved diagnostic test is to admit the patient, place a lumbar drain, and monitor the patient over the course of a couple days for improvement in gait, bladder function, or cognitive status. Unfortunately there is no definitive, confirmatory test to make the diagnosis. Therapy requires CSF diversion either via a shunt (typically a ventriculoperitoneal [VP] shunt) or endoscopic third ventriculostomy, a surgical procedure where the ventricular system is opened up endoscopically to enhance drainage. Classically, the symptoms will improve in the same order in which they appear (i.e., improvement in gait followed by improved continence followed by improvement in mental status, which is rarely complete).

Alzheimer disease is usually a progressive global dementia, with very late motor findings. A brain tumor can present with mental status changes, but the neurologic examination usually is more focal and the patient is likely to have headache. Chronic subdural hematoma is unlikely to present with incontinence unless the patient is obtunded.

BIBLIOGRAPHY

Black PMcL. Hydrocephalus in adults. In: Youman JR (ed.), *Neurological Surgery*, 4th ed. Philadelphia, PA: Lippincott-Raven; 1996:930–937.

Muhonen MG, Wellman BJ. Hydrocephalus and benign intracranial cysts. In: Grossman RG, Loftus CM (eds.), *Principles of Neurosurgery*, 2nd ed. Philadelphia, PA: Lippincott-Raven; 1999:99–100.

Paidakakos N, Borgarello S, Naddeo M. Indications for endoscopic third ventriculostomy in normal pressure hydrocephalus. *Acta Neurochir Suppl* 2012;113:123–127.

27. **(A)** Although this patient has multiple medical problems, her presentation is classic for spontaneous aneurysmal SAH. The CT scan reveals blood in the basilar cisterns and subarachnoid spaces. The most common cause of SAH is trauma, although this is usually managed conservatively (depending on the other injuries). Of the types of spontaneous, nontraumatic SAH, aneurysm rupture is the most common etiology. This can be detected with an initial CT angiogram but can be confirmed on four-vessel cerebral arteriography in 85% of cases. Other potential etiologies for spontaneous SAH include other vascular malformations (i.e., arteriovenous malformations), tumors, or benign perimesencephalic SAH, which is a completely benign entity that presents with blood in the subarachnoid space near the brainstem. This latter entity is thought to occur secondary to small venous bleeds, but the exact cause is unknown.

Definitive treatment for a ruptured aneurysm can be pursued via craniotomy and clip application to the vessel, endovascular treatment, or a combination of the two. Endovascular options include coil application, embolization, or deployment of intracranial flow-diverting stents. Whether or not endovascular treatment is employed usually depends on the anatomy of the aneurysm, the width of its neck, and nearby perforator vessels. Any coils or stents usually require long-term anticoagulation. Treatment is usually carried out soon after the diagnosis is made to prevent a second hemorrhage. Risk factors for aneurysmal SAH include smoking, family history, female gender, and possibly hypertension. SAH carries significant morbidity and mortality. Approximately one-third of patients die in the first 24 hours after hemorrhage, and only one-third of patients will have a good outcome. A lumbar puncture is the most sensitive test for SAH, but need only be performed in the rare patient with suspicious history and normal head CT.

There are ECG abnormalities and laboratory findings consistent with cardiac ischemia (elevated CK isoenzymes and troponin) in up to 70% of cases of patients with SAH. Many patients will even have cardiac wall motion abnormalities on echocardiography. This phenomenon, referred to as a demand ischemia or Takotsubo cardiomyopathy, is a transient stress on the myocardium associated with SAH. Although it has been known for nearly 100 years that insults to the brain have cardiac effects, the phenomena are not well understood. Altered hypothalamic control of the autonomic nervous system may account for some of the pathophysiology. There can also be flash pulmonary edema either from the SAH or the cardiomyopathy.

Carcinomatous meningitis (breast and lung cancer and melanoma are most common primaries) can present with headache and neck pain but usually is associated with cranial neuropathies and will not have the appearance of SAH on CT. MRI with contrast and lumbar puncture assist with the diagnosis. Patients with migraine who present with SAH will almost always report that the headache is different from the usual migraine. Septic emboli from valvular heart disease will usually present with fever and stroke-like symptoms but are a rare problem in the patient with other manifestations of endocarditis. Patients with bacterial endocarditis can develop bacterial (sometimes called mycotic) aneurysms of the cerebral arteries. These aneurysms are usually located in the distal branches and present more often with intraparenchymal hemorrhage than SAH.

BIBLIOGRAPHY

Elrifai AM, Dureza C, Bailes JE. Cardiac and systemic complications of subarachnoid hemorrhage. In: Bederson JB (ed.), *Neurosurgical Topics: Subarachnoid Hemorrhage: Pathophysiology and Management*. Park Ridge, IL: American Association of Neurological Surgeons; 1997:87–105.

Froehler MT. Endovascular treatment of ruptured intracranial aneurysms. *Curr Neurol Neurosci Rep* 2013;13:326.

Greenberg MS. *Handbook of Neurosurgery*, 5th ed. New York, NY: Thieme; 2001:1034–1038, 1057–1060.

Lanzino G, Kongable GL, Kassell NF. Electrocardiographic abnormalities after nontraumatic subarachnoid hemorrhage. *J Neurosurg Anesthesiol* 1994;6:156–162.

Yao KC, Bederson JB. Subarachnoid hemorrhage. In: Andrews BT (ed.), *Intensive Care in Neurosurgery*. New York, NY: Thieme; 2003:161–171.

28. **(A)** This patient is suffering from cerebral venous sinus thrombosis. It can present as in this case with elevated ICP without focal neurologic deficits or as a focal deficit with or without increased ICP (implying occlusion of a cortical vein). Risk factors are extremes of age, especially men over 60, women between the ages of 20 and 35, and various states of abnormal blood flow (dehydration, congestive heart failure, polycythemia, or other hematologic disorder). It is also associated with trauma and infection of the paranasal and mastoid sinuses and can be a result of obstruction of flow in the venous sinus from a meningioma. In young women, most cases are associated with pregnancy, the postpartum period, or oral contraceptives.

CT scan may reveal clot in the venous sinuses or cortical veins, venous infarcts, parenchymal hemorrhages, and small ventricles. Angiography will show prolonged circulation times and lack of filling of the affected venous sinuses. MRI is the imaging modality of choice for venous sinus thrombosis, as it is noninvasive, multiplanar, and can evaluate flow (or lack of) in the sinuses in addition to the effects on the brain parenchyma (in particular, via the venous phase or the magnetic resonance venography). This patient's images reveal thrombosis in the superior

sagittal sinus, thrombosis of cortical veins, and bilateral venous infarctions with hemorrhage on the left.

Goals of treatment are to prevent extension of the thrombosis, control symptoms from elevated ICP or seizures until recanalization, and remove any causative factor. Anticoagulation should be instituted immediately, even if there is evidence of hemorrhagic venous infarction, to prevent extension of thrombus until recanalization or formation of collaterals. Anticoagulation has been shown to improve the patient's condition without significant risk of increased hemorrhage. Endovascular treatment has been used to mechanically disrupt the thrombus and also to deliver thrombolytic medications. Adequate hydration is also important and should be monitored with central venous pressure catheter. Antibiotics are given if there is an infectious cause, and surgical treatment of the infected site (e.g., mastoid sinus) is occasionally indicated. Surgery on the venous sinuses is reserved for thrombosis caused by mass lesion such as a tumor. Ventriculostomy may be required to treat elevated ICP, but it is not first-line therapy. Steroids have no proven benefit.

BIBLIOGRAPHY

Iskandar BJ, Kapp JP. Nonseptic venous occlusive disease. In: Wilkins RH, Rengachary SS (eds.), *Neurosurgery*, 2nd ed. New York, NY: McGraw-Hill; 1996:2177–2190.

Soleau SW, Schmidt R, Stevens S, et al. Extensive experience with dural sinus thrombosis. *Neurosurgery* 2003;52:534–544.

Southwick FS, Swartz MN. Inflammatory thrombosis of major dural venous sinuses and cortical veins. In: Wilkins RH, Rengachary SS (eds.), *Neurosurgery*, 2nd ed. New York, NY: McGraw-Hill; 1996:3307–3311.

29. **(D)**

30. **(B)**

Explanations for questions 29 and 30

Trigeminal neuralgia (TN) is usually a disorder of older individuals, but it is not rare in middle age. A small percentage of patients may have MS or a neoplasm as the cause of TN. Many neurosurgeons feel that the majority of cases of TN are probably due to compression of the trigeminal nerve by a normal blood vessel near the exit zone of the trigeminal nerve from the brainstem. Typically, the vessel is the superior cerebellar artery, and it forms a "vessel loop" that compresses the trigeminal nerve in the region known as "Meckel's cave." MRI is obtained to rule out other causes of TN (tumor, MS, vascular malformation), but occasionally will reveal the offending vessel, especially in the T2 sequences. One of the most successful procedures for treating TN is a posterior fossa craniectomy with microvascular decompression. This entails examining the trigeminal nerve under the microscope in search of vascular compression and decompressing the nerve by placing a sponge between the vessel and nerve; however, drug therapy is first-line treatment, and the most effective medication is carbamazepine. The initial response to carbamazepine is so good that it can be considered as a diagnostic test for TN; however, there is eventually a 50% relapse rate. The patient should be instructed to take the lowest dose that relieves symptoms. The medication induces its own metabolism and must be started gradually in order to avoid toxic symptoms. Rare idiosyncratic reactions can result in aplastic anemia or liver necrosis. Mild abnormal liver function tests and leukopenia can be observed, and these abnormalities usually reverse when the medication is discontinued. An occasional patient will develop acute hyponatremia shortly after starting carbamazepine. Gabapentin and phenytoin also can be used in treating TN but are less effective. Posterior fossa microvascular decompression has the lowest rate of recurrence and causes minimal sensory loss but has the greatest risk profile and is usually reserved for younger patients. Percutaneous procedures (e.g., injection of glycerol) via a needle through the foramen ovale cause partial damage to the trigeminal nerve root and cause some facial sensory loss. The trigeminal root can also be partially injured by stereotactic radiation (gamma knife). Although this is the least invasive surgical technique, there is significant recurrence and some sensory loss, and it is the treatment least likely to allow patients to be off all medication.

BIBLIOGRAPHY

Greenberg, MS. *Handbook of Neurosurgery*, 7th ed. New York, NY: Thieme; 2010:551–560.

Wilkins R. Trigeminal neuralgia. In: Wilkins R, Rengachary S (eds.), *Neurosurgery*, 2nd ed. New York, NY: McGraw-Hill; 1996:3921–3929.

31. **(C)**

32. **(C)**

Explanations for questions 31 and 32

This patient is suffering from optic neuritis. It has been described as a syndrome in which "the patient can't see anything and the doctor can't see anything," due to a lack of findings on examination. This may lead the examiner to believe the patient is hysterical. The patient will have a relative afferent papillary defect (RAPD or Marcus-Gunn pupil), which is diagnosed with the swinging light test. The pupils are equal at baseline and constrict in the light; however, when swinging the light from the normal eye to the affected eye, the pupils will dilate. This is due to a relative decrease in afferent stimulation of the affected eye. Significant monocular vision loss does not occur without an RAPD.

Optic neuritis is the initial presentation of MS in 15% of cases, and 50% of patients with MS will develop optic neuritis at some point in their course. MS is a chronic demyelinating disease that is usually diagnosed in young adulthood and affects women twice as often as men. Its cause is unknown. The diagnosis is made based on the history of neurologic symptoms combined with MRI evidence of lesions explaining the deficits. Lumbar puncture is performed for elevated IgG index and oligoclonal bands. It can be a relapsing-remitting or chronic-progressive disease.

TN usually presents in the sixth decade. Its diagnosis in a young person should prompt a workup for MS.

Amaurosis fugax is usually very transient (minutes) and painless, and the vision loss is often altitudinal, described by the patient as a shade being pulled over the eye.

BIBLIOGRAPHY

Corbett JJ. Approach to the patient with visual loss. In: Biller J (ed.), *Practical Neurology*. Philadelphia, PA: Lippincott-Raven; 1997:97–107.

DeMyer WE. *Technique of the Neurologic Examination*, 4th ed. New York, NY: McGraw-Hill; 1994:143–144.

Greenberg MS. *Handbook of Neurosurgery*, 7th ed. New York, NY: Thieme; 2010:61–65.

Miller JR. Multiple sclerosis. In: Rowland LP (ed.), *Merritt's Neurology*, 10th ed. Philadelphia, PA: Lippincott Williams & Wilkins; 2000:773–792.

33. **(C)** SE is usually defined as a seizure of more than 5 minutes in duration or multiple consecutive seizures without recovery from the postictal state. The seizure activity is usually generalized tonic-clonic, but may be nonconvulsive in rare circumstances. Morbidity and mortality are due to continuous electrical discharges causing neuronal membrane damage and metabolic derangements from convulsive activity causing stress on cardiac, respiratory, renal, and nervous systems. Emergency treatment includes ensuring airway, breathing, and circulation (ABCs), thiamine and D50 (hypoglycemia is a life-threatening cause of seizures), and lorazepam (in adults, 4 mg over 2 minutes, may repeat in 5–10 minutes if necessary) or diazepam (10 mg over 2 minutes, may repeat in 3–5 minutes) early in the course. Regardless of response to benzodiazepine medications, the patient should be loaded with phenytoin (20 mg/kg) or fosphenytoin (which can be administered more quickly). Treatment should be aggressive because there is irreversible damage to the central nervous system in less than

20 minutes of SE. If uncontrolled within 30 minutes, the patient should be intubated and treated with barbiturates, midazolam, or even inhalation anesthetics.

The most common cause of SE in a patient with a seizure disorder is noncompliance or subtherapeutic anticonvulsant levels, but treatment should be instituted before serum glucose and anticonvulsant levels have returned from the laboratory. Other common causes include stroke and alcohol (intoxication or withdrawal) in adults and febrile illness in children.

BIBLIOGRAPHY

Costello DJ, Cole AJ. Treatment of acute seizures and status epilepticus. *J Intensive Care Med* 2007;22:319–347

Greenberg MS. *Handbook of Neurosurgery*, 7th ed. New York, NY: Thieme; 2010:402–408.

Pedley TA, Bazil CW, Morrell MJ. Epilepsy. In: Rowland LP (ed.), *Merritt's Neurology*, 10th ed. Philadelphia, PA: Lippincott Williams & Wilkins; 2000:829–830.

34. **(D)** This patient has a type I Chiari malformation (also known as hindbrain herniation syndrome) with resultant syringomyelia, a cavitary CSF collection in the spinal cord. There are four types of Chiari malformations, and all of them entail some extent of hindbrain abnormalities. Most are either type I (commonly referred to as a Chiari malformation) or type II (referred to as an Arnold-Chiari malformation). Type I malformations are usually less severe than type II. They commonly present with headache in young adults and usually have mild cerebellar tonsillar herniation (>5 mm) but rarely have medullary involvement or hydrocephalus. Type II malformations in contrast are more severe, are usually associated with a myelomeningocele and hydrocephalus, and present in infancy with more severe symptoms like respiratory distress or dysphagia. Type III is the most severe, entails cerebellar herniation through the foramen magnum, and is usually incompatible with life. Type IV is cerebellar hypoplasia without herniation.

Most if not all of the patient's symptoms and physical examination findings are directly referable to the syrinx. In over 70% of cases, the cause of a cystic cavity in the spinal cord is a hindbrain abnormality. Multiple theories of the pathophysiology exist, and most deal with alterations in the CSF dynamics at the cervicomedullary junction. Therefore, definitive treatment is directed at the posterior fossa.

Surgical treatment of the Arnold-Chiari malformation with syringomyelia is with posterior fossa craniectomy and often requires upper cervical laminectomy. The dura is opened, arachnoid adhesions are taken down, and the dura is then patched with cervical fascia, fascia lata, or artificial dural substitute. The syrinx is followed with serial images. If the symptoms or the syrinx do not improve after adequate posterior fossa decompression, fenestration or shunting of the syrinx into the subarachnoid or pleural space can be performed.

Syringomyelia can also be the result of any compressive lesion of the spinal cord (intramedullary or extramedullary tumor, prior trauma), or any tethering of the spinal cord (spina bifida, arachnoiditis). Appropriate imaging studies with contrast should be performed to rule out tumor. Even in these cases, initial treatment is still directed at the causative pathologic process and not the syrinx.

BIBLIOGRAPHY

Greenberg MS. *Handbook of Neurosurgery*, 7th ed. New York, NY: Thieme; 2010:233–240.

Piper JG, Menezes AH. The relationship between syringomyelia and the Chiari malformations. In: Anson JA, Benzel EC, Awad IA (eds.), *Neurosurgical Topics: Syringomyelia and the Chiari Malformations*. Park Ridge, IL: American Association of Neurological Surgeons; 1997:91–104.

Williams B. Management schemes for syringomyelia: surgical indications and nonsurgical management. In: Anson JA, Benzel EC, Awad IA (eds.), *Neurosurgical Topics: Syringomyelia and the Chiari Malformations*. Park Ridge, IL: American Association of Neurological Surgeons; 1997:125–143.

35. **(B)** Patients with VP shunts can and often do have medical problems that are completely unrelated to their shunt. Even though the foreign body is an easy scapegoat, once a VP shunt has been in place for more than a year, the chances of it being a source of fever or infection are extremely low. The exception is the shunted patient with the acute abdomen, because the shunt often is the culprit for the symptoms. Small bowel obstructions, enterocutaneous fistulae, and even bowel perforations have been reported. Ultrasound can be very important in assisting with the diagnosis.

The patient in this example has a classic case of appendicitis, and if there were no VP shunt, his management would be very straightforward. If the appendix were unruptured, surgical treatment is no different than in the patient without a shunt. The patient should undergo appendectomy and receive appropriate antibiotics. The shunt tubing should not be sought and should be left undisturbed if in the surgical field. If there is gross peritonitis, the neurosurgeon should bring the abdominal catheter out through a separate incision and connect it to a drainage bag. The spinal fluid should be cultured. The risk of ascending infection of the shunt in this patient is extremely low. If the shunt tubing becomes infected, the entire shunt system will be removed and replaced after elimination of the infection and resolution of peritonitis. Postoperative complications include CSF pseudocyst due to decreased peritoneal absorption and are rare. Conversion to a ventriculoatrial or ventriculopleural shunt may be performed in the uninfected shunt even before the peritonitis has resolved.

In patients without obvious cause for peritonitis, it is usually recommended that the distal portion of the shunt be externalized and antibiotics started. Abdominal symptoms related to shunt infection will usually resolve within 6 hours.

BIBLIOGRAPHY

Hadani M, Findler G, Muggia-Sullam M, et al. Acute appendicitis in children with a ventriculoperitoneal shunt. *Surg Neurol* 1982;18:69–71.

Pumberger W, Löbl M, Geissler W. Appendicitis in children with a ventriculoperitoneal shunt. *Pediatr Neurosurg* 1998;28:21–26.

Rekate HL, Yonas H, White RJ, et al. The acute abdomen in patients with ventriculoperitoneal shunt. *Surg Neurol* 1979;11:442–445.

36. **(D)** The funduscopic pictures reveal retinal hemorrhages, which are seen in significant head trauma, traumatic birth, or acute altitude sickness. They have been rarely reported with other significant central nervous system insults such as aneurysmal SAH. They resolve quickly, so their presence is indicative of an acute injury. The head CT reveals bilateral subdural hematomas. They appear less dense (darker) than expected in this patient due to anemia as well as their chronic state (this child likely has had multiple traumatic insults accumulate). Nonaccidental trauma is the most common cause of subdural hematoma in infants and young children. MRI is better for differentiating acute from subacute or chronic blood because the intensity is based on the oxidative state of hemoglobin. This child has classic presentation for shaken baby syndrome (also referred to as shaken impact syndrome), and the CT and funduscopy are nearly pathognomonic. Due to legal ramifications, a thorough evaluation is warranted and should include a skeletal survey for fractures (acute or old), a workup for coagulopathy, and metabolic/genetic screen for glutaric aciduria (a rare metabolic disorder that causes neurologic decline and brain atrophy and can be associated with subdural hematoma).

Any physician or caregiver that suspects child abuse is required by state and federal law to report these suspicions to the appropriate child protective services or to law enforcement personnel.

BIBLIOGRAPHY

Duhaime A, Christian C. Child abuse. In: McLone DG (ed.), *Pediatric Neurosurgery: Surgery of the Developing Nervous System*, 4th ed. Philadelphia, PA: W.B. Saunders; 2001:593–600.

Greenberg MS. *Handbook of Neurosurgery*, 7th ed. New York, NY: Thieme; 2010:917–919.

37. **(D)** The axial T1-weighted MRI with contrast (see Fig. 35-14) reveals a lesion in the posterior fossa, obliterating the fourth ventricle. Headache in a child is always a cause for concern because brain tumors are the most common solid tumor in children, and this patient's history of postural headache is even more concerning. When lying down, the tumor obstructs flow of CSF through the cerebral aqueduct or through the foramina of Magendie and Luschka in the fourth ventricle, causing symptomatic hydrocephalus. Sitting or standing up relieves the obstruction and the hydrocephalus.

The differential diagnosis for a posterior fossa tumor in the pediatric population includes medulloblastoma, cerebellar astrocytoma, ependymoma, and brainstem glioma. These four account for about 90% of pediatric posterior fossa tumors. Presenting symptoms are usually related to hydrocephalus because most of these are slow-growing tumors. Focal deficits typically appear late and are caused by infiltration of structures by the tumor or metastatic spread via the subarachnoid spaces. This tumor would be resected via posterior fossa craniotomy. If there is hydrocephalus, a ventriculostomy could be placed at the time of tumor resection or earlier if the patient became symptomatic. This would be removed after resolution of hydrocephalus and tumor resection, or it can be converted to a VP shunt if the hydrocephalus does not resolve. MRI of the entire neuraxis and lumbar puncture are indicated for medulloblastomas and ependymomas due to their propensity for drop metastases, and the information obtained from these studies is used in staging and determination of adjunctive therapy.

Medulloblastomas compose 29% of pediatric posterior fossa tumors, arise from the roof of the fourth ventricle, and are usually midline. They enhance with gadolinium-contrasted MRI. Postoperative treatment is with chemotherapy and radiation depending on age, stage, and extent of resection. The overall 5-year survival is approximately 60%. Cerebellar astrocytomas compose over 25% of posterior fossa tumors in children, are often cystic, and enhance with contrast on MRI. They typically do not require postoperative adjunctive therapy and may have over 95% 25-year survival rates with complete resection. Ependymomas arise from the floor or lateral recesses of the fourth ventricle, variably enhance on contrasted MRI, and account for 10% of posterior fossa tumors in children. Postoperatively, they are treated with radiation. Unfortunately, ependymomas are relatively chemotherapy resistant. The 5-year survival rate is approximately 50%. Brainstem gliomas account for 27% of posterior fossa tumors. They are further subclassified by their appearance on imaging studies and have different treatments and outcomes based on this subclassification.

Choroid plexus papilloma is a tumor of the choroid plexus, most commonly seen in the lateral ventricles of adults. A choroid plexus papilloma can occur in the fourth ventricle of a child, but it would be far less common than any of the above tumors.

BIBLIOGRAPHY

Choux M, Lena G, Gentet JC, et al. Medulloblastoma. In: McLone DG (ed.), *Pediatric Neurosurgery: Surgery of the Developing Nervous System*, 4th ed. Philadelphia, PA: W.B. Saunders; 2001:804–818.

Reddy AT, Mapstone TB. Cerebellar astrocytoma. In: McLone DG (ed.), *Pediatric Neurosurgery: Surgery of the Developing Nervous System*, 4th ed. Philadelphia, PA: W.B. Saunders; 2001:835–842.

Tomita T. Ependymomas. In: McLone DG (ed.), *Pediatric Neurosurgery: Surgery of the Developing Nervous System*, 4th ed. Philadelphia, PA: W.B. Saunders; 2001:822–832.

38. **(A)**

39. **(D)**

Explanations for questions 38 and 39

The MRI and clinical history are most compatible with glioblastoma multiforme (GBM). This tumor is the most common primary brain tumor in adults and unfortunately the most malignant of all of the gliomas. Gliomas are tumors that arise from glial cells, which are the supporting cells of the brain. Some GBMs develop from malignant progression of low-grade gliomas (which usually occur in younger adults), but most GBMs appear *de novo* in older patients and are associated with a shorter, devastating clinical history. MRI scans show an irregularly ring-enhancing lesion (indicating breakdown of the blood–brain barrier) with a dark, necrotic center and surrounding edema. The histology consists of malignant-appearing astrocytes, vascular hyperplasia, and areas of necrosis. A biopsy will not relieve the mass effect and could precipitate hemorrhage or further swelling of the tumor, leading to transtentorial herniation. That said, often tumor tissue is sent for frozen pathologic diagnosis intraoperatively to confirm diagnosis. Also, because the nondominant hemisphere is involved, aggressive therapy should be undertaken to prolong life. The immediate threat to the patient is death from increased ICP secondary to the large mass effect. This patient needs a craniotomy with debulking of as much tumor as possible. Prior to the craniotomy, pretreatment with steroids to decrease cerebral edema is appropriate.

Because this patient is young, his prognosis is better than an elderly patient with a similar lesion. The extent of resection is best estimated by performing an MRI scan in the very early postoperative period. Enhancing areas probably represent residual tumor. In later scans, it may be difficult to distinguish scar from tumor. Even though the tumor may seem circumscribed, tumor cells always infiltrate beyond the enhancing margin.

The median survival for this lesion with surgery, radiation, and chemotherapy is 9 to 15 months, and this has unfortunately not increased despite significant efforts in biomedical research. Radiation therapy is the most important adjuvant therapy for GBM and should be given to the patient following resection. A dose of 60 Gy is usually given in 33 fractions. Chemotherapy with alkylating agents such as carmustine and temozolomide (Temodar, an oral agent) is now standard of care as well. The antineoplastic agents are weak though. It is difficult for them to penetrate the blood–brain barrier to reach neoplastic cells. Also, tumor cells can develop drug resistance, and there is risk to normal brain. There are currently multiple active clinical trials evaluating efficacy for molecular inhibitors and vaccines targeted against tumor antigens.

BIBLIOGRAPHY

Binder D, Keles G, Aldape K, et al. Aggressive glial neoplasms. In: Batjer H, Loftus C (eds.), *Textbook of Neurological Surgery*. Philadelphia, PA: Lippincott Williams & Wilkins; 2003:1270–1280.

Mrugala MM. Advances and challenges in the treatment of glioblastoma: a clinician's perspective. *Discov Med* 2013;15:221–230.

Shrieve D, Alexander E, Black P, et al. Treatment of primary glioblastoma multiforme with standard radiotherapy and radiosurgical boost: prognostic factors and long-term outlook. *J Neurosurg* 1999;90:72–77.

40. **(A)** This patient has lung cancer with a single metastasis to the brain, as is the case in approximately one-third of patients with brain metastases. The most common primaries of metastasis to the brain are lung, breast, colon, kidney, and melanoma. In general, the prognosis is poor, and an untreated patient will have a median life expectancy of approximately 1 month. Brain radiation therapy alone can be expected to add 3–6 months of life and is used in all patients with metastases, single or multiple and operative or not.

Indications for surgery and outcomes depend on location of the metastases, extent of systemic disease, and type of primary. Randomized, prospective studies of surgery followed by whole-brain radiation versus radiation alone reveal statistically significant increases in life expectancy and quality of life. Therefore, the patient with a surgically accessible single brain metastasis will usually undergo craniotomy for resection, followed by whole-brain radiation therapy. The patient in this example may have an even better prognosis, because there is evidence that patients undergoing a curative procedure for a primary lung cancer have a statistically significant increased survival compared to those undergoing only palliative surgery or no resection of the primary. Radiosurgery (stereotactic-focused high-dose radiation) of a metastasis may be considered as an alternative to craniotomy in the patient with the surgically inaccessible lesion, the patient who is not medically able to undergo craniotomy, or the patient who refuses to consider craniotomy. Radiosurgery does not impact on the patient's ability to receive adjuvant radiation therapy. Finally, radiosurgery in addition to whole-brain radiation has not been shown to have any statistically significant benefit.

BIBLIOGRAPHY

Galicich JH, Arbit E, Wronski M. Metastatic brain tumors. In: Wilkins RH, Rengachary SS (eds.), *Neurosurgery*, 2nd ed. New York, NY: McGraw-Hill; 1996:807–821.

Patchell RA, Tibbs PA, Walsh JW. A randomized trial of surgery in the treatment of single metastases to the brain. *N Engl J Med* 1990;322:494–500.

Patil CG, Pricola K, Sarmiento JM, Garg SK, Bryant A, Black KL. Whole brain radiation therapy (WBRT) alone versus WBRT and radiosurgery for the treatment of brain metastases. *Cochrane Database Syst Rev* 2012;9:CD006121.

Wrónski M, Arbit E, Burt M, et al. Survival after surgical treatment of brain metastasis from lung cancer. A follow up study of 231 patients treated between 1976–1991. *J Neurosurg* 1995;83:605–616.

Young B, Patchell RA. Surgery for a single brain metastasis. In: Wilkins RH, Rengachary SS (eds.), *Neurosurgery*, 2nd ed. New York, NY: McGraw-Hill; 1996:823–828.

41. **(C)** This patient most likely has radiation myelopathy. In a patient with lung carcinoma who presents with paraplegia, spinal cord compression from vertebral or epidural compression from metastasis is the most likely cause, but with extradural compression, there is almost always severe pain. This patient has no pain. Radiation myelopathy results from inclusion of the spinal cord in the radiation field. It is usually painless and becomes symptomatic in about 18 months after the radiation therapy is completed. The upper level of spinal cord dysfunction is usually at the level of radiation. Although all the other diagnoses listed are possible, the time course from radiation and the rarity of other disorders make radiation the likely culprit. In most cases of radiation myelopathy, the MRI is normal, but occasionally, as in this case, the cord can be swollen with signal change. The imaging studies can look similar in all of the above and may not absolutely establish the diagnosis. Eventually, the spinal cord will atrophy. There is no proven effective treatment, but in some cases, the neurologic deficits will stabilize. There are anecdotal reports of response to steroids. The risk of developing radiation myelopathy increases with the total dose, the dose per fraction, and the length of the spinal cord radiated.

BIBLIOGRAPHY

Black P, Nair S, Giannakopoulos G. Spinal epidural tumors. In: Wilkins R, Rengachary S (eds.), *Neurosurgery*, 2nd ed. New York, NY: McGraw-Hill; 1996:1791–1804.

Cahill D. Malignant tumors of the boney spine. In: Batjer H, Loftus C (eds.), *Textbook of Neurological Surgery*. Philadelphia, PA: Lippincott Williams & Wilkins; 2003:1401–1421.

Dropcho E. Neurologic complications of radiation therapy. In: Biller J (ed.), *Iatrogenic Neurology*. Boston, MA: Butterworth-Heinemann; 1998:469–470.

Eyster E, Wilson C. Radiation myelopathy. *J Neurosurg* 1970;32:414–420.

42. **(C)** Toxoplasmosis, lymphoma, and PML are the three most common cerebral lesions seen on imaging studies in a patient with acquired immunodeficiency syndrome (AIDS). When an MRI scan is obtained with contrast, *Toxoplasma* abscesses and lymphoma may ring enhance and may be indistinguishable with any degree of certainty. Rather than perform a biopsy, some neurosurgeons prefer to treat the patient empirically with pyrimethamine and sulfadiazine for 2–3 weeks. If there is radiographic improvement, the patient should be maintained on these drugs for the remainder of life to control the infection. If there is no response to these drugs, biopsy is indicated. Other intracranial infections that can occur less frequently in AIDS are caused by *Cryptococcus neoformans, Candida, Coccidioidomycosis, Treponema pallidum* (syphilis), *M tuberculosis*, and *Aspergillus*.

Primary central nervous system lymphoma associated with AIDS is treated with radiation therapy, and the prognosis is worse than the lymphoma without AIDS.

PML is an infection of white matter in the immunocompromised patient caused by a papovavirus. The lesions of PML characteristically do not enhance and often do not act like a mass. There is no satisfactory treatment. The AIDS virus can cause a subacute encephalitis manifested by dementia. Herpes simplex or herpes zoster encephalitis as well as a viral myelitis can also occur.

BIBLIOGRAPHY

Greenberg M. *Handbook of Neurosurgery*, 7th ed. New York, NY: Thieme; 2010:364–367.

Levy R, Russell E, Yungbluth M, et al. The efficacy of image-guided stereotactic brain biopsy in neurologically symptomatic acquired immuno-deficiency syndrome patients. *Neurosurgery* 1992;30:186–190.

43. **(B)** Cyclosporin toxicity can result in the posterior leukoencephalopathy syndrome. There are a variety of acute illnesses that can result in a reversible encephalopathy secondary to edema of the cerebral white matter, most prominently in the occipital and posterior parietal and temporal regions of the brain. Clinically the syndrome is manifested by the subacute onset of headache, lethargy, confusion, altered mental status, seizures, and difficultly with vision. The white matter edema is visible as decreased attenuation on CT scans and hypointensity on T1 and hyperintensity on T2 MRI scans. Originally described in encephalopathy associated with malignant hypertension and eclampsia of pregnancy, the syndrome also occurs secondary to toxicity of cyclosporin and other immunosuppressants. White matter edema results from disruption of the blood–brain barrier. The mechanism for this disturbance is not entirely clear in cases of immunosuppression. The syndrome can occur with levels of drug in the therapeutic range and is probably the result of a vasculopathy caused by the medication. The syndrome is reversible by discontinuing or lowering the drug level. The radiologic abnormalities often resolve completely within several weeks.

Creutzfeldt-Jakob disease is a prion (proteinaceous infectious particle) disease that results in an invariably fatal encephalopathy manifested by dementia, ataxia, myoclonic jerks, and visual symptoms. Creutzfeldt-Jakob disease is not associated with immunosuppression. PML is a white matter infection of the brain caused by the polyomavirus in patients who are immunosuppressed and with certain malignancies. Mental symptoms and blindness can occur. The disease is rapidly progressive. Imaging studies show areas of white matter hypointensity on CT and low signal on T1 and high signal on T2 images. There is no enhancement and little, if any, mass effect. Primary central nervous system lymphoma occurs in patients with AIDS and in patients who have had organ transplantation and are immunosuppressed.

BIBLIOGRAPHY

Hinchey J, Chaves C, Appignana B, et al. A reversible posterior leukoencephalopathy syndrome. *N Engl J Med* 1996;334:494–500.

Truwit C, Denaro C, Lake J, et al. MR imaging of reversible cyclosporin A-induced neurotoxicity. *Am J Neuroradiol* 1991;12:651–659.

CHAPTER 36

INTRACRANIAL AND SPINAL TRAUMA

JOSH ABECASSIS AND AMY LEE

1. A 23-year-old man presents to the emergency department after being involved in a motor vehicle crash. On physical examination, he opens his eyes to painful stimulation, he occasionally mumbles incomprehensible sounds, he localizes to painful stimulation with his right upper extremity, and he withdraws his left upper extremity to pain. His pupils are 4 mm bilaterally and reactive. What is this patient's Glasgow Coma Scale (GCS) score?
   (A) 7
   (B) 9
   (C) 8
   (D) 10

2. Cerebral perfusion pressure (CPP) is equal to
   (A) Systolic blood pressure (SBP) – Intracranial pressure (ICP)
   (B) Diastolic blood pressure (DBP) – ICP
   (C) Mean arterial pressure (MAP) + ICP
   (D) MAP – ICP

3. All of the following are physical signs of a basal skull fracture *except*
   (A) Dilated and nonreactive pupil
   (B) Bilateral periorbital ecchymosis (raccoon eyes)
   (C) Ecchymosis over mastoids (Battle's sign)
   (D) Hemotympanum

4. Generally accepted criteria for elevating a depressed skull fracture in the operating room include all of the following *except*
   (A) Open fracture
   (B) Coexistence of other traumatic lesion (i.e., hematoma) underlying fragment
   (C) Dural tear with cerebrospinal fluid (CSF) leak
   (D) Involvement of the anterior wall of the frontal sinus

5. Cardinal signs of intracranial hypertension include all of the following *except*
   (A) Flexor (decorticate) posturing
   (B) Papilledema
   (C) Aphasia
   (D) Dilated and nonreactive pupil

6. A 42-year-old man presents to the emergency department after being involved in a motor vehicle crash. On initial examination, the patient has a GCS score of 7 (localizes to pain, no eye opening, and no verbal response) and multiple injuries including a long bone fracture. The patient's vital signs are normal. You consult orthopedic surgery, and they want to take the patient to the operating room (OR) to repair his fracture. A computed tomography (CT) scan of the head shows mild-to-moderate diffuse cerebral edema. What is the most appropriate course of action to take with this patient?
   (A) Allow the patient to go the OR immediately for repair of his fracture.
   (B) Consult neurosurgery to evaluate for placement of an ICP monitor prior to his going to the OR.
   (C) Consult neurosurgery to evaluate for placement of an ICP monitor after he returns from the OR.
   (D) Delay surgery indefinitely until the patient's neurologic status improves.

7. Initial routine measures for controlling ICP in a patient with a closed head injury include all of the following *except*
   (A) Hyperventilation
   (B) Elevate head of bed to 30–45 degrees
   (C) Avoid hypotension
   (D) Keep head midline

8. A 22-year-old woman presents to the emergency department after falling off a horse and hitting her head on the ground. She had brief loss of consciousness and is now oriented to name and place only. A CT scan of the head shows mild generalized cerebral edema. What is the most appropriate intravenous fluid for this patient?
   (A) Ringer's lactate
   (B) 0.225% normal saline (NS) with 20 mEq potassium chloride (KCl)
   (C) 0.45% NS with 20 mEq KCl
   (D) 0.9% NS with 20 mEq KCl

9. Late complications of traumatic brain injury may include all of the following *except*
   (A) Seizures
   (B) Communicating hydrocephalus
   (C) Primary brain tumors
   (D) Memory impairment

10. A 24-year-old man is taken to the emergency department after being involved in a motor vehicle crash approximately 3 hours ago. The patient was the unrestrained driver, and he cannot recall the crash. He complains of a left-sided headache, and you notice on physical examination that he has a palpable deformity over the left side of his skull and a boggy temporalis muscle. You order a CT scan of the head. The nurse calls you 20 minutes later to see the patient because he has suddenly become unresponsive. A CT scan of the head is most likely to reveal what type of lesion?
    (A) Chronic subdural hematoma
    (B) Diffuse subarachnoid hemorrhage
    (C) Intraventricular hemorrhage
    (D) Epidural hematoma

11. What category of subdural hematoma appears isodense to brain on CT scans?
    (A) Acute
    (B) Subacute
    (C) Chronic
    (D) None of the above

12. A 19-year-old man presents to the emergency department after being shot in the head with a handgun. Appropriate initial steps in managing this patient include all of the following *except*
    (A) Begin Solumedrol (methylprednisolone) protocol
    (B) Control scalp bleeding
    (C) Elevate head of bed to 30–45 degrees
    (D) Give mannitol 1 g/kg bolus

13. A mother brings her 14-month-old son into the emergency department because he is difficult to arouse. The mother states that the infant accidentally fell off a changing table that is approximately 3 ft tall. On physical examination, you find that the infant has multiple bruises and bilateral retinal hemorrhages. Skull radiographs show a right frontal and a left parietal linear fracture. A CT scan of the head shows a left convexity chronic subdural hematoma. The most likely diagnosis is
    (A) Coagulopathy
    (B) Accidental trauma
    (C) Child abuse
    (D) Neglect

14. All of the following examination findings are consistent with a diagnosis of brain death *except*
    (A) Dilated and nonreactive pupils
    (B) Absent oculocephalic reflex
    (C) Extensor (decerebrate) posturing
    (D) Absent gag reflex

15. Diffuse axonal injury (DAI) results from what type of force acting on the brain?
    (A) Direct impact
    (B) Axial loading
    (C) Linear acceleration
    (D) Rotational acceleration

For Questions 16 through 20, match the following CT scans with the appropriate diagnosis.
    (A) Chronic subdural hematoma
    (B) Subarachnoid hemorrhage
    (C) Acute subdural hematoma
    (D) Intracerebral hemorrhage
    (E) Epidural hematoma

16. Figure 36-1

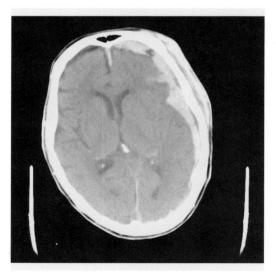

FIGURE 36-1. Computed tomography scan.

17. Figure 36-2

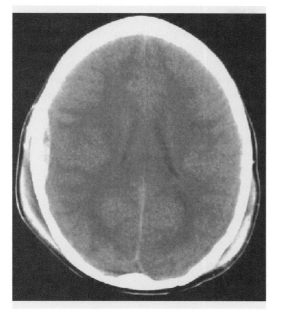

FIGURE 36-2. Computed tomography scan.

18. Figure 36-3

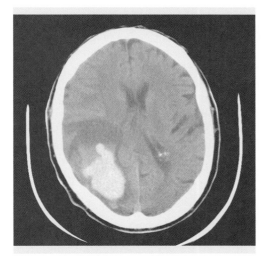

FIGURE 36-3. Computed tomography scan.

19. Figure 36-4

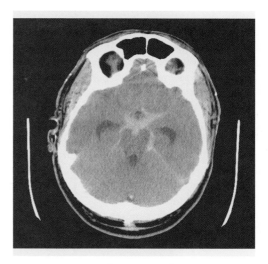

FIGURE 36-4. Computed tomography scan.

20. Figure 36-5

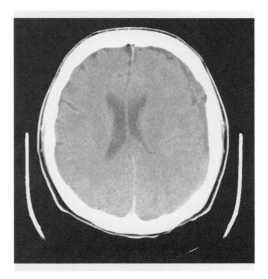

FIGURE 36-5. Computed tomography scan.

21. What percentage of patients who present with a major spinal injury will have a second spinal injury at another level?
    (A) 2%
    (B) 10%
    (C) 20%
    (D) 40%

22. A 20-year-old woman presents to the emergency department after being involved in an all-terrain vehicle crash. Her initial vital signs are normal. Her only complaint is back pain, but she is unable to move her legs and has no sensation below her nipples. On physical examination, she has a step-off deformity in her upper thoracic spine. Her abdominal examination is benign. Chest and pelvis x-rays are normal. Ten minutes later, her blood pressure suddenly falls to 75/35 mmHg. A focused assessment with sonography for trauma (FAST) exam shows no fluid in the abdomen, and her blood pressure does not respond to boluses of intravenous fluids. The most likely cause of the hypotension is
    (A) Spinal shock
    (B) Myocardial infarction
    (C) Intra-abdominal hemorrhage
    (D) Neurogenic shock

23. The most appropriate treatment for refractory hypotension related to neurogenic shock is
    (A) Aggressive intravenous hydration
    (B) Dopamine
    (C) Trendelenburg position
    (D) Phenylephrine

24. Appropriate steps in the initial management of a patient with a suspected spinal cord injury include all of the following *except*
    (A) Maintain on backboard until cervical spine is cleared
    (B) Regulate temperature
    (C) Place nasogastric tube to suction
    (D) Place bladder catheter

25. Which of the following statements regarding the use of methylprednisolone for the treatment of acute spinal cord injuries is correct?
    (A) Greatest benefits are noted when it is given greater than 8 hours after the time of injury.
    (B) The appropriate dose is a 2-g bolus followed by 350 mg/h for 23 hours.
    (C) It is not recommended for treatment of spinal cord injury.
    (D) Complications from its use are rare.

26. A 32-year-old man presents to the emergency department after being involved in a low-velocity motor vehicle crash. He is wearing a cervical collar that was placed by paramedics. He is awake; alert; oriented to name, place, and time; and sober and does not complain of neck pain. On physical examination, he has no cervical tenderness and no other significant injury. He has full range of motion in his neck without any pain. The most appropriate x-rays to order are
    (A) Lateral cervical spine only
    (B) CT scan of the cervical spine

(C) Anteroposterior (AP) and lateral cervical spine
(D) No imaging is necessary

27. An inebriated 62-year-old man presents to the emergency department after a motor vehicle crash. He has ecchymosis and a small laceration on his forehead. His strength is 3/5 in his upper extremities and 4+/5 in his lower extremities. Sensation to pain and temperature is mildly decreased in his upper extremities, and he has urinary retention. The most likely diagnosis is
    (A) Brown-Sequard syndrome
    (B) Anterior cord syndrome
    (C) Central cord syndrome
    (D) Cervical herniated disk

28. All of the following are true statements regarding spinal cord injury without radiographic abnormality (SCIWORA) *except*
    (A) Higher incidence in children <9 years of age
    (B) Radiographs including flexion/extension views are normal
    (C) Immobilization for up to 3 months is often recommended
    (D) Magnetic resonance imaging (MRI) studies are normal

29. Death related to an atlanto-occipital dislocation is most often the result of
    (A) Respiratory arrest
    (B) Cardiac arrest
    (C) Spinal shock
    (D) Hemorrhagic shock

30. A fracture through the arches of the atlas, usually resulting from an axial load, is referred to as a
    (A) Hangman's fracture
    (B) Odontoid fracture
    (C) Jefferson fracture
    (D) Avulsion fracture

31. A fracture through the base of the odontoid is classified as
    (A) Type I
    (B) Type II
    (C) Type III
    (D) Type IV

32. How should locked or perched facets in the cervical spine be treated initially?
    (A) Open reduction and internal fixation
    (B) Closed reduction with cervical traction
    (C) Keep patient immobilized in cervical collar
    (D) No treatment is necessary

33. A clay-shoveler fracture is a fracture of what part of the vertebra?
    (A) Pedicle
    (B) Odontoid process
    (C) Body
    (D) Spinous process

34. A 20-year-old man presents to the hospital with a spine fracture and a complete spinal cord injury. Potential benefits of early surgical stabilization would include all of the following *except*
    (A) Earlier mobilization
    (B) Psychological benefit
    (C) Improved neurologic function
    (D) Reduced comorbidities

35. Which of the following types of thoracolumbar spine fractures is considered unstable?
    (A) Burst fracture
    (B) Transverse process fracture
    (C) Articular process fracture
    (D) Spinous process fracture

36. According to the three-column model of the spine, a seat belt–type fracture involves disruption of which columns?
    (A) All three
    (B) Anterior and middle
    (C) Anterior and posterior
    (D) Middle and posterior

37. Indications for operating on gunshot wounds to the spine include all of the following *except*
    (A) Persistent CSF leak
    (B) Neurologic deterioration
    (C) Compression of a nerve root
    (D) All gunshot injuries require surgical exploration

38. The overall mortality rate from deep venous thromboses in patients with spinal cord injuries is
    (A) 1%
    (B) 5%
    (C) 10%
    (D) 20%

39. A 22-year-old man presents after being in a motor vehicle accident. Imaging is concerning for a spinal cord injury at the T10 level. He is moving his lower extremities but with significant weakness, such that he cannot resist gravity. He has decreased sensation from the navel down. His American Spinal Injury Association (ASIA) grade is
    (A) A
    (B) B
    (C) C
    (D) D
    (E) E

ANSWERS AND EXPLANATIONS

1. **(B)** The GCS is the most widely used scale for predicting outcome following head trauma. It was developed by Teasdale and Jennett as a practical means of assessing and categorizing a patient's level of arousal and neurologic function. The scale is divided into three categories: eye opening, best verbal response, and best motor response. Eye opening is rated on a scale of 1–4, verbal response is rated on a scale of 1–5, and motor response is rated on a scale of 1–6 (Table 36-1). Therefore, the lowest possible score is 3, and the highest possible score is 15. The patient in this question receives 2 points for opening his eyes to painful stimulation, 2 points for verbalizing incomprehensible sounds, and 5 points for localizing to stimulation since this represents his best motor response. Pupillary size and reactivity do not factor into the GCS score. Therefore, the patient's total score in this question is 9. A major disadvantage of using the GCS is that endotracheal intubation prevents the use of the best verbal response category. In such cases, the letter "T" follows the combined score of the remaining two categories. For example, if the patient in this case had been intubated, then his score would have been 7T. When using the GCS, one must keep in mind that although it is an effective

TABLE 36-1 Glasgow Coma Scale

Measure	No. of Points
Eye opening	
Spontaneous	4
To speech	3
To pain	2
No eye opening	1
Best verbal response	
Oriented and appropriate	5
Confused	4
Inappropriate words	3
Incomprehensible sounds	2
No verbal response	1
Best motor response	
Obeys commands	6
Localizes to pain	5
Withdraws to pain	4
Flexor (decorticate) posturing	3
Extensor (decerebrate) posturing	2
No motor response	1

tool for rapidly assessing neurologic function and assisting with outcome predictions, it only shows general trends in the patient's status over time. It is not an accurate or valuable means of following a patient's specific clinical status, and it should not replace a thorough neurologic examination.

2. **(D)** Cerebral blood flow remains relatively constant in the normal brain over a wide range of CPPs, a process that is termed autoregulation. When a patient suffers a severe head injury, however, this autoregulation may be disrupted. One study has suggested that approximately 50% of patients sustaining a severe head injury will have disrupted autoregulation. This causes cerebral blood flow to become dependent on CPP. Because CPP is equal to the difference between the ICP and the MAP, even small or transient drops in blood pressure could translate into decreased cerebral blood flow and lead to ischemia. Therefore, both hypotension and elevated ICP should be avoided in the head-injured patient. A problem arises in monitoring such patients because cerebral blood flow is difficult to measure. Fortunately, CPP may be obtained by simply knowing the blood pressure and ICP. Historically, most physicians taking care of patients with traumatic brain injuries focused on ICP alone. Several reports have now suggested that maintaining an adequate CPP is more important than controlling ICP alone. It is now believed that a CPP of >70 is associated with improved long-term outcome after severe head injury.

BIBLIOGRAPHY

Bouma G, Muizelaar J. Cerebral blood flow, cerebral blood volume, and cerebrovascular reactivity after severe head injury. *J Neurotrauma* 1992;9:S333–S348.

Caron M, Kelly D, Shalmon E, et al. Intensive management of traumatic brain injury. In: Wilkins R, Rengachary S (eds.), *Neurosurgery*, 2nd ed. New York, NY: McGraw-Hill; 1996:2706.

Greenberg M, Greenberg MS. *Handbook of Neurosurgery*, 7th ed. New York, NY: Thieme; 2010:279.

3. **(A)** Basal skull fractures are usually diagnosed by clinical signs. CT scan findings include linear lucencies through the skull base, pneumocephalus, and opacification of air sinuses. Clinical signs vary depending on the site of fracture. Anterior skull base fractures may cause anosmia, CSF rhinorrhea, and periorbital ecchymosis (raccoon eyes). Middle fossa or temporal bone fractures may result in ecchymosis over the mastoids (Battle's sign, see Fig. 36-6), hemotympanum, CSF otorrhea or rhinorrhea, and cranial nerve VII or VIII palsies. A dilated and nonreactive pupil is often the result of compression of cranial nerve III, causing interruption of the sympathetic

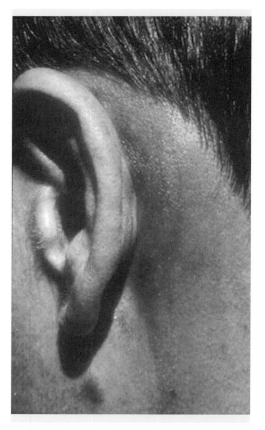

FIGURE 36-6. Ecchymosis overlying the mastoid is known as Battle's sign. This is a sign of a basal skull fracture.

fibers traveling along this nerve. This is most often a sign of elevated ICP and not of a basal skull fracture, although related trauma to the orbit could result in a dilated and nonreactive pupil. Other consequences of basal skull fractures include optic nerve injury, abducens nerve injury, traumatic carotid artery aneurysms, carotid-cavernous fistulae, CSF fistulae, meningitis, and cerebral abscess.

Temporal bone fractures may be divided into two categories based on the relationship between the fracture line and the long axis of the petrous portion of the temporal bone. The longitudinal pattern entails a fracture that is parallel to the long axis of petrous bone. The fracture is usually through the petrosquamosal suture and often passes between the cochlea and semicircular canals, sparing cranial nerves VII and VIII. It is more common (70–90% of all cases) than the transverse fracture pattern, which is, in contrast, perpendicular to long axis of petrous bone (see Figs. 36-7 and 36-8).

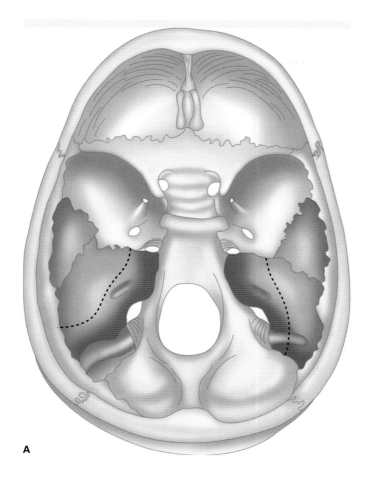

A

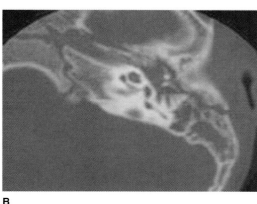

B

FIGURE 36-7. **A.** View of cranial surface of skull base. Longitudinal (left) and transverse (right) temporal bone fractures. **B.** Computed tomography scan showing a longitudinal temporal bone fracture. **(A)** From Brunicardi FC, Andersen DK, Billiar TR, et al. (eds.), *Schwartz's Principles of Surgery*, 9th ed. New York, NY: McGraw-Hill; 2009: Fig. 18-20.

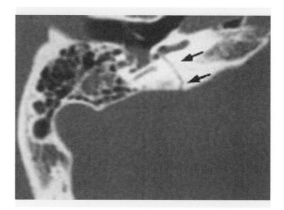

FIGURE 36-8. Computed tomography scan showing a transverse temporal bone fracture (*arrows*).

Damage to cranial nerves VII and VIII occurs more frequently with transverse fractures, whereas longitudinal fractures are more likely to disrupt the ossicular chain and result in hearing loss. Treatment of basal skull fractures almost always involves expectant management, but surgery may be indicated to treat one of the secondary complications of these fractures.

BIBLIOGRAPHY

Geisler F. Skull fractures. In: Wilkins R, Rengachary S (eds.), *Neurosurgery*, 2nd ed. New York, NY: McGraw-Hill; 1996:2753–2754.
Greenberg M, Greenberg MS. *Handbook of Neurosurgery*, 7th ed. New York, NY: Thieme; 2010:887–888.

4. **(D)** Depressed skull fractures are caused by a significant force being applied to a relatively small area of the head. They can be further classified as either closed (i.e., a simple fracture) or open (i.e., a compound fracture). The modality of choice for diagnosing depressed skull fractures is a CT scan of the head (see Fig. 36-9). Although somewhat controversial, there are generally accepted criteria for elevating a depressed skull fracture in the operating room, and this includes open depressed fractures, coexistence of an underlying intracranial hematoma, evidence of a dural tear with CSF leak, depression thickness that is larger than thickness of the calvarium, sinus involvement, or gross cosmetic deformity. Fractures involving the frontal sinus are divided into those that disrupt the anterior wall and those that disrupt the posterior wall. A fracture of the anterior wall of the frontal sinus would only require surgical repair if it caused a significant cosmetic deformity, and this could be done on an elective basis. A fracture through the posterior wall, however, is in a different category because communication between the sinus and the brain increases the risk of developing meningitis or a cerebral abscess.

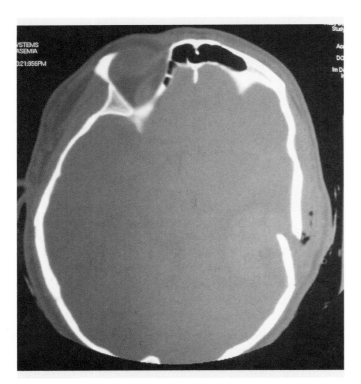

FIGURE 36-9. Bone-window axial head computed tomography of a patient who presented aphasic after being struck with the bottom of a beer bottle. From Brunicardi FC, Andersen DK, Billiar TR, et al. (eds.), *Schwartz's Principles of Surgery*, 9th ed. New York, NY: McGraw-Hill; 2009: Fig. 42-7.

Traditionally, the treatment of choice for fractures through the posterior wall of the frontal sinus involved removing the posterior wall, repairing any dural tear, removing all of the mucous membrane lining the sinus, and plugging the nasofrontal ducts (a process referred to commonly as *cranializing* the sinus). Removing every portion of the mucous membrane is necessary to prevent the formation of a mucocele. Recent studies, however, are proposing a more conservative approach to treating many types of depressed skull fractures, citing the improvements in diagnosis by CT scanning, antibiotic therapy, and rapid transfer to neurosurgical care. Moreover, there is no evidence that elevating a depressed skull fracture will reduce the incidence of posttraumatic seizures, because this is probably related to the initial brain insult.

Most practitioners caring for head-injured patients would consider an open depressed skull fracture to be an emergent situation secondary to the risk of intracranial infection. The goals of surgery are to remove contaminated material, debride devitalized tissue, and close the dura. Irrigation of the wound at bedside is often inadequate for thorough debridement. Overall though,

all of these recommendations (including early timing of surgery) are fairly weak (level III) due to a paucity of randomized controlled studies.

BIBLIOGRAPHY

Avery N, Cheak T. Treatment of cranial vault fractures: recent trends toward a more conservative approach. *J Craniomaxillofac Trauma* 1998;4(3):42–48.

Bullock MR, Chesnutt RM, Ghajar J, et al. Surgical management of depressed cranial skull fractures. *Neurosurgery* 2006;58:S56–560.

Curry D, Frim D. Delayed repair of open depressed skull fracture. *Pediatr Neurosurg* 1999;31(6):294–297.

Greenberg M, Greenberg MS. *Handbook of Neurosurgery*, 7th ed. New York, NY: Thieme; 2010:885–887.

Jennet B. *Epilepsy After Non-Missile Head Injuries*, 2nd ed. London, United Kingdom: William Heinemann; 1975:179.

5. **(C)** Intracranial hypertension may be defined as an ICP greater than 20 cmH$_2$O. Any process that increases the volume within the intracranial compartment may cause intracranial hypertension, such as hydrocephalus, cerebral edema, or a space-occupying lesion. The most consistent and one of the only early signs of intracranial hypertension is papilledema. The other common signs of elevated ICP usually develop late and are related to brain herniation. There are five common categories of brain herniation. These include cingulate (subfalcine) herniation, uncal herniation, central transtentorial herniation, cerebellar tonsillar herniation, and upward cerebellar herniation. Note that the last two are infratentorial and the prior two are supratentorial.

Cingulate herniation results when an expanding mass in one of the cerebral hemispheres forces the cingulate gyrus under the falx cerebri. This may cause compression of the anterior cerebral arteries and internal cerebral veins leading to further ischemia of the herniating hemisphere, although if not, this syndrome is usually asymptomatic. The utility of recognizing this syndrome is that it can be a sign of impending transtentorial herniation. Uncal herniation is caused by an expanding lesion in a hemisphere that pushes the uncus and hippocampus over the edge of the tentorium cerebelli. The medial temporal lobe then compresses the posterior cerebral artery and oculomotor nerve lying within the ambient cistern, and continued herniation results in compression of the midbrain. The hallmarks of this type of herniation are an ipsilateral dilated, nonreactive pupil and contralateral hemiparesis. Of special note, a false localizing sign may occur if herniation causes grooving of the opposite cerebral peduncle against the tentorial edge (referred to as Kernohan's notch), resulting in ipsilateral hemiparesis. Therefore, always rely on the side of papillary involvement when in doubt. As uncal herniation progresses, distortion of the midbrain leads to decorticate and decerebrate posturing, coma, and midbrain hemorrhage, leading to brain death. Central transtentorial herniation occurs usually as a much more chronic process (i.e., a progressively growing brain tumor) and entails herniation of the diencephalon through the tentorial incisura. There can be entrapment of the posterior cerebral arteries and resultant bilateral occipital lobe ischemia, resulting in cortical blindness. This herniation syndrome has multiple stages (diencephalic, midbrain–upper pons, lower pons–upper medullary, and lower medullary) that gradually produce a comatose state. Upward transtentorial herniation occurs when an expanding mass in the posterior fossa forces the cerebellum and lower brainstem up through the tentorial opening.

The final two categories of brain herniation syndromes are cerebellar tonsillar herniation, which is usually the result of an expanding mass in the posterior fossa forcing its contents down through the foramen magnum, and upward cerebellar herniation, where the cerebellar vermis ascends above the tentorium, causing compression of the midbrain.

A discussion of the signs of intracranial hypertension would not be complete without mentioning the triad of symptoms first described by Cushing in 1902. He noted that intracranial hypertension resulted in respiratory irregularity, bradycardia, and hypertension. These responses have been shown to be the result of damage to the medial pons, most likely the reticular formation, and to paramedian areas on the floor of the fourth ventricle. An additional common result of intracranial hypertension is pulmonary edema. This likely results from increased sympathetic tone, which leads to left heart strain and pulmonary congestion. Aphasia is usually the result of ischemia or a focal mass lesion interfering with the temporoparietal area of the dominant hemisphere. It is not regarded as a hallmark of intracranial hypertension.

BIBLIOGRAPHY

Cohen D, Quest D. Increased intracranial pressure, brain herniation, and their control. In: Wilkins R, Rengachary S (eds.), *Neurosurgery*, 2nd ed. New York, NY: McGraw-Hill; 1996:345–353.

Cushing H. Some experimental and clinical observations concerning states of increased intracranial tension. *Am J Med Sci* 1902;124:375–400.

Greenberg M, Greenberg MS. *Handbook of Neurosurgery*, 7th ed. New York, NY: Thieme; 2010:284–287.

6. **(B)** Although there is much debate regarding the precise indications for and benefit of ICP monitoring, several recent studies have suggested that an aggressive stance toward monitoring head-injured patients is associated with a reduced risk of mortality. In 2000, the American Association of Neurological Surgeons Joint Section on Neurotrauma and Critical Care in association with the Brain Trauma Foundation published guidelines relating to the indications for ICP monitoring. In this review, it was noted that ICP monitoring helps in the early detection of intracranial mass lesions, limits the indiscriminate use of therapies to control ICP that may be potentially harmful, helps in determining prognosis, and may improve outcome. Therefore, the Brain Trauma Foundation guidelines state that a comatose head-injured patient (GCS 3–8) with an abnormal CT scan should undergo ICP monitoring. Additionally, comatose head-injured patients with normal CT scans should undergo ICP monitoring if they have two or more of the following features at admission: age over 40, unilateral or bilateral motor posturing, or an SBP of less than 90 mmHg. A review of the Ontario Trauma Registry from 1989 to 1995 was completed to test the hypothesis that insertion of ICP monitors in patients with traumatic brain injuries is not associated with a decrease in the death rate. The conclusions were that monitor insertion rates varied widely from hospital to hospital and that, after controlling for injury scale and injury mechanism, insertion of an ICP monitor was associated with statistically significant decrease in the death rate among patients with severe traumatic brain injury. Finally, a retrospective review of data for consecutive patients with severe closed head injury (GCS ≤8) and long bone fracture admitted over an 8-month period in 34 academic trauma centers in the United States revealed that, in addition to considerable variation in the rates of ICP monitoring, management at an aggressive center (defined as those placing ICP monitors in >50% of patients meeting the Brain Trauma Foundation criteria) was associated with a significant reduction in the risk of mortality. That said, a recent study published in the *New England Journal of Medicine* showed that close clinical exam with CT imaging fared similar to the use of ICP monitors, although the trial was conducted in a third-world country and has generated some controversy regarding its applicability to neurointensive care units in the United States. The overall trend in the United States is to use an ICP monitor in patients with GCS ≤8 (severe brain injury) with either an abnormal CT scan or a normal CT scan with two or more risk factors for intracranial hypertension, including age over 40 years, SBP less than 90 mmHg, or decerebrate or decorticate posturing on neurologic exam.

Another consideration regarding the patient in this case is the anticipated use of intravenous fluids in the operating room under the situation of general anesthesia in which the neurologic examination is compromised. Worsening cerebral edema and secondary neurologic injury may progress unnoticed without the ability to monitor ICP and CPP. With all of these factors in mind, the most appropriate course of action is to consult neurosurgery to evaluate the patient for placement of an ICP monitor prior to his going to the operating room.

BIBLIOGRAPHY

Brain Trauma Foundation, American Association of Neurological Surgeons, Joint Section on Neurotrauma and Critical Care. Indications for intracranial pressure monitoring. *J Neurotrauma* 2000;17(6–7):479–491.

Bulger E, Nathens A, Rivara F, et al. Management of severe head injury: institutional variations in care and effect on outcome. *Crit Care Med* 2002;30(8):1870–1876.

Chesnut RM, Temkin N, Carney N, et al. A trial of intracranial-pressure monitoring in traumatic brain injury. *N Engl J Med* 2012;367:2471–2481.

Lane P, Skoretz T, Doig G, et al. Intracranial pressure monitoring and outcomes after traumatic brain injury. *Can J Surg* 2000;43(6):406.

7. **(A)** When a patient presents with a head injury, several initial routine measures may be instituted to help prevent intracranial hypertension. These include correct positioning of the patient, avoiding hypotension, controlling hypertension, light sedation, preventing hyperglycemia, and avoiding excessive hyperventilation. Correct positioning of the patient means elevating the head of the bed to 30–45 degrees and keeping the head midline. Elevating the head of the bed even 30 degrees has been shown to reduce ICP without reducing CPP or cerebral blood flow. Keeping the head midline prevents kinking of the jugular veins and subsequent reduced venous outflow, which could lead to venous congestion and increased ICP. Hypotension is a predictor of poor outcome in a head-injured patient. Because autoregulation is likely disrupted, cerebral blood flow decreases as the blood pressure decreases. SBPs of less than 90 mmHg will result in inadequate perfusion of the brain. Likewise, hypertension must be controlled, because this may elevate ICP and increase the risk of hemorrhage. Light sedation is used to calm the head-injured patient. Caution should be used when administering sedatives, however, so that the patient is not too sedated to give a reliable neurologic examination. Another routine measure for controlling ICP is avoiding hyperglycemia because this aggravates cerebral edema and cell damage. With regard to ventilatory status, both hyperventilation and hypoventilation should be avoided. Hypoventilation will elevate partial pressure of carbon dioxide (PCO_2), causing vasodilation of cerebral vessels, increased intracranial blood volume, and elevated ICP.

Hyperventilation was once used as a first-line defense against intracranial hypertension. Initiating hyperventilation prior to the appearance of signs of intracranial hypertension and prior to documenting the failure of other methods to reduce this has been associated with a worse outcome. Hyperventilation reduces ICP by reducing the PCO_2, which causes cerebral vasoconstriction and results in decreased cerebral blood volume. The danger arises in that this also reduces cerebral blood flow. In head-injured patients with disrupted autoregulation, this may result in cerebral ischemia. Therefore, hyperventilation should not be used routinely in the first 24 hours following head injury. The indications for hyperventilation include using it for brief periods when signs of intracranial hypertension appear prior to placement of an ICP monitor or after insertion of a monitor if there is a sudden increase in the ICP or there is acute neurologic deterioration. Hyperventilation may be used for longer periods if intracranial hypertension proves to be unresponsive to other aggressive measures. The appropriate goal for hyperventilation when initiated is a PCO_2 of 30–35 mmHg. The PCO_2 should never drop below 25 mmHg because this carries a high risk of cerebral ischemia.

BIBLIOGRAPHY

Feldman Z, Kanter M, Robertson C, et al. Effect of head elevation on intracranial pressure, cerebral perfusion pressure, and cerebral blood flow in head-injured patients. *J Neurosurg* 1992;76(2):207–211.

Greenberg M, Greenberg MS. *Handbook of Neurosurgery*, 7th ed. New York, NY: Thieme; 2010:860–869.

8. **(D)** Management of intravenous fluids in head-injured patients is one area where trauma surgeons and neurosurgeons often disagree. Although reasons to convert to hypotonic solutions may develop, the initial choice for head-injured patients is isotonic solution. Hypotonic solutions should be avoided if possible, because they may impair cerebral compliance and worsen cerebral edema. With an intact blood-brain barrier, hypertonic solutions can establish an osmotic gradient that actually drives water out of the brain and into plasma. This is the principal method of action of mannitol, the most well-studied and proven osmotic diuretic for lowering ICP. In addition to mannitol, hypertonic saline has been shown in recent studies to lower ICP. A recent literature review concluded that hypertonic saline has favorable effects on both systemic hemodynamics and ICP. The most deleterious side effect of these agents is renal failure secondary to a hyperosmolar state and renal hypoperfusion. Therefore, urine output, serum osmolality, and serum sodium must be monitored closely when using hypertonic agents.

Other basic fluid management principles to keep in mind when treating a head-injured patient include the following: provide adequate resuscitation to avoid hypotension, maintain patient in euvolemia, and consider pressors over repeated fluid boluses.

BIBLIOGRAPHY

Greenberg M, Greenberg MS. *Handbook of Neurosurgery*, 7th ed. New York, NY: Thieme; 2010:876–885.

Qureshi A, Suarez J. Use of hypertonic saline solutions in treatment of cerebral edema and intracranial hypertension. *Crit Care Med* 2000;28(9):3301–3313.

9. **(C)** Well-documented late complications of head injury include seizures, communicating hydrocephalus, postconcussion syndrome, and varying degrees of cognitive impairment. Other documented late complications include hypogonadotropic hypogonadism and the deposition of amyloid proteins, which may be related to the development of Alzheimer disease. Posttraumatic seizures are divided into early (occurring within 1 week of injury) and late (occurring after 1 week of injury) types. The incidence of early seizures ranges from 2.5 to 7%, and the incidence of late seizures ranges from 5 to 7.1%. The risk of developing early posttraumatic seizures is related to the type of injury, with subdural and intracerebral hemorrhages being associated with the greatest risk. Approximately 25% of patients with early seizures will develop late seizures. Late seizures require around 8 weeks to develop. This seems to be related to the time it takes for the brain to develop an epileptogenic focus. The incidence of late seizures is directly proportional to the severity of the initial head injury. Although helpful in preventing early seizures in patients at high risk, prophylactic anticonvulsant administration does not reduce the frequency of late seizures.

Postconcussive syndrome is a constellation of symptoms that occurs after a minor head injury. The most common symptoms are headache, dizziness, and memory impairment. Other symptoms may include impaired concentration, anxiety, balance difficulties, tinnitus, loss of libido, impaired judgment, photophobia, and personality changes. In addition, one review notes that traumatic brain injury increases the risk for depression by a factor of 5–10, for psychotic disorders by a factor of 2–5, and for dementia by a factor of 4–5. The precise cause for these symptoms is often difficult to determine. Organic dysfunction, psychological factors, and even secondary gain issues may contribute to a patient's symptomatology. As a recent Swedish study supports, there is no association between traumatic head injury and primary brain tumors.

BIBLIOGRAPHY

Annegers J, Grabow J, Groover R, et al. Seizures after head trauma: a population study. *Neurology* 1980;30:683–689.

Greenberg M, Greenberg MS. *Handbook of Neurosurgery*, 7th ed. New York, NY: Thieme; 2010:906, 910–912.

Gualtieri T, Cox D. The delayed neurobehavioral sequelae of traumatic brain injury. *Brain Injury* 1991;5(3):219–232.

Jennet B. *Epilepsy After Non-missile Head Injuries*, 2nd ed. Chicago, IL: Year Book; 1975.

Nygren C, Adami J, Ye W, et al. Primary brain tumors following traumatic brain injury a population-based cohort study in Sweden. *Cancer Causes Control* 2001;12(8):733–737.

Young B. Sequelae of head injury. In: Wilkins R, Rengachary S (eds.), *Neurosurgery*, 2nd ed. New York, NY: McGraw-Hill; 1996:2841–2843.

10. **(D)** Epidural hematomas compose about 1% of all head trauma admissions. An epidural hematoma is defined as a blood clot that forms between the dura and the inner table of the skull. The classic presentation of an epidural hematoma, only occurring a minority of the time, is a young adult who has a brief loss of consciousness followed by a lucid interval for several hours. This is then followed by obtundation, contralateral hemiparesis, and ipsilateral pupillary dilation (signs of uncal herniation as described in Question 5). Death may result from continued compression of the midbrain causing bradycardia and respiratory distress. Overall mortality from epidural hematomas ranges from 20 to 55%, with prompt diagnosis and treatment lowering this rate to 5–10%.

The most common location for an epidural hematoma is temporoparietal, and the most common cause is a tear in a branch of the middle meningeal artery. A temporoparietal skull fracture is the usual offending injury. Other sources of bleeding include meningeal veins and dural sinuses. The classic CT finding for an epidural hematoma is a biconvex, hyperdense area adjacent to the skull. The hematoma is usually limited to a small area of the skull and does not cross suture lines. Generally accepted indications for removing an epidural hematoma in the operating room include any symptomatic epidural hematoma or an acute asymptomatic epidural hematoma that is greater than 1 cm at its widest portion because these tend not to resorb. Additionally, the threshold for operating on pediatric patients is lower than for adults because children have less available intracranial space to accommodate a blood clot.

BIBLIOGRAPHY

Greenberg M, Greenberg MS. *Handbook of Neurosurgery*, 7th ed. New York, NY: Thieme; 2010:894–896.

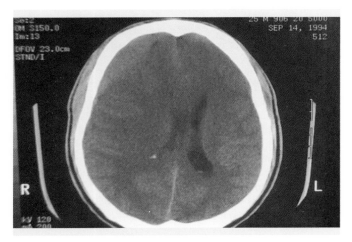

FIGURE 36-10. Computed tomography scan showing a subacute subdural hematoma in the right frontal area. Note that the hemorrhage appears isodense to brain. Also note the midline shift from right to left.

11. **(B)** The brain is covered by the meninges, which include pia (a thin membrane tightly adherent to the brain), arachnoid, and dura. A subdural hematoma is a hemorrhage that occurs between the dura and arachnoid membrane. Subdural hematomas may be divided radiographically into three categories: acute, subacute, and chronic. An acute subdural hematoma is seen within 3 days of the initial hemorrhage and appears hyperdense to brain on CT scans. A subacute subdural hematoma forms between 4 days and 3 weeks following the initial hemorrhage and appears isodense to brain on CT scans (see Fig. 36-10). A chronic subdural hematoma may be seen after 3 weeks following the initial hemorrhage and appears hypodense to brain on CT scans. All categories of subdural hematomas usually appear as concave fluid collections that spread out over the convexity of the brain. Subdural hematomas may also occur along the tentorium cerebelli, along the interhemispheric fissure, and in the posterior fossa.

Clinically, a distinction is made between the acute and chronic categories of subdural hematomas, because these two categories differ so markedly in their presentation, treatment, and outcome. Subacute subdural hematomas are typically lumped into one of these categories based on the patient's presentation and symptoms. Acute subdural hematomas most often result from trauma and are commonly associated with a primary underlying brain injury. The actual hemorrhage may be the result of a parenchymal laceration or tearing of a vein that bridges the brain surface with the dura. The overall mortality with acute subdural hematomas is higher than with epidural hematomas and much higher than with chronic subdural hematomas, ranging from approximately 50 to 90%. Surgical evacuation of the hematoma should be considered for any symptomatic hematoma that is greater than 1 cm at its thickest point. Treatment of acute subdural hematomas involves making a large craniotomy to allow for removal of clotted blood over a large surface area of brain. Smaller subdural hematomas may be watched and will usually resorb over time. Time to surgery has been held as an important factor influencing mortality and functional survival, with evacuation within 4 hours resulting in improved outcome.

On the other hand, chronic subdural hematomas typically occur in the elderly and are linked to trauma in only a minority of cases. Risk factors include coagulopathy, seizures, ventricular shunts, alcohol abuse, and any condition that increases the risk of falling. Symptoms of a chronic subdural hematoma may be mild (i.e., headache, lethargy, confusion), and diagnosis is often delayed. Treatment most commonly consists of drilling burr holes over the hematoma and irrigating the subdural space until it is clear. This is possible because the old blood has liquefied into a fluid with the appearance of motor oil. The outcome for patients following evacuation of a chronic subdural hematoma is generally good, although complications may include seizures or acute hemorrhage.

BIBLIOGRAPHY

Greenberg M, Greenberg MS. *Handbook of Neurosurgery*, 7th ed. New York, NY: Thieme; 2010:896–902.

12. **(A)** Gunshot wounds to the head represent the most lethal type of brain injury, with two-thirds of victims dying at the scene and death ultimately resulting in greater than 90% of victims. Although previously held as the most critical determinant of tissue injury, projectile velocity is no longer thought to be the primary factor related to wounding potential. According to recent literature, the major determinant of brain injury is the behavior of the projectile within the tissue, such as its deformation, yaw, and fragmentation. These projectile characteristics result in varying degrees of primary and secondary brain injury. The impact of the projectile with the skull and its path through the brain results in primary injury that may include scalp laceration, skull fractures, tracking of debris into the brain, brain cavitation, and intracerebral hemorrhage (see Fig. 36-11). A major goal of treating gunshot wounds to the head is to prevent secondary injury, which may include cerebral edema, intracranial hypertension, disseminated intravascular coagulopathy, seizures, cerebral abscess, and traumatic aneurysm.

Initial steps in the management of a patient with a gunshot wound to the head include cardiopulmonary resuscitation as needed, endotracheal intubation if airway is compromised, cervical spine precautions, control

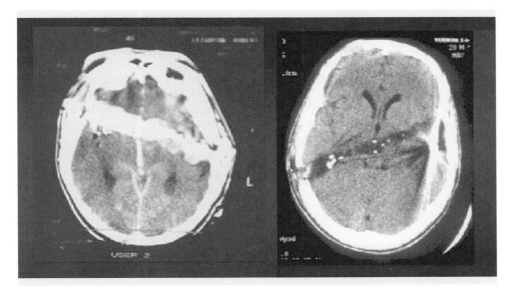

FIGURE 36-11. Two computed tomography scans showing gunshot wounds to the head. Note that the track of the bullet is filled with debris.

scalp bleeding, shave the scalp, and obtain a noncontrast CT scan of the brain. In addition, one must assume that the ICP is elevated in a patient with a gunshot wound to the head. Therefore, initial measures must be taken to control the patient's ICP. These steps are elevating the head of bed to 30–45 degrees, keeping the head in midline position, administering a 1-g/kg bolus of mannitol as blood pressure permits, and mild hyperventilation (PCO_2 = 35 mmHg). The efficacy of steroids in penetrating head injuries is unsubstantiated and is therefore not recommended. Further medical management of this patient includes the use of prophylactic antibiotics, anticonvulsants, and antacids. Cerebral angiography is indicated in patients with a delayed hemorrhage or when the trajectory of the projectile is believed to involve named vessels or a dural venous sinus in a salvageable patient.

The most important prognostic indicator of outcome in patients with a gunshot wound to the head is the presenting GCS score. Additional risk factors for poor outcome are suicide attempts, intracranial hemorrhage, bullet traversing through ventricles or geographic center of brain, bihemispheric injury, and multilobar injury. One prospective study suggests a paradigm in which surgery is reserved for the following patients: those with a GCS score of 3–5 with a large extra-axial hematoma; those with a GCS score of 6–8 without bihemispheric, transventricular, or multilobar dominant hemisphere injury; and those with a GCS score of 9–15. In general, patients sustaining a gunshot wound to the head will either do relatively well or die.

BIBLIOGRAPHY

Brain Trauma Foundation. The use of mannitol in severe head injury. *J Neurotrauma* 1996;13(11):705–709.

Fackler M. Wound ballistics. A review of common misconceptions. *JAMA* 1988;259:2730–2736.

Grahm T, Williams F, Harrington T, et al. Civilian gunshot wounds to the head: a prospective study. *Neurosurgery* 1990;27:696–700.

Greenberg M, Greenberg MS. *Handbook of Neurosurgery*, 7th ed. New York, NY: Thieme; 2010:912–916.

Kaufman H. Civilian gunshot wounds to the head. *Neurosurgery* 1993;32:962–964.

Rosenberg W, Harsh G. Penetrating wounds of the head. In: Wilkins R, Rengachary S (eds.), *Neurosurgery*, 2nd ed. New York, NY: McGraw-Hill; 1996:2813–2819.

13. **(C)** Homicide is the most frequent cause of death in children between the ages of 1 month and 1 year (17%). Common histories given by abusive caregivers include no known trauma, a presumed but unwitnessed fall, seizure, or respiratory arrest. Many studies have looked at the differences in injuries between abused children and children sustaining accidental injuries. In general, these studies have shown that abuse should be suspected when a child has retinal hemorrhages, bilateral chronic subdural hematomas if less than 2 years of age, multiple skull fractures, or skull fractures associated with intracranial injury. A recent retrospective review of cases further delineated several key differences between accidental and nonaccidental trauma in children. First, the mean age of the accident group in this study was 2.5 years, whereas the mean age for the definite abuse group was 0.7 years.

Distinctions in frequencies of various types of injuries included the following: subdural hematomas were found in 10% of the accident group and in 46% of the definite abuse group, subarachnoid hemorrhages were seen in 8% of the accident group and in 31% of the abuse group, retinal hemorrhages were documented in 2% of the accident group and in 33% of the abuse group, and associated cutaneous injuries were found in 16% of the accident group and in 50% of the definite abuse group. Although retinal hemorrhages are nearly pathognomonic for child abuse, these may also be seen following traumatic parturition, with benign subdural effusions in infants, and with acute high altitude sickness. In addition, mortality rates were 2% in the accident group and 13% in the definite abuse group. The increased mortality rate associated with abused children may often be related to a delay in seeking medical attention. Following an episode of abuse, the caregiver may place the unconscious child back in her crib or bed. Subsequently, the infant may develop cerebral edema and show signs of elevated ICP such as respiratory arrest or seizures. In other instances, the child may not wake up for many hours. In either case, the child presents to the hospital too late to reverse the existing brain damage.

Radiographically, there appear to be certain skull fracture characteristics that suggest a diagnosis of abuse. Fracture characteristics seen more commonly in abused children are multiple or complex configuration, involvement of more than a single cranial bone, depressed fracture, wide or growing fracture, nonparietal fracture, and associated intracranial injury. Accidents typically cause single, narrow, linear fractures of the parietal bone without associated intracranial injury. With these differences in mind, a clinician will be better able to distinguish between accidental trauma and cases of abuse.

BIBLIOGRAPHY

Greenberg M, Greenberg MS. *Handbook of Neurosurgery*, 7th ed. New York, NY: Thieme; 2010:917–919.

Hobbs C. Skull fractures and the diagnosis of abuse. *Arch Dis Child* 1984;59(3):246–252.

Reece R, Sege R. Childhood head injuries: accident or inflicted? *Arch Pediatr Adolesc Med* 2000;154(1):11–15.

Waller A, Baker S, Szocka A. Childhood injury deaths: national analysis and geographic variations. *Am J Public Health* 1989;79:310–315.

14. **(C)** There are two reasons to declare that a patient is brain dead. The first is to allow for organ donation, and the second is to allow for removal of life support mechanisms once it is deemed that further medical treatment is futile. Most state governments and hospitals refer to the guidelines established by the President's Commission for the determination of brain death. For older children and adults, the physical examination must show absence of cerebral and brainstem function, no response to deep central pain, and absence of complicating conditions such as hypothermia or hypotension. Findings consistent with absence of brainstem function are dilated and nonreactive pupils, absent corneal reflexes, absent oculocephalic (doll's eyes) reflex, absent oculovestibular reflex, and absent oropharyngeal (gag) reflex. In addition to these, the apnea test is used to assess the function of the medulla. Brain death is confirmed if the patient has no spontaneous respirations after allowing the partial pressure of arterial carbon dioxide ($PaCO_2$) to reach greater than 60 mmHg (hypercapnia of this degree will always produce spontaneous respirations in a patient with a functioning brainstem). If a patient has extensor (decerebrate) or flexor (decorticate) posturing in response to deep central pain, then information from the brainstem is still being transmitted down through the spinal cord, which is incompatible with a diagnosis of brain death. Additionally, a patient should be free of any complicating condition that may simulate brain death. Such conditions include hypothermia, hypotension, intoxication, anoxia, immediate postresuscitation state, and emergence from a pentobarbital coma. Certain observation periods ranging from 6 to 24 hours may also be warranted depending on the specific circumstances.

For children less than 5 years of age, coma and apnea must coexist, and there must be absence of brainstem function on physical examination. Additional criteria include two examinations and two negative electroencephalograms (EEGs) 48 hours apart for children age 7 days to 2 months, two examinations and two negative EEGs 24 hours apart for children age 2 months to 12 months, and an interval of 12 hours between examinations and EEGs for children age 12 months to 5 years. Besides EEG, other confirmatory tests for diagnosing brain death include cerebral angiography and radionuclide blood flow studies. These studies may be helpful in patients with severe congestive heart failure or chronic obstructive pulmonary disease where the apnea test is invalid, in patients with severe facial trauma that would preclude cranial nerve testing, in patients coming out of a pentobarbital coma, and in allowing more expedient organ donation.

BIBLIOGRAPHY

President's Commission for the Study of Ethical Problems in Medicine. Guidelines for the determination of death. *JAMA* 1981;246:2184–2186.

Task Force for the Determination of Brain Death in Children. Guidelines for the determination of brain death in children. *Arch Neurol* 1987;44:587–588.

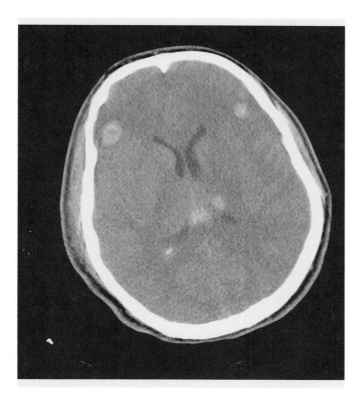

FIGURE 36-12. Computed tomography scan showing diffuse axonal injury resulting from a motor vehicle accident. Note the multiple areas of hemorrhage within the brain.

15. **(D)** DAI refers to a characteristic brain injury pattern. The patient presents with unconsciousness and a lack of a focal mass lesion on CT scanning (see Fig. 36-12). Patients who suffer from DAI typically do not present with a lucid interval. Neuronal damage results from shearing of the axons that is caused by rotational acceleration forces. These same forces cause shearing of small blood vessels as well. Skull fractures are less common in patients with DAI than in those with a focal lesion. The rotational forces necessary to cause DAI most commonly occur in motor vehicle accidents. In motor vehicle accidents, the head makes contact with a relatively soft, broad surface such as a padded dashboard or energy-absorbing steering column, resulting in a long period of acceleration within the skull. This longer period of acceleration translates into greater shearing and deformation of brain tissue.

There are three classic pathologic lesions seen in the brains of patients with DAI. The first is focal necrosis and/or hemorrhage in the corpus callosum. This may vary in size from microscopic to involving the entire corpus callosum. The second classic finding is hemorrhagic necrosis in the dorsolateral rostral pons. The third lesion is reactive axonal swelling from tearing of the axon (aka retraction balls). This is a microscopic finding that may develop as early as 3 hours after injury.

Direct impact forces cause injuries such as skull fracture, epidural hematomas, and coup contusions. These injuries are primarily the result of deformation of the skull. Linear acceleration forces are associated with subdural hematomas and contrecoup contusions. Differential movement between the skull and the brain causes tearing of bridging veins resulting in a subdural hematoma. In addition, brain movement away from the skull results in areas of low pressure creating sufficient tensile strain to produce a contrecoup contusion on the surface of the brain. Axial loading is associated with cervical spine fractures.

16. **(C)**, 17. **(E)**, 18. **(D)**, 19. **(B)**, 20. **(A)** Because subdural and epidural hematomas are discussed in other questions, the focus now will be on subarachnoid hemorrhage and intracerebral hemorrhage. A subarachnoid hemorrhage is defined as bleeding into the space between the pia and the arachnoid membranes. Trauma is the most common cause of a subarachnoid hemorrhage, and this occurs as a result of tearing of a superficial cortical vessel. The management and prognosis of a traumatic subarachnoid hemorrhage are far different than those of a spontaneous subarachnoid hemorrhage that is most often the result of a ruptured intracranial aneurysm (as shown in this question). On CT scan, a traumatic subarachnoid hemorrhage is typically less dense and is more often seen along the surface of the cerebral hemispheres (i.e., the convexity) rather than in the cisterns known to harbor major cerebral blood vessels (as would be seen with a ruptured aneurysm). In addition, other related brain injuries such as cerebral contusions are more commonly seen with traumatic subarachnoid hemorrhages. Finally, the morbidity and mortality of a traumatic subarachnoid hemorrhage are much less compared with those of a subarachnoid hemorrhage related to a ruptured aneurysm. Spontaneous subarachnoid hemorrhages resulting from a ruptured aneurysm have a significant risk of vasospasm and hydrocephalus. Patients who present with a small amount of traumatic subarachnoid hemorrhage and are neurologically intact may be discharged safely to home after an overnight period of observation.

Although not as common, trauma may cause an intracerebral hemorrhage as well. This results from tearing of a blood vessel that lies within the brain parenchyma. These tend to occur in a lobar fashion (in cortex or subcortical white matter) rather than in the deeper basal ganglia region, as seen in hemorrhages related to hypertension. It is important to remember that an intracerebral hemorrhage in a trauma patient may have preceded and led to the trauma rather than being the result of the trauma. Other important causes of lobar intracerebral hemorrhages to keep in mind are tumor, arteriovenous malformations, distal aneurysms that are adherent to the brain, and hemorrhagic transformation of an ischemic infarct. Intracerebral hemorrhages may need to be surgically evacuated if they are large and producing significant mass effect on surrounding brain.

The CT scan in Fig. 36-1 shows an acute subdural hematoma on the left. The blood is hyperdense to brain and is concave to brain.

The CT scan in Fig. 36-2 shows an epidural hematoma on the right side. The blood is hyperdense to brain and is convex to brain.

The CT scan in Fig. 36-3 shows an acute, right occipital lobar intracerebral hemorrhage.

The CT scan in Fig. 36-4 shows a diffuse subarachnoid hemorrhage. Note that the blood is tracking within the cisternal spaces at the base of the brain. This was the result of a ruptured berry aneurysm. Also note the acute hydrocephalus as evidenced by the enlarged temporal horns of the lateral ventricles.

The CT scan in Fig. 36-5 shows a chronic subdural hematoma in the left frontal area. The blood is hypodense to brain.

BIBLIOGRAPHY

Gennarelli T, Meaney D. Mechanisms of primary head injury. In: Wilkins R, Rengachary S (eds.), *Neurosurgery*, 2nd ed. New York, NY: McGraw-Hill; 1996:2611–2621.

21. **(C)** One in five patients with a major spinal injury will have a second spine injury at another level. Most of these injuries will be to the cervical spine, and many of these patients will also have injuries to other systems. It is critical that patients suspected of having a spine injury have their entire spine immobilized during transport. Likewise, it is essential that the entire spine be examined when the patient is seen in the emergency department. All victims of trauma who are unconscious, or those conscious who complain of back pain should be treated as having a spinal cord injury until proven otherwise and be immobilized accordingly. Whereas this was considered an "option" in the 2002 Spinal Cord Injury guidelines, this is now a level II recommendation in the 2012 guidelines. Clinical criteria that can be used to verify cervical spine stability include an awake patient with no mental status changes (including no intoxication), no neck pain, no other injuries that might distract from the neurologic exam, no neurologic deficits, and full range of motion. These patients do not need imaging.

Although the medical management of patients with spinal cord injuries has improved over time, the prognosis for functional recovery in patients with severe spinal cord injuries remains poor. The prognosis for functional recovery in these patients is directly related to the patient's neurologic condition at admission. In other words, a patient who presents with minimal weakness will have a very good chance of improving, whereas a patient who presents with no motor function will have almost no chance of improvement. Approximately 3% of patients with complete spinal cord injuries will show some sign of improvement within 24 hours. If there is no improvement in 24 hours, then it is almost certain that no recovery of function will occur. Therefore, it is important at the time of presentation to determine whether a patient has a complete (no motor or sensory function below level of injury) or incomplete spinal cord injury. Additionally, patients with incomplete spinal cord injuries improve the greatest amount within the first year after injury, although improvement may continue for several years.

BIBLIOGRAPHY

Greenberg M, Greenberg MS. *Handbook of Neurosurgery*, 7th ed. New York, NY: Thieme; 2010:933–935.

Hadley MN, Walters BC. Introduction to the guidelines for the management of acute cervical spine and spinal cord injuries. *Neurosurgery* 2013;72(3):S5–S16.

22. **(D)** The term neurogenic shock refers to hypotension that commonly follows certain types of spinal cord injury. A cervical or high thoracic spinal cord injury (typically above T6) may interrupt the sympathetic pathways to the body. This results in a loss of vascular tone in much of the body causing pooling of blood in the vascular system. Loss of muscle tone below the level of injury contributes to the hypotension as well. In the absence of any significant coexisting injury or worrisome examination findings, the most likely cause of this patient's hypotension is spinal shock. Of note, however, hypovolemia is the most common cause of hypotension in a trauma patient, and treatment should first be aimed at restoring euvolemia.

The term spinal shock is used is to describe the immediate, transient loss of all spinal reflexes below the level of spinal cord injury. This results in a flaccid paralysis that lasts approximately 2 weeks to 2 months. After this period of time, the patient will develop hyperreflexia and increased spasticity below the level of injury as the spinal cord damage becomes chronic in nature.

23. **(B)** Hypotension is a common finding in patients following acute spinal cord injury. As is the case with traumatic brain injury, hypotension may contribute to worsening neurologic function following spinal cord injury because of decreased perfusion to the spinal cord. Therefore, it is now recommended that hypotension (SBP <90 mmHg) be avoided or corrected as soon as possible following spinal cord injury. In addition, maintaining a MAP of 85–90 mmHg for the first 7 days after acute spinal cord injury is recommended. Many clinicians even support

invasive monitoring (i.e., placement of an arterial line and central line for possible pressors) within an intensive care unit setting in the first 7 days following acute spinal cord injury because of the increased risk of cardiac and pulmonary disturbances in these patients. These practices are supported by investigators who have demonstrated improvements in neurologic outcome seemingly as a result of early, aggressive volume resuscitation and blood pressure augmentation alone. In regard to the treatment of hypotension in the face of acute spinal cord injury, pressors are recommended once volume resuscitation is completed because this counteracts the underlying physiologic disturbance (i.e., provides sympathetic tone). Dopamine is the agent of choice because it has a lower incidence of reflex bradycardia than pure α-agonist agents like phenylephrine. Intravenous fluids should be used to maintain a state of euvolemia, but these are usually inadequate to treat hypotension resulting from spinal shock. As such, there is a propensity to cause pulmonary edema if intravenous fluids alone are used for treating this disorder. Although it may be helpful in the initial resuscitation period, the Trendelenburg position should not be used as the definitive treatment for hypotension.

BIBLIOGRAPHY

Blood pressure management after acute spinal cord injury. Guidelines for the management of acute cervical spine and spinal cord injuries. *Neurosurgery* 2002;50(3):S58–S62.
Vale F, Burns J, Jackson A, et al. Combined medical and surgical treatment after acute spinal cord injury: results of a prospective pilot study to assess the merits of aggressive medical resuscitation and blood pressure management. *J Neurosurg* 1997;87:239–246.

24. **(A)** A patient presenting to the emergency department with an acute spinal cord injury will have several unique problems that should be addressed early in his or her management. First, the patient may present with poikilothermia (inability to regulate body temperature) as a result of vasomotor paralysis. Appropriate warming or cooling should be instituted early. Second, many patients with spinal cord injury will have paralytic ileus that may last for several days. Therefore, a nasogastric tube should be placed to suction to prevent emesis and aspiration. Aspiration poses a significant risk to a patient with a cervical or high thoracic cord injury, because the paralyzed abdominal musculature is unable to develop a forceful cough. Third, many patients with spinal cord injury will have disrupted bowel and bladder function. These patients are at increased risk of developing severe bladder distension. This is especially important in patients who develop autonomic dysreflexia. This condition occurs in patients with spinal cord injury above the T6 level and is characterized by an exaggerated autonomic

response (sympathetic usually dominates) secondary to a stimulus that is usually only mildly noxious. Common stimuli include bladder distension, fecal impaction, administration of enemas, skin infections, and urinary tract infections. The response to such stimuli may be severe hypertension, flushing, tachycardia, headache, hyperhidrosis, or diaphoresis. The hypertension resulting from this illness has been reported to have caused a fatal intracerebral hemorrhage. Therefore, it is very important to place a bladder catheter in patients with a spinal cord injury. Additional initial measures include rapid treatment of hypotension with pressors and maintaining adequate oxygenation. All patients with a suspected spinal cord injury should be immobilized on a backboard in the field. Patients should remain on the backboard, however, only while it is beneficial in assisting with patient transfers such as onto and off of the CT scanner. As soon as this period has passed, the backboard should be removed. It only takes a few hours on a backboard for a patient to develop pressure sores.

BIBLIOGRAPHY

Greenberg M, Greenberg MS. *Handbook of Neurosurgery*, 7th ed. New York, NY: Thieme; 2010:933–936.

25. **(C)** The use of methylprednisolone for treating patients with acute spinal cord injury remains one of the most controversial topics in trauma and neurosurgical literature. The most commonly cited guidelines for the use of methylprednisolone in spinal cord injury are derived from the second and third National Acute Spinal Cord Injury Studies (NASCIS). According to the results of NASCIS II, patients who were given a 30-mg/kg bolus of methylprednisolone in the first 15 minutes of the first hour followed by a 5.4-mg/kg/h infusion over the next 23 hours had improvement in motor function and in sensation at the 6-month follow-up. Because this study included patients with complete and incomplete injuries, many clinicians use this regimen for both types of patients.

More recently, NASCIS III results showed benefits using a slightly altered regimen. In this study, patients could receive methylprednisolone for a total of 24 or 48 hours. The results showed improvement in motor function for patients in both groups if treated within 3 hours of injury and in the 48-hour group if treatment began between 3 and 8 hours after injury. Therefore, the investigators recommended giving a 48-hour methylprednisolone regimen to patients if administration of the drug began in the 3- to 8-hour postinjury window and limiting the regimen to 24 hours when the drug could be started within 3 hours of injury. This study also noted the increased incidence of severe sepsis and severe pneumonia with the 48-hour methylprednisolone treatment group. Several other studies have demonstrated an increased risk of gastrointestinal bleeding and poor wound healing with both of these regimens.

Along with many concerns regarding the harmful side effects of using high-dose steroids, many investigators have questioned the significance of the NASCIS II and NASCIS III results. A thorough review of the published data on the use of methylprednisolone is provided in the recent American Association of Neurological Surgeons/Congress of Neurological Surgeons–sponsored Guidelines for the Management of Acute Cervical Spine and Spinal Cord Injuries. In contrast to the prior recommendations from 2002 (that treatment with steroids for 24–48 hours was recommended with the knowledge that the side effects likely outweigh the benefits), the new position statement is that the administration of methylprednisolone is *not recommended*, because it is not Food and Drug Administration approved, and there is no level I or level II evidence supporting its clinical benefit in the use of acute spinal cord injury. This is a level I recommendation. Thus, steroids are not given in acute spinal cord injury.

BIBLIOGRAPHY

Bracken M, Shepard M, Collins W, et al. A randomized, controlled trial of methylprednisolone or naloxone in the treatment of acute spinal cord injury: results of the second National Acute Spinal Cord Injury Study (NASCIS II). *N Engl J Med* 1990;322:1405–1411.

Bracken M, Shepard M, Holford T, et al. Administration of methylprednisolone for 24 or 48 h or tirilazad mesylate for 48 h in the treatment of acute spinal cord injury: results of the third National Acute Spinal Cord Injury Randomized Controlled Trial—NASCIS. *JAMA* 1997;277:1597–1604.

Hadley MN, Walters BC. Introduction to the guidelines for the management of acute cervical spine and spinal cord injuries. *Neurosurgery* 2013;72(3):S5–S16.

Hurlbert RJ, Hadley MN, Walters BC, et al. Pharmacological therapy for acute spinal cord injury. *Neurosurgery* 2013;72:93–105.

26. **(D)** It is now standard care for emergency medical services (EMS) personnel to immobilize a patient's cervical spine with a collar following trauma. It is the physician's role to rule out spinal column or spinal cord injury in a patient before removing the cervical collar. In an effort to reduce expense and prevent unnecessary exposure to radiation, it is important to know which patients truly need to have plain radiographs of their cervical spine. One of the largest studies to address this issue looked at over 34,000 patients evaluated in 21 different emergency departments in the United States. Of the 576 patients who were deemed to have clinically significant injuries,

two were originally assigned to the asymptomatic group (based on history and physical examination). Of these two patients, one developed paresthesias in an arm and underwent surgery. Therefore, the results showed that the negative predictive value of an asymptomatic examination was 99.9%. Several other well-developed investigations have had similar results. After reviewing numerous pertinent studies, the American Association of Neurological Surgeons and the Congress of Neurological Surgeons found the data convincing enough to publish a treatment standard. According to this standard, radiographic assessment of the cervical spine is not recommended in trauma patients who meet the following criteria: awake, alert, not intoxicated, without neck pain or tenderness, without a significant distracting injury, and with full range of motion. The patient in this question meets these criteria and, therefore, needs no radiographs before clearing his cervical spine.

For patients who are symptomatic or do not meet the above criteria, the same published guidelines recommend as a treatment standard obtaining a three-view cervical spine series (AP, lateral, and odontoid views). In addition, supplemental CT scanning should be performed to further define suspicious areas or areas that are not well visualized on plain radiographs. Only treatment options are recommended for symptomatic patients who end up having normal x-rays and CT scans. Awake patients with neck pain or tenderness may have their cervical collars removed once they have either a normal and adequate dynamic flexion/extension series or a normal MRI study within 48 hours of injury. Cervical collars on obtunded patients may be removed following the acquisition of a normal dynamic flexion/extension study performed under fluoroscopic guidance, after a normal MRI study obtained within 48 hours of injury, or at the discretion of the treating physician. Of course, not every patient falls neatly into one of these categories. Much variation remains across hospitals and regions in the process used to clear cervical spines in trauma patients. Many hospitals will have algorithms for clearing cervical spines in place for physicians to reference.

BIBLIOGRAPHY

Hadley M, Walters B, Section on Disorders of the Spine and Peripheral Nerves, American Association of Neurological Surgeons and the Congress of Neurological Surgeons. Blood pressure management after acute spinal cord injury. Guidelines for the management of acute cervical spine and spinal cord injuries. *Neurosurgery* 2002;50(3):S63–S72.

Hadley M, Walters B, Section on Disorders of the Spine and Peripheral Nerves, American Association of Neurological Surgeons and the Congress of Neurological Surgeons. Radiographic assessment of the cervical spine in asymptomatic trauma patients.

Guidelines for the management of acute cervical spine and spinal cord injuries. *Neurosurgery* 2002;50(3):S30–S35.

Hoffman J, Mower W, Wolfson A, et al. Validity of a set of clinical criteria to rule out injury to the cervical spine in patients with blunt trauma: National Emergency X-Radiography Utilization Study Group. *N Engl J Med* 2000;343:94–99.

Theodore N, Hadley MN, Aarabi B, et al. Prehospital cervical spinal immobilization after trauma. *Neurosurgery* 2013;72:22–34.

27. **(C)** The central cord syndrome is a common type of incomplete spinal cord injury. This syndrome usually results from hyperextension of the cervical spine such as when a person falls and hits his forehead or in a motor vehicle accident when a person's forehead strikes the windshield. It occurs most commonly in elderly patients who have preexisting cervical spinal spondylosis with a narrowed spinal canal. On hyperextension of the cervical spine, the spinal cord is compressed by bony spurs anteriorly or by buckling of the ligamentum flavum posteriorly. The arterial supply of the spinal cord is divided such that several radially oriented circumferential branches supply the outer white matter while a central anterior sulcal branch supplies the deep white and gray matter. This arrangement produces both a watershed area between the two arterial supplies and a greater susceptibility for disruption of blood flow into the central area of the spinal cord. As a result, blunt trauma to spinal cord is more likely to damage the central portion of the cord. Because the fibers in the corticospinal tract that supply the upper extremities are more medial than those supplying the lower extremities, this syndrome results in disproportionate weakness of the upper extremities. Sensory loss is usually minimal and may occur in any distribution. Urinary retention is common, especially in more severe cases.

Another type of incomplete spinal cord injury is the Brown-Sequard syndrome. This refers to hemisection of the cord. It is usually caused by penetrating trauma such as stab wounds, although it may also be caused by lateral cord compression. This syndrome or a similar pattern is seen in 2–4% of traumatic spinal cord injuries. Clinically, the patient presents with ipsilateral paralysis (corticospinal tract) and loss of vibration and position sense (posterior columns) with contralateral loss of pain and temperature sensation (lateral spinothalamic tract). This syndrome carries a more favorable prognosis than the central cord syndrome.

The anterior cord syndrome is an infarction of the spinal cord in the territory supplied by the anterior spinal artery. This may result from anterior spinal artery occlusion or from anterior compression of the cord. The classic presentation is a patient who has no motor function below the level of the lesion, no pain and temperature sensation below the level of the lesion, and preservation of vibration and position sense. This occurs because the anterior spinal artery supplies the anterior two-thirds of the cord, thus sparing the posterior columns if this region becomes ischemic. The anterior cord syndrome is thought to carry the worst prognosis of the incomplete spinal cord injury syndromes, with only 10–20% of patients ever recovering functional motor control.

Finally, a cervical herniated disk presents most commonly as a radiculopathy. The typical presentation is a patient who complains of pain and/or numbness down one arm in a specific nerve root distribution. Weakness of the muscles supplied by this nerve root may occur as well. On occasion, a herniated disk will be large enough to compress the spinal cord and cause a myelopathy. The hallmark of this entity is hyperreflexia with the presence of abnormal reflexes such as clonus, plantar extensor response, and Hoffman's sign. Pain, paresthesias, and weakness are variable with myelopathy. Rarely, a traumatic acute central disk herniation can cause an acute central cord syndrome as well.

BIBLIOGRAPHY

Greenberg M, Greenberg MS. *Handbook of Neurosurgery*, 7th ed. New York, NY: Thieme; 2010:948–951.

Roth E, Park T, Pang T, et al. Traumatic cervical Brown-Sequard and Brown-Sequard plus syndromes: the spectrum of presentations and outcomes. *Paraplegia* 1991;29:582–589.

28. **(D)** The term SCIWORA was coined in 1982 by Pang and Wilberger to describe cases in which there were objective signs of myelopathy as a result of trauma with no evidence of fracture, subluxation, or instability on plain radiographs or tomography. Most physicians extend this definition to include patients with symptoms, as well as signs, of spinal cord injury. SCIWORA occurs more commonly in children younger than 9 years of age. In addition, younger children are more likely to have more severe injuries than older children. This is largely the result of younger children sustaining more upper cervical injuries than older children. In younger children, the maximal level of flexion occurs at C2/3 and C3/4. As a child ages, the maximal point of flexion migrates caudally to settle at the adult level of C5/6 around 8 years. This point helps explain the increased incidence of upper cervical spine injuries in young children, but how can such injuries occur without producing evidence of fracture or instability?

In addition to having a proportionately larger head and weaker neck muscles, children possess certain characteristics in their spine that make them more susceptible to excess intersegmental motion than an adult. First, children have a more horizontal orientation of their facet joints. Second, there is anterior wedging of the superior aspect of the vertebral bodies in children. Third, children have more elastic ligaments and joint capsules than adults. These characteristics allow for greater intersegmental instability without overt disruption of the ligaments, bones, or disk spaces. Spinal cord injury thus results from a transient compression of the spinal cord. The clinical presentation varies from transient paresthesias to complete spinal cord injury, and recurrent SCIWORA may occur as well (often after trauma of less magnitude than in the original injury).

As alluded to earlier, the diagnosis of SCIWORA is made after all x-rays, including flexion-extension views, and tomograms are read as normal. An MRI scan, however, may be abnormal in a child diagnosed with SCIWORA. An MRI scan is helpful for detecting compressive lesions and for identifying transection, hemorrhage, or edema within the cord. In addition, MRI is a valuable prognostic indicator of outcome, with any visible injury to the cord signaling a worse prognosis than having no abnormality on MRI. In addition to obtaining an MRI at the level of concern, assessment of spinal stability via flexion-extension radiographs is recommended in both the acute setting and at late follow-up, even in the presence of a normal MRI.

Treatment of SCIWORA is focused on preventing a recurrent spinal cord injury. Because spinal laxity with excessive motion is the cause of SCIWORA, immobilization of the spine is the mainstay of treatment. Although the time period of immobilization may vary depending on the patient's symptoms and MRI findings, the current guidelines suggest a period of up to 12 weeks. Children with cervical injuries are often placed in a Guilford brace (harder to remove than a collar), and children with thoracic injuries are often placed in a thoracolumbosacral orthosis (TLSO). Limiting activity from contact sports for up to 6 months is recommended as well.

BIBLIOGRAPHY

Grabb P, Albright A. Spinal cord injury without radiographic abnormality in children. In: Wilkins R, Rengachary S (eds.), *Neurosurgery*, 2nd ed. New York, NY: McGraw-Hill; 1996:2867–2870.

Hadley MN, Walters BC. Introduction to the guidelines for the management of acute cervical spine and spinal cord injuries. *Neurosurgery* 2013;72(3):S5–S16.

Pang D, Pollack I. Spinal cord injury without radiographic abnormality in children the SCIWORA syndrome. *J Trauma* 1989;29:654–664.

Pang D, Wilberger J Jr. Spinal cord injury without radiographic abnormalities in children. *J Neurosurg* 1982;57:114–129.

Rozzelle CJ, Aarabi B, Dhall SS, et al. Spinal cord injury without radiographic abnormality. *Neurosurgery* 2013;72:227–233.

29. **(A)** Traumatic atlanto-occipital dislocation represents approximately 1% of patients who present to the emergency department with cervical spine injuries. Most of these injuries are related to a motor vehicle accident or a pedestrian versus automobile accident. Anatomically, the dislocation is most often the result of disruption of the tectorial membrane (continuation of posterior longitudinal ligament that connects dorsal surface of dens to ventral surface of basion) and the alar ligaments (connect lateral portions of dens to occipital condyles and lateral mass of atlas). Hyperextension may cause tearing of the tectorial membrane, and lateral flexion may cause disruption of the alar ligaments. Hyperflexion may also produce this injury by causing separation of the posterior elements of the atlas and axis. Children are more susceptible to atlanto-occipital dislocation than adults, because children have a more horizontal articulation between the skull and atlas and have less developed occipital condyles. Patients may present as neurologically intact or with spinal cord injury, cervical root injury, or brainstem injury. The most common cause of death in patients with atlanto-occipital dislocation is respiratory arrest secondary to brainstem injury.

The diagnosis of atlanto-occipital dislocation may be made with a lateral cervical spine x-ray (see Fig. 36-13). Although there are many measurements used to diagnose this injury including the Power's ratio and x-line method, the American Association of Neurological Surgeons and the Congress of Neurological Surgeons recommend as an option using the basion-axial interval–basion-dental interval (BAI-BDI) method because of its increased sensitivity in diagnosing this injury. In this method, a displacement of more than +12 mm or more than –4 mm between the basion and the posterior axis line or a displacement of more than 12 mm from the basion to the dens is considered diagnostic of a dislocation. Additionally, the presence of prevertebral soft tissue swelling should raise suspicion for this injury. CT and MRI imaging are recommended to further characterize the injury and assist with preoperative planning.

Treatment of atlanto-occipital dislocations may vary depending on the type of dislocation. One group of investigators divided these dislocations into three types based on the direction of separation between the occiput and atlas: type I refers to anterior displacement of the occiput in relation to the atlas, type II refers to longitudinal distraction of the occiput away from the atlas, and type III refers to posterior displacement of the occiput in relation to the atlas. In this report, the authors suggest that light traction may be used for type I and type III injuries to realign the bones and decompress the spinal cord. Traction for type II dislocations is contraindicated, because a longitudinal force would only worsen the longitudinal distraction injury. Because of the high association of worsening neurologic condition and late instability with no treatment, cervical traction, and external immobilization alone, the American Association of Neurological Surgeons and the Congress of Neurological

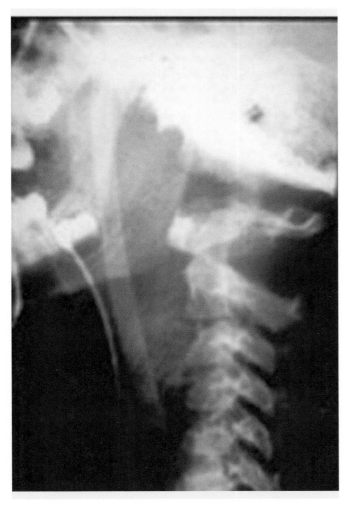

FIGURE 36-13. Lateral cervical spine radiograph showing atlanto-occipital dislocation. Note the increased distance between the base of the skull and the atlas.

Surgeons recommend against traction and cite a 10% risk of neurologic deterioration. Craniocervical fusion with internal fixation can be considered for patients with atlanto-occipital dislocation.

BIBLIOGRAPHY

Greenberg M, Greenberg MS. *Handbook of Neurosurgery*, 7th ed. New York, NY: Thieme; 2010:951–954.

Harris J Jr, Carson G, Wagner L, et al. Radiologic diagnosis of traumatic occipitovertebral dislocation: Part 2. Comparison of three methods of detecting occipitovertebral relationships on lateral radiographs of supine subjects. *Am J Radiol* 1994;162:887–892.

Lee C, Woodring J, Goldstein S, et al. Evaluation of traumatic atlantooccipital dislocations. *Am J Neuroradiol* 1987;8:19–26.

Powers B, Miller M, Kramer R, et al. Traumatic anterior atlantooccipital dislocation. *Neurosurgery* 1979;4:12–17.

Theodore N, Aarabi B, Dhall SS, et al. The diagnosis and management of traumatic atlanto-occipital dislocation injuries. *Neurosurgery* 2013;72:114–126.

Traynelis V, Marano G, Dunker R, et al. Traumatic atlanto-occipital dislocation: case report. *J Neurosurg* 1986;65:863–870.

30. **(C)** Sir Geoffrey Jefferson reviewed several cases of atlas fractures in 1920 and characterized a burst fracture of the atlas ring (now known as a "Jefferson fracture"). An axial load to the head causes this type of fracture by forcing the occipital condyles down onto the lateral masses of the atlas. Enough force applied in this manner will result in fractures through the anterior and posterior arches of the atlas (see Fig. 36-14). Treatment of atlas fractures varies depending on whether or not the fracture is considered to be stable. The critical structure providing stability to the atlas is the transverse atlantal ligament. There are several ways to determine radiographically if the transverse atlantal ligament is intact. First, the rules of Spence state that the transverse atlantal ligament is likely torn if the sum of the lateral mass displacement (LMD) of C1 over C2 on an AP x-ray is greater than 6.9 mm. Second, more recent studies have supported using an atlantodens interval of greater than 3 mm on a lateral x-ray to predict disruption of the transverse atlantal ligament. Finally, MRI is a sensitive indicator of transverse atlantal ligament injury. If the above criteria are not met and the fracture appears to be stable, then the American Association of Neurological Surgeons

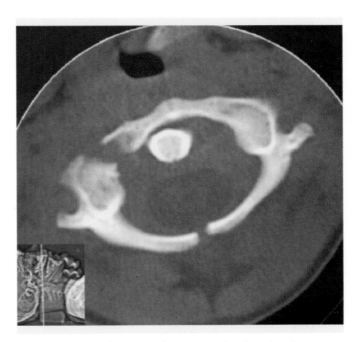

FIGURE 36-14. Computed tomography showing fractures through the anterior and posterior arches of the atlas. This is known as a Jefferson fracture.

and the Congress of Neurological Surgeons recommend as a treatment option cervical immobilization alone. If the above criteria are met and the transverse atlantal ligament appears to be disrupted, then cervical immobilization alone or surgical fixation and fusion is recommended. Many surgeons support C1–C2 transarticular screw fixation with a posterior fusion for the treatment of unstable atlas fractures.

A hangman's fracture is a fracture through the pars interarticularis of both pedicles of the axis that results in a traumatic spondylolisthesis (see Fig. 36-15). The fracture was named after a similarity was noted between these fractures and those that occurred as a result of judicial hangings. The mechanism of injury is hyperextension and compression, often associated with a motor vehicle accident. Most patients with this fracture are neurologically intact and may be treated with cervical immobilization alone. Surgical stabilization may be considered for cases with severe angulation of C2 on C3, disruption of the C2–C3 disk space, or inability to establish or maintain alignment with external immobilization.

BIBLIOGRAPHY

Jefferson G. Fractures of the atlas vertebra: report of four cases and a review of those previously reported. *Br J Surg* 1920;7:407–422.
Ryken TC, Aarabi B, Dhall SS, et al. Management of isolated fractures of the atlas in adults. *Neurosurgery* 2013;72:127–131.
Ryken TC, Hadley MN, Aarabi B, et al. Management of isolated fractures of the axis in adults. *Neurosurgery* 2013;72:132–150.
Spence K Jr, Decker S, Sell K. Bursting atlantal fracture associated with rupture of the transverse ligament. *J Bone Joint Surg Am* 1970;52A:543–549.

31. **(B)** Axis fractures account for about 17% of cervical spine fractures, and most of these are odontoid fractures. The mechanism of injury is usually flexion, and this is often associated with anterior subluxation of C1 on C2. Anderson and D'Alonzo developed a classification system in 1974 for odontoid fractures based on location of the fracture. Type I odontoid fractures involve the tip of the odontoid process, and they are the rarest type. These fractures are caused by an avulsion of the attachment of the alar ligament. Type II odontoid fractures involve the base of the odontoid process at the synchondrosis where the dens fuses with the body of C2 (see Fig. 36-16). This is the most common type of odontoid fracture. Type III

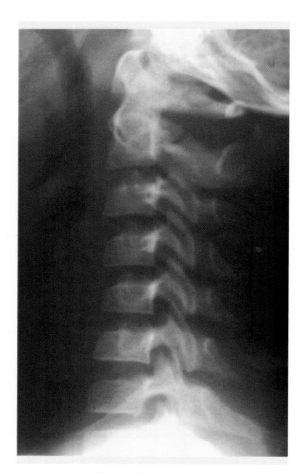

FIGURE 36-15. Radiograph showing a fracture through the pedicles of C2, also known as a hangman's fracture.

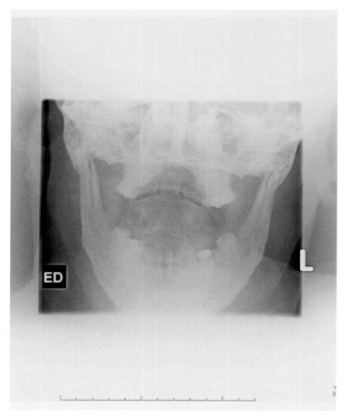

FIGURE 36-16. Odontoid view cervical spine radiograph showing a type II fracture of the odontoid process.

odontoid fractures are those that involve the base of the odontoid but extend into the body of C2. An addition to this classification system was made by Hadley and colleagues in 1988. They added a type IIA subtype fracture that represents a comminuted fracture through the base of the dens with associated free fragments of bone. In general, type II fractures are the least stable and have the highest nonunion rates. In addition, advanced age and dens displacement of >5 mm is associated with lower rates of fusion. After careful review of the literature, the current recommended guidelines in the neurosurgical literature are to consider surgical fixation and fusion for patients over the age of 50 years with type II odontoid fractures. Additionally, type II and type III fractures should be considered for surgical fixation in cases of dens displacement of 5 mm or greater, comminution of the fracture (type IIA), and inability to achieve or maintain alignment with external immobilization. Options for surgical treatment include posterior fusion with C1–C2 transarticular screw fixation and anterior odontoid screw fixation. The advantage of the latter procedure is that it provides greater preservation of cervical rotation. Other odontoid fractures may be successfully treated with halo brace immobilization.

BIBLIOGRAPHY

Anderson L, Alonzo R. Fractures of the odontoid process of the axis. *J Bone Joint Surg* 1974;56-A:1663–1674.
Hadley M, Browner C, Liu S, et al. New subtype of acute odontoid fractures (type IIA). *Neurosurgery* 1988;22:67–71.
Hadley M, Browner C, Sonntag V. Axis fractures: a comprehensive review of management and treatment in 107 cases. *Neurosurgery* 1985;17:281–290.
Ryken TC, Hadley MN, Aarabi B, et al. Management of isolated fractures of the axis in adults. *Neurosurgery* 2013;72:132–150.

32. **(B)** Severe flexion injuries of the cervical spine may cause unilateral or bilateral locked facets. Typically, unilateral locked facets result from flexion plus rotation injuries, and bilateral locked facets result from hyperflexion injuries. Anatomically, locked facets refer to the condition when the inferior articular facets of the upper dislocated vertebra slide forward over the superior facets of the vertebra below (see Fig. 36-17). Bilateral locked facets are extremely unstable given the extensive amount of ligamentous injury involved. The forces applied in this type of injury rupture the posterior ligamentous complex, the joint capsules, the intervertebral disk, and, usually, the posterior and anterior longitudinal ligaments. In about 80% of these cases, patients will present with complete spinal cord injuries. Nerve root injuries are common as well. Unilateral locked facets are more stable than bilateral, and these patients are usually neurologically intact. Patients in either of these groups should be

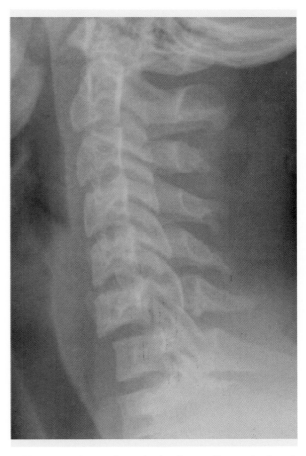

FIGURE 36-17. Lateral cervical spine radiograph showing unilateral locked facets of C6 on C7.

treated initially with closed reduction using cervical traction. Once reduction of the cervical spine is achieved, patients may be stabilized by immobilization in a halo vest or by internal fixation and fusion. Surgical management is often preferred given the high incidence of unsatisfactory fusion when using a halo vest alone. Surgical management should be used if attempts at closed reduction are unsuccessful.

MRI is helpful in evaluating for a herniated disk and determining the extent of damage to the spinal cord (see Fig. 36-18). It is also useful for preoperative planning. Perched facets refer to facets that have just reached the point of locking without actually doing so. These injuries are treated in a similar manner to locked facets.

BIBLIOGRAPHY

Hadley M, Fitzpatrick B, Sonntag V, et al. Facet fracture-dislocation injuries of the cervical spine. *Neurosurgery* 1992;31:661–666.
Sears W, Fazl M. Prediction of stability of cervical spine fracture managed in the halo vest and indications for surgical intervention. *J Neurosurg* 1990;72:426–432.

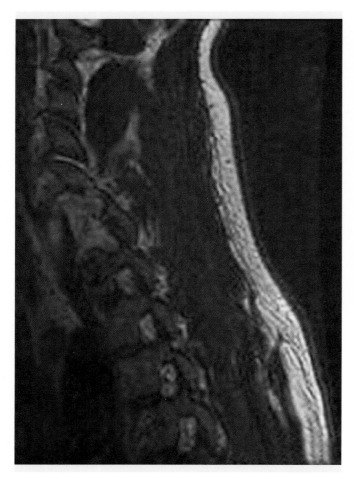

FIGURE 36-18. Magnetic resonance imaging scan of the cervical and upper thoracic spine showing locked facets of C6 on C7.

Sypert G, Arpin E. Management of lower cervical spinal instability. In: Wilkins R, Rengachary S (eds.), *Neurosurgery*, 2nd ed. New York, NY: McGraw-Hill; 1996:2927–2937.

33. **(D)** A clay-shoveler fracture is an avulsion fracture of a spinous process that usually occurs at C6, C7, or T1, with C7 being the most common vertebra involved (see Fig. 36-19). The mechanism of injury is flexion of the head combined with an opposing force of the posterior musculature attached to the spinous processes of the lower cervical and upper thoracic vertebra. This was originally described as occurring when clay stuck to the end of a shovel during the throwing phase, causing the arms to be jerked upward. These fractures may also be caused by neck hyperflexion or by blunt trauma to the back of the neck. Patients presenting with these fractures are usually neurologically intact. These are stable fractures, and treatment involves placing the patient in

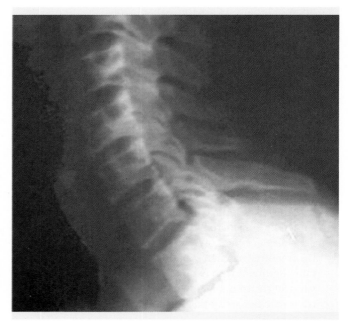

FIGURE 36-19. Lateral cervical spine radiograph showing a clay-shoveler fracture of T1.

a cervical collar for 6–8 weeks. Of course, clay-shoveler fractures may be associated with other cervical injuries. A CT scan is helpful to exclude other fractures, and flexion-extension radiographs or an MRI are required to exclude significant ligamentous injury.

34. **(C)** Although the spine will usually fuse on its own in 8–12 weeks, this often requires the patient to remain on bed rest. Besides being difficult on the patient psychologically, prolonged bed rest carries a relatively high risk of several comorbidities such as deep venous thrombosis, pneumonia, pulmonary embolus, and decubitus ulcers. Early surgical fixation and fusion allows for early mobilization and expedites rehabilitation. It also helps prevent delayed kyphotic angulation deformity. Early surgery, however, does not improve neurologic function in a patient with a complete spinal cord injury.

A difficult question to answer is when is the best time to operate on a patient who has an incomplete spinal cord injury. Although it may seem most appropriate to decompress and fixate the spine as quickly as possible, studies have shown that emergency surgery produces the greatest amount of neurologic deterioration in patients with spinal cord injury. Other studies support the position that timing of surgery has no effect on neurologic function. Still others dispute the validity of these investigations and support emergent surgery for patients with incomplete spinal cord injury. Further research will be required before a consensus can be reached on this issue.

BIBLIOGRAPHY

Benzel E, Larson S. Functional recovery after decompressive operation for thoracic and lumbar spine fractures. *Neurosurgery*
1986;19:772–778.

Greenberg M, Greenberg MS. *Handbook of Neurosurgery*, 7th ed.
New York, NY: Thieme; 2010:944.

Hall R. Clay-shoveller's fracture. *J Bone Joint Surg* 1940;22:63–75.

Marshall L, Knowlton S, Garfin S, et al. Deterioration following spinal
cord injury: a multicenter study. *J Neurosurg* 1987;66:400–404.

35. **(A)** Approximately two-thirds of all spine fractures occur
at the thoracolumbar junction, and 70% of these present
without neurologic injury. Many thoracolumbar fractures
are considered minor injuries and are stable fractures.
Fractures that fit into this category include transverse
process, articular process, and spinous process fractures.
Transverse process fractures may be associated with neurologic injury if they occur at T1 or T2 where the applied
force might damage the brachial plexus or at L4 or L5
where the force might damage the lumbosacral plexus
or the kidneys. Although no specific treatment of these
fractures is usually warranted, many clinicians will treat
these fractures with a lumbar or thoracolumbar brace for
several weeks.

A burst fracture, on the other hand, is considered an
unstable fracture. It occurs as a result of an axial load
that causes disruption of the anterior and posterior
portions of the vertebral body (see Fig. 36-20). These

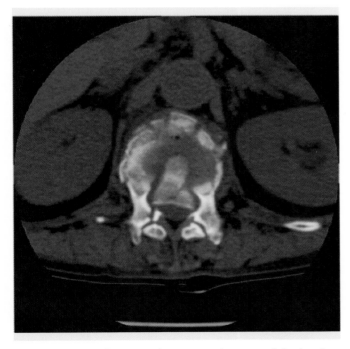

FIGURE 36-20. Computed tomography scan of the lumbar
spine showing a burst fracture of L1. Note the disruption of
both the anterior and posterior portions of the vertebral
body with retropulsion of bone into the spinal canal.

fractures usually occur between T10 and L2. Lateral
x-ray will almost always show some degree of loss of
posterior vertebral body height and retropulsion of bone
into the spinal canal. An AP x-ray will demonstrate
an increased interpeduncular distance. About half the
patients presenting with a burst fracture will be neurologically intact. Burst fractures of thoracic vertebra tend
to be more severe than fractures of the lumbar vertebra.
Patients who present with no neurologic injury and have
minor vertebral body disruption may be treated with a
rigid thoracolumbar sacral orthosis (TLSO brace), but
most burst fractures will require surgical decompression
with stabilization.

BIBLIOGRAPHY

Greenberg M, Greenberg MS. *Handbook of Neurosurgery*, 7th ed.
New York, NY: Thieme; 2010:986–990.

36. **(D)** In an attempt to define radiographic characteristics
that would predict instability in thoracolumbar spine
fractures, Denis created a three-column model of the
spine. According to this model, the anterior column
includes the anterior half of the vertebral body and
disk along with the anterior longitudinal ligament. The
middle column is made up of the posterior half of the
vertebral body and disk as well as the posterior longitudinal ligament. The posterior column is comprised of the
posterior bony complex (all structures posterior to the
vertebral body) and the posterior ligamentous complex
(interspinous and supraspinous ligaments, facet joint and
capsule, and ligamentum flavum).

Using the three-column model of the spine as a
foundation, Denis proposed three degrees of instability
associated with thoracolumbar fractures. Instability of
the first degree, or mechanical instability, occurs when
there is disruption of the anterior and posterior columns,
as in a severe compression fracture with distraction of
the posterior elements, or when there is disruption of
the middle and posterior columns, as in a seat belt–type
fracture. A seat belt fracture is caused by flexion as would
occur when the spine is flexed over a lap belt. These fractures are considered mechanically unstable, because they
are at risk for either further compression or angulation
with increasing kyphotic deformity. External immobilization is usually adequate, although surgical stabilization
may be required for severe cases. Although compression
fractures that cause only anterior column disruption are
usually considered stable, instability should be suspected
if there are three or more compression fractures in a row
or if there is greater than 50% loss of height of the
vertebral body with angulation.

Instability of the second degree, or neurologic instability, occurs with burst fractures with no neurologic injury where there is disruption of the anterior and middle columns. These fractures are considered neurologically unstable, because there is a risk for further collapse of the vertebral body with further encroachment of free bone fragments into the spinal canal.

Instability of the third degree, or mechanical and neurologic instability, occurs with severe burst fractures with neurologic injury or with fracture-dislocations where there is disruption of all three columns. These fractures are at risk for further neurologic deterioration and deformity. Fractures with this degree of instability almost always require surgical reduction, decompression, and stabilization.

BIBLIOGRAPHY

Denis F. The three column spine and its significance in the classification of acute thoracolumbar spinal injuries. *Spine* 1983;8:817–831.

37. **(D)** Most penetrating wounds of the spine in the United States today are caused by gunshot wounds. These are more common in urban areas where the rates of violent crimes are relatively high. Civilian gunshot wounds cause direct injury to the spinal cord by the bullet, whereas high-velocity military weapons tend to cause more indirect damage from cavitation and shock waves. Although debated, surgery has been shown to have little effect on recovery for patients with spinal cord injury secondary to gunshot wounds to the spine. For this reason, the trend now seems to be to treat patients with gunshot wounds to the spine without surgery unless they have a specific indication to do so. One of the historically cited reasons for operating on all gunshot wounds to the spine was to prevent infection. This may likely remain pertinent with military gunshot wounds because these cause massive tissue injury. With the creation of new antibiotics, however, infections may be prevented in civilian gunshot wounds with adequate courses of antibiotics alone.

The more commonly accepted indications for operating on gunshot wounds to the spine include neurologic deterioration, compression of a nerve root, and persistent cerebrospinal fluid leak or fistula. In addition, there are a few late complications that may develop that require surgical treatment. First, an abscess could develop that requires surgical drainage, especially if there is compression of the spinal cord. Second, a syrinx may develop and be the cause of late neurologic deterioration. This could require a shunting procedure to alleviate the symptoms. Third, lead intoxication may result if the bullet is lodged in a disk space or joint capsule. The treatment for this would include removing the bullet fragment and administering a chelating agent. Finally, spinal deafferentation following spinal cord injury may result in intractable dysesthetic pain. Placement of a dorsal column stimulator or dorsal root entry zone lesioning may help in these cases.

38. **(C)** Patients with spinal cord injuries have a relatively high risk for developing deep venous thrombosis, especially with higher levels of injury. The overall mortality from deep venous thromboses in patients with spinal cord injury is approximately 10%. Death may result from pulmonary embolus or embolic stroke if the patient has a patent foramen ovale. Because of this risk, patients with spinal cord injury should be on some form of deep venous thrombosis prophylaxis. This may include passive lower extremity motion, pneumatic compression boots, and heparin delivered subcutaneously. Additionally, physicians caring for patients with spinal cord injuries should have a high index of suspicion and a low threshold for diagnosing and treating deep venous thromboses in these patients. Current guidelines suggest initiating thromboembolism prophylaxis within 72 hours of presentation, and advise *against* placement of inferior vena cava filters as prophylaxis, unless of course the patient is not a candidate for or fails anticoagulation.

39. **(C)** Per the new 2012 Guidelines for the Management of Acute Cervical Spine and Spinal Cord Injury, there is now level II evidence to suggest using the American Spinal Injury Association (ASIA) grading scale as an international standard for evaluating a patient's spinal cord function. Within this scale, a class A injury has a complete motor and sensory level. Class B has complete motor loss but incomplete sensory loss. Class C has incomplete motor loss below the level of injury with more than half of the key muscles having a strength of less than grade 3 (meaning less than antigravity). Class D injuries have an incomplete motor loss (similar to class C), but more than half of the key muscles below the level are at a strength of 3 or higher (can resist gravity). Finally class E has normal sensory and motor function.

BIBLIOGRAPHY

Dhall SS, Hadley MN, Aarabi B, et al. Deep venous thrombosis and thromboembolism in patients with cervical spinal cord injuries. *Neurosurgery* 2013;72:244–254.

Greenberg M, Greenberg MS. *Handbook of Neurosurgery*, 7th ed. New York, NY: Thieme; 2010:947, 998.

Hadley MN, Walters BC. Introduction to the guidelines for the management of acute cervical spine and spinal cord injuries. *Neurosurgery* 2013;72(3):S5–S16.

CHAPTER 37

ORTHOPEDICS

SHERIF RICHMAN, ALEXANDRA I. STAVRAKIS, AND NICHOLAS M. BERNTHAL

1. A 31-year-old man is involved in a motor vehicle crash and transported to the emergency department. On arrival, his hemodynamics are normal, but he is unable to flex or extend his left hip, and there is concern for a possible posterior hip dislocation. The anteroposterior (AP) pelvis radiograph is shown in Fig. 37-1. On clinical examination, the left lower extremity would most likely be in which of the following positions?
   (A) Flexed, adducted, internal rotation
   (B) Flexed, abducted, internal rotation
   (C) Flexed, adducted, external rotation
   (D) Flexed, adducted, external rotation
   (E) Flexed, adducted, neutral rotation

2. A 25-year-old man has severe pain and is unable to ambulate on his left lower extremity following a car accident. A posterior knee dislocation was diagnosed at a referring hospital and reduced. An initial AP radiograph is shown in Fig. 37-2A, and a postreduction lateral radiograph is shown in Fig. 37-2B. The patient is now evaluated 6 hours after injury following the transfer. The examination now reveals an extremely swollen and painful knee and evidence of ischemia. Posterior tibial and dorsalis pedis pulses are absent. What is the next best course of action?
   (A) Obtain an emergent arteriogram.
   (B) Obtain emergent magnetic resonance imaging (MRI) to assess the ligamentous injuries.
   (C) Perform a comprehensive examination to assess the ligamentous stability.
   (D) Perform surgical repair or bypass of the injured popliteal vessels.
   (E) Perform surgical repair or ligamentous reconstruction.

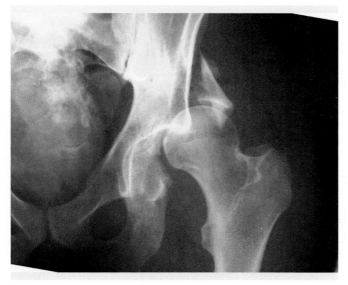

FIGURE 37-1. Anteroposterior pelvis radiograph. From Doherty GM (ed.). *Current Diagnosis & Treatment: Surgery*, 13th ed. New York, NY: McGraw-Hill; 2010: Fig. 40-13.

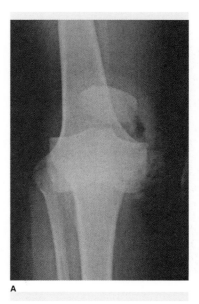

FIGURE 37-2. Anteroposterior (AP) radiograph of knee **A.** before reduction and **B.** after reduction.

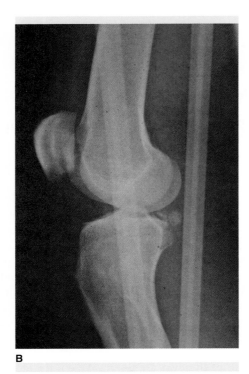

B

FIGURE 37-2. (Continued)

3. A 19-year-old patient sustained a left arm injury in a motorcycle crash. Initial examination in the emergency department reveals a Glasgow Coma Scale (GCS) score of 15 and no hemodynamic abnormality. Radiographs of the closed, isolated injury to the right arm are shown in Fig. 37-3. Which of the following deficits are most likely to be identified on a detailed physical assessment?

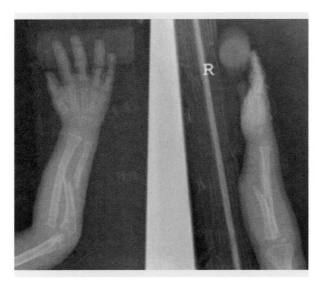

FIGURE 37-3. Monteggia fracture-dislocation. Used with permission from M. Brygel.

(A) Extension of the wrist and radial deviation
(B) Flexion of the thumb interphalangeal joint
(C) Abduction and adduction of the fingers
(D) Sensory loss over the dorsal web space of the thumb with no motor deficits
(E) Sensory loss over the tip of the thumb and index finger with no motor deficits

4. A 16-year-old student-athlete reported sudden onset of low back pain while weight training for football. The initial examination revealed no abnormalities in muscle strength, sensation, or reflexes; however, muscle spasms and a positive straight leg raise test were noted. The x-rays were unremarkable. Now, several weeks later, the symptoms have persisted. The next course of action should include
(A) Electromyogram (EMG) and nerve conduction studies
(B) MRI scan
(C) Repeat x-rays
(D) Physical therapy
(E) Bed rest followed by decreased activity

5. A 35-year-old man who sustained a blow to the anterior region of his left shoulder in a car crash is unable to abduct the arm above shoulder level. The examination also reveals pain and limitation in external rotation. Figure 37-4 reveals the initial radiograph.
Which of the following would be the next appropriate course of action?
(A) Physical therapy
(B) Bone scan
(C) MRI
(D) EMG
(E) Axillary radiograph

6. Figure 37-5 shows the radiograph of a 40-year-old man who was riding a bicycle and was struck by a car. Treatment should consist of
(A) Cemented total hip arthroplasty
(B) Protected weight bearing until union
(C) Bed rest until union
(D) Open reduction and internal fixation (ORIF)
(E) Cemented hemiarthroplasty

7. An 18-year-old man injured his left shoulder playing rugby. He has his left arm supported by his right hand. Radiograph is shown in Fig. 37-6. What would be the best course of treatment for this patient's injury?
(A) Surgical stabilization with plate and screws
(B) Surgical stabilization with a percutaneous intramedullary screw
(C) Closed reduction and cast treatment
(D) Sling for comfort and restricted activity with the extremity
(E) Biopsy and culture, followed by appropriate antibiotics

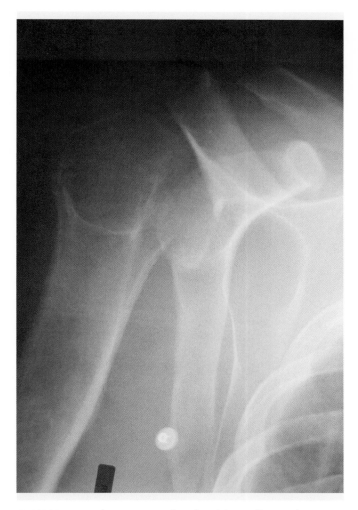

FIGURE 37-4. Anteroposterior shoulder radiograph.

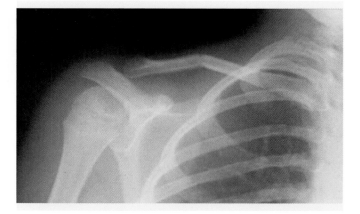

FIGURE 37-6. Anteroposterior shoulder radiograph. Used with permission from M. Brygel.

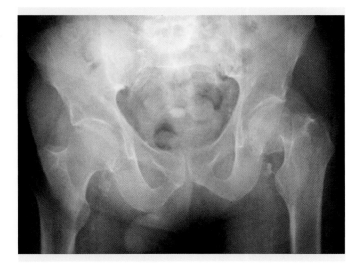

FIGURE 37-5. Anteroposterior pelvis radiograph. Used with permission from M. Brygel.

8. A 20-year-old man injured his left shoulder while playing football. Physical examination reveals decreased external rotation and inability to abduct his shoulder. A neurovascular examination determines the patient has numbness over the proximal-lateral aspect of his upper arm. What is the explanation for the numbness on the arm?
   (A) Injury to the axillary nerve
   (B) Injury to the musculocutaneous nerve
   (C) Injury to the ulnar nerve
   (D) Injury to the medial brachial cutaneous nerve
   (E) Injury to the lateral antebrachial cutaneous nerve

9. A 28-year-old man is brought to the emergency department (ED) 2 hours after a motor vehicle crash. He is unable to move his lower extremities. Radiographs reveal a flexion-distraction injury. A subsequent MRI is shown in Fig. 37-7 and confirms cord injury at the level of the fracture. Which of the following is the most appropriate course of pharmacologic treatment for this patient's spinal cord injury?
   (A) Methylprednisolone bolus 30 mg/kg, then infusion of 5.4 mg/kg/h for 72 hours
   (B) Methylprednisolone bolus 30 mg/kg, then infusion of 5.4 mg/kg/h for 24 hours
   (C) Methylprednisolone bolus 30 mg/kg, then infusion of 5.4 mg/kg/h for 48 hours
   (D) No benefit from treatment with methylprednisolone
   (E) Naloxone infusion for 48 hours

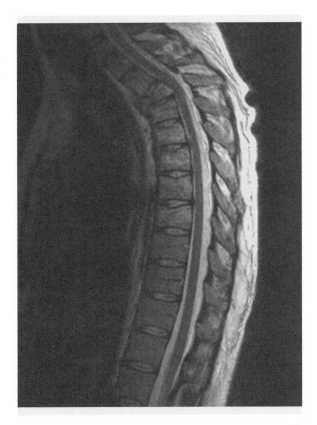

FIGURE 37-7. Sagittal magnetic resonance imaging of thoracic spine.

10. The radiograph and computed tomography (CT) scan shown in Figs. 37-8A and 37-8B are from the right hip of a 20-year-old woman who has been having pain in her groin. Although she has not had any fevers or night sweats, the pain seems to be worse at night. She has been taking aspirin with some relief of the pain. The most likely diagnosis is
    (A) Osteosarcoma
    (B) Osteoblastoma
    (C) Multiple myeloma
    (D) Myositis ossificans
    (E) Osteoid osteoma

11. What type of spinal fracture is shown in Figs. 37-9A and 37-9B?
    (A) Compression fracture
    (B) Flexion-distraction
    (C) Fracture-dislocation
    (D) Extension injury
    (E) Burst fracture

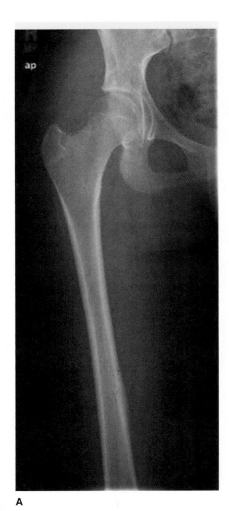

A

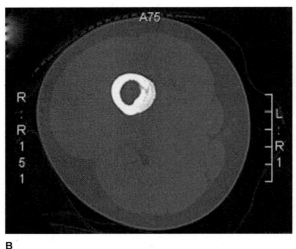

B

FIGURE 37-8. A. Femur radiograph and **B.** computed tomography. From Skinner H. *Current Diagnosis and Treatment in Orthopedics*, 5th ed. New York, NY: McGraw-Hill; 2013: Figs. 5-89A and 5-89C.

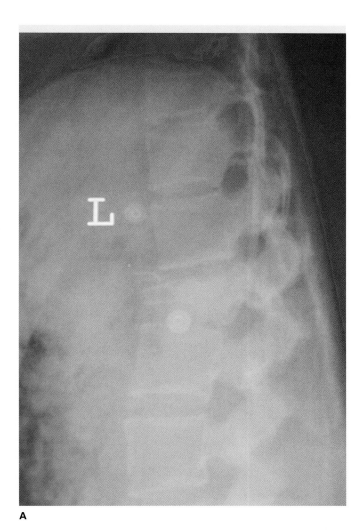

A

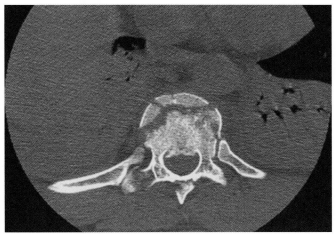

B

FIGURE 37-9. A. Lateral lumbar radiograph. **B.** Axial computed tomography scan of the thoracic spine.

12. A 28-year-old man is seen following a gunshot wound to the back. Examination reveals 5/5 strength in both upper extremities. He has 5/5 strength in the left lower extremity; however, there is decreased sensation in the left lower extremity. The right lower extremity has normal sensation but significant motor weakness. Which of the following conditions best describes his neurologic injury?
    (A) Central cord syndrome
    (B) Anterior cord syndrome
    (C) Brown-Sequard syndrome
    (D) Cauda equina syndrome
    (E) Complete spinal cord syndrome

13. A lesion on MRI reveals a very homogeneous characteristic. It reveals bright signal intensity on T1, and there is high signal with no increase on T2 images. Based on these characteristics, the lesion most likely represents a
    (A) Lipoma
    (B) Normal muscle
    (C) Synovial sarcoma
    (D) Liposarcoma
    (E) Desmoid tumor

14. Which Salter-Harris fracture type best describes a transverse fracture through the entire length of the growth plate without involving the metaphysis?
    (A) Type I
    (B) Type II
    (C) Type III
    (D) Type IV
    (E) Type V

15. An 11-year-old boy injured his left leg while tackling an opponent in a football game. He was treated to stabilize the fracture, and postoperative radiographs are shown in Fig. 37-10.
    What is the most likely diagnosis?
    (A) Unicameral bone cyst
    (B) Metastatic tumor
    (C) Ewing tumor
    (D) Nonossifying fibroma
    (E) Osteosarcoma

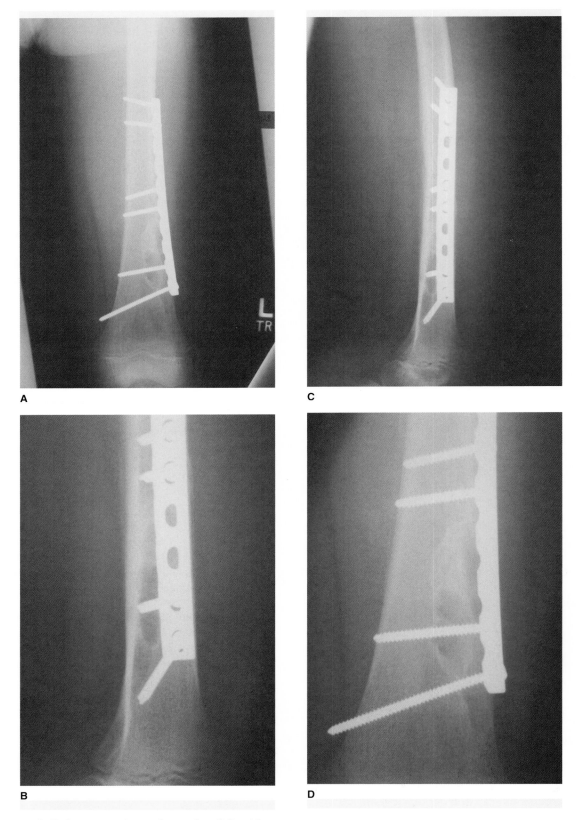

FIGURE 37-10. A–D. Postoperative radiographs of distal femur.

16. A 28-year-old man sustains a laceration and degloving to the volar and ulnar surface of his dominant left forearm. Figure 37-11 shows the clinical photo prior to surgical debridement.

Preoperatively, the median nerve is best evaluated initially by

(A) Checking reflexes in the right arm compared to the uninjured left arm
(B) Asking the patient to cross his fingers
(C) Ordering urgent nerve conduction studies and an EMG
(D) Asking the patient to extend his thumb at the interphalangeal (IP) joint
(E) Assessing the thumb for abduction and opposition

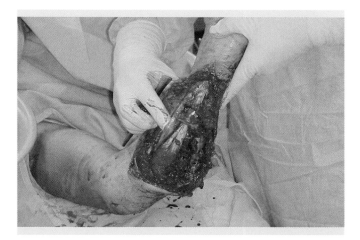

FIGURE 37-11. Degloving injury of left forearm.

17. A 39-year-old woman was involved in a motor vehicle crash and sustained multiple injuries including a splenic laceration, left forearm fracture, and a closed right midshaft femur fracture. At initial evaluation, she was hemodynamically normal, alert, and oriented. The patient was transferred from a referring hospital for definitive care. Later that evening, the patient becomes confused and petechiae are noted in the conjunctiva and on the chest. An arterial blood gas (ABG) reveals a partial pressure of arterial oxygen (PaO_2) of 51 mmHg, and vital signs include a heart rate of 125 bpm and a respiratory rate of 25 breaths/min. Management should include

(A) Emergent stabilization of the femur fracture with intramedullary nailing
(B) Ventilatory support
(C) Emergent Doppler ultrasound examination of both lower extremities
(D) Treatment with albuterol nebulizers as needed
(E) Urgent helical CT scan of the chest followed by low-molecular-weight heparin

18. A 19-year-old man is injured in an industrial accident. He sustains a closed femur fracture and a distal radius fracture. Radiograph is shown in Fig. 37-12. The chest radiograph reveals a pneumothorax and multiple rib fractures. He has a GCS of 15 and a normal neurovascular examination in his extremities. Vital signs reveal a pulse rate of 100 bpm, respirations of 24 breaths/min, and a blood pressure of 144/92 mmHg. An ABG reveals a PaO_2 of 75 mmHg, a partial pressure of arterial carbon dioxide ($PaCO_2$) of 33 mmHg, and a normal pH. The femoral shaft fracture is best managed with

(A) External fixation as definitive treatment
(B) Skeletal traction only
(C) Intramedullary nailing
(D) Skeletal traction until stable and then external fixation
(E) Skeletal traction until stable and then intramedullary nailing

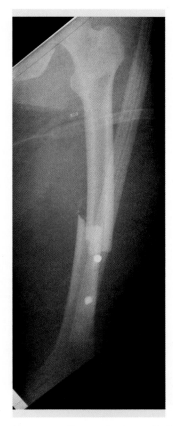

FIGURE 37-12. Femur radiograph. From Doherty GM (ed.). *Current Diagnosis & Treatment: Surgery*, 13th ed. New York, NY: McGraw-Hill; 2010: Fig. 40-16A.

19. A 47-year-old man sustains an injury to his right arm in a work-related fall. You are asked to consult for a left humerus fracture, and there is concern for potential injury to his radial nerve at the fracture site. A radiograph of the right humerus is shown in Fig. 37-13. Clinical findings supporting an injury to the radial nerve would include
    (A) Inability to flex the thumb at the IP joint
    (B) Decreased sensation over the volar surface of the index finger and thumb
    (C) Loss of sensation over the ulnar border of the ring and small fingers
    (D) Loss of sensation over the lateral border of the arm extending from the fracture site to the wrist
    (E) Inability to extend the wrist and fingers

20. A 22-year-old man sustained pelvic injuries in a motor vehicle crash. An AP pelvis radiograph and an outlet pelvis radiograph are shown in Figs. 37-14A and 37-14B. Examination reveals perineal swelling, a scrotal hematoma, and blood at the meatus. The patient complains of inability to void and pelvic pain.
    The next step in management would include
    (A) Intravenous pyelogram
    (B) External fixation to stabilize the pelvis
    (C) Careful insertion of a Foley catheter
    (D) CT scans of the abdomen
    (E) Retrograde urethrogram

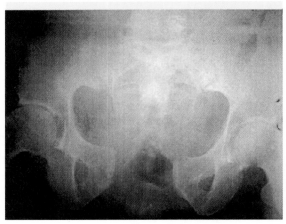

A

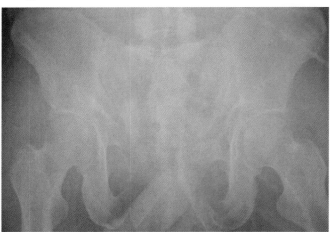

B

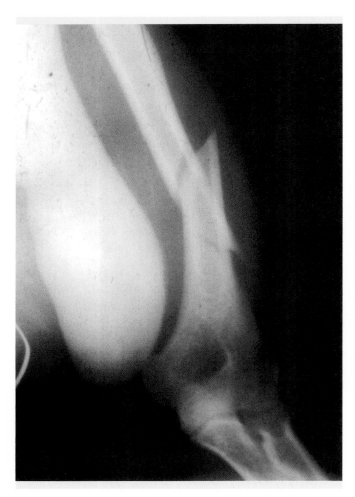

FIGURE 37-13. Right humerus radiograph. From Mattox K, Moore E, Feliciano D (eds.), *Trauma*, 7th ed. New York, NY: McGraw-Hill; 2012: Fig. 39-7.

FIGURE 37-14. A. Anteroposterior pelvis radiograph. From Hall JB, Schmidt GA, Wood LH (eds.), *Principles of Critical Care*, 3rd ed. New York, NY: McGraw-Hill; 2005: Fig. 96-4A. **B.** Outlet pelvis radiograph.

21. A 25-year old man presents with a posterior hip dislocation and associated femoral head dislocation. Following closed reduction, there is 4-mm displacement on a postreduction CT scan. The next course in treatment should include

(A) MRI
(B) Closed reduction under anesthesia
(C) ORIF
(D) Excision of the fragment
(E) Protective progressive weight bearing

22. A 40-year-old man is transported to the ED with bilateral tibia fractures. He is combative and requires sedation and subsequent intubation. You are called to evaluate the patient and notice the left lower leg is tense and swollen, but the posterior tibial and dorsalis pedis pulses are palpable. Radiographs of the left proximal tibia are shown in Fig. 37-15.
    Which of the following is the next best step in management of this patient?
    (A) Measurement of compartment pressures
    (B) Elevation above heart level to reduce swelling
    (C) Serial observation for improvement of soft tissue and swelling
    (D) ORIF of tibia fracture with plates and screws
    (E) Closed reduction and casting of tibia fracture

23. A 32-year-old man injures his left ankle while snowboarding. The initial AP and lateral radiographs are shown in Figs. 37-16A and 37-16B. A subsequent CT scan is shown in Fig. 37-16C.
    The next best course of treatment for this patient is
    (A) ORIF
    (B) Closed reduction and casting
    (C) Treatment with an external fixator spanning the ankle
    (D) Delayed internal fixation to allow swelling to subside
    (E) Air cast and gradual mobilization

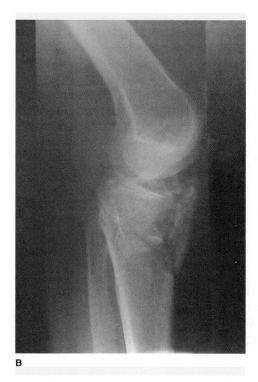

B

FIGURE 37-15. (Continued)

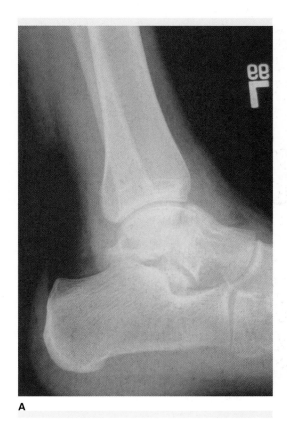

A

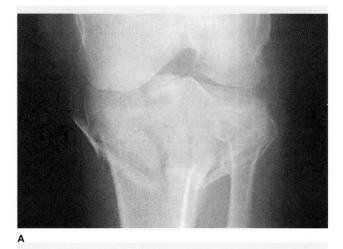

A

FIGURE 37-15. **A.** Anteroposterior and **B.** lateral knee radiographs.

FIGURE 37-16. **A.** Anteroposterior and **B.** lateral ankle radiographs. **C.** Computed tomography scan of ankle.

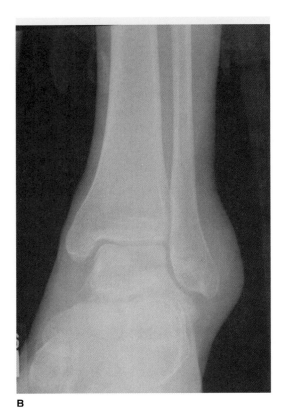

B

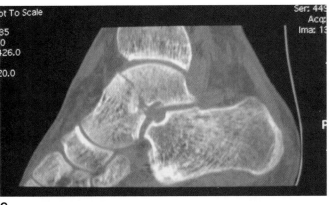

C

FIGURE 37-16. (Continued)

24. A pathologic fracture secondary to metastasis from which of the following common primary tumors requires a preoperative angiogram prior to surgical stabilization?
    (A) Kidney
    (B) Lung
    (C) Breast
    (D) Thyroid
    (E) Prostate

25. A patient sustains a complete cervical cord injury secondary to a cervical burst fracture. The radiographs reveal injury at the C6–C7 level. Assuming a complete cord injury at this level, which of the following findings on physical examination would not correlate with this level of injury?
    (A) Absent patellar tendon reflexes
    (B) Weakness with ankle plantar flexion
    (C) Weakness with elbow flexion
    (D) Weakness with finger abduction/adduction
    (E) Weakness with shoulder abduction

ANSWERS AND EXPLANATIONS

1. **(A)** Hip dislocations are generally the result of a high-energy injury, commonly a motor vehicle crash in which the knee strikes the dashboard and forces the hip out of the acetabulum. This may often be associated with an acetabulum fracture as well, specifically a posterior wall fracture. Hip dislocations can be diagnosed based on physical examination. Posterior hip dislocation will present with a hip that is flexed, adducted, and internally rotated, whereas anterior hip dislocations will present with a hip that is flexed and abducted. In most cases, a plain pelvic radiograph, which typically shows a smaller femoral head in posterior dislocations and a larger head in anterior dislocations, is sufficient to confirm the diagnosis.

   The key structures at risk during dislocation of a hip are the circulation to the femoral head and the sciatic nerve. The posterior vascular supply to the femoral head provides the majority of the circulation. An extracapsular ring originates at the base of the neck and traverses the capsule to the head (see Fig. 37-17). Injury to this region can result in acute disruption of the vessels that are closely associated with the capsule, stretching or compression of the vessels, and venous occlusion of the vascular outflow. All of these may contribute to the risk of developing subsequent avascular necrosis.

   The sciatic nerve is in close proximity to the posterior capsule and can be injured directly as the femoral head displaces posteriorly out of the acetabulum. A complete sciatic nerve injury can result, or more commonly the peroneal distribution is affected. A varied clinical outcome can range from isolated dorsal foot numbness to complete motor and sensory loss for the entire foot.

   Hip dislocations are considered an orthopedic emergency. The incidence of osteonecrosis has been reported in 1–20% of hip dislocations. Prompt reduction, within 6 hours, can reduce the incidence of osteonecrosis. This should be performed under conscious sedation with adequate muscle relaxation. If reduction is not completed on the first attempt, repeated attempts are not indicated, and reduction should be performed under general anesthesia to ensure adequate muscle relaxation. Following

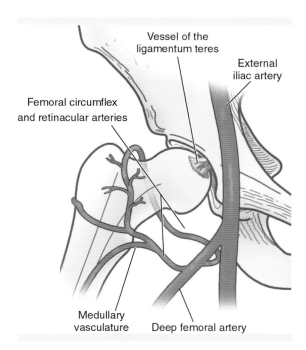

FIGURE 37-17. Vascular ring at the base of the femoral neck. From Sherman S. *Simon's Emergency Orthopedics*, 7th ed. New York, NY: McGraw-Hill; 2014: Fig. 18-2.

reduction, patients should be allowed to weight bear as tolerated to the limits of pain. There is currently no evidence to support the belief that delayed weight bearing has any impact on the outcome of isolated hip dislocations. Extremes of motion should be avoided to allow capsular healing. Acute sciatic nerve injuries occur in 8–20% of hip dislocations. Most of these are neurapraxias, and 60–80% of patients will recover to a level in which good function can be obtained; however, full recovery of strength is unusual, and use of an appropriate ankle-foot orthosis and a rehabilitation program are critical during the recovery phase. Development of post-traumatic arthritis is the most common long-term complication. This is more likely after posterior dislocations than anterior and is related to age, severity of the injury, and activity of the patient.

BIBLIOGRAPHY

Goulet JA, Levin PE. Hip dislocations. In: Browner BD, Jupiter JB, Levine AM, et al. (eds.), *Skeletal Trauma*, 3rd ed. Philadelphia, PA: W.B. Saunders; 2003:1657–1690.

Heckman JD (ed.), *Rockwood and Green's Fractures in Adults*, 5th ed. Philadelphia, PA: Lippincott Williams & Wilkins; 2001:1547–1576.

Leighton RK, Lammens P. Hip dislocations and fractures of the femoral head. In: Kellam JF, Fischer TJ, Tornetta P III (eds.), *Orthopaedic Knowledge Update: Trauma 2*. Rosemont, IL: American Academy of Orthopaedic Surgeons; 2000:311–314.

Motley GS, Eddings TH III, Moore RS. Adult trauma. In: Miller MD, Brinker MR (eds.), *Review of Orthopaedics*, 3rd ed. Philadelphia, PA: W.B. Saunders; 2000:476–477.

Mullis B, Anglen J. Hip trauma. In: Flynn JM (ed.), *Orthopaedic Knowledge Update 10*. Rosemont, IL: American Academy of Orthopaedic Surgeons; 2011:399–411.

2. **(D)** The traumatic dislocation of the knee is uncommon but should be considered an orthopedic emergency. Capsular disruption often prevents a tense hemarthrosis from developing, and spontaneous reductions are common. Both of these contribute to occasional missed diagnosis. A normal radiograph with obvious knee instability and soft tissue swelling should alert the physician to consider traumatic knee dislocation. It is critical to closely evaluate and document the neurovascular status of the limb during examination. Emergent reduction should be performed with appropriate sedation and analgesia. The limb should then be immobilized in the position of greatest stability, usually 15–20 degrees of flexion. The goals of treatment are a painless, stable knee, with normal strength and range of motion. Associated injuries are common, and injury to the popliteal artery has been reported in up to 30% of dislocations. It is most common in anterior and posterior dislocations because of the course of the popliteal artery as it traverses the popliteal fossa of the knee. It is tethered at the adductor hiatus proximally and by the soleal arch distally.

Clinical signs associated with vascular injury include diminished pulses or capillary refill, neurologic deficit, hypotension, or hematoma. More obvious signs include absent pulses, coolness or cyanosis, active bleeding, expanding hematoma, and bruits or thrill. The knee does not have the collateral circulation to remain viable in the presence of a popliteal artery injury. Therefore, vascular spasm is not a valid clinical assessment, and any vascular insufficiency, including diminished pulses, implies arterial injury until proven otherwise. The ankle-brachial index is an excellent noninvasive tool to screen for vascular injury, with a negative predictive value approaching 100%. In the presence of satisfactory perfusion following reduction, obtaining an arteriogram on an urgent basis may be an acceptable option. However, as in this patient, surgical repair or restoration of flow to the extremity should not be delayed to obtain an arteriogram. If necessary, an arteriogram can be obtained in the operating room (OR). This particular patient has evidence of ischemia that is approaching 6 hours. This should be considered a vascular emergency. The risk of muscle necrosis, contracture, and amputation rises significantly when ischemia exceeds 6 hours. Amputation rates approach 30% if repair is not accomplished within the first 7–12 hours and approach 0% when done within the first 6 hours. No delays are acceptable in this patient.

Ligamentous assessment can be assessed clinically and confirmed by MRI, following the arterial repair. Ligamentous reconstruction should be delayed until vascular stability and soft tissue healing have been achieved. Peroneal nerve injuries can be associated with knee dislocations as well and have been reported in 14–35% of cases. This injury carries a poor prognosis, and primary or secondary repairs and grafting have resulted in poor results. Bracing or tendon transfers are often required.

BIBLIOGRAPHY

Kaar SG, Stuart MJ, Levy BA. Soft-tissue injuries about the knee. In: Flynn JM (ed.), *Orthopaedic Knowledge Update 10*. Rosemont, IL: American Academy of Orthopaedic Surgeons; 2011:457–458.

Motley GS, Eddings TH III, Moore RS. Adult trauma. In: Miller MD, Brinker MR (eds.), *Review of Orthopaedics*, 3rd ed. Philadelphia, PA: W.B. Saunders; 2000:484–485.

Schenck RC. Injuries of the knee. In: Bucholz RW, Heckman JD (eds.), *Rockwood and Green's Fractures in Adults*, 5th ed. Philadelphia, PA: Lippincott Williams & Wilkins; 2001:1914–1928.

Siliski JM. Dislocations and soft tissue injuries of the knee. In: Browner BD, Jupiter JB, Levine AE, et al. (eds.), *Skeletal Trauma*, 3rd ed. Philadelphia, PA: W.B. Saunders; 2003:2045–2073.

Wascher DC. High velocity knee dislocation with vascular injury: treatment principles. *Clin Sports Med* 2000;19:457–477.

3. **(A)** This patient's x-rays reveal a fracture pattern commonly referred to as a Monteggia fracture. In 1814, Monteggia described a fracture of the proximal third of the ulna and dislocation of the radial head at the proximal radioulnar joint. Bado has classified these into four types (see Fig. 37-18):

Type I: Anterior (65%) radial head dislocation–anterior ulna angulation

Type II: Posterior (18%) radial head dislocation–posterior angulation

Type III: Lateral (16%) radial head dislocation–ulna fracture just distal to coronoid

Type IV: Both bone fracture (1%) radial head dislocation–anterior dislocation and proximal fracture of both radius and ulna

Monteggia fractures that are open, unstable, or comminuted require early ORIF of the ulna. Closed reduction of the forearm generally leads to reduction of the radial head. The arm is immobilized in the proper position to allow healing of the radioulnar joint. This is based

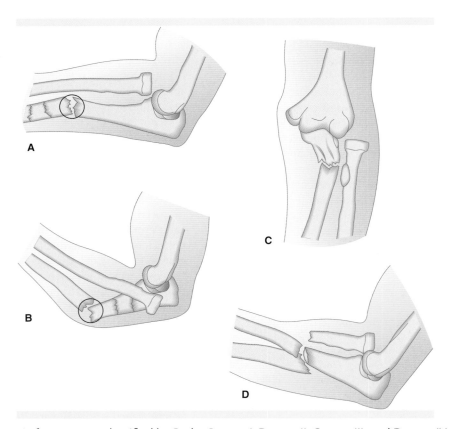

FIGURE 37-18. Monteggia fractures, as classified by Bado: **A.** type I, **B.** type II, **C.** type III, and **D.** type IV. Reproduced with permission from Browner B et al: *Skeletal Trauma*. Saunders, 1992.

on the degree of stability during examination and is usually a position of flexion and supination. If closed reduction is not possible, then open reduction via a lateral approach is indicated. If there is an associated fracture of the radial head or neck, all attempts to reconstruct or to replace the radial head should be made. There is often an injury to the interosseous membrane, and simple excision can lead to proximal migration of the radius.

It is logical that the radial nerve is the most commonly injured because of its proximity to the radial neck. Specifically this would involve the motor component or posterior interosseous nerve (PIN). On examination, this would manifest as extensor weakness of the wrist and fingers. Flexion of the thumb is the result of the flexor pollicis brevis, which is innervated by the median nerve. Flexion at the IP joint of the thumb specifically is from the flexor pollicis longus, which is innervated by the anterior interosseous nerve. Finger adduction and abduction are powered by the interossei and lumbricals. The ulnar nerve innervates all the interossei and the ulnar two lumbricals. The median nerve innervates the radial two lumbricals. The sensory branch of the radial nerve provides sensation to the dorsal web space of the thumb; however, this branches prior to the nerves passing around the radial neck. The PIN is closely associated with the radial neck, and isolated injury to the sensory branch is much less common than motor involvement. The median nerve provides the sensory distribution over the tips of the thumb and index fingers.

BIBLIOGRAPHY

Jupiter JB, Kellam JF. Diaphyseal fractures of the forearm. In: Browner BD, Jupiter JB, Levine AE, et al. (eds.), *Skeletal Trauma*, 3rd ed. Philadelphia, PA: W.B. Saunders; 2003:1381–1387.

Richards RR. Fractures of the shafts of the radius and ulna. In: Bucholz RW, Heckman JD (eds.), *Rockwood and Green's Fractures in Adults*, 5th ed. Philadelphia, PA: Lippincott Williams & Wilkins; 2001:900–916.

Wattenbarger JM, Frick SL. Shoulder, upper arm, and elbow trauma: pediatrics. In: Flynn JM (ed.), *Orthopaedic Knowledge Update 10*. Rosemont, IL: American Academy of Orthopaedic Surgeons; 2011:681–682.

4. **(B)** The majority of cases of low back pain and back-related leg pain are generally self-limited and respond favorably to a short period of 24–48 hours of rest, decreased activity, and physical therapy. Herniated lumbar disks most commonly affect the L4–L5 disk space, followed by the L5–S1 disk. Most herniated disks are posterolateral. The nerve root affected is the lower nerve root, or traversing root. The root from the upper level is already exiting beneath the pedicle at the level of the disk herniation. Central herniations are often only accompanied by pain. In any individual with back pain who fails to respond to rest and activity restriction, nonspinal etiologies for back or radiating pain must always be considered, especially in children. These include abdominal or pelvic pathology, sciatic joint pathology, and hip pathology. A positive contralateral straight leg-raising test is the most specific test for a herniated disk, and although nerve root tension signs are generally very reliable in patients younger than age 30 years, they are not absolute.

The natural history of lumbar disk herniation is progressive resolution of symptoms without the need for surgical intervention. Approximately 50% of patients recover in 1 week, and up to 90% of patients recover within 1–3 months. Activities that load the spine with significant shear stresses, such as weight lifting, are associated with a higher rate of central disk herniation, and lumbar herniated disks in adolescents may not present with the more typical findings in adults such as radicular symptoms, sensory deficits, or even motor deficits. Therefore, when an adolescent who lifts weights has low back pain that has failed to respond to rest and activity restriction, an MRI scan is the next study of choice to evaluate for a herniated disk. Regular x-rays are generally not helpful in the initial evaluation of low back pain or in the diagnosis of a herniated disk and can be deferred for 6 weeks. However, x-rays are warranted in a patient with greater than 6 weeks of symptoms and in those with a history of cancer, constitutional symptoms, or significant trauma. Repeat x-rays in a short time span are certainly of no benefit. The use of physical therapy is part of the initial phase of treatment, combined with rest and decreased activity. These would be continued as part of the treatment plan once other causes have been eliminated.

BIBLIOGRAPHY

Lauerman WC, Goldsmith ME. Spine. In: Miller MD, Brinker MR (eds.), *Review of Orthopaedics*, 3rd ed. Philadelphia, PA: W.B. Saunders; 2000:359–362.

Spivak JM, Bendo JA. Lumbar degenerative disorders. In: Koval KJ (ed.), *Orthopaedic Knowledge Update 7*. Rosemont, IL: American Academy of Orthopaedic Surgeons; 2002:630–634.

5. **(E)** The shoulder has little intrinsic stability. The capsuloligamentous structures provide static stability and the muscles provide dynamic stability. The anterior shoulder dislocation is the most common shoulder dislocation. Most of these injuries are the result of athletic-related trauma or a fall. The arm is usually in an abducted and externally rotated position, resulting in disruption of the anterior capsule and labral complex. This is referred to as the Bankart lesion. Acute anterior dislocations are initially managed

with gentle, closed reduction in the ED. If reduction cannot be achieved, it can be tried under general anesthesia. Those who fail conservative treatment are candidates for surgical repair of the torn capsulabral complex. Although acute surgical stabilization can be considered for young high-demand patients, conservative treatment remains the standard for first-time dislocations. The need and duration for postreduction immobilization remains controversial. Some studies associate a clinically greater reduction of the labrum to its anatomically correct position with immobilization in external rotation versus internal rotation, whereas other studies find no difference. Associated injuries may include fractures, rotator cuff tears, or neurovascular injury. It is important to assess for these associated injuries because their presence may require surgical management.

An AP radiograph may be adequate to initially diagnose a shoulder dislocation; however, an axillary view should be part of the standard radiographic assessment of any shoulder injury. The recommended series is three views in the plane of the scapula including AP, axillary, and scapular lateral (Y view) views (see Fig. 37-19).

Complete radiography assessment is extremely important in patients, such as this one, with a posterior shoulder dislocation. The history of an anterior blow and the limitation in rotation and abduction on clinical examination are classic for a posterior shoulder dislocation. Clinically, there may also be posterior prominence and anterior flattening of the shoulder, and the coracoid is also often prominent. The diagnosis of a posterior dislocation is often delayed and can be missed on an

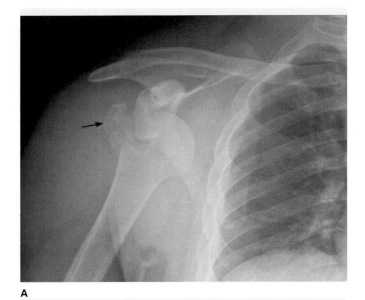

A

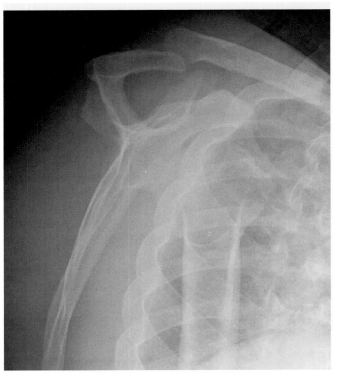

B

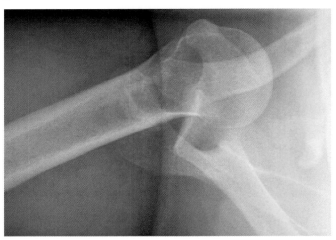

C

FIGURE 37-19. (Continued)

FIGURE 37-19. Anterior shoulder dislocation: **A.** antero-posterior, **B.** axillary, and **C.** scapular (Y view). From Block J, Jordanov M, Stack L, Thurman RJ. *Atlas of Emergency Radiology*. New York, NY: McGraw-Hill; 2013: Fig. 9.9.

AP radiograph. An AP radiograph, such as that in Fig. 37-19, does reveal some signs that suggest the injury, however. The normal elliptical shadow and overlap of the humeral head on the glenoid are distorted. Normally on an AP radiograph, the humeral head will fill an even portion of the glenoid fossa. In this case, the majority of the glenoid is vacant and there is an apparent increase in the space between the anterior rim of the glenoid and the medial aspect of the humeral head. This is referred to as the "vacant glenoid" or "positive rim sign." The AP radiograph may reveal significant internal rotation, and the margins of the greater tuberosity are no longer visible; however, it fails to reveal the displacement, which is directly posterior. An axillary radiograph is the most effective means to assess the position of the humeral head relative to the glenoid. Axial CT scans could also be useful but are less cost-effective. They would be helpful in the case of suspected fractures to help quantify displacement. Similarly, an MRI may be helpful later in the course of treatment to assess for intra-articular pathology. MRI is of limited use acutely, however. The other options would not help to confirm the diagnosis. Although the majority of shoulder dislocations are anterior, a posterior dislocation should be suspected with a history of an anterior blow, electrocution, or seizure disorder. These dislocations can often become locked on the posterior glenoid, and force or excessive internal rotation at the time of reduction can result in an iatrogenic humerus fracture. Immobilization in a position of stability, which may include slight extension and limited internal rotation is used in the initial healing phase followed by range of motion and strengthening. Fractures of the glenoid rim or proximal humerus are relatively common with posterior dislocations. Compression of the anteromedial aspect of the humeral head is referred to as a "reverse Hill-Sachs lesion." Fractures of the lesser tuberosity may also occur. These should be identified at the time of injury and addressed if they are related to recurrent instability.

BIBLIOGRAPHY

Getz CL, Buzzell JE, Krishnan SG. Shoulder instability and rotator cuff tears. In: Flynn JM (ed.), *Orthopaedic Knowledge Update 10*. Rosemont, IL: American Academy of Orthopaedic Surgeons; 2011:301–302.

Green A, Norris TR. Glenohumeral dislocations. In: Browner BD, Jupiter JB, Levine AE, et al. (eds.), *Skeletal Trauma*, 3rd ed. Philadelphia, PA: W.B. Saunders; 2003:1598–1614.

Schmidt AH. Fractures of the proximal humerus and dislocation of the glenohumeral joint. In: Kellam JF, Fischer TJ, Tornetta P III (eds.), *Orthopaedic Knowledge Update: Trauma 2*. Rosemont, IL: American Academy of Orthopaedic Surgeons; 2000:19–20.

Wirth MA, Rockwood CA. Subluxations and dislocations about the glenohumeral joint. In: Bucholz RW, Heckman JD (eds.), *Rockwood and Green's Fractures in Adults*, 5th ed. Philadelphia, PA: Lippincott Williams & Wilkins; 2001:1109–1162.

6. **(D)** The radiographs reveal a displaced femoral neck fracture. Femoral neck fractures are found in two different clinical scenarios: the elderly patient who sustains a low-energy fall, and the patient (usually younger than age 50) who sustains an injury from a high-energy traumatic event. Femoral neck fractures can be categorized as displaced, nondisplaced, or impacted fractures.

Treatment of nondisplaced or impacted fractures is generally performed using multiple lag screws, or occasionally with a large compression screw and side plate. Nonunion and avascular necrosis (AVN) are uncommon following nondisplaced fractures, occurring in less than 5 and 10% of cases, respectively. Nonunion and AVN are more common following displaced fractures. The incidence of nonunion ranges from 10–30%, and the incidence of AVN ranges from 15–33%. The treatment of displaced fractures remains somewhat controversial; however, achieving anatomic reduction is the most critical factor in maintaining reduction and avoiding nonunion or AVN. It is critical to perform surgery within 2–4 days of the injury because delayed surgery is an independent risk factor for mortality and other complications. Treatment of displaced fractures in the elderly patient traditionally consists of cemented hemiarthroplasty. However, in more mobile patients, total hip arthroplasty is gaining more traction as the treatment of choice. Total hip arthroplasty is also indicated in patients with significant preexisting arthritis. In younger patients with high-energy injuries, ORIF with a fixed-angle device is typically done.

A network of vascularity that includes the lateral and medial femoral circumflex arteries and the obturator artery supplies the femoral head. Some individuals advocate performing a capsulotomy or aspiration at the time of ORIF to release the hemarthrosis that develops. They feel this elevated pressure may be the pathophysiologic mechanism that may influence the circulation to the femoral head and contribute to the development of AVN. This has been shown to improve femoral head blood flow in laboratory animal models; however, this has not been conclusively proven in clinical trials.

BIBLIOGRAPHY

Baumgaertner MR, Higgins TF. Femoral neck fractures. In: Bucholz RW, Heckman JD (eds.), *Rockwood and Green's Fractures in Adults*, 5th ed. Philadelphia, PA: Lippincott Williams & Wilkins; 2001:1583–1602, 1609–1610.

Mullis B, Anglen J. Hip trauma. In: Flynn JM (ed.), *Orthopaedic Knowledge Update 10*. Rosemont, IL: American Academy of Orthopaedic Surgeons; 2011:403–404.

Swiontkowski MF. Intracapsular hip fractures. In: Browner BD, Jupiter JB, Levine AE, et al. (eds.), *Skeletal Trauma*, 3rd ed. Philadelphia, PA: W.B. Saunders; 2003.

7. **(D)** This man has an isolated clavicle fracture. Fractures of the clavicle are among the most common seen among adults. These fractures are classified based on the location of injury (see Fig. 37-20).

The most common fracture location is the middle onethird (85% of fractures) of the clavicle. This portion of the clavicle is vulnerable because it is in a subcutaneous

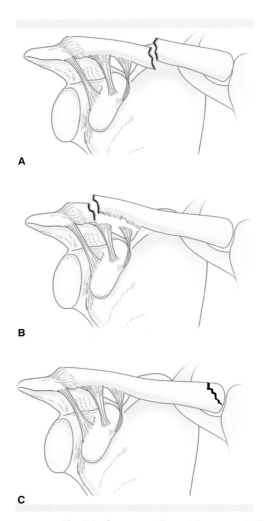

FIGURE 37-20. Clavicle fractures. From Sherman S. *Simon's Emergency Orthopedics*, 7th ed. New York, NY: McGraw-Hill; 2014: Fig. 16-29.

position and has no muscular attachments. Lateral-third fractures occur distal to the coracoclavicular ligaments, which are often ruptured in the setting of displaced fractures. Medial-third fractures are uncommon and have a high likelihood of associated injuries due to the extent of force required.

A cephalic and caudal tilt radiograph can be obtained to supplement the standard AP radiograph used to diagnose a clavicle fracture. Most of these injuries are managed nonsurgically with a figure-of-eight bandage or sling for up to 6 weeks with gradual increases in range of motion. Healing is usually evident on radiographs by 6 weeks; however, up to 12 weeks may be needed for full return to function. There has been no difference shown between use of a sling or figure-of-eight bandage. The long-term results of isolated clavicle fractures managed with sling or immobilizer are excellent. Full functional return is expected, and the incidence of nonunion is

between 0.1 and 5%. More recent studies have shown a link between displaced fracture and nonunion. Shortening can occur in displaced fractures; however, this has been shown to not affect functional outcome.

Indications for acute surgical management include open fractures, associated vascular injury, polytrauma, and ipsilateral scapula fracture. Fractures that are tenting the skin and for which it appears that skin compromise is imminent are also considered in this group. Some have advocated displacement of greater than 2 cm as an indication for surgery to avoid the higher risk of nonunion is this select group. If surgery is indicated, attempts are made to avoid the supraclavicular nerves, which cross the incision. Plate fixation is the most commonly used method, which requires precise contouring of the plate to match the shape of the clavicle. Intramedullary fixation with larger diameter threaded pins is another alternative. Small diameter, smooth K-wires, however, should never be used. Complications include infection, nonunion, damage to the underlying neurovascular structures, and hardware migration. A higher complication rate has been reported following internal fixation of acute fractures (over 20% in one study), and routine ORIF of isolated middle one-third clavicle fractures is not supported by the literature.

BIBLIOGRAPHY

Abboud JA, Boardman ND III. Shoulder trauma: bone. In: Flynn JM (ed.), *Orthopaedic Knowledge Update 10*. Rosemont, IL: American Academy of Orthopaedic Surgeons; 2011:271–284.

Blachut PA, Broekhuyse HM. Fractures of the scapula and clavicle and injuries of the acromioclavicular and sternoclavicular joints. In: Kellam JF, Fischer TJ, Tornetta P III (eds.), *Orthopaedic Knowledge Update: Trauma 2*. Rosemont, IL: American Academy of Orthopaedic Surgeons; 2000:8–9.

Lazarus M. Fractures of the clavicle. In: Bucholz RW, Heckman JD (eds.), *Rockwood and Green's Fractures in Adults*, 5th ed. Philadelphia, PA: Lippincott Williams & Wilkins; 2001:1044–1054.

Malik S, Pirotte A. Shoulder. In: Sherman SC (eds.), *Simon's Emergency Orthopedics*, 7th ed. New York, NY: McGraw-Hill; 2014.

8. **(A)** This patient has an anterior shoulder dislocation. Most of these injuries are the result of athletic-related trauma or a fall. The injury usually occurs when the arm is in an abducted and externally rotated position, resulting in disruption of the anterior capsule and labral complex. The shoulder has little intrinsic stability. The capsuloligamentous structures provide static stability, and the muscles provide dynamic stability. Acute anterior dislocations are managed with gentle, closed reduction. Other shoulder girdle injuries can be associated with dislocations. Among these are fractures, rotator cuff tears, and nerve and vascular injuries. The position of the brachial plexus and peripheral nerves in the axilla places them at risk at the time of injury (see Fig. 37-21).

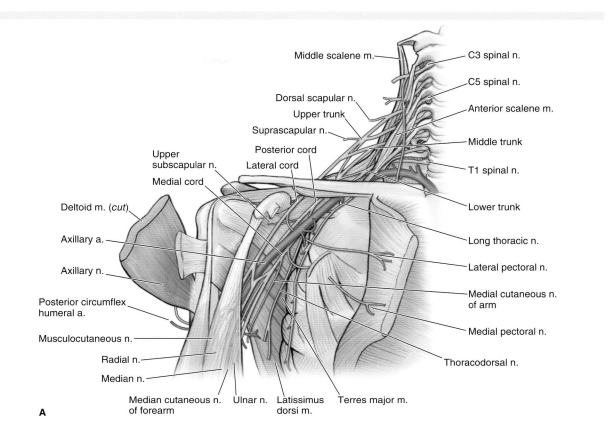

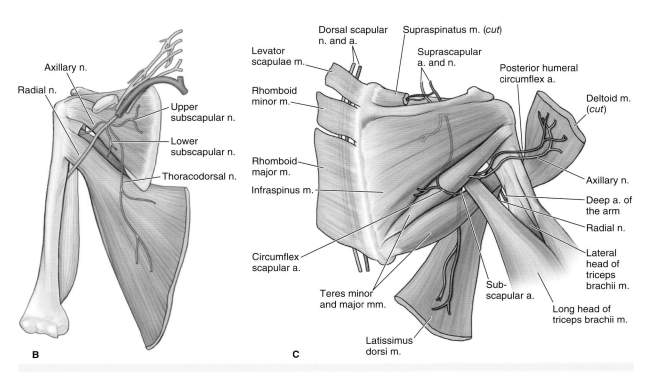

FIGURE 37-21. Brachial plexus of the shoulder. From Morton DA, Foreman KB, Albertine KH. *The Big Picture: Gross Anatomy.* New York, NY: McGraw-Hill; 2011: Fig. 30-4.

Brachial plexus and axillary nerve injuries are the most common. The axillary nerve arises from the posterior cord of the brachial plexus. It is tethered both anteriorly and posteriorly to the glenohumeral joint and is vulnerable to injury as it passes through the quadrangular space in conjunction with the posterior humeral circumflex artery. The nerve divides into a superior and inferior branch. The superior branch passes around the humeral neck to innervate the deltoid muscle. The inferior branch supplies the teres minor muscle and some posterior fibers of the deltoid. It then continues on to provide cutaneous innervation to the lateral arm as the superior lateral brachial cutaneous nerve.

The musculocutaneous nerve provides only motor innervation in the upper arm. It continues into the forearm as the lateral antebrachial cutaneous nerve providing sensory innervation to the anterolateral forearm. The ulnar nerve has no innervation in the upper arm. In the forearm, the ulnar sensory components involve the small finger and the ulnar border of the ring finger. The medial brachial cutaneous nerve is a branch off the medial cord of the brachial plexus. It travels beside the brachial artery to the middle arm where it pierces the fascia and provides sensation to the posterior surface of the lower third of the upper arm extending to the olecranon. These sensory innervations are easily summarized in Fig. 37-22.

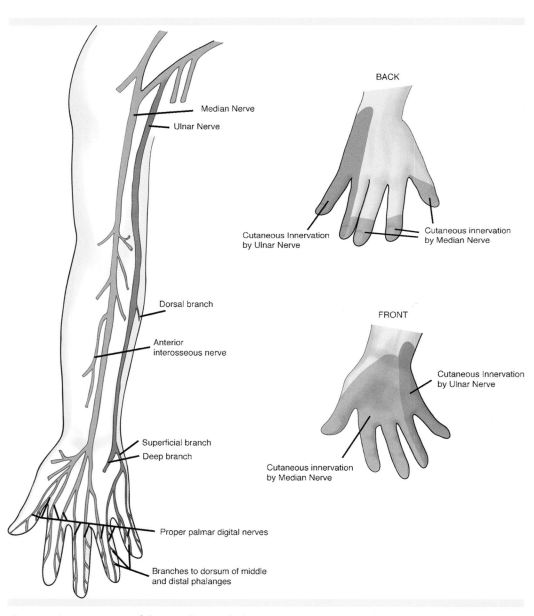

FIGURE 37-22. Sensory innervations of the median and ulnar nerves.

BIBLIOGRAPHY

Green A, Norris TR. Glenohumeral dislocations. In: Browner BD, Jupiter JB, Levine AE, et al. (eds.), *Skeletal Trauma*, 3rd ed. Philadelphia, PA: W.B. Saunders; 2003:1598–1614.

Netter FH. *The Ciba Collection of Medical Illustrations. Volume 8—Musculoskeletal System, Part I: Anatomy Physiology and Metabolic Disorders*. Summit, NJ: Ciba-Geigy; 2001:20–26.

Schmidt AH. Fractures of the proximal humerus and dislocation of the glenohumeral joint. In: Kellam JF, Fischer TJ, Tornetta P III (eds.), *Orthopaedic Knowledge Update: Trauma 2*. Rosemont, IL: American Academy of Orthopaedic Surgeons; 2000:19–20.

Wirth MA, Rockwood CA. Subluxations and dislocations about the glenohumeral joint. In: Bucholz RW, Heckman JD (eds.), *Rockwood and Green's Fractures in Adults*, 5th ed. Philadelphia, PA: Lippincott Williams & Wilkins; 2001:1109–1162.

9. **(B)** Up to 65% of spinal cord injuries occur in the cervical region. Common mechanisms include motor vehicle accidents, falls, and gunshot wounds. Spinal cord injury occurs from two distinct processes. The primary injury is the result of the mechanical injury at the time of the initial insult. This primary injury is followed by a cascade of events, which leads to secondary injury and increased cell death as a result of the pathophysiologic response. Surgical stabilization of the spine can prevent further mechanical injury to the cord. Additionally, removing compression such as a herniated disk or encroaching fragments of bone might further assist in the functional recovery. Over the past several years, the pharmacologic treatment of spinal cord injury has been used in an attempt to reduce or minimize the secondary injury. It is felt that interrupting the cascade of events that leads to the secondary injury has the potential to limit cell damage and improve functional outcome. Methylprednisolone is the only agent in randomized clinical trials that has been shown to have favorable effects on the neurologic recovery following injury. It has, therefore, become the standard for acute care of the patient with a spinal cord injury. The National Acute Spinal Cord Injury Study (NASCIS) trials were large-scale, randomized clinical trials that evaluated the use of methylprednisolone in spinal cord injury patients. The most recent NASCIS III trial recommendations are as follows: methylprednisolone bolus of 30 mg/kg followed by infusion of 5.4 mg/kg for 24 hours when the bolus is given within 3 h of injury or for 48 hours when the bolus is given between 3 and 8 hours from time of injury. There is no benefit when methylprednisolone is started more than 8 hours after injury. There is no benefit from naloxone or tirilazad.

BIBLIOGRAPHY

Bracken MB. Steroids for acute spinal cord injury. *Cochrane Database Syst Rev* 2012;1:CD001046.

Mirza SK, Chapman JR, Grady MS. Spinal cord injury: pathophysiology and current treatment strategies. In: Kellam JF, Fischer TJ, Tornetta P III (eds.), *Orthopaedic Knowledge Update: Trauma 2*. Rosemont, IL: American Academy of Orthopaedic Surgeons; 2000:359–368.

Tay B, Eismont F. Cervical spine fractures and dislocations. In: Fardin DF, Garfin SR, Abitbol J, et al. (eds.), *Orthopaedic Knowledge Update: Spine 2*. Rosemont, IL: American Academy of Orthopaedic Surgeons; 2002:251–253.

10. **(E)** Osteoid osteoma is one of three lesions in which the tumor cells produce osteoid. It is a self-limiting, benign, painful vascular lesion of uncertain etiology. It occurs most commonly in patients age 5–30. The pain usually increases with time, and most patients have pain at night. Common sites include the proximal femur, tibial diaphysis, and spine. The lesion may be difficult to identify on plain radiographs; however, findings include reactive bone and a radiolucent nidus. For this reason, special studies may be warranted. Bone scans are always positive, and MRI or CT scan can help to further define the location. By definition, the nidus is less than 1.5 cm; however, the reactive area of bone may be larger. Microscopically, there is a distinct differentiation between the nidus and the reactive bone. The nidus consists of osteoid trabeculae with varied mineralization. The organization is haphazard, and the greatest mineralization is in the center of the lesion.

Nonoperative treatment with the use of aspirin or nonsteroidal anti-inflammatory drugs (NSAIDs) may alleviate the pain in some patients. However, resolution of pain with NSAIDs may take up to 36 months. Up to 50% of these patients treated medically will have the pain resolve secondary to burn out of the lesion. A newer technique of percutaneous radiofrequency ablation under CT guidance is gaining popularity. This has resulted in treatment success rates of approximately 90%. Surgical removal of the complete lesion through excision of the entire legion or curettage of the nidus is indicated if medical management fails and the location is not amenable to percutaneous radiofrequency ablation.

Osteoblastoma is similar to osteoid osteoma; however, it is not self-limited like osteoid osteoma and can attain a large size. As noted earlier, osteoid osteoma is by definition less than 1.5 cm. Osteosarcoma is a malignant bone-forming tumor. Multiple myeloma is a plasma cell disorder and not a bone-forming tumor. Although it does present with pain, it occurs more commonly in older patients between 50 and 80 years of age. In addition, the classic radiographic appearance is that of a punched-out lytic lesion. Myositis ossifians occurs following a traumatic event. It is most common over long bones in the midportion of muscles. This should not be confused with osteoid osteoma. Radiographically, there is no similarity, and the microscopic pattern, which reveals mature, trabecular bone at the periphery and immature tissue at the center, is the opposite of that found in osteoid osteoma.

BIBLIOGRAPHY

Daffner SD. Spinal tumors. In: Flynn JM (ed.), *Orthopaedic Knowledge Update 10*. Rosemont, IL: American Academy of Orthopaedic Surgeons; 2011:555–557.

Frassica FJ, Frassica DA, McCarthy EF. Orthopaedic pathology. In: Miller MD, Brinker MR (eds.), *Review of Orthopaedics*, 3rd ed. Philadelphia, PA: W.B. Saunders; 2000:379–440.

11. **(E)** The Denis classification divides the vertebra into three columns: anterior column (anterior longitudinal ligament, anterior annulus and disk, and anterior half of vertebral body), middle column (posterior disk and annulus, posterior longitudinal ligament, and posterior half of vertebral body), and posterior column (posterior bony arch including lamina, pedicles, facets, and spinous process). Lumbar spine fractures generally occur from four mechanisms or a combination of them. These forces include compression, flexion, distraction, and shear. The resulting injuries include compression, burst, flexion-distraction, and fracture-dislocation.

Compression fractures are the result of axial loading and flexion forces on the anterior column with an intact middle column (see Fig. 37-23). They most commonly result from flexion and distraction. Compression fractures are generally stable injuries because of the intact middle and posterior structures, and most are managed nonoperatively with a brace for up to 3 months or longer.

An intact posterior cortex distinguishes a compression fracture from a burst fracture, which involves axial compression failure of the anterior and middle columns with either an intact or disrupted posterior column

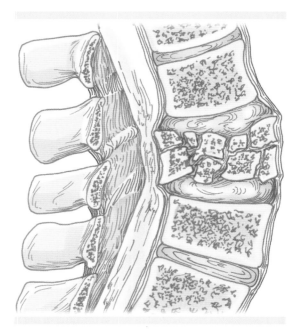

FIGURE 37-24. Burst fracture. From Sherman S. *Simon's Emergency Orthopedics*, 7th ed. New York, NY: McGraw-Hill; 2014: Fig. 10-4.

(see Fig. 37-24). Burst fractures most commonly result from falls and high-energy motor vehicle crashes. Important factors to consider in the treatment of burst fractures are spinal canal compromise, the degree of angulation, and presence or absence of neurologic deficit; however, all burst fractures are considered unstable. Controversy still exists regarding the most beneficial means of management of these fractures. Surgical treatment is generally preferred if there is greater than 50% canal compromise or more than 30 degrees of kyphosis at the level of injury, even if there are no neurologic deficits. If a neurologic deficit is present, surgical management is again usually preferred. Neurologic deficit must consider not only lower extremity motor and sensory function, but also perineal sensation, and bladder and bowel function must be evaluated. Nonoperative management can be considered, even if a neurologic deficit is present, only if the fracture pattern is stable and there is no spinal cord compression.

Fracture-dislocations are high-energy injuries involving failure of all three columns from a combination of forces, usually involving a shearing mechanism (see Fig. 37-5). They are unstable injuries and are associated with the highest incidence of neurologic injury. These injuries require surgical stabilization.

The seat belt injury is the classic flexion-distraction injury, which involves tension failure of the middle and posterior columns and either tension or compressive

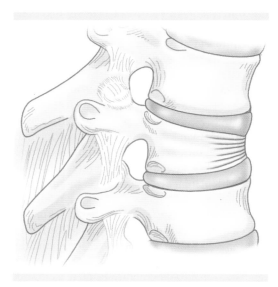

FIGURE 37-23. Wedge compression fracture. Sherman S. *Simon's Emergency Orthopedics*, 7th ed. New York, NY: McGraw-Hill; 2014: Fig. 10-2.

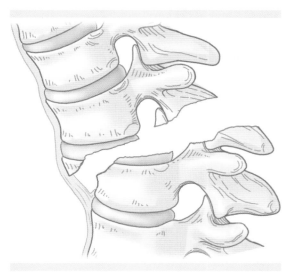

FIGURE 37-25. Fracture-dislocation. From Sherman S. *Simon's Emergency Orthopedics*, 7th ed. New York, NY: McGraw-Hill; 2014: Fig. 10-8.

failure of the anterior column depending on the site of the axis of rotation. These injuries can occur through either the bony or soft tissue elements (see Fig. 37-26). The fractures through bone have a better prognosis for healing, whereas the injuries through the ligamentous or soft tissue structures are less predictable and should be considered unstable. The radiographs of the lumbar spine show obvious involvement of the anterior and middle columns, and therefore, this injury is consistent with a lumbar burst fracture.

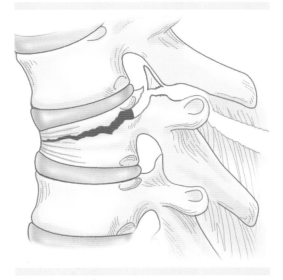

FIGURE 37-26. Flexion-distraction injury. From Sherman S. *Simon's Emergency Orthopedics*, 7th ed. New York, NY: McGraw-Hill; 2014: Fig. 10-7.

BIBLIOGRAPHY

Bolesta MJ, Rechtine GR III. Fractures and dislocations of the thoracolumbar spine. In: Bucholz RW, Heckman JD (eds.), *Rockwood and Green's Fractures in Adults*, 5th ed. Philadelphia, PA: Lippincott Williams & Wilkins; 2001:1405–1415.

Kwok DC. Thoracolumbar injuries: the posterior approach. In: Kellam JF, Fischer TJ, Tornetta P III (eds.), *Orthopaedic Knowledge Update: Trauma 2*. Rosemont, IL: American Academy of Orthopaedic Surgeons; 2000:393–400.

Motley GS, Eddings TH III, Moore RS. Adult trauma. In: Miller MD, Brinker MR (eds.), *Review of Orthopaedics*, 3rd ed. Philadelphia, PA: W.B. Saunders; 2000:469–470.

Vaccaro AR, Jacoby SM. Thoracolumbar fractures and dislocations. In: Fardin DF, Garfin SR, Abitbol J, et al. (eds.), *Orthopaedic Knowledge Update: Spine 2*. Rosemont, IL: American Academy of Orthopaedic Surgeons; 2002:273–276.

Vaccaro AR, Singh K. Thoracolumbar injuries: nonsurgical treatment. In: Kellam JF, Fischer TJ, Tornetta P III (eds.), *Orthopaedic Knowledge Update: Trauma 2*. Rosemont, IL: American Academy of Orthopaedic Surgeons; 2000:383–387.

12. **(C)** It is the responsibility of the physician to perform a thorough neurologic evaluation in every patient and especially in a patient with a suspected spinal cord injury. The extent of injury must be determined, because a patient with an incomplete injury has a reasonable prognosis for some gains in functional recovery; however, a functional recovery is only seen in 3% of patients with complete injuries in the first 24 hours and never after 24–48 hours.

According to the American Spinal Injury Association (ASIA), a complete nerve injury is one in which no motor and/or sensory function exists more than three segments below the neurologic level of injury. An incomplete injury is one in which some neurologic function is spared more than three levels below the level of injury. The level of injury is defined as the most caudal segment that tests at least grade 3 (antigravity) out of 5 for motor and the next level above is graded 4 out of 5. Sacral sparing is defined as perianal sensation, great toe flexor activity, and rectal tone. Sacral sparing is important because it indicates that there is at least partial continuity of the spinal tracts within the cord. This presence indicates an incomplete cord injury. This may be the only finding on initial examination, so documentation of this finding is important. It is vital, however, to rule out spinal shock. Spinal shock is that initial period of complete spinal areflexia that develops after severe spinal cord injuries. This is evaluated by testing the bulbocavernosus reflex. The completeness of a spinal cord injury cannot be determined until the bulbocavernosus reflex returns, usually within the first 24 hours.

This patient's clinical examination is consistent with an incomplete spinal cord injury. Incomplete spinal cord syndromes have a variable prognosis for recovery.

Greater recovery can be expected in patients in whom there is greater initial sparing of function below the level of injury. Brown-Sequard syndrome is a lesion caused by hemitransection of the cord usually from penetrating trauma. It results in ipsilateral motor and proprioception loss below the level of injury and contralateral loss of pain and temperature sensation beginning one to two levels below the injury level. This carries the best prognosis for recovery of all the incomplete syndromes. Central cord syndrome occurs essentially in the cervical region and involves injury to the central portion of the cord. This results in sacral sparing (preservation of perianal sensation and rectal tone) and greater weakness in the upper extremities with sparing of the motor function in the lower extremities. This injury pattern reflects the topographic organization of the motor tracts within the spinal cord in which the upper extremity tracts are located in a more central position within the cord. Overall, this carries the second best prognosis for recovery, with the lower extremities often recovering better function than the upper extremities. Anterior cord syndrome results from damage to the anterior spinal artery and involves damage to the anterior two-thirds of the cord and sparing of the posterior columns. Patients will have minimal if any motor function distally, and pain and temperature sensation is lost as well; however, proprioception, deep pressure, and vibratory sensation are preserved. The prognosis for motor recovery is poor. Cauda equina syndrome involves injury to the lumbosacral nerve roots within the spinal canal resulting in areflexic bladder, bowel, and lower limbs.

BIBLIOGRAPHY

Vaccaro AR, Jacoby SM. Thoracolumbar fractures and dislocations. In: Fardin DF, Garfin SR, Abitbol J, et al. (eds.), *Orthopaedic Knowledge Update: Spine 2.* Rosemont, IL: American Academy of Orthopaedic Surgeons; 2002:239–253.

13. **(A)** MRI is the most useful modality for the definition of soft tissue masses. Tissues display different signal intensity (SI) on T1 and T2 images. The MRI provides excellent definition of normal muscle, fascial boundaries, and the tumor mass. Both T1- and T2-weighted sequences are essential to detect and characterize soft tissue lesions. MRI cannot accurately predict the histology or whether a lesion is benign or malignant. Two exceptions to this rule are lipomas and hemangiomas. Lipomas are often very homogeneous and have signal characteristics that exactly match the surrounding fat, thus establishing the diagnosis. They show bright SI on T1 and do not increase in SI on T2 or fat suppression images. Hemangiomas contain numerous blood vessels and present with a recognizable pattern. Synovial sarcoma is low to intermediate on T1 and homogeneously bright on T2. Desmoid tumors are characterized by low SI fibrous bands, which demonstrate low to intermediate SI on T1 images and high SI on T2 images. Malignant fibrous histiocytoma features on MRI are nonspecific. Inhomogeneity with low to intermediate SI on T1 and high SI on T2 is found. Liposarcomas are more inhomogeneous than lipomas. The focal areas of malignant change demonstrate low to intermediate SI on T1 and high SI on T2.

BIBLIOGRAPHY

Brinker MR. Basic sciences: section 7—imaging and special studies. In: Miller MD, Brinker MR (eds.), *Review of Orthopaedics,* 3rd ed. Philadelphia, PA: W.B. Saunders; 2000:115–116.
Jones KB. Musculoskeletal oncology. In: Flynn JM (ed.), *Orthopaedic Knowledge Update 10.* Rosemont, IL: American Academy of Orthopaedic Surgeons; 2011:193–212.

14. **(A)** Physeal fractures make up 15–30% of all childhood fractures. Injury to the physis is rare before age 5 years and peaks in early adolescence, around age 11–12. Boys are affected twice as often as girls. Salter and Harris developed a classification system of fractures that involve the physeal plate. The five types in this system can be very useful in predicting the effects of the fracture on the physis and the effect on future growth.

Type I fractures involve a transverse fracture through the entire length of the growth plate without involvement of the metaphysis. Prognosis is generally excellent with the exception of the distal femur, or after severely displaced fractures, which are subsequently difficult to reduce.

Type II injuries account for 75% of all physeal fractures. A type II fracture passes through the growth plate, but then exits through the metaphysis prior to passing the full length, as in a type I fracture. This results in a metaphyseal bone fragment attached to the epiphyseal segment. The prognosis for these fractures is good, with growth disturbances occurring in 10–30% of cases.

Type III injuries involve a transverse fracture extending through part of the growth plate and then crossing the epiphysis to exit the articular surface. Anatomic reduction is indicated, and prognosis is dependent on the vascularity of the physis and damage to the germinal zone.

Type IV fractures are vertical fractures that cross all regions of the physis. These traverse the metaphysis, physis, and epiphysis and exit the articular surface. Despite an anatomic reduction, the prognosis for normal growth is poor.

Type V involves a compressive mechanism with a crushing force. Growth arrest is common. This injury can occur in combination with any of the other patterns.

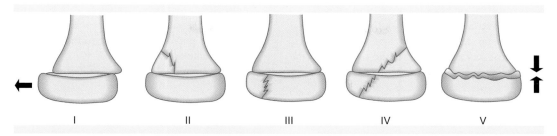

FIGURE 37-27. Salter-Harris classification. From Doherty GM (ed.). *Current Diagnosis & Treatment: Surgery*, 13th ed. New York, NY: McGraw-Hill; 2010: Fig. 40-22.

Type VI has been added by Rang. This is a peripheral injury to the perichondrial ring. Localized growth disturbances can occur. Fractures through the physis tend to pass through the hypertrophic zone. This region consists of cartilage, which is weaker than bone. Although this region is responsible for conversion of cartilage to bone, it is not the site of growth and cell multiplication. This occurs in the regions nearer the epiphysis; however, any trauma to the region surrounding or involving the physis can result alteration in growth. This may be from damage to the vascularity, damage to the germinal cells, or formation of a physeal bar or bony bridge that tethers the epiphysis to the metaphysis.

Figure 37-27 shows the different Salter-Harris classifications. In summary, type I and II fractures are the least likely to interfere with growth because they do not pass through the growth zone; however, all bones respond differently, and the mechanism of injury may involve a compression component to the injury not initially appreciated. This may account for some of the higher-than-expected growth disturbances seen with some type II injuries. Type III and IV fractures cross the growth zone, are intraarticular, and are more likely to develop growth disturbances. Type IV fractures are more likely to develop a bony bridge; therefore, these fractures must be anatomically reduced. Type V fractures can occur in association with any other pattern, as implied earlier, or they may occur independently. Type V fractures may not always be easily recognized on initial radiographs. This classification provides assistance in predicting the potential of growth disturbance, but definitive prediction is not possible. For this reason, close clinical follow-up with radiographs is mandatory for these patients.

BIBLIOGRAPHY

Price CT, Phillis JH, Devito DP. Management of fractures. In: Morrissy RT, Weinstein SL (eds.), *Lovell and Winter's Pediatric Orthopaedics*, 5th ed. Philadelphia, PA: Lippincott Williams & Wilkins; 2001:1323–1326.

15. **(D)** Nonossifying fibroma or metaphyseal fibrous defect is a common benign lesion in young patients. Most patients are asymptomatic, and lesions are found incidentally. The vast majority (90%) are located in the distal femur and proximal and distal tibia. It can be diagnosed by its characteristic appearance on x-ray (see Fig. 37-28). The lesion is metaphyseal, lytic, and eccentric. It is scalloped and surrounded with a sclerotic rim, and the cortex may be slightly thinned or expanded. Treatment

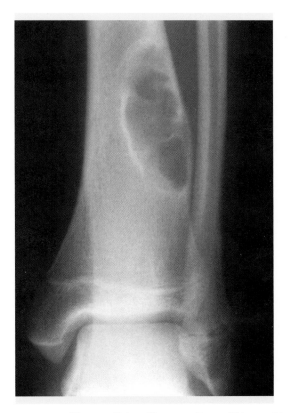

FIGURE 37-28. Nonossifying fibroma. From Skinner H. *Current Diagnosis and Treatment in Orthopedics*, 5th ed. New York, NY: McGraw-Hill; 2013: Fig. 5-22.

of this lesion is observation because most of them will resolve. Surgery, curettage, and bone grafting are indicated if there is risk for pathologic fracture, if the patient is symptomatic, or if more than 75% of the cortex is involved.

Ewing tumor is a small round cell sarcoma. It is a malignant tumor found in children and young adults, who usually present with pain and may have fevers. The most common locations include the pelvis, distal femur, proximal tibia, femoral diaphysis, and proximal humerus. The radiographs reveal a destructive lesion that may be purely lytic or have some reactive new bone (see Fig. 37-29). There is often a large soft tissue component, and the periosteum may be lifted off in layers, creating the classic radiographic onionskin appearance. Treatment involves multiagent chemotherapy, irradiation, and surgical resection. Ewing tumor is associated with a translocation of chromosomes 11 and 22, resulting in a fusion protein EWS-FLI 1, which is a transcription factor.

Giant cell tumor is a benign tumor; however, it can be locally aggressive and can rarely metastasize to the lungs. It is most common in the third and fourth decades of

life. It is most commonly found in the epiphysis of long bones. Patients may present with pain, and radiographs reveal a purely lytic, well-circumscribed lesion within the metaphysis (see Fig. 37-30). Treatment involves careful removal of the lesion, with preservation of the

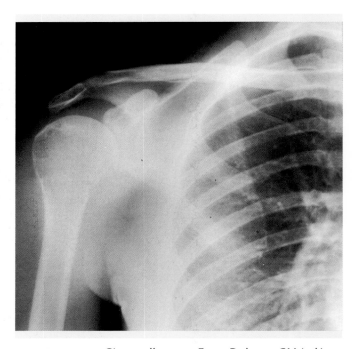

FIGURE 37-30. Giant cell tumor. From Doherty GM (ed.). *Current Diagnosis & Treatment: Surgery*, 14th ed. New York, NY: McGraw-Hill; 2015: Fig. 40-39.

surrounding joint. Giant cell tumor has a high incidence of local recurrence.

Osteosarcoma is a malignant primary bone tumor, second only to multiple myeloma. It most commonly occurs around the knee (distal femur and proximal tibia) in children and young adults. Osteosarcoma can also occur in older patients who have received radiotherapy in the past or in patients with Paget disease. Most patients will present with pain. Most tumors are high-grade, destructive, bone-forming lesions. They often penetrate the cortex early and form a large soft tissue component. Radiographs reveal a poorly defined lesion with bone destruction and bone formation. Lesions involve the medullary canal and have periosteal reaction, such as Codman's triangle or sunburst pattern, which is indicative of rapid growth (see Fig. 37-31). On microscopic examination, there is osteoid production, and the cells are obviously malignant. Following appropriate staging, treatment involves multiagent chemotherapy and surgical resection.

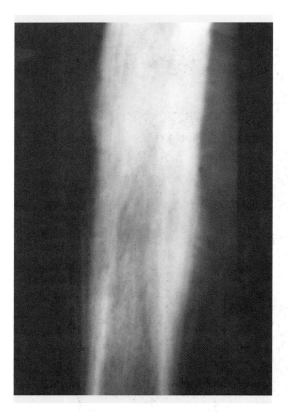

FIGURE 37-29. Ewing sarcoma. From Skinner H. *Current Diagnosis and Treatment in Orthopedics*, 5th ed. New York, NY: McGraw-Hill; 2013: Fig. 5-52.

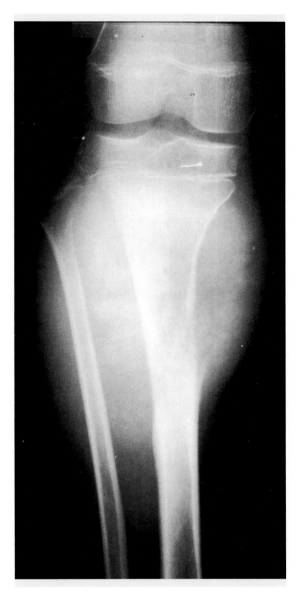

FIGURE 37-31. Osteosarcoma with Codman's triangle. From Doherty GM (ed.). *Current Diagnosis & Treatment: Surgery*, 14th ed. New York, NY: McGraw-Hill; 2015:40-38.

Fibrosarcoma is a malignant soft tissue sarcoma or fibrous tumor. Patients usually present with a mass that is enlarging and relatively painless. Plain radiographs are often normal except in advanced cases where there is involvement of the bone resulting in destructive changes. Treatment involves wide local excision and radiation therapy for larger tumors greater than 5 cm. These particular radiographs reveal a lesion that has a typical appearance for a nonossifying fibroma/metaphyseal fibrous defect. It has sclerotic, scalloped margins and has a benign appearance. It is not aggressive in

appearance as would be expected with osteosarcoma or Ewing sarcoma. The fact that the patient presented with a pathologic fracture and no prior symptoms supports the slow-growing, less aggressive nature of this lesion. Giant cell tumors are epiphyseal in location and uncommon in children with open physes. Fibrosarcoma is similar in appearance to osteosarcoma and is found in patients age 30–80 years.

BIBLIOGRAPHY

Frassica FJ, Frassica DA, McCarthy EF. Orthopaedic pathology. In: Miller MD, Brinker MR (eds.), *Review of Orthopaedics*, 3rd ed. Philadelphia, PA: W.B. Saunders; 2000:379–440.

Jones KB. Musculoskeletal oncology. In: Flynn JM (ed.), *Orthopaedic Knowledge Update 10*. Rosemont, IL: American Academy of Orthopaedic Surgeons; 2011:193–212.

Milbrandt T, Iwinski HJ, Talwakar VR. Pediatric tumors and hematologic diseases. In: Flynn JM (ed.), *Orthopaedic Knowledge Update 10*. Rosemont, IL: American Academy of Orthopaedic Surgeons; 2011:825–835.

16. **(E)** Any time there is soft tissue injury or fracture of an extremity, a thorough neurologic assessment of the peripheral nerves is critical once the appropriate advanced trauma life support (ATLS) protocols have been followed. This should include a detailed assessment of motor, sensory, and vascular status. This particular patient has a significant soft tissue injury involving the volar and ulnar aspects of the forearm. This creates suspicion for injury to the median nerve as well as the ulnar nerve based on their locations within the forearm. The median nerve enters the forearm by splitting the heads of the pronator teres muscle. It then runs down the forearm deep to the flexor digitorum superficialis and on the surface of the flexor digitorum profundus muscle. It provides sensory distribution to the hand as outlined in Fig. 37-32.

Motor innervation is provided proximally to the flexor carpi radialis (FCR), flexor digitorum superficialis (FDS), and flexor digitorum profundus (FDP; index and long). Distally, the motor innervation continues to the thenar eminence including the abductor pollicis brevis, flexor pollicis brevis, and opponens pollicis. The anterior interosseous is an important branch from the median nerve in the proximal aspect of the forearm. This courses distally to innervate the flexor pollicis longus, pronator quadratus, and flexor digitorum profundus to the index and long fingers. The median nerve function cannot be evaluated by specific reflex testing. The ulnar nerve travels along the medial aspect of the forearm on the flexor digitorum profundus muscle and deep to the flexor carpi ulnaris muscle. It lies in close proximity to the ulnar artery, which is just lateral. A dorsal cutaneous branch emerges from the ulnar nerve approximately 5–10 cm

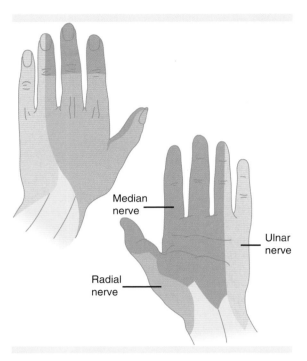

FIGURE 37-32. Sensory innervation of the hand. From Doherty GM (ed.). *Current Diagnosis & Treatment: Surgery,* 14th ed. New York, NY: McGraw-Hill; 2015: Fig. 42-9.

above the wrist. The intrinsic muscles of the hand allow the patient to cross his fingers and are innervated by the ulnar nerve. Urgent nerve conduction studies and an EMG are not practical in the ED and are unnecessary. Asking the patient to extend his thumb at the IP joint specifically involves the extensor pollicis longus, which is innervated by the radial nerve. Only by assessing the most distal innervation of the median nerve, the abductor pollicis brevis, and by assessing sensation in the appropriate distribution can the integrity of the median nerve be evaluated.

BIBLIOGRAPHY

Netter FH. *The Ciba Collection of Medical Illustrations. Volume 8— Musculoskeletal System, Part I: Anatomy Physiology and Metabolic Disorders.* Summit, NJ: Ciba-Geigy; 2001:45–58.

17. **(B)** Fat embolism is the unexpected development of hypoxia, confusion, and petechiae within a few days after long bone fractures. It is usually seen 24–72 hours following trauma. It occurs in 3–4% of patients with long bone fractures and can be fatal in 10–15% of patients. Fat embolism syndrome (FES) seems to affect young adult patients with lower extremity fractures. Often the fractures are closed. FES consists of the triad of symptoms described earlier. Additional symptoms include tachypnea and tachycardia. Sixty percent of cases are seen in the first 24 hours, and 90% appear within 72 hours. Gurd and Wilson's criteria for FES are commonly referenced (Table 37-1). The diagnosis is made when one major and four minor signs are present in addition to macroglobulinemia. Use of these criteria is often criticized for not considering blood gas in the criteria. Clinically when partial pressure of oxygen (PO_2) is less than 60 mmHg, the patient is in the early stages of FES. Embolization of fat and marrow contents is part of the inciting events in FES; however, other events occur to cause the injury to the lungs, brain, and other tissues. Although the exact pathomechanics of FES have not been completely defined, two prevailing theories exist. The mechanical theory suggests that fat droplets enter the circulation and create a mechanical obstruction of the pulmonary vasculature because the droplets are larger than the small vessels in the lungs. The biomechanical theory postulates that mediators from the fracture site create a cascade of events that leads to activation of the clotting cascade and chemical injury to the vascular endothelial cells and subsequent increased pulmonary permeability. Prevention of FES is critical because it can be fatal. Proper fracture splinting, use of oxygen in the postinjury period, and early surgical stabilization of long bone fractures are three measures that can reduce the incidence of FES. Large doses of steroids immediately after injury may have a beneficial effect on FES, most likely by reducing damage from free fatty acids; however, routine use of steroids is not without significant risks, which may outweigh the benefits. Therefore, currently, treatment methods are mainly with oxygen and ventilatory support. High levels of positive end-expiratory pressure (PEEP) are frequently required, and early recognition is the key to preventing a potential devastating course of events.

TABLE 37-1 Lumbar Disc Herniations

Level	Nerve Root	Motor	Sensory	Reflex
L3-L4	L4	Quadriceps, Tibialis anterior	Medial calf	Knee Jerk
L4-5	L5	EHL, EDL	Dorsal foot, medial calf	None
L5-S1	S1	Gastroc/Soleus	Plantar foot, Posterior calf	Ankle Jerk

BIBLIOGRAPHY

Brinker MR. Basic sciences: section 6—perioperative problems. In: Miller MD, Brinker MR (eds.), *Review of Orthopaedics*, 3rd ed. Philadelphia, PA: W.B. Saunders; 2000:109.

Roberts CS, Gleis GE, Seligson D. Diagnosis and treatment of complications. In: Browner BD, Jupiter JB, Levine AE, et al. (eds.), *Skeletal Trauma*, 3rd ed. Philadelphia, PA: W.B. Saunders; 2003:437–441.

Schemitsch EL, Bhandari M. Complications. In: Bucholz RW, Heckman JD (eds.), *Rockwood and Green's Fractures in Adults*, 5th ed. Philadelphia, PA: Lippincott Williams & Wilkins; 2001:479–489.

18. **(C)** Femoral shaft fractures most commonly occur in young patients secondary to high-energy trauma. They are classified into three types: spiral, transverse, or oblique shaft fractures; comminuted femoral shaft fractures; and open femoral shaft fractures. Displaced femoral shaft fractures are best treated with antegrade intramedullary nailing. Closed intramedullary nailing involves minimal soft tissue dissection and provides stable fixation. An intramedullary nail is a load-sharing device and has union rates of 99% with few complications. The nails should be locked statically. This does not impact fracture healing. Reaming of the femoral canal results in pulmonary embolization of fat and bone marrow contents. This leads to concern regarding exacerbation of an underlying pulmonary injury; however, technique, reamer design, and reamer sharpness all affect this degree of embolization, and the clinical significance is debated. This patient's pneumothorax, multiple rib injuries, and findings consistent with a pulmonary contusion, although consistent with underlying pulmonary injury, should not prohibit the treatment of this patient's femoral shaft fracture with an intramedullary nail.

A delay in stabilization of the femur limits mobilization of the patient, prolongs the hospital stay, and may subsequently worsen the pulmonary injury. Skeletal traction is rarely indicated as the only form of treatment. It is a rapid means to provide length and stability as a temporizing measure in unstable trauma patients. Definitive treatment with traction predisposes a patient to the added risks of remaining in bed and is rarely indicated unless the patient has many significant medical comorbidities. These risks are even magnified in the trauma patient. External fixation, likewise, is rarely indicated as definitive treatment. It is generally used acutely only as a temporary method of stabilization in a patient who has a vascular injury or may be hypothermic or coagulopathic and requires further resuscitation. Once the patient is stabilized, the external fixator is removed and converted to intramedullary fixation. External fixation may be used definitively in children, where open physes preclude the use of intramedullary nails.

BIBLIOGRAPHY

Nelson R. General principles. In: Sherman SC (ed.), *Simon's Emergency Orthopedics*, 7th ed. New York, NY: McGraw-Hill; 2014.

Siegel J, Tornetta P III. Femoral fractures. In: Flynn JM (ed.), *Orthopaedic Knowledge Update 10*. Rosemont, IL: American Academy of Orthopaedic Surgeons; 2011:431–442.

19. **(E)** Humeral shaft fractures are a relatively common orthopedic occurrence. A variety of methods are available for the treatment of these fractures with good results. Increased concern develops when there is an associated neurovascular injury. The proximity of the brachial plexus and vascular structures of the shoulder make them vulnerable in an injury to the shoulder girdle. The radial nerve is the most vulnerable nerve in a shaft fracture because of its location as it spirals around the humerus and descends through the upper arm. Radial nerve injury with a shaft fracture occurs in up to 18% of patients. The distal-third oblique shaft fracture (Holstein-Lewis) is the most widely associated with radial nerve injury; however, it is the middle-third fracture that actually has the highest incidence of radial nerve palsy. Most nerve injuries are true "palsies" or neurapraxias. EMG studies can help evaluate the degree of nerve injury and follow the recovery; however, most patients recover in 3–4 months. For this reason, the treatment of a closed fracture with a nerve palsy is not an indication for surgery, and most fractures will heal with nonoperative treatment and most of the nerve deficits will resolve. Historically, a nerve palsy that develops following manipulation has been considered an indication for open treatment; however, observation is currently recommended.

The only absolute indication for surgical treatment is an open fracture with a nerve injury. Surgical exploration of a nerve injury is generally recommended after 3–4 months if there has been no recovery. An accurate understanding of radial nerve anatomy and innervation allows a thorough examination and subsequent management if a deficit is identified. The radial nerve begins as the terminating branch of the posterior cord of the brachial plexus. It contains nerve bundles from nerve roots C5 to T1, the entire brachial plexus. It passes with the deep brachial artery through the triangular interval formed by the long and lateral heads of the triceps and the lower border of the teres major muscles. It then comes in close proximity to the bone as it lies in the groove for the radial nerve on the posterior aspect of the humerus. It is here where it can become lacerated by fracture fragments or become entrapped between fracture fragments. The radial nerve provides no innervation in the proximal arm. The sensory distribution is most reliably tested in the dorsal web space between the thumb and index finger. The motor innervation generally involves all extensors of the wrist and hand, and any deficit in extension of the wrist or fingers is indicative of injury to the radial nerve. Inability to flex the thumb at the IP joint indicates anterior interosseous nerve injury and loss of the flexor pollicis longus. This is seen in supracondylar humerus fractures in children. Decreased sensation over the volar aspect of the thumb and index finger represents the median nerve distribution. The ulnar nerve innervates the small finger and ulnar border of the ring finger. Injury to this nerve may occasionally be seen in injuries around the elbow. The lateral antebrachial cutaneous nerve, the terminal branch of the musculocutaneous nerve, innervates the lateral border of the forearm.

BIBLIOGRAPHY

Abboud JA, Boardman ND III. Shoulder trauma: bone. In: Flynn JM (ed.), *Orthopaedic Knowledge Update 10*. Rosemont, IL: American Academy of Orthopaedic Surgeons; 2011:271–284.

Gregory PR Jr. Fractures of the shaft of the humerus. In: Bucholz RW, Heckman JD (eds.), *Rockwood and Green's Fractures in Adults*, 5th ed. Philadelphia, PA: Lippincott Williams & Wilkins; 2001:991–992.

Netter FH. *The Ciba Collection of Medical Illustrations. Volume 8— Musculoskeletal System, Part I: Anatomy Physiology and Metabolic Disorders*. Summit, NJ: Ciba-Geigy; 2001:28–31, 38–39, 53.

Schemitsch EL, Bhandari M. Complications. In: Browner BD, Jupiter JB, Levine AE, et al. (eds.), *Skeletal Trauma*, 3rd ed. Philadelphia, PA: W.B. Saunders; 2003:1504–1505.

20. **(E)** High-energy pelvic injuries are associated with significant injury to the surrounding soft tissues and can lead to disruption of the pelvic floor. These patients should also be carefully assessed for a urethral injury. Associated urologic injury occurs in up to 15% of pelvic fractures and is more common in males. The most common physical findings of urethral disruption are high-riding prostate and blood at the meatus. Hematuria may also be found but is more indicative of bladder injury. Occasionally inability to freely pass a Foley catheter may be the first sign of injury. In a hemodynamically normal male patient, a retrograde urethrogram should be obtained prior to placing a Foley catheter. In a hemodynamically abnormal male patient, one attempt at placement of a Foley catheter is appropriate. Placement of a Foley catheter can be attempted in females without obtaining an urethrogram because the urethra is short. This patient has a pelvic fracture with associated perineal swelling, a scrotal hematoma, and blood at the meatus; therefore, a retrograde urethrogram should be obtained prior to inserting a Foley catheter. Inserting a Foley catheter should only be performed after a urethral injury has been ruled out, and this is most accurately done through a retrograde urethrogram.

This patient's retrograde urethrogram (see Fig. 37-33) confirms the suspected genitourinary injury. An intravenous

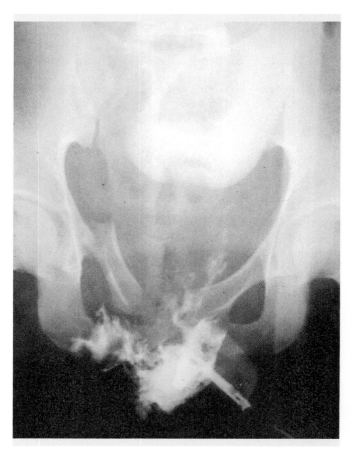

FIGURE 37-33. Retrograde urethrogram. From Mattox K, Moore E, Feliciano D (eds.), *Trauma*, 7th ed. New York, NY: McGraw-Hill; 2012: Fig. 36-14A.

pyelogram would not provide sufficient information about the lower genitourinary tract. A pelvic external fixator is a key component of management of a hemodynamically unstable patient, but would not assist in evaluating the lower genitourinary tract. It would provide stability to the pelvis; however, this could be temporarily performed with use of a sheet or pelvic binder. The placement of an external fixator or definitive open reduction and fixation of the pelvic fracture should be coordinated with the urologist. Proper communication will allow simultaneous management and hopefully definitive care of the urologic injury and the fracture. CT scans of the abdomen without contrast do not adequately image general urinary tract trauma.

BIBLIOGRAPHY

Jones AL, Burgess AR. Fractures of the pelvic ring. In: Bucholz RW, Heckman JD (eds.), *Rockwood and Green's Fractures in Adults*, 5th ed. Philadelphia, PA: Lippincott Williams & Wilkins; 2001:1495–1496.

Kellam JF, Mayo K. Pelvic ring disruptions. In: Browner BD, Jupiter JB, Levine AE, et al. (eds.), *Skeletal Trauma*, 3rd ed. Philadelphia, PA: W.B. Saunders; 2003:1102.

Sagi HC, Liporace FA. Fractures of the pelvis and acetabulum. In: Flynn JM (ed.), *Orthopaedic Knowledge Update 10*. Rosemont, IL: American Academy of Orthopaedic Surgeons; 2011:379–398.

21. **(E)** Patients with hip dislocations must be carefully assessed for a femoral head fracture. Posterior femoral head dislocations are associated with a 7% incidence of femoral head fracture. Although much less common, anterior dislocations are associated with a higher rate of fracture. Radiographs should include an AP pelvis and AP and lateral views of the injured hip. By uncovering some overlap of the hip and pelvis, Judet views may uncover a fracture not easily visible on the initial films. The most important task is prompt reduction of the femoral head. Like hip dislocations, femoral head reduction should be considered an orthopedic emergency, and reduction should be accomplished as quickly and atraumatically as possible. This may be performed with adequate conscious sedation in the ED; however, generally anesthesia is warranted if any difficulty is encountered. Care must also be taken to avoid possible displacement of an associated nondisplaced femoral neck fracture. If a hip dislocation is irreversible and associated with a femoral head fracture, treatment requires open reduction, usually from the direction of the dislocation. Following reduction, an AP radiograph can evaluate concentricity of the hip joint. A CT scan is necessary to assess the quality of reduction and to evaluate any potential loosed body within the joint.

The most commonly used classification system for femoral head fractures is that of Pipkin. This system divides the femoral head fractures at the fovea and identifies the location of the fracture, which correlates with initial treatment. The preferred treatment is anatomic reduction. Closed reduction may be used for Pipkin type I fractures, because they do not involve the weight-bearing portion of the femoral head. ORIF is otherwise the standard for Pipkin types II, III, and IV, as opposed to excision of the fragment. Any step off or deformity at the fracture is not well tolerated and can lead to increased risk of posttraumatic arthritis. Type III fractures, which have an associated femoral neck fracture, require fixation of the femoral neck fracture, followed by ORIF of the femoral head. Type IV fractures, which have an associated acetabular fracture, can be managed surgically with a posterior approach with a digastric osteotomy. The risk of posttraumatic arthritis and osteonecrosis is high. Type I fractures and type II fractures have rates similar to simple dislocations. Type III fractures have a poor prognosis with 50% rate of posttraumatic osteonecrosis. Type IV fractures have about the same prognosis as acetabular fractures.

BIBLIOGRAPHY

Leighton RK, Lammens P. Hip dislocations and fractures of the femoral head. In: Kellam JF, Fischer TJ, Tornetta P III (eds.), *Orthopaedic Knowledge Update: Trauma 2*. Rosemont, IL: American Academy of Orthopaedic Surgeons; 2000:314–316.

Motley GS, Eddings TH III, Moore RS. Adult trauma. In: Miller MD, Brinker MR (eds.), *Review of Orthopaedics*, 3rd ed. Philadelphia, PA: W.B. Saunders; 2000:477.

Mullis B, Anglen J. Hip trauma. In: Flynn JM (ed.), *Orthopaedic Knowledge Update 10*. Rosemont, IL: American Academy of Orthopaedic Surgeons; 2011:399–411.

Swiontkowski MF. Intracapsular hip fractures. In: Browner BD, Jupiter JB, Levine AE, et al. (eds.), *Skeletal Trauma*, 3rd ed. Philadelphia, PA: W.B. Saunders; 2003:1700–1714.

Tornetta P III. Hip dislocations and fractures of the femoral head. In: Bucholz RW, Heckman JD (eds.), *Rockwood and Green's Fractures in Adults*, 5th ed. Philadelphia, PA: Lippincott Williams & Wilkins; 2001:1547–1576.

22. **(A)** Acute compartment syndrome (ACS) is defined as elevated tissue pressures within a closed, nondistensible space or compartment. This can reduce muscle and nerve tissue perfusion below levels necessary for tissue viability. The most common causes are fractures, soft tissue trauma, arterial injury, limb compression, burns, and bleeding disorders. Chronic exertional compartment syndrome (CECS) is a reversible elevation of tissue pressure brought on by exercise that returns to normal between periods of activity. It is most common in long-distance runners and military recruits. Iatrogenic ACS can result from tight closure of fascial defects, excessive traction of fractured limbs, intravenous (IV) infiltration, and circumferential casts/splints. Although the mechanisms of ACS and CECS may differ, the pathogenesis is similar. Swelling and edema within the compartment cause increased tissue pressure. Increased tissue pressure leads to increased local venous pressure. As venous pressure increases, the A-V pressure gradient is decreased and can result in decreased local blood flow. Capillary basement membranes may become leaky, compounding the problem. If blood flow drops below metabolic demands, the tissues become ischemic, and viability is compromised. Clinically, this results in pain, dysfunction, dysesthesia, and potentially muscle necrosis.

ACS is primarily a clinical diagnosis; severe pain out of proportion to injury is the hallmark. A swollen and tense compartment that is painful to palpation is also a finding. Pain with passive stretch is a reliable sign in an alert patient. Paresthesia or weakness because of nerve or muscle ischemia is a late finding. Intracompartmental pressures rarely exceed systolic blood pressure, so peripheral pulses are present, and an absent pulse is never a finding unless there is an associated arterial injury. In addition, digital capillaries may drain into extracompartmental veins, so capillary refill is not a good indicator of tissue perfusion within a compartment. Capillary refill may be slow but is often normal. Diagnosis becomes more difficult in an unconscious or obtunded patient.

Without the benefit of appropriate history and physical examination, measurement of compartment pressures becomes the only means to diagnose the condition. There are several methods of measurement available; however, uniform consensus as to when fasciotomy is warranted is lacking. Normal pressures range from 0–10 mmHg, and pressures of 30–45 mmHg have been recommended as the threshold for decompression. However, the difference between the diastolic and compartment pressures is more reliable, with decompression recommended when pressures are within 10–30 mmHg of the patient's diastolic pressure. The use of 30–35 mmHg as an absolute pressure may be adequate; however, the patient's clinical status and diastolic blood pressure must be considered. It is critical to remove any tight or constricting dressings on a patient with symptoms of ACS. Limb position should be at the level of the heart to promote arterial inflow. It has been shown that elevation reduces mean arterial pressure and, as a result, reduces blood flow to the compartment. ACS is most common in the leg but may occur in the forearm, hand, foot, thigh, arm, shoulder, and buttocks. Management is by surgical decompression of the involved compartments. Skin, fat, and fascial layers must all be decompressed. Fasciotomy wounds should be left open, and repeat inspection and debridement are performed after 48 hours. There are various mechanical methods available to assist with closure, but this is ultimately by delayed skin closure or split-thickness skin grafts. Pain associated with a tense and swollen compartment and worsening pain with passive stretch are the earliest findings in ACS. Surgical decompression is the standard treatment for ACS, and if delayed, irreversible damage to muscle or nerves may occur.

BIBLIOGRAPHY

Amendola A, Twaddle BC. Compartment syndromes. In: Browner BD, Jupiter JB, Levine AE, et al. (eds.), *Skeletal Trauma*, 3rd ed. Philadelphia, PA: W.B. Saunders; 2003:268–290.

Gardner MJ. Fractures about the knee. In: Flynn JM (ed.), *Orthopaedic Knowledge Update 10*. Rosemont, IL: American Academy of Orthopaedic Surgeons; 2011:443–452.

Heppenstall RB, McCombs PR, DeLaurentis DA. Vascular injuries and compartment syndromes. In: Bucholz RW, Heckman JD (eds.), *Rockwood and Green's Fractures in Adults*, 5th ed. Philadelphia, PA: Lippincott Williams & Wilkins; 2001:331–350.

Lang GJ. Fractures of the tibial diaphysis. In: Kellam JF, Fischer TJ, Tornetta P III (eds.), *Orthopaedic Knowledge Update: Trauma 2*. Rosemont, IL: American Academy of Orthopaedic Surgeons; 2000:185–186.

Miller MD. Sports medicine. In: Miller MD, Brinker MR (eds.), *Review of Orthopaedics*, 3rd ed. Philadelphia, PA: W.B. Saunders; 2000:213.

Motley GS, Eddings TH III, Moore RS. Adult trauma. In: Miller MD, Brinker MR (eds.), *Review of Orthopaedics*, 3rd ed. Philadelphia, PA: W.B. Saunders; 2000:463.

Netter FH. *The Ciba Collection of Medical Illustrations. Volume 8—Musculoskeletal System, Part I: Anatomy Physiology and Metabolic Disorders*. Summit, NJ: Ciba-Geigy; 2001:98–103.

23. **(A)** There are no muscles that attach to the talus, and more than 60% of the surface is covered with articular cartilage. It is supported by its bony architecture and ligamentous restraints between the tibia and the calcaneus. Three major arteries supply the talar body by forming a vascular ring at the neck of the talus. The artery of the tarsal canal arises from the posterior tibial artery. The deltoid artery also arises from the posterior tibial artery and may be the only remaining circulation in many fractures of the talus. The third, the sinus tarsi artery, arises from the anterior and peroneal arteries. The circulation to the talar body is vulnerable in fractures and dislocations. This is in part because of the retrograde flow that must occur to supply the body from the circulation at the neck. Fractures may occur in any part of the talus, but more than 50% involve the neck. The Hawkins classification system is the most commonly used.

Displaced talar neck fractures are an orthopedic emergency, and urgent reduction is required to restore circulation. Anatomic alignment of the fracture is one of the most important factors affecting outcome. The preferred approach uses medial and lateral incisions to restore anatomic alignment, assess the degree of comminution, explore, debride the subtalar joint of any debris, and finally insert hardware. Early range of motion is encouraged, and patients are kept non–weight bearing until union at the fracture site. Complications encountered include delayed union and nonunion, arthritis, malunion, and osteonecrosis. Delayed union occurs when there is no healing evident at 6 months, and nonunion occurs when there is no healing at 12 months. Arthritis has been reported to occur in 50% of cases in the subtalar joint, 33% in the tibiotalar joint, and 25% in both. Malunion involves varus malposition, which results in hindfoot varus and forefoot adduction. Patients are forced to walk on the lateral border of their foot. A custom orthosis may relieve the subsequent pain, but often osteotomy or fusions are required and can be unpredictable. Finally, osteonecrosis is related to the severity of the injury and subsequent disruption of circulation. During follow-up, an AP radiograph of the ankle at 6–8 weeks may reveal subchondral lucency (Hawkins sign) within the talus. This is a positive finding indicating there is restoration of circulation to the talar body. Absence of the sign, however, does not absolutely indicate osteonecrosis. If osteonecrosis is diagnosed after 3 months, patients are not kept non–weight bearing. There is no evidence indicating that outcome is improved with prolonged non–weight bearing. If patients go on to develop collapse, salvage is usually with a tibiotalar or tibiocalcaneal fusion.

BIBLIOGRAPHY

DiGiovanni CW, Benirschke SK, Hansen ST. Foot injuries. In: Browner BD, Jupiter JB, Levine AE, et al. (eds.), *Skeletal Trauma*, 3rd ed. Philadelphia, PA: W.B. Saunders; 2003:2379–2397.

Heckman JD. Fractures of the talus. In: Bucholz RW, Heckman JD (eds.), *Rockwood and Green's Fractures in Adults*, 5th ed. Philadelphia, PA: Lippincott Williams & Wilkins; 2001:2091–2128.

Motley GS, Eddings TH III, Moore RS. Adult trauma. In: Miller MD, Brinker MR (eds.), *Review of Orthopaedics*, 3rd ed. Philadelphia, PA: W.B. Saunders; 2000:491–493.

Stephen DJG. Ankle and foot injuries. In: Kellam JF, Fischer TJ, Tornetta P III (eds.), *Orthopaedic Knowledge Update: Trauma 2*. Rosemont, IL: American Academy of Orthopaedic Surgeons; 2000:210–213.

Yoo BJ, Giza E. Foot trauma. In: Flynn JM (ed.), *Orthopaedic Knowledge Update 10*. Rosemont, IL: American Academy of Orthopaedic Surgeons; 2011:507–522.

24. **(A)** A pathologic fracture is one that occurs in abnormal bone. These fractures often result from minimal to no trauma and may even occur during events of everyday normal activity. Osteoporosis is the most common condition associated with pathologic fractures. Other conditions include Paget disease, osteomalacia, osteogenesis imperfecta, osteopetrosis, a primary bone lesion, and metastatic bone lesions. Plain radiographs should be closely evaluated. While the lesion may be obvious, the entire extent of the bone should be examined; the remainder of the skeleton should also be examined with plain radiographs if the lesion appears metastatic. The spine, ribs, pelvis, femur, and humerus are the most common sites of metastasis to bone. Further identification of the primary lesion is important. A bone scan is the most efficient means to identify occult metastatic sites. A chest radiograph, breast examination, and mammogram can assess for metastatic breast and lung carcinoma, the two most common metastases to bone. Renal, thyroid, and prostate are the other three cancers that commonly produce metastatic lesions to bone. A careful physical examination, baseline laboratory studies, prostate-specific antigen, and abdominal ultrasound or chest CT scan will further identify most of these primary sites. In treatment of pathologic fractures, the goal is to provide surgical stabilization. This is more difficult in the diseased bone due to slowed healing relative to normal bone. All patients should also receive adjuvant irradiation beginning about 3 weeks after surgery, which does not increase the incidence of nonunions. Long bone fractures are generally stabilized with an intramedullary implant when available, as this provides a load-sharing construct as well as prophylactic fixation for the entire length of the bone. Another component of preoperative assessment includes the need for embolization. Renal cell carcinoma is extremely vascular and can result in significant intraoperative blood loss. In this situation, a known primary or suspicion of renal cell carcinoma requires an angiogram and embolization.

BIBLIOGRAPHY

Springfield DS. Pathologic fractures. In: Bucholz RW, Heckman JD (eds.), *Rockwood and Green's Fractures in Adults*, 5th ed. Philadelphia, PA: Lippincott Williams & Wilkins; 2001:557–580.

25. **(E)** This patient has a burst fracture at the C6–C7 level with complete cord injury. A complete cord injury indicates loss of motor and sensory function at all levels below the level of injury (Table 37-2). Therefore, patellar tendon reflexes and ankle plantar flexion would be lost. Finger

TABLE 37-2 Functional Level after Spinal Cord Injury

Functioning Level	Working	Not Working	Mobility/ADLs
Above C4		Diaphragm, Upper extremity muscles	Respirator dependent
C4	Diaphragm, Trapezius	Upper extremity muscles	Wheelchair, chin/puff
C5	Elbow flexors	Below elbow	Electric wheelchair
C6	Wrist extensors	Elbow extensors	Manual wheelchair, flexor hinge
C7	Elbow extensors	Grasp	Manual wheelchair–independent, Cut meat
L2	Iliopsoas	Knee/ankle	KAFO, Household ambulation
L3	Quadriceps	Ankle	AFO, Community ambulation

abduction and adduction are primarily functions of T1, so these would also be lost. Elbow flexion is primarily derived from C5 and C6, so some weakness could be detected with resisted testing. Shoulder abduction, however, is primarily from C5, so this likely would be spared.

BIBLIOGRAPHY

Netter FH. *The Ciba Collection of Medical Illustrations. Volume 8— Musculoskeletal System, Part I: Anatomy Physiology and Metabolic Disorders*. Summit, NJ: Ciba-Geigy; 2001:29.

CHAPTER 38

UROLOGIC SURGERY

TANYA DAVIS, GINA LOCKWOOD, AND CARLEY DAVIS

QUESTIONS

1. A 19-year-old man undergoes a left radical orchiectomy for a painless left testicular mass. Pathology reveals embryonal carcinoma (40%), yolk sac tumor (20%), and teratoma (40%). Serum α-fetoprotein (AFP) and β-human chorionic gonadotropin (β-hCG) were both elevated preoperatively. A computed tomography (CT) scan reveals moderate para-aortic lymphadenopathy, and the patient receives three courses of platinum-based chemotherapy. Following chemotherapy, his tumor markers normalize, and a follow-up CT is shown in Fig. 38-1. What is the most appropriate next step?

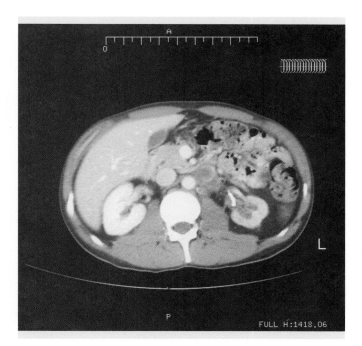

FIGURE 38-1. Abdominal computed tomography scan showing para-aortic lymphadenopathy.

(A) Observation
(B) Repeat tumor markers and CT in 3 months
(C) Administer one additional cycle of platinum-based chemotherapy
(D) Administer two additional cycles of platinum-based chemotherapy
(E) Retroperitoneal lymph node dissection (RPLND)

2. Which of the following is the most important prognostic indicator for patients with renal cell carcinoma?
(A) Tumor size
(B) Tumor grade
(C) Histologic subtype
(D) Performance status
(E) Pathologic stage

3. A 32-year-old man presents for evaluation prior to a vasectomy. Physical examination reveals a normal phallus, and the testicles are descended bilaterally without any palpable masses. The right vas deferens is normal, but the left is absent. What is the most appropriate next step?
(A) Scrotal ultrasound
(B) Renal ultrasound
(C) CT of abdomen
(D) Transrectal ultrasound
(E) Right vasogram

4. A 20-year-old man sustains a gunshot wound to the abdomen. He undergoes an emergent laparotomy and is found to have a complete transection of the left ureter at the pelvic brim. Which technique of repair is most appropriate?
(A) Ureteral reimplantation
(B) Primary reanastamosis
(C) Transureteroureterostomy
(D) End cutaneous ureterostomy
(E) Ureteral reimplantation with Boari flap

5. A 12-year-old boy presents to the emergency department with acute scrotal pain and swelling for 4 hours. On examination, his left hemiscrotum is edematous, erythematous, and exquisitely tender to touch. Vital signs are as follows: temperature (T) 99.9°F, heart rate (HR) 125 bpm, and blood pressure (BP) 126/60 mmHg. An ultrasound with Doppler is obtained and is shown in Fig. 38-2. What is the most likely diagnosis?
   (A) Epididymitis
   (B) Testicular cancer
   (C) Acute testicular torsion
   (D) Torsion of the appendix testis
   (E) Orchitis

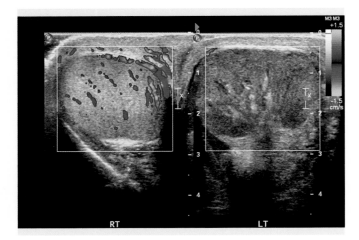

FIGURE 38-2. Scrotal ultrasound. From Schrope B. *Surgical and Interventional Ultrasound.* New York, NY: McGraw-Hill; 2013:Fig. 13-14.

6. A 60-year-old man with a history of diverticulitis presents with complaints of recurrent urinary tract infections and passing air when he urinates. He has no recent history of catheterization or genitourinary tract instrumentation. What is the most sensitive and specific modality to make the diagnosis?
   (A) CT scan
   (B) Cystoscopy
   (C) Colonoscopy
   (D) Oral administration of active charcoal
   (E) Bourne test (first voided urine following a barium enema is immediately centrifuged and then examined radiographically for radiodense particles)

7. Which of the following bacteria is most commonly associated with infected renal calculi?
   (A) *Escherichia coli*
   (B) *Ureaplasma urealyticum*
   (C) *Staphylococcus epidermidis*
   (D) *Klebsiella pneumonia*
   (E) *Proteus mirabilis*

8. A 50-year-old woman undergoes a radical hysterectomy for invasive endometrial carcinoma. The operation was complicated by excessive bleeding during division and ligation of the right uterine artery. On postoperative day 3, she develops persistent right flank pain, nausea, and vomiting. Physical examination reveals significant discomfort in the right upper quadrant and severe costovertebral angle (CVA) tenderness. Vital signs are as follows: T 102.1°F, HR 119 bpm, and BP 91/46 mmHg. CT urogram is performed and shows right hydroureteronephrosis with abrupt termination of contrast drainage in the mid to distal ureter on delayed images. What is the most appropriate next step?
   (A) Percutaneous nephrostomy tube
   (B) Observation
   (C) Reexploration and open repair
   (D) Ureteroscopy
   (E) Pain medication and antiemetics

9. A 50-year-old man presents with complaints of acute-onset scrotal pain and vague abdominal discomfort. Physical examination demonstrates a new grade III varicocele on the right. The remainder of the genitourinary exam is normal. What is the most appropriate next step?
   (A) Observation
   (B) Varicocelectomy
   (C) Scrotal ultrasound
   (D) CT scan of the abdomen and pelvis
   (E) Percutaneous embolization of varicocele

10. An 18-year-old man presents after a high-speed motor vehicle crash. On physical examination, he has severe pelvic pain but the abdomen is nontender. Plain radiograph demonstrates a pelvic fracture. A Foley catheter is inserted with return of 75 mL of bloody urine, and a fluoroscopic cystogram is obtained including postdrainage films (see Fig. 38-3). What is the appropriate management in this patient?
   (A) Continued catheter drainage for 10–14 days
   (B) CT cystogram
   (C) Flexible cystoscopy
   (D) Suprapubic cystostomy tube placement
   (E) Open operative repair

11. A 55-year-old G3P3 woman undergoes an abdominal perineal resection for rectal malignancy. She returns for a follow-up visit complaining of urinary incontinence multiple times daily. The incontinence is not associated with coughing, sneezing, or laughing and is not preceded by a strong urge to urinate. Postvoid residual on bladder scan in the office shows 500 mL in the bladder. What type of incontinence is this patient most likely experiencing?
   (A) Stress incontinence
   (B) Urge incontinence

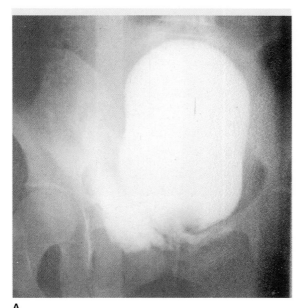

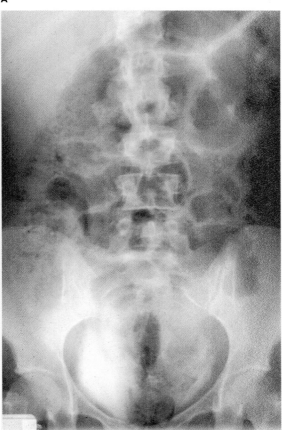

A

B

FIGURE 38-3.   A and B. Fluoroscopic cystograms. From Mattox K, Moore E, Feliciano D (eds.), *Trauma*, 7th ed. New York, NY: McGraw-Hill; 2012:Fig. 36-10.

(C)   Incontinence associated with a fistula
(D)   Overflow incontinence
(E)   Incontinence from a congenital abnormality

12.   A 17-year-old male patient presents to the emergency department with right flank pain after being kicked in the flank during soccer practice. On exam, he is found to be hemodynamically normal, and urinalysis is unremarkable. Hemoglobin and hematocrit are normal. Abdominal exam is normal, and right CVA tenderness is present. CT scan is obtained (see Fig. 38-4). What is the most likely diagnosis?
(A)   Renal mass
(B)   Renal laceration, grade 4, with perinephric hematoma
(C)   Renal laceration, grade 3
(D)   Urinoma
(E)   Ureteropelvic junction obstruction

13.   A 7-year-old girl is diagnosed with bilateral grade III vesicoureteral reflux after developing a urinary tract infection. A renal ultrasound reveals normal kidneys bilaterally, and she is started on prophylactic antibiotics. Three months later, she develops a temperature of 39°C. A urine culture done at that time grows >100,000 colony-forming units of *E coli*. The most appropriate management is treatment of the active infection and
(A)   Observation
(B)   Unilateral vesicoureteral reimplant
(C)   Bilateral vesicoureteral reimplants
(D)   Bilateral cutaneous ureterostomies until she is old enough to undergo reimplants
(E)   Bilateral percutaneous nephrostomy tubes to decompress the kidneys

14.   Which of the following statements concerning undescended testicles (cryptorchidism) is *false*?
(A)   In diagnostic laparoscopy, the observation of blind ending testicular vessels indicates a vanishing testis and requires no further exploration.
(B)   The risk of testis cancer does not decrease to that of normal controls even when orchidopexy is performed at an early age.
(C)   Ultrasound is an important adjunct in evaluating boys with cryptorchidism.
(D)   Testicles that remain undescended by 6 months (corrected for gestational age) are unlikely to descend spontaneously.
(E)   Hormonal therapy should not be used to induce testicular descent.

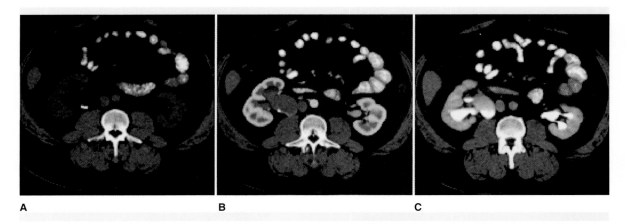

A   B   C

FIGURE 38-4. Abdominal computed tomography scan with contrast. From McDougal WS, Wein AJ, Kavoussi LR, et al. *Campbell-Walsh Urology*, 10th ed. New York, NY: Elsevier; 2011.

15. A 71-year-old man with a known solitary left kidney presents with a 3-week history of intermittent painless gross hematuria. His medical history is significant for hypertension and non–insulin-dependent diabetes mellitus. His serum creatinine is 2.0 mg/dL. Cystoscopy is performed and is negative. A retrograde pyelogram is performed at that time (see Fig. 38-5) and shows multiple small filling defects in the left ureter. Biopsy of the lesion during ureteroscopy is consistent with a low-grade superficial urothelial carcinoma. Which of the following is the most appropriate management?
    (A) Open radical nephroureterectomy with bladder cuff excision
    (B) Laparoscopic radical nephroureterectomy with bladder cuff excision
    (C) Segmental ureterectomy with ureteroureterostomy
    (D) Subtotal ureterectomy with psoas hitch ureteroneocystostomy
    (E) Ureteroscopy with endoscopic resection and laser ablation of the tumor

16. A 36-year-old woman with Crohn disease requires a partial small bowel resection. Six months following her surgery, she develops left flank pain. A CT scan reveals a 3-mm calculus in the left midureter. What is the most likely composition of the ureteral stone?
    (A) Calcium oxalate
    (B) Uric acid
    (C) Struvite
    (D) Cystine
    (E) Ammonium acid urate

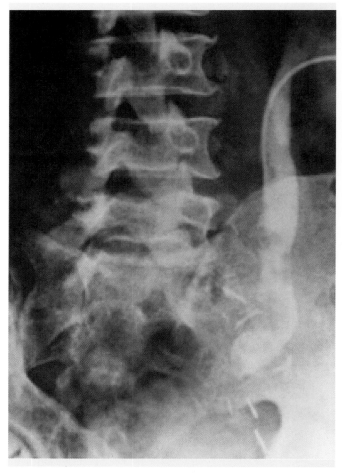

FIGURE 38-5. Retrograde pyelogram. From McDougal WS, Wein AJ, Kavoussi LR, et al. *Campbell-Walsh Urology*, 10th ed. New York, NY: Elsevier; 2011.

17. A hypertensive 10-month-old boy presents with a large, fixed abdominal mass as shown in the CT in Fig. 38-6. What is his most likely diagnosis?
   (A) Wilms tumor
   (B) Neuroblastoma
   (C) Multicystic dysplastic kidney
   (D) Ureteropelvic junction obstruction
   (E) Sacrococcygeal teratoma

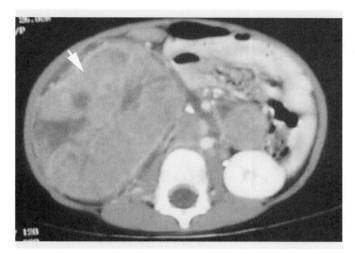

FIGURE 38-6. Abdominal computed tomography scan. From Brunicardi FC, Andersen DK, Billiar TR, et al. (eds.), *Schwartz's Principles of Surgery*, 9th ed. New York, NY: McGraw-Hill; 2009:Fig. 39-38.

18. A 50-year-old woman presents with right flank pain following blunt abdominal trauma. She is hemodynamically stable with BP 120/70 mmHg, HR 82 bpm, and respiratory rate (RR) of 13. Physical examination reveals mild right flank tenderness but is otherwise unremarkable. Her urine is grossly clear, but urinalysis reveals 15 red blood cells (RBCs) per high-powered field (HPF). What is the most appropriate next step?
   (A) CT of abdomen and pelvis
   (B) Renal ultrasound
   (C) Observation
   (D) Magnetic resonance imaging (MRI)
   (E) Surgical exploration

19. A 53-year-old man with a history of tobacco use has 10 RBCs/HPF on routine urinalysis. Culture shows no evidence of urinary tract infection, and the patient is asymptomatic. Which of the following is the most appropriate next step?
   (A) Repeat urinalysis in 6 months
   (B) CT urogram and cystoscopy
   (C) Cystogram

   (D) Observation
   (E) Prostate needle biopsy

20. A newborn is delivered by spontaneous vaginal delivery at 39 weeks' gestation. The mother is a healthy 26-year-old woman who reports normal prenatal care. The child is discharged home on the second day of life and represents 4 days later with lethargy, vomiting, and poor oral intake. Physical examination reveals clitoromegaly and labial fusion. No testicles are palpable.

   Laboratory evaluation reveals:
   Na: 119 mEq/L
   K: 6.5 mEq/L
   CO_2: 16 mEq/L

   What is the most likely diagnosis?
   (A) 21-hydroxylase deficiency
   (B) 11-β-hydroxylase deficiency
   (C) 3-β-hydroxylase deficiency
   (D) Cholesterol side chain cleavage enzyme
       € 17-α-hydroxylase deficiency

21. A 61-year-old man presents for evaluation of an elevated prostate-specific antigen (PSA) of 6.2. The patient is a poorly controlled type 2 diabetic and has a history of coronary artery disease status post coronary artery bypass grafting (CABG). Digital rectal examination (DRE) reveals a normal prostate with no nodules or induration. Transrectal ultrasound-guided prostate needle biopsy reveals Gleason grade 3 + 3 = 6 and prostate adenocarcinoma in <5% of 1 of 12 biopsy cores. What is the most appropriate treatment option for this patient?
   (A) Androgen deprivation/hormonal therapy
   (B) Immediate repeat prostate needle biopsy
   (C) Radical prostatectomy
   (D) Active surveillance
   (E) Chemotherapy

22. A 24-year-old African American man presents to the emergency department with a painful erection that has been present for 8 hours. Aspiration of the corpora reveals dark blood with a pH of 7.23, partial pressure of oxygen (PO_2) of 26 mmHg, and a partial pressure of carbon dioxide (PCO_2) of 65 mmHg. Which of the following choices least likely represents the etiology of this patient's priapism?
   (A) Sickle cell disease
   (B) Intracavernosal injection therapy
   (C) Total parenteral nutrition
   (D) Perineal trauma
   (E) Trazodone therapy

CHAPTER 38   UROLOGIC SURGERY

23. Which of the following best describes the mechanism of action of sildenafil citrate (Viagra)?
    (A) Inhibition of phosphodiesterase-5 (PDE-5)
    (B) 5-α-reductase inhibition
    (C) A-adrenergic antagonist
    (D) Aromatase inhibition
    (E) B-adrenergic agonist

24. A healthy 60-year-old man was evaluated for microscopic hematuria. CT scan with intravenous (IV) contrast was obtained (see Fig. 38-7). What is the most appropriate management of this lesion?
    (A) Observation
    (B) Percutaneous biopsy
    (C) Left partial nephrectomy
    (D) Left radical nephrectomy
    (E) Left radical nephroureterectomy with excision of bladder cuff

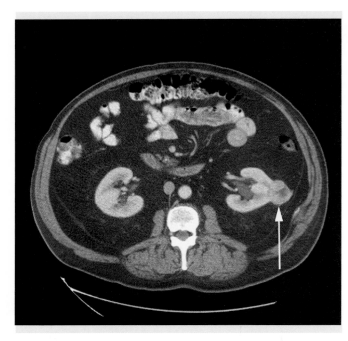

FIGURE 38-7. Abdominal computed tomography with left renal mass. From Doherty GM (ed.). *Current Diagnosis & Treatment: Surgery*, 13th ed. New York, NY: McGraw-Hill; 2010:Fig. 38-12.

25. A 51-year-old woman is evaluated for severe hypertension and headaches. As part of the workup, a significant elevation in plasma-free metanephrines was discovered. A CT of the abdomen and pelvis is obtained and is illustrated in Fig. 38-8. Which of the following familial syndromes *is not* associated with this neoplasm?
    (A) Autosomal dominant polycystic kidney disease
    (B) Multiple endocrine neoplasia type 2a (MEN2A)
    (C) Multiple endocrine neoplasia type 2b (MEN2B)

    (D) Von Hippel-Lindau
    (E) Tuberous sclerosis

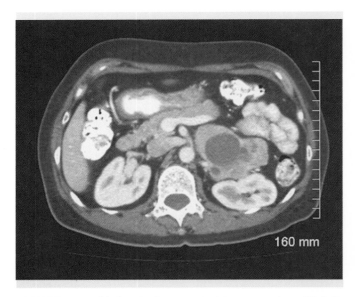

FIGURE 38-8. Abdominal computed tomography with left adrenal mass. From Morita S, Dackiw A, Zeiger M. *McGraw-Hill Manual: Endocrine Surgery*. New York, NY: McGraw-Hill; 2010:Fig. 15-1.

26. A 46-year-old man presents with complaints of right flank pain. Urinalysis reveals 100 RBCs/HPF and 75 white blood cells (WBCs)/HPF. An abdominal x-ray is obtained and is shown in Fig. 38-9. Which of the following is the most appropriate definitive management?
    (A) Extracorporeal shock wave lithotripsy (ESWL)
    (B) Ureteroscopy and laser lithotripsy
    (C) Chemolysis with sodium bicarbonate
    (D) Percutaneous nephrolithotomy (PCNL)
    (E) Anatrophic nephrolithotomy

27. An 18-year-old woman presents after a high-speed motor vehicle crash. On physical examination, she has severe pelvic pain but the rest of her abdomen is nontender. Plain radiograph demonstrates a pelvic fracture. A Foley catheter is inserted with return of 75 mL of bloody urine, and a CT cystogram is obtained (see Fig. 38-10). What is the appropriate management in this patient?
    (A) Continued catheter drainage for 10–14 days
    (B) CT cystogram
    (C) Flexible cystoscopy
    (D) Suprapubic cystostomy tube placement
    (E) Open operative repair

28. A 38-year-old man is involved in a motor vehicle crash. Initial radiographs reveal bilateral inferior pubic rami fractures. On physical examination, he is noted to have

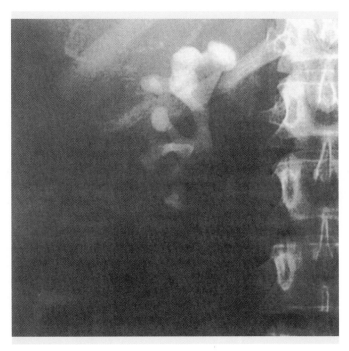

FIGURE 38-9. Abdominal plain film with renal calculus. From McAnich JW, Lue TF. *Smith & Tanagho's General Urology*, 18th ed. New York, NY: McGraw-Hill; 2012:Fig. 17-21.

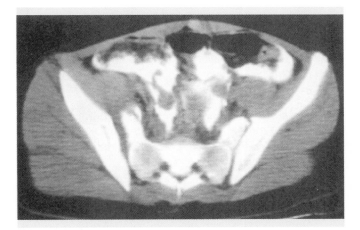

FIGURE 38-10. Abdominal computed tomography. From Mattox K, Moore E, Feliciano D (eds.), *Trauma*, 7th ed. New York, NY: McGraw-Hill; 2012:Fig. 36-11A.

blood at the urethral meatus, and a retrograde urethrogram is obtained (see Fig. 38-11). Which of the following is the best next step in management?
(A) Observation with serial bladder scans
(B) Urethral Foley catheter placement
(C) Suprapubic tube placement
(D) Cystoscopy
(E) Immediate open repair

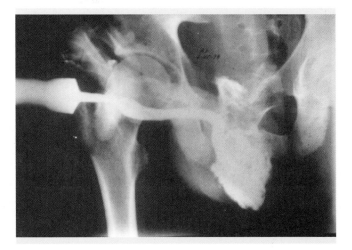

FIGURE 38-11. Retrograde urethrogram with posterior urethral injury.

29. An 18-year-old man with developmental delay and history of seizures presents to the emergency department with vague abdominal pain. Physical exam reveals a palpable right flank mass. He is also noted to have multiple angiofibromas in the malar region of his face. A CT is obtained and illustrated in Fig. 38-12. What is the most likely diagnosis?
(A) Von Hippel-Lindau (VHL) disease
(B) Sturge-Weber syndrome
(C) Beckwith-Wiedemann syndrome
(D) Prune belly syndrome
(E) Tuberous sclerosis

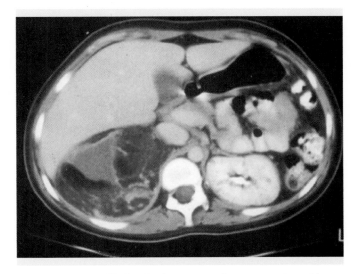

FIGURE 38-12. Abdominal computed tomography with renal masses. From Wein A, Kavoussi L, Novick A, et al. (eds.), *Campbell's Urology*, 10th ed. Philadelphia, PA: W.B. Saunders; 2012:Chapter 137.

30. What is the mechanism of action of α-blockers in the treatment of benign prostatic hypertrophy?
    (A) Relaxation of prostate smooth muscle
    (B) 5-α-reductase inhibition
    (C) Inhibition of androgen binding
    (D) Aromatase inhibition
    (E) B-adrenergic agonist

31. A 46-year-old man presents after a high-speed motor vehicle collision. He is hemodynamically stable (BP 110/70 mmHg, HR 100 bpm, RR 13). Physical exam reveals diffuse abdominal tenderness and left flank ecchymosis. A CT of the abdomen and pelvis is obtained and shown in Fig. 38-13.

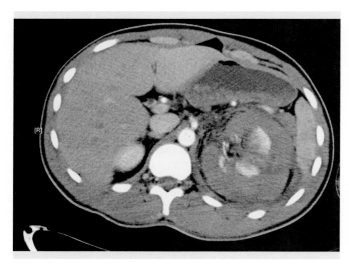

FIGURE 38-13. Abdominal computed tomography with renal injury. From Brunicardi FC, Andersen DK, Billiar TR, et al. (eds.), *Schwartz's Principles of Surgery*, 9th ed. New York, NY: McGraw-Hill; 2009:Fig. 40-6A.

Lab data include the following:

Hct: 30%

Na: 136 mEq/L

K: 4.1 mEq/L

Cl: 110 mmoL/L

CO_2: 22 mmol/L

BUN: 11 mg/dL

Cr: 1.3 mg/dL

Which of the following is the most appropriate management strategy for this patient?
(A) Hospital admission, bedrest, serial complete blood count (CBC)
(B) Selective left renal arteriogram

(C) Selective segmental artery embolization
(D) Cystoscopy and left ureteral stent placement
(E) Surgical exploration

32. A 42-year-old man is a restrained driver in a head-on motor vehicle collision. Physical exam reveals left upper quadrant and left flank tenderness. A CT scan is obtained and illustrated in Fig. 38-14. What is the most likely diagnosis?
    (A) Segmental renal artery injury
    (B) Segmental renal vein injury
    (C) Main renal artery injury
    (D) Main renal vein injury
    (E) Ureteropelvic junction (UPJ) disruption

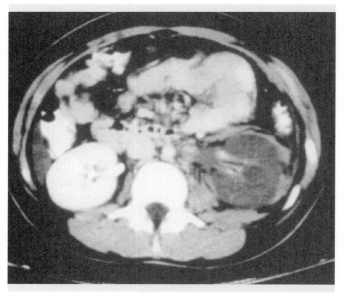

FIGURE 38-14. Abdominal computed tomography with renal injury. From Brunicardi FC, Andersen DK, Billiar TR, et al. (eds.), *Schwartz's Principles of Surgery*, 9th ed. New York, NY: McGraw-Hill; 2009:Fig. 36-8A.

33. A 7-year-old girl is struck by a motor vehicle. She is hemodynamically normal. Physical examination reveals point tenderness over the L1 and L2 vertebrae. A CT scan with delayed images is shown in Fig. 38-15. What is the most likely diagnosis?
    (A) Renal artery injury
    (B) Renal vein injury
    (C) Renal contusion
    (D) Renal cortical laceration
    (E) UPJ disruption

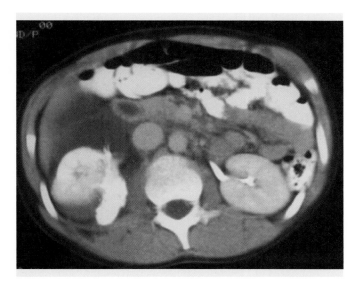

FIGURE 38-15. Abdominal computed tomography with right ureteral injury. From McDougal WS, Wein AJ, Kavoussi LR, et al. *Campbell-Walsh Urology*, 10th ed. New York, NY: Elsevier; 2011.

34. Which of the following is a potential complication of using intestinal segments in urinary diversion procedures?
    (A) Electrolyte abnormalities
    (B) Conduit stone formation
    (C) Osteomalacia
    (D) Sepsis
    (E) All of the above

35. A 65-year-old man is evaluated for gross hematuria and is found to have two small bladder tumors on cystoscopy. CT urogram reveals no abnormalities of the kidneys or ureters. Transurethral resection demonstrates low-grade urothelial carcinoma confined to the bladder mucosa. What is the next most appropriate step in this patient's management?
    (A) Bone scan
    (B) Repeat cystoscopy in three months
    (C) External-beam radiation
    (D) Radical cystectomy with urinary diversion
    (E) MRI of abdomen/pelvis

36. Which of the following statements regarding risk factors for the development of urothelial carcinoma (UC) of the bladder is *false*?
    (A) Females are three to four times more likely than males to develop bladder cancer.
    (B) Occupational exposure to aromatic amines increases the risk of developing UC of the bladder.
    (C) Treatment with cyclophosphamide increases the risk of developing UC of the bladder.

(D) Cigarette smoking is the main known cause of UC of the bladder.
(E) Long-term indwelling catheters increase the risk of developing squamous cell carcinoma of the bladder.

37. Which of the following factors contributes to postoperative urinary retention?
    (A) Bladder overdistention
    (B) Traumatic instrumentation
    (C) Postoperative pain
    (D) Preexistent bladder outlet obstruction
    (E) All of the above

38. A 46-year-old man presents after a low-speed motorcycle collision with superficial lower extremity lacerations and abrasions but also with complaints of severe left scrotal pain. On physical examination, his abdomen is soft, nondistended, and nontender to palpation. The left hemiscrotum is moderately edematous, and palpation of the testicle is extremely tender. The testicle is palpable and normal in size and consistency. Urinalysis is normal. What is the most appropriate next step?
    (A) Scrotal ultrasonography
    (B) CT of the abdomen and pelvis with IV contrast
    (C) Scrotal exploration
    (D) Retrograde urethrogram
    (E) Observation

39. A male infant is born at 37 weeks' gestational age. His mother had no prenatal care. On initial physical exam, his abdomen is noted to be large, flaccid, and wrinkled. On further exam, he is noted to have bilaterally undescended testicles. He has a normal phallus. What other clinical finding would be most likely given this clinical presentation?
    (A) Wilms tumor
    (B) Urinary tract calculi
    (C) Urothelial carcinoma of the bladder
    (D) Dilated and tortuous ureters
    (E) Pyloric stenosis

ANSWERS AND EXPLANATIONS

1. **(E)** The CT reveals persistent para-aortic lymphadenopathy following chemotherapy. Ninety-five percent of testicular cancers are germ cell tumors (GCTs), and these are further subdivided into seminomas and nonseminomas. Nonseminomatous tumors are often mixed in terms of their histology and can be comprised of embryonal carcinoma, choriocarcinoma, yolk sac tumor, and teratomas.

   Patients with nonseminomatous testicular cancer who are treated with primary chemotherapy and subsequently have negative tumor markers but have a residual retroperitoneal mass ≥1 cm should proceed to bilateral RPLND.

After chemotherapy, approximately 30% of patients will have residual disease on imaging. Of that 30%, approximately 40% will have necrosis in the specimen, 45% will have teratoma, and 15% will have viable malignancy. Therefore, RPLND provides both staging and therapeutic benefits. If viable malignancy is found, then additional chemotherapy is indicated. If teratoma is present, surgical resection is therapeutic because teratoma is not chemotherapy sensitive. It can transform into a malignancy or can cause morbidity secondary to rapid growth and mass effect.

The technique of RPLND has also evolved to decrease morbidity. A full bilateral RPLND is not always necessary, and a modified nerve-sparing RPLND allows for the preservation of retroperitoneal sympathetic fibers and virtually eliminates the risk of anejaculation.

BIBLIOGRAPHY

Stephenson A, Gilligan T. Neoplasms of the testis. In: Wein A, Kavoussi L, Novick A, et al. (eds.), *Campbell's Urology*, 10th ed. Philadelphia, PA: W.B. Saunders; 2012.

2. **(E)** Pathologic stage has been proven to be the single most important prognostic factor for renal cell carcinoma (RCC). Five-year survival for organ-confined RCC is estimated at 70–90%. Survival drops to 50–70% with invasion of the perinephric or renal sinus fat.

BIBLIOGRAPHY

Campbell S, Lane B. Malignant renal tumors. In: Wein A, Kavoussi L, Novick A, et al. (eds.), *Campbell's Urology*, 10th ed. Philadelphia, PA: W.B. Saunders; 2012.

3. **(B)** Absence of the vas deferens occurs in less than 1% of males and is often discovered during evaluation for infertility or vasectomy. The mesonephric or Wolffian duct is the precursor of both the ureteral bud and the vas deferens, seminal vesicles, and epididymis. Therefore, both the kidney and reproductive tract can be affected by anomalous development. Ipsilateral renal agenesis is present in up to 85% of males with unilateral absence of the vas deferens but is variable. Of note, congenital bilateral absence of the vas deferens is expected in patients with cystic fibrosis, as cystic fibrosis transmembrane regulator (*CFTR*) gene mutations often contribute to maldevelopment of the vas deferens.

BIBLIOGRAPHY

MacDonald M, Barthold JS, Cass E. Abnormalities of the penis and scrotum. In: Docimo S, Canning D, Khoury A (eds.), *Clinical Pediatric Urology*, 5th ed. London, England: Informa Healthcare; 2007:1261.

Pope JC. Renal dysgenesis and cystic disease of the kidney. In: Wein A, Kavoussi L, Novick A, et al. (eds.), *Campbell's Urology*, 10th ed. Philadelphia, PA: W.B. Saunders; 2012.

Ritchey M, John S. Renal anomalies. In: Docimo S, Canning D, Khoury A (eds.), *Clinical Pediatric Urology*, 5th ed. London, England: Informa Healthcare; 2007:294–295.

4. **(B)** Ureteral injuries represent less than 1% of genitourinary trauma, and patients often have significant concomitant injuries. If the ureteral injury occurs in the upper two-thirds of the ureter (i.e., above the pelvic brim), options for repair include ureteroureterostomy (i.e., primary reanastomosis), transureteroureterostomy, bowel interposition, and autotransplant of the kidney. Most proximal and mid ureteral injuries are amenable to ureteroureterostomy, which is the least morbid of the previously listed options. If the injury involves the lower one-third of the ureter, ureteroneocystostomy (reimplant of the ureter into the bladder, typically at the dome) can be performed. Additional techniques that can be employed in the setting of longer ureteral defects include a psoas hitch and/or Boari flap. A psoas hitch involves suturing the bladder to the psoas tendon to "hitch" the bladder proximally. A Boari flap is a pedicle of bladder that is tubularized to bridge the gap to the injured ureter.

General surgical principles that apply to all ureteral repairs include: (1) careful handling of the ureter to prevent devascularization; (2) debridement of nonviable tissue; (3) adequate mobilization to facilitate a tension-free anastomosis; and (4) ureteral spatulation with creation of a watertight anastomosis over a double-J ureteral stent. Retroperitonealization of the repaired ureter and drainage of the retroperitoneum are also advised.

Due to concomitant life-threatening injury, it may be necessary to defer definitive repair of the ureter. In this scenario, ureteral stenting or percutaneous nephrostomy tube can temporarily provide urinary drainage.

BIBLIOGRAPHY

Santucci R, Doumanian L. Upper urinary tract trauma. In: Wein A, Kavoussi L, Novick A, et al. (eds.), *Campbell's Urology*, 10th ed. Philadelphia, PA: W.B. Saunders; 2012.

5. **(C)** Testicular torsion is a urologic emergency requiring prompt diagnosis and treatment. Although a high index of suspicion should be maintained for all adolescent boys, the peak age of incidence ranges from 12–16 years of age. The anatomic variant that predisposes a patient to testicular torsion is referred to as the bell-clapper deformity. This abnormality results from an incomplete attachment of the testicle and epididymis to the scrotum due to a failure of fusion of the tunica vaginalis to the epididymis.

The classic presentation of a patient with testicular torsion includes acute onset of severe scrotal pain occurring both at rest and with activity. Clinical exam findings include absence of the cremasteric reflex and varying scrotal edema and erythema. Elevation of the testis and lateral lie may be present but are nonspecific findings. Patients may also complain of nausea and vomiting.

The differential diagnosis in a patient presenting with acute scrotal pain or swelling includes epididymo-orchitis, testicular torsion, torsion of the appendix testis, testicular trauma, testicular malignancy, indirect inguinal hernia, and hydrocele. Although ultrasound can differentiate between testicular torsion and other etiologies of acute scrotum, scrotal exploration is appropriate based on a clinical exam consistent with testicular torsion. Doppler ultrasound will show an absence of blood flow to the torsed testis. Patients with epididymo-orchitis differ from patients with testicular torsion in that they often complain of urinary symptoms and/or a positive urinalysis. Epididymitis will present on ultrasound as increased blood flow to the epididymis and normal blood flow to the testicle. A patient with a torsed appendix testis may be differentiated from a patient with testicular torsion with the physical exam finding of a "blue dot sign." This blue dot correlates with necrosis of the appendix testis. Testicular cancer typically presents as a painless testicular mass.

Treatment of testicular torsion consists of scrotal exploration, detorsion of the affected testicle, and orchidopexy of the contralateral testis to prevent future torsion. The affected testicle should be assessed for viability after detorsion intraoperatively. Testis survival is best if detorsion occurs within 6 hours of the onset of pain, with only 5% requiring orchiectomy for a nonviable testis if operated on in this time frame. Manual detorsion or rotating the testis laterally, like opening a book, has been described, but this does not preclude surgical exploration.

BIBLIOGRAPHY

Barthold JS. Abnormalities of the testis and scrotum and their surgical management. In: Wein A, Kavoussi L, Novick A, et al. (eds.), *Campbell's Urology*, 10th ed. Philadelphia, PA: W.B. Saunders; 2012.

6. **(A)** The diagnosis in this scenario is an enterovesical fistula. Enterovesical fistulae are most commonly caused by diverticular disease, colorectal carcinoma, and Crohn disease. Diverticulitis is the most common cause of colovesical fistulae, accounting for approximately 70% of diagnoses. Other less common etiologies include radiation, infection, and trauma.

The most common presenting symptoms include pneumaturia, recurrent urinary tract infections, suprapubic pain, hematuria, dysuria, urinary frequency, and urgency. Gastrointestinal symptoms may include fecaluria and tenesmus.

Of all the answer choices provided, CT scan is the most sensitive and specific modality for the diagnosis of enterovesical fistulae. CT scan demonstrates the classic radiologic findings of a colovesical fistula: (1) air in the urinary bladder; (2) bladder wall thickening adjacent to a thickened loop of colon; and (3) colonic diverticula (see Fig. 38-16). If air is present within the urinary bladder, it important to consider the possibility of an iatrogenic cause such as catheterization or instrumentation of the urinary tract, as well as active infection with a gas-forming organism.

In the setting of an enterovesical fistula, cystoscopy is likely to identify the abnormality. However, findings are typically nonspecific (e.g., localized erythema, papillary, or bullous change). Cystoscopy allows for biopsy of a suspicious area to rule out malignancy as the etiology of the fistula. Colonoscopy, the Bourne test, and oral administration of active charcoal (if a fistula is present, black particles can be visualized in the urine) are useful adjuncts in confirming the diagnosis of enterovesical fistula but are not as sensitive or specific as a CT scan.

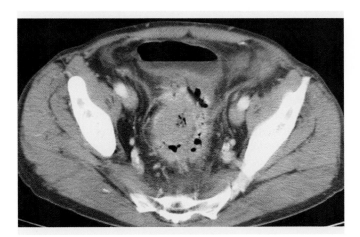

FIGURE 38-16. Abdominal computed tomography with enterovesicular fistula. From Kaiser A. *McGraw-Hill Manual: Colorectal Surgery*. New York, NY: McGraw-Hill; 2008: Fig. 4-19.

BIBLIOGRAPHY

Rovner E. Urinary tract fistulae. In: Wein A, Kavoussi L, Novick A, et al. (eds.), *Campbell's Urology*, 10th ed. Philadelphia, PA: W.B. Saunders; 2012.

7. **(E)** Struvite (magnesium ammonium phosphate) calculi are notoriously associated with urinary tract infections caused by urease-producing bacteria. As urea is split by

urease, the byproduct of ammonia is created, alkalinizing the urine (most patients have a urinary pH >6.5) with the subsequent precipitation of struvite stones. Patients may present with pyelonephritis-like symptoms and recurrent urinary tract infections (UTIs) with the same organism isolated from urinary culture. Struvite calculi may fill the calyces and renal pelvis, creating a staghorn calculus. These stones can often be seen on plain film alone, although noncontrast CT scan is important for surgical planning. Percutaneous nephrolithotomy is typically the most appropriate treatment modality in this scenario because patients will often continue to suffer from recurrent UTIs until all stone burden is cleared.

Urease-producing bacteria include some species of *Klebsiella*, *Pseudomonas*, and *Staphylococcus*; however, the most common species associated with infection and calculi is *P mirabilis*. *E coli* is not a urea-splitting organism.

BIBLIOGRAPHY

Ferrandino M, Pietrow P, Preminger G. Evaluation and medical management of urinary lithiasis. In: Wein A, Kavoussi L, Novick A, et al. (eds.), *Campbell's Urology*, 10th ed. Philadelphia, PA: W.B. Saunders; 2012.

8. **(A)** The majority of iatrogenic ureteral injuries occur during hysterectomy as the ureter passes deep to the uterine vessels see Fig. 38-17. After gynecologic surgery, iatrogenic ureteral injury occurs most frequently during colorectal surgery with the rate of ureteral injury in abdominoperineal resection (APR) ranging from approximately 0.3 to almost 6%. For this reason, many advocate placement of ureteral catheters to assist in intraoperative identification of the ureter or a ureteral injury.

Ideally, ureteral injury is identified immediately and repaired. If the injury is caused by ligation with a clip or suture, the ligature should be removed with observation of the ureter for viability. If repair is indicated, options are identical to those used in ureteral trauma. Placement of a ureteral stent is also an option.

Patients with a missed diagnosis of a ureteral injury can present with anuria, urogenital or urocutaneous fistula, hydronephrosis, hematuria, fevers/urosepsis, and flank or abdominal pain. If the diagnosis of ureteral injury is delayed, options for management include ureteral stent placement or nephrostomy tube to allow for drainage of urine until open repair can be pursued. In some cases, ureteral stenting alone may resolve the obstruction. If the patient is septic or clinically unstable at presentation, urinary diversion with a stent or nephrostomy tube is the appropriate next step.

BIBLIOGRAPHY

Santucci R, Doumanian L. Upper urinary tract trauma. In: Wein A, Kavoussi L, Novick A, et al. (eds.), *Campbell's Urology*, 10th ed. Philadelphia, PA: W.B. Saunders; 2012.

9. **(D)** Varicoceles are dilated veins of the pampiniform plexus of the spermatic cord and present in 15% of normal males. Varicoceles are graded by size on the following scale:

Grade I: Detectable only during the Valsalva maneuver

Grade II: Palpable without Valsalva

Grade III: Visible on inspection of the scrotum

On exam, varicoceles are classically described as a "bag of worms." The vast majority (~90%) present on the left side, likely due to the 90-degree insertion of the left gonadal vein into the renal vein. New-onset grade III unilateral right-sided varicoceles may be indicative of retroperitoneal or caval pathology (e.g., renal cell carcinomas with extension into the inferior vena cava).

BIBLIOGRAPHY

Sabanegh E, Agarwal A. Male infertility. In: Wein A, Kavoussi L, Novick A, et al. (eds.), *Campbell's Urology*, 10th ed. Philadelphia, PA: W.B. Saunders; 2012.

10. **(A)** The cystogram reveals an extraperitoneal bladder rupture. Classically this appears as a "flame-shaped" collection of contrast that has extravasated within the pelvis. The most common associated injury is pelvic fracture, and this is present in up to 95% of bladder injuries.

Diagnosis and delineation of type of injury (intra- versus extraperitoneal) can be made with fluoroscopic or CT cystogram. It important that the bladder is adequately filled during the study (350 mL or when patient feels as though their bladder is full). Additionally, if fluoroscopic cystogram is the study used, postdrainage films are important in identifying posterior injuries.

If bladder injury is suspected, catheterization is the appropriate step followed by imaging as discussed earlier. If concern for urethral injury exists (blood at the urethral meatus, inability to place the Foley catheter), a retrograde urethrogram may need to be obtained. Urethral injuries occur in approximately 10–30% of patients with concomitant bladder injury. Management of an extraperitoneal bladder rupture consists of catheter drainage for 10–14 days. Cystography should be performed to ensure bladder healing prior to removal of Foley catheter.

BIBLIOGRAPHY

Morey AF, Dugi DD. Chapter 88: genital and lower urinary tract injury. In: Wein A, Kavoussi L, Novick A, et al. (eds.), *Campbell's Urology*, 10th ed. Philadelphia, PA: W.B. Saunders; 2012.

11. **(D)** The pelvic autonomic nerves consist of the paired hypogastric (sympathetic), sacral (parasympathetic), and inferior hypogastric nerves (see Fig. 38-17). Sympathetic activity causes relaxation of the bladder muscle and contraction of the bladder outlet and urethra, contributing to urine storage. Parasympathetic activity causes contraction of the bladder muscle and relaxation of the bladder outlet and urethra, contributing to bladder emptying. The sympathetic and parasympathetic nerves join anterior and lateral to the rectum to form the pelvic plexus. The inferior hypogastric nerve plexus arises from both sympathetic and parasympathetic fibers and is located on the lateral pelvic side wall. Fibers from these nerve bundles innervate the rectum as well as the bladder, ureter, prostate, seminal vesicles, membranous urethra, and corpora cavernosa. Therefore, injuries to these nerves in pelvis surgery can lead to impotence, bladder dysfunction, and fecal incontinence.

This patient is retaining a large volume of urine in her bladder after voiding, suggesting overflow incontinence secondary to incomplete bladder emptying. Clean intermittent catheterization may be necessary to treat her

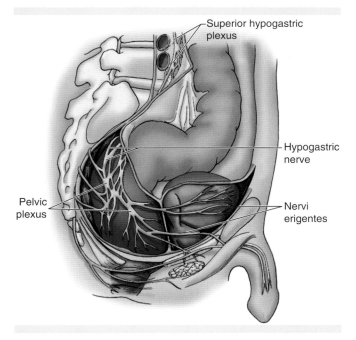

FIGURE 38-17. Pelvic autonomic nerves. From Zinner MJ, Ashley SW. *Maingot's Abdominal Operations*, 12th ed. New York, NY: McGraw-Hill; 2013:Fig. 40-5.

incontinence, in order to prevent urinary tract infection, bladder stones, and renal dysfunction.

Stress urinary incontinence is involuntary leakage of urine associated with exertion, sneezing, or coughing. Up to 20% of all women experience recurrent symptoms of stress incontinence. Risk factors include age, obesity, and vaginal childbirth. Urge urinary incontinence is involuntary leakage of urine immediately preceded by urinary urgency. Continuous leakage of urine is associated with vesicovaginal fistula. In the industrialized world, 75% of vesicovaginal fistulae are secondary to injury of the bladder at the time of gynecologic, urologic, or other pelvic surgery. This most commonly occurs in the setting of hysterectomy.

BIBLIOGRAPHY

Chapple C, Milson I. Urinary incontinence and pelvic prolapse: epidemiology and pathophysiology. In: Wein A, Kavoussi L, Novick A, et al. (eds.), *Campbell's Urology*, 10th ed. Philadelphia, PA: W.B. Saunders; 2012.
Goldberg J, Bleday R. Cancer of the rectum. In: Zinner M, Ashley S (eds.), *Maingot's Abdominal Operations*, 12th ed. New York, NY: McGraw-Hill; 2013.
Rovner E. Urinary tract fistulae. In: Wein A, Kavoussi L, Novick A, et al. (eds.), *Campbell's Urology*, 10th ed. Philadelphia, PA: W.B. Saunders; 2012.

12. **(E)** CT with contrast demonstrates ureteropelvic junction (UPJ) obstruction. Although presentation may not occur until later in life, UPJ obstruction is typically congenital, arising from an aperistaltic segment of ureter. Other potential etiologies include crossing blood vessels and a high insertion of the ureter into the renal pelvis leading to inadequate drainage of urine.

Diagnosis of UPJ obstruction as an infant is increasingly common due to the detection of hydronephrosis on prenatal ultrasound. In older children, adolescents, and adults, presentation can be intermittent abdominal pain accompanied by nausea and vomiting. In this scenario, CT scan is often the initial imaging modality. Diuretic renal scan is a useful adjunctive study because it provides data about differential renal function as well as differentiates between obstructive versus nonobstructive hydronephrosis.

The procedure of choice for surgical intervention in the setting of a UPJ obstruction is pyeloplasty, although endourologic procedures may be an appropriate alternative in some scenarios. In the setting of a minimally functioning or nonfunctioning kidney secondary to long-standing obstruction, nephrectomy may also be an appropriate option.

BIBLIOGRAPHY

Nakada SY, Hsu T. Chapter 41: management of upper urinary obstruction. In: Wein A, Kavoussi L, Novick A, et al. (eds.), *Campbell's Urology*, 10th ed. Philadelphia, PA: W.B. Saunders; 2012.

13. **(C)** Vesicoureteral reflux (VUR) is not normal at any age, and UTI is the most common presenting symptom. Reflux is the retrograde flow of urine from the bladder proximally into the ureters or renal collecting system. Congenital VUR occurs due to an inadequate flap valve mechanism along the intramural ureter as it inserts into the urinary bladder. In addition to abnormal ureteral development seen in congenital VUR, bowel and bladder dysfunction can cause development of secondary reflux (or contribute to the severity of congenital VUR). The grading of VUR is based on voiding cystourethrogram (VCUG) and ranges from grade 1 (reflux into ureter) to 5 (reflux into the kidney with severe dilation of the ureter, renal pelvis, and calyces, as well as a tortuous ureter). Lower grades of reflux are more likely to resolve over time than higher grades of reflux.

    Surgical intervention is indicated in patients with high-grade reflux, recurrent UTIs despite optimal medical management, and concern for or evidence of renal injury due to scarring (often caused by recurrent UTIs). Ureteral reimplantation is the gold standard and serves to increase the length of the intramural ureteral tunnel within the urinary bladder, thereby providing an antireflux mechanism.

BIBLIOGRAPHY

Martin A, Peters C. *Vesicoureteral Reflux*. American Urologic Association Update Series, Volume 32, Lesson 18, 2013.

14. **(C)** Cryptorchidism, or undescended testicle, is a failure of the testis to descend into the scrotum. The prevalence is approximately 1–3% in full-term and 15–30% in premature male infants. Testes that remain undescended by 6 months (corrected for gestational age) are unlikely to descend spontaneously, and referral to an appropriate surgical specialist should occur in anticipation of orchidopexy. Hormonal therapy should not be used to assist in testicular descent.

    Assessment of the testicles should occur at each well-child exam, and in the hands of an experienced provider, more than 70% of cryptorchid testes are palpable by physical examination alone. The American Urologic Association recommends against routine imaging with ultrasound or other imaging modalities (CT, MRI), because no radiologic test can conclude with 100% accuracy that a testis is absent. Additional concerns include cost, the need for anesthesia, and radiation exposure. Diagnostic laparoscopy (or open exploration) remains the gold standard to assess for the presence or absence of a nonpalpable unilateral testis. If a testis is found during the diagnostic portion of the procedure, the surgeon can immediately proceed to orchidopexy, thereby providing diagnosis and therapy simultaneously.

    Patients with a history of cryptorchidism are at increased risk of testicular malignancy and infertility. The increased incidence of malignancy in cryptorchid testes ranges from 0.05–1%. Boys undergoing orchidopexy *prior to* puberty are felt to have a decreased risk of testis cancer compared to boys who undergo orchidopexy *after* puberty; however, the risk of testis cancer remains elevated. Formerly bilateral cryptorchid men have greatly reduced fertility compared with men with a history of unilateral cryptorchidism and the general male population.

BIBLIOGRAPHY

Kolon TF, Herndon CD, Baker LA, et al. Evaluation and treatment of cryptorchidism: AUA guideline. 2014. www.auanet.org.

15. **(E)** Upper urinary tract urothelial carcinoma accounts for only 5% of all urothelial tumors (95% involve the bladder/lower urinary tract). Ureteral tumors occur most commonly in the lower ureter, comprising 70% of all ureteral tumors. Smoking is the most important modifiable risk factor for development of an upper tract urothelial carcinoma.

    The most common presenting symptom is microscopic or gross hematuria. The imaging modality most commonly used in the workup of hematuria is a CT urogram. In a CT urogram, IV contrast is administered and a delayed phase captures contrast excreted from the kidney highlighting the collecting system. Any filling defects identified during this phase are suggestive of tumor. Given this patient's creatinine of 2.0, IV contrast is not possible, and therefore, a retrograde pyelogram (contrast medium injected into the collecting system in a retrograde fashion via a ureteral catheter) was performed at the time of cystoscopy. Cystoscopy would be required in this patient regardless of ureteral imaging because concomitant lower tract urothelial carcinomas can exist simultaneously.

    The treatment of upper tract malignancies is a work in progress due to the relatively low incidence of this type of malignancy and lack of prospective randomized control trials. Nephroureterectomy with excision of a bladder cuff is the gold standard for large, high-grade, invasive upper tract urothelial carcinoma. Radical surgery may also be appropriate in low-grade superficial upper tract urothelial carcinomas that are recurrent, are multifocal, or have progressed despite attempts at more conservative approaches.

The patient in this scenario is an ideal candidate for an attempt at a conservative, nephron-sparing approach, given his solitary kidney, already compromised renal function, and low stage, low-grade ureteral tumor. Nephron-sparing approaches include endoscopic resection and/or ablation, both antegrade and retrograde, segmental ureterectomy with ureteroureterostomy, and subtotal ureterectomy with reimplantation. A ureteroscopic approach is less morbid than an open approach in this elderly patient with multiple comorbidities. Multiple series have shown the safety and efficacy of an endoscopic approach with the primary concern being recurrence of disease. A wide range of recurrence rates have been reported (20–90%), and close follow-up is required.

BIBLIOGRAPHY

Sagalowski AI, Jarrett TW, Flanigan RC. Urothelial tumors of the upper urinary tract and ureters. In: Wein A, Kavoussi L, Novick A, et al. (eds.), *Campbell's Urology*, 10th ed. Philadelphia, PA: W.B. Saunders; 2012.

16. **(A)** Inflammatory bowel disease can lead to the formation of calcium oxalate stones, especially in those who have undergone bowel resection, by causing varying degrees of fat malabsorption. Fatty acids and calcium form soaps in the bowel lumen, decreasing the normal binding of calcium and oxalate that occurs there. Increased oxalate is reabsorbed into the blood and excreted into the urine. Hyperoxaluria secondary to chronic diarrheal states is termed enteric hyperoxaluria. There is also evidence that the poorly absorbed fatty acids and bile salts in these patients may increase enteric permeability to oxalate, exacerbating the problem.

    Enteric hyperoxaluria is the most common form of acquired hyperoxaluria, but dietary habits can also lead to calcium oxalate stone formation. High intake of oxalate-rich foods like nuts, chocolate, tea, spinach, and strawberries can result in hyperoxaluria in otherwise normal individuals. Also implicated is the intestinal bacterium *Oxalobacter formigenes*, which degrades oxalate in the gut. Reduced levels of this flora are associated with higher urinary oxalate levels.

    Primary hyperoxaluria is a rare autosomal recessive disorder of metabolism leading to overproduction of oxalate. Renal failure can ensue with this disorder secondary to recurrent calcium oxalate stones and severe nephrocalcinosis.

BIBLIOGRAPHY

Pearle M, Lotan Y. Urinary lithiasis: etiology, epidemiology, and pathogenesis. In: Wein A, Kavoussi L, Novick A, et al. (eds.), *Campbell's Urology*, 10th ed. Philadelphia, PA: W.B. Saunders; 2012.

17. **(B)** Neuroblastoma is the third most common pediatric malignancy. Eighty percent of cases present before the age of 4 years, and most patients have advanced disease at presentation (70% have metastasis at diagnosis), with an overall survival rate of less than 30%. These tumors arise from neural crest cells and arise most frequently from the adrenal glands, posterior mediastinum, neck, or pelvis, but can arise anywhere in the sympathetic ganglia. Tumors are most often initially identified as an asymptomatic abdominal mass, which can cross the midline. Initial evaluation should include abdominal CT and measurement of serum or urine vanillylmandelic acid and homovanillic acid. Because these tumors derive from the sympathetic nervous system, serum catecholamine release can sometimes mimic symptoms frequently associated with pheochromocytoma, including paroxysmal hypertension, palpitations, flushing, and headache. Despite the overall poor prognosis, children of any age with localized disease and children <1 year of age even with advanced disease have a high likelihood of disease-free survival. Because complete resection is often not possible at presentation given extensive local tumor extension, a biopsy is usually performed and neoadjuvant chemotherapy given based on tumor stage. The main goal of subsequent surgery is 95% tumor resection without compromising adjacent structures.

    Neuroblastoma is often difficult to distinguish from Wilms tumor, which is the most common primary malignant tumor of the kidney in children. However, median age of diagnosis is less than with neuroblastoma, with a median age of 3.5 years. It is rarely diagnosed in infants. It also usually presents as an asymptomatic abdominal mass and can cause hypertension (secondary to elevated renin), hematuria, and weight loss. The finding of intratumor calcifications or vascular encasement on CT may help distinguish neuroblastoma from Wilms. Unlike neuroblastoma, the overall cure rate for Wilms tumor, even in the presence of metastatic spread, is >90%.

    Multicystic dysplastic kidney is a common cause of abdominal mass in neonates, but on imaging, it appears as a severely dysplastic kidney filled with multiple noncommunicating cysts. Ureteropelvic junction obstruction does not present as a solid mass. Sacrococcygeal teratoma presents as a large mass extending from the sacrum.

BIBLIOGRAPHY

Hackham D, Grikscheit T, Wang K, et al. Pediatric surgery. In: Brunicardi FC, Andersen D, Billiar T, et al. (eds.), *Schwartz's Principles of Surgery*, 9th ed. New York, NY: McGraw-Hill; 2010.

Ritchey M, Shamberger R. Pediatric urologic oncology. In: Wein A, Kavoussi L, Novick A, et al. (eds.), *Campbell's Urology*, 10th ed. Philadelphia, PA: W.B. Saunders; 2012.

18. **(C)** The kidney is the most common urologic organ injured from trauma. The best indicators for injury to the urinary tract are the presence of microscopic hematuria (>5 RBCs/HPF), gross hematuria, and hypotension (systolic blood pressure <90 mmHg). The degree of hematuria does not correlate well with severity of injury. For example, in a recent analysis, hematuria was absent in 7% of grade 4 renal injuries as well as 36% of renal vascular injuries from blunt trauma. However, several studies have confirmed that patients with microscopic hematuria who are hemodynamically stable can safely be observed clinically (<0.0016% of these patients will have significant renal injury).

    If renal trauma is suspected, the criteria for radiologic imaging of the kidney include (1) all penetrating trauma in the abdomen, flank, or low chest, regardless of presence and degree of hematuria; (2) blunt trauma with significant mechanism of injury including rapid deceleration or fall from heights; (3) blunt trauma with gross hematuria; (4) blunt trauma with hypotension; and (5) pediatric patients with microscopic hematuria. CT is the gold standard for imaging renal trauma. All patients who remain hemodynamically unstable after initial resuscitation require surgical exploration.

BIBLIOGRAPHY

Santucci R, Doumanian L. Upper urinary tract trauma. In: Wein A, Kavoussi L, Novick A, et al. (eds.), *Campbell's Urology*, 10th ed. Philadelphia, PA: W.B. Saunders; 2012.

Shariat SF, Jenkins A, Roehrborn CG, et al. Features and outcomes of patients with grade IV renal injury. *BJU Int* 2008;102:728–733.

19. **(B)** The most common urologic causes of microhematuria are benign prostatic hypertrophy (BPH), UTI, and urinary calculi. Asymptomatic microhematuria (AMH) is defined as ≥3 RBCs/HPF on one properly collected urine specimen in the absence of a benign cause like infection, menstruation, vigorous exercise, trauma, or recent urologic instrumentation. Once a benign cause has been ruled out, urologic evaluation should proceed. Those incidentally diagnosed with AMH during a regular medical encounter like a check-up have an overall malignancy rate of approximately 4%.

Important risk factors for urinary tract malignancy are male gender, age >35 years, past or current smoking history, occupational exposure to chemicals or dyes (aromatic amines), and history of gross hematuria, pelvic irradiation, or indwelling foreign body (Foley catheter).

A cystoscopy should be performed in all patients over age 35 or any patient with risk factors for urinary tract malignancy, regardless of age. CT urography (CTU) is also needed to rule out renal tumors and evaluate the urothelium of the upper tracts (renal pelvis and ureters). CTU is the initial imaging of choice because it has the highest sensitivity and specificity to detect upper tract disease. If contrast administration is contraindicated, magnetic resonance urography, ultrasonography, and retrograde pyelography are suitable alternatives. The use of voided urine cytology is not initially indicated in the AMH patient. If the hematuria workup is negative and the patient has two consecutive negative annual urinalyses, then no further urinalyses for surveillance are necessary. If AMH persists after negative workup, yearly analyses should be considered, and a repeat workup should be considered within 3–5 years of the original evaluation.

BIBLIOGRAPHY

Davis R, Jones S, Barocas D, et al. Diagnosis, evaluation and follow-up of asymptomatic microhematuria (AMH) in adults: AUA guideline. American Urological Association Education and Research, Inc., 2012. https://www.auanet.org/education/guidelines/asymptomatic-microhematuria.cfm.

20. **(A)** This infant has the salt-wasting form of congenital adrenal hyperplasia (CAH). CAH accounts for the vast majority of masculinized females (46,XX disorders of sexual differentiation). Patients who fall in this category have a normal female karyotype (46,XX) and have ovaries, but their external genitalia are masculinized to varying degrees.

    At its most basic, CAH results from an error in steroid synthesis due to the deficiency of any one of a number of enzymes involved. 21-Hydroxylase deficiency accounts for 95% of cases, with the second most common being 11-β-hydroxylase deficiency. Low cortisol production leads to increased secretion of adrenocorticotrophic hormone (ACTH) and subsequently increased production of precursor steroids proximal to the enzymatic defect. These precursors are then metabolized into testosterone, and the result is virilization of the fetus. In addition to virilization, some patients also have an aldosterone deficiency, and these patients are considered "salt wasters." CAH patients with salt wasting present with hyperkalemia, dehydration, failure to gain weight, and vomiting within the first few weeks of life.

Without treatment, this can be life-threatening. Diagnosis of 21-hydroxylase deficiency is made by markedly elevated levels of plasma 17-hydroxyprogesterone on radioimmunoassay. Treatment consists of corticosteroid supplementation.

BIBLIOGRAPHY

Diamond DA, Yu RN. Sexual differentiation: normal and abnormal. In: Wein A, Kavoussi L, Novick A, et al. (eds.), *Campbell's Urology*, 10th ed. Philadelphia, PA: W.B. Saunders; 2012.

21. **(D)** It is known that many men may not benefit from treatment of localized prostate cancer, because it usually follows an indolent course. It is estimated that 60–70% of men die with at least a small focus of prostate cancer, yet there is only a 3% lifetime risk of death from prostate cancer. The most widely used and accepted system to classify prostate cancer aggressiveness and risk for progression is the D'Amico risk classification system, as follows:

    - **Low risk:** PSA ≤10 ng/mL and a Gleason score of 6 or less and clinical stage T1c or T2a
    - **Intermediate risk:** PSA >10–20 ng/mL or a Gleason score of 7 or clinical stage T2b but not qualifying for high risk
    - **High risk:** PSA >20 ng/mL or a Gleason score of 8 to 10 or clinical stage T2c

    Life expectancy is a critical factor when considering treatment options. If life expectancy is <10 years, treatment for cure should not be a goal. In these patients, a watchful waiting regimen is advocated in which definitive treatment is avoided and palliative treatment is enacted for local or metastatic progression should it occur.

    The patient in this question has what is considered low-risk prostate cancer, and although he has significant comorbidities, his life expectancy is >10 years. Although definitive treatment with radical prostatectomy or external-beam radiation could be considered options for his disease, they could incur complications such as impotence, urinary incontinence, and radiation cystitis/proctitis. Studies have shown that patients with low-grade, localized prostate cancer have a low risk for progression within the first 10–15 years of diagnosis. An active surveillance regimen with periodic PSA, DRE, and repeat prostate needle biopsy would be best suited for this patient. Active surveillance strives to provide definitive treatment for men whose cancer is likely to progress and to reduce the risk of treatment-related complications in men whose disease is not likely to progress. Men on active surveillance have the ability to choose definitive treatment at any time during their therapy, usually if biochemical progression (rise in PSA) or histopathologic progression (upstaging of Gleason grade or tumor volume) occurs.

    Androgen deprivation therapy, although accepted treatment for metastatic prostate cancer and as an adjuvant to radiation with locally advanced prostate cancer, is not appropriate for treatment of clinically localized prostate cancer. Chemotherapy is an adjunct for prostate cancer that no longer responds to hormonal therapy (castrate-resistant prostate cancer) and is appropriate for treatment of small cell carcinoma of the prostate.

BIBLIOGRAPHY

Thompson I, Thrasher JB, Aus G, et al. Guidelines for the management of clinically localized prostate cancer: 2007 update. *J Urol* 2007;177(6):2106–2131.

22. **(D)** Priapism is defined as an erection lasting longer than 4 hours in the absence of sexual stimulation. Priapism is classified as ischemic or nonischemic. This distinction is critical, given management differs significantly, and ischemic priapism is considered a medical emergency. If left untreated, it can lead to irreversible penile ischemia, necrosis, and scarring of the erectile tissue.

    Ischemic priapism is similar to a compartment syndrome in which there is occlusion of venous outflow and cessation of arterial inflow. Causes include intracavernosal therapy with various agents, use of psychotropic medications (including chlorpromazine, clozapine, and trazodone), use of lipid-rich total parenteral nutrition, and hematologic disease like sickle cell disease/trait and leukemia. Physical examination will typically reveal a rigid and painful erection with a soft glans penis. Corporal blood gas can aid in diagnosis, revealing hypoxia and acidosis, as is the case with this patient. Initial management consists of corporal aspiration and irrigation with saline and an α-adrenergic agonist. If this does not result in detumescence, surgical shunting is performed.

    Nonischemic priapism almost exclusively results from penile or perineal trauma. Injury to branches of the cavernosal artery result in a fistula to the corporal body sinusoids. Because the tissue is well-oxygenated, patients present with a semi-erect penis that is not painful. If diagnosis is unclear, Doppler ultrasound can be obtained. In the nonischemic type, unregulated blood flow and pooling may be seen, whereas in the ischemic type, no cavernosal arterial flow is visualized. Patients can often be followed conservatively for months while awaiting spontaneous fistula closure, but in some cases, arterial embolization or surgical ligation is necessary.

BIBLIOGRAPHY

Brant W, Bella A, Garcia M, Tantiwongse K, et al. Priapism: etiology, diagnosis and management. *AUA Update Series* 2006;25:11.

23. **(A)** Sildenafil is a competitive inhibitor of PDE-5. This enzyme breaks down cyclic guanosine monophosphate (cGMP), which is an intracellular messenger responsible for corporal smooth muscle relaxation. The inhibition of PDE-5 allows for accumulation of cGMP, which, in turn, promotes smooth muscle relaxation, arterial dilation, and increased penile blood flow needed for an erection (see Fig. 38-18). PDE-5 inhibitors augment, but do not induce, an erection; this requires the release of nitric oxide (NO) from penile nerves and penile vascular endothelium.

    PDE-5 inhibitors should be offered as a first-line therapy for erectile dysfunction unless contraindicated. Absolute contraindications include patients taking organic nitrates, due to the potential worsening of hypotension. Other side effects related to peripheral vasodilation include facial flushing, nasal congestion, and headache. It is important to note that these symptoms can be aggravated by concomitant α-blocker therapy. Some PDE-5 inhibitors have cross-reactivity with PDE-6, and therefore, reversible visual side effects can occur.

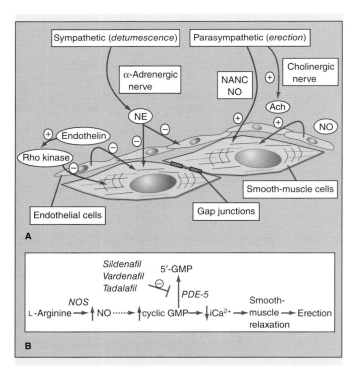

FIGURE 38-18. Pathways that control erection and detumescence. From Longo D, Fauci A, Kasper D, et al. *Harrison's Principles of Internal Medicine*, 18th ed. New York, NY: McGraw-Hill; 2011:Fig. 48-1.

BIBLIOGRAPHY

Burnett AL. Evaluation and management of erectile dysfunction. In: Wein A, Kavoussi L, Novick A, et al. (eds.), *Campbell's Urology*, 10th ed. Philadelphia, PA: W.B. Saunders; 2012.

Montague DK, Jarow JP, Broderick GA, et al. The management of erectile dysfunction: an AUA update. *J Urol* 2005;174(1):230–239.

24. **(C)** The CT scan reveals a small enhancing mass in the interpolar region of the left kidney. Any renal mass that enhances with IV contrast administration on CT scan is a renal cell carcinoma (RCC) until proven otherwise.

    Enhancing, small renal masses are benign in 20% of cases, 60% are indolent RCC, and 20% are potentially aggressive RCC. Although historically renal mass biopsy was not routinely performed due to a high false-negative rate, the actual false-negative rate has since been found to be significantly lower. As a result, renal biopsy is becoming increasingly used, particularly if the biopsy result will impact management. This is particularly true in patients with findings suggestive of lymphoma, metastases, or renal abscess.

    Partial nephrectomy is now the standard of care for small renal masses, even if the contralateral kidney is normal. Oncologic outcomes between partial and radical nephrectomy are equivalent, and the morbidity of a partial nephrectomy has decreased significantly with increasing experience. Patients with RCC treated with partial nephrectomy have overall survival of greater than 90% and local recurrence rates of 1–2%. Furthermore, the importance of a nephron-sparing approach in an attempt to avoid chronic kidney disease is now well recognized.

BIBLIOGRAPHY

Campbell SC, Lane BR. Malignant renal tumors. In: Wein A, Kavoussi L, Novick A, et al. (eds.), *Campbell's Urology*, 10th ed. Philadelphia, PA: W.B. Saunders; 2012.

25. **(A)** The CT illustrates a large left pheochromocytoma. This is a catecholamine-producing tumor of the cells of the adrenal medulla and accounts for approximately 5% of incidental adrenal masses. One-third of pheochromocytomas are hereditary. Associated genes include the *RET* proto-oncogene (responsible for MEN2A and MEN2B, VHL, and neurofibromatosis type 1). Pheochromocytoma is not a component of autosomal dominant polycystic kidney disease.

    The classic presenting symptom of a pheochromocytoma is paroxysmal hypertension. Headaches and episodic palpitations or perspiration are also reported. On MRI, pheochromocytomas demonstrate a bright signal intensity of T2-weighted imaging due to their low lipid content. Of note, CT washout studies are considered the gold standard for adrenal imaging with adenomas demonstrating more rapid washout. On laboratory evaluation, patients will have elevated serum and urine metanephrines. Treatment is surgical. Patients require a preoperative catecholamine blockade either with α-blockers (phenoxybenzamine) or calcium channel blockers to prevent severe hypertension and/or cardiac arrhythmias. Postoperatively long-term follow-up is necessary; recurrences have been documented even 15 years after resection of a localized lesion.

BIBLIOGRAPHY

Kutikov A, Crispin PL, Uzzo RG. Pathophysiology, evaluation, and medical management of adrenal disorders. In: Wein A, Kavoussi L, Novick A, et al. (eds.), *Campbell's Urology*, 10th ed. Philadelphia, PA: W.B. Saunders; 2012.

26. **(D)** This figure depicts a staghorn calculus, or a stone that fills a major part of the renal collecting system, typically occupying the renal pelvis and branching into most calyces. Most are composed of struvite (magnesium ammonium phosphate), but cystine, calcium oxalate monohydrate, and uric acid crystals can also form staghorn configurations. These stones are often difficult to treat and, if left untreated, can cause pain, recurrent UTI, sepsis, renal failure, and mortality up to 30%.

The treatment of staghorn calculi is multifactorial. First, complete surgical removal of all stone burden is mandatory, as urea-splitting bacteriuria can persist and lead to stone regrowth if a nidus remains. Next, metabolic abnormalities must be appropriately treated. Last, anatomic variations that may contribute to urine stasis should be addressed.

Both PCNL and anatrophic nephrolithotomy are treatment options for staghorn calculi. However, studies have shown a similar stone-free rate between the treatment methods but less convalescence, morbidity, hospital stay, and blood transfusion in patients undergoing PCNL. ESWL monotherapy has been shown to yield a poor stone-free rate, but it is advocated by some to use ESWL in combination with PCNL for "sandwich therapy." When sandwich therapy is used, PCNL must always be the final procedure in the series. Ureteroscopy is appropriate for smaller stone burden but, in this setting, would likely necessitate multiple procedures.

BIBLIOGRAPHY

Matlaga B, Lingeman J. Surgical management of upper urinary tract calculi. In: Wein A, Kavoussi L, Novick A, et al. (eds.), *Campbell's Urology*, 10th ed. Philadelphia, PA: W.B. Saunders; 2012.

Pearle M, Lotan Y. Urinary lithiasis: etiology, epidemiology and pathogenesis. In: Wein A, Kavoussi L, Novick A, et al. (eds.), *Campbell's Urology*, 10th ed. Philadelphia, PA: W.B. Saunders; 2012.

27. **(E)** The CT cystogram reveals an intraperitoneal bladder rupture. After filling of the bladder with contrast, the abdomen is scanned. Here, extravasated contrast can be visualized in the colic gutters and the true pelvis, as well as outlining the ovaries. Intraperitoneal bladder ruptures tend to occur at the dome of the bladder.

In contrast to extraperitoneal bladder rupture, intraperitoneal bladder rupture should be managed with open operative repair. These injuries are unlikely to heal spontaneously, and chemical peritonitis, urinary ascites, ileus, and sepsis can occur if the bladder is not repaired. After repair, a drain should be utilized as well as bladder decompression with a Foley catheter, suprapubic tube, or both depending on the complexity of the injury and the need for maximal drainage of the bladder. Repeat imaging of the bladder, either fluoroscopic cystogram or CT cystogram, should be performed in 10–14 days after repair to ensure no further leakage exists.

BIBLIOGRAPHY

Morey AF, Duggi DD. Genital and lower urinary tract trauma. In: Wein A, Kavoussi L, Novick A, et al. (eds.), *Campbell's Urology*, 10th ed. Philadelphia, PA: W.B. Saunders; 2012.

28. **(C)** The retrograde urethrogram (RUG) demonstrates a posterior urethral injury, specifically a prostatomembranous urethral disruption. The majority of posterior urethral injuries occur in the setting of blunt trauma and pelvic fracture. The proposed mechanism is that shearing forces are generated separating the membranous urethra from the prostatic apex.

Anterior urethral injuries may be caused by blunt (urethra crushed against the pubic bone, e.g., straddle injury) or penetrating trauma (gunshot wound, knife wound). The classic presentation of a urethral injury includes blood at the meatus, inability to urinate, and a palpably full bladder. All patients with a suspected urethral injury should undergo a retrograde urethrogram prior to catheter placement; however, urethral disruption is often first suspected when a urethral Foley catheter is unable to be placed.

In the setting of a posterior urethral injury in a male, repair is deferred due to high rates of incontinence and impotence with immediate repair. Suprapubic tube placement to provide bladder drainage is therefore the appropriate next step in management. Of note, if the patient is clinically stable, primary realignment of the urethra may be attempted by the consulting urologist in some circumstances. If successful, the urethral Foley catheter is ultimately removed in approximately 4–6 weeks. In this circumstance, suprapubic drainage of the bladder is still necessary as many patients will develop a urethral stricture. In women, immediate repair, or at a minimum alignment of the urethra over a catheter, is important to avoid obliteration of the urethra and to prevent fistula formation.

Anterior urethral injuries due to penetrating trauma can be closed primarily when possible. Some circumstances may require bladder drainage and deferred repair.

BIBLIOGRAPHY

Morey AF, Duggi DD. Genital and lower urinary tract trauma. In: Wein A, Kavoussi L, Novick A, et al. (eds.), *Campbell's Urology*, 10th ed. Philadelphia, PA: W.B. Saunders; 2012.

29. **(E)** The classic triad of tuberous sclerosis (TS) consists of epilepsy, mental retardation, and adenoma sebaceum (facial angiofibromas). Central nervous system hamartomas are also common. Adenoma sebaceum are firm, discrete, red or brown telangiectatic papules located in the nasolabial folds, chin, and cheeks. Angiomyolipomas (AML) develop in up to 80% of patients with this autosomal dominant disorder. Those with TS are more likely to develop AML at a young age (mean age, 30 years) and have multiple, bilateral, and symptomatic tumors. Renal cysts also develop in 20% of patients with TS, and 2% will develop RCC.

AML is a benign renal tumor composed of blood vessels, smooth muscle, and adipose tissue. These are the only tumors that can be confidently diagnosed on cross-sectional imaging. The presence of fat (as confirmed on the nonenhanced phase as areas within the lesion measuring –10 to –50 Hounsfield units) confirms the diagnosis. Care must be taken not to misdiagnose liposarcoma or fat-poor AML. Although benign, it is the most common renal neoplasm associated with perirenal hemorrhage. Lesions greater than 4 cm in size are more prone to hemorrhage, and many advocate prophylactic selective embolization or partial nephrectomy for larger AMLs. Standard of care for acute hemorrhage is renal angioembolization.

VHL is also an autosomal dominant syndrome manifesting as cerebellar and retinal hemangioblastomas; pancreatic, kidney, and epididymal cysts; pheochromocytoma; and clear cell RCC. Beckwith-Wiedemann syndrome is associated with pediatric Wilms tumor and would be exceedingly rare after 15 years of age. Prune belly syndrome and Sturge-Weber syndrome are not associated with solid renal masses.

BIBLIOGRAPHY

Margulis V, Matin S, Wood C. Benign renal tumors. In: Wein A, Kavoussi L, Novick A, et al. (eds.), *Campbell's Urology*, 10th ed. Philadelphia, PA: W.B. Saunders; 2012.
Pope J. Renal dysgenesis and cystic disease of the kidney. In: Wein A, Kavoussi L, Novick A, et al. (eds.), *Campbell's Urology*, 10th ed. Philadelphia, PA: W.B. Saunders; 2012.
Ritchey M, Shamberger R. Pediatric urologic oncology. In: Wein A, Kavoussi L, Novick A, et al. (eds.), *Campbell's Urology*, 10th ed. Philadelphia, PA: W.B. Saunders; 2012.

30. **(A)** The mechanism of action of α-blockers is via relaxation of the prostatic smooth muscle. Studies have shown that over 90% of α-receptors in the prostate are localized to the prostatic stroma. Relaxation of the prostate smooth muscle decreases bladder outlet obstruction with subsequent improvement in the symptoms of BPH. The clinical response to therapy with α-blockers is rapid and dose dependent. Most α-blockers have the effect of lowering blood pressure, and therefore, it is important to counsel patients, particularly the elderly, on the side effects of dizziness and orthostatic hypotension.

Another class of drugs used in the treatment of BPH are the 5-α-reductase inhibitors (finasteride). Their mechanism of action is to block the conversion of testosterone to dihydrotestosterone (DHT) by competitive inhibition of the enzyme 5-α-reductase. The development of BPH is an androgen-dependent process, and therefore, lowering DHT levels ultimately reduces prostatic size and thus bladder outlet obstruction. Maximal reduction of prostate volume after initiation of androgen suppression is achieved within 6 months; thus, there may be a substantial delay for a patient to experience maximal clinical benefit. Side effects associated with 5-α-reductase inhibitors are minimal and are related primarily to sexual function (e.g., decreased libido, impotence, decreased volume of ejaculate). Of interest, finasteride is effective in the management of gross hematuria associated with BPH.

Combination therapy with α-blockers and 5-α-reductase inhibitors has been shown to prevent progression of BPH better than either agent alone in a prospective, randomized, double-blind, multicenter, placebo-controlled trial (Medical Therapy of Prostatic Symptoms Trial [MTOPS]).

BIBLIOGRAPHY

McNichols TA, Kirby RS, Lepor H. Evaluation and non-surgical management of benign prostatic hypertrophy. In: Wein A, Kavoussi L, Novick A, et al. (eds.), *Campbell's Urology*, 10th ed. Philadelphia, PA: W.B. Saunders; 2012.

31. **(A)** This scan reveals a grade 1 renal injury with several deep lacerations of the kidney into the collecting system as well as a perirenal hematoma. The most widely used and accepted classification system for staging and management of renal trauma is that of the American Association for the Surgery of Trauma Organ Injury Severity Scale for the Kidney (Table 38-1).

Significant renal injuries (grades 2–5) are found in only 5% of renal trauma scenarios. It is widely accepted that grade 1–3 injuries can be managed conservatively in the stable patient, regardless of mechanism. Patients with grades 4 and 5 injuries will more often require surgical exploration, but select patients can be managed nonoperatively.

TABLE 38-1 American Association for the Surgery of Trauma Renal Injury Scale

Grade	Injury Type	Description
1	Contusion	Microscopic or gross hematuria with normal imaging
	Hematoma	Subcapsular, nonexpanding without parenchymal laceration
2	Hematoma	Nonexpanding perirenal hematoma confined to renal retroperitoneum
		<1 cm in depth without urinary extravasation
3	Laceration	>1 cm in depth without collecting system rupture or urinary extravasation
4	Laceration	Parenchymal laceration through cortex, medulla, and collecting system
4	Vascular	Main renal artery or vein injury with contained hemorrhage
5	Laceration	Completely shattered kidney
5	Laceration	Avulsion of renal hilum leading to devascularized kidney

Source: From Brunicardi FC, Andersen D, Billiar T, et al. (eds.), *Schwartz's Principles of Surgery*, 9th ed. New York, NY: McGraw-Hill; 2010:Table 38-1.

Ninety-eight percent of blunt kidney injury can be managed nonoperatively, as can many renal stab wounds and even selective renal gunshot wounds. Absolute indications for renal exploration after trauma include (1) hemodynamic instability (shock); (2) expanding and/or pulsatile renal hematoma (indicative of renal artery avulsion); (3) suspected renal pedicle avulsion; and (4) ureteropelvic junction disruption. Relative indications are urinary extravasation together with nonviable tissue, concomitant colon or pancreatic injury, and a delayed arterial injury, which will likely necessitate delayed nephrectomy.

If conservative management is decided upon, hospital admission and bedrest in patients with gross hematuria are required. Ambulation should not be allowed until gross hematuria clears. The patient should know about the possibility of renovascular hypertension and delayed bleeding.

BIBLIOGRAPHY

La Rochelle J, Shuch B, Belldegrun A. Urology. In: Brunicardi FC, Andersen D, Billiar T, et al. (eds.), *Schwartz's Principles of Surgery*, 9th ed. New York, NY: McGraw-Hill; 2010.

Santucci R, Doumanian L. Upper urinary tract trauma. In: Wein A, Kavoussi L, Novick A, et al. (eds.), *Campbell's Urology*, 10th ed. Philadelphia, PA: W.B. Saunders; 2012.

32. **(C)** The left kidney is not perfused in this scan, with poor renal sinus vascular enhancement and good cortical rim enhancement from capsular vessels. This is consistent with renal artery occlusion secondary to intimal disruption from deceleration injury. For major renovascular injuries (laceration and thrombosis), there are often concomitant injuries requiring surgery. In most instances, rapid nephrectomy is advocated.

Before renal exploration, it is necessary to confirm contralateral renal function. In this case, CT verifies parenchymal uptake of contrast in the contralateral kidney. If an unstable patient is taken to the operating room without preoperative imaging, an "on-table" or one-shot IV pyelogram (IVP) can be performed 10 minutes after a 2-mL/kg bolus of IV contrast is given.

When immediate repair is possible, salvage rates for the kidney are low (33% salvage rate for main renal artery reconstruction). There are case reports of renal revascularization with the use of endovascular stents during angiography for renal artery thrombosis. With delayed diagnosis >8 hours, the kidney can rarely be salvaged. Additionally, hypertension often develops in patients with renal artery thrombosis, regardless of management.

Segmental renal arterial injuries should generally be managed nonoperatively.

BIBLIOGRAPHY

Santucci R, Doumanian L. Upper urinary tract trauma. In: Wein A, Kavoussi L, Novick A, et al. (eds.), *Campbell's Urology*, 10th ed. Philadelphia, PA: W.B. Saunders; 2012.

33. **(E)** This CT shows medial contrast extravasation on a delayed film indicating disruption of the collecting system at the UPJ. Ureteral injury is rare in blunt trauma, but it occurs more often in children, owing to the increased flexibility of their spinal columns. The mechanism of injury usually involves hyperextension and sudden deceleration with ureteral compression against a vertebral body.

    Classic findings on CT with delayed images include (1) medial perirenal/periureteral contrast extravasation; (2) contrast extravasation in the absence of parenchymal laceration; and (3) no visualization of the ipsilateral distal ureter. Immediate diagnosis can often be difficult, because 30% of patients with this injury will have a normal urinalysis.

    In stable patients in whom this diagnosis is made within 5 days of injury, immediate surgical repair is advocated. The type of repair is based on the location and extent of injury. After that time, placement of a ureteral stent or a nephrostomy tube with delayed repair after 12 weeks is preferred.

BIBLIOGRAPHY

Husmann D. Pediatric genitourinary trauma. In: Wein A, Kavoussi L, Novick A, et al. (eds.), *Campbell's Urology*, 10th ed. Philadelphia, PA: W.B. Saunders; 2012.

Husmann D. Upper urinary trauma. In: Docimo S, Canning D, Khoury A (eds.), *Clinical Pediatric Urology*, 5th ed. London, England: Informa Healthcare; 2007:536–537.

34. **(E)** All of the listed complications may be seen with the use of intestinal segments in urinary diversion. Metabolic complications arise from altered absorption in the repurposed intestinal segment, and the type of metabolic abnormality is directly related to which segment of intestine is used. The use of a gastric segment leads to the development of a hypochloremic, hypokalemic metabolic acidosis. Use of jejunum results in a hyponatremic, hypochloremic, hyperkalemic metabolic alkalosis. The more proximal the segment of jejunum, the more likely these electrolyte abnormalities are to occur. Ileum and colon cause a hyperchloremic, hypokalemic metabolic acidosis. This occurs due to reabsorption of renally excreted ammonium by the intestinal segment. Symptoms include fatigue/lethargy and anorexia. Treatment involves potassium citrate (to address the hypokalemia and acidosis) and, in some cases, blockers of chloride

transport (nicotinic acid, chlorpromazine), which will limit reabsorption of ammonium.

    Several factors lead to conduit stone formation including chronic infection with urease-producing bacteria, mucus production, and incomplete drainage of the conduit (particularly true in continent urinary diversions). The presence of a metabolic acidosis also increases the risk of stone formation primarily due to hypercalciuria.

    Osteomalacia occurs as a result of the chronic metabolic acidosis created typically by a ureterosigmoidostomy or ileal or colonic urinary diversion. Bone demineralization occurs as the body attempts to buffer the additional acid. Treatment involves correction of the acidosis and dietary supplementation of calcium.

    Patients with intestine in contact with the urinary tract have a higher rate of UTI, pyelonephritis, and sepsis. Of note, patients with conduits have a high incidence of bacteriuria and will have positive urine cultures. If asymptomatic and clinically well, these patients can often be managed with observation alone.

BIBLIOGRAPHY

Dahl DM, McDougal MA. Use of intestinal segments in urinary diversion. In: Wein A, Kavoussi L, Novick A, et al. (eds.), *Campbell's Urology*, 10th ed. Philadelphia, PA: W.B. Saunders; 2012.

35. **(B)** Approximately 70–75% of newly diagnosed bladder cancers present as tumors that do not invade the muscularis propria of the bladder wall. Of these, 70–75% are confined to the bladder mucosa (stage Ta). Most of these are low grade, or considered low risk for disease progression. Ta low-grade urothelial carcinoma only has a 5–10% chance of progression to muscle invasive disease, but 50–70% will recur. There is consensus that many small, low-grade tumors can be observed with surveillance cystoscopy and endoscopic resection, until they exhibit significant growth because of the minimal risk of progression.

    T1 tumors are also considered non-muscle-invasive, but unlike Ta lesions they invade the lamina propria of the urinary bladder. In patients with multifocal or large-volume, low-grade Ta cancer or in patients with high-grade Ta, T1, or carcinoma-in-situ (Tis) of the bladder, further treatment is warranted including possible repeat resection, intravesical chemotherapy, or intravesical immunotherapy (bacillus Calmette-Guérin). In contrast to low-grade Ta lesions, high-grade T1 lesions recur in 80% of cases and progress in 50% of patients within 5 years. Radical cystectomy may even be considered in select patients with the above characteristics and most patients with muscle-invasive (T2) disease unless comorbidity precludes this surgical option. Chemoradiation is an alternative bladder-sparing option.

BIBLIOGRAPHY

Hall MC, Chang SS, Dalbagni G, et al. Guideline for the management of nonmuscle invasive bladder cancer (stages Ta, T1, and Tis): 2007 update. *J Urol* 2007;178(6):2314–2330.

Jones JS, Larchian W. Non-muscle-invasive bladder cancer (Ta, T1, and CIS). In: Wein A, Kavoussi L, Novick A, et al. (eds.), *Campbell's Urology*, 10th ed. Philadelphia, PA: W.B. Saunders; 2012.

36. **(A)** Males are three to four times more likely to develop urothelial carcinoma (UC) of the bladder than females, and this is felt to be secondary to increased occupational exposure and an increased incidence of smoking in the past. The incidence rate of UC of the bladder is currently decreasing more rapidly in men than women because of the recent decrease in the percentage of men smoking as compared to women. The lifetime risk of developing UC in a white male has been calculated as 3.7%; this is approximately 3 times the probability of white females or black males and approximately 4.5 times the probability of black females developing UC in their lifetimes.

Environmental risk factors associated with the development of UC of the bladder include smoking, occupational exposure to carcinogens, and exposure to certain chemotherapeutic agents. As previously stated, tobacco, and in particular cigarette smoking, is the main known cause for development of UC of the bladder. The increase in risk in a smoker is approximately two to six times that of a nonsmoker, and this risk continues to increase with increased number of cigarettes smoked and years of smoking. Smoking cessation decreases the risk for UC.

Approximately 20–30% of all UC of the bladder is associated with occupational exposure, with aromatic amines being the most frequently implicated. Rubber workers have been found to be at the highest risk for development of bladder cancer.

Cyclophosphamide is a chemotherapeutic agent associated with development of UC of the bladder.

Chronic inflammation and infection as seen in patients with chronic indwelling bladder catheters predispose patients to squamous, not urothelial, cell carcinoma of the bladder.

BIBLIOGRAPHY

Wood D. Urothelial tumors of the bladder. In: Wein A, Kavoussi L, Novick A, et al. (eds.), *Campbell's Urology*, 10th ed. Philadelphia, PA: W.B. Saunders; 2012.

37. **(E)** The incidence of postoperative urinary retention is reported as being anywhere from 4–25%, occurring frequently after pelvic surgery. Other contributing factors include decreased awareness of bladder sensation, decreased bladder contractility, and increased bladder outlet resistance. Anesthesia, analgesia, and postoperative pain are all implicated in causing it, but the mechanisms are poorly understood. Studies have shown that bladder decompression with a Foley catheter for 18–24 hours postoperatively decreases the incidence of retention dramatically when compared with clean intermittent catheterization. Prophylactic treatment with phenoxybenzamine, an α-adrenergic blocker, has also been shown to decrease the incidence of postoperative retention.

BIBLIOGRAPHY

Wein A, Dmochowski R. Neuromuscular dysfunction of the lower urinary tract. In: Wein A, Kavoussi L, Novick A, et al. (eds.), *Campbell's Urology*, 10th ed. Philadelphia, PA: W.B. Saunders; 2012.

38. **(A)** Seventy-five percent of injuries to the testicle occur from blunt trauma. Rupture of the testicle with a laceration of the tunica albuginea is the most serious concern with blunt scrotal trauma and requires a high index of suspicion. Differential diagnoses include hematocele without rupture, testicular or appendage torsion, reactive hydrocele, hematoma of the epididymis or spermatic cord, and intratesticular hematoma. Swelling and bruising are variable in these cases, and the degree of hematoma present does not necessarily correlate with the severity of injury. Ultrasonography can assist in making a definitive diagnosis.

Testicular rupture can be seen as heterogeneous echotexture of the testicular parenchyma and disruption of the tunica albuginea. However, if ultrasound is equivocal and rupture is suspected, immediate surgical intervention should not be delayed.

Surgical exploration should strive to achieve testicular salvage, prevention of infection, control of bleeding, and decreased recuperation. Even small defects in the tunica should be closed. Intratesticular hematoma, even without rupture, should be explored and drained, to prevent further necrosis and subsequent atrophy. All penetrating scrotal trauma should be surgically explored to rule out vascular and vasal injury. Minor scrotal injuries without direct testicular damage can be managed conservatively with ice, elevation, and analgesics.

BIBLIOGRAPHY

Morey A, Dugi D. Genital and lower urinary tract trauma. In: Wein A, Kavoussi L, Novick A, et al. (eds.), *Campbell's Urology*, 10th ed. Philadelphia, PA: W.B. Saunders; 2012.

39. **(D)** Prune belly (Eagle-Barrett) syndrome is classically defined as a deficiency of the abdominal wall musculature, bilateral cryptorchidism, and a dilated and dysmorphic urinary tract. The majority of cases are sporadic with a normal karyotype. Most infants diagnosed with the disorder are males (95–97%), but cases in females have been reported (clearly without cryptorchidism). The lack of abdominal wall musculature can lead to delays in sitting and walking, as well as chronic respiratory infections and poor body image issues. Patients with prune belly syndrome can have many associated conditions, including pulmonary hypoplasia, renal dysplasia, hydronephrosis and insufficiency, cardiac anomalies, lower extremity musculoskeletal malformations, imperforate anus, and intestinal malrotation.

Diagnosis in the newborn is easily made because of the abdominal wall appearance. Presence and degree of pulmonary hypoplasia and renal insufficiency will most greatly affect immediate and ultimate prognosis, so this should be the focus of initial evaluation. Once stabilized, a thorough urologic examination and ultrasonography of the urinary tract are required to assess the degree of urinary tract dilation.

Overall goals of patient management are preservation of renal function and prevention of infection. These goals can be attained through a variety of treatment approaches, including watchful waiting and surgical reconstruction (immediate or delayed) tailored to the specific patient abnormalities.

BIBLIOGRAPHY

Hudson RG, Skoog S. Prune belly syndrome. In: Docimo S, Canning D, Khoury A (eds.), *Clinical Pediatric Urology*, 5th ed. London, England: Informa Healthcare; 2007:1081–1098.

CHAPTER 39

OBSTETRICS AND GYNECOLOGY

CECILY A. CLARK-GANHEART AND ELIZABETH M. COVIELLO

1. A 50-year-old, gravida 2 para 2, woman status post total abdominal hysterectomy (TAH), bilateral salpingo-oophorectomy (BSO) for a myomatous uterus presents with a 6-month history of pelvic pain and pressure. What is the most likely diagnosis?
   (A) Bartholin gland duct cyst
   (B) Vaginal vault prolapse
   (C) Urethral diverticulum
   (D) Vaginal neoplasm

2. A mother presents to your office with her 14-year-old daughter who has been experiencing monthly cyclical abdominal pain. Menarche has not yet occurred. During physical examination, an introital opening could not be identified. Rectal examination revealed a palpable anterior vaginal fullness and a palpable uterus. The correct diagnosis is
   (A) Vaginal agenesis
   (B) Imperforate hymen
   (C) Vaginal septum
   (D) Leiomyoma

Questions 3 and 4 refer to the following scenario.
A 33-year-old, gravida 2 para 1, pregnant obese woman at 26 weeks' gestation presents complaining of increasing nausea for 3 days with decreased appetite and one episode of emesis this morning. She also admits to abdominal pain but denies similar symptoms with her first pregnancy. Past medical history is significant only for obesity. Past obstetric history includes one prior spontaneous vaginal delivery at full term without complications. Physical examination reveals a temperature of 100°F and normal fetal heart tones at 140 bpm without uterine contractions.

3. Abdominal examination reveals right upper quadrant tenderness without uterine tenderness. Fundal height is appropriate to gestational age, and cervical examination reveals a normal, nondilated, firm cervix. Your next step in evaluation is
   (A) Serial cervical examinations
   (B) Abdominal ultrasound

(C) Urinalysis
(D) Antiemetic therapy with observation

4. Abdominal ultrasound, and specifically right upper quadrant ultrasound, reveals multiple small gallstones with biliary sludge present. The best treatment for this patient should include
   (A) Hospitalization with parenteral nutrition
   (B) Oral bile acid therapy
   (C) Laparoscopic cholecystectomy
   (D) Extracorporeal shock wave lithotripsy

Questions 5 and 6 refer to the following scenario.
You are the general surgeon on call at a community hospital and are paged to labor and delivery to assist the obstetrician with a cesarean delivery for a 32-year-old, gravida 5 para 5, woman with arrest of labor. A live-born 4000-g male infant was delivered, followed by extraction of the placenta. After delivery of the infant and placenta, increased hemorrhage is noted with greater than 1 L of blood loss. Vital signs are as follows: pulse rate, 100 bpm; blood pressure, 140/96 mmHg; and temperature, 99°F.

5. The most likely etiology for postpartum hemorrhage in this case scenario is
   (A) Uterine atony
   (B) Vaginal laceration
   (C) Chorioamnionitis
   (D) Prolonged labor

6. The next step in management is
   (A) Abdominal hysterectomy
   (B) Methylergonovine maleate (Methergine 0.2 mg intramuscularly)
   (C) Uterine massage
   (D) Intramuscular prostaglandin 15-methyl $F_{2\alpha}$ ($PGF_{2\alpha}$) 0.25 mg
   (E) Interventional radiology for arterial embolization

Questions 7 through 10 refer to the following scenario.

A 26-year-old nulliparous woman presents to the emergency room with sudden onset of right lower quadrant pain. She recently stopped her oral contraceptives as she desires pregnancy. Her last menstrual period was 5 weeks ago. She reports nausea and vomiting but denies any vaginal bleeding or fever. Her past medical history is otherwise unremarkable.

On physical examination, she is noticeably uncomfortable, but physical examination reveals no abdominal rebound tenderness. Bimanual examination reveals marked voluntary guarding and a fullness in the right lower quadrant as well as cervical motion tenderness.

7. Differential diagnosis in this patient does not include
   (A) Ectopic pregnancy
   (B) Adnexal torsion
   (C) Mittelschmerz
   (D) Acute appendicitis
   (E) Acute pancreatitis

8. Appropriate next steps include
   (A) Complete blood count (CBC)
   (B) Urine pregnancy test
   (C) Pelvic ultrasound
   (D) All of the above

9. The results of the pelvic ultrasound demonstrate an 8-cm right adnexal mass with minimal fluid in the cul-de-sac. CBC is normal, and urine pregnancy test is negative. Abnormal (markedly decreased) right ovarian arterial blood flow is noted on Doppler ultrasound. The most likely diagnosis now is
   (A) Adnexal/ovarian torsion
   (B) Ruptured hemorrhagic cyst
   (C) Tubo-ovarian abscess
   (D) Fallopian tube carcinoma

10. The most appropriate management of the patient described in Question 9 at this time is
    (A) Laparoscopic evaluation of the adnexa
    (B) Inpatient intravenous antibiotics
    (C) Exploratory laparotomy
    (D) Obtaining a serum CA-125 level

11. Leiomyosarcomas
    (A) Are malignant sarcomas that can mimic benign leiomyomas
    (B) Are diagnosed by pathologic and histologic examination
    (C) Are characterized by rapid uterine enlargement
    (D) Have a worse prognosis if the patient is postmenopausal
    (E) Are all of the above

12. Which of the following is *not* a risk factor for endometrial adenocarcinoma?
    (A) Early menarche
    (B) Diabetes
    (C) Obesity
    (D) Use of combination oral contraceptives, either presently or in the past

13. A 42-year-old para 3 woman presents for her routine yearly physical examination. She is having no problems. She recently had a normal mammogram and reports regular menses with slightly lessening flow. Her close friend was recently diagnosed with ovarian cancer. She expresses concern about her own chances of having ovarian cancer and wants to be thoroughly screened for it. Which of the following information do you share with her?
    (A) Ovarian cancer is the most common gynecologic malignancy.
    (B) Ovarian cancer is the leading cause of death among gynecologic malignances.
    (C) Transvaginal ultrasound has a limited role in ovarian cancer screening because of its inability to accurately visualize the ovaries in pre- and postmenopausal women.
    (D) The prevalence of ovarian cancer decreases after age 50 years.

Questions 14 through 16 refer to the following scenario.

A 28-year-old gravida 1 woman presents to the emergency room with vaginal bleeding and right lower quadrant pain. Last menstrual period was 8 weeks ago, and she had a positive home urine pregnancy test 2 weeks ago. Her past medical history is noncontributory except that she and her husband have been trying to conceive for 6 months. Past surgical history is significant for a laparoscopic right ovarian cystectomy 2 years ago for a mature teratoma. Physical examination reveals stable vital signs and a palpable right adnexal fullness with voluntary guarding. Mild cervical motion tenderness is noted, especially when moving the cervix to the patient's left. The cervix is closed and thick. There is a small amount of dark blood in the vagina but no acute active bleeding.

14. Appropriate workup at this point includes
    (A) Type and screen
    (B) Quantitative serum β-human chorionic gonadotropin (β-hCG)
    (C) CBC
    (D) Pelvic ultrasound
    (E) All of the above

15. The β-hCG is 6000 mIU/mL, CBC is within normal limits, blood type is A negative, and pelvic ultrasound shows no intrauterine pregnancy, minimal amount of fluid in the cul-de-sac, and a 3.0-cm mass in the right adnexa. The most likely diagnosis at this point is
    (A) Incomplete abortion
    (B) Threatened abortion
    (C) Hemorrhagic cyst
    (D) Ectopic pregnancy

16. Management options of a patient with a confirmed ectopic pregnancy include

    I. Intramuscular methotrexate

    II. Uterine dilation and curettage

    III. Laparoscopic salpingostomy

    IV. Expectant management

    (A) I, II, and III
    (B) I and III
    (C) II and IV
    (D) IV only
    (E) All of the above

Questions 17 and 18 refer to the following scenario.
A 53-year-old gravida 0 postmenopausal woman is referred to you for evaluation of a labial lump. She reports two prior episodes that spontaneously resolved within a few days. She states she noticed this present labial fullness after intercourse 1 day ago. Past medical and surgical history is significant only for a lipoma excision. On physical examination, she is afebrile, and you note a unilateral, tense, nonpainful 3-cm mass located at the region of the left labia minora.

17. The most likely diagnosis is
    (A) Bartholin gland abscess
    (B) Gartner duct cyst
    (C) Bartholin gland cyst
    (D) Vaginal mesonephric cyst

18. The preferred treatment option for this patient is
    (A) Obtain an intravenous pyelogram (IVP) to assess the urinary collecting system
    (B) Incision and drainage of mass
    (C) Excision or biopsy
    (D) Expectant management because spontaneous resolution is more common in older patients

ANSWERS AND EXPLANATIONS

1. **(B)** Pelvic organ prolapse is a common diagnosis affecting millions of American women. Risk factors in the development of pelvic organ prolapse include the following: childbirth, smoking, menopause, chronic medical conditions such as collagen vascular diseases, chronic obstructive pulmonary disease, obesity, prior pelvic surgery, and other social or environmental factors associated with chronic increased abdominal pressure. The common exposure in these conditions is increased abdominal pressure, which leads to nerve and muscle devascularization along with ligamentous stretching and tearing, resulting in pelvic floor laxity and dysfunction.

The vagina is a fibromuscular tube extending from the vestibule to the uterus in the standing position. The upper vagina runs horizontally. It is commonly at a 90-degree angle with the uterus. The vagina is held in its position by the surrounding endopelvic fascia and ligaments. Endopelvic fascia is a fine meshwork of collagen, elastin, and neural fibers.

The uterus is a thick-walled, hollow muscular organ located centrally in the female pelvis. Anterior to the uterus is the bladder with the rectum posteriorly and broad ligaments laterally. The dome-shaped upper portion of the uterus is termed the fundus. The short area of constriction in the lower uterus is termed the isthmus below which is the uterine cervix, which extends into the upper portion of the vagina.

Extending from the uterus are five pairs of ligaments (see Fig. 39-1). The pelvic ligaments, however, are not classic ligaments but are thickenings of retroperitoneal fascia and consist primarily of blood and lymphatic vessels, nerves, and fatty connective tissue. The retroperitoneal fascia is referred to by surgeons as endopelvic fascia. Extending from the superior portion of the uterus are the paired round ligaments and utero-ovarian ligaments. The round ligament provides minimal support to the uterus but is an important surgical landmark in making the initial incision into the parietal peritoneum, allowing access to the retroperitoneal space. The round ligament is composed of fibrous tissue and muscle fibers and runs via the broad ligament to the lateral pelvic side wall, entering into the inguinal canal and terminally inserting into the labia majora. The utero-ovarian ligament is one of three ligaments that provide anatomic mobility to the ovary. This is a narrow, short, fibrous band extending from the lower pole of the ovary to the uterus. The broad ligaments are a double reflection of peritoneum, stretching the lateral pelvic side wall to the uterus, which becomes contiguous with the uterine serosa. These peritoneal folds enclose a loose connective tissue termed the parametrium. The broad ligaments provide minor support to the uterus but are conduits to many important anatomic structures of the pelvis. The uterosacral ligaments extend from the upper portion of the cervix posteriorly to the third sacral vertebra. They are thickened anteriorly near the cervix and run a curved course around the lateral aspect of the rectum. Along with the cardinal ligaments, the uterosacral ligaments provide the major support to

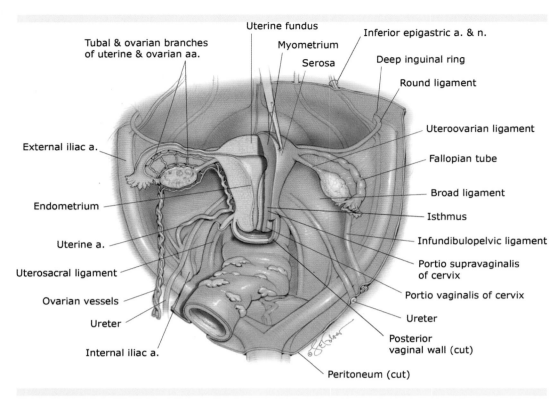

FIGURE 39-1. Uterine ligaments. From Corton MM, Cunningham FG: Anatomy. In Hoffman BL, Schorge JO, Schaffer JI, et al (eds): *Williams Gynecology*, 2nd ed. New York, McGraw-Hill, 2012, p 943.

the uterus and cervix. The cardinal ligaments extend from the lateral aspect of the upper portion of the cervix and vagina to the pelvic side wall.

Support to the uterus, cervix, and vagina is often described in three levels as described by DeLancey. Level I support includes the uterus and upper vagina as provided by the uterosacral cardinal ligament complex. Level II support includes the middle third of the vagina, including the lateral attachment of the vagina with the endopelvic fascia to the arcus tendineus fascia pelvis. Level III is the distal or lower third vaginal support associated with the urethral attachment in apposition with the pelvic and urogenital diaphragms.

In this case presentation, the patient's surgical history is the risk factor toward development of pelvic organ prolapse. Clinical presentations of pelvic organ prolapse include cystocele, rectocele, enterocele, uterine prolapse, and vaginal vault prolapse. These terms describe the relaxation of the anterior, posterior, and middle or superior compartments, respectively. Numerous surgical procedures have been described in order to restore the pelvic support anatomy. As seen in this case presentation, symptoms of discomfort, pain, and pressure in the vaginal area are common and may also be associated with bowel and bladder dysfunction including urinary and fecal incontinence and urinary retention (Table 39-1).

TABLE 39-1 Clinical-Anatomic Correlation

Level	Structure	Function	Effect of Damage
Level I: Suspension	Upper paracolpium	Suspends apex to pelvic walls	Prolapse of vaginal apex
Level II: Attachment	Lower paracolpium Pubocervical fascia Rectovaginal fascia	Supports bladder and vesical neck Prevents anterior expansion of rectum	Cystocele-urethrocele Rectocele
Level III: Fusion	Fusion to perineal membrane, perineal body, musculus levator ani	Fixes vagina to adjacent structures	Urethrocele or deficient perineal body

BIBLIOGRAPHY

DeLancey J. Anatomic aspects of vaginal eversion after hysterectomy. *Am J Obstet Gynecol* 1992;166:1717–1724.

Droegemueller W. Reproductive anatomy. In: Stenchever MA, Droegemueller W, Herbst AL, Mishell DR Jr (eds.), *Comprehensive Gynecology*, 4th ed. St. Louis, MO: Mosby; 2001.

2. **(B)** Congenital anomalies of the female reproductive tract are often caused by genetic error or by a teratologic event during embryonic development. Minor abnormalities are often of little consequence, but major abnormalities may lead to severe impairment of menstrual and reproductive functions.

One of the common abnormalities of the external genitalia includes imperforate hymen. The hymen is a thin membrane at the vaginal orifice covered by stratified squamous epithelium and consisting of fibrous tissue. It represents the junction of the sinovaginal bulbs with the urogenital sinus. Perforation of the hymen ordinarily occurs during embryonic life to establish connection between the vaginal canal and vestibule. Because this is an abnormality of the external genitalia, the internal genitalia are intact.

In the pediatric patient, the diagnosis of imperforate hymen is rarely made before puberty, because primary amenorrhea is the major symptom. At puberty, the patient may experience cyclic cramping; however, because of outflow obstruction, no menstrual flow is evident. This may result in hematocolpos, menstrual blood trapped behind the hymen, and/or hematometrium, menstrual blood trapped in the uterus, as is seen in this case scenario with a palpable vaginal fluid collection. Diagnosis is often made by history and clinical examination demonstrating a bulging membrane at the introitus. Therapy is surgical and consists of a cruciate incision into the hymen extending to the 10, 2, and 6 o'clock positions.

Vaginal agenesis occurs with both Rokitansky-Küster-Hauser syndrome and testicular feminization syndrome. In both syndromes, there is complete absence of the uterus, thus ruling out these diagnoses in this case scenario. Rokitansky-Küster-Hauser syndrome is the congenital absence of both vagina and uterus and is associated with the genotype of 46,XX. The ovaries and fallopian tubes are usually present. Twenty-five percent of these patients may have a short vaginal pouch. This disorder does not appear to be an inherited condition.

Testicular feminization syndrome (also known as androgen insensitivity) demonstrates a 46,XY karyotype. This is usually associated with complete vaginal agenesis or the presence of a short vaginal pouch. These patients have undescended testicles and male sex ducts, and therefore, no internal female genitalia are present. The testes in these patients should be removed after puberty to prevent the risk of seminomas. These disorders are often associated with additional urologic and skeletal abnormalities and should, therefore, be screened.

Vaginal septum is incorrect as this is associated with incomplete canalization of the vaginal canal and would be associated with a shortened vaginal pouch.

BIBLIOGRAPHY

Stenchever MA. Congenital anomalies of the female reproductive tract. In: Stenchever MA, Droegemueller W, Herbst AL, Mishell DR Jr (eds.), *Comprehensive Gynecology*, 4th ed. St. Louis, MO: Mosby; 2001:254.

Wilson EE. Pediatric gynecology. In: Schorge JO, Schaffer JI, Halvorson LM, Hoffman BL, Bradshaw KD, Cunningham FG (eds.), *Williams Gynecology*. New York, NY: McGraw-Hill; 2009:317–318.

3. **(B)**

4. **(C)**

Explanations for questions 3 and 4

Gallbladder disease including cholelithiasis is common in the United States and affects upward of 20% of women over the age of 40. Gallstones are most commonly cholesterol predominant, and oversecretion into the bile is a major factor in pathogenesis. Biliary sludge, which has been shown to increase during pregnancy, is also an important precursor to gallstone formation. As the cumulative risk for surgery remains low at approximately 1–2% per year, prophylactic cholecystectomy is not recommended for asymptomatic gallstones. Similarly, in pregnancy and the puerperium, the incidence of asymptomatic gallstones on ultrasound approaches 10%; therefore, as in the nonpregnant patient, cholecystectomy is not recommended for silent stones.

Pregnancy is associated with an increased risk of gallstones. Multiple nonsurgical approaches for gallstone disease are available. These options include oral bile acid therapy, extracorporeal shock wave lithotripsy, and contact dissolution; however, no experience with these methods during pregnancy is available. Therefore, they are not recommended in the obstetric patient.

Cholecystitis holds a high recurrence rate during the same pregnancy. With recurrence later in gestation, complications of this disease including preterm labor and biliary pancreatitis are more likely. Similarly, surgical management including cholecystectomy becomes technically more difficult. Because of these factors, more aggressive surgical approach is recommended. Cholecystectomy, both open and laparoscopic, has been demonstrated to be equally safe throughout pregnancy. In the patient with concomitant pancreatitis, cholecystectomy should be considered after inflammation subsides.

Of note, several serious obstetrical complications can present with nausea, vomiting, and right upper quadrant pain. Although the case scenario is consistent with cholecystitis, clinicians should also consider hypertensive disorders of pregnancy (preeclampsia/HELLP [hemolysis, elevated liver enzymes, low platelet count] syndrome), acute fatty liver of pregnancy, and thrombotic thrombocytopenic purpura (TTP)/hemolytic uremic syndrome (HUS). The following examinations should be performed: review of the patient's history (for presence of headache or other cerebral disturbances), vital signs (looking for the presence of hypertension), a physical exam (for presence of hyperreflexia or petechiae, which could signal disseminated intravascular coagulation), comprehensive metabolic panel (for the presence of transaminitis, bilirubin, and glucose), and a CBC (for the presence of thrombocytopenia). If abnormalities are present, consideration of an obstetrical cause is warranted, even in the presence of cholelithiasis on ultrasound. Consultation with an obstetrician or maternal fetal medicine specialist to assist in management is critical, because in the case of preeclampsia, HELLP, and acute fatty liver of pregnancy, delivery is typically indicated for treatment, whereas plasmapheresis is required in TTP/HUS.

BIBLIOGRAPHY

Cunningham FG, Leveno KJ, Bloom SL, et al. (eds.), Hepatic, biliary and pancreatic disorder. In: *Williams Obstetrics*, 24th ed. New York, NY: McGraw-Hill Education; 2014.

5. **(A)**

6. **(C)**

Explanations for questions 5 and 6

The female reproductive organs are supplied by a network of arteries. The arteries are generally paired bilaterally and have multiple, collateral connections resulting in an extensive anastomotic network. The arteries generally enter their respective organs laterally and unite with the vessels from the contralateral side near the midline. Venous drainage is complex and accompanies the arterial system.

The ovarian arteries originate from the aorta just below the renal vessels (see Fig. 39-2). During their course in the

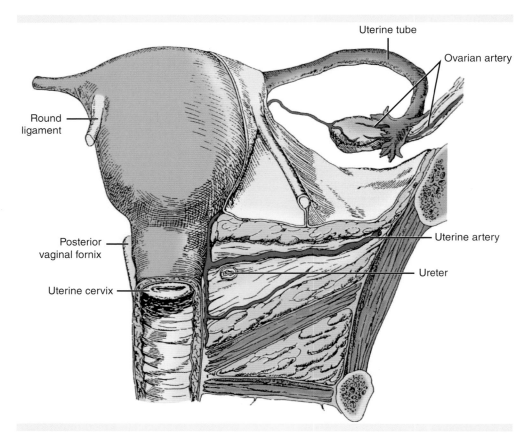

FIGURE 39-2. Ovarian and uterine arteries. From Skandalakis JE, Colborn GL, Weidman TA, et al. *Skandalakis' Surgical Anatomy*. New York, NY: McGraw-Hill; 2004:Fig. 28-11.

retroperitoneal space, the ovarian arteries will cross anterior to the ureter and enter the infundibulopelvic ligament to supply the ovary and oviduct. The ovarian artery will then unite with the ascending branch of the uterine artery just under the suspensory ligament of the ovary.

After the bifurcation, the common iliac artery divides into the external iliac and hypogastric (internal iliac) arteries (see Fig. 39-3). The hypogastric arteries are approximately 3–4 cm in length and throughout their course are in close association with the ureters. Each hypogastric artery branches into an anterior and posterior division. The posterior division divides into three parietal branches: iliolumbar, lateral sacral, and superior gluteal arteries. The anterior division has nine branches including three parietal and six visceral branches: the obturator, internal pudendal, and inferior gluteal comprise the parietal branches, whereas the umbilical, medial vesical, inferior vesical, middle hemorrhoidal, uterine, and vaginal arteries comprise the visceral branches. The superior vesical artery often arises from the umbilical artery. In situations of hemorrhage, surgical ligation of the anterior division of the hypogastric arteries distal to the posterior parietal branch either unilaterally or bilaterally is effective in controlling hemorrhage. Because of the extensive collateral circulation, this procedure results in reduction of pulse pressure, which allows clot formation without producing hypoxia.

Postpartum hemorrhage is a serious complication of labor and delivery and requires a coordinated and rapid response. Possible etiologies for postpartum hemorrhage are uterine atony, retained placenta, genital tract lacerations, maternal coagulopathy, uterine inversion or rupture, and low-lying placenta. General risk factors for the development of postpartum hemorrhage include both obstetric and medical disorders. Obstetric risk factors include multiparity, prolonged labor, preeclampsia, use of antepartum oxytocin, chorioamnionitis, low-lying or retained placenta, uterine overdistention secondary to polyhydramnios or multifetal pregnancy, and operative vaginal delivery. Similarly, the use of uterine relaxants for tocolysis in the setting of preterm labor or halogenated inhalation agents for anesthesia has also been associated with increased hemorrhage.

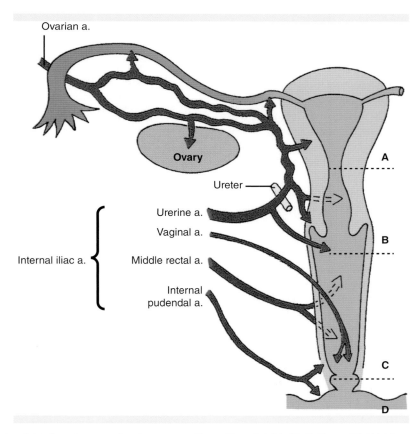

FIGURE 39-3. Blood supply of the female reproductive system. From Skandalakis JE, Colborn GL, Weidman TA, et al. *Skandalakis' Surgical Anatomy*. New York, NY: McGraw-Hill; 2004:Fig. 26-6.

This patient has uterine atony for which she has three risk factors. She has had five obstetric deliveries (multiparity) and delivered a large neonate after a probable prolonged labor that resulted in arrest. Vaginal laceration in this patient is unlikely because her child was delivered by cesarean section. Similarly, chorioamnionitis in the afebrile patient is less likely. Prolonged labor is a risk factor for uterine atony and not an etiology for postpartum hemorrhage. Inspection of the surgical field should be performed to verify hemostasis at all suture lines. In addition, lacerations or extension of the uterine incision should be identified and repaired.

Initial treatment for uterine atony should include vigorous uterine bimanual massage along with intravenous oxytocin (20 units in 1000 mL of lactated Ringer's or normal saline at 10 mL/min). Rapid infusion of oxytocin is not recommended due to increased risk for water intoxication. To perform a bimanual massage following a cesarean delivery, one hand is placed on the lower uterine segment, while the other hand is placed on the uterine fundus. The uterus is then compressed between the two hands and continuously massaged until the uterus becomes firm. When the uterus is no longer atonic, finger indentation should not be possible or, if present, should be minimal. This method can be performed following a vaginal delivery by placing one hand into the vagina to reach the lower uterine segment, while the other hand is placed onto the patient's abdomen at the level of the fundus.

If inadequate response is noted, ergot derivatives may be used to stimulate uterine contraction. The agent most commonly used is methylergonovine maleate (Methergine) 0.2 mg intramuscularly. Methylergonovine is contraindicated in the hypertensive patient and should not be given intravenously. If no response persists, prostaglandin derivatives including $PGF_{2\alpha}$ (Hemabate) can be given either intramuscularly or intramyometrially and is the best next step. The initial recommended dose is 250 µg. $PGF_{2\alpha}$ is contraindicated in patients with asthma because it can precipitate bronchospasm. Misoprostol (Cytotec) is another agent that is highly useful in the treatment of postpartum hemorrhage as a result of uterine atony. The standard dose is 1000 µg administered rectally (preferred route), although oral or intrauterine administration has been tried. Common side effects include GI distress and fever. The agent is especially useful when administration of other agents is contraindicated.

If bleeding continues to be unresponsive to uterotonic agents, reevaluation for lacerations or retained placenta is necessary. Additional resuscitative efforts including two large-bore intravenous catheters should be used to administer intravenous crystalloid and/or blood. Coagulation profile should also be evaluated.

Surgical management is then indicated for failed medical therapy. This may include initially uterine artery ligation, compression sutures (such as B-lynch), hypogastric artery ligation, or hysterectomy. If available, consideration for interventional radiologic treatment with arterial embolization may be considered but only in the hemodynamically stable patient.

Although hypogastric artery ligation can be effective at controlling hemorrhage, it is rarely performed by most clinicians. This maneuver should be reserved for someone familiar with pelvic surgery because ligation of the posterior division (as opposed to the anterior division) can result in necrosis of the buttock.

BIBLIOGRAPHY

Cunningham FG, Leveno KJ, Bloom SL, et al. (eds.), Obstetrical hemorrhage. In: *Williams Obstetrics*, 24th ed. New York, NY: McGraw-Hill Education; 2014:781–788.

Schorge JO, Schaffer JI, Halvorson LM, Hoffman BL, Bradshaw KD, Cunningham FG (eds.), Anatomy. In: *Williams Gynecology*. New York, NY: McGraw-Hill; 2009:791–793.

7. **(E)**

8. **(D)**

9. **(A)**

10. **(A)**

Explanations for questions 7 to 10

The differential diagnosis of a sexually active female patient presenting with right lower quadrant (RLQ) pain is vast. Differential diagnosis includes ectopic pregnancy, adnexal torsion, mittelschmerz/ovarian cyst rupture, hydrosalpinx, pelvic inflammatory disease (PID)/tubo-ovarian abscess, and acute appendicitis.

PID, also known as acute salpingitis, is an upper reproductive tract infection. PID is a clinical diagnosis. The most recently recommended guidelines for diagnosis by the Centers for Disease Control and Prevention (CDC; 2010) are as follows: sexually active patients with cervical motion tenderness or uterine or adnexal tenderness along with one of the following: oral temperature >101°F, abnormal cervical or vaginal mucopurulent discharge, presence of vaginal white blood cells (WBC) on microscopy, elevated erythrocyte sedimentation rate (ESR) or C-reactive protein, and presence of cervical *Neisseria gonorrhoeae* or *Chlamydia trachomatis* infection. Patients with a high suspicion of PID should be treated immediately to prevent potential complications including tubo-ovarian abscesses and infertility. Patients with mild to moderate disease can be treated with as outpatients; however, if symptoms do not resolve in 72 hours, inpatient management with parenteral broad-spectrum antibiotics is indicated in accordance with CDC recommendations.

There is an increased prevalence of sexually transmitted diseases leading to PID/pelvic adhesions. Advanced technology of and increased access to artificial reproductive technology and increased use of IUD with failures have all contributed to an increase in ectopic pregnancy. Patients commonly present with a history of amenorrhea and pelvic pain. Patients may present with hypotension and tachycardia consistent with a ruptured ectopic pregnancy, which is a surgical emergency. Diagnosis is made by a quantitative β-hCG level and a transvaginal ultrasound. A normal pregnancy should have a β-hCG level that doubles every 48 hours with visualization of a gestational sac on transvaginal ultrasound with a β-hCG level of 1500–2000 IU/L; however, this is institutional dependent. Once confirmed, ectopic pregnancy can be managed medically with methotrexate (MTX), if there are no absolute contraindications to MTX therapy, or surgically.

Adnexal torsion most commonly occurs in women of reproductive age with ovarian cysts. Both ovarian torsion and rupture of ovarian cysts can also cause sudden-onset lower abdominal pain. However, torsion is a surgical emergency, whereas ruptured ovarian cysts can be managed with supportive treatment and ovarian suppression with oral contraceptive pills. Cysts that are greater than 5 cm more commonly cause adnexal torsion with the tube and ovary twisting around the round ligament. Patients commonly present with sudden lower quadrant pain with radiation to flank or thigh. Sometimes this is accompanied by a low-grade fever or nausea and vomiting. Diagnosis is commonly made with Doppler studies on ultrasound. Management includes a diagnostic laparoscopy or laparotomy. The goal of surgery is detorsion, cystectomy, and salvage of the tube and ovary if possible.

Mittelschmerz is midcycle pain believed to be because of ovarian follicular rupture during ovulation; however, the actual mechanism is not clearly understood. Both mittelschmerz and a ruptured ovarian cyst can present with acute onset of pelvic pain; however, following the results of the pelvic ultrasound, mittelschmerz or a ruptured hemorrhagic ovarian cyst is unlikely, as the patient is noted to have a right adnexal mass and minimal fluid in the cul-de-sac. Typically, there is marked fluid in the cul-de-sac following a ruptured ovarian cyst, and an adnexal mass or cyst is not present.

The diagnosis of appendicitis is difficult in pregnant women due to both the occurrence of mild leukocytosis with pregnancy and the movement of the appendix upward and outward as the uterus enlarges. Abdominal pain and tenderness are common findings, and ultrasound can assist in the diagnosis. Despite this, suspected appendicitis is one of the most frequent causes of abdominal exploration during pregnancy. When the diagnosis is uncertain and other possibilities have been ruled out, exploration is appropriate given the high rates of fetal loss in cases of rupture.

BIBLIOGRAPHY

Centers for Disease Control and Prevention. Sexually transmitted diseases treatment guidelines. *MMWR Recomm Rep* 2010;59(No. RR-12):63–67.

Cunningham F, Leveno KJ, Bloom SL, et al. Gastrointestinal disorders. In: Cunningham F, Leveno KJ, Bloom SL, (eds.), *Williams Obstetrics*, 24th ed. New York, NY: McGraw-Hill; 2013.

Hemsell DL. Gynecologic infection. In: Schorge JO, Schaffer JI, Halvorson LM, Hoffman BL, Bradshaw KD, Cunningham FG, (eds.), *Williams Gynecology*. New York, NY: McGraw-Hill; 2009:73–76.

Schorge JO, Schaffer JI, Halvorson LM, Hoffman BL, Bradshaw KD, Cunningham FG (eds.), Ectopic pregnancy. In: *Williams Gynecology*. New York, NY: McGraw-Hill; 2009:157–169.

Schorge JO, Schaffer JI, Halvorson LM, Hoffman BL, Bradshaw KD, Cunningham FG (eds.), Pelvic mass. In: *Williams Gynecology*. New York, NY: McGraw-Hill; 2009:215–217.

11. **(E)** Leiomyosarcoma is a smooth muscle malignancy of the uterus. Of all the uterine sarcomas that can occur, leiomyosarcomas are the most common, but the overall incidence is very rare. Approximately 0.1% of uterine leiomyomas are noted to have a malignant change consistent with a leiomyosarcoma. The signs and symptoms of a leiomyosarcoma are similar to those of a leiomyoma—abnormal bleeding, pressure, and abdominal fullness. However, rapid enlargement of a presumed benign leiomyoma, particularly in a perimenopausal or postmenopausal patient, should heighten the clinician's suspicion for a leiomyosarcoma. Leiomyosarcomas often occur in patients in their fifties and in conjunction with leiomyomas. Once thought to be a result of malignant degeneration of benign leiomyomas, leiomyosarcomas are now thought to arise *de novo*.

One study by Leibsohn and colleagues evaluated hysterectomy specimens from 1423 patients with a uterine size 12 weeks or greater. The incidence of sarcoma was 0.4% for patients in their thirties. The incidence increased for patients in their fifties to 1.4%. In addition to the increased incidence of leiomyosarcomas in postmenopausal patients, the prognosis and survival are decreased in the postmenopausal population. Histologically, a triad of hypercellularity, nuclear atypia, and numerous mitotic figures is seen in leiomyosarcomas. Differentiation between a leiomyoma and leiomyosarcoma is based on the microscopic evaluation of the level of mitotic activity and the cellular atypia. Five mitotic figures per 10 high-powered fields (HPF) with cytologic atypia confirms the diagnosis of leiomyosarcoma. Vascular invasion, extrauterine spread, and >10 mitotic figures/10 HPF all worsen the prognosis. The overall 5-year survival is 20% but increases to approximately 40% in patients with stage I or II disease.

TAH/BSO is the most important treatment for leiomyosarcomas, and in reality, diagnosis is made and confirmed at the time of hysterectomy. Distant metastases to the lung, liver, and bone do occur, but lymph node metastases are uncommon. Radiotherapy and chemotherapy have been used with fair results.

BIBLIOGRAPHY

Burrows LJ, Elkins TE. Leiomyoma. In: Ransom SB, Dombrowski MP, McNeeley SG, et al. (eds.), *Practical Strategies in Obstetrics and Gynecology*. Philadelphia, PA: W.B. Saunders; 2000:53.

Herbst AL. Neoplastic diseases of the uterus. In: Stenchever MA, Droegemueller W, Herbst A, et al. (eds.), *Comprehensive Gynecology*, 4th ed. St. Louis, MO: Mosby; 2001:943.

Miller DS. Uterine sarcoma. In: Schorge JO, Schaffer JI, Halvorson LM, Hoffman BL, Bradshaw KD, Cunningham FG, (eds.), *Williams Gynecology*. New York, NY: McGraw-Hill; 2009:707–713.

Whelan JG, Vlatios NE, Wallach EE. Contemporary management of leiomyomas. In: Ransom SB, Dombrowski MP, Evans MI, et al. (eds.), *Contemporary Therapy in Obstetrics and Gynecology*. Philadelphia, PA: W.B. Saunders; 2000:367.

12. **(D)** Endometrial carcinoma is the most common gynecologic malignancy in the United States. One out of 50 women in the United States will develop endometrial cancer in her life. This is 1.3 times the likelihood of developing ovarian cancer and twice that of developing cervical cancer.

Postmenopausal bleeding is the presenting symptom in approximately 90% of patients with endometrial adenocarcinoma. By definition, postmenopausal bleeding is vaginal bleeding that occurs 1 year after the last normal menstrual period. In the premenopausal patient, endometrial cancer can be associated with menorrhagia, metrorrhagia, or menometrorrhagia. Sampling of the endometrium (either via endometrial biopsy or dilatation and curettage) is indicated. Transvaginal ultrasound to evaluate the thickness of the endometrial lining in a postmenopausal patient is helpful in the diagnosis of endometrial hyperplasia or adenocarcinoma. A thickness greater than 5 mm on transvaginal ultrasound warrants histologic evaluation in a postmenopausal patient not taking hormone therapy.

The main risk factor for endometrial adenocarcinoma is endometrial stimulation by unopposed estrogen. The postmenopausal patient taking estrogen alone has a four- to eightfold increased risk of developing endometrial adenocarcinoma. Patients with breast cancer taking tamoxifen are also at an increased risk. Tamoxifen is a selective estrogen receptor modulator with both estrogen and antiestrogen properties. The use of a progestin

in addition to estrogen therapy decreases the risk of endometrial cancer. Likewise, there is a decreased risk of endometrial adenocarcinoma in patients taking combination oral contraceptives. Other risk factors include obesity, nulliparity, late menopause (after age 52 years), and diabetes. Hypertension has often been reported as a risk factor but has not been established as an independent risk factor; obesity and hypertension are frequently seen in the same patient.

The staging of endometrial adenocarcinoma is based on surgical and pathologic findings. The primary therapy for endometrial adenocarcinoma is exploratory laparotomy, pelvic washings, and TAH/BSO. High-grade lesions (grade 2 or 3), depth of myometrial invasion, cervical involvement, and histology consistent with papillary serous or clear cell carcinoma increase the risk of lymphatic spread. The benefit of complete surgical staging has been debated, and lymph node sampling may be reserved for the above high-risk findings.

BIBLIOGRAPHY

Herbst AL. Neoplastic diseases of the uterus. In: Stenchever MA, Droegemueller W, Herbst A, et al. (eds.), *Comprehensive Gynecology*, 4th ed. St. Louis, MO: Mosby; 2001:919–921.

Miller DS. Endometrial cancer. In: Schorge JO, Schaffer JI, Halvorson LM, Hoffman BL, Bradshaw KD, Cunningham FG (eds.), *Williams Gynecology*. New York, NY: McGraw-Hill; 2009:687–700.

Ransom SB, Dombrowski MP, McNeeley SG, et al. (eds.), *Practical Strategies in Obstetrics and Gynecology*. Philadelphia, PA: W.B. Saunders; 2000.

13. **(B)** Ovarian cancer is the deadliest gynecologic malignancy. Endometrial cancer is the most common gynecologic malignancy. Ovarian cancer accounts for 4% of all new cancers diagnosed in women, and 14,000 deaths occur each year from ovarian cancer.

Seventy-five percent of all ovarian cancers are diagnosed at an advanced stage, and survival is based on histologic grade and extent of disease at time of diagnosis. Overall 5-year survival for all stages of ovarian cancer is 50%, but decreases to 28% with stage III or IV disease at initial diagnosis. If detected and treated at stage I, 5-year survival approaches 95%. Early diagnosis is the key to survival and successful treatment; however, early clinical symptoms rarely occur. For this reason, ovarian cancer screening using ultrasound and serum tumor markers has gained increased attention.

Ultrasonography can detect early morphologic changes in ovarian cancer and has been used as a screening tool. Transvaginal ultrasound has improved the resolution of ovarian imaging because the transvaginal transducer is in a closer proximity to the ovaries than a transabdominal transducer. Transvaginal ultrasonography can accurately visualize the ovaries in approximately 95% of premeno-pausal women and 85% of postmenopausal women. However, high-false positive rates of abnormal ovarian ultrasound findings and an inability to show a decrease in ovarian cancer deaths by screening for ovarian cancer with ultrasound have limited the usefulness of ovarian ultrasound as a universal screening tool.

A radioimmunoassay is used to detect serum tumor marker CA-125. It is elevated in over 80% of stage III and IV ovarian cancers, but an elevated CA-125 is not specific for ovarian cancer. Other conditions such as endometriosis, leiomyomas, smoking, PID, inflammatory bowel disease, diverticulitis, and several nongynecologic malignancies are also associated with an elevated CA-125. When combining elevated serum CA-125 with abnormal pelvic ultrasound findings, surgical intervention yielded an ovarian cancer specificity of 99.9% and a positive predictive value of 26.8%.

The lifetime risk of a woman developing ovarian cancer is 1:70 and increases to 1:20 with one affected first-degree relative and 1:14 with two or more affected first-degree relatives. Focusing on high-risk populations may improve the yield of ovarian cancer screening. A family history consistent with hereditary ovarian cancer syndrome puts a woman at the highest risk for developing ovarian cancer. Women with site-specific familial ovarian cancer, breast ovarian cancer syndrome, or a predisposition to developing ovarian, endometrial, and/or colon cancer (Lynch syndrome II) have been reported to develop ovarian cancer as early as age 30–40 years.

The prevalence of ovarian cancer is highest in women over age 50. There is a greater than threefold increase in risk for ovarian cancer between the age of 40 years compared to 75 years. There is also an increase in ovarian cancer mortality in women over 65 years of age.

BIBLIOGRAPHY

Platt LD, Karlan BY, Greene NH, et al. Screening for ovarian cancer. In: Ransom SB, Dombrowski MP, Evan EI, et al. (eds.), *Contemporary Therapy in Obstetrics and Gynecology*. Philadelphia, PA: W.B. Saunders; 2002:399.

14. **(E)**

15. **(D)**

16. **(B)**

Explanations for questions 14 to 16

With a β-hCG of 6000 mIU/mL in this patient, transvaginal ultrasound should demonstrate an intrauterine pregnancy if, in fact, it exists (see Fig. 39-4). Minimal fluid in the cul-de-sac suggests that oviduct rupture and profuse blood loss have not occurred. The 3-cm mass in the right

adnexa most likely represents an ectopic pregnancy in the fallopian tube. Based on the patient's positive β-hCG and her ultrasound findings, the most likely diagnosis is ectopic pregnancy; specifically, a right fallopian tube ectopic pregnancy. Incomplete and threatened abortion are very unlikely because no intrauterine pregnancy or sac is visualized.

The incidence of ectopic pregnancy has steadily increased in the United States. Currently, approximately 20 per 1000 pregnancies are ectopic. Despite the increase in incidence, maternal mortality has decreased. This is mainly because of increased diagnostic modalities and an earlier diagnosis prior to rupture. Risk factors for ectopic pregnancy include a history of PID, particularly PID caused by *C trachomatis*, prior ectopic pregnancy, cigarette smoking, and prior tubal surgery. Increasing age is also associated with an increased incidence of ectopic pregnancy.

The classic triad of ectopic pregnancy includes the following symptoms: abdominal pain, absence of menses, and irregular vaginal bleeding. Abdominal pain is present in approximately 90–100% of patients with an ectopic pregnancy. The location may be unilateral, bilateral, or generalized, and can be severe or colicky in nature. If rupture of the oviduct occurs, the pain usually becomes intense. Syncope occurs in approximately one-third of patients who experience tubal rupture with an ectopic pregnancy. Approximately half of the women with ectopic pregnancies will have a palpable adnexal mass on bimanual examination. Temperature elevation is rare, and tachycardia and hypotension are usually seen only with oviduct rupture and profuse blood loss.

Quantitative β-hCG helps confirm the state of pregnancy, date the pregnancy, and direct the use of ultrasonography. For patients with a quantitative β-hCG greater than 6500 mIU/mL and no gestational sac seen in the uterus on abdominal ultrasound, nearly all women had an ectopic pregnancy. When no intrauterine sac is seen with hCG levels exceeding this value, a pathologic pregnancy—either an ectopic or a nonviable intrauterine pregnancy—is most likely present. Of note, nearly two-thirds of women presenting with symptoms consistent with an ectopic pregnancy will have β-hCG levels greater than 2500 mIU/mL. With this level of β-hCG, the diagnosis of ectopic pregnancy can usually be made using transvaginal ultrasonography when no intrauterine sac is identified. Type and screen is also imperative not only if oviduct rupture has occurred and blood loss is profuse, but also to determine based on the patient's Rh status if RhoGAM is required. Rh-negative pregnant patients with abnormal bleeding or an ectopic pregnancy are required to receive RhoGAM.

Standard treatment of ectopic pregnancy had been surgical; however, medical management of tubal

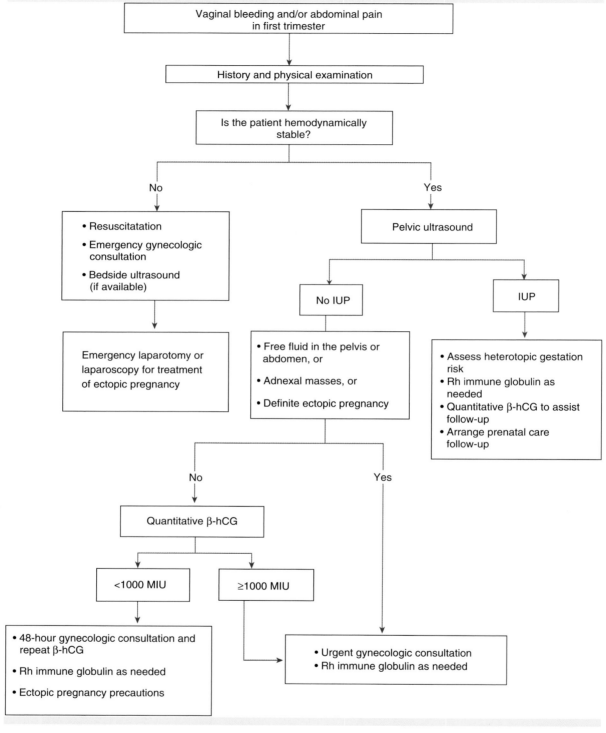

FIGURE 39-4. IUP, intrauterine pregnancy. From Stone CK, Humphries R. *Current Diagnosis & Treatment: Emergency Medicine*, 7th ed. New York, NY: McGraw-Hill; 2011:Fig. 38-3.

pregnancy has become an option using intramuscular methotrexate for selected ectopic pregnancies. This option allows outpatient treatment of ectopic pregnancies and allows avoidance of surgery. Patients who receive methotrexate should be counseled to expect to experience vaginal bleeding or spotting and mild abdominal pain, as well as medication-related side effects including nausea, vomiting, stomatitis, diarrhea, gastric distress, and dizziness. Patients who experience sudden onset of severe abdominal pain or worsening of current abdominal pain should be evaluated immediately by the physician because rupture of an ectopic pregnancy has been reported following methotrexate injection. Likewise, dizziness, syncope, or tachycardia also warrants evaluation of the patient. Additionally, patients should be instructed to avoid alcoholic beverages, nonsteroidal anti-inflammatory drugs, and sexual intercourse. Because methotrexate is a folinic acid antagonist that inhibits dihydrofolic acid reductase, thereby interfering with DNA synthesis repair and cellular replication, patients should also be instructed to avoid vitamins containing folic acid, particularly their prenatal vitamins.

Optimal management options for this patient include intramuscular methotrexate and laparoscopic salpingostomy or salpingectomy. A definitive diagnosis of ectopic pregnancy by direct visualization of the pelvis with laparoscopy can nearly always be made. Difficulty in visualizing the pelvic organs may be because of hemoperitoneum, adhesions, or obesity, which the surgeon should anticipate depending on the clinical scenario. Diagnostic laparoscopy with either laparoscopic salpingostomy or salpingectomy is a treatment option for this patient. Exploratory laparotomy is generally reserved for patients who are hemodynamically unstable, oviduct rupture with profuse blood loss, inability to adequately visualize the pelvic organs with laparoscopy, or lack of expertise in laparoscopic surgery.

BIBLIOGRAPHY

American College of Obstetricians and Gynecologists. ACOG Practice Bulletin 94: Medical management of ectopic pregnancy. *Obstet Gynecol* 2008;111(6):1479–1485.

Schorge JO, Schaffer JI, Halvorson LM, Hoffman BL, Bradshaw KD, Cunningham FG. Ectopic pregnancy. In: *Williams Gynecology*. New York, NY: McGraw-Hill; 2009:157–169.

17. **(C)**

18. **(C)**

Explanations for questions 17 and 18

A Bartholin gland cyst is an obstruction of the duct usually secondary to trauma or nonspecific inflammation.

Following obstruction of the duct, there is continued secretion of fluid by the gland, and this results in cystic dilation. The incidence of adult women who develop Bartholin gland cyst is approximately 2%. When present, it is commonly seen in women during their reproductive years.

Normally, the Bartholin glands cannot be palpated. They are located deep in the perineum at the 5 and 7 o'clock position at the entrance of the vagina. When ductal obstruction occurs, Bartholin gland cysts are located in the labia majora near the hymen.

Most women who develop a Bartholin cyst are asymptomatic with the exception of them noticing a fullness in the labia. On physical examination, a nontender, unilateral, ovoid, and tense cyst can be appreciated.

Obstruction of the duct and formation of the Bartholin cyst usually occur without an infection or abscess; however, an abscess of the cyst may develop rapidly over 2–4 days. Physical findings of a Bartholin gland abscess differ from that of a simple Bartholin gland cyst in that patients report acute pain and tenderness. On physical examination, there is marked erythema, pain on palpation of the mass, and occasionally cellulitis in the adjacent subcutaneous tissues. In this patient, the physical findings and the patient's history are most consistent with a Bartholin gland cyst because findings of an abscess are not present.

Treatment options for a Bartholin gland duct cyst include warm soaks and expectant management, insertion of a Word catheter, or a marsupialization of the duct to create a fistulous tract. However, in this patient, because the Bartholin gland cyst is recurrent, expectant management with warm soaks is not appropriate. Simple incision and drainage of the cyst will immediately alleviate the fullness; however, the tendency for recurrence is high. Because this patient has had recurrent Bartholin gland duct cysts, insertion of a Word catheter or marsupialization of the duct is the most appropriate treatment.

A Word catheter is a short catheter with an inflatable Foley balloon at the distal end that is inserted into the cyst after a stab incision is made. This can be performed under local anesthesia. Ideally, the Word catheter is left in place for 4–6 weeks, during which time a tract will form that will help prevent further duct obstruction and recurrence of a Bartholin gland duct cyst. Commonly, the Word catheter will spontaneously fall out prior to the 4- to 6-week time period. Care must be taken when inserting a Word catheter to keep the stab incision of a size just big enough to insert the tip of the Word catheter. This will help with premature extraction of the catheter before the 4- to 6-week time frame. Marsupialization is performed in the operating room and is the classical surgical treatment. Marsupialization of the duct will help develop a fistulous tract in an attempt to prevent recurrence. An elliptical incision is made overlying the protruding Bartholin cyst, and the tissue is removed. Marsupialization is then performed by suturing the edges of the everted duct to the surrounding skin. This has a success rate of approximately 90% in preventing recurrent Bartholin gland duct cysts.

Because this patient does not have an obvious Bartholin gland abscess, broad-spectrum antibiotics are not indicated; however, in the case of Bartholin gland abscess, broad-spectrum antibiotics with aerobic and anaerobic coverage are indicated. Cultures from Bartholin gland abscess contain anaerobic, aerobic, and facultative anaerobic organisms and typically are classified as polymicrobial. It was once believed that Bartholin gland cysts or abscesses were pathognomonic with a gonococcal infection. This is no longer believed to be true because bacterial cultures of Bartholin cysts and abscess have revealed polymicrobial infections. In fact, in the majority of patients, Bartholin gland cysts or infection is not felt to be caused by a sexually infection.

Although asymptomatic Bartholin gland cysts in women under age 40 do not require treatment, excision of a Bartholin gland duct cyst is indicated in women over the age of 40. If complete excision is not possible, biopsy of the gland is required to rule out adenocarcinoma of the Bartholin gland. Excision of the Bartholin gland is also indicated for persistent deep infection, multiple recurrences of Bartholin gland cyst or abscess, and despite marsupialization. Although very rare, histology of a recurrent Bartholin gland cyst in patients older than 40 may reveal squamous carcinoma or adenocarcinoma.

BIBLIOGRAPHY

Schorge JO, Schaffer JI, Halvorson LM, Hoffman BL, Bradshaw KD, Cunningham FG. Benign disorders of the lower reproductive tract. In: *Williams Gynecology*. New York, NY: McGraw-Hill; 2009:96–97.

Schorge JO, Schaffer JI, Halvorson LM, Hoffman BL, Bradshaw KD, Cunningham FG. Surgeries for benign gynecological conditions. In: *Williams Gynecology*. New York, NY: McGraw-Hill; 2009:874–878.

CHAPTER 40

BIOSTATISTICS

ALEXANDRA BROWN AND KATHRYN JACKSON

This is a review of basic statistical concepts. Statistical analysis involves two main processes: summarizing the data and hypothesis testing. Summarizing the data means describing the data to inform the reader of central tendency and variation. Summary data include estimates of the mean, median, range, standard deviation, frequency, and proportions. Hypothesis testing includes comparing means and proportions and model building. With a growing emphasis on evidence-based medicine, a basic understanding of statistics is critical in order for physicians and/or researchers to make informed decisions and conclusions about research. The goal of this chapter is to present the more prevalent statistical concepts with which every physician should be familiar.

The following questions and answers focus on the overall understanding of statistical terms and concepts. Therefore, no mathematical calculations are necessary.

Please note that researchers typically work very closely with skilled statisticians throughout the entirety of the research process. If you plan to conduct a research study, it would be helpful to form a collaborative relationship with a statistician and involve him or her at the beginning of the project when the study objective is being defined, because the statistician has the expertise and knowledge to optimize design, conduct analysis, interpret results, and make informed conclusions.

QUESTIONS

1. Which of the following correctly describes categorical data?
   - (A) Data that can be any numeric value within a specified range
   - (B) Data that have a finite number of categories
   - (C) Data that have a finite number of categories with an implied order
   - (D) Data that can have only one of two specified values

2. Which of the following correctly describes ordinal data?
   - (A) Data that can be any numeric value within a specified range
   - (B) Data that have a finite number of categories
   - (C) Data that have a finite number of categories with an implied order
   - (D) Data that can have only one of two specified values

3. Which of the following correctly describes continuous data?
   - (A) Data that can be any numeric value within a specified range
   - (B) Data that have a finite number of categories
   - (C) Data that have a finite number of categories with an implied order
   - (D) None of the above

4. Which of the following correctly pairs a summary statistic for central tendency with its definition?
   - (A) Mean: the most frequently occurring value
   - (B) Median: the middle value when the data are ordered from smallest to largest
   - (C) Mode: the arithmetic average of a set of numbers
   - (D) Confidence interval: The area of variation between upper and lower limits on a particular scale

5. Which of the following summary statistics is defined as the proportion of cases at a given point in time?
   - (A) Percent
   - (B) Rate
   - (C) Prevalence
   - (D) Incidence

6. Which of the following measures of variability is defined as the difference between the 25th and 75th percentiles?
   - (A) Standard deviation
   - (B) Standard error
   - (C) Interquartile range (IQR)
   - (D) Confidence interval (CI)

7. Which of the following correctly pairs the probability used with hypothesis testing with its definition?
   (A) Alpha (α): 1 – probability of a type II error
   (B) Beta (β): the probability of a type I error
   (C) Power: the probability of a type II error
   (D) *P* value: the observed significance level

8. Which of the following is the correct definition of sensitivity?
   (A) The strength of the linear association between two variables
   (B) The ratio of the odds of disease between two groups
   (C) The probability of testing negative when the condition is not present
   (D) The probability of testing positive when the condition is present

9. True or false? Two variables that are associated with each other are always correlated.
   (A) True
   (B) False

Questions 10 to 12 refer to the following case study.
A study is conducted to investigate the effectiveness of a new analgesic in relieving headache (HA) pain. A subject's HA intensity is recorded at baseline and subsequently at 15-minute intervals after treatment administration for up to 1 hour. HA intensity is measured using a 0- to 100-mm visual analog scale (VAS) with 0 representing no HA and 100 representing worst pain imaginable. The initial analysis consists of comparing various outcomes between the treatment group and the control group.

10. Which statistical test would you use to measure HA intensity at 30 minutes?
    (A) Pearson's chi-square (χ^2) test
    (B) Student's *t* test
    (C) Log-rank test
    (D) Mann-Whitney *U* test

11. Which statistical test would you use to measure the percentage of subjects with at least 50% reduction in HA intensity at 30 minutes?
    (A) Pearson's χ^2 test
    (B) Student's *t* test
    (C) Log-rank test
    (D) Mann-Whitney *U* test

12. Which statistical test would you use to measure time to complete HA relief (subjects are observed for up to 2 hours)?
    (A) Pearson's χ^2 test
    (B) Student's *t* test
    (C) Log-rank test
    (D) Mann-Whitney *U* test

13. Which study design is most appropriate for conducting a survey on people's use and attitudes toward seat belts?
    (A) Randomized clinical trial
    (B) Meta-analysis
    (C) Case-control
    (D) Observational
    (E) Crossover

14. Which study design is most appropriate for comparing the effectiveness of two analgesics in relieving headache pain in patients presenting to the emergency department with severe headaches?
    (A) Randomized clinical trial
    (B) Meta-analysis
    (C) Case-control
    (D) Observational
    (E) Crossover

15. Which study design is most appropriate for comparing pain intensity of instillation in two ophthalmic anesthetics where each subject gets both treatments?
    (A) Randomized clinical trial
    (B) Meta-analysis
    (C) Case-control
    (D) Observational
    (E) Crossover

16. Which study design is most appropriate for determining factors associated with skeletal fluorosis in sibling pairs (one sibling with skeletal fluorosis and one without)?
    (A) Randomized clinical trial
    (B) Meta-analysis
    (C) Case-control
    (D) Observational
    (E) Crossover

17. Which study design is most appropriate for reviewing previously published papers on the effectiveness of hyperdynamic therapy for cerebral vasospasm?
    (A) Randomized clinical trial
    (B) Meta-analysis
    (C) Case-control
    (D) Observational
    (E) Crossover

Questions 18 to 22 refer to the following case study.
A study is conducted to investigate the effectiveness of a new analgesic in relieving headache (HA) pain. A subject's HA intensity is recorded at baseline and subsequently at 15-minute intervals after treatment administration up to 1 hour. HA intensity is measured using a 0- to 100-mm VAS with 0 representing no HA and 100 representing worst pain imaginable. Select the most appropriate statistical model to use to analyze the data for each outcome below.

Outcome	Factors
18. HA intensity at 30 minutes	HA intensity at baseline (mm VAS), age (in years), body mass index (BMI; kg/m^2)
19. Subject has at least 50% relief in HA intensity at 30 minutes	Treatment group (treatment/control), gender, history of severe headaches (yes/no)
20. Change in HA intensity at 30 minutes	Treatment group (treatment/control), gender, history of severe headaches (yes/no)
21. Rate of change of HA intensity—measured at baseline and at 15, 30, 45, and 60 minutes	Treatment group (treatment/control), gender, history of severe headaches (yes/no)
22. Time to complete HA relief—subjects are observed for all most 2 hours	Treatment group (treatment/control), gender, history of severe headaches (yes/no)

(A) Analysis of variance (ANOVA)
(B) Logistic regression
(C) Linear regression
(D) Proportional hazards regression
(E) Repeated measures ANOVA

ANSWERS AND EXPLANATIONS

1. **(B)** Examples of categorical data include gender (male/female), randomization group (treatment/control), and mortality (dead/alive).
2. **(C)** Likert-type scales (no pain, some pain, terrible pain) and the New York Heart Association classification of congestive heart failure are examples of ordinal data.
3. **(A)** Continuous data examples are age and body mass index (BMI).

   It is important to know the type of data that is being collected and/or presented. For instance, blood pressure can be captured as the actual systolic blood pressure in mmHg, or it may be dichotomized into hypertensive or nonhypertensive. How the data are captured influences the summary measures and statistical tests that can be used. Certain statistical measures and tests can only be used on categorical data, whereas other measures and tests can only be used on continuous data.

4. **(B)** The mean is perhaps the most common measure of central tendency for continuous or ordinal data and cannot be used with categorical data. It is found by adding all of the data values together and then dividing by the

sample size. A limitation of using the mean is that it is very sensitive to extreme values—particularly when the sample size is small. For example, suppose the length of stay in days for seven patients is as follows (1, 2, 2, 1, 30, 1, and 3). The mean of these values is 5.7 days. But most of the patients were in the hospital less than 3 days. Hence, the mean in this case is not giving accurate information. It is overestimating the number of days a patient would expect to stay.

   The median is less sensitive to extreme values and is most often used when the data are left or right skewed. Data are said to be skewed if when plotted they no longer have a nice bell-shape curve. If the left tail is elongated, then the data are left skewed, and vice versa. The median is found by ordering all of the data from smallest to largest and then finding the middle data value. It is balanced in that 50% of the observations are below the median and 50% are above. Because 50% of the data are less than the median, another name for the median is the 50th percentile. Other percentiles can also be found. For example, the 25th percentile is the data point where 25% of the data are below it. In the example of length of stay, the median is found to be 2 days. This is a more reasonable estimate of the true length of stay.

   The mode is the most frequently occurring value in a set of data and is best used to summarize ordinal and categorical data. In the length of stay example, the mode is 1 day. The mode is a seldom used summary statistic.

5. **(C)** Mathematically, percentages and prevalences are defined the same way. They are the number of cases of interest divided by the total number of samples (multiplied by 100 to convert to a percentage). However, they differ in semantics. For example, we never say the prevalence of females in a study is 45%; rather, we say the *percentage* of females is 45%. Prevalence is used to define the proportion of cases in a population. Similarly, rates and incidences are mathematically similar but differ in how the terms are used. The key difference between percentages/prevalences and rates/incidences is the inclusion of a time factor in the divisor.

   Additionally, we often use the term *rate* to express prevalence in a more convenient format. For instance, suppose the prevalence of a disease is 0.014% (i.e., 0.00014). We often report this prevalence or *rate* as 14 out of 100,000. It is not a rate *per se* because there is not a defined time period in the denominator, but we use the term anyway, most often in epidemiology or population-based studies.

6. **(C)** The range, simply the difference between the maximum and minimum values of data, conveys little information about how the data are distributed. The interquartile range (IQR) describes the spread of the middle 50% of the data.

The standard deviation and standard error are two terms that are often confused. The standard deviation is a summary statistic (like the mean) used to describe the variability of continuous data. Mathematically, it is the square root of the average squared deviation of each data point about the sample mean. The standard error, however, describes the variability of a statistic and can be thought of as being the standard deviation of a statistic. The standard error of a measure depends on the statistic and can often be cumbersome to calculate (even more difficult than the standard deviation!). It should be noted that even the standard deviation has a standard error.

A confidence interval (CI) can be estimated for any statistic. Although the method used to determine each is quite different, they are all similar in that they are measures of the uncertainty in a parameter estimate. We usually report a 95% CI. It is important to note that, when we say that we are 95% confident, we are commenting on the *procedure* used, and not on the specific value calculated. That is, if we were to perform an experiment a large number of times and estimate a 95% CI in each of these trials, 95% of these CIs would contain the true population parameter.

In presenting summary statistics to describe the data collected, both a measure of central tendency and its associated measure of variability should be presented. In general, if the mean is reported, then the standard deviation or the standard error of the mean should be reported. If the median is reported, then the range, or preferably the IQR, should also be reported. For all statistical measures, a 95% CI should be reported.

7. **(D)** In statistical hypothesis testing, we have a null hypothesis (H_0) and an alternative hypothesis (H_A). In general, assume null hypothesis of "no difference." For example, we assume the effects of two different treatments are the same. In the alternative hypothesis, we believe that a difference exists (i.e., the two effects are different from each other). In hypothesis testing, the assumption is that the null hypothesis is true, and there must be overwhelming evidence to reject the null hypothesis and conclude that a difference exists (Table 40-1).

Evidence to reject or not reject the null hypothesis is obtained by performing an appropriate statistical test and assessing the P value. We conclude a difference exists if this P value is less than our predefined significance level α. In most situations, α is set at 0.05, although an α of 0.10 is often used in exploratory analyses. Most medical journals now require investigators to report confidence intervals instead of (or in addition to) P values.

The P value can be viewed as the *observed* significance level. It is the probability of getting a more extreme result assuming under the null hypothesis that no difference exists. It is not the probability that the null hypothesis is true.

A problem with hypothesis testing is that an incorrect conclusion can be reached. Hypothesis testing can be thought of in terms of a diagnostic test and is in fact conceptually equivalent. With any diagnostic test, we can make an error—such as concluding that a patient has a disease when in fact they do not (i.e., a false positive). A type I error is made when we reject the null hypothesis when in fact the null hypothesis is true. A type II error occurs when we fail to reject the null hypothesis when we should. Power ($1 - \beta$) is the probability that we correctly reject the null hypothesis when the null hypothesis is, in fact, false.

In diagnostic testing, sensitivity measures a test's ability to correctly identify a condition, whereas specificity measures the test's ability to correctly exclude a condition. The sensitivity of a diagnostic test is analogous to ($1 - \alpha$) in hypothesis testing, and specificity is analogous to power ($1 - \beta$). However, keep in mind that the two have very different calculations.

8. **(D)** Sensitivity measures a test's ability to correctly identify a condition, whereas specificity measures the test's ability to correctly exclude a condition. The sensitivity and specificity are just two of many measures that are used to describe the characteristics of a diagnostic test (see Fig. 40-1). Other measures include the accuracy, the positive and negative predictive values, the positive and negative errors, the positive and negative likelihood ratios, and the likelihood ratio. All of these measures estimate the error rates that are inherent in all diagnostic tests.

TABLE 40-1 Correct Decisions and Errors in Hypothesis Testing

		True Situation	
		Difference Exists (H_1)	No Difference (H_0)
Conclusion from Hypothesis Test	Difference Exists (Reject H_0)	*(Power or $1-\beta$)	I (Type I error, or α error)
	No Difference (Do not reject H_0)	II (Type II error, or β error)	*
From Dawson B, Trapp RG. *Basic and Clinical Biostatistics*, 4th ed. New York, NY: McGraw-Hill; 2004.			

Disease

	Present	Absent
Positive	*a* True positives	*b* False positives
Negative	*c* False negatives	*d* True negatives

EST

Sensitivity (Sn) = $\dfrac{a}{a+c}$ 　　Specificity (Sp) = $\dfrac{b}{b+d}$

Positive predictive value 　　Negative predictive value

(PPV) = $\dfrac{a}{a+b}$ 　　　　(NPV) = $\dfrac{d}{a+d}$

FIGURE 40-1. The 2 × 2 table: sensitivity, specificity, positive predictive value, and negative predictive value. From LeBlond RF, Brown DD, Suneja M, Szot JF. *DeGowin's Diagnostic Examination*, 10th ed. New York, NY: McGraw-Hill; 2014:Fig. 17-2.

9. **(B)** Statistically, correlation and association are not synonymous terms. These terms are often misused by study investigators much to the disdain of statisticians. Correlation is a measure of the strength of the association between two variables and is a mathematically defined quantity. Association describes the nature of the relationship between two variables. For instance, an investigator may state that the objective of a study is to assess the *correlation* between use of a treatment and some outcome of interest, but what is really being assessed is the *association* between the treatment and outcome. Two variables that are highly correlated are associated with each other, but two variables that are associated with each other may not be correlated.

10. **(B)**

11. **(A)**

12. **(C)**

Explanation for Questions 10 through 12

These basic tests are also called univariate tests of association. They are called univariate because the effect of one factor is being assessed on one outcome variable. They are usually performed first to identify factors that

are associated with the outcome of interest or to compare demographic characteristics of the two groups. Once factors are identified, a more sophisticated model can be developed that uses all of the factors in one model.

The student's *t* test is not always the most appropriate test to use when comparing continuous data. One of the underlying assumptions made with the student's *t* test is that the data follow a normal distribution. The other and more critical assumption that is made with the *t* test is that the variances (i.e., the square of the standard deviation) between the two groups are equal, and if they are not equal, then a correction must be made. If both of these assumptions are violated, the Wilcoxon rank-sum test should be used. The Wilcoxon rank-sum test (also called the Mann-Whitney *U* test) is a nonparametric test. In nonparametric tests, we relax many of the assumptions that we make in using the more common parametric tests. The Wilcoxon test is in essence comparing the medians of the two groups. It should be noted that there is no such thing as nonparametric data. Statistical tests are parametric or nonparametric; whole data are simply data.

The Pearson's χ^2 test is what is called a large-sample test. That is, it holds when there is a large sample size, but it may give spurious results when the sample size is small or when the outcome of interest has a small probability of occurring. In either of these cases, Fisher's exact test should be used. The Fisher's exact test is like a nonparametric test in that it makes no assumptions but the distribution of the data. Another test that can be used instead of Pearson's χ^2 test is the *Z*-test. The *Z*-test compares two proportions but is only applicable when there is a large number of subjects in each group. The χ^2 test and the *Z*-test are mathematically related to each other.

The log-rank test is a basic nonparametric test used in survival analysis to compare the survival curves of two or more groups. When comparing survival times, a plot of the survival curves should be made. The Kaplan-Meier method is the most commonly used nonparametric method of estimating survival curves. Along with estimates of the survival curves, estimates of the median survival times should also be reported. The log-rank test compares the survival curves and is not a direct comparison of median survival times.

The Mann-Whitney *U* test is a nonparametric test of the null hypothesis that two populations are the same against an alternative hypothesis, especially when a particular population tends to have larger values than the other.

It has greater efficiency than the *t* test on nonnormal distributions, such as a mixture of normal distributions, and it is nearly as efficient as the *t* test on normal distributions. While the *P* value is traditionally reported in manuscripts, an estimate of the effect size (i.e., the difference between groups) is preferred by many medical journals. That is, instead of reporting the *P* value from a *t* test comparing two means, the difference in the group means should be estimated along with a 95% CI for the difference.

13. **(D)**

14. **(A)**

15. **(E)**

16. **(C)**

17. **(B)**

Explanation for Questions 13 through 17

All study designs have their own strengths and weaknesses. The appropriate design for a study depends on many factors, including the outcome of interest, availability of a patient population to sample, and investigator resources (time, money, and manpower). A study should not be criticized or dismissed based merely on its design if the design used is the most appropriate to meet the study objectives. Although a prospective randomized clinical trial is considered the gold standard for study designs, in many research projects, this type of study design is not feasible because of resource constraints or ethical concerns.

Knowing the study design is essential for statistical analysis and interpretation of the results. The correct statistical analysis is dependent on the study design. An investigator should consider the advantages and disadvantages of the study design when it is selected, and a reader should also consider them when interpreting the results. Consulting with a statistician when planning the study design should be the first step in every investigator's plan of action. A good study design will yield a good study—whether or not the results obtained are what the investigator expects.

The strength of the results of a study is dictated by the study design and the stage of the research process. Usually new ideas or investigations start out as case studies. Case studies then lead to observational (exploratory) studies to see if there is evidence that what was seen in the case studies holds in a larger set of subjects. From an observational study, an investigator may generate a hypothesis that can then be tested with a randomized clinical trial. Observational study designs are shown in Fig. 40-2.

Once several clinical trials have been conducted and published, a meta-analysis can be performed to synthesize the results reported in each of these trials. A meta-analysis is considered to be the most definitive clinical research study because it combines the results of several trials, regardless of whether the results are "positive" or "negative"; hence, it is just as important to report negative studies as it is to report positive studies. Both add to the knowledge base of researchers and are indispensable to the physician when making an informed decision on patient care.

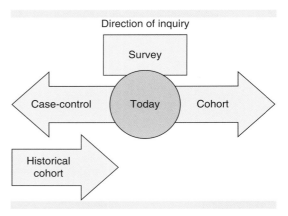

FIGURE 40-2. Schematic diagram of the time relationship among different observational study designs. The arrows represent the direction of the inquiry. From Dawson B, Trapp RG. *Basic and Clinical Biostatistics*, 4th ed. New York, NY: McGraw-Hill; 2004:Fig. 2-5.

18. **(D)**

19. **(A)**

20. **(E)**

21. **(C)**

22. **(B)**

Explanation For Questions 18 through 22

All statistical models have the same basic form. There is an outcome variable, and we wish to explain the variability in this outcome as a function of independent factors. In fact, most statistical models come from a general class of statistical models called general linear models (GLMs). The key point to knowing which statistical model is most appropriate is to know the data type of the outcome variable.

Repeated measures analysis of variance (ANOVA) is used when an outcome measure is recorded at multiple time points on each subject. These repeated outcome measures are correlated with each other within a subject. This correlation of the outcome within a subject must be taken into account when modeling the outcome. It should be noted that the student's paired *t* test is really a simplified form of a repeated measures ANOVA using only two time points and no other factors in the model.

Proportional hazards regression is a statistical model used in analysis of survival data. Survival data occur when the outcome of interest is the time to an event occurrence (e.g., time to death, time to reinfection, fistula patency). If the subject does not experience the event by the end of the study observation period, the subject's survival time is said to be censored. Proportional hazard models take into account this censoring of the data.

A regression analysis can be simple, multiple, or multivariate. A simple regression model means that there is one and only one independent factor. A multiple regression model means that there are two or more independent factors. A multivariate regression model means there are two or more dependent factors with one or more independent factors. The terms multiple and multivariate are often mistakenly interchanged, but statistically speaking, they imply two very different models.

BIBLIOGRAPHY

Campbell MJ, Machin D, Walters SJ. *Medical Statistics: A Textbook for the Health Sciences*, 4th ed. Chichester, England: John Wiley & Sons; 2007.

Dawson B, Trapp RG. *Basic & Clinical Biostatistics*, 4th ed. New York, NY: McGraw-Hill; 2004.

Kirkwood BR, Sterne J. *Essentials of Medical Statistics*, 2nd ed. Malden, MA: Blackwell Science; 2001.

Norman GR, Streiner DL. *Biostatistics: The Bare Essentials*, 3rd ed. St. Louis, MO: BC Decker; 2007.

INDEX

Note: Page numbers followed by *f* or *t* denote figures and tables, respectively.